NATIONALLY NOTIFIABLE INFECTIOUS DISEASES (See also Chapter 17)

- Acute Flaccid Paralysis
- Acquired Immunodeficiency Syndrome
- Amebiasis
- Anthrax
- Botulism
- Brucellosis
- Campylobacteriosis
- Chancroid
- Chicken Pox
- Chlamydia, Genital
- Cholera
- Creutzfeldt-Jakob Disease
- Cryptosporidiosis
- Cyclosporiasis
- Diphtheria
- Giardiasis
- Gonococcal Ophthalmia Neonatorum
- Gonorrhea
- Group B Streptococcal Disease of the Newborn
- Hantavirus Pulmonary Syndrome
- Hepatitis A
- Hepatitis B
- Hepatitis C
- Hepatitis Non-A, Non-B
- Human Immunodeficiency Virus
- Influenza, Laboratory Confirmed
- Invasive Group A Streptococcal Disease
- Invasive *Haemophilus Influenzae* Type B Disease
- Invasive Meningococcal Disease
- Invasive Pneumococcal Disease
- Legionellosis
- Leprosy
- Listeriosis (all types)

Continued

WINDSHIELD/WALKING SURVEY COMPONENTS (See also Chapter 9)

Element	Areas to Consider
History	Appearance, e.g., old, established neighbourhoods or new subdivision. Ask residents, especially any "old-timer(s)" for the history of the area.
Demographics	What sorts of people do you see, e.g., young, old, homeless, alone, families? Is the population homogeneous?
Ethnicity	What evidence is there of different cultural and ethnic groups (e.g., restaurants, festivals, etc.)?
Values and beliefs	Are there churches, mosques, or temples? Is there an appearance of homogeneity? Are homes and public spaces cared for? What values are indicated by the art, culture, heritage, or historical markers?
Physical environment	What are the air quality, flora, housing, zoning, space, green areas, animals, people, human-made structures, natural beauty, water, and climate like? Can you find or develop a map of the area? What is the size (e.g., kilometres, blocks)?
Health and social services	What medical, nursing, and other health-related services are evident? Are there resources outside the community but readily accessible?
Economy	Are there industries, stores, or other places of employment? Where do people shop? Is there a food bank being used? What is the unemployment rate?
Transportation and safety	What types of private and public transportation are available? Are there sidewalks and walking and bike trails? Is getting around in the community possible for people with disabilities? What types of protective services are there (e.g., fire, police, sanitation)? Is air quality monitored? What types of crimes are committed? Do people feel safe?

Continued

COMMON EPIDEMIOLOGICAL RATES (See also Chapter 8)

GENERAL MORTALITY RATES

Crude mortality rate

$$\frac{\text{Number of deaths occurring during 1 year}}{\text{Mid-year population}} \times 100{,}000$$

Cause-specific mortality rate

$$\frac{\text{Number of deaths from a stated cause during 1 year}}{\text{Mid-year population}} \times 100{,}000$$

Case-fatality rate

$$\frac{\text{Number of deaths from a specific disease}}{\text{Number of cases of the same disease}} \times 100$$

Proportional mortality ratio

$$\frac{\text{Number of deaths from a specific cause within a given time period}}{\text{Total deaths in the same time period}} \times 100$$

Age-specific mortality rate

$$\frac{\text{Number of persons in a specific age-group dying during 1 year}}{\text{Mid-year population of the specific age group}} \times 100{,}000$$

Continued

SIGNS OF ABUSE AND NEGLECT (See also Chapter 11)

Emotional Abuse/Neglect		Physical Abuse	
Physical Findings	**Suggestive Behaviours**	**Physical Findings**	**Suggestive Behaviours**
• Failure to thrive • Feeding disorders • Enuresis • Sleep disorders • Speech disorders • Delays in physical development • Physical symptoms, such as headaches and nausea	• Self-stimulatory behaviours, finger sucking, rocking, biting • Withdrawal, aggressive behaviour, or depression • Unusual fearfulness • Antisocial behaviour • Excessively compliant, obsessive-compulsive behaviours • Sleep disorders and learning disorders • Lags in emotional or intellectual development • Suicide attempts	• Numerous bruises and welts, wounds at different stages of recovery or healing • Burns, especially on feet, palms of hands, back, and buttocks; absence of splash mark • Bites, burns, bruises, and welts that conform to the shape of an object • Fractures and dislocations—skull, nose, facial fracture with spiral fracture or dislocation • Any injury not consistent with history • Lacerations and abrasions on back of arms, torso, face, or external genitalia • Bites or hair pulled out • Unexplained poisonings or chemical exposures	• Fear of contact with adults • Cannot explain or remember injuries or explanations are inconsistent • Believes that punishment is deserv • Apparent fear of pare or of going home • Inappropriate reacti to injury, such as failure to cry from pa • Flinches when touched unexpectec • Superficial relationships • Apprehension when other children cry • Extremely aggressiv or withdrawn

Con

WINDSHIELD/WALKING SURVEY COMPONENTS—cont'd

Element	Areas to Consider
Politics and government	Are there signs of political activity (e.g., posters, meetings)? What party affiliation predominates? What is the governmental jurisdiction of the community? Are people involved in decision making in their local governmental unit?
Communication	Are there "common areas" where people gather? What newspapers do you see in the stands? Do people have televisions and radios? What do residents watch and listen to?
Education	How do the schools in the area look and function? What is their reputation? What are major educational issues? What are the dropout rates? Are extracurricular activities available? Is there a school health service or nurse?
Recreation	Where do children play? What are the major forms of recreation? Who participates? Are recreation fees affordable?
The residents	How do several people (from different groups, e.g., young, old, workers, professional, clergy, housewives, etc.) feel about their community? What do they identify as its strengths? Problems? (Record who gives what answers.)
Your perceptions	What are your general statements about the "health" of this community, its strengths, concerns, or potential concerns?

Modified from Vollman, A. R., Anderson, E. T., & McFarlane, J. M. (2008). *Canadian community as partner: Theory and multidisciplinary practice in nursing* (2nd ed., pp. 248–249). Philadelphia PA: Lippincott.

NATIONALLY NOTIFIABLE INFECTIOUS DISEASES—cont'd

Malaria
Measles
Meningitis, Other Bacterial
Meningitis, Pneumococcal
Meningitis, Viral
Mumps
Paratyphoid
Pertussis
Plague*
Poliomyelitis
Rabies
Rubella
Rubella, Congenital
Salmonellosis
Shigellosis
Smallpox
Syphilis, All
Syphilis, Congenital
Syphilis, Early Latent
Syphilis, Early Symptomatic (Primary and Secondary)
Syphilis, Other
Tetanus
Trichinosis
Tuberculosis
Tularemia
Typhoid
Verotoxigenic *Escherichia coli*
Viral Hemorrhagic Fevers (Crimean Congo, Ebola, Lassa, Margurg)
West Nile Virus Asymptomatic Infection
West Nile Virus Fever
West Nile Virus Neurological Syndromes
West Nile Virus Unclassified/Unspecified
Yellow Fever*

*The notifiable disease database has never received a report of plague or yellow fever.

SIGNS OF ABUSE AND NEGLECT—cont'd

Sexual Abuse		Physical Neglect	
Physical Findings	**Suggestive Behaviours**	**Physical Findings**	**Suggestive Behaviours**
• Bruises, bleeding, lacerations, or irritation to external genitalia, vagina, and anus • Stained, bloody underclothing • Pain on urination or pain, swelling, and excessive itching of genital area • Vaginal/penile discharge • Sexually transmitted infections • Difficulty walking or sitting • Recurrent urinary tract infection • Evidence of semen • Excessive masturbation • Pregnancy in young adolescent	• Sexual knowledge or play is not appropriate for age • Seductive behaviour and prostitution • Withdrawn behaviour, excessive daydreaming • Change to poor school performance • Poor relationship with peers • Sudden changes—anxiety, weight loss/gain, clinging behaviour • Regressive behaviours—wets bed, sucks thumb • Sleeping disorders, aggressive and abusive behaviours, and self-mutilation • Running away from home and/or delinquent behaviours • Profound personality change • Suicide attempts or ideation	• Poor growth pattern, underweight, failure to thrive • Constant hunger • Malnutrition, lack of subcutaneous fat • Poor personal hygiene • Unclean and/or inappropriate dress • Unmet physical and medical health care needs	• Unkempt, inappropriate dress for the weather, pale, listless, excessively tired • Seeking inappropriate affection • Begging/stealing food • Frequently absent from school • Drug/alcohol abuse • Delinquent behaviour, e.g., vandalism/shoplifting • States there is no caretaker

Modified from Ontario Ministry of Children and Youth Services. (2010). Recognizing the signs of child abuse and neglect. Retrieved from http://www.children.gov.on.ca/(S(yuqv033quey01k55i4eual55))/htdocs/English/topics/childrensaid/reportingabuse/recognisingabuse.aspx. Royal Canadian Mounted Police. (2008). What is child abuse? Retrieved from http://www.rcmp-grc.gc.ca/pubs/ccaps-spcca/chi-enf-eng.htm.

COMMON EPIDEMIOLOGICAL RATES—cont'd

MATERNAL AND INFANT RATES

Crude birth rate
$$\frac{\text{Number of live births during 1 year}}{\text{Mid-year population}} \times 1000$$

General fertility rate
$$\frac{\text{Number of live births during 1 year}}{\text{Number of females aged 15–44 at mid-year}} \times 1000$$

Maternal mortality rate
$$\frac{\text{Number of deaths from puerperal causes during 1 year}}{\text{Number of live births during same year}} \times 100{,}000$$

Infant mortality rate
$$\frac{\text{Number of deaths of children under 1 year of age during 1 year}}{\text{Number of live births during same year}} \times 1000$$

Perinatal mortality rate
$$\frac{\text{Number of fetal deaths plus infant deaths under 7 days of age during 1 year}}{\text{Number of live births plus fetal deaths during same year}} \times 1000$$

Neonatal mortality rate
$$\frac{\text{Number of deaths of children under 28 days of age during 1 year}}{\text{Number of live births during same year}} \times 1000$$

Fetal mortality rate
$$\frac{\text{Number of fetal deaths during 1 year}}{\text{Number of live births plus fetal deaths during same year}} \times 1000$$

DAVIDHIZAR AND GIGER'S TRANSCULTURAL ASSESSMENT MODEL CATEGORIES (See also Chapter 7)

This tool can help community health nurses (CHNs) provide culturally competent care for clients in all aspects of community health nursing practice.

1. **Culturally Unique Individual:** Each individual is culturally unique, and CHNs need to elicit client cultural data—such as place of birth, how the client defines his or her own culture and race, and length of time in the country—in order to interact sensitively with the client.
2. **Communication:** Understanding the differences in communication patterns can help overcome communication barriers due to culture and improve quality of client care.
3. **Space:** The physical distance between client and CHN is an important consideration in promoting the comfort level of the client during interactions.

Continued

FAMILY ASSESSMENT GUIDE (See also Chapter 12 and Appendix 9)

This Branching Diagram from the Calgary Family Assessment Model outlines the categories and subcategories to be used when conducting a holistic approach to assessment of family health.

Family Assessment (Structural, Developmental, and Functional)		
Structural	**Developmental**	**Functional**
Internal Family composition Gender Sexual orientation Rank order Subsystems Boundaries External Extended family Larger systems Context Ethnicity Race Social class Religion or spirituality Environment	Stages Tasks Attachments	Instrumental Activities of Daily Living Expressive Emotional communication Verbal communication Nonverbal communication Circular communication Problem solving Roles Influence and power Beliefs Alliances and coalitions

THE TWELVE DETERMINANTS OF HEALTH

Determinant	Relevance
1. Income and social status	The most important determinant of health nationally. However, it is the distribution, rather than the actual amount of wealth, that is associated with healthier people among the population.
2. Social support networks	The effects of social support may be as important as identified risk factors, such as smoking, physical activity, obesity, and high blood pressure. It is not the quantity of relations that matter but the quality.
3. Education	Education provides skills useful for daily tasks, employment (income and job security), and community participation.
4. Employment and working conditions	Health status is improved with increased control of work circumstances and lower levels of stress. Unemployment is highly correlated with poorer health.
5. Physical environment	Factors in the natural environment, such as air, water, and soil quality, are key influences on health. Human-built factors, such as housing, workplace, community, and road design, are also important. Many of the writings from a population health promotion perspective do not account for environmental implications.
6. Biology and genetic endowment	The functioning of body systems and genetic endowment contribute to health status and to the process of development.
7. Personal health practices and coping skills	Psychological characteristics, such as personal competence, locus of control, and mastery over one's life, contribute to mental and physical health; however, the focus on personal health practices has been characterized as blaming the victims instead of societal factors.

Continued

CANADIAN COMMUNITY HEALTH NURSING STANDARDS, 2008 (See also Chapters 1 and 3 and Appendix 1)

Standard 1:	Promoting Health A. Health Promotion B. Prevention and Health Protection C. Health Maintenance, Restoration, and Palliation
Standard 2:	Building Individual/Community Capacity
Standard 3:	Building Relationships
Standard 4:	Facilitating Access and Equity
Standard 5:	Demonstrating Professional Responsibility and Accountability

Source: Community Health Nurses Association of Canada. (2003 [Revised 2008]). *Canadian Community Health Nursing Standards of Practice.* Retrieved from http://www.chnc.ca/documents/chn_standards_of_practice_mar08_english.pdf. Reproduced with permission.

PRIMARY HEALTH CARE PRINCIPLES

1. Accessibility to Health Services
2. Increased Emphasis on Health Promotion and Disease Prevention
3. Public Participation
4. Intersectoral Collaboration in Health
5. Appropriate Utilization of Resources

World Health Organization. (1978). *Declaration of Alma-Ata*. Retrieved from http://www.who.int/hpr/NPH/docs/declaration_almaata.pdf.

THE VALUES AND BELIEFS OF COMMUNITY HEALTH NURSES

The community health nurse values and believes in

- Caring
- The principles of primary health care
- Multiple ways of knowing
- Individual/Community partnership
- Empowerment

Source: Community Health Nurses Association of Canada. (2003 [Revised 2008]). *Canadian Community Health Nursing Standards of Practice*. Retrieved from http://www.chnc.ca/documents/chn_standards_of_practice:mar08_english.pdf. Reproduced with permission.

DAVIDHIZAR AND GIGER'S TRANSCULTURAL ASSESSMENT MODEL CATEGORIES—cont'd

4. **Social Organization:** There are various types of family forms, such as traditional nuclear family, one-parent family, reconstructed or blended family, gay family, and communal family. CHNs need to incorporate the family cultural beliefs and concerns into a client care plan.
5. **Time:** It may be frustrating when people arrive late for a group meeting, but a culturally sensitive nurse is aware that this lateness is not an avoidance of the topic but, rather, the groups' cultural view of time.
6. **Biological Variations:** To provide culturally competent and safe nursing care, CHNs need to be familiar with the biological variations associated with racial groups and consider that biological parameters are usually based on Caucasian standards and these norms may not be applicable to non-Caucasian clients.

THE TWELVE DETERMINANTS OF HEALTH—cont'd

Determinant	Relevance
8. Healthy child development	A wide range of chronic conditions seem to have their origins in fetal and infant life. Prenatal and early childhood experiences are also important in the development of coping skills and competence.
9. Health and social services	These services contribute to creating healthier people. However, increased expenditures on health care seem to be less successful in improving the health of Canadians.
10. Gender	Biological differences in men and women and socially constructed gender roles influence health and health care service use.
11. Culture	Culture may influence the way people interact with health care systems, their participation in prevention activities, health-related lifestyle choices, and understanding of health and illness. Racism, language barriers, prejudice, and misunderstandings may cause reduced access to health care.
12. Social environment	Low availability of emotional support and low social participation have a negative impact on health and well-being. Questions have been raised about any value added by including "social environment" as a health domain, since it already exists within at least seven of the determinants.

Adapted from Health Canada. (2002). *Chronic diseases in Canada, 23*(4), 124. Reproduced with permission of the Minister of Public Works and Government Services Canada, 2007.

Community Health Nursing in Canada

Second Canadian Edition

Marcia Stanhope, RN, DSN, FAAN
The Good Samaritan Professor and Chair in
Community Health Nursing
College of Nursing, University of Kentucky
Lexington, Kentucky

Jeanette Lancaster, RN, PhD, FAAN
Visiting Professor, Department of Nursing Studies
The University of Hong Kong
Professor, University of Virginia
Formerly, Sadie Heath Cabaniss Professor and Dean
School of Nursing, University of Virginia
Charlottesville, Virginia

Heather Jessup-Falcioni, RN, BScN, BEd, MN
Associate Professor
School of Nursing, Laurentian University
Sudbury, Ontario

Gloria A. Viverais-Dresler, RN, MHSc
Associate Professor (retired)
School of Nursing, Laurentian University
Sudbury, Ontario

ELSEVIER
MOSBY

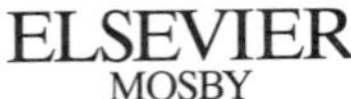

Notice

Knowledge and best practice in this field are constantly changing. As new research and expertise broaden our knowledge, changes in practice, treatment, and drug therapy may become necessary or appropriate. Readers are advised to check the most current information provided (i) on procedures featured or (ii) by the manufacturer of each product to be administered, to verify the recommended dose or formula, the method and duration of administration, and contraindications. It is the responsibility of the practitioner, relying on their own experience and knowledge of the patient, to make diagnoses, to determine dosages and the best treatment for each individual patient, and to take all appropriate safety precautions. To the fullest extent of the law, neither the Publisher nor the Authors assumes any liability for any injury and/or damage to persons or property arising out of or related to any use of the material contained in this book.

The Publisher

Library and Archives Canada Cataloguing in Publication
Community health nursing in Canada / Marcia Stanhope ... [et al.]. – 2nd ed.
Includes index.
ISBN 978-1-926648-09-5
1. Community health nursing–Canada–Textbooks.
I. Stanhope, Marcia
RT98.C664 2010 610.73'430971 C2010-903803-7

Vice President, Publishing: Ann Millar
Developmental Editor: Dawn du Quesnay
Managing Developmental Editor: Martina van de Velde
Publishing Services Manager: Jeff Patterson
Senior Project Manager: Anne Konopka
Cover Design: Jessica Williams
Interior Design: Monika Kompter/Jessica Williams

Elsevier Canada
905 King Street West, 4th Floor, Toronto, ON, Canada M6K 3G9
Phone: 1-866-896-3331
Fax: 1-866-359-9534

Printed in the United States of America

3 4 5 15 14 13

Community Health Nursing in Canada

Detailed Contents

This book is dedicated to my husband, Ken, and to our daughters, Shannyn and Cortney. Their love and support for me have never faltered despite the time commitment to this scholarly activity. Thanks and appreciation also to my numerous extended family and friends for their interest and support. A special memorial dedication to my mother, Doris Jessup, who passed away peacefully on November 11, 2010, at the age of 93. She was my inspiration, being a compassionate, strong, and caring person.

—HJF

This book is dedicated to my husband, Werner, for his continued love, incredible encouragement, and support, and to my sisters and their families: Linda (Marino and Natasha) and Shirley (David, James Joseph [JJ], and Brett) for their continued interest and support. Also, thanks to my extended family and friends for their ongoing encouragement.

—GVD

About the Authors

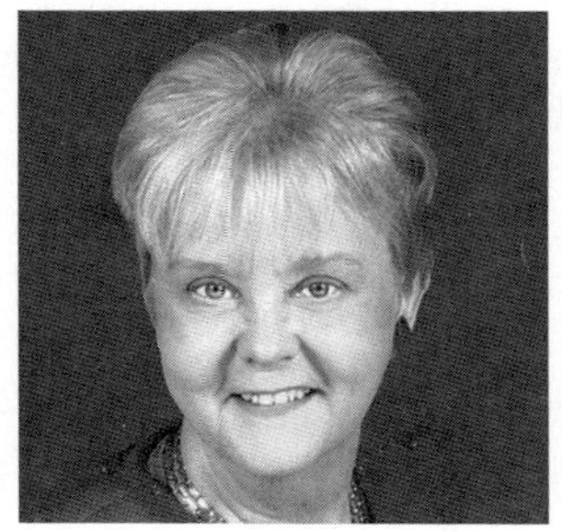

Marcia Stanhope, RN, DSN, FAAN

Marcia Stanhope is currently The Good Samaritan Professor and Chair in Community Health Nursing at the University of Kentucky College of Nursing in Lexington, Kentucky. She has practised community and home health nursing, has served as an administrator and consultant in home health, and has been involved in the development of multiple nurse-managed centres. She has taught public and community health, primary care nursing, and administration courses. Dr. Stanhope formerly served as associate dean at the University of Kentucky College of Nursing, also directed the Division of Community Health Nursing and Administration, and co-directed the Doctorate of Nursing Practice program from its inception. She has been responsible for both undergraduate and graduate courses in public and community health nursing. She also has taught at the University of Virginia and the University of Alabama, Birmingham. Her presentations and publications have been in the areas of home health, community health and community-based nursing practice, primary care nursing, and nurse-managed centres with emphasis on vulnerable populations. Dr. Stanhope holds a diploma in nursing from the Good Samaritan Hospital in Lexington, Kentucky, and a bachelor of science in nursing from the University of Kentucky. She has a master's degree in public health nursing from Emory University in Atlanta and a doctorate of science in nursing from the University of Alabama, Birmingham. Dr. Stanhope is the co-author of four other Mosby/Elsevier publications: *Public Health Nursing* (also with Dr. Lancaster), *Handbook of Community-Based and Home Health Nursing Practice, Public and Community Health Nurse's Consultant,* and *Case Studies in Community Health Nursing Practice: A Problem-Based Learning Approach.* Dr. Stanhope received the 2000 Public Health Nursing Creative Achievement Award from the Public Health Nursing Section of the American Public Health Association. She was inducted into the University of Kentucky Distinguished Alumni Hall of Fame, May 2005, joining 257 other graduates of the University of Kentucky who have received this honour. Other honours include recognition as an Edgerunner by the American Academy of Nursing, October 2006, for her work with nurse-managed centres.

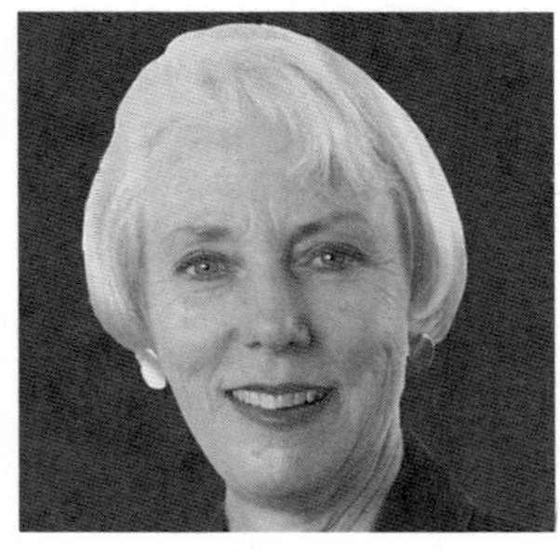

Jeanette Lancaster, RN, PhD, FAAN

Jeanette Lancaster is currently a visiting professor in the Department of Nursing Studies at the University of Hong Kong. She served for 19 years as the Sadie Heath Cabaniss Professor of Nursing and Dean at the University of Virginia School of Nursing in Charlottesville, Virginia. Dr. Lancaster also served as president of the American Association of Colleges of Nursing. She has practised psychiatric nursing and taught both psychiatric and community health nursing. She formerly directed the master's program in community health nursing at the University of Alabama, Birmingham, and served as dean of the School of Nursing at Wright State University in Dayton, Ohio. Her publications and presentations have been largely in the areas of community and public health nursing, leadership and change, and the significance of nurses to effective primary health care. Dr. Lancaster is a graduate of the University of Tennessee, Memphis, College of Nursing. She holds a master's degree in psychiatric nursing from Case Western Reserve University in Cleveland and a doctorate in public health from the University of Oklahoma. Dr. Lancaster is the author of another Mosby/Elsevier publication, *Nursing Issues in Leading and Managing Change,* and co-author (with Dr. Stanhope) of *Public Health Nursing.* She edits the interdisciplinary journal *Family & Community Health.* She most recently has taught undergraduate and graduate courses in public health nursing and health promotion in the Department of Nursing Studies, Faculty of Medicine at the University of Hong Kong.

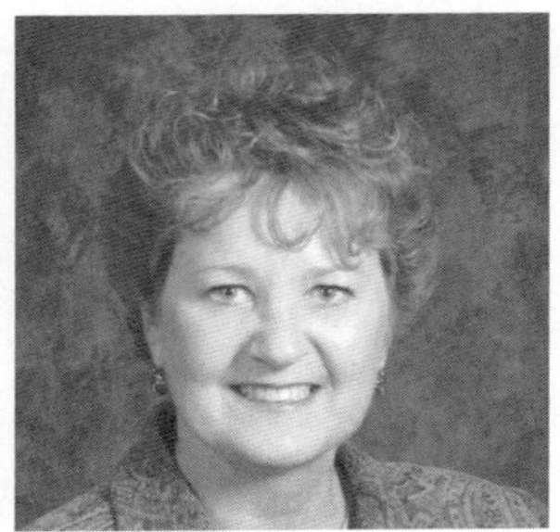

Heather Jessup-Falcioni, RN, BScN, BEd, MN

Heather Jessup-Falcioni is currently Associate Professor at the School of Nursing, Laurentian University, Sudbury, Ontario. She has more than 35 years of experience in health care and academia in several provinces. Her experiences include community and public health nursing, community development, project management, and program planning and evaluation. Her scholarly activities, including presentations and publications, encompass such areas as women's health, cultural health, heart health, gerontological health, team work, and smoking cessation. Professor Jessup-Falcioni's other interests include ergonomic and environmental health issues. In 2006, she was the recipient of the Ontario Heather Crowe Award for her work related to issues concerning smoking and the 2006 Ontario Volunteer Services Award for her work as a long-time volunteer with the Sudbury Heart Health Project. In 2008, 2009, and 2010, she co-facilitated a roundtable discussion at the National Community Health Nurses Conferences (CHNC).

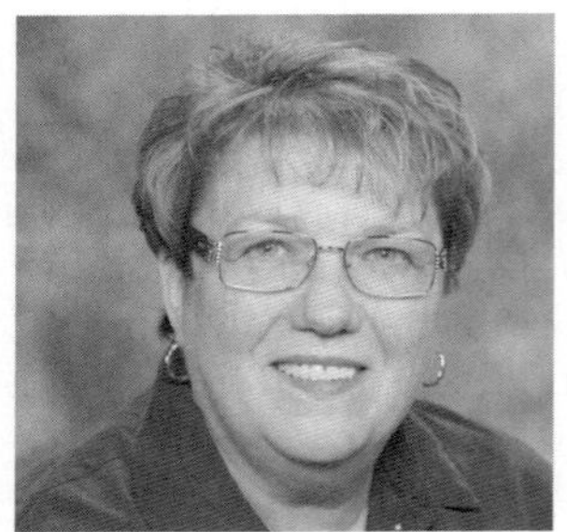

Gloria A. Viverais-Dresler, RN, MHSc

Gloria Viverais-Dresler is a health care professional with many years of varied nursing experience both in nursing practice and in academia. Her nursing practice background includes experience as a staff nurse in maternity care, psychiatry, public health, and advanced practice. She has recently retired from her position as Associate Professor at the School of Nursing, Laurentian University, Sudbury, Ontario. She was an educator in the undergraduate and graduate nursing programs and a tutor in the nurse practitioner program. She was also the program liaison at Laurentian University for the Ontario Primary Health Care Nurse Practitioner Program. Professor Viverais-Dresler was a panel member of a Registered Nurses' Association of Ontario committee for the development of the best practice guideline for nurses, titled "Caregiving Strategies for Older Adults with Delirium, Dementia, and Depression." Her research interests are in the areas of gerontology, community health nursing practice, and distance education. She has presented papers at several regional, national, and international conferences and workshops and has published numerous articles in health care and nursing journals.

CREDIT LINES FOR PERFORATED CARDS

Nationally Notifiable Infectious Diseases
Adapted from Public Health Agency of Canada. (2003). *Notifiable diseases on-line.* Retrieved from http://dsol-smed.phac-aspc.gc.ca/dsol-smed/ndis/list_e.html#tab1.

Windshield Survey Components
Modified from Vollman, A. R., Anderson, E. T., & McFarlane, J. M. (2008). *Canadian community as partner: Theory and multidisciplinary practice in nursing* (2nd ed., pp. 248–249). Philadelphia, PA: Lippincott.

Signs of Abuse and Neglect
Modified from Ontario Ministry of Children and Youth Services. (2010). *Recognizing the signs of child abuse and neglect.* Retrieved from http://www.children.gov.on.ca/(S(yuqv033quey01k55i4eual55))/htdocs/English/topics/childrensaid/reportingabuse/recognisingabuse.aspx; and Royal Canadian Mounted Police. (2008). *What is child abuse?* Retrieved from http://www.rcmp-grc.gc.ca/pubs/ccaps-spcca/chi-enf-eng.htm.

Davidhizar and Giger's Transcultural Assessment Model Categories
Adapted from Davidhizar, R. E., & Giger, J. N. (1998). *Canadian transcultural nursing: Assessment and intervention.* St. Louis, MO: Mosby.

Family Assessment Guide
Source: Wright, L., & Leahey, M. (2009). *Nurses and families: A guide to family assessment and intervention.* (5th ed., p. 124). Philadelphia, PA: F. A. Davis.

Primary Health Care Principles
Source: World Health Organization. (1978). *Declaration of Alma-Ata.* Retrieved from http://www.who.int/hpr/NPH/docs/declaration_almaata.pdf.

Determinants of Health
Adapted from Health Canada. (2002). *Chronic diseases in Canada,* 23(4), 124. Reproduced with permission of the Minister of Public Works and Government Services Canada, 2007.

Canadian Community Health Nursing Standards
Source: Community Health Nurses Association of Canada. (2003 [Revised 2008]). *Canadian community health nursing standards of practice.* Retrieved from http://www.chnc.ca/documents/chn_standards_of_practice_mar08_english.pdf. Reproduced with permission.

The Values and Beliefs of Community Health Nurses
Community Health Nurses Association of Canada. (2003 [Revised 2008]). *Canadian community health nursing standards of practice.* Retrieved from http://www.chnc.ca/documents/chn_standards_of_practice_mar08_english.pdf. Reproduced with permission.

Canadian Contributors

Catherine Aquino-Russell, RN, PhD
Associate Professor
University of New Brunswick
Faculty of Nursing, Moncton Campus

Mary Louise Batty, RN, BA, MN
District Site Manager
Victorian Order of Nurses
Fredericton, New Brunswick

Elizabeth (Liz) Diem, RN, PhD
Assistant Professor
Faculty of Health Sciences
School of Nursing
University of Ottawa
Ottawa, Ontario

Nancy Horan, BScN, RN, SANE-A, SANE-P
Coordinator
Domestic Violence/Sexual Assault Treatment Program
Sudbury Regional Hospital
Sudbury, Ontario

Manon Lemonde, RN, PhD
Associate Professor
Faculty of Health Sciences
University of Ontario Institute of Technology
Oshawa, Ontario

Victoria Morley, RN, BScN, MEd
Faculty Clinical Advisor
Laurentian University

Alwyn Moyer, RN, PhD
Adjunct Professor
University of Ottawa
Ottawa, Ontario
Self-employed Health Consultant

Bonnie Myslik, RN(EC), MScN, NP-PHC
Primary Health Care Nurse Practitioner
Adjunct Course Professor
University of Windsor
Windsor, Ontario

Lisa Perley-Dutcher, RN
Director
Aboriginal Health Human Resources Initiative
University of New Brunswick
Fredericton, New Brunswick

Ivana Zuliani, RN, BScN, MScN
Nurse Consultant
Workplace Safety and Insurance Board
Sudbury, Ontario

Contributors to the U.S. 3rd Edition

We gratefully acknowledge the following individuals who wrote chapters for the U.S. 3rd edition of *Foundations of Nursing in the Community,* upon which the chapters in this book are based.

Monty Gross, PhD, RN, CNE
Associate Professor
Department of Nursing
James Madison University
Harrisonburg, Virginia

Cynthia Z. Gustafson, PhD, APRN-BC
Chair and Associate Professor
Department of Nursing
Director of the Parish Nurse Center
Carroll College
Helena, Montana

Patty J. Hale, RN, PhD, FNP, FAAN
Professor and Graduate Program Coordinator
Department of Nursing
James Madison University
Harrisonburg, Virginia

Susan B. Hassmiller, PhD, RN, FAAN
Senior Advisor for Nursing
The Robert Wood Johnson Foundation
Former Chair
Disaster Services
American Red Cross
Princeton, New Jersey

Diane C. Hatton, DNSc, RN
Professor
Community Health Nursing Concentration Chair
San Diego State University
San Diego, California

Bonnie Jerome-D'Emilia, PhD, RN
Professor
Department of Nursing
Rutgers Camden College of Arts and Sciences
Camden, New Jersey

Joanna Rowe Kaakinen, PhD, RN
Associate Professor
School of Nursing
University of Portland
Portland, Oregon

Lisa M. Kaiser, RN, MSN, PhD(c)
Associate Faculty
National University
LaJolla, California

Kären M. Landenburger, RN, PhD
Professor
Nursing Program
University of Washington, Tacoma
Tacoma, Washington

Susan C. Long-Marin, DVM, MPH
Epidemiology Manager
Mecklenburg County Health Department
Charlotte, North Carolina

Karen S. Martin, RN, MSN, FAAN
Health Care Consultant
Martin Associates
Omaha, Nebraska

Mary Lynn Mathre, RN, MSN, CARN, CLNC
President
Patients Out of Time
Sole Proprietor of Medical Legal Management
Howardsville, Virginia

Robert E. McKeown, PhD
Professor of Epidemiology, Department Chair
Arnold School of Public Health
University of South Carolina
Columbia, South Carolina

DeAnne K. Hilfinger Messias, RN, PhD, FAAN
Associate Professor
College of Nursing and Women's and Gender Studies Program
University of South Carolina
Columbia, South Carolina

Lillian H. Mood, RN, MPH, FAAN
Retired
State Director of Public Health Nursing, Assistant Commissioner, and Community Liaison for Environmental Quality Control
South Carolina Department of Health and Environmental Control
Chapin, South Carolina

Marie Napolitano, RN, PhD, FNP
Associate Professor
School of Nursing
University of Portland
Portland, Oregon

Lisa L. Onega, PhD, RN, FNP, GNP
Professor
Waldron College of Health and Human Services
Radford University
Radford, Virginia

Bonnie Rogers, DrPH, COHN-S, LNCC, FAAN
Director
North Carolina Occupational Safety and Health Education and Research Center
Director
Public Health/Occupational Health Nursing Programs
University of North Carolina
Chapel Hill, North Carolina

Barbara Sattler, RN, DrPH, FAAN
Professor, Family and Community Health
School of Nursing
University of Maryland
Baltimore, Maryland

Juliann G. Sebastian, ARNP, PhD, FAAN
Dean and Professor
College of Nursing
University of Missouri—St. Louis
St. Louis, Missouri

George F. Shuster, RN, DNSc
Associate Professor
College of Nursing
University of New Mexico
Albuquerque, New Mexico

Mary Cipriano Silva, RN, PhD, FAAN
Professor Emeritus
College of Nursing and Health Science
George Mason University
Fairfax, Virginia

Jeanne Merkle Sorrell, PhD, RN, FAAN
Professor
College of Nursing and Health Science
George Mason University
Fairfax, Virginia

Francisco S. Sy, MD, DrPH
Director
Division of Extramural Activities and Scientific Programs
National Center on Minority Health and Health Disparities
National Institutes of Health
Bethesda, Maryland

Anita Thompson-Heisterman, MSN, RN, CS, FNP
Assistant Professor
University of Virginia
School of Nursing
Charlottesville, Virginia

Heather Ward, MSN, ARNP
Master's Student
University of Kentucky
College of Nursing
Lexington, Kentucky

Carolyn A. Williams, RN, PhD, FAAN
Professor and Former Dean
College of Nursing
University of Kentucky
Lexington, Kentucky

Judith Lupo Wold, PhD, RN
Associate Professor Emeritus
School of Nursing
College of Health and Human Sciences
Georgia State University
Atlanta, Georgia

Janet T. Ihlenfeld, RN, PhD[†]
[†]Before her death, Dr. Ihlenfeld was a professor of nursing at D'Youville College where she taught both child health and community health nursing.

Canadian Reviewers

Megan Aston, RN, PhD
Assistant Professor
School of Nursing
Dalhousie University
Halifax, Nova Scotia

Mary Lou Batty, RN, BN, MN
Senior Instructor
Faculty of Nursing
University of New Brunswick
Fredericton, New Brunswick

Sally Dampier, RN, BScN, MMedSc, RSM, RSCN, PGDE (DNP student)
Faculty
School of Health and Community Services
Confederation College
Thunder Bay, Ontario

Corinne Hart, RN, MHSc, PhD
Assistant Professor
Daphne Cockwell School of Nursing
Ryerson University
Toronto, Ontario

Michelle Hogan, RN, MSc
Academic Associate
Faculty of Health Sciences
University of Ontario Institute of Technology
Oshawa, Ontario

Nina Hrycak, RN, PhD
Associate Professor
Faculty of Nursing
University of Calgary
Calgary, Alberta

Claudette Kelly, RN, BScN, MA, PhD
Nursing Department
Thompson Rivers University
Kamloops, British Columbia

Marie Dietrich Leurer, RN, BSN, MBA, PhD
Assistant Professor
College of Nursing (Regina Site)
University of Saskatchewan
Regina, Saskatchewan

Aliyah Mawji, RN, BN, MPH
Instructor
Faculty of Nursing
University of Calgary
Calgary, Alberta

Roberta Mercier, RN, BSN, MEd
Instructor, Faculty of Health Sciences
Bachelor of Science in Nursing Program
Douglas College
Coquitlam, British Columbia

Preface

For a developed country, the population of Canada is not as healthy as one might expect. Social determinants of health, such as socioeconomic status, social environment, and social support networks, are recognized as significantly affecting the health of Canadians. Macro-level factors, such as poverty and unemployment, and micro-level factors, such as lifestyle, influence the health of Canadians. Therefore, to improve the health of Canadians, there is a need to deal with the social, political, and economic conditions that negatively influence health and contribute to disease and disability.

Community health nursing plays a major role in focusing on the health of populations, aggregates, groups, communities, and individuals, as well as that of families, in order to change the health of society as a whole. Community health nursing considerations include health promotion, health protection, disease prevention, health maintenance, health education, cultural sensitivity, advocacy, restoration, coordination, management, and evaluation of care to clients. Community health nurses (CHNs) deliver health services to all age groups in a variety of public and private settings. One of the challenges for community health nursing is to initiate change. To meet the demands of a constantly changing health care system, CHNs need to be visionary in designing their roles and identifying their practice areas. To do this effectively, they need to understand the concepts and theories of public health, the changing health care system, the actual and potential roles and responsibilities of CHNs and other health care providers, the importance of a health promotion and disease prevention orientation, and the need to involve other health care providers and consumers as partners in the assessment, planning, implementation, and evaluation of community health care efforts.

Disease prevention and health promotion strategies designed to address the determinants of health are most effective when they are developed through partnerships among government, businesses, voluntary organizations, consumers, communities, and health care providers. These partnerships aim to eliminate health disparities among Canadians by focusing on health care for children, minorities, older adults, and other vulnerable groups in order to increase the lifespan and quality of Canadians' lives. To develop healthy populations, therefore, individuals, families, and communities must all commit to meeting these health disparity goals. In addition, through the development of healthy public policy, society must support better health care, the design of improved health education, and the financing of strategies to address the issues related to the identified determinants of health and thereby positively alter health status.

Compared with many other developed countries, in Canada the practice of community health nursing places a greater emphasis on the determinants of health as factors influencing health; on the Ottawa Charter, specifically on equity in health and health promotion strategies; on Epp's health promotion framework; on population health; on the *Canadian Community Health Nursing Standards;* and on the development of the certification process for community health nursing. Unfortunately, in recent years Canada has been falling behind in addressing the determinants of health and health inequities.

In this text, the term *community health nursing* encompasses a variety of practitioners, such as public health nurses (PHNs), home health care nurses (HHNs), occupational health nurses (OHNs), and primary health care nurse practitioners (PHCNPs), who practise in a variety of settings in the community. This text focuses on the processes and practices for promoting health used principally by CHNs. CHNs are ideally positioned to work with communities to promote health, as they have an awareness that many factors interact to influence health. The current "upstream focus" on working with groups and communities involves such activities as setting health care policies that address the determinants of health. CHNs strive to use the essential strategies and approaches for health promotion outlined in the Ottawa Charter for Health Promotion to promote and preserve the health of Canadians.

This Second Edition of *Community Health Nursing in Canada* provides a comprehensive approach to community health nursing concepts, skills, and practice. This text presents readers with historical, conceptual, and theoretical perspectives in content areas that are necessary for novice practitioners in community health nursing practice. It also identifies the increasing awareness of social justice and the impact of society on individual health, with a shift from individual-centred care to population- and community-centred care.

This edition has been extensively revised. Examples have been updated using the most current research, and readers are directed to the most current Canadian Web sites. This edition maintains a population-based approach; a socioenvironmental, equity, and social justice perspective; and a behavioural perspective.

A list of additional resources for more in-depth exposure to certain topics is provided in each chapter. Students are required to incorporate prior learning in such areas as physiology, psychology, sociology, research, and ethics. Nursing program graduates can further develop their knowledge and skills in community health nursing practice as they apply the *Canadian Community Health Nursing Standards of Practice.*

It is our belief that learning is a lifelong adventure, and it is our hope that graduates will continue to develop their knowledge and skills in community health nursing through experience, through continuing education, and, for some, through further academic learning, such as master's and doctoral programs.

TEXT ORGANIZATION

This book's 18 chapters are organized for easy use by students and faculty. The ordering of the chapters is a suggestion only. Each chapter stands alone, so the ordering can be modified by individual faculty.

Chapters begin with a list of **Objectives** that guide student learning and assist faculty in knowing what students should gain from the content and reflect what are sometimes referred to in the field of nursing education as "ends in view." The **Chapter Outline** alerts students to the structure and content of the chapter. **Key Terms** are identified at the beginning of the chapter, and the definitions are provided, in alphabetical order for quick reference, in a glossary of terms at the end of the text to assist the student in understanding unfamiliar terminology. The key terms are bolded in the text.

CLASSIC FEATURES

- **Critical View** boxes present questions on a contemporary issue that are intended to stimulate debate and discussion. They have been strengthened to include a social justice and equity lens.
- **Determinants of Health** boxes, found in selected chapters, relate the chapter content to the determinants of health as supported by the literature. Ideas about the meaning of the facts presented expand on their possible impact. The information presented in these boxes is intended to stimulate further class discussion about the determinants of health, their impact, and further implications.
- **How To...** boxes provide specific, application-oriented information.
- **Evidence-Informed Practice** boxes illustrate the application of the latest research findings in nursing and community health nursing and include critical thinking questions for reflection and discussion.
- **Levels of Prevention** boxes provide examples of primary, secondary, and tertiary prevention related to community health nursing practice specific to the chapter.
- The **Remember This!** list at the end of each chapter provides a summary of the most important points made in the chapter.
- The term *reflective praxis* refers to the transfer of theory to practice using critical thinking to deliberate, plan, intervene, implement, and evaluate nursing practice. The **Reflective Praxis** section at the end of each chapter consists of Case Studies and "What Would You Do" questions. Both types of exercises help students develop their assessment and critical thinking skills and provide an opportunity to reflect on chapter content and gain an understanding of how to apply it in the practice setting.
  - evolve The **Case Studies** include questions students need to think about as they analyze a case. (Answers to the Case Studies are now provided on the Evolve Web site accompanying the text.)
  - *What Would You Do* questions encourage learning through a variety of suggested activities that involve both independent and collaborative efforts. These activities can be used for classroom discussions, assignments, or student projects.
- evolve The **Tool Box** section at the end of each chapter directs students to excellent sources of supplemental information, including appendices that are relevant to the chapter content and specific links to Web sites with practical tools, such as checklists or guides, that will assist students in applying chapter-related content.
- evolve The **Weblinks** include an extensive list of annotated Web resources that will provide a wealth of additional information on specific chapter topics.
  - Both the Tool Box links and the Weblinks can be accessed on the text's accompanying Evolve site at http://evolve.elsevier.com/Canada/Stanhope/community/. At the time of publication, these links were active and were selected on the basis of such factors as source, authorship, affiliation, and currency.
  - Users are encouraged to evaluate Web resources for these and other factors. One example of a resource that could be used to evaluate Web resources is http://www.lib.berkeley.edu/TeachingLib/Guides/Internet/Evaluate.html.

- Students are reminded that when typing in a URL, be sure not to type in a period (.) at the end of the URL.

- evolve **Appendices:** There are 13 appendices at the end of the text, and five more can be accessed on the Evolve Web site. The majority of these appendices are Canadian and are referred to in the chapters throughout the text. They provide a more in-depth look at primary sources, such as the Canadian Community Health Nursing Standards of Practice, the Ottawa Charter for Health Promotion, Giger and Davidhizar's Transcultural Assessment Model, and the Calgary Family Assessment Model. Several Canadian Nurses Association (CNA) position statements on such topics as the environment, as well as social justice, and the determinants of health, are also included, as is the Government of Ontario's fact sheet, "What You Should Know About an Influenza Pandemic."
- Many acronyms and abbreviations are used throughout the chapters, and a **List of Commonly Used Abbreviations** is provided on the inside back cover of this text for easy reference.

NEW FEATURES

- New **Ethical Considerations** boxes appear in most chapters and provide examples of ethical situations and the relevant principles involved. Questions are raised for student and faculty reflection and discussion.
- New **Student Experience** boxes assist students to apply and reflect on specific content areas in each chapter. Questions encourage students to use their critical thinking skills and, often, to share findings for discussion and debate with fellow classmates.
- **Chapter 18, Applications in Working with Specific Aggregates,** is a new chapter designed to promote application of content covered throughout the earlier chapters. Two approaches are used. The first part consists of a single case study with a step-by-step application of the community health nursing process with an Aboriginal community; the second uses several case studies on mental illness with questions for students to address. Both approaches include examples of nurses' reflections.
- A more critical lens has been used in the expanded Determinants of Health boxes with respect to the impact of the statistical information.
- The social justice and equity lens of the book has been strengthened through the addition of questions in the Critical View boxes.
- There is a greater focus on the social determinants of health throughout the text.
- evolve The information available at the text's Evolve Web site has been expanded and is denoted with an Evolve icon in the margin, where applicable. Students and instructors are advised to establish access to the Evolve site as soon as they purchase their textbook. At Evolve, you will find additional resources such as access to the links in the Tool Box and Weblinks sections for each chapter, additional appendices, and answers to the case studies in the text.

ACKNOWLEDGMENTS

First and foremost, we want to thank our immediate and extended families for their interest, love, and support, particularly during all the times they had to adjust plans for family gatherings in order to accommodate our writing schedule. We also thank our friends for their words of encouragement.

We wish to give special thanks to the many health professionals who made contributions to the textbook: Catherine Aquino-Russell, Mary Louise Batty, Liz Diem, Nancy Horan, Manon Lemonde, Victoria Morley, Alwyn Moyer, Bonnie Myslik, Lisa Perley-Dutcher, and Ivanna Zuliani.

We would like to acknowledge and thank our nursing colleagues at Laurentian University, who supported us during the writing of this text by sharing textbook resources upon request. We especially extend our thanks to Sharolyn Mossey and Ivana Zuliani for their thoughtful contributions; Catherine Aquino-Russell for her revisions and additions to the Evidence-Informed Practice boxes within the text; Joyce MacQueen for sharing her historical nursing collection; and Joan Reiter for the provision of resources for the history of nursing. We greatly appreciate the contributions from our research assistants, David Razao and Mark Collins, and Patricia Kitching for her technical support. A special thank you to Mary-Catherine Taylor for her photography contributions and assistance, and to others, too numerous to mention, for being photo subjects.

We wish to thank Marcia Stanhope and Jeanette Lancaster and acknowledge their contributions over many years and many editions of community health nursing texts and the contributors to *Foundations of Nursing in the Community,* the U.S. text upon which this Canadian edition is based. We also want to thank the staff at Elsevier, especially Ann Millar, Publisher, for her excellent leadership; Martina van de Velde for her capable direction, and Dawn du Quesnay, developmental editor, for her dedication to the task and her unfailing patience, continued support, and encouragement.

LIST OF BOXED FEATURES*

Chapter 1: Community Health Nursing

Chapter 2: The Evolution of Community Health Nursing in Canada

Chapter 3: Community Health Nursing in Canada: Settings, Functions, and Roles

Chapter 4: Health Promotion

*(does not contain Critical View boxes)

Chapter 5: Evidence-Informed Practice in Community Health Nursing

Chapter 6: Ethics in Community Health Nursing Practice

Chapter 7: Diversity

Chapter 8: Epidemiological Applications

Chapter 9: Working with Community

Chapter 10: Health Program Planning and Evaluation

Chapter 11: Working with Vulnerable Populations

Chapter 12: Working with Family

Chapter 13: Working with Client as Individual: Health and Wellness Across the Lifespan

Chapter 14: Working with Groups, Teams, and Partners

Chapter 15: Environmental Health

Chapter 16: Disaster Management

Chapter 17: Communicable and Infectious Disease Prevention and Control

Chapter 18: Applications in Working with Specific Aggregates

CHAPTER 1

Community Health Nursing

OBJECTIVES

After reading this chapter, you should be able to:

1. Explain the concepts of community health nursing, primary health care, health promotion, levels of disease prevention, population health, and public health.
2. Describe the population health promotion model.
3. Explain the determinants of health.
4. Identify the social determinants of health.
5. Explain the relationship between primary health care, social justice, and global health.
6. Discuss the *Canadian Community Health Nursing Standards of Practice.*
7. Discuss the roles and functions of the community health nurse.
8. Explain community health nursing practice.

CHAPTER OUTLINE

KEY TERMS

See Glossary on page 593 for definitions.

In recent years, the visibility of community health nursing in Canada has increased. Community health nurses (CHNs) have increasingly become a more vital part of the Canadian health care landscape. The number of recognized community health nursing specialties has increased. The variety of settings in which CHNs practice has expanded, as has the scope of their role. The 2003 adoption of the *Community Health Nursing Standards of Practice* (refer to Appendix 1) has further reinforced the status of community health nursing as a specialty nursing practice within the discipline of nursing.

One result of this new focus on community health nursing is its shift into some nontraditional specialties such as primary health care nurse practitioner and nurse entrepreneur in independent practice. CHNs as entrepreneur nurses may, for example, be self-employed providers of foot care services in their community or, as in some parts of Canada, registered psychiatric nurses engaged in independent community nursing practice. Increasingly, CHNs are also employed as community leaders in nongovernmental organizations such as the Young Men's Christian Association (YMCA) and the Young Women's Christian Association (YWCA).

The settings in which CHNs practise have changed and continue to evolve. For example, more CHNs are employed in correctional and school settings, and increasing numbers are becoming involved in international and global health activities.

Some aspects of the CHN's role have also been evolving. For example, there is now a greater emphasis than ever before on the role of CHN as advocate for policy change or as activist on issues pertaining to the social determinants of health. Recognizing that health status is influenced by determinants such as income, employment, education, gender, and social environment, to name but a few, CHNs aim to improve the health of all persons by addressing these determinants and minimizing health disparities wherever possible. They also consider that lifestyle choices (e.g., tobacco, alcohol, and drug use, diet, physical activity, sexual practices, etc.) influence health as well. The consideration of policy strategies to address the complex issues of vulnerable populations, those who have the poorest health status, will continue to be a priority for CHNs but will require further development.

In Canada, community health nursing practice emphasizes population health promotion, disease prevention, and health protection. CHNs work with various types of clients, as illustrated in Figure 1-1. (Throughout this book, the term **client** refers to individuals, families, groups or aggregates, communities, populations, or society.) CHNs bring people together, such as community members who know what it takes to make their community healthy, at the same time always ensuring that they are responsive to the current available evidence relevant to CHN practice.

It is critical that CHNs continue to be partners in knowledge generation and exchange and are not only observers of these processes. In order to gain a better

FIGURE 1-1 The Community Health Nursing Client

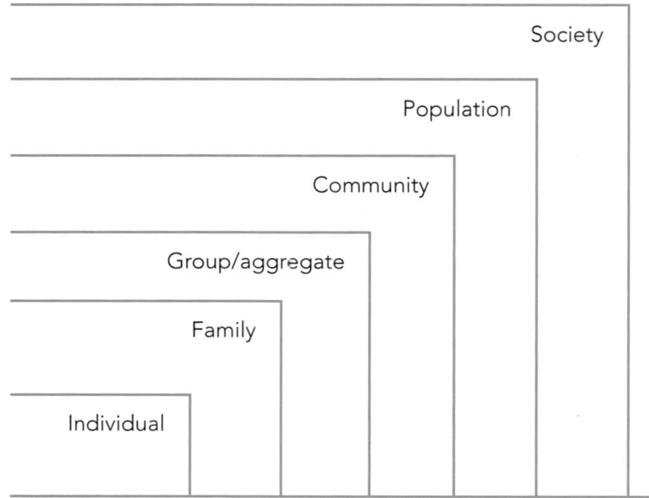

understanding of factors affecting the health of clients, as well as be cognizant of trends relating to the transformation of health care, CHNs need to know how to access and use resources, associations, and agencies, such as the Canadian Population Health Initiative, the Public Health Agency of Canada, Health Canada, the Canadian Nurses Association, provincial and territorial nurses' associations, and the Community Health Nurses of Canada.

CHNs cannot be expected to be experts in all areas; thus, interdisciplinary collaboration and partnership development are important in community health nursing. It is critical that clear boundaries be in place to ensure positive, successful, and collaborative partnerships and that CHNs and other health care professionals become comfortable with a blurring of roles and responsibilities (always within CHNs' scope of practice).

At the same time, it is important for CHNs to recognize the value of their generalist health care knowledge, which enables them to address diverse and complex community health care concerns. The *Community Health Nursing Standards of Practice* guide and facilitate the practice of CHNs in Canada as they work within the principles of primary health care to promote and preserve the health of populations (Community Health Nurses of Canada [CHNC], 2009).

The community health nursing students of today are the community health nursing practice leaders of tomorrow. CHNs will continue to make a difference through a focus on areas such as population health, "upstream thinking," evidence-informed nursing practice, the determinants of health, and the Ottawa Charter health promotion strategies, concepts that will be explored in this text. Chapter 1 introduces the reader to some of the key community health nursing concepts, such as public health, primary health care, and community health nursing and its settings and roles, and briefly discusses health care in Canada.

CONCEPTS WITHIN COMMUNITY HEALTH NURSING IN CANADA

Health Care in Canada

Canada is a bilingual country that is geographically vast, covering diverse types of terrain over 10 provinces and three territories and comprising many cultures residing in both urban and rural settings. In order to guarantee an equitable national health care system for all Canadians, the *Canada Health Act* was developed in 1984. The five principles of this Act are (1) universality, (2) accessibility, (3) comprehensiveness of services, (4) portability, and (5) public administration (refer to the Health Canada Web site listed in the Evolve Weblinks at the end of the chapter).

For the past decade, health care reform has been initiated at various levels in the health care system across Canada, and different restructuring models have been adopted in the provinces and territories (Public Health Agency of Canada [PHAC], 2006). One example of these changes has been the establishment of community health centres across Canada with the goal of improving access to health care and, in underserviced regions, providing such access. Although there are some similarities among these centres, differences do exist (refer to the Association of Ontario Health Centres Web site listed in the Evolve Weblinks). CHNs need to be prepared to address health concerns and population health care issues locally or regionally, provincially or territorially, nationally, and globally within the context of the health care reform initiatives.

Roles and Functions of Community Health Nurses

Community health nursing is an umbrella term used to define nursing specialties and applies to all nurses who work in and with the community in a variety of practice areas, such as public health, home health, occupational health, and other similar fields. Figure 1-2 lists the most common specialties encompassed by the term and some of the usual roles assumed by community health nurses. Table 1-1 provides some examples of the most common community health nursing practice areas based on areas of specialty. Table 1-2 provides examples of clients that CHNs may work with and examples of their roles based on some of the specialty areas. Client types and community specialty areas are discussed in Chapter 3.

Community health nursing includes various functions. It is a specialty nursing practice that involves working with clients to preserve, protect, promote, and maintain health. Community health nurses work *with* the client, not just *for* the client, in their approach to assessment, planning, intervention, and evaluation. Working *with* the client involves establishing partnerships with clients.

FIGURE 1-2 Community Health Nursing Umbrella: Specialties and Roles

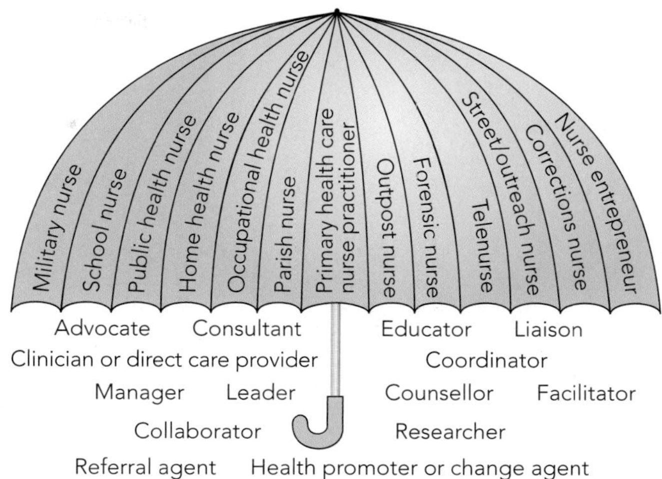

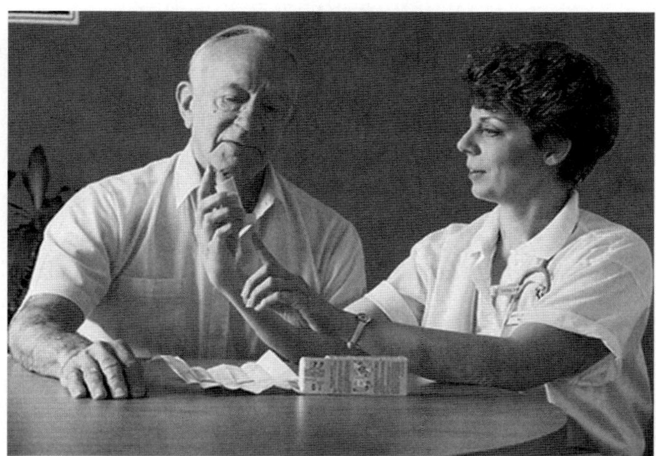

Community health nurses work with clients in many different practice settings. Here, a community health nurse visits with a client in his home to teach him how to use his medication.

This will become evident to you as you work through the content in this text. Although CHNs work independently as they practise in the community, they also work with other health care providers in community partnerships and as members of various teams.

It is important to consider the word *community* in the term *community health nursing*. **Community** may be defined as people and the relationships that emerge among them as they develop and commonly share agencies, institutions, or a physical environment. Members of a community can be defined in terms of either geography (e.g., a city or town, a group of cities or towns that form a region, district, or province) or a group who shares a common interest or focus (e.g., children attending a particular school). Is the CHN working *in* the community or *with*

TABLE 1-1 Examples of Community Health Nursing Practice Areas

Community Health Nurses (CHNs)	Definition	Practice Settings	Client Group	Educational Preparation	Examples of Roles and Activities	Funding
Public health nurse (PHN)	Public health nurses use knowledge of nursing, social sciences, and public health sciences for the promotion and protection of health and for the prevention of disease among populations.	• Community groups • Community health centres • Workplaces • Street clinics • Schools • Outpost settings • Homes	• Population • Aggregates or groups • Communities • Families • Individuals	Baccalaureate degree in nursing or registered or licensed practical nurse (RPN or LPN)*	• Health promotion • Disease prevention • Client advocacy • Education • Direct care in clinics	Provincial and municipal government funding
Home health nurse (HHN)	Home health nurses use their knowledge and skills to provide direct care and treatment for individuals to maintain and restore health or to provide palliation during illness.	• Clients' homes • Schools • Clinics • Workplaces	• Individuals • Families • Caregivers	Registered nurse (RN) or RPN or LPN*	• Direct client care • Disease prevention • Health promotion with individual clients	Public or private funding
Occupational health nurse (OHN)	An RN who specializes in workplace health and safety, health promotion, disease prevention, and rehabilitation for workers	• Workplace	• Employees (individuals, groups)	RN with certificate in occupational health	• Direct care • Assessment of the workplace • Education of employees on health and safety issues	Employer
Parish nurse	An RN who serves the health and wellness needs of faith community members	• Clients' homes • Places of worship • Hospitals	• Individuals • Families • Groups	RN	• Health promotion • Health counsellor • Liaison • Health advocate • Integrator of faith and health	Place of worship funding

Primary health care nurse practitioner (PHCNP)	An RN with advanced practice education, which allows for an expanded role, such as diagnosing episodic illnesses, prescribing medication, and ordering diagnostic tests	• Community health centres • Clinics • Physicians' offices • Emergency departments in hospitals • Nursing stations • Long-term care facilities	• Individuals • Families • Groups • Communities	Baccalaureate degree in nursing, minimum of post-baccalaureate diploma with licensing in extended class (EC)	• Direct care (i.e., health assessment; diagnosis and treatment of episodic illness) • Health promotion • Disease prevention • Community development and planning	Public or private funding
Outpost nurse	An RN who works in an outpost or rural setting that is often geographically separated from face-to-face physician contact	• Nursing stations • Clients' homes • Community	• Individuals • Families • Groups • Rural communities	RN	• Direct care • Health promotion • Liaison with other health professionals • Referral	Provincial or federal funding
Military nurse	An RN, nursing officer, employed by the Canadian Forces Health Services	• Military hospitals • Military outpatient centres • Civilian tertiary care facilities • Military operational units	• Individuals • Families	Baccalaureate degree in nursing	• Direct client care • Disease prevention • Occupational health care • Environmental health care	Federal funding
Forensic nurse	An RN who has completed continuing education programs in the area of forensic science	• Sexual assault treatment setting, often in hospital emergency departments	• Adults and children who are victims of acute sexual assault and survivors of domestic violence or intimate partner abuse	RN	• Direct client care for collection of physical evidence • Crisis response, such as counselling and referral	Provincial funding

(Continued)

TABLE 1-1 Examples of Community Health Nursing Practice Areas—Cont'd

Community Health Nurses (CHNs)	Definition	Practice Settings	Client Group	Educational Preparation	Examples of Roles and Activities	Funding
Telenurse	An RN who provides nursing service over the telephone	• Community agencies	• Individuals • Families • Caregivers	RN	• Telephone advice • Telehealth network (live video links for nurse-led telehealth clinics)	Provincial funding provided to private companies
Corrections nurse	An RN who works in a correctional facility	• Correctional facilities	• Inmates (individuals, groups) • Correctional facility staff	RN	• Direct care • Health promotion • Disease prevention • Inmate advocate • Crisis intervention	Provincial or federal funding
Nurse entrepreneur	An RN who is self-employed in the provision of nursing services	• Home • Variety of workplace settings	• Individuals • Families • Groups • Communities	RN or RPN or LPN*	• Direct client care as contracted • Consultant • Advocate • Health promotion • Disease prevention	Private funding
Street or outreach nurse	An RN who serves the health and wellness needs of marginalized populations living on the streets	• Community streets	• Individuals • Families • Communities	RN	• Direct client care (i.e., wound care; drug overdose treatment) • Disease prevention • Health promotion • Client advocate • Political activist	Provincial or municipal funding

*Some Canadian provinces and territories designate registered practical nurses (RPNs) or licensed practical nurses (LPNs) to work in some settings such as home health nursing and public health nursing. Note: In some provinces, *RPN* refers to *registered psychiatric nurse;* however, in this table, the abbreviation designates *registered practical nurse.*

TABLE 1-2 Community Health Nursing Roles and Practice Examples

Client as:	Role Example	Practice Example
Society **Society** is defined as the systems that incorporate the social, political, economic, and cultural infrastructure to address issues of concern.	Advocate	A street nurse advocates for affordable housing for the homeless in Canada.
Population A population is a large group of people who have at least one characteristic in common and who reside in a community (e.g., adolescents residing in Regina, mothers with newborns).	Advocate	A team of community health nurses consisting of a parish nurse, a public health nurse, and a nurse practitioner have identified the need for options in the community that would provide adolescents enhanced opportunities for physical activity. The team has approached the city council requesting designated times for "adolescent-only" access to the facilities at the local sports complex.
Community Community may be defined as people and the relationships that emerge among them as they develop and commonly share agencies, institutions, or a physical environment. Members of a community can be defined in terms of either geography (e.g., residents of Regina, Sask.) or a shared status or special interest group (e.g., single parents).	Educator	A group of public health nurses (PHNs) organize a community health fair at the local shopping centre to inform the community about diabetes.
Group or Aggregate Aggregates are defined as groups within a population (e.g., adolescents with diabetes mellitus, high-risk newborns).	Educator	A nurse practitioner (NP), employed at a local diabetic education centre, holds monthly diabetes education sessions with a small group of adolescents with diabetes mellitus. These interactive sessions provide an opportunity for group members to share challenges related to having diabetes as a teenager and ideas on how to manage these challenges.
Family **Family** is defined as two or more individuals who depend on one another for emotional, physical, or financial support or a combination of these (e.g., Sally, adolescent diabetic, and her family).	Counsellor	A home health nurse (HHN) visits Sally and her family (parents and younger brother). At this visit, the HHN talks with the family to explore their concerns about their ability to support Sally in the management of her diabetes.
Individual An individual is one human being (e.g., Sally, adolescent diabetic).	Liaison and referral agent	Sally is a 13-year-old newly diagnosed with type 1 diabetes mellitus. John, a community care case manager, assesses Sally in the hospital and determines that she requires assistance with the management of her diabetes. John makes a referral to a home health care agency requesting that an HHN visits Sally within 24 hours of her discharge to address her health care needs.

the community? When providing health care to individuals and families, the CHN maintains a focus on health promotion and disease prevention and views the community as a resource; therefore, the CHN is said to be working *in* the community. The CHN views the community itself as the client and applies the community health nursing process to the whole community; therefore, the CHN is working *with* the community and also focuses on health promotion and disease prevention. This concept of working with the community is explored further in Chapter 9.

Populations and Aggregates

Although it is hoped that all direct care providers contribute to the community's health, in the broadest sense, not all are primarily concerned with the population focus, or the "big picture." All CHNs in a given community, including those working in hospitals, physicians' offices, and health clinics, contribute positively to the health of the community. Examples of community settings for health promotion, disease prevention, and treatment for individuals include ambulatory surgery, outpatient clinics, physician and advanced-practice nursing clinics, employment and school sites, preschool programs, housing projects, and summer camps. These sites often provide individual-focused health care services, in contrast to population-focused services.

The terms *populations* and *aggregates* are sometimes used interchangeably, but differences do exist. A **population** refers to a large group of people who have at least one characteristic in common and who reside in a community. Generally, **subpopulations** are referred to as *aggregates* within the larger community population (Clark, 2003; Porche, 2004). Therefore, **aggregates** are defined as groups within a population. Examples of a subpopulation, or aggregate, within a population include high-risk infants younger than 1 year of age, unmarried pregnant adolescents, and individuals exposed to a particular harmful incident, such as a chemical spill.

Population health refers to the health of a population using as measurements the determinants of health and health status indicators. Examples of health status indicators are measures of well-being, life expectancy, incidence and prevalence rate, crude death rate, mortality rate, burden of illness, and case fatality rate (Shah, 2003). CHNs, other health care providers, and government policymakers use health status indicators and health patterns to determine the health of a community (McEwen & Nies, 2007). Population health is covered in more depth in Chapter 4.

Community Health Nursing Practice Considerations

Community health nursing practice has as one area of focus disease prevention, which is divided into three levels: primary, secondary, and tertiary. **Primary prevention** is a type of intervention or activity that seeks to prevent disease from the beginning, before people have a disease, and relates to the natural history of a disease. Examples of primary prevention for CHNs include individual and mass immunizations, the organization of community vaccination programs for influenza, and the education of the community through mass media about the importance of handwashing to prevent the spread of infection. **Secondary prevention** is a type of intervention or activity that seeks to detect disease early in its progression (early pathogenesis), before clinical signs and symptoms become apparent, in order to make an early diagnosis and begin treatment. For example, in secondary prevention, mass screening programs to assess vision and hearing or to detect breast cancer, cervical cancer, hypertension, and scoliosis would be conducted for early case finding. **Tertiary prevention** is a type of intervention or activity that begins once the disease has become obvious; its aim is to interrupt the course of the disease, reduce the amount of disability that might occur, and begin rehabilitation. An example of tertiary prevention would be cardiac rehabilitation at a local wellness centre for groups of clients who have been recently discharged from hospital following a cardiovascular event. Another example is the CHN providing education for a group of children who have experienced abuse. The "Levels of Prevention" box above illustrates the three levels as they relate to public health.

LEVELS OF PREVENTION

Related to Public Health Nursing

PRIMARY PREVENTION

A community health nurse provides an influenza vaccination program in a community retirement village.

SECONDARY PREVENTION

A community health nurse, in partnership with the local police, organizes an infant and child car seat safety screening program for a group of parents in a low-income housing complex.

TERTIARY PREVENTION

A community health nurse helps set up a rehabilitation clinic for middle-aged adults residing in an apartment complex who have type 2 diabetes and have experienced a cerebral vascular accident.

The primary, secondary, and tertiary levels of prevention are categorized into two levels of care: episodic care and distributive care. *Episodic care* refers to the curative and restorative aspect of practice (secondary and tertiary prevention), and *distributive care* refers to health maintenance, disease prevention, and health promotion (Pizzuti, 2006). The following clinical example illustrates the application of these two aspects in community health nursing, specifically home health care:

Mr. Smith, a 75-year-old retired miner, was discharged from the hospital with a referral through a community care access centre for home nursing services. This referral was made to assess his respiratory status following a diagnosis of chronic obstructive pulmonary disease (COPD). Episodic care involves teaching Mr. and Mrs. Smith about his medications and how to implement healthy lifestyle patterns, such as smoking cessation and exercise. The CHN will also assess Mr. Smith's rehabilitation to help him reach his optimal level of functioning. The CHN will conduct a family assessment to determine their current health status as well as health-enhancing behaviours, such as smoking cessation, nutrition, physical activity, stress management, and immunization, especially flu vaccines. A family assessment framework could be used for this assessment [discussed in Chapter 12]. The family's psychosocial adaptation and health concerns, as well as the client's level of self-care and adjustment, will also be assessed. Distributive care will involve the CHN teaching Mr. Smith ways to prevent an exacerbation of his condition (e.g., medical follow-up and lifestyle adaptations to increase his adherence to the programs set up for him) so that he can achieve his optimal level of functioning.

When working with clients and their health concerns, CHNs need to determine whether upstream or downstream solutions—or both—are required. **Downstream thinking** refers to taking a microscopic individual curative focus, a view that does not consider the economic, sociopolitical, and environmental variables (Butterfield, 2007; McKinley & Marceau, 2000). CHNs need to ask the question, "How can the illness and its consequences be treated?" Whereas downstream thinking focuses on the individual, **upstream thinking** looks beyond the individual to take a macroscopic, big-picture population focus. It also includes a primary prevention perspective and is a population health approach. A population health approach "aims to improve the health of the entire population and reduce health inequalities among population groups by embracing the full range of protection, prevention and promotion strategies" (Leeds, Grenville & Lanark District Health Unit, 2006, p. 1). When working with clients, CHNs using upstream thinking would consider the determinants of health and other relevant economic, sociopolitical, and environmental factors that may influence the health of the client (Butterfield, 2007; Young & Higgins, 2008).

Additionally, CHNs need to ask the question, "How could this have been prevented?" In most situations, CHNs need to take an upstream thinking approach. The following story, frequently shared in public health, helps to illustrate the difference between downstream and upstream thinking.

As the story goes, several people have fallen in a river. A physician at the side of the river hears their cries for help. The physician rescues one of the people and resuscitates the person. Shortly after, the physician hears another cry for help and rescues that person. The cries for help and the rescues by the physician continue all day long. The physician is so busy rescuing people and dealing with the acute crisis situation that he cannot go upstream to identify exactly why people are continually needing to be rescued—for example, whether a bridge requires repair, a walkway over the water is unsafe, or slippery rocks present danger at the river's edge. If the physician had been able to go upstream, he might have identified the reasons for the people falling in the river and been able to initiate interventions early and thereby prevent unnecessary deaths, injuries, and depletion of his resources. Furthermore, by using this approach, he would have dealt with the problem as a group problem and not had to deal with the problems of each individual.

Although this story has a medical perspective, the analogy of the situation can be applied by all health care professionals in their approach to care.

Numerous definitions of *health* exist. The definition a health care professional chooses to use will direct that person's practice. For instance, a health care provider who defines *health* as the absence of disease will practise with a medical focus involving downstream thinking. The more commonly used definition of *health* in community health, however, involves upstream thinking. Community health nursing practice supports the World Health Organization (WHO) definition, which views health positively as a resource for everyday living that is holistic and includes physical, social, and personal capabilities (World Health Organization [WHO], 2006).

Collaborating in Interdisciplinary Teams

Within their practice, CHNs often work with other health care team members in an interdisciplinary approach. Team members could include physicians, social workers, nutritionists, physiotherapists, occupational therapists, epidemiologists, researchers, and other health care professionals. The client, the focus of care, is also a team member and participates in shared decision making with regard to his or her health concerns. All team members are valued for their individual expertise, and trust among them is essential, as is sharing of power in the decision-making process. Such collaboration among members of the interdisciplinary team contributes to ensuring that the client receives the best care possible (D'Amour, Ferrada-Videla, San Martin Rodriguez, & Beaulieu, 2005). Groups and teams are discussed further in Chapter 14.

Collaboration refers to the commitment of two or more parties (partners such as agency, client, and professional) who set goals to address identified client health concerns. D'Amour et al. (2005), in their review of the relevant literature, found proposals for many different models of collaboration and identified seven theoretical frameworks that would help clarify the collaboration process. These authors found that not all of the frameworks were based on empirical data and that not all had been tested. However, a common element among most of the models was that interactions form an essential part of collaborative processes (D'Amour et al., 2005).

Researchers Orchard, Curran, and Kabene (2005) supported interdisciplinary collaborative practice but found insufficient research on the progressive stages that interdisciplinary teams need to develop for collaborative practice. So they proposed a conceptual framework to guide the development of interdisciplinary collaborative professional teams in primary health care. Their framework addresses some of the processes involved in collaboration, such as decision making, role clarification and socialization, value sharing, development of trust, and power sharing. This framework also explores the

CRITICAL VIEW

1. To what extent do you think that the concepts of collaboration and cooperation can be used interchangeably? Support your thinking.
2. What are the similarities and differences between collaboration and cooperation?

CRITICAL VIEW

1. What agencies and departments come under the umbrella of Health Canada? Locate an existing organizational chart or develop one to show this structure.
2. Locate an organizational chart of your local public health authority, department, or unit. How does public health nursing fit within this organization?

barriers to team development and discusses strategies to convert these barriers into enablers using a change process (Orchard et al., 2005). When team members respect interdisciplinary differences in values and beliefs and establish a power balance, they are more likely to collaborate effectively (Orchard et al., 2005).

A Canadian collaboration called the Enhancing Interdisciplinary Collaboration in Primary Health Care (EICP) Initiative provides a "collaboration tool kit" (see the Tool Box at the end of the chapter and on Evolve). This tool kit provides information gathered from across Canada about how organizations practise interdisciplinary care in a collaborative manner and also includes practical tools and advice. Another example of collaborative activity is that of the Canadian Collaborative Mental Health Initiative (CCMHI), whose mission is to enhance collaboration between mental health care providers and primary care providers (see the Tool Box on Evolve). A number of projects within this latter initiative employ a collaborative model, with a focus on improving access to services, mental health care, disease prevention, and health promotion.

The Canadian Nurses Association (CNA, 2005a) has formulated its position on collaboration on the basis of the six principles and framework for interdisciplinary collaboration in primary health care. The six principles are (1) focus on the patient/client, (2) population health approach, (3) quality care and services, (4) access, (5) trust and respect, and (6) communication. For the complete CNA position statement, see Appendix 2.

Health Canada and the Public Health Agency of Canada

Health Canada, which has regional offices across Canada, is a Canadian umbrella agency for many other health portfolios, such as the Public Health Agency of Canada (PHAC); Canadian Institutes of Health Research (CIHR); Health Products and Food Branch; First Nations, Inuit, and Aboriginal Health; Healthy Environments and Consumer Safety Branch; and others. Health Canada safeguards the population's health through surveillance, prevention, legislation, and research in such areas as environmental health, disease outbreaks, drug products, and food safety. The Health Canada Web site (listed in the Evolve Weblinks) provides access to its resources and links to other agencies.

Following the 2003 severe acute respiratory syndrome (SARS) outbreak, the PHAC was established in 2004 to revitalize the public health system in Canada and to support a sustainable health care system. Led by a chief public health officer, this new agency has provided opportunities for further collaboration between the federal government and the provinces and territories. The chief public health officer communicates important public health issues in an annual report. These annual reports are comprehensive and will be referred to throughout this text to inform the reader about key issues that affect the health of Canadians. The PHAC Web site (listed in the Evolve Weblinks) provides a wealth of information on various federal branches, centres, and directorates, as well as links to other excellent resources.

COMMUNITY HEALTH NURSING STANDARDS OF PRACTICE

The *Canadian Community Health Nursing Standards of Practice* were initially adopted by the Community Health Nurses Association of Canada (CHNAC) in 2003 and edited and translated in March 2008. The CHNAC underwent a name change in June 2009 and is now known as the Community Health Nurses of Canada (CHNC). The five standards of practice according to CHNC are listed in Box 1-1, and the complete text of the standards is provided in Appendix 1. CHNC has developed a conceptual model of the Canadian community health nursing practice standards, the context of practice, the foundational values and beliefs, and the community health nursing process (see Figure 1-3). Further explanation of this model is available at the CHNC Weblink on Evolve.

The terms *community health nurse* and *public health nurse* (PHN) have often been used interchangeably;

BOX 1-1 Canadian Community Health Nursing Standards of Practice

The five Canadian Community Health Nursing Standards of Practice are as follows:

1. Promoting health*
2. Building individual and community capacity
3. Building relationships
4. Facilitating access and equity
5. Demonstrating professional responsibility and accountability

*Includes disease prevention, health protection, health maintenance, restoration, and palliation.

SOURCE: Community Health Nurses Association of Canada. (2008). *Canadian community health nursing standards of practice* (p. 9). Retrieved from http://www.chnc.ca/documents/chn_standards_of_practice:mar08_english.pdf.

however, the *Canadian Community Health Nursing Standards of Practice* have helped to differentiate among the various community health nursing specialties. The differences among all community health nursing specialties, such as public health nursing, home health nursing, and parish nursing, are their unique practice settings, roles, beliefs, and philosophies about community health nursing practice. Refer to Table 1-1, which lists some of the most commonly encountered CHN practice areas in Canada. Community health nurses working as home health nurses (HHNs) and PHNs practise in diverse settings. These specialties share many similarities in their community health nursing practice, including use of strategies for health promotion, prevention, and protection (CHNAC, 2008). Even though the location and unit of care, the practice and goals of care, and specific nursing activities may vary, all CHNs are expected to meet the five standards of practice. In fact, CHNs are expected to function beyond the level of the standards in order to become experts in this field of nursing (CHNAC, 2008).

Whatever their practice title and setting, within 2 years of beginning community nursing practice, CHNs are expected to meet the requirements in knowledge, skills, and abilities outlined in the *Standards of Practice* (CHNAC, 2008). Since 2006, the CNA has offered certification for Canadian community health nurses (CHNC, 2009; CNA, 2009a). This certification is voluntary and provides an opportunity for further professional development and the demonstration of competency and currency in community health nursing. Table 1-3 provides community health nursing practice examples applied to each of the standards in the *Standards of Practice* for PHNs, HHNs, and some CHNs working in other community health settings. The standards of practice are referred to throughout this text.

FIGURE 1-3 The Canadian Community Health Nursing Practice Model

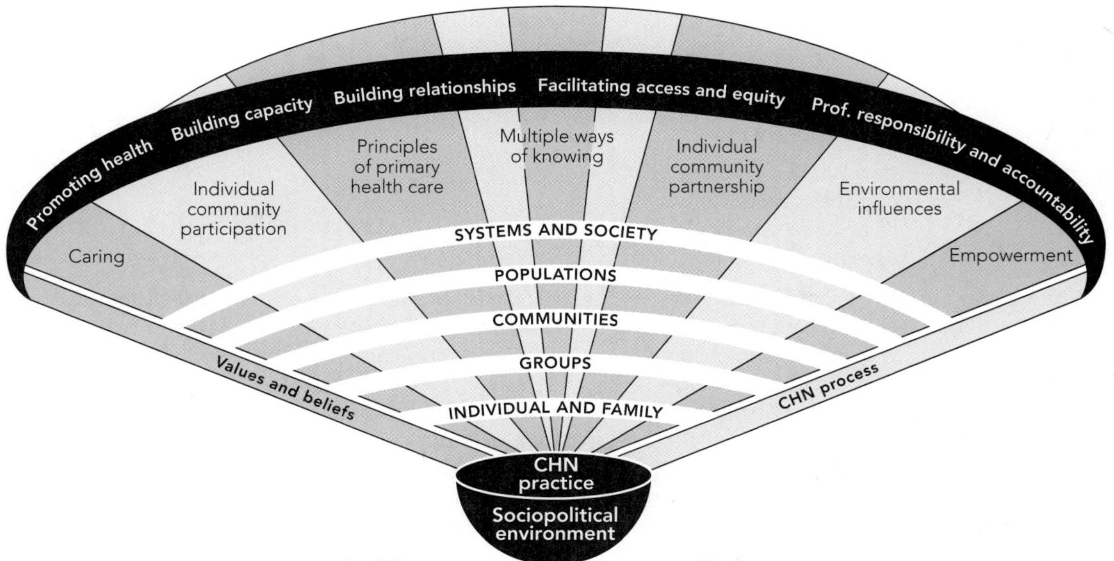

Community Health Nurses Association of Canada. (2003) [Revised 2008]. *Canadian community health nursing standards of practice*, p. 9. Retrieved from http://www.chnc.ca/documents/chn_standards_of_practice:mar08_english.pdf. Reproduced with permission.

TABLE 1-3 Practice Examples of Application of the Canadian Community Health Nursing Standards of Practice[1]

Standard	Public Health Nurses (PHNs)	Home Health Nurses (HHNs)	Nurses Working in Health Promotion in the Community (NHP)[2]
Standard 1: Promoting Health			
A) Health Promotion	• PHNs work with a community and use social marketing to promote the development of more recreational spaces and activities for families. • PHNs promote physical activity and healthy eating through such programs as the Supermarket Safari and the Schools Awards Program.	• HHNs encourage families dealing with a chronic illness to participate in regular physical and social activities.	• NHPs encourage families dealing with a chronic illness to participate in regular physical and social activities.
B) Prevention and Health Protection	• PHNs track immunization schedules for each child so that families and practitioners can access information when needed (in case of an outbreak, travel, school records, etc.). • PHNs work with HHNs and NHPs to develop and distribute information that is appropriate in terms of culture and reading level on identifying and reducing risk factors, such as falls, medication errors, and communicable diseases. • PHNs work with parents' organizations, parent resource centres, and the police to promote proper installation of car seats through the media and conduct several clinics to provide one-on-one assessment and teaching.	• HHNs work with PHNs to develop and distribute information that is appropriate in terms of culture and reading level on identifying and reducing risk factors, such as falls, communicable diseases, and low immunization rates. • When HHNs observe high rates of smoking among caregivers and clients, they raise a concern, and a task group is formed to find ways to address the issue.	• NHPs work with PHNs to develop and distribute information that is appropriate in terms of culture and reading level on identifying and reducing risk factors, such as falls, communicable diseases and low immunization rates. • When NHPs observe high rates of smoking within a particular client group, they bring it to the attention of the practice team, and a plan is developed to find ways to address the issue.
C) Health Maintenance, Restoration, and Palliation	• PHNs provide ongoing nursing care to families with infants and children who are experiencing difficulties. Care may be provided directly or through supervised unregulated workers. This may include telephone follow-up, home visits, or referrals to other community-based services.	• HHNs adapt the care provided to acute-care and long-term care clients and their families based on the clients' choices, their own personal skills, and the resources available in the setting and community.	• NHPs provide ongoing nursing care or care coordination to individuals and families who are experiencing poor health. Care may be provided directly or through telephone follow-up, home visits, or referrals to other community-based services.

TABLE 1-3 Practice Examples of Application of the Canadian Community Health Nursing Standards of Practice—Cont'd

Standard	Public Health Nurses (PHNs)	Home Health Nurses (HHNs)	Nurses Working in Health Promotion in the Community (NHP)[2]
		• HHNs provide long-term nursing care—in the home, school, or work—for children, youth, and adults for conditions such as acquired brain injury. Collaboration is required with the client, unregulated care providers, family, teachers, and/or employers to promote capabilities, prevent secondary illness, and improve response to treatment.	
Standard 2: Building Individual/Community Capacity	• PHNs encourage a school to form a school health committee that includes students, parents, teachers, administrators, and community partners. Committee members identify the school community's strengths and needs and prioritize, plan, implement, evaluate, and celebrate action for a healthier school. The school community's capacity to take its own action for health is enhanced by the formation of a sustainable structure (the committee), with the PHN as a partner in the process.	• HHNs provide training and encouragement for people in the home to carry out care for a family member. For example, a mother and teenaged children would be supported in developing and carrying out a schedule for range-of-motion (ROM) exercises for a grandmother living with them. • HHNs teach clients and family members how to change dressings and assess for deterioration and healing of a wound. Within a short period, the clients and the families take over the dressing changes and report steady improvement.	• NHPs initiate mother-to-mother groups for women in a specific linguistic group so that they can share resources and experiences in raising children. • NHPs ensure that clients and family members living with diabetes receive education and ongoing support on monitoring blood sugar, taking medication, exercising, and moderating diet. Depending on the individual and family, they may provide the service themselves on an individual basis or in a group, or refer them to another community program.
Standard 3: Building Relationships	• PHNs are selected to coordinate heart health coalitions because they are able to communicate effectively and regularly with community members and are able to help find a goal that everyone believes in.	• HHNs working in palliative care listen to the concerns of stressed and exhausted caregivers and support them in making decisions about respite and hospice care.	• NHPs in the primary health care team ask to be assigned to work with a defined case load of clients rather than being assigned each day to different tasks. This arrangement will allow them more opportunity to develop an ongoing relationship with clients.

(Continued)

TABLE 1-3 Practice Examples of Application of the Canadian Community Health Nursing Standards of Practice—Cont'd

Standard	Public Health Nurses (PHNs)	Home Health Nurses (HHNs)	Nurses Working in Health Promotion in the Community (NHP)[2]
	• PHNs working with families experiencing child care difficulties identify that postnatal visits based on issues or tasks do not allow them to develop a continuing relationship with families. They bring their concern to the attention of management.	• HHNs and management work together to provide "continuity of care" so that the majority of clients have the same nurse most of the time.	• NHPs provide options and ask clients and caregivers how they want to learn about coping with an acute or long-term illness or disability.
Standard 4: Facilitating Access and Equity	• PHNs identify that new immigrants are especially vulnerable to communicable diseases, such as tuberculosis, and make limited use of prevention services. The PHNs decide to work with the teachers in the English as a Second Language (ESL) classes and the staff in immigrant assistance centres to develop and provide health information and services at those locations. • A PHN works with business owners and volunteer community groups to promote breastfeeding-friendly businesses and public places.	• HHNs and case managers work together to advocate for families caring for medically fragile children by: – seeking respite care for families exhausted by the required intense care – contacting the local provincial/territorial member of parliament (MP) to encourage enhanced funding for respite services – planning for a resolution through the provincial/territorial registered nurses association • HHNs are joined by PHNs and NHPs to lobby for retaining home visits and case management by registered nurses for people living with mental illness.	• NHPs and case managers work together to support immigrant families by: – hosting multicultural celebrations featuring foods from different cultural groups served by their organization – lobbying municipal councillors for funding for community gardens and food banks – planning for a resolution on health literacy at the provincial/territorial registered nurses association • NHPs organize exercise classes at suitable times and places for workers, caregivers, or seniors.
Standard 5: Demonstrating Professional Responsibility and Accountability	• PHNs are assigned to work in needle exchange programs based on harm reduction. When a PHN has difficulty accepting the tenets of harm reduction, reflective practice alone and with the supervisor can help the PHN understand the program and change assumptions.	• When an HHN is asked by an amyotrophic lateral sclerosis (ALS) client to be present during removal of the bi-level positive airway pressure (Bi-PAP) machine, which will result in death, the nurse explores the client's reasons for this decision and discusses the ethics of responding to this request with the health care team as well as the nursing practice advisor at their provincial/territorial Registered Nurses association.	• NHPs work in clinics serving the homeless. When an NHP has difficulty accepting the harm reduction approach adopted by the clinic, the NHP uses reflective practice alone and with the supervisor to understand the approach and change assumptions.

TABLE 1-3 Practice Examples of Application of the Canadian Community Health Nursing Standards of Practice—Cont'd

Standard	Public Health Nurses (PHNs)	Home Health Nurses (HHNs)	Nurses Working in Health Promotion in the Community (NHP)[2]
	• PHNs work together to identify how they can incorporate the CCHN Standards in their provincial/territorial Registered Nurses association continuing competence or quality assurance program.	• HHNs work together to identify how they can incorporate the CCHN Standards in their provincial/territorial Registered Nurses association continuing competence or quality assurance program.	• NHPs work together to identify how they can incorporate the CCHN Standards in their provincial/territorial Registered Nurses association continuing competence or quality assurance program.
	• The Nursing or Professional Practice Council initiates action on integrating the Standards by following the steps in the CHNC's Standards Toolkit (2007): (1) forming a committee to work on the initiative, (2) conducting a stakeholder and environmental scan, (3) developing a plan after determining that staff and management want an orientation, policies, and professional development based on the Standards.	• A group of nurses in the organization initiates action on integrating the Standards by following the steps in the CHNC's Standards Toolkit (2007): (1) organizing themselves, (2) conducting a stakeholder and environmental scan, (3) developing a plan after determining that staff and management want an orientation, policies, and professional development based on the Standards.	• A group of NHPs in the organization initiates action on integrating the Standards by following the steps in the CHNC's Standards Toolkit (2007): (1) organizing themselves, (2) conducting a stakeholder and environmental scan, (3) developing a plan after determining that staff and management want an orientation, policies, and professional development based on the Standards.

[1]The Canadian Community Health Nursing (CCHN) Standards, 2003, revised 2008, have been promoted throughout Canada by the Community Health Nurses of Canada (CHNC). Part of the promotion strategy was the development of a tool kit in March 2006 by Elizabeth Diem and Alwyn Moyer and fellow investigators Ruth Schofield, Cheryl Reid Haughian, and Jo Ann Tober. This tool kit was developed for CHNC and PHAC with funding received from PHAC. Promotion of the tool kit occurred during an introductory workshop in Cornwall in October 2006 and three subsequent teleconferences, attended by CHNs from across Canada. Further promotion of the tool kit occurred in a preconference workshop session during the First National Conference for Community Health Nurses, titled "Mapping the Future for Better Health," which was held in Toronto in May 2007. Table 1-3 was developed by Elizabeth Diem for the teleconference sessions held in early 2007 and was updated in 2009.

[2]The term "nurses working in health promotion" (NHP) was coined to include nurses who practise health promotion in a variety of community settings. The settings could include community health care centres, primary care clinics, family practice, care or case management centres, streets, schools, workplaces, and churches.

SOURCE: Diem, E. (2007) [Revised 2009]. *Practice examples of application of the Canadian community health nursing standards of practice.* Table presented at the First National Conference for Community Health Nurses, Toronto, ON. Reprinted with permission.

DETERMINANTS OF HEALTH

The Lalonde Report (Lalonde, 1974), titled *A New Perspective on the Health of Canadians,* first identified four of the determinants of health—human biology, lifestyle, health care organization, and environment. This report initiated the shift from primarily curative aspects of care to holistic health care and provided the foundation for health promotion (Canadian Policy Research Networks, 2000; Fricke, 2005). The WHO's *Ottawa Charter for Health Promotion* (2006) identified the prerequisites for health as peace, shelter, education, food, income, a stable ecosystem, sustainable resources, social justice, and equity, which established the roots of the current determinants of health in Canada. The Epp Report, titled *Achieving Health for All* (Epp, 1986), identified reducing inequities, increasing prevention, and enhancing coping skills as specific challenges to achieving health; these challenges are also included in the determinants of health. The ecosystem health approach, adopted by some health care researchers and practitioners, hypothesized that there is interconnectedness among the health determinants (Institute of Health Promotion Research, 2005). Hamilton and Bhatti (1996), in their population health promotion model (discussed later in this chapter and in Chapter 4), identify nine determinants of health (see Figure 1-4). This model does not include gender and culture (nonmodifiable factors) among the determinants, nor does it include the broad term *environment.* The PHAC identifies 12 determinants of health because it includes these two nonmodifiable factors and separates "environment" into social and physical environments.

FIGURE 1-4 Population Health Promotion Model

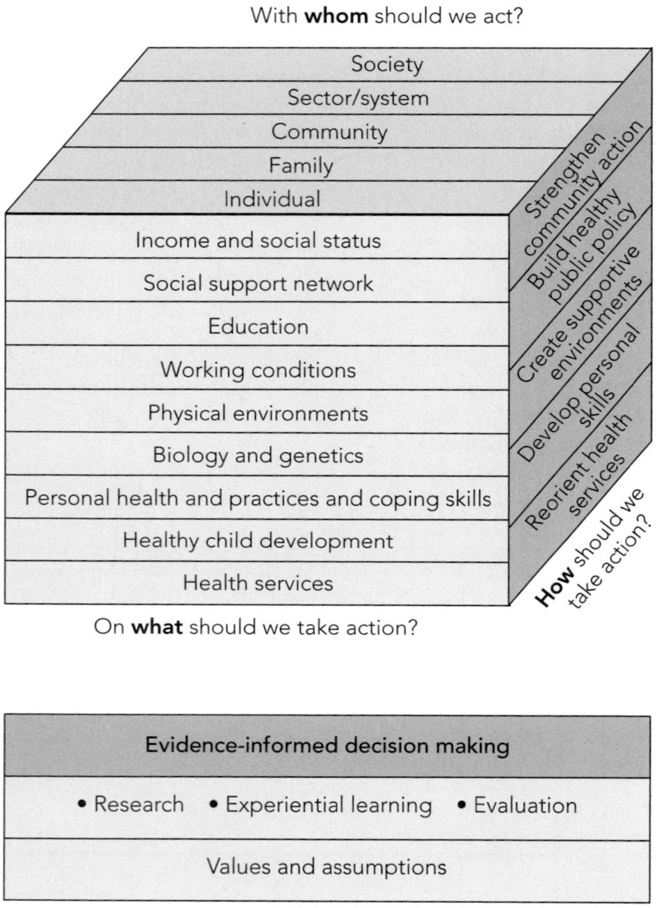

Adapted from Hamilton, N., and Bhatti, T. (2001). *Population health promotion: An integrated model of population health and health promotion.* Ottawa, ON: Public Health Agency of Canada. Retrieved from http://www.phac-aspc.gc.ca/ph-sp/php-psp/php3-eng.php#Values.

The 12 **determinants of health** (DOH) that affect the health of clients as listed by the PHAC (2006) are provided above. These health-determining factors directly relate to such outcomes as disability, disease, and death, and CHNs need to consistently consider these factors in their day-to-day work.

1. *Income and social status* have consistently been shown in the literature to be the most important determinants of health (Labonte, 2003). As income and social status are raised, the health status of Canadians improves (Labonte, 2003). With increased income, healthy, affordable housing and more nutritious food purchases become possible. For example, the CHN working with low-income families could lobby for access to subsidized housing.
2. *Social support networks* are associated with improved health; it has been suggested that poor social relationships may, in fact, be as important a risk factor as smoking or obesity. For example, the CHN working with self-help groups provides support to the group members through group facilitation.
3. *Education and literacy* are part of socioeconomic status (SES) and significantly contribute to better health outcomes since health status improves with higher levels of education. For example, the CHN working with clients who have literacy challenges could refer these clients to community literacy programs.
4. *Employment and working conditions* are associated with improved health because of the better economic conditions that support health and the psychological satisfaction of being gainfully employed. For example, the CHN working with the unemployed in the community could refer clients to job retraining programs.
5. *Social environments* include the support and resources available in the community, region, province or territory, and country that help individuals avoid potential risks that negatively influence health. For example, the CHN working with communities could participate in coalitions to influence social public policy.
6. *Physical environments* refer to human-built environments (e.g., housing, playgrounds, workplaces, communities) as well as the pollutants in the environment that affect the quality of air, water, food, and soil. For example, the CHN working with schools could advocate for safe playground equipment on school property.
7. *Personal health practices and coping skills* include lifestyle choices and the ability to cope with health outcomes. For example, the CHN working with certain populations could partner with other health care professionals to provide stress management group sessions.
8. *Healthy child development* implies consideration of prenatal and early childhood exposures and experiences that may contribute to a variety of chronic conditions and also to the development of physical

and emotional health outcomes later in life. For example, the CHN working with a group of first-time mothers could help them identify concerns that they may have about parenting and provide educational support and referral when necessary.

9. *Biology and genetic endowment* predispose some individuals to certain illnesses, such as Tay-Sachs disease, Huntington's disease, and sickle cell anemia. For example, the CHN working with families with genetic conditions could refer them for genetic counselling.

10. *Health services* must be accessible to all for health maintenance, promotion, protection, disease prevention, and treatment if population health is to be achieved. For example, the CHN could assist a low-income family to gain access to health services, such as eye care, by using service clubs in the community to pay for eye examinations and eyeglasses.

11. *Gender* indicates that some health problems and health practices are gender specific; for example, men are more likely than women to die prematurely from heart disease. For example, the CHN working with women in shelters who have just come out of abusive relationships could work with these women and the shelter staff to develop and conduct group sessions to enhance self-esteem and coping.

12. *Culture* may predispose some groups to certain diseases, such as sickle cell anemia and thalassemia. Also, culture may have implications for access to care. For example, the CHN working with new Canadians could partner with multicultural associations in the community to provide access to interpreters when new immigrant groups are trying to use community health services.

Social Determinants of Health

More recent literature indicates that some of these determinants, known as the *social* determinants of health (SDOH), now have a greater influence on client health (PHAC, 2008a; Raphael, 2009; WHO, 2009). **Social determinants of health** are defined as "the economic and social conditions that shape the health of individuals, communities, and jurisdictions as a whole.... Social determinants of health are about the quantity and quality of a variety of resources that a society makes available to its members" (Raphael, 2009, p. 3). Various conceptualizations of the social determinants of health have been proposed. Table 1-4 presents some of these conceptualizations found nationally and internationally. Note that Aboriginal status, social safety net, and health services are not found in most conceptualizations (Raphael, 2009). Table 1-5 provides seven different discourses on the

TABLE 1-4 Various Conceptualizations of the Social Determinants of Health

Ottawa Charter	Dahlgren & Whitehead (1992)	Health Canada (1998)	World Health Organization	Centers for Disease Control and Prevention (2005)	Raphael, Bryant, & Curry-Stevens (2004)
Peace	Agriculture and food production	Income and social status	Social gradient	Socioeconomic status	Aboriginal status
Shelter	Education	Social support networks	Stress	Transportation	Early life education
Education	Work environment	Education, employment, and working conditions	Early life	Housing	Employment and working conditions
Food	Unemployment	Physical and social environments	Social exclusion	Access to services	Food security
Income	Water and sanitation	Healthy child development	Work	Discrimination by social grouping	Gender
Stable ecosystem	Health care services	Health services	Unemployment	Social or environmental stressors	Health care services
Sustainable resources	Housing	Gender	Social support		Housing
Social justice		Culture	Addiction		Income and its distribution
Equity			Food		Social safety net
(WHO, 1986)			Transport		Social exclusion
			(Wilkinson & Marmot, 2003)		Unemployment and employment security

SOURCE: Raphael, D. (in press). Critical perspectives on the social determinants of health. In E. McGibbon (Ed.), *Oppression as a determinant of health.* Halifax, NS: Fernwood Publishers.

TABLE 1-5 Various Discourses of the SDH Among Health Researchers and Professionals

SDH Discourse	Key Concept	Dominant Research and Practice Paradigms	Practical Implications of the Discourse	Literature Sources Supporting the Discourses
1. SDH* as identifiers of Canadians requiring specific health and social services.	Health and social services should be responsive to people's material living circumstances.	Develop and evaluate services for those experiencing adverse living conditions.	Focus is limited to service provision with the assumption that this will improve health.	(Benoit, Carroll, & Chaudhry, 2003; Hwang & Bugeja, 2000; Saxena, Majeed, & Jones, 1999; Sword, 2000)
2. SDH as identifiers of Canadians with modifiable medical and behavioural risk factors.	Health behaviours (e.g., alcohol and tobacco use, physical activity, diet) are shaped by living circumstances.	Develop and evaluate lifestyle programming that targets individuals experiencing adverse living conditions.	Focus is limited to health behaviours with the assumption that targeting for behaviour change will improve health.	(Allison, Adlaf, Ialomiteanu, & Rehm, 1999; Choi & Shi, 2001; Choiniere, Lafontaine, & Edwards, 2000; Potvin, Richard, & Edwards, 2000)
3. SDH as indicators of material living conditions that shape health.	Material living conditions operating through various pathways—including biological—shape health.	Identify the processes by which adverse living conditions come to determine health.	Identifying SDH pathways and processes reinforces the concept and strengthens evidence base.	(Brunner & Marmot, 2006; Dunn & Hayes, 1999; Hertzman & Frank, 2006; Keating & Hertzman, 1999)
4. SDH as indicators of material living circumstances that differ as a function of group membership.	Material living conditions systematically differ among those in various social locations such as class, disability status, gender, and race.	Carry out class-, race-, and gender-based analysis of differing living conditions and their health-related effects.	Providing evidence of systematic differences in life experiences among citizen groups forms the basis for further antidiscrimination efforts.	(Dunn & Dyke, 2000; Galabuzi, 2004; McMullin, 2008; Ornstein, 2000; Pederson & Raphael, 2006; Wallis & Kwok, 2008)
5. SDH and their distribution as results of public policy decisions made by governments and other societal institutions.	Public policy analysis and examination of the role of politics should form the basis of SDH analysis and advocacy efforts.	Carry out analyses of how public policy decisions are made and how these decisions affect health (i.e., health impact analysis).	Attention is directed toward governmental policymaking as the source of social and health inequalities and the role of politics.	(Armstrong, 1996; Bryant, 2006; Bryant, Raphael, Schrecker, & Labonte, 2010; McIntyre, 2008; Shapcott, 2008; Tremblay, 2008)
6. SDH and their distribution as results of economic and political structures and justifying ideologies.	Public policy that shapes the SDH reflects the operation of jurisdictional economic and political systems.	Identify how the political economy of a nation fosters particular approaches to addressing the SDH.	Political and economic structures that need to be modified in support of the SDH are identified.	(Bambra, 2006; Bambra, Fox, & Scott-Samuel, 2005; Coburn, 2004; Navarro & Shi, 2002; Raphael & Bryant, 2006)
7. SDH and their distribution as results of the power or influence of those who create and benefit from health and social inequalities.	Specific classes and interests both create and benefit from the existence of social and health inequalities.	Research and advocacy efforts should identify how imbalances in power and influence can be confronted and defeated.	Identifying the classes and interests that benefit from social and health inequalities mobilizes efforts toward change.	(Chernomas & Hudson, 2009; Kerstetter, 2002; Langille, 2008; Navarro, 2009; Scambler, 2001; Wright, 2003; Yalnizyan, 2007)

SOURCE: Raphael, D. (in press). Critical perspectives on the social determinants of health. In E. McGibbon (Ed.), *Oppression as a determinant of health.* Halifax, NS: Fernwood Publishers.
*SDH refers here to *social determinants of health.*

social determinants of health (Raphael, in press), as well as sources in the literature supporting each discourse. As you refer to this table, consider that the definition of the social determinants of health that is used will result in definite assumptions that lead to specific focuses within the research and practice areas. These focuses, in turn, contribute to service, research, policy, and economic actions.

Raphael, Bryant, and Curry-Stevens (2004) and Raphael (2009) have conducted extensive scholarly work in the examination of the social determinants of health and their application within health care policy, particularly in Canada. Despite the fact that Canada is a recognized leader in the health promotion movement, specifically regarding the impact of the social determinants of health on populations, Canada has been slow to develop public health policy based on the research evidence (Raphael, 2009).

The WHO publication by Wilkinson and Marmot (2003), *Social determinants of health: The solid facts* (see the Evolve Weblinks), provides an excellent review of the social determinants of health identified at that time and evidence to explain each of these with discussion of policy considerations. In 2005, the WHO established the Commission on Social Determinants of Health to provide recommendations on how to address the social factors contributing to health inequities (WHO, 2009). The final WHO report, titled *Closing the Gap in a Generation: Health Equity Through Action on the Social Determinants of Health,* put forward the following three recommendations with corresponding principles of action: improve daily living conditions; tackle the inequitable distribution of power, money, and resources; and measure and understand the problem and assess the impact of action (WHO, 2008). For further information on the global issues in reference to the social determinants of health, and to review the corresponding principles of action for these recommendations, see the Evolve Weblink.

Another document, *The Chief Public Health Officer's Report on the State of Public Health in Canada: Addressing Health Inequalities* (Butler-Jones, 2008), provides further information on the determinants of health, with examples of their application to client care (see the Evolve Weblinks). Specifically, see Chapter 4 of the report, "Social and Economic Factors That Influence Our Health and Contribute to Health Inequalities."

The determinants of health will be discussed throughout the text, including in "Determinants of Health" boxes in select chapters highlighting the influences of some of the determinants on the health of Canadians. The determinants are also highlighted in specific appendices found in this book. For example, the Canadian Nurses Association (2005b) backgrounder titled *Social Determinants of Health and Nursing: A Summary of the Issues* (see Appendix 3) explains why social determinants are an important factor directly related to the health of individuals, groups, and all Canadians. The backgrounder also lists and explains some of the most important social determinants of health as provided by the WHO—poverty, economic inequality, social status, stress, education and care in early life, social exclusion, employment and job security, social support, and food security. It also identifies cardiovascular disease and diabetes as being most closely linked to the social determinants of health; why this issue is important to nurses; what the CNA has done to address it; and what nurses can do about it. Of relevance specifically to community health nurses is to ensure that the social determinants of health form an integral component of their nursing practice, that they recognize that the social determinants can predict the health of populations, and that healthy public policy includes the social determinants of health.

CRITICAL VIEW

Read the following critique:
Kirkpatrick, S. I., & McIntyre, L. (2009). The chief public health officer's report on health inequalities: What are the implications for public health practitioners and researchers? *Canadian Journal of Public Health, 100*(2), 93–95.

1. What criticisms of the report do the authors present?
2. What are your thoughts on the chief public health officer's report and on the critique by Kirkpatrick and McIntyre?

PRIMARY HEALTH CARE

In the early 1970s, the medical model, which focused on treatment and cure in institutions, was the most commonly used model in health care. The Lalonde Report (Lalonde, 1974) started the shift in thinking toward a population health promotion approach that considered factors influencing health, such as lifestyle. In 1978, at the International Conference on Primary Health Care held in Alma-Ata, USSR, participating countries, organizations, and the World Health Organization (WHO) committed to a goal to achieve "health for all" by the year 2000 (WHO, 1978). Primary health care, as the health care delivery system, was the international strategy chosen to achieve this goal. The Lalonde Report and the Alma-Ata conference and their influence on health promotion are discussed further in Chapter 4. The WHO (see the Evolve Weblinks), an umbrella organization of the United Nations established in 1948, aims to achieve the optimal level of health for all peoples globally. This organization, which has played a key role in the development of health and health promotion approaches, provides many primary health care resources. The "Ethical Considerations" box raises questions about achieving health for all in difficult circumstances.

ETHICAL CONSIDERATIONS

In the course of their practice, CHNs will sometimes find themselves confronted with difficult ethical decisions. Chapter 6, Ethics in Community Health Nursing Practice, discusses ethical issues, principles, and theories in detail. "Ethical Considerations" boxes like this one appear throughout the text to help raise awareness of topical ethical issues and the principles involved in making informed, ethical community health nursing decisions.

Achieving "health for all," particularly through the reduction of inequities, remains a subject of discussion. Take the case of a CHN working with a homeless client unable to afford medication to treat his diabetes. The ideal of "health for all" meets the reality of inequity. The CHN must consider the ethical principles involved.

The following ethical principles (see Box 6-2 on p. 168 for a more detailed discussion of these principles) apply to the above case:

- *Beneficence.* This ethical principle states that CHNs are ethically bound to do good, within the limitations of time, place, and talent. CHNs uphold principles of beneficence by safeguarding human rights, by promoting the public good, and by working with people to enable them to attain their highest possible level of health and well-being.
- *Distributive justice.* This ethical principle requires that there be a fair distribution of the benefits and burdens in society based on the needs and contributions of its members, and, consistent with the dignity and worth of its members and within the limits imposed by its resources, a society must determine a minimal level of goods and services to make available to its members. CHNs uphold principles of distributive justice by working for fairness and equality in health services.

Question to Consider

1. As a CHN, how would you apply the ethical principles of beneficence and distributive justice for homeless clients who cannot afford the medications they require?

It is necessary to distinguish between primary health care and primary care. **Primary care** refers to the first contact between individuals and the health care system (health care providers) and usually relates to the curative treatment of disease (CNA, 2005c), rehabilitation, and preventive measures, such as immunization, smoking cessation, and dietary changes. Primary care is not necessarily comprehensive care, nor is it necessarily intersectoral. *Primary health care,* on the other hand, has a broader meaning. WHO has defined primary health care as "essential health care based on practical, scientifically sound, and acceptable methods and technology made universally accessible to individuals and families in the community through their full participation and at a cost that the community and country can afford to maintain at every stage of their development in the spirit of self-reliance and self-determination" (WHO, 1978, p. 2). Currently, **primary health care** is comprehensive care that includes disease prevention, community development, a wide spectrum of services and programs, working in interdisciplinary teams, and intersectoral collaboration for healthy public policy (CNA, 2005c). This comprehensive primary health care model addresses issues of social justice and equity.

Primary Health Care and Social Justice

Social justice in the context of primary health care refers to ensuring fairness and equality in health services so that all members of society have equal access to health care (Austin, 2008; CNA, 2009b). Political, social, and economic actions are necessary to promote social justice. "Taking action for social justice means attempting to reduce system-wide differences that disadvantage certain groups and prevent equal access to determinants of health and to health-care services" (CNA, 2009b, p. 2). For example, social justice is an important consideration in the care of persons with mental health issues. Inequality in resource allocation for mental health services does exist, causing difficulty for persons with mental illnesses to access health services in their community. In light of such issues, CHNs need to adopt the primary health care model and principles and also partner with others in the community to promote universal and equitable access to health services (CHNAC, 2008). The Canadian Nurses Association document titled *Ethics in Practice for Registered Nurses: Social Justice in Practice* (see Appendix 4) provides a more detailed discussion of the social justice and ethical considerations for nurses. Take note of the first scenario, which depicts a community health nurse working in a rural setting and the application of social justice to this environment.

Social Justice and Global Health

The Canadian Nurses Association, in its position statement on international health partnerships (see the Evolve Weblinks), supports global health and equity within the context of social justice (CNA, 2005d). Brown, Cueto, and Fee (2006) provide a historical perspective on the development of the term *international health* to *global health.* These authors indicate that global health "implies consideration of the health needs of the people of the whole planet above the concerns of particular nations" (p. 62). Koplan et al. (2009) define **global health** as "an area for study, research, and practice that places a priority on improving health and achieving equity in health for all people worldwide" (p. 1995). Koplan et al. (2009) provide an excellent comparison of global health, international health, and public health and emphasize that global health addresses transnational health issues such as climate change, human immunodeficiency virus (HIV), acquired immune deficiency syndrome (AIDS), and determinants of health such as poverty and education; involves an interdisciplinary approach with populations; and includes prevention, treatment, and care. Community health nurses are becoming more involved in working in global health and international development. See Box 1-2 for some key organizations involved in global health efforts.

CRITICAL VIEW

Read the following article:
Raphael, D., Curry-Stevens, A., & Bryant, T. (2008). Barriers to addressing the social determinants of health: Insights from the Canadian experience. *Health Policy, 88*(2), 222–235.

1. What are the strengths associated with viewing health concerns as "population based" compared to "individual based"?
2. How do the authors' suggested policy options relate to social justice?

The CHNC standards of practice have their underpinnings in the primary health care principles. Refer specifically to Standard 4: Facilitating Access and Equity. As members of a primary health care interdisciplinary team, CHNs are well positioned to address the social determinants of health and health inequalities that affect their

BOX 1-2 Some Key Organizations Involved in Global Health Efforts

The following sources can assist CHNs in understanding global health issues. (These links are also available at the Evolve Web site for this text.)

1. **World Health Organization (WHO)** is a leading international health organization involved in global health issues. Refer to its Web site at http://www.who.int/about/en. WHO produces an annual global health report. The 2008 report, titled *Primary Health Care: Now More Than Ever,* can be found at http://www.who.int/whr/2008/whr08_en.pdf.
2. **World Bank** assists with economic and technical development in developing countries globally. Its mission is to deal with issues related to poverty, such as water and sanitation systems. Refer to its Web site at http://web.worldbank.org.
3. **Global Health Council** is a group of health care professionals and government and nongovernment organizations and institutions that work to achieve equity in global health. They address global health issues such as women's health, children's health, HIV/AIDs, infectious diseases, and health systems. Refer to its Web site at http://www.globalhealth.org/.
4. **United Nations Children's Emergency Fund (UNICEF)** is an international organization that focuses mainly on children and their family's health for disease prevention, care, and treatment. Refer to its Web site at http://www.unicef.org/whatwedo/index.html.
5. **Canadian International Development Agency (CIDA)** is a leading Canadian organization involved in international policy development that provides support and assistance to developing countries to address global health. CIDA works in partnership with other countries and national nongovernmental organizations and international organizations such as WHO and UNICEF to address global health issues. Refer to its Web site at http://www.acdi-cida.gc.ca/home.
6. **International Council of Nurses (ICN)** represents more than 125 national nursing associations worldwide. This organization represents nursing as a profession internationally and influences health policy globally. Its vision is to improve health for all. Refer to its Web site at http://www.icn.ch/abouticn.htm.
7. **Canadian Nurses Association** is the national voice for provincial and territorial Canadian nursing associations and colleges. One of its goals is to influence global health and equity. Refer to its Web site at http://www.cna-nurses.ca/CNA/international/involved/default_e.aspx.

BOX 1-3 Six Principles of Interdisciplinary Collaboration in Primary Health Care

1. Patient/client engagement
2. Population health approach
3. Best possible care and services
4. Access
5. Trust and respect
6. Effective communication

SOURCE: Enhancing Interdisciplinary Collaboration in Primary Health Care (EICP) Initiative Steering Committee. (2005). *The principles and framework for interdisciplinary collaboration in primary health care.* Ottawa, ON: Author. Retrieved from http://www.eicp.ca/en/principles/sept/EICP-Principles%20and%20Framework%20Sept.pdf.

clients. Six principles grounded in interdisciplinary collaboration in primary health care are listed in Box 1-3. CHNs need to consider these principles as a whole when participating in interdisciplinary collaborative efforts in primary health care in Canada (Enhancing Interdisciplinary Collaboration in Primary Health Care [EICP] Initiative Steering Committee, 2005). These principles are detailed on the EICP Web site (see the Tool Box on Evolve).

Principles of Primary Health Care

Primary health care, as a philosophy of health care, includes five principles, adopted at the Alma-Ata international conference (WHO, 1978):

1. Equitable distribution of essential health services to all populations
2. Increased emphasis on services that are preventive and promotive rather than curative only
3. Maximum individual and community involvement in the planning and operation of health care services
4. The integration of health development with social and economic development
5. The use of appropriate technology

Principle 1 refers to *accessibility for all* to health services, including those living in rural, remote, and urban communities (Calnan & Lemire Rodger, 2002; CNA, 2003). Essential health care services must be equitably shared among all persons, regardless of such factors as geographical location, culture, and income. This principle indicates that vulnerable groups (e.g., the homeless,

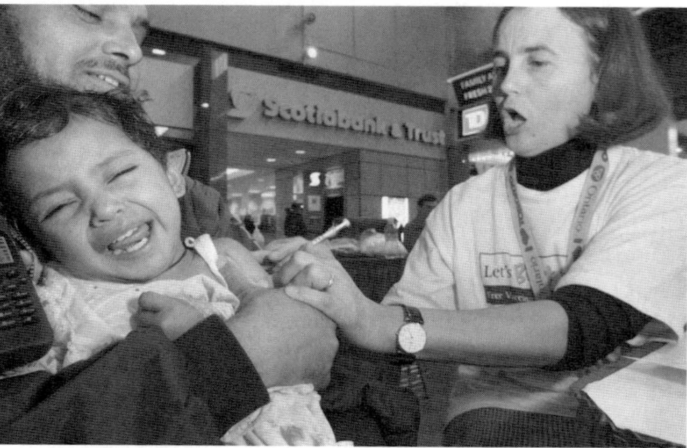

Public health nurses are frequently involved in organizing flu clinics for the public, one of the activities that fall under disease prevention.

persons with HIV/AIDS, persons with hepatitis) should have access to the health care system on an equal basis. However, many people do not have equal access at present. CHNs provide care in the community to such vulnerable populations and play a vital role in facilitating access to needed health care services in their communities. For example, Cathy Crowe, a CHN who works as a PHN, advocates for the homeless in Toronto.

Principle 2 refers to *health promotion and disease prevention* activities, such as health education and immunization (Calnan & Lemire Rodger, 2002), and emphasizes the need for health systems to focus on promoting health and preventing disease so that the focus is on maintaining health rather than a curative approach after disease has occurred. For example, CHNs work with low-income families and groups to help them maintain good health by, for instance, educating them on how to eat healthily on their restricted budgets.

Principle 3 is often referred to as *public participation* in decision making on issues of personal and community health (Calnan & Lemire Rodger, 2002; CNA, 2003). Communities need to be encouraged and supported to participate in developing and managing their health care (community partnering and empowerment). For example, CHNs partner with other health care professionals and the community to develop community-initiated programs, such as school breakfast, heart health, and safe walking.

Principle 4 is frequently referred to as *intersectoral collaboration,* which involves interdisciplinary teams working together to identify and develop sustainable health programs supported by policy (Calnan & Lemire Rodger, 2002; CNA, 2003). Professionals from the health sector will work interdependently with professionals from other sectors, such as agriculture, food, industry, and housing, as well as with community members to promote the health of the community. For example, CHNs have worked with businesses, community institutions, and professionals from other sectors to develop and implement a policy regarding smoking in public at the municipal and provincial government levels.

Principle 5 is the *appropriate use of health care resources,* including human resources and technology (CNA, 2003). This principle calls for finding the most cost-effective ways to provide appropriate health care to everyone in the community. For example, primary health care nurse practitioners can help reduce demands on the health care system by using their skills and abilities in the prevention and treatment of common conditions encountered in the clinic. Another example is CHNs using telehealth technology to respond to client health care concerns. The use of this technology often reduces the strain on emergency departments.

In recent years, federal financial support has been provided to encourage primary health care reform, especially using a team approach and delivering comprehensive services to clients (PHAC, 2009). For example, in 2000, the Canadian federal government provided $800 million to a Primary Health Care Transition Fund for the development of primary health care models in the provinces and territories (Shah, 2003; Health Council of Canada, 2006). The Health Council of Canada (2006) report (see Weblink on Evolve) recommends the setting of three goals for primary health care renewal: improve access to needed health care, improve quality of care, and improve population health.

Two examples of health care reform initiatives that have used some of the transition funding are "Enabling Primary Health Care in the North Through Traditional Knowledge" and "Rainbow Health: Improving Access to Care." The first initiative received $494,761 in funding to develop a DVD titled *A Different Way of Living.* Through interviews, elders in their respective communities shared the history, the culture, and the health and healing practices of Aboriginal people in Yukon, Northwest Territories, and Nunavut communities. The DVD serves to educate health care and social service providers about the culture and the diverse health needs of Aboriginal peoples living in the remote and northern communities of Canada (Health Canada, 2006a). The second initiative, a coalition representing members from the east coast to the west coast and with some representation from the First Nations, received $2,307,000 to address inequities in health status and provide equal access to primary health care to gay, lesbian, bisexual, and transgendered (GLBT) Canadians. The purposes of this initiative were to develop partnerships among GLBT communities and various health professional associations, national health care associations, and health delivery associations to eliminate barriers to health services; to build capacity among health care providers and GLBT communities; and to encourage members of the GLBT community to actively participate in their own health care (Health Canada, 2006b).

CRITICAL VIEW

1. What are the differences and connections among the concepts of primary care, primary health care, health promotion, and population health?
2. How would you explain WHO's role in primary health care?

Primary health care is especially relevant to CHNs for some of the following reasons (CNA, 2005c):

- It provides essential health care services in the community.
- It considers the determinants of health.
- It focuses on health promotion, disease prevention, and protection.
- It includes therapeutic, curative, and rehabilitative care.
- It promotes coordination and interdisciplinary collaboration.
- It focuses on the client as an equal partner in health with health professionals.

CHNs should be aware of the principles and issues surrounding primary health care as they conduct their practice.

PUBLIC HEALTH PRACTICE

Within the framework of "health for all," Canada has set the broad goal of holistic health—that every person will be as physically, mentally, emotionally, and spiritually healthy as he or she can be (PHAC, 2009). To reach this goal, the following requirements have been identified: (1) basic needs, including social and physical environments; (2) belonging and engagement; (3) healthy living; and (4) a system for health (PHAC, 2009). According to the PHAC, **public health** is

> *an organized activity of society to promote, protect, improve, and when necessary, restore the health of individuals, specified groups, or the entire population. It is a combination of sciences, skills, and values that function through collective societal activities and involves programs, services, and institutions aimed at protecting and improving the health of all people. The term 'public health' can describe a concept, a social institution, a set of*

scientific and professional disciplines and technologies, and a form of practice. It is a way of thinking, a set of disciplines, an institution of society, and a manner of practice. It has an increasing number and variety of specialized domains and demands of its practitioners an increasing array of skills and expertise. (PHAC, 2008, p. 13)

This definition was developed to complement the Core Competencies for Public Health in Canada (PHAC, 2008). Thirty-six core competencies that capture the "essential knowledge, skills and attitudes" required to practise in the public health workforce sector were developed within seven categories to provide direction to the public health workforce for effective service delivery (PHAC, 2008). (See the Core Competency Statement listed in the Evolve Weblinks.)

Chapter 2 of *The Chief Public Health Officer's Report on the State of Public Health in Canada* (Butler-Jones, 2008) portrays the richness of Canada's public health history, the scope of public health activities, and the commitment of public health efforts to the health of Canadians, as shown through early interventions, such as immunization development, tobacco use prevention, and seat belt legislation, and responses to current infectious diseases, such as severe acute respiratory syndrome (SARS).

Public health aims to keep communities and populations healthy and safe by employing the following six major public health functions: health protection, health promotion, population health assessment, public health surveillance, injury and disease prevention, and emergency preparedness and response (Butler-Jones, 2008). The dramatic increase in life expectancy among Canadians from the early 1900s to the present has been the result primarily of improvements in sanitation, control of infectious diseases through education and immunization, and other preventive population health activities. These activities have also significantly reduced health care costs for Canadians (Butler-Jones, 2008).

The emphasis in public health has shifted from the management of communicable diseases to the prevention and management of chronic disease (Butler-Jones, 2008). At least 33% of Canadians (approximately nine million) are affected by one or more of the following seven chronic diseases (Broemeling, Watson, & Prebtani, 2008; Health Council of Canada, 2007): arthritis, hypertension, heart disease, cancer, chronic obstructive pulmonary disease, diabetes mellitus, and mood disorders. The number of chronic diseases experienced per individual increases with age (Butler-Jones, 2008). However, Broemeling et al. (2008) report that the first two of the seven listed chronic diseases are the most prevalent chronic diseases found in youths and adults. Chapter 3 of *The Chief Public Health Officer's Report on the State of Public Health in Canada,* "Our Population: Our Health," (Butler-Jones, 2008) offers an in-depth discussion of the health of the Canadian population with specific mention of Canada's Aboriginal peoples. This chapter also identifies life expectancy changes, morbidity and mortality rates throughout the lifespan, and patterns of disease and disability. The increased prevalence of chronic diseases and increased life expectancy have major implications for primary health care teams (Health Council of Canada, 2009). Behavioural risk factors, such as smoking, unhealthy eating habits, obesity, and physical inactivity; societal forces, such as improved life expectancy; and some unfavourable determinants of health contribute to the development of many chronic illnesses. In summary, public health has as a primary focus the health care of communities and populations rather than of individuals, groups, and families. Its goal is to prevent disease and preserve, promote, and protect the health of the community and the population within it. Further discussion of the determinants affecting health and leading to chronic diseases appears later in this text.

Community health nurses who work in public health are called *public health nurses.* Public health nurses acquire specialized knowledge and skills for working with populations. **Public health nursing** is community health nursing with a distinct focus and scope of practice. (See the "How To" box, which outlines the distinguishing features of public health nursing.) The knowledge and skills necessary for public health nursing are outlined in the 2009 Canadian competencies for public health nursing practice Version 1.0. These competencies, elaborated upon in Chapter 3, are discipline-specific and identify the skills, knowledge, attitudes, beliefs, and values necessary for competent public health nursing practice in Canada.

CRITICAL VIEW

Log on to the following website:
http://www.chnc.ca/documents/PublicHealth-CommunityHealthNursinginCanadaRolesandActivities2010.pdf

1. Compare the terms *standard* and *competency.*
2. Outline the differences between regulatory standards and specialty standards.
3. Identify three reasons for believing standards and competencies are important.

CRITICAL VIEW

1. What are the public health programs and services for public health care delivery in your city or town, province or territory?
2. How are the determinants of health included in these programs and services?

How To... Distinguish Public Health Nursing

- *Population-focused:* Primary emphasis on *populations* that live in the community, as opposed to those that are institutionalized
- *Community as context:*
  - Concern for the connection between the health status of the population and the environment in which the population lives (physical, biological, sociocultural)
  - An imperative to work *with* the members of the community to carry out public health functions
- *Health- and prevention-focused:* Emphasis on strategies for health promotion, health maintenance, and disease prevention, particularly primary and secondary prevention
- *Interventions at the community or population level:* The use of political processes to influence public policy as a major intervention strategy for achieving goals
- *Concern for the health of all members of the population or community, particularly vulnerable subpopulations*
- *Consideration of the influence of the determinants on the health of clients*

SOURCE: Williams, C. A. (2010). Community-oriented nursing and community-based nursing. In M. Stanhope & J. Lancaster (Eds.), *Foundations of nursing in the community: Community-oriented practice* (3rd ed., pp. 2–14). St. Louis, MO: Mosby Elsevier.

Evidence-Informed Practice

The purpose of a study of CHNs (N = 1,044) conducted in Ontario was to explore (a) work-related concerns, (b) satisfaction with certain aspects of their jobs, and (c) factors influencing their decision to remain in community health nursing. The CHNs who participated in this study were PHNs, home care nurses, and community care access centre (CCAC) nurses. The findings on work-related concerns indicated that CHNs, as a group, identified as their greatest concerns inadequate staffing and certain client-related factors, such as injuries in the client work environment and unsafe client homes. Some of the positive aspects reported by the group in the study were that they liked their jobs, felt pride in their work, and liked their employers.

Although the group members expressed similar concerns, the extent of their concerns varied. For example, CCAC and home care nurses were more concerned about aspects of their work than were the PHNs. CCAC nurses were also more concerned than the others about the emotional effect their work had on them. Job satisfaction varied among the group, with CCAC nurses expressing the most dissatisfaction due to continual change in clientele and programs as well as inadequate staffing. Home care nurses were most dissatisfied with their salaries and benefits. PHNs expressed concern about inadequate office spaces. The researchers concluded that CHNs must be considered as a heterogeneous group and not as a homogenous group and also that work settings must be considered, especially when addressing work-related and client-related concerns.

Application for CHNs: Retention of nursing staff is an issue often connected to job satisfaction. The wide variety of practice settings makes each type of community health nursing unique, with differing work environments and organization supports. Community health nurses, within their practice setting, need to work together as a group to address work-related and client-related concerns. Improved job satisfaction among CHNs should lead to more positive client–nurse relationships.

Questions for Reflection & Discussion

1. What are the major concerns of the CHNs in this study?
2. How would you address these concerns if you were one of these CHNs?

REFERENCE: Armstrong-Stassen, M., & Cameron, S. J. (2005). Concerns, satisfaction, and retention of Canadian community health nurses. *Journal of Community Health Nursing, 22*(4), 181–194.

POPULATION-FOCUSED PRACTICE

In traditional health care, the individual is the focus, and the approach is curative or rehabilitative, whereas in population health, the population or aggregates are the focus, and importance is given to the influence of the determinants of health. Thus, traditional health care provides treatment to individuals with an illness, whereas population health advocates disease prevention and health promotion among groups or populations (Nova Scotia Health Promotion and Protection, 2007).

Population-focused practice directs community health nursing practice with an emphasis on reducing health inequalities to a defined population or aggregates compared with individual-level care. The following scenario demonstrates population-focused practice applied to a community health nursing situation:

A CHN visiting an older adult centre conducts blood pressure screening and determines that a group of older adults are hypertensive based on certain clinical signs. The CHN also considers the determinants of health relevant to each client's situation, such as his or her culture, income, education, gender, biology and genetic endowment, and social support network. Any of these determinants of health can contribute to the client's situation. For example, low income may cause a client's inability to purchase antihypertensive medications; cultural beliefs and practices may influence food preferences, use of herbs, and health practices, such as consulting traditional healers. Using income as a determinant of health, the CHN could evaluate different intervention options with the older adult group to identify the best available options for this client group; partner with them to implement interventions such as changes in diet; conduct group sessions on strategies to reduce hypertension; review budgeting practices to determine ways to obtain more expensive, healthier foods; and refer them for budget counselling if needed and if the client agrees. CHNs who engage in population-focused practice and identify health indicators and health patterns pertaining to hypertension would also ask the following questions:

- Based on age, race, and gender, what is the prevalence rate of hypertension?
- In Canada, which aggregates have the highest rates of untreated hypertension?
- What community educational strategies could address the health concern of untreated hypertension?
- What programs for the aggregates with untreated hypertension could reduce this health concern and contribute to the prevention of future cardiovascular diseases and death?
- What community environmental supports are available to promote the health of persons with hypertension?
- What, if any, policy changes need to be developed or initiated for both diagnosed and undiagnosed hypertension?

Evidence-Informed Practice

In Carrière's article (see reference), a description of a client-centred population health approach was developed and tested to address the needs of a specific target group (disenfranchised, vulnerable women) in Kamloops, British Columbia. The approach involved completing a needs assessment by asking the women what was important to them and what they felt they needed; creating a community-based health conference entitled *It's All 'Bout You* for the target group of women; and developing an educational awareness program for health and social service providers, including storyboards, which were used for sharing the women's stories. The storyboards were valuable in providing information in a different way to individuals in the nonhealth sector, the community at large, and policymakers. The information also demonstrated linkages and barriers to women's health. The paradigm shift in this outreach program was from an individual service approach to a population health approach. Guided by the determinants of health, this population health approach reached a greater percentage of the target group and led to empowering strategies. This program resulted in capacity building for this target group of women, their family members, service providers, and community members at large.

Application for CHNs: It is important for CHNs to consider the population in any assessment and to customize the planning and implementation of community action projects for various aggregates in the community. A population health approach and storyboards are important considerations in addressing the health care concerns of clients in their communities.

Questions for Reflection & Discussion

1. Which determinants of health are evident in this study? What other determinants could influence the health of these clients?
2. What other actions might the CHN implement to ensure improved outcomes?

REFERENCE: Carrière, G. L. (2008). Linking women to health and wellness: Street outreach takes a population health approach. *International Journal of Drug Policy, 19*, 205–210.

COMMUNITY HEALTH NURSING PRACTICE

The role of the CHN has changed over the years, mainly in response to changes in health care, priorities for health care funding, the needs of the population, the educational preparation of CHNs, and the community health nursing standards of practice.

Health Promotion, Empowerment, Capacity Building, and Population Health

Community health nursing practice places emphasis on health promotion and disease prevention. **Health promotion** is a process of empowering people to increase control over and improve their health (WHO, 2006). In community health nursing, **empowerment** refers to actively engaging the client to gain greater control and involves "political efficacy, improved quality of community life and social justice" (CHNAC, 2008, p. 7). CHNAC (2008) describes empowerment as "not something that can be done 'to' or 'for' people—it involves people discovering and using their own strengths" (p. 7). CHNs partner with clients to build capacity. When clients are empowered, the power shifts from health care providers to clients in the identification, prioritization, and addressing of their own health concerns. The strategies of advocacy and empowerment contribute, in turn, to capacity building (CHNAC, 2008). The PHAC offers a "Community Capacity Building Tool" that CHNs working with health promotion projects can use to determine the current project status and options for building community capacity for the project. The tool has nine categories, with specific questions in each category that relate to planning for building community capacity (see the Tool Box on Evolve). Empowerment and capacity building will be discussed in greater detail in Chapters 4 and 9. The *Canadian Community Health Nursing Standards of Practice* in Appendix 1 provide examples of the actions CHNs take in their advocacy role.

Canada has been a leader in population health research and policymaking, which is reflected in its attempts at various government levels to improve the health of Canadians (Johnson et al., 2008; PHAC, 2008a; Senate Canada, 2009). Hamilton and Bhatti (1996) developed the population health promotion model for Health Canada (see Figure 1-4), which illustrates the various forces and factors that influence health, the strategies required to promote the health of populations, and answers to the questions of who, what, and how in health-related matters. This model, as well as the concept of health promotion, will be discussed in more depth in Chapter 4. Another model that incorporates components of population health promotion is the Expanded Chronic Care Model by Barr et al. (2003) (see the Evolve Weblinks). Developed for the prevention and management of chronic disease, this model integrates the five health promotion strategies as outlined in the Ottawa Charter.

Community Health Nursing Roles

The primary focus of public health nursing is on populations and the health of the community, whereas home health care nursing tends to focus on the health of individuals and families. The CHN practising as an HHN is therefore more likely to give direct care to people than are other CHNs. The HHN assesses client health concerns as well as the services that are available in order to plan the most appropriate course of action for a particular client as individual and family. Throughout care delivery, the HHN educates and counsels clients so that they can learn better ways of taking care of themselves. Many private agencies, such as the Victorian Order of Nurses (VON) Canada, employ HHNs in the community. For historical and current information on the VON, a Canadian national nonprofit organization, see the VON Weblink on the Evolve Web site.

Other examples of CHNs are occupational health nurses, parish nurses, nurse practitioners, outpost nurses, military nurses, forensic nurses, telenurses, corrections nurses, nurse entrepreneurs, and street or outreach nurses. Refer to Table 1-1 for further information on all of these and some additional community health nursing practice areas. Chapter 3 provides in-depth information on each of these community health nursing specialties, their practice settings, and their roles.

CHNs have various opportunities for assuming many different roles at different times depending on the client and practice settings. Not every CHN will actually take on all of these roles during his or her practice. The activities within each of these roles often depend on the resources available to the CHN and may vary depending on such factors as client availability, commitment, culture, and health beliefs. Refer to Table 1-6 for an introduction to the diverse roles played by CHNs, such as advocate, collaborator, educator, facilitator, and researcher. Many CHNs have a considerable amount of professional autonomy as they perform these diverse roles in a variety of community practice settings. While this professional autonomy can be very exciting, it is accompanied by responsibility and accountability, as indicated in Standard 5 of the *Canadian Community Health Nursing Standards of Practice:* "Demonstrating professional responsibility and accountability" (CHNAC, 2008).

CHNs are mostly involved in providing family-centred care to individuals, families, and groups across the lifespan of clients, but their practice also includes identifying high-risk groups in the community. Once such

TABLE 1-6 Common Roles, Functions, and Examples in Community Health Nursing

Role	Function/Activities	Examples
Advocate	Provides a voice to client concerns when necessary	• Networking with other community members on behalf of homeless people • Participating in a community action group for provision of accessible transit choices • Initiating contact with community stakeholders
Clinician or direct care provider	Provides hands-on care to the client	• Providing wound care on a diabetic client's foot • Doing a prenatal assessment • Working in sexually transmitted infections (STI) clinics • Working in immunization clinics
Collaborator	Involves the client and interdisciplinary team members or inter-agency groups working together toward improving client health	• Working with nutritionist, physiotherapist, and client to address client obesity • Working with health care providers in a long-term care facility to explore feeding options • Being a member of coalitions, such as heart health groups
Consultant	Provides advice and information to client, health care providers, and agencies to assist in meeting client's health care concerns	• Providing information to a family that is considering the use of complementary therapies • Providing information to school administrators about bullying
Counsellor	Provides support to clients to facilitate their decision making in reference to emotional challenges	• Working with a family and the family member with a new diagnosis of cancer • Working with a pregnant adolescent to explore birth choices
Educator	Facilitates client learning through teaching that is appropriate to a client's situation to meet his or her cognitive, affective, and psychomotor needs	• Educating a worker about back safety in the workplace • Educating a new mother on the care of her newborn
Facilitator	Works with clients and others to set and fulfill health goals	• Facilitating a self-help group for smoking cessation • Facilitating a community focus group to improve neighbourhood safety
Health promoter or change agent	Assists clients to acknowledge need for lifestyle changes and take responsibility for working toward identified change	• Working with children with obesity problems to identify the physical activity changes required • Helping clients identify stressors and stress management strategies to deal with these stressors
Leader	Guides and encourages clients to take the initiative to explore options and make decisions to enable goal achievement	• Helping a low-income neighbourhood formulate a plan to present traffic safety proposals to a local municipal council • Assisting a school board in developing a school policy on food vending machine options
Liaison	Acts as an intermediary between clients and agencies and other health care providers	• Organizing referrals to cardiac rehabilitation after surgery • Working with hospital staff to arrange for home support and follow-up for a high-risk mother

TABLE 1-6 Common Roles, Functions, and Examples in Community Health Nursing—Cont'd

Role	Function/Activities	Examples
Manager	Plans and directs client care	• Organizing home care support for a newly discharged older adult client • Organizing a family planning clinic • Organizing sexual health clinics
Referral agent	Directs clients to additional appropriate resources in the community	• Referring community stakeholders to a health promotion consultant • Referring clients to a child car seat safety inspection clinic
Researcher	Investigates phenomena related to health and identifies opportunities for research	• Identifying increased cases of measles in a specific community • Identifying increased numbers of snowmobile injuries

groups are identified, the CHN can work with others to develop appropriate policies and interventions to reduce the risk and to provide beneficial services. In the course of their practice, CHNs must remain constantly aware of diversity in the community and provide care that is appropriate to address the health care needs of diverse clients.

CRITICAL VIEW

1. Some of the concepts of community health and related skills are transferable to other nursing practice settings. For example, if you are a nurse working in an emergency department and are providing care to a homeless patient, how would applying a community lens set the context for your nursing care for this patient?
2. To what extent do you think concepts and skills of community health nursing are transferable to other nursing practice settings?

CRITICAL VIEW

Identify a current health issue in your local community (e.g., childhood obesity, diabetes, HIV/AIDS).

1. What primary, secondary, and tertiary prevention interventions relate to this health issue?
2. As a CHN, how would you improve the effectiveness of the prevention activities related to this health issue?

STUDENT EXPERIENCE

The Canadian Partnership for Children's Health & Environment (CPCHE) has developed a game that provides an opportunity for players to explore the health determinants of a hypothetical child. As players, students will be able to identify that some health determinants are not modifiable and others are modifiable through personal choices and sociopolitical activities.

ACTIVITY

1. Log on to the following Web site: http://www.healthyenvironmentforkids.ca/english/resources/card_file.shtml?x=3991.
2. Download the pdf file found under Determinants of Health Worksheet.
3. Follow the directions for the game.

QUESTIONS

1. What have you learned from playing this game?
2. How would you use this information as a community health nurse?

REMEMBER THIS!

- The concepts of community health nursing such as client, community, community health, upstream thinking, downstream thinking, health, primary health care, health promotion, disease prevention, determinants of health, population health, public health practice, and collaboration are key to understanding community health nursing practice.
- The social determinants of health as identified by Raphael (in press) are as follows: Aboriginal status, early life education, employment and working conditions, food security, gender, health care services, housing, income and its distribution, social safety net, social exclusion, and unemployment and employment security.
- *Community health nursing* is an umbrella term used to define nursing specialties and applies to all nurses who work in and with the community.
- Community health nursing is a specialty nursing practice that involves working with clients to preserve, protect, promote, and maintain health.
- CHNs work in diverse settings and perform many different roles.
- Population-focused practice emphasizes health protection, health promotion, and disease prevention.
- The three levels of prevention are primary, secondary, and tertiary.
- Primary prevention is a type of intervention or activity that seeks to prevent disease from the beginning, before people have a disease, and relates to the natural history of a disease.
- Secondary prevention is a type of intervention or activity that seeks to detect disease early in its progression (early pathogenesis), before clinical signs and symptoms become apparent, in order to make an early diagnosis and initiate treatment.
- Tertiary prevention is a type of intervention or activity that begins once the disease has become obvious; its aim is to interrupt the course of the disease, reduce the amount of disability that might occur, and begin rehabilitation.
- *Population* is defined as a large group of people who have at least one characteristic in common and who reside in a community. The terms *population* and *aggregate* should not be used interchangeably. Aggregates are subpopulations within the larger population.
- The *Canadian Community Health Nursing Standards of Practice* guide and facilitate the practice of CHNs in Canada as they work within the principles of primary health care to promote and preserve the health of populations
- *Primary health care* refers to comprehensive care and addresses issues of social justice and equity. It is a philosophy of care and is composed of five important principles for CHNs to consider.
- *Social justice* refers to ensuring fairness and equality in health services.
- Community health nurses are becoming more involved in global health and international development.
- In all interactions and on a daily basis, CHNs need to consider the influence of the determinants of health, especially the social determinants of health, on the health status of their clients.
- Public health is the collective effort of the members of a society to ensure that existing conditions promote health for all in the community.

REFLECTIVE PRAXIS

Case Study

You are Stan, the new public health nurse for the rural community of Treeville, Canada. All communities have some health inequities. What aggregates and other information would you need to explore in your community in order to identify the possibility of health inequities? Provide rationales for your choices.

Answers are on the Evolve Web site at http://evolve.elsevier.com/Canada/Stanhope/community/.

What Would You Do?

1. Locate one article from a refereed (i.e., scholarly, peer-reviewed) journal for each of the following community health nursing practice areas:
   - Home health nursing (VON and one private agency)
   - Parish nursing
   - Occupational health nursing
   - Outpost nursing
   - Primary health care nurse practitioner and acute care nurse practitioner (tertiary care)
   - School nursing
   - Telehealth nursing
   - Public health nursing

   In chart form, identify for each of these community health nursing practices the nursing roles and functions that relate to community health nursing. Bring your findings to class for further discussion.

TOOL BOX

evolve

The Tool Box contains useful instruments that can be applied in community health nursing practice. These related resources are found either in the appendices at the back of this book or on the Evolve Web site at http://evolve.elsevier.com/Canada/Stanhope/community/.

Appendices

- Appendix 1: Canadian Community Health Nursing Standards of Practice
- Appendix 2: CNA Position Statement: "Interprofessional Collaboration"
- Appendix 3: CNA Backgrounder: "Social Determinants of Health and Nursing: A Summary of the Issues"
- Appendix 4: Ethics in Practice for Registered Nurses: Social Justice in Practice

Tools

Alberta Health Services. Canadian Collaborative Mental Health Initiative (CCMHI).
This Web site provides access to a general tool kit titled "Collaboration Between Mental Health and Primary Care Services: A Planning and Implementation Toolkit for Health Care Providers and Planners" and eight specific tool kits on populations such as Aboriginal peoples, children and adolescents, rural and isolated populations, and urban marginalized populations.

The Enhancing Interdisciplinary Collaboration in Primary Health Care (EICP) Initiative. *Collaboration Toolkit.*
This Web site contains a tool kit that provides practical tools and advice, as well as information gathered from across Canada about how various organizations practise interdisciplinary care in a collaborative manner.

Health Canada. *The Population Health Template Working Tool.*
This tool consolidates information regarding key elements of population health and determinants of health.

Public Health Agency of Canada. *Community Capacity Building Tool.*
This tool can be used by health promotion project groups to determine current project status and options for growth in building community capacity for the project. The tool contains nine categories, with specific questions in each category that encompass planning for building community capacity.

WEBLINKS

evolve

Direct links to these resources can be found on the text's accompanying Evolve Web site at http://evolve.elsevier.com/Canada/Stanhope/community.

Association of Ontario Health Centres. ***A Scan of the Effects of Regionalization on Community Health Centres in Selected Regions Across Canada.*** This document provides information about the focus on community health centres across Canada and the effects of regionalization. The reader will gain an understanding of how services are being integrated in primary health care.

Barr, V. J., Robinson, S., Marin-Link, B., Underhill, L., Dotts, A., Ravensdale, D., & Salivaras, S. ***The Expanded Chronic Care Model: An Integration of Concepts and Strategies From Population Health Promotion and the Chronic Care Model.*** This document provides information on the development of the expanded chronic care model. This model was developed for the prevention and management of chronic disease and integrates the five health promotion strategies as outlined in the Ottawa Charter.

Canadian Nurses Association. ***Social Justice … A Means to an End, an End in Itself.*** This document provides an overview of social justice concepts, defines social justice attributes, and identifies the guiding assumptions of social justice as applied to nurses.

Community Health Research Unit: Perspectives. At this Web site, you can access monthly publications titled *Perspectives,* which provide a summary of developments in the field of community health. Each monthly edition has a main research topic focus. For example, the December 2006 issue focused on faculty research studies on HIV/AIDS, and the November 2006 issue focused on fall prevention for seniors, with additional links provided. The site also provides access to discussion papers and publications.

CNA Relevant Position Statements and Backgrounders

- CNA Position Statement: "The Nurse Practitioner"
- CNA Position Statement: "Interprofessional Collaboration"
- CNA Backgrounder: "Social Determinants of Health and Nursing: A Summary of the Issues"
- CNA Backgrounder: "Primary Health Care: A Summary of the Issues"

Other CNA Resources

- The Canadian Nurse Practitioner Initiative
- Fact sheets pertaining to the nurse practitioner role

Core Competency Statements. This site provides, within the seven categories, the 36 core competencies with examples for the public health practitioner.

Enhancing Interdisciplinary Collaboration in Primary Health Care (EICP) Initiative Steering Committee. ***The Principles and Framework for Interdisciplinary Collaboration in Primary Health Care.*** This site defines *primary health care* and discusses the underlying principles of interdisciplinary collaboration and primary health care.

Health Canada. Health Canada is a Canadian umbrella agency for many other health institutions, such as the PHAC; Canadian Institutes of Health Research; Canadian Food Inspection Agency; First Nations, Inuit, and Aboriginal Health; Healthy Living; and others. The Health Canada Web site provides access to many health care resources.

Health Canada: About Health Canada. This site is the home page for Health Canada and provides information on its mission and values, and links to various associated agencies and partners.

Health Canada: Canada's Health Care System (Medicare). This site provides current information on Canada's national health insurance program and the *Canada Health Act.* The reader can navigate the various topics to acquire complete information on the Act.

Health Canada: Funded Initiatives: Provincial/Territorial Envelope. This site provides links to the projects for provinces and territories that received funding through the Primary Health Care Transition Fund.

Health Canada: Primary Health Care. This site provides information on primary health care, past and present, and responses to frequently asked questions.

Health Canada. Population and Public Health Branch, Manitoba and Saskatchewan Region. ***How Our Programs Affect Population Health Determinants: A Workbook for Better Planning and Accountability.*** This document provides an excellent description of the determinants of health with their application to programs in health care.

Health Council of Canada. ***Primary Health Care: Health Care Renewal in Canada—Clearing the Road to Quality.*** This document is an excerpt from *Health*

Care Renewal in Canada: Clearing the Road to Quality. The document depicts fictional families in reference to their experiences with health care in Canada and also offers information about the progress that has been made across Canada in reforming primary health care.

Public Health Agency of Canada: About the Agency. This site outlines the mission and vision of this agency and provides excellent links to its branches, centres, and directorates, which individually explain each of their responsibilities and provide many resources that focus on topics pertaining to public health issues.

Public Health Agency of Canada: Background to the Public Health Human Resources Strategy. This site provides a historical record of the development of public health in the past 30 years and includes direct links to Web sites that contain important reports, such as those of Lalonde, Romanow, Kirby, and Naylor, plus recent events affecting health care system reform.

Public Health Agency of Canada. *The Chief Public Health Officer's Report on the State of Public Health in Canada: Addressing Health Inequalities.* This report from Canada's chief public health officer describes public health in Canada and the factors that affect it, including the determinants of health, actions to address inequalities, and future directions of public health care in Canada.

Public Health Agency of Canada: Health Goals for Canada: A Federal, Provincial & Territorial Commitment to Canadians. This site provides information on the federal, provincial, and territorial discussions on the health goals for Canada.

Victorian Order of Nurses Canada: About VON Canada. This site provides information on the programs and services offered by VON.

World Health Organization: About WHO. This site provides information about the organization and provides links to its history, access to information on other countries, research tools, and information about collaboration endeavours.

World Health Organization. *Closing the Gap in a Generation: Health Equity Through Action on the Social Determinants of Health.* This document is the final report by the Commission on Social Determinants of Health. It makes recommendations for addressing the inequities in health internationally and promotes a global movement to achieve its goals.

World Health Organization: Social Determinants of Health: The Solid Facts. This Web site provides an excellent review of the social determinants of health identified by WHO in 2003 as well as evidence to explain each of these, with discussion of policy considerations.

REFERENCES

Allison, K., Adlaf, E., Ialomiteanu, A., & Rehm, J. (1999). Predictors of health risk behaviours among young adults: Analysis of the national population health survey. *Canadian Journal of Public Health, 90*(2), 85–89.

Armstrong, P. (1996). Unravelling the safety net: Transformations in health care and their impact on women. In J. Brodie (Ed.), *Women and Canadian public policy* (pp. 129–150). Toronto, ON: Harcourt Brace.

Armstrong-Stassen, M., & Cameron, S. J. (2005). Concerns, satisfaction, and retention of Canadian community health nurses. *Journal of Community Health Nursing, 22*(4), 181–194.

Austin, W. (2008). Ethical psychiatric and mental health nursing practice. In W. Austin & M. A. Boyd (Eds.), *Psychiatric nursing for Canadian practice* (pp. 49–65). Philadelphia, PA: Lippincott Williams & Wilkins.

Bambra, C. (2006). Health status and the worlds of welfare. *Social Policy and Society, 5*, 53–62.

Bambra, C., Fox, D., & Scott-Samuel, A. (2005). Towards a politics of health. *Health Promotion International, 20*(2), 187–193.

Barr, V. J., Robinson, S., Marin-Link, B., Underhill, L., Dotts, A., Ravensdale, D., & Salivaris, S. (2003). The expanded chronic care model: An integration of concepts and strategies from population health promotion and the chronic care model. *The Hospital Quarterly, 7*(1), 73–82.

Benoit, C., Carroll, D., & Chaudhry, M. (2003). In search of a healing place: Aboriginal women in Vancouver's Downtown Eastside. *Social Science & Medicine, 56*(4), 821–833.

Broemeling, A., Watson, D. F., & Prebtani, F. (2008). Population patterns of chronic health conditions, co-morbidity and healthcare use in Canada: Implications for policy and practice. *Healthcare Quarterly, 11*(3), 70–76.

Brown, T. M., Cueto, M., & Fee, E. (2006). The World Health Organization and the transition from international to global public health. *American Journal of Public Health, 96*(1), 62–72.

Brunner, E., & Marmot, M. (2006). Social organization, stress, and health. In M. Marmot & R. G. Wilkinson (Eds.), *Social determinants of health.* (2nd ed., pp. 6–30). Oxford, UK: Oxford University Press.

Bryant, T. (2006). Politics, public policy, and population health. In D. Raphael, T. Bryant, & M. Rioux (Eds.), *Staying alive: Critical perspectives on health, illness, and health care* (pp. 193–216). Toronto, ON: Canadian Scholars' Press.

Bryant, T., Raphael, D., Schrecker, T., & Labonte, R. (2010). Canada: A land of missed opportunity for addressing the social determinants of health. *Health Policy.*

Butler-Jones, D. (2008). *The chief public health officer's report on the state of public health in Canada: Addressing health inequalities*. Retrieved from http://www.phac-aspc.gc.ca/publicat/2008/cphorsphc-respcacsp/index-eng.php.

Butterfield, P. G. (2007). Thinking upstream: Nursing theories and population-focused nursing practice. In M. A. Nies & M. McEwen (Eds.), *Community/public health nursing: Promoting the health of populations* (4th ed.). St. Louis, MO: W. B. Saunders.

Calnan, R., & Lemire Rodger, G. (2002). *Primary health care: A new approach to health care reform*. Ottawa, ON: Canadian Nurses Association.

Canadian Nurses Association. (2003). Primary health care—the time has come. *Nursing Now*, *6*, 1–4.

Canadian Nurses Association. (2005a). *Position statement: Interprofessional collaboration*. Retrieved from http://cna-aiic.ca/CNA/documents/pdf/publications/PS84_Interprofessional_Collaboration_e.pdf.

Canadian Nurses Association. (2005b). CNA Backgrounder. *Social determinants of health and nursing: A summary of the issues*. Retrieved from http://www.cna-nurses.ca/CNA/documents/pdf/publications/BG8_Social_Determinants_e.pdf.

Canadian Nurses Association. (2005c). CNA Backgrounder. *Primary health care: A summary of the issues*. Retrieved from http://www.cna-nurses.ca/CNA/documents/pdf/publications/BG7_Primary_Health_Care_e.pdf.

Canadian Nurses Association. (2005d). *Position statement: International health partnerships*. Retrieved from http://www.cna-aiic.ca/CNA/documents/pdf/publications/PS82_Intl_Health_Partnerships_e.pdf.

Canadian Nurses Association. (2009a). *Obtaining CNA certification*. Retrieved from http://www.cna-aiic.ca/CNA/nursing/certification/default_e.aspx.

Canadian Nurses Association. (2009b). *Ethics in practice for registered nurses: Social justice in practice*. Retrieved from http://www.cna-nurses.ca/CNA/documents/pdf/publications/Ethics_in_Practice_April_2009_e.pdf.

Canadian Policy Research Networks. (2000). *Non-medical determinants of health often neglected: Historical study*. Retrieved from http://www.cprn.com/en/doc.cfm?doc=425.

Carrière, G. L. (2008). Linking women to health and wellness: Street outreach takes a population health approach. *International Journal of Drug Policy*, *19*, 205–210.

Centers for Disease Control and Prevention (2005). *Social determinants of health*. Retrieved from http:/www.cdc.gov/sdoh/.

Chernomas, R., & Hudson, I. (2009). Social murder: The long-term effects of conservative economic policy. *International Journal of Health Services*, *39*(1), 107–121.

Choi, B. C. K., & Shi, F. (2001). Risk factors for diabetes mellitus by age and sex: Results of the national population health survey. *Diabetologia*, *44*(10), 1221–1231.

Choiniere, R., Lafontaine, A., & Edwards, A. (2000). Distribution of cardiovascular disease risk factors by socioeconomic status among Canadian adults. *Canadian Medical Association Journal*, *162*, S13–S18.

Clark, M. J. (2003). *Nursing in the community: Dimensions of community health nursing*. (4th ed.). Upper Saddle River, NJ: Prentice Hall.

Coburn, D. (2004). Beyond the income inequality hypothesis: Globalization, neo-liberalism, and health inequalities. *Social Science & Medicine*, *58*, 41–56.

Community Health Nurses Association of Canada. (2003). *Canadian Community Health Nursing Standards of Practice*. Retrieved from http://www.communityhealthnursescanada.org/Standards/Standards%20Practice%20jun04.pdf.

Community Health Nurses Association of Canada. (2008). *Canadian community health nursing standards of practice*. Retrieved from http://www.chnc.ca/documents/chn_standards_of_practice_mar08_english.pdf.

Community Health Nurses of Canada. (2009). *Nursing certification*. Retrieved from http://www.chnc.ca/nursing-certification.cfm.

Dahlgren, G., & Whitehead, M. (1992). *Policies and strategies to promote equity in health*. Copenhagen, Denmark: WHO Regional Office for Europe.

D'Amour, D., Ferrada-Videla, M., San Martin Rodriguez, A., & Beaulieu, M. (2005). The conceptual basis for interprofessional collaboration: Core concepts and theoretical frameworks. *Journal of Interprofessional Care*, *19*(Suppl. 1), 116–131.

Diem, E. (2007). *Practice examples of application of the Canadian community health nursing standards of practice*. Table presented at the First National Conference for Community Health Nurses, Toronto, ON. [Revised 2009].

Dunn, J., & Dyke, I. (2000). Social determinants of health in Canada's immigrant population: Results from the national population health survey. *Social Science and Medicine*, *51*(11), 1573–1593.

Dunn, J., & Hayes, M. (1999). Identifying social pathways for health inequalities. The role of housing. *Annals of the New York Academy of Sciences*, *896*, 399–402.

Enhancing Interdisciplinary Collaboration in Primary Health Care (EICP) Initiative Steering Committee. (2005). *The principles and framework for interdisciplinary collaboration in primary health care*. Ottawa, ON: Author. Retrieved from http://www.eicp.ca/en/principles/sept/EICP-Principles%20and%20Framework%20Sept.pdf.

Epp, J. (1986). *Achieving health for all: A framework for health promotion*. Ottawa, ON: Minister of Supply & Services.

Fricke, M. (2005). *Physiotherapy and primary health care: Evolving opportunities*. Retrieved from http://www.mbphysio.org/docs/PHC.pdf.

Galabuzi, G. E. (2004). Social exclusion. In D. Raphael (Ed.), *Social determinants of health: Canadian perspectives* (pp. 235–251). Toronto, ON: Canadian Scholars' Press.

Hamilton, N., & Bhatti, T. (1996). *Population health promotion: An integrated model of population health and health promotion*. Ottawa, ON: Health Promotion Development Division, Health Canada. Retrieved from http://www.phac-aspc.gc.ca/ph-sp/php-psp/index-eng.php.

Health Canada. (1998). *Taking action on population health: A position paper for health promotion and programs branch staff*. Ottawa, ON: Health Canada.

Health Canada. (2006a). *Primary health transition fund: Enabling primary health care in the north through traditional knowledge*. Retrieved from http://www.apps.hc-sc.gc.ca/hcs-sss/phctf-fassp.nsf/WebProject/0039?OpenDocument&lang=eng&.

Health Canada. (2006b). *Primary health transition fund: Rainbow health—improving access to care*. Retrieved from http://www.apps.hc-sc.gc.ca/hcs-sss/phctf-fassp.nsf/WebProject/0025?OpenDocument&lang=eng&.

Health Council of Canada. (2006). *Primary health care: Health care renewal in Canada—clearing the road to quality*. Toronto, ON: Author. Retrieved from http://www.healthcouncilcanada.ca/docs/rpts/2006/EX_PrimaryCare_EN.pdf.

Health Council of Canada. (2007). *Canadians' experiences with chronic illness care in 2007: A data supplement to why health care renewal matters: Learning from Canadians with chronic health conditions*. Toronto: Health Council. Retrieved from http://www.healthcouncilcanada.ca/docs/rpts/2007/outcomes2/Outcomes2ExperiencesFINAL.pdf.

Health Council of Canada. (2009). *Getting it right: Case studies of effective management of chronic disease using primary health care teams*. Retrieved from http://www.healthcouncilcanada.ca/docs/rpts/2009/CaseStudies_FINAL.pdf.

Hertzman, C., & Frank, J. (2006). Biological pathways linking the social environment, development, and health. In J. Heymann, C. Hertzman, M. Barer, & R. G. Evans (Eds.), *Healthier societies: From analysis to action* (pp. 35–57). Toronto, ON: Oxford University Press.

Hwang, S., & Bugeja, A. (2000). Barriers to appropriate diabetes management among homeless people in Toronto. *Canadian Medical Association Journal*, *163*(2), 161–165.

Institute of Health Promotion Research. (2005). *History and evolution of world knowledge on determinants of health and health promotion*. Retrieved from http://www.ihpr.ubc.ca/?section_copy_id = 741§ion_id = 491.

Johnson, S., Abonyi, S., Jeffery, B., Hackett, P., Hampton, M., McIntosh, T., & Sari, N. (2008). Recommendations for action on the social determinants of health: A Canadian perspective. *Lancet*, *372*(9650), 1690–1693.

Keating, D. P., & Hertzman, C. (Eds.). (1999). *Developmental health and the wealth of nations*. New York, NY: Guilford Press.

Kerstetter, S. (2002). *Rags and riches: Wealth inequality in Canada*. Ottawa, ON: Canadian Centre for Policy Alternatives.

Koplan, J. P., Bond, T. C., Merson, M. H., Reddy, K. S., Rodriguez, M. H., Sewankambo, N. K., Wasserheit, J. (2009). Towards a common definition of global health. *Lancet*, *373*(9679), 1993–1995.

Labonte, R. (2003). *How our programs affect population health determinants: A workbook for better planning and accountability*. Regina, SK: Health Canada. Retrieved from http://www.phac-aspc.gc.ca/ph-sp/progphd-progdsp/pdf/progphd_work_e.pdf.

Lalonde, M. (1974). *A new perspective on the health of Canadians: A working document*. Ottawa, ON: Government of Canada.

Langille, D. (2008). Follow the money: How business and politics shape our health. In D. Raphael (Ed.), *Social determinants of health: Canadian perspectives*. (2nd ed., pp. 305–317). Toronto, ON: Canadian Scholars' Press.

Leeds, Grenville and Lanark District Health Unit. (2006). *Moving upstream: The strategic plan of the Leeds, Grenville & Lanark District Health Unit for 2006–2010*. Retrieved from http://www.healthunit.org/reportpub/strategic/strategic_plan2006-2010_final_report-revised_April_13-06.pdf.

McEwen, M., & Nies, M. A. (2007). Health: A community view. In M. A. Nies, & M. McEwen (Eds.), *Community/public health nursing: Promoting the health of populations* (4th ed., pp. 3–18). St. Louis, MO: W. B. Saunders.

McIntyre, L. (2008). Food insecurity in Canada. In D. Raphael (Ed.), *Social determinants of health: Canadian perspectives*. (2nd ed., pp. 188–204). Toronto, ON: Canadian Scholars' Press.

McKinley, J., & Marceau, L. (2000). US public health in the 21st century: Diabetes mellitus. *The Lancet*, *356*(9231), 757–761.

McMullin, J. (2008). *Understanding social inequality: Intersections of class, age, gender, ethnicity and race in Canada*. (2nd ed.). Toronto, ON: Oxford University Press.

Navarro, V. (2009). What we mean by social determinants of health. *Global Health Promotion*, *16*(1), 5–16.

Navarro, V., & Shi, L. (2002). The political context of social inequalities and health. In V. Navarro (Ed.), *The political economy of social inequalities: Consequences for health and quality of life* (pp. 403–418). Amityville, NY: Baywood.

Nova Scotia Health Promotion and Protection. (2007). *Public health 101: An introduction to public health*. Retrieved from http://www.gov.ns.ca/ohp/publications/PH-101.pdf.

Orchard, C. A., Curran, V., & Kabene, S. (2005). Creating a culture for interdisciplinary collaborative professional practice. *Medical Education Online*, *10*(11), 1–13. Retrieved from http://www.med-ed-online.org/pdf/T0000063.pdf.

Ornstein, M. (2000). *Ethno-racial inequality in the city of Toronto: An analysis of the 1996 census*. Toronto, ON: Access and Equity Unit, Strategic and Corporate Policy Division, Chief Administrator's Office.

Pederson, A., & Raphael, D. (2006). Gender, race, and health. In D. Raphael, T. Bryant, & M. Rioux (Eds.), *Staying alive: Critical perspectives on health, illness, and health care*. Toronto, ON: Canadian Scholars' Press.

Pizzuti, D. G. (2006). The nurse in home health and hospice. In M. Stanhope & J. Lancaster (Eds.), *Foundations of nursing in the community: Community-oriented practice*. St. Louis, MO: Mosby Elsevier.

Porche, D. J. (2004). *Public & community health nursing practice: A population-based approach*. Thousand Oaks, CA: Sage.

Potvin, L., Richard, L., & Edwards, A. (2000). Knowledge of cardiovascular disease risk factors among the Canadian population: Relationships with indicators of socioeconomic status. *Canadian Medical Association Journal*, *162*, S5–S12.

Public Health Agency of Canada. (2006). *Determinants of health*. Retrieved from http://www.phac-aspc.gc.ca/media/nr-rp/2006/2006_06bk2-eng.php.

Public Health Agency of Canada. (2008). *Core competencies for public health in Canada: Release 1.0*. Ottawa, ON: Author. Retrieved from http://www.phac-aspc.gc.ca/ccph-cesp/pdfs/cc-manual-eng090407.pdf.

Public Health Agency of Canada. (2009). *Health goals for Canada: A federal, provincial & territorial commitment to Canadians*. Retrieved from http://www.phac-aspc.gc.ca/hgc-osc/new-1-eng.html.

Raphael, D. (2009). *Social determinants of health: Canadian perspective*. (2nd ed.). Toronto, ON: Canadian Scholars' Press, Inc.

Raphael, D. (in press). Critical perspectives on the social determinants of health. In E. McGibbon (Ed.), *Oppression as a determinant of health*. Halifax, NS: Fernwood Publishers.

Raphael, D., & Bryant, T. (2006). Maintaining population health in a period of welfare state decline: Political economy as the missing dimension in health promotion theory and practice. *Promotion and Education*, *13*(4), 12–18.

Raphael, D., Bryant, T., & Curry-Stevens, A. (2004). Toronto charter outlines future health policy directions for Canada and elsewhere. *Health Promotion International*, *19*, 269–273.

Saxena, S., Majeed, A., & Jones, M. (1999). Socioeconomic differences in childhood consultation rates in general practice in England and Wales: Prospective cohort study. *British Medical Journal*, *318*(7184), 642–646.

Scambler, G. (2001). *Health and social change: A critical theory* (Vol. 52). Buckingham, UK: Open University Press.

Senate Canada. (2009). *A healthy, productive Canada: A determinant of health approach*. Retrieved from http://www.parl.gc.ca/40/2/parlbus/commbus/senate/com-e/popu-e/rep-e/rephealth1jun09-e.pdf.

Shah, C. P. (2003). *Public health and preventive medicine in Canada* (5th ed.). Toronto, ON: W. B. Saunders.

Shapcott, M. (2008). Housing. In D. Raphael (Ed.), *Social determinants of health: Canadian perspectives*. (2nd ed., pp. 221–234). Toronto, ON: Canadian Scholars' Press.

Sword, W. (2000). Influences on the use of prenatal care and support services among women of low income. *National Academies of Practice Forum*, *2*(2), 125–133.

Tremblay, D. G. (2008). Precarious work and the labour market. In D. Raphael (Ed.), *Social determinants of health: Canadian perspectives* (2nd ed., pp. 75–87). Toronto, ON: Canadian Scholars' Press.

Wallis, M., & Kwok, S. (Eds.), (2008). *Daily struggles: The deepening racialization and feminization of poverty in Canada*. Toronto, ON: Canadian Scholars' Press.

Wilkinson, R., & Marmot, M. (2003). *Social determinants of health: The solid facts*. (2nd ed.). Copenhagen, Denmark: WHO Regional Office for Europe. Retrieved from http://www.euro.who.int/document/e81384.pdf.

Williams, C. A. (2010). Community-oriented nursing and community-based nursing. In M. Stanhope & J. Lancaster (Eds.), *Foundations of nursing in the community: Community-oriented practice*. (3rd ed., pp. 2–14). St. Louis, MO: Mosby Elsevier.

World Health Organization. (1978). *Declaration of Alma-Ata*. Retrieved from http://www.who.int/hpr/NPH/docs/declaration_almaata.pdf.

World Health Organization. (1986). *Ottawa charter for health promotion*. Retrieved from http://www.who.dk/policy/ottawa.htm.

World Health Organization. (2006). *Ottawa charter for health promotion, 1986*. Retrieved from http://www.euro.who.int/AboutWHO/Policy/20010827_2.

World Health Organization. (2008). *Closing the gap in a generation: Health equity through action on the social determinants of health*. Retrieved from http://whqlibdoc.who.int/publications/2008/9789241563703_eng.pdf.

World Health Organization. (2009). *The determinants of health*. Retrieved from http://www.who.int/hia/evidence/doh/e.

Wright, E. O. (2003). Class analysis, history and emancipation. In R. J. Antonio (Ed.), *Marx and modernity: Key readings and commentary*. Oxford, UK: Blackwell Publishers.

Yalnizyan, A. (2007). *The rich and the rest of us: The changing face of Canada's growing gap*. Toronto, ON: Canadian Centre for Policy Alternatives.

Young, L. E., & Higgins, J. W. (2008). Concepts of health. In L. L. Stamler & L. Yiu (Eds.), *Community health nursing: A Canadian perspective* (pp. 80–92). Toronto, ON: Pearson Education Canada.

The Evolution of Community Health Nursing in Canada

CHAPTER 2

OBJECTIVES

After reading this chapter, you should be able to:

1. Explain significant historical events leading to the development of the modern conception of public health.
2. Discuss historical events in Canada relevant to the development of public health efforts in this country.
3. Discuss some of the milestones specific to the development of community health nursing in Canada.
4. Describe the developments in the profession of nursing in the Western world during the nineteenth and early twentieth centuries.
5. Outline the events since 1920 that have led to the development of community health nursing in Canada.

CHAPTER OUTLINE

Historical Roots of Public Health

Public Health in Canada

Early Development of Community Health Nursing in Canada

Nursing in the Nineteenth and Early Twentieth Centuries

Community Health Nursing From the 1920s to the Present

KEY TERMS

Canadian Nurses Association (CNA) 50

Canadian Public Health Association (CPHA) 41

Canadian Red Cross 41

demonstration project 50

district nursing 47

Eunice Dyke 48

Florence Nightingale 42

Lillian Wald 47

Metropolitan Life Insurance Company 47

occupational health nursing 53

outpost nursing 50

visiting nurse associations 47

visiting nurses 47

William Rathbone 47

See Glossary on page 593 for definitions.

The Canadian authors thank Ivana Zuliani for her contribution in updating the chapter tables.

Gaining a better understanding and appreciation of community health nursing today requires a review of the past. Lessons learned through history provide direction for current and future community health nursing practice. For example, lessons learned from the global outbreak of severe acute respiratory syndrome (SARS) in 2003 led to a renewed emphasis on public health and efforts to deal with the pandemic threats of avian flu and the recent H1N1 virus to prevent these diseases from assuming severe global proportions. As well, having an understanding of the evolution of the profession of nursing allows community health nurses (CHNs) to function most effectively in the current sociopolitical and economic environments (see the CNA position statement "Promoting Nursing History" available on the CNA Web site listed in the Evolve Weblinks at the end of this chapter).

The Canadian Nurses Association (CNA), a national advocacy body for registered nurses, encourages nurses to understand, consider, collect, and preserve their nursing history. The Web site of the Canadian Association for the History of Nursing (CAHN), an affiliate group of the CNA, also offers information about the history of nursing (see the Evolve Weblinks). Some of the links at this Web site provide access to nursing archives and the histories of some provincial nursing associations, such as those of New Brunswick and British Columbia.

As noted in Chapter 1, the term *community health nursing,* as it is used today, encompasses all registered nurses working in a variety of practice areas in the community with focuses on primary, secondary, and tertiary prevention and health promotion. In the past, public health nursing, for example, was considered separate from home visiting nursing. Public health nurses and visiting nurses (e.g., Victorian Order of Nurses [VON] and Saint Elizabeth Visiting Nurses) (renamed Saint Elizabeth Health Care in 1995) provided a variety of different nursing services but both provided care in the home. However, historically, at times, the care provided by each of these nurses overlapped depending on available resources and community needs.

For more than 100 years, public health nurses (PHNs) in Canada have made significant contributions to solving public health problems. Although only a few such historical figures are highlighted in this chapter, many nurses have played a part in building organizations and providing services to improve public health. Effective planning for the future is thus built on the foundation that they have laid.

Over the years, CHNs have been flexible, creative, and able to work with people from many backgrounds and with varied skills. Leaders in community health nursing have worked to improve the health status of individuals, families, and populations. They have spent time, energy, and effort working with high-risk or vulnerable groups. Part of the appeal of community health nursing is the autonomy of practice and independence in problem solving and decision making that it affords, as well as its interdisciplinary nature. Many of the varied and challenging community health roles that exist today can be traced to the late 1800s, when public health efforts focused on environmental factors, such as sanitation and control of communicable diseases, as well as on education for health promotion, for the prevention of disease and disability, and for the care of sick persons in their homes. This chapter provides an introduction to the history of community health nursing, public health, and public health nursing.

HISTORICAL ROOTS OF PUBLIC HEALTH

Events surrounding birth, death, and illness hold great importance for all peoples and all cultures. Worldwide, people work to prevent, understand, and control disease. Their ability to preserve health and treat illnesses has depended on their knowledge of science, use and availability of technologies, and degree of social organization. For example, ancient Babylonians understood the importance of hygiene, and historical records indicate they also had some medical skills and knew how to use medicine to treat the sick. The Egyptians of circa 1000 B.C. developed a variety of pharmaceutical preparations and became known for their remarkable construction of earth privies and public drainage systems. The Mosaic Law, as described in the Old Testament, talked about many aspects of health, including maternal health, communicable disease control, protection of food and water, and waste and sanitary disposal (Rosen, 1958).

The ancient Greeks were more concerned with personal health than community health. They practised many health-promoting behaviours that are considered vital for good health, even today. The Greeks linked health to the environment; wealthy Greeks valued personal cleanliness, exercise, diet, and sanitation—considered luxuries by the less privileged, who led difficult lives and struggled to survive. The classical Roman civilization viewed medicine from the perspective of community health and social medicine. It placed great emphasis on the regulation of medical practice and punishment for negligence; provision of pure water through a complex system of settling basins, aqueducts, and reservoirs; establishment of sewage systems and drainage of swamps; and supervision of street cleaning and public food preparation. During the period of the Roman Empire, women visited and cared for sick persons in their homes (Pellegrino, 1963).

The decline of the Greco–Roman civilization led to the decay of urban culture and disintegration of community health organization and practice (Rosen, 1958). As cities grew, people built large walls around the cities to protect themselves from invasions. These walls, although sheltering the citizens from attacks, led to crowding and poor sanitary conditions.

The spread of Christianity brought with it the idea of personal responsibility for others; care of the sick was considered one way of fulfilling this responsibility. During the Middle Ages, between 500 and 1500 A.D., European cities suffered high population density, lacked clean water, and had inefficient systems to dispose of refuse and body wastes. Poor sanitary conditions and residential crowding caused increases in communicable diseases, such as cholera, smallpox, and bubonic plague. Most people had to secure their own health care services; however, religious institutions, such as convents and monasteries, began to establish hospitals to care for the sick, poor, and neglected, including the aged, disabled, and orphaned (Rosen, 1958). During the later years of the Middle Ages, an interest in health education and the promotion of personal hygiene and healthy living grew, and moderate eating was encouraged. In the eleventh century, similar forces guided the work of Muslim nurses in what is now Saudi Arabia. Rufaida Al-Asalmiya cared for injured soldiers, established a school of nursing for women, and developed a code for nursing conduct and ethics (Jan, 1996).

During the Renaissance (from the fourteenth through the sixteenth centuries), health practices were influenced by a recognition of human dignity and worth (Kalisch & Kalisch, 1995). In England, the Elizabethan Poor Law of 1601 guaranteed medical care for poor, blind, and "lame" individuals. This minimal care was generally provided in almshouses supported by local governments, with a goal of regulating the lives of the poor and providing care during illness. Table 2-1 summarizes milestones in public health efforts, public health nursing, and community health nursing that occurred during the seventeenth, eighteenth, and nineteenth centuries.

The Industrial Revolution in nineteenth-century Europe led to social changes, including great advances in transportation, communication, and other forms of technology. Previous caregiving structures, which relied on families, neighbours, and friends, had by then become inadequate because of increased migration, urbanization, and higher populations. During this period, small numbers of Roman Catholic and Protestant religious women provided nursing care in institutions and sometimes in the home. For example, Mary Aikenhead, also known by her religious name, Sister Mary Augustine, started the order of Irish Sisters of Mercy in 1812 in Dublin. These nuns visited poor people in their homes (Kalisch & Kalisch, 1995).

Many laywomen who performed nursing functions in almshouses and early hospitals in Great Britain were poorly educated and untrained. As the practice of medicine became more complex in the mid-1800s, hospital work required a more skilled caregiver, and physicians and hospital administrators sought to improve the quality of nursing services. Early experimental efforts led to some improvement in care, but it was because of the groundbreaking work of Florence Nightingale, discussed later in this chapter, that health care was revolutionized and the discipline of nursing actually came into its own.

TABLE 2-1 International Historical Milestones in Public Health, Public Health Nursing, and Community Health Nursing: 1600–1895

Year	Milestone
1601	Elizabethan Poor Law enacted
1617	Sisterhood of the Dames de Charité organized in France by St. Vincent de Paul
1789	Baltimore Health Department established
1798	Marine Hospital Service established in the United States; later became Public Health Service
1812	Sisters of Mercy established in Dublin; nuns visited the poor
1813	Ladies Benevolent Society of Charleston, South Carolina, founded
1836	Lutheran deaconesses made home visits in Kaiserswerth, Germany
1851	Florence Nightingale visited Kaiserswerth, Germany, for 3 months of nurse training
1855	Quarantine Board established in New Orleans; beginning of tuberculosis eradication campaign in the United States
1859	District nursing established in Liverpool by William Rathbone
1860	Florence Nightingale Training School for Nurses established at St. Thomas Hospital in London
1864	Founding of American Red Cross
1895	Founding of Canadian Red Cross

PUBLIC HEALTH IN CANADA

Early public health efforts in Canada were driven by the need to deal with epidemics. Before 1900, Canada did not have Europe's problems of overcrowded cities and had the advantage of alternating hot and cold seasons, which helped reduce disease-causing organisms in the

Evidence-Informed Practice

MacDougall (2009) describes the deep historical roots involved in the creation of twenty-first century pandemic preparation plans—for example, allocating personnel, facilities, vaccines, and equipment; addressing and discussing ethical issues; and determining whether preventive or curative measures will be the most effective.

The first cholera epidemic, in 1832 in Ontario and Quebec, provided guidelines for disease prevention and control when cholera reoccurred in 1834, 1849, 1854, and 1866. The governing bodies identified the importance of the following: strong leadership at central and local levels; clear communication about the disease and nature of it; and description of the steps required to prevent or control it. As well, adequate legal and financial support was required for front-line workers and volunteers. There was also recognition that each outbreak would spawn a response from society based on the society's cultural values and perceptions of danger. These guiding principles and courses of action remain the foundation for current programs and policies pertaining to disease prevention.

Application for CHNs: This article supports the importance of history to present-day community health nursing practice. CHNs need to use what has been learned in the past and apply that knowledge as relevant to current-day practice. When considering changes to health care practices, it is often valuable to conduct a historical review to identify past lessons learned.

Questions for Reflection & Discussion

1. Think about the H1N1 pandemic that occurred in 2009. What was the societal response to this potential danger?
2. What roles did CHNs assume in the H1N1 pandemic?
3. With the knowledge you have gained from MacDougall's article, how would you frame your question to search for the most recent and available evidence on strategies for pandemic planning?

REFERENCE: MacDougall, H. (2009). "Truly alarming": Cholera in 1832. *Canadian Journal of Public Health, 100*(5), 333–336.

environment. However, devastating epidemics did occur, nearly always coinciding with the arrival of new immigrants from Europe on crowded, unsanitary ships carrying such highly contagious diseases as smallpox, typhus, cholera, and influenza. The diseases spread quickly and wrought havoc among the Aboriginal populations, in particular, who had no natural defences against the new pathogens that multiplied quickly (Cadotte, 2006).

From the seventeenth to the nineteenth centuries, various epidemics ravaged towns and cities in Canada, killing tens of thousands of people. In order to prevent the devastation caused by such outbreaks, Canadian authorities began to take action to protect public health. Vaccination programs were introduced as early as the end of the eighteenth century (e.g., for smallpox) and, in some cases, made mandatory. In 1882, Ontario passed legislation for the establishment of the first Board of Health, which reported to municipal councils and assumed responsibility for educating the public about health matters (Allemang, 2000). Following this, Boards of Health were established in other provinces to deal with the problem of frequent epidemics and the incidence and prevalence of communicable diseases and to ensure support and enforcement of public health efforts.

With industrialization, the rapid population growth in the cities led to inadequate housing and poor sanitation, thus causing epidemics of diseases such as smallpox, yellow fever, cholera, typhoid, and typhus (Allemang, 2000). Tuberculosis (TB) was always present (Allemang, 2000), and infant mortality rates continued to rise (McKay, 2008); therefore, concern regarding the health of the public was continuous.

The early 1900s marked the introduction of organized public health nursing as a major component of public health programs. For example, PHNs employed by the Toronto Department of Health made home visits for all positive and suspected cases of TB, then called consumption, unless the physicians-in-charge indicated visits were not necessary (Royce, 1983). The purpose of these home visits was to teach those affected self-care as well as to teach family members ways to prevent the spread of infection throughout the household. The Department of Health maintained records of children who had been exposed to TB in the home. In some areas of the city, summer schools, held in parks, were opened for TB-exposed children to protect other children. When people infected with TB had to be moved away from their homes, the PHN had to arrange and oversee complete fumigation of the house.

In 1906, the Montreal Board of Health implemented a program of medical inspection of schoolchildren, and nurses from the Victorian Order of Nurses (VON) were assigned to work with children in schools and conduct home visits to families with newborns (Duncan, Leipert, & Mill, 1999). It was around this time that school nurses were first hired to work in Hamilton and Toronto schools. Just prior to World War I, the focus shifted to maternal–child health, resulting in expanded roles for PHNs. However, some specialized nursing roles, such as that of the "TB nurse," were maintained.

After World War I, several voluntary organizations, including the **Canadian Red Cross** (the national organization conducting various health, safety, and disaster-relief programs), in affiliation with the International Red Cross, worked with PHNs to ensure the availability of services in communities to prevent disease, promote health, and provide support for those experiencing stress and suffering (Allemang, 2000; Duncan et al., 1999). The VON also contributed to public health development in Canada. The VON, through its home health nurse visiting program and preventive work, was able to demonstrate that nursing care in the community effectively addressed public health concerns (Pringle & Roe, 1992). In Canada, the VON recognized the importance of and opportunities for health promotion by nurses in all nursing work settings (Allemang, 2000). In 1910, the **Canadian Public Health Association (CPHA)** was founded in order to deliver and support national and international health and social service programs (CPHA, 2009).

In the post–World War I era, 1918 to 1939, "screening programs to detect disease at an early stage, to activities to assist and maintain a healthy environment and to offer personal nursing health services" (Ross-Kerr, 2006, p. 11) became the focus of public health nursing responsibilities. The economic depression of the 1930s led to two significant realizations: (1) that Canadian citizens were demanding that government take responsibility for health care and (2) that poverty was a result of sociopolitical factors and not of individual character weaknesses (McKay, 2008). As an outcome of these sociopolitical and economic realizations, the federal government initiated social assistance, while provincial governments focused on public health programs, such as immunization, improved sewage systems, and clean water (Allemang, 2000; McKay, 2008).

After World War II, from 1945 to 1970, the vision for public health expanded beyond the maintenance and control of the physical environment and, thus, public hygiene to include prevention of diseases and health education (Duncan et al., 1999). At the same time, significant advances were being made in pharmacology, especially in the development of antibiotics to treat many infectious diseases, vaccines to prevent some of the communicable diseases, and other highly effective drugs to treat various illnesses. These pharmacological advances shifted the previous focus on prevention and "care" to a medical focus of "cure" (Allemang, 2000).

In the mid-1970s, the Lalonde Report (Lalonde, 1974) initiated the health promotion movement in Canada. Health promotion focuses on achieving a high level of wellness through a healthy lifestyle. At international conferences and in the form of written documents, such as the Epp Report (Epp, 1986), Canada led the worldwide efforts in health promotion initiatives. These health promotion initiatives, as well as the development of population health and the determinants of health, are discussed further in Chapter 4.

More than 100 years of combined efforts in the field of public health have resulted in improved health for individual Canadians, their families, and their communities. The development and availability of vaccinations, clean water, the pasteurization process, and improved living conditions in the past century have resulted in a markedly increased life expectancy and improved health status and quality of life for Canadians. These efforts have also led to the development of community health nursing practice. In recent years, health promotion efforts have contributed to a decrease in suffering as well as in costs related to the treatment of illnesses. It is worth noting that relative to many other nations, Canada has a healthier population (Public Health Agency of Canada [PHAC], 2005a).

EARLY DEVELOPMENT OF COMMUNITY HEALTH NURSING IN CANADA

Interestingly, in Canada, nursing first developed in the community, then later emphasized acute care, and now, in more recent years, has begun to shift its focus back to the community. Villeneuve and MacDonald (2006) propose that by 2020 approximately 66% of all nurses in Canada will be practising in the community.

In the early years of North American settlement, the nursing care of the sick was usually informal and provided in the home by the women of the household. These women provided care during times of sickness and childbirth; also, throughout the year, they cultivated or gathered herbs for their "healing" properties. From the early seventeenth century onward, these women and also other groups, such as religious orders and wealthy philanthropists, began to see the need to take care of the sick who could not afford to hire caregivers; these compassionate caregivers laid the foundations for modern

TABLE 2-2 Milestones in the Early Evolution of Community Health Nursing in Canada: 1617 to 1900

Year	Milestone
1617	Marie Rollet Hébert became the first laywoman to care for the sick in her own home and in other homes in the community in Quebec.
1629	First nurses (male attendants) worked with the sick in what resembled a modern community clinic in Acadia. Jesuit priests also cared for the sick.
1639	The Duchesse d'Aiguillon arranged for three nuns to settle in Quebec and establish a mission (later known as Quebec's first hospital—Hôtel-Dieu); these nuns also cared for the sick in the community.
1641	Jeanne Mance arrived in Ville Marie (later Montreal) and established the first Hôtel-Dieu hospital there. Being the first lay nurse in North America, she cared for those wounded in battles and also took on a major leadership role in the community and became very involved in political activities to improve life within the colony. In recognition of this pioneer in nursing, the Canadian Nurses Association established the Jeanne Mance Award (Ross-Kerr, 2009), granted biennially to nurses who have made remarkable contributions to the health of Canadians (Canadian Nurses Association, 2006).
1737	Marguerite d'Youville founded the order of the Grey Nuns; in Canada, they became the first nurses who visited and cared for the sick in their own homes and developed community hospitals for the care of the acutely and chronically ill regardless of their race, culture, religion, or social status. Hardill (2007) identifies these home visits as the initiation of community visits to the sick poor and states that this was the beginning of "the practical origins of modern Canadian outreach nursing" (p. 91).
1845–1895	The Grey Nuns founded community hospitals and made home visits to the poor in Ottawa, Ontario; St. Boniface, Manitoba; Edmonton, Alberta; and northern native settlements in Saskatchewan.
1859	Florence Nightingale published her "Notes on Nursing," which influenced the philosophy of nursing, including community health nursing, in Canada.
1898	Lady Aberdeen, wife of the governor general of Canada, recognized the need for specialized health services for women, especially during childbirth, and for health care for the poor living near the railways and in the mining areas in isolated communities. She founded the Victorian Order of Nurses (VON) in Canada. The VON nurses provided home care in urban as well as in isolated rural areas.

SOURCES: Allemang, M. M. (2000). Development of community health nursing in Canada. In M. J. Stewart (Ed.), *Community nursing: Promoting Canadians' health* (pp. 4–32). Toronto, ON: Saunders; Potter, P. A., Perry, A. G., Ross-Kerr, J. C., & Wood, M. J. (2006). *Canadian Fundamentals of nursing* (3rd ed.). Toronto, ON: Elsevier.

community health nursing. Refer to Table 2-2 for the significant milestones in the development of community health nursing practice in Canada from its beginnings to 1898.

NURSING IN THE NINETEENTH AND EARLY TWENTIETH CENTURIES

Many of the changes to the profession of nursing in general during the nineteenth and twentieth centuries affected and shaped the development of community health and public health nursing. Refer to Table 2-3 for a summary of select milestones in public health, public health nursing, and community health nursing. **Florence Nightingale**'s vision of trained nurses and her model of nursing education influenced the development of professional nursing and, indirectly, community health nursing in the United States as well as in Canada. During 1850–1851, Nightingale carefully studied the "system and method" of nursing instituted by visiting pastor Theodor Fliedner at his School for Deaconesses in Kaiserswerth, Germany. Her work with Pastor Fliedner and the Kaiserswerth Lutheran deaconesses and with their systems of district nursing led Nightingale to later promote her model for nursing care for the sick in their homes.

During the Crimean War (1854–1856), the British military established hospitals for the sick and wounded soldiers in Scutari in Asia Minor. These hospitals were cramped; plagued by poor sanitation, lice, and rats; provided insufficient food; had inadequate medical supplies; and, overall, offered poor care (Kalisch & Kalisch, 1995; Palmer, 1983). The British public demanded improved conditions, and Florence Nightingale asked to be sent to work in Scutari. Her personal wealth, social and political connections, and knowledge of hospitals influenced the British government, and along with 40 other ladies, 117

TABLE 2-3 Select Milestones in the History of Public Health, Public Health Nursing, and Community Health Nursing

Era	Public Health	Public Health Nursing	Community Health Nursing
1800s	• Recurrent and devastating epidemics, e.g., smallpox and tuberculosis (TB), killed thousands in Canada. • 1832: Cholera epidemic killed millions worldwide and thousands in Canada. • 1882: First permanent provincial Board of Health was established in Ontario. • 1884: *Public Health Act* was introduced to establish municipal Boards of Health in Ontario; other provinces followed suit. • In the late 1800s, discovery of disease-causing bacteria led to a focus on disease prevention, including vaccination of school-aged children.	• 1860s: William Rathbone instituted district nursing in Liverpool, England, by dividing the city into districts and hiring nurses to work in them. • 1874: William Rathbone and Florence Nightingale hired Florence Lee to study nursing needs in London; she highlighted the need for district nursing training. • Florence Nightingale, in England, between 1861 and 1897, developed the early principles of public health nursing: disease prevention through teaching cleanliness and sanitation. • Pioneer PHNs were dependent on assistance from communities.	• Compassionate women and men cared for sick in their homes. • 1840: Elizabeth Fry founded a Protestant order of visiting nurses in London. • 1887: Florence Nightingale founded the Queen's Nursing Institute of visiting nurses; she fought for specific training and appropriate salaries for nurses. • Rathbone, Nightingale, and Lee established community health nursing, initially in England, based on the district nursing concepts of professionalism, accountability, and use of research in the late 1800s. • Religious orders helped with care of "destitute immigrants." • 1897: Victorian Order of Nurses (VON) in Canada founded by Lady Aberdeen; the VON focused on public health, TB prevention and care, and maternity care. • Private-duty nurses lived with patients in their homes and were paid well by the patients.
1900s	• In 1901, TB was the leading cause of death in Canadian cities, especially among the poor, with a mortality rate of 180 per 100,000 Canadians. • Major threats to public health included TB, influenza, and syphilis. • 1906: Montreal became the first city in Canada to legislate medical inspection of schoolchildren. • 1911: *School Medical Inspection Act* was passed in British Columbia. • Infant mortality rates continued to climb in Canadian cities. • 1918: Spanish influenza epidemic affected one-sixth of the Canadian population and killed approximately 30,000 Canadians.	• 1905: Ms. E. C. Rayside became the first home visiting TB nurse in Ottawa. • 1907: Christina Mitchell became the first home visiting TB nurse employed by Toronto health department. • 1908: The first public health nursing training program began at University of British Columbia with the financial support of the Canadian Red Cross. • 1909: Canada's first school nurse was appointed in Hamilton. • 1913: Ms. Blanche Swan became the first provincial school nurse in British Columbia. • 1910: Well-baby clinics were established in Toronto. • 1911: Eunice Dyke became the first director of public health nursing in Toronto.	• 1907: Elizabeth Lindsay became the first city nurse on the city of Toronto, Ontario payroll. • 1911–1918: Metropolitan Life Insurance Company proved the effectiveness of visiting nurses in decreasing infant mortality rates. • 1920: VON and Metropolitan Life nurses provided home nursing for the sick, education for prevention, prenatal and postnatal care, and well-baby clinics across Ontario. • 1920: In Ontario, the Red Cross established nursing outposts. • 1920s: Private-duty nurses in Nova Scotia worked autonomously in the community.

(Continued)

TABLE 2-3 Select Milestones in the History of Public Health, Public Health Nursing, and Community Health Nursing—Cont'd

Era	Public Health	Public Health Nursing	Community Health Nursing
	• 1919: Federal Department of Health was established in Canada. • 1919: British Columbia was the first province to have a health centre with public health nurses.	• 1914: Metropolitan Life insisted that public health and visiting nurses be included on health research teams funded by the agency. • The University of Alberta offered its first public health nursing course. • 1919: UBC established the first baccalaureate nursing program. • The Canadian Red Cross offered financial assistance to universities and scholarships to nurses to study public health nursing. • 1920: School boards across Ontario employed nurses, usually as PHNs, in the school setting. • 1920: Urban public health departments employed nurses as specialists in school nursing, TB nursing, and maternal–child nursing areas; public health nursing was well established in major cities. • 1920s: The VON stopped training its own nurses to support the development of Canadian public health nursing programs. • 1921: UBC graduated 56 PHNs. • 1928: British Columbia Provincial Board of Health ruled all PHNs must complete university course in public health nursing.	
	• 1930s: Beginning of the Great Depression—no unemployment insurance or social assistance; outbreaks of communicable disease.	• 1930s: Public health nursing programs provided most preventive and educative public health work. • 1932: The Weir Report raised concerns and made recommendations for public health nursing (e.g., doubling the number of PHNs and raising their salaries); it also recognized public health nursing as a specialty area requiring advanced education. • 1930s: In Canada, Edna L. Moore, a nurse, advocated for generalized, rather than specialized, public health nursing, which led to the acceptance of generalized activities (as opposed to specialized activities such as TB care) for all age groups in public health nursing.	• The VON focused on home nursing care of the sick. • Most private-duty nurses were unemployed.

	• 1940: World War II; men and women join military service or work in war-related industries—unemployment ceased. • Post–World War II: There was a rise in industrialization and population growth in urban centres, which provided conditions conducive to the spread of contagions. • 1950–60s: Nursing shortage evident. • 1973: Pickering Report recommended that the VON be mandated to deliver home care programs. • 1974: Lalonde introduced elements that determined the health of Canadians in a document titled *A New Perspective on the Health of Canadians*—these elements were human biology, environment, lifestyle, and health care organization; over time, additional determinants of health have been added. • 1978: Primary health care was defined by Alma-Ata Declaration. • 1980s: Sexually transmitted diseases became a concern. • 1984: *Canada Health Act* was adopted. • 1986: The Ottawa Charter for Health Promotion identified the prerequisites for health. • 1990s: TB re-emerged as a leading threat to global health.	• 1943: PHNs assumed full responsibility for prenatal, postnatal, and child health programs from the VON. • 1945: PHNs were the first nurses in Canada to administer immunization. • 1946: Registered Nurses of British Columbia (RNBC) became the first provincial nursing association certified under the *Labor Relations Act* as the bargaining agent for nurses. • 1948: *Hospital Insurance Act* gave hospital care to all British Columbia residents. • The Baillie–Creelman Report, a Canada-wide study, examined the roles of nurses and physicians and explored recruitment and retention of public health staff. • Prevention programming became the focus of PHN attention. • Nursing programs began including public health nursing content. • 1970s: In Canada, PHNs increased their focus on health promotion, in addition to disease prevention. • 1980s: Health care spending constraints began to lead to reduction in programs. • 1990s: With public health reorganization, public health nursing visits to client homes were greatly reduced.	• 1941: In Manitoba, the Buck Commission recommended reorganization of visiting nurse programs. • 1943: Prenatal, postnatal, and child health programs were transferred from the VON to the provincial health department/authority. • In 1967, Dalhousie University in Nova Scotia offered the first program to train northern nurses as nurse practitioners. • Early 1970s: The VON evolved to include home care for older adults and the chronically ill. • Mid-1970s: McMaster University in Ontario offered a primary health care nurse practitioner program. • 1974: The VON became the first publicly funded provincial home care program in Manitoba; this trend continued throughout Canada as a result of the Pickering Report. • 1982: Occupational health nursing was established. • 1990s: Primary health care nurse practitioner programs were established in most provinces across Canada.
2000 to present	• 2000: *Escherichia coli* outbreak in Walkerton, Ontario. • 2003: SARS outbreak in Toronto, Ontario. • 2004: A 10-year action plan to establish public health goals for Canada was signed by the prime minister and the premiers. • 2004: Creation of the Public Health Agency of Canada and the position of Canada's chief public health officer.	• 2003: Public health nursing now came under the umbrella term "community health nursing." • 2009: Release of core competencies for public health nurses.	• 2001: Studies demonstrated that providing home care to older adults costs less than institutional care. • 2002: Romanow Report identified home care as the most rapidly growing area of community health nursing. • 2003: *Canadian Community Health Nursing Standards of Practice* were implemented.

(Continued)

TABLE 2-3 Select Milestones in the History of Public Health, Public Health Nursing, and Community Health Nursing—Cont'd

Era	Public Health	Public Health Nursing	Community Health Nursing
	• 2006: Research continued to support the extent of contributions to the 12 determinants of health. • 2006: A joint task force released its report on public health human resources; identified the presence of many planning challenges. • 2007: Core competencies for public health workforce in Canada were introduced. • 2008: The chief public health officer's report released on the state of public health in Canada addressed health inequities. • 2008: Listeriosis outbreak linked to packaged meat products in Canada. • 2009: H1N1 (swine flu) outbreak in Canada.		• PHNs, within community health nursing, anticipated and planned for handling tropical diseases, SARS, and influenza. • PHNs continued health promotion and re-established home visiting to all mothers and their newborns. • Health care cutbacks led to a shift back to home care. • Untrained family members often cared for the ill. • The Canadian Institute for Health Information (CIHI), based on research and consultation, developed a common set of home care indicators. • 2006: The Ontario Community Health Nursing Study found that fewer CHNs were working in the community sector despite the shift to community care. • 2006: Canadian community health nurses certification became available. • 2009: Community Health Nurses Association of Canada (CHNAC) changed its name to Community Health Nurses of Canada (CHNC).

Sources: Allemang, 2000; Duncan et al., 1999; Green, 1984; Hebert et al., 2001; Hollander, 2001; Keddy & Dodd, 2005; MacQueen, 1997; Mansell, 2003; McKay, 2005, 2008; Mount Saint Vincent University Archives, 2005; Romanow, 2002; Royce, 1983; Vollman, Anderson, & McFarlane, 2004.

hired nurses, and 15 paid servants, Nightingale went to Scutari. There, she succeeded in significantly improving the soldiers' health using a population-focused approach that included better environmental conditions and excellent nursing care. Using simple epidemiological measures, she documented a mortality rate that decreased from 415 per 1,000 at the beginning of the war to 11.5 per 1,000 at the end (Cohen, 1984; Palmer, 1983). Following the example of Florence Nightingale in Scutari, nurses who practise community health care start by identifying health care needs that affect the entire population. They then organize themselves and the community and mobilize resources to meet these needs.

After the Crimean War, Florence Nightingale returned to England in 1856 with her fame established. She went on to organize hospital nursing practice and nursing education in hospitals in England, replacing untrained lay nurses with trained "Nightingale nurses." She focused on both hospital nursing and community nursing. Believing that nursing should not only promote health but also prevent illness, she emphasized the importance of proper nutrition, rest, sanitation, and hygiene (Nightingale, 1894, 1946). Florence Nightingale's work marks the beginning of community health nursing practice as we know it today. In Canada, some of the hospital nursing programs established in the late 1950s and early 1960s adopted the Nightingale philosophy of nursing—that is, that healing processes can be facilitated or hindered by nursing interventions (Allemang, 2000).

In 1859, in Liverpool, England, British philanthropist **William Rathbone** founded the first association for **district nursing,** a system in which a nurse was assigned to each district in a town to provide a wide variety of health services to people in need. On the basis of the success of these "friendly visitors" (Kalisch & Kalisch, 1995),

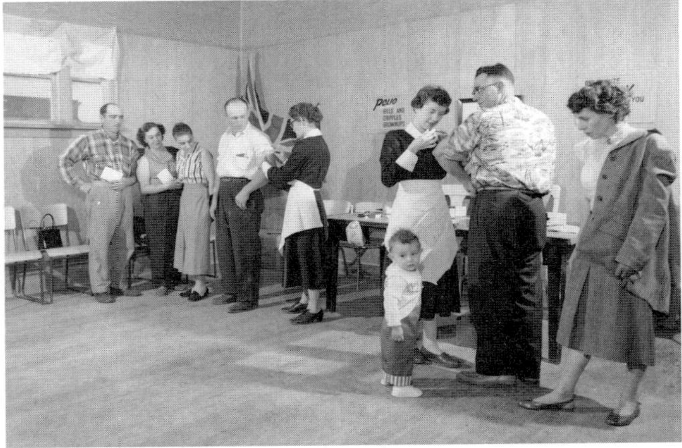

After World War II, public health in Canada expanded to include disease prevention and health education. In this photo, public health nurses are giving polio vaccinations to residents of Southey, Saskatchewan, in the 1950s.

Florence Nightingale and William Rathbone made recommendations for providing nursing in the home. As a result, district nursing and the VON became established throughout England (Nutting & Dock, 1935).

In Canada, the first "training school" (hospital diploma school) for nurses opened in 1874 at the St. Catharines General and Marine Hospital in St. Catharines, Ontario (Ross-Kerr, 2009). By 1930, there were nearly 330 hospital diploma schools of nursing in Canada (Canadian Nurses Association [CNA], 1968). In the early days, trained graduate nurses worked in private-duty nursing or held the few hospital administrator or instructor positions that were available. Private-duty nurses often lived with the families of clients receiving care. Because it was expensive to hire private-duty nurses, only the affluent could afford their services. Subsequently, the introduction of community health nursing and home visits would contribute toward meeting health care needs in urban communities, especially for the disadvantaged.

It was recognized that the additional responsibilities of visiting PHNs required their obtaining more education and training than the hospital nursing diploma course provided. Initially, in-services and continuing education courses were offered to fill this gap. In 1920, Kathleen Russell, director of the Department of Public Health Nursing at the University of Toronto, was instrumental in establishing the first integrated basic degree nursing program, a major milestone in nursing education, including public health nursing education.

Following World War I, greater emphasis was placed on the health of aggregates, particularly infants and children. **Visiting nurses,** who provided care wherever the client was located—at home, work, or school—took care of several families in 1 day (rather than only one client or family, as the private-duty nurse did), making their care more economical. The movement grew, and the next few years saw the establishment of **visiting nurse associations,** agencies that provided visiting nurses.

Public health nursing made significant strides in the United States in the late nineteenth and early twentieth centuries, largely because of the work of a nurse and social reformer named **Lillian Wald.** Wald recognized that sickness should be considered within its social and economic context. Her accomplishments included visionary work in three critical areas: the invention of public health nursing; the establishment of an American system of insurance payments for home-based care, and the creation of an American public health nursing service (Buhler-Wilkerson, 1993).

In 1909, Wald, along with her friend Lee Frankel, who was in charge of the welfare department of the **Metropolitan Life Insurance Company,** established the first public health nursing program for the life insurance policyholders of that company, believing that keeping workers healthier would increase their productivity.

Wald also proposed that nurses assess illness, teach health practices, and effectively collect data from policyholders (Hamilton, 1992). Wald convinced the company that it would be more economical to use the services of public health nurses than to employ its own nurses. According to Frachel (1988),Wald also convinced the company to:

- Provide home nursing care on a fee-for-service basis
- Establish an effective cost accounting system for visiting nurses
- Use advertisements in newspapers and on the radio to recruit nurses
- Reduce mortality from infectious diseases

In 1909, largely because of Wald's groundbreaking work, the Metropolitan Life Insurance Company implemented a program using visiting nurse organizations to provide care for sick policyholders. In 1918, Metropolitan Life calculated an average 7% decrease in the mortality rate of policyholders and almost a 20% decrease in the mortality rate of children younger than 3 years. The insurance company attributed this improvement, as well as its own reduced costs, to the work of visiting nurses. In the 1920s, the Canadian Metropolitan Life Insurance Company also provided home nursing services for policyholders who became ill and required in-home care.

In Canada, in the early 1900s, a nurse named **Eunice Dyke** became interested in the public health issues in Ontario. Working at the Department of Health in Toronto, she implemented her vision for public health nursing and emerged as a leading Canadian figure in the field for several decades (see Box 2-1).

Eunice Dyke kept a journal, referred to as the "Brown Book." On page 317 of the "Brown Book," she described the contents of a PHN's black bag, a useful aid that she initiated and that would become a symbol of public health nursing. The contents of the bag, organized in such a manner as to ensure cleanliness, included equipment required for assessment and care of the client in the home. The PHN black-bag contents, as described by Eunice Dyke, were as follows (Royce, 1983, p. 317):

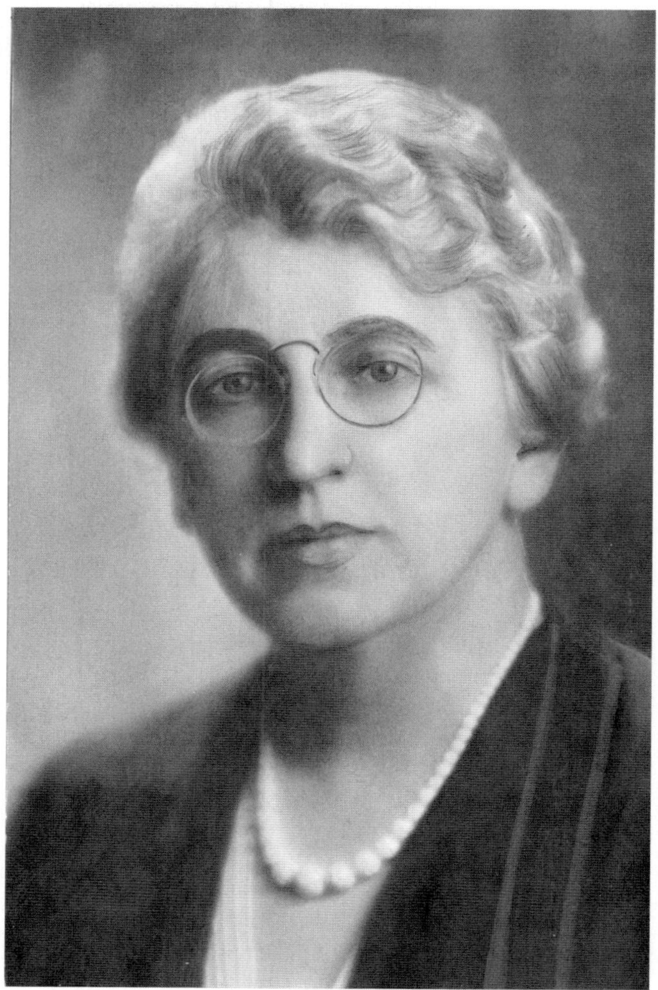

Eunice Dyke.

Nursing Supplies

- Castor oil
- Green soap
- Mouthwash
- Vaseline tube
- Thermometers: rectal and mouth
- Instruments: scissors and forceps
- Bags: absorbent cotton, rectal tube and funnel
- Hand towel
- Gown
- Book
- Bichloride tablets
- Olive oil
- Alcohol
- Talcum powder
- Basin
- Safety pins
- Bandages—1" and 2"

Literature on TB & Child Welfare

- Care of baby—2
- Diet slips—2

BOX 2-1 Eunice Dyke: Public Health Nurse Pioneer in Canada

Public health nursing evolved in Canada in the late nineteenth and early twentieth centuries, largely because of the pioneering work of Eunice Henrietta Dyke. Born in Toronto in 1883, she was one of six children. Florence Nightingale's work had cemented nursing as a viable employment option for women, and Dyke decided to become a nurse, choosing to attend the Johns Hopkins Training School for Nurses in Baltimore, Maryland. There, she received a strict, disciplined nursing education that moulded her into a high achiever on the hospital wards. Her district nursing experiences as a student incited in her a deep interest in public health issues. In 1911, she took on the position of first director of public health nursing in Toronto. She was committed to public health nursing, especially the care of those with TB, the main communicable disease of the time, as well as baby and child welfare.

Many noteworthy developments in public health nursing occurred during the time of Eunice Dyke's nursing leadership. Other public health officials supported Dyke in bringing about these developments, which included structural changes to nursing district offices once she became superintendent of public health nurses. In 1914, Eunice Dyke played a key role in the decentralization of public health nursing. Before this time, public health nurses worked in specialized areas of nursing (e.g., tuberculosis care), but they now became generalists (though they did not provide bedside nursing care in the home as CHNs or visiting nurses would). Dyke's philosophy was that the family, home, and community composed essential parts of the work of PHNs, so public health nursing should be generalized. In addition, Eunice Dyke's philosophy recognized the importance of referral to, and working with, community agencies. This represented a paradigm shift from specialist public health nursing, which put focus on the individual. Eunice Dyke also ensured better care for new immigrants by hiring two nurses who could speak foreign languages. Finally, she introduced the placement of PHNs in Toronto schools through the Board of Health. In other parts of Ontario and in other provinces, however, school nurses worked for the Board of Education, not for the Board of Health (MacQueen, 1997).

- Prenatal care—2
- City order papers—2
- Birth registration cards—2

Sanitary Supplies

- Spectum outfit
- Refills
- Handkerchiefs
- Paper bags

For a recent discussion on the historical significance of a public health nurse's bag, refer to the article by Abrams (2009) titled "The Public Health Nursing Bag as Tool and Symbol."

In 1917, Manitoba became the first province in Canada to establish a public health nursing service (Stewart, 1979). In 1919, after completing a 2-month diploma program in public health nursing from the University of Alberta, along with seven other nurses who made up the first graduating class, Kate Brighty Colley started working as a public health district nurse with Alberta's Department of Public Health (Glenbow Museum, 2009; Stewart, 1979). District nurses worked in isolated rural communities where no other medical services were available. Colley temporarily left that position to return in 1923 to establish a district nursing centre in Alberta in two areas without road access. She travelled to the communities via horse-drawn carriage or sled. She later was appointed superintendant of public health nurses in Alberta. Colley contributed to community health nursing by establishing many district nursing centres in Alberta. Additionally, she provided invaluable health information to community residents through radio broadcasts. This method of delivering health information was especially effective for those living in isolated communities.

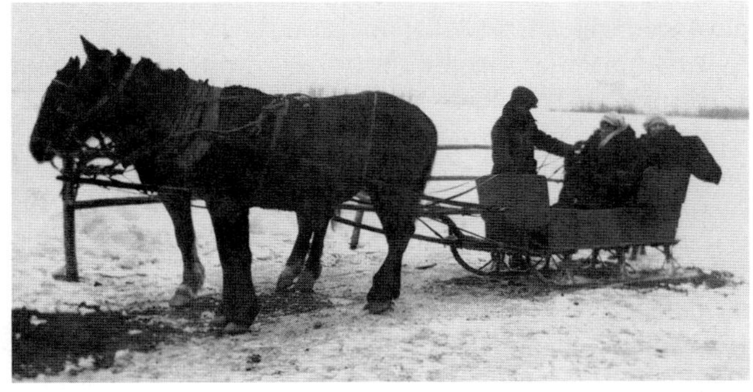

District nurses starting out on visit (Kate Brighty Colley is driving the horse-drawn sled), Onaway, Alberta, 1919.

The remarkable legacies of the early leaders, such as Florence Nightingale, Lillian Wald, Eunice Dyke, and Kate Brighty Colley, continue to inspire ideas for the present and the future. These women demonstrated an exceptional ability to develop approaches and programs to solve the health care as well as the social problems of their times. The emphasis of community health nursing has changed over the years; however, from its inception, community health nursing practice has included health teaching as well as prevention of diseases. In fact, "it was when prevention became a goal that home nursing became public health nursing" (MacQueen, 1997, p. 51). Proactive interventions by community members led to improvements in sanitation, economic conditions, and nutrition, and these interventions were credited with reducing the incidence of acute communicable diseases.

The years 1918 to 1932 marked several major milestones in the development of public health nursing in Canada. It was recognized that nurses working in communities needed more knowledge and skills in disease prevention and health promotion and that PHNs required specialized skills and knowledge beyond their basic education and training (Duncan et al., 1999). E. Kathleen Russell, director of public health nursing at the University of Toronto, proposed that such additional knowledge and skills could best be provided through university education. In 1918, the University of Alberta offered the first Canadian university course in public health nursing, which entailed 2 months of study. Then, in the early 1920s, the Canadian Red Cross provided financial support for public health nursing certificate courses at Dalhousie University, McGill University, University of Alberta, University of British Columbia (UBC), University of Toronto, and University of Western Ontario. In 1919, UBC launched Canada's first 5-year baccalaureate degree program in nursing, with the last year of the program including a specialty course in public health nursing (Allemang, 2000). In 1932, Professor G. M. Weir of UBC released a report on nursing education and public health nursing titled *Survey of Nursing Education in Canada* (Weir, 1932). One of this landmark study's most significant recommendations was that public health nursing become a specialty area in advanced education (Allemang, 2000).

Another area of community health nursing, **outpost nursing**—that is, care provided in rural and remote communities—began in Canada in the late 1800s and gained momentum in the 1920s as a growing number of PHNs chose to work in this field. In the 1920s, the Canadian Red Cross established outpost nursing stations in Canada's north to meet the needs of Aboriginal Canadians and new settlers in remote parts of Canada (Canadian Museum of Civilization Corporation, 2004). Demonstration projects, in which the Canadian Red Cross provided financial support to PHNs, made it possible for public health nursing services to be provided in rural communities in Nova Scotia and New Brunswick (Allemang, 2000). A **demonstration project** is a project that is funded externally to promote the testing of ideas and hunches. The Red Cross–funded projects were so successful that government, public, and private funding was made available to continue them.

Historically, outpost nurses worked autonomously and had the responsibility of looking after populations in areas where residents had only minimal access to medical care. These nurses encountered many challenges, such as having to travel long distances and dealing with language barriers. Outpost nursing is still provided in some of Canada's remote regions today (Dodd, Elliott, & Rousseau, 2005). Currently, even though nurses working in isolated areas continue to face many challenges, technological advances and the introduction of medical directives (the delegation of certain medical acts to nurses working in outpost settings) have made their work more rewarding and somewhat less overwhelming and isolated.

A significant development in the nursing profession during the late nineteenth and early twentieth centuries was the institution of various professional nursing bodies. The International Council of Nurses (ICN) was founded in 1899, becoming the first professional nursing organization. Britain, the United States, and Germany were charter members; Canada was also represented in the organization. In 1908, a national organization of nurses was established in Canada as the Provisional Society of the Canadian National Association of Trained Nurses (CNATN), which became a member of the ICN in 1909. By 1924, the CNATN membership had expanded considerably, and the association was renamed the **Canadian Nurses Association (CNA)**. In 1930, the CNA brought provincial nursing associations under its umbrella (Ross-Kerr & Wood, 2003). These and other nursing organizations continue to develop and advance the profession of nursing and advocate the importance of nursing in the community. In 1975, the Registered Nurses of Canadian Indian Ancestry was formed to provide an opportunity for Aboriginal nurses to come together as a professional group and play a key role in dealing with issues that affect the health of First Nations communities. In 1992, this professional association was renamed the Aboriginal Nurses Association of Canada. In 1987, the Community Health Nurses Association of Canada (CHNAC), an interest group of the CNA, was formed (CHNAC, 2003). In 2003, it developed and released the national standards of practice for CHNs, as discussed in Chapter 1. These standards of practice have helped clarify the term *community health nursing* as the umbrella term for all nurses working in and with the community and defined the minimum scope of practice for CHNs. As well, in 2006, a group of CHNs wrote the first community health nursing certification examination. This association was renamed in June 2009 and is now known as the Community Health Nurses of Canada.

CRITICAL VIEW

The percentage of male registered nurses (RNs) is increasing; in 1985, men made up only 2.6% of RNs, compared with 5.6% in 2005 (Health Canada, 2007). The number of male nurses in community health nursing practice, however, remains low.

1. What sociopolitical (or other) factors do you think influence men's choice of not taking on community health nursing as a career?

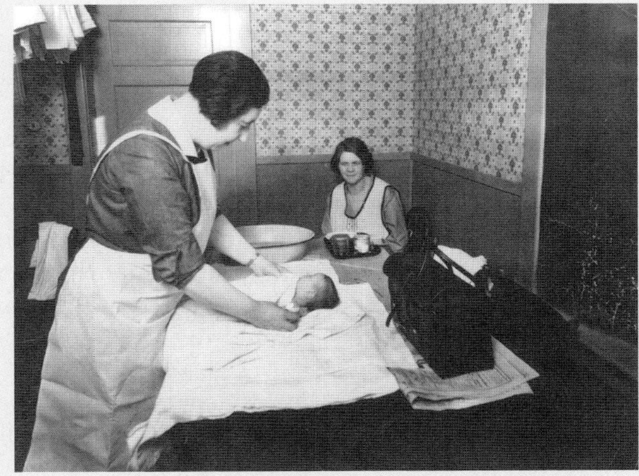

Visiting nurses, such as the Victorian Order of Nurses, were first established in Canada during the early 1900s.

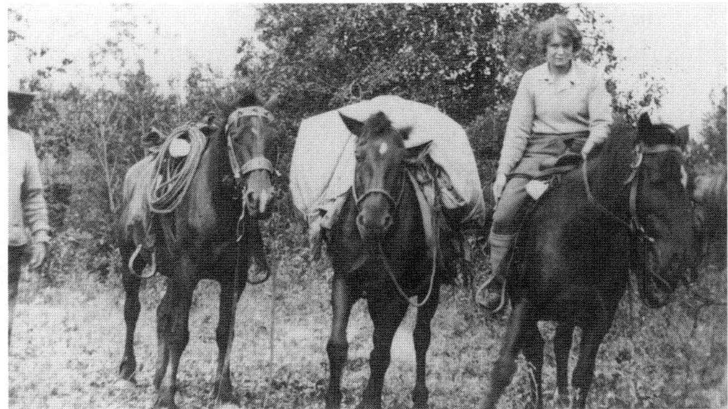

Early Canadian outpost nurses had to contend with many challenges, such as travelling long distances to visit sick patients. On the left, a nurse uses pack horses to bring supplies to her station in Slave Lake, Alberta, during the 1930s.

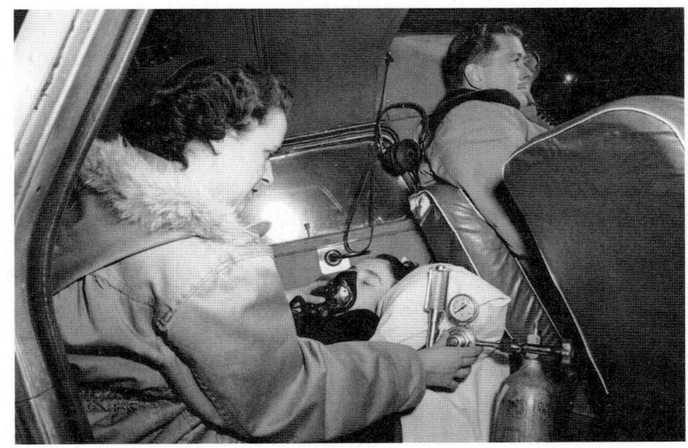

The outpost nurse on the right is shown accompanying a young patient to hospital by air ambulance in 1952.

CRITICAL VIEW

Refer to the Aboriginal Nurses Association of Canada Web site (see the Weblinks on the Evolve Web site).

1. What brought about the development of the Registered Nurses of Canadian Indian Ancestry, which later became the Aboriginal Nurses Association of Canada?
2. Which of the sociopolitical and economic factors in Aboriginal nursing and health care have had implications for community health nursing?

COMMUNITY HEALTH NURSING FROM THE 1920s TO THE PRESENT

As previously mentioned, in the early 1920s, a public health nursing practice section of the CNATN was formally recognized (Duncan et al., 1999). This association had leadership representation from across the country that included Ms. Dyke from the Toronto Department of Health, Ms. DeLaney from VON Montreal, Ms. Russell from the Manitoba Department of Public Health, Ms. Brown from the Department of Education of Saskatchewan, and Ms. Breeze, superintendent of the School Nurses of British Columbia. These public health nurse leaders and other nurses published articles in the journals *Canadian Nurse* and *Public Health* to keep their fellow nurses abreast of developments in public health nursing.

The Weir Report of 1932 discussed and proposed solutions for several important issues in public health nursing practice. In Canada at that time, there were 1,521 PHNs (Allemang, 2000), who held positions such as staff nurse, supervisor, visiting nurse, school nurse, industrial nurse, and VON nurse. The report indicated that some of the challenges these nurses faced included transportation to rural and remote areas; some physician resistance due to lack of understanding of the PHN's role; poor compensation; and lack of advanced skill and nursing experience for working in rural settings. This report also concluded that too many of the graduating nurses focused on hospital nursing rather than public health nursing, which was experiencing an extreme shortage. In fact, the Weir Report projected that between the years 1937 and 1942, the number of PHNs would have to double to meet the needs of the Canadian population (Allemang, 2000).

From the 1920s to the 1940s, nurses specializing in TB care were replaced by PHNs because of the belief that visiting nurses would be more effective and efficient if they moved to general nursing care (Toth, Fackelmann, Pigott, & Tolomeo, 2004). Therefore, PHNs became specialists in TB education, prevention, and treatment.

During the 1950s and 1960s, PHNs moved from specialized services in the community to generalized services. The responsibilities of the PHN were often described as caring for clients from "womb to tomb," through all developmental ages and stages starting with prenatal care. PHNs regularly visited clients in their homes, in schools, and in clinics (e.g., immunization clinics and well-baby clinics) and provided other services (e.g., hospital liaison to arrange for continuity of care). The focus of public health nursing was disease prevention and promotion of health, especially through health education. PHNs did not provide direct nursing care; the VON, rather, provided nursing services in the home. In some areas of Canada, various boards of education hired nurses to provide school health programs. These school nurses worked 5 days a week in the schools and delivered such services as screening for vision and hearing problems, checking for and monitoring communicable diseases, counselling, and individual and classroom teaching.

In 1967, Dalhousie University in Halifax, Nova Scotia, offered the first nurse practitioner program for northern nurses (Worster, Sarco, Thrasher, Fernandes, & Chemeria, 2005). During the 1970s, nurses made many contributions to improving the health care of communities, including participating in the hospice movement and the development of birthing centres, day care for older adults and disabled persons, drug abuse treatment programs, and rehabilitation services in long-term care. During this period, in Ontario, the nurse practitioner model for alternative health care delivery was initiated with an educational program offered by McMaster University; however, its existence was short-lived because of a perceived duplication of services and a lack of career opportunities for nurse practitioners, partly due to an overabundance of primary care physicians in urban areas (Harper-Femson, 1998). However, the Burlington Trial (1974), a randomized control study in Ontario, reported that nurse practitioners were a safe and effective alternative in primary health care and that patients were satisfied with this model of care (Spitzer et al., 1974).

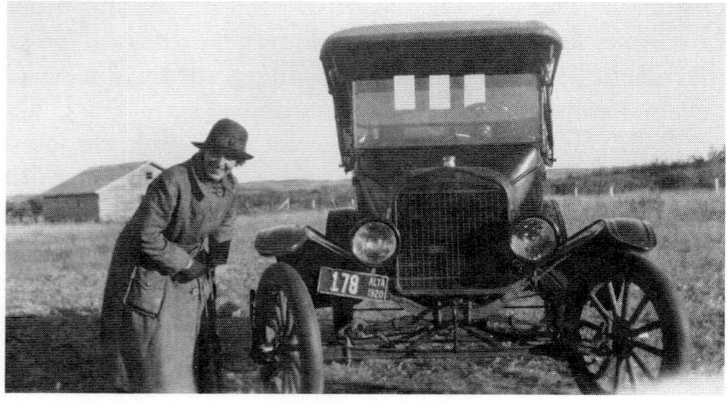

Helen Anderson, a district nurse, is shown here in 1921 beside her automobile, which she used to conduct school visits.

Nurses' frustration because of their lack of power resulted in the emergence of nursing unions and collective bargaining agents in the 1970s (Mansell, 2003). It was a time of discontent and division between unions and professional associations, between degree-prepared and diploma-prepared nurses. Currently, each of the 10 provinces has a nursing union separate from its professional nursing association.

Also in the 1970s, public health departments focused on reducing morbidity and mortality from chronic illnesses and injuries, representing a shift from traditional programs (McKay, 2008). At various times during the 1970s, Canada's provinces and territories placed greater emphasis on home care because of the shift from institutional care to community care (Romanow, 2002) brought on by such factors as fiscal concerns, patient preferences, and early hospital discharge (Shah, 2003).

In the 1980s, mothers and their newborns were discharged from hospitals sooner after birth, making the PHN's liaison role more prominent because of the need for close interaction between hospital health care staff and community programs to ensure effective follow-up care (McKay, 2005). The PHN's role in the prevention of chronic illnesses resulted in community development and community-based health promotion activities becoming part of public health strategies. This emphasis marked a change in the focus from illness prevention to health promotion in the community. PHNs contributed to community development by working with other community members to develop, facilitate, and implement health programs. In the late 1980s and into the 1990s, PHNs further expanded their skills in community development, capacity building, and group work by developing and supporting relevant partnerships and coalitions. At this time, there was an identified need to develop public health research to support and guide the practice of public health professionals, including PHNs. One example of this applied research is the Public Health Research, Education, & Development (PHRED) program, which was established in 1986 at five sites in Ontario. This nationally recognized program has contributed to public health policy changes in Ontario (PHRED, 2002).

Escalating health care costs in the 1980s resulted in some significant changes. Health promotion and disease prevention programs received less financial support while more funding was directed to acute hospital care, medical procedures, and institutional long-term care. Reduced federal and provincial funds led to decreases in the number of nurses in some public health agencies. Despite the risk of reduction in the reimbursements of costs, the role of home care increased. Individuals and families began to assume more responsibility for their own health; thus, health education—always a part of community health nursing—became more popular. Also at this time, Ontario established a new position in public health units for the coordination of the province's health promotion initiatives. Persons in this role, often titled "health educators," were generally given a middle-management position. Possibly in response to such initiatives, consumer and professional advocacy groups urged the enactment of laws to prohibit health-harming practices (e.g., smoking, driving under the influence of alcohol) in public.

During this time, another form of community health nursing began to take shape—occupational health nursing, earlier called "industrial nursing." The Canadian Occupational Health Nurses Association, formally established in 1982, has developed standards of practice for occupational health nurses (OHNs) (Canadian Occupational Health Nurses Association [COHNA], 2003). These standards help ensure quality nursing care in the workplace. Currently, **occupational health nursing** is a specialty area within community health nursing with a focus on disease prevention, including rehabilitation, and health promotion activities in the workplace. In Canada, OHNs are RNs with a diploma or degree in nursing as well as additional qualifications and work experience. Related to OHN certification, the CNA grants a specialty designation. For example, a Canadian occupational health nurse who meets the certification requirements would have the designation of COHN(C) (COHNA, 2003).

In the late 1980s and early 1990s, debates surfaced about the terms *community health nursing* and *public health nursing* being used interchangeably, at times causing confusion. King, Harrison, and Reutter (1995) helped clarify that *community health nursing* was the broader term and encompassed "subspecialties," such as public health nursing, home care nursing, and occupational health nursing. Also in the 1990s, the primary health care nurse practitioner role and designation were established in most Canadian provinces.

Evidence-Informed Practice

The health of Canadians is changing, and so is the focus for nursing. The Canadian Nurses Association has proposed that by the year 2020, 60% of nurses will be working in the community. In the Underwood et al. study, community health nurses, sometimes referred to as community nurses, are those nurses who work outside of hospitals and long-term care facilities. The objectives of this national comprehensive research study were as follows: (1) to describe the Canadian community health nursing workforce; (2) to compare provinces related to what helps or hinders community health nurses; and (3) to identify what attributes of organizations in the public health sector would support community health nurses to work to their full capacity.

The researchers used mixed research methods including the following: a demographic analysis of Canadian Institute for Health Information (CIHI) databases (1996–2007); a survey of 13,000 registered and licensed practical nurses working in the community; and 23 focus groups of public health policymakers and practising public health nurses.

Canada's community health nurses in 2007 included more than 53,000 registered and licensed practical nurses, who were demographically older than the rest of those in the nursing profession. Titles held by community health nurses were inconsistent among the various sectors. The practice settings in which they worked included health centres, home care, and public health units or departments. CHNs reported that in order for them to practise effectively, they required professional confidence, supportive workplaces with good team relationships, and community support. The community health nurses felt confident in their practice and relationships, although they often felt less confident with physicians than with other professionals. CHNs wanted more learning opportunities, more information related to policy and practice, and more opportunities to debrief about work-related issues. They reported that their communities could do more to provide quality resources and opportunities to address social determinants of health.

(Continued)

Evidence-Informed Practice—Cont'd

To succeed, public health nurses are reported to require the following: a comprehensive government policy; good management and an organizational culture that is supportive and offers flexible funding and program design and thorough job descriptions; an organizational vision that is driven by shared values and the ability to address community needs; and strong leadership that invests in education and training of the workforce. Additionally, community health nurses perform best in a work environment that encourages creativity and autonomy of practice; that is involved in and in harmony with the organizational mission and vision; and that provides time and other organizational supports to facilitate the building of community relationships, collaboration, and team building.

Application for CHNs: Community health nursing has changed and continues to evolve to ensure the following: the social determinants of health are addressed; health care is provided in the community to address the needs of more complex clients, often a result of early hospital discharges; collaboration and team building is essential to community health nursing practice; and the workplace environment can influence CHN practice.

Questions for Reflection & Discussion

1. Considering the history of community health nursing in Canada, what do you think have been the most significant changes in its development?
2. How has community health nursing developed in your community?
3. What search words would you use to find out more about the history of community health nursing?

REFERENCE: Underwood, J. M., Mowat, D. L., Meagher-Stewart, D. M., Deber, R. B., Baumann, A. O., MacDonald, M. B., et al. (2009). Building community and public health nursing capacity: A synthesis report of the national community health nursing study. *Canadian Journal of Public Health, 100*(5), I-1–13.

In 2001, researchers demonstrated that home care for older adults costs less than institutional care (Hebert et al., 2001; Hollander, 2001). The Romanow Report (Romanow, 2002) identified home care as the most rapidly growing area of community health care. In 2003, the Community Health Nurses Association of Canada identified *community health nursing* as the descriptor for community health nursing specialties such as home health nursing public health nursing, occupational health nursing, forensic nursing, parish nursing, and nurse practitioners. The approach taken in the United States differs in that community health nursing and public health nursing are discussed as two distinct entities. Also, in the United States, reference is often made to community-*oriented* care vis-à-vis community-*based* care.

Recently, interest in the planning and direction of community health care in Canada has grown. In 2005, a joint task force released a report pertaining to the Canadian public health workforce. The report identified many unique health human resources planning challenges, such as the overlapping of functions among a variety of public health care providers and the fact that public health has more regulated as well as nonregulated care providers than do other health care workforces (Public Health Agency of Canada, 2005b). The report also stressed the importance of a collaborative planning process to facilitate the tasks of the public health workforce across Canada. As a result, core competencies for public health workers were developed and launched in 2007 across Canada. In 2009, public health nursing discipline-specific core competencies (Version 1.0) that apply to all public health nurses across Canada were released.

The community health nursing profession is currently receiving a lot of attention. This mounting interest may be a result of recent major public health events such as SARS, avian flu, listeriosis, and the H1N1 outbreak; the creation in 2004 of the Public Health Agency of Canada with the appointment of a chief medical officer of health; and the visibility of the Community Health Nurses Association. Additionally, increased chronic illness and an aging population with increased demands for home health nursing care, along with the emphasis on population health and the social determinants of health, have contributed to the stronger focus on community health care. Villeneuve and MacDonald (2006), in their report titled *Toward 2020: Visions for Nursing* (see the Evolve Weblinks), predict that by the year 2020 most of health care, including nursing care, will take place in the client's home or in the community on an outpatient basis. This vision is supported by the use of advanced technology and the enhancement of resources to better support families to care for the client at home. Interdisciplinary care teams will become increasingly essential and will put a greater focus on primary services and preventive programs.

In 1993, the CNA wrote a policy statement on health information to highlight the unique contribution that nurses make to the health of Canadians and the importance of capturing essential nursing information that will inform educators, researchers, policymakers, governments, and clients about nursing's role in a changing health care system (CNA, 1993). Since that time, nursing informatics has been implemented in health care agencies to assist nurses to process the enormous volume of information required to work with clients. This enhanced process of organizing health information facilitates an environment for improved and faster health assessment and interventions to address client health care concerns and challenges.

Today, CHNs look to their history for inspiration, explanation, and prediction. For a pictorial and descriptive review of some of the historical community health nursing positions held across Canada, refer to the B.C. History of Nursing Group Weblink on the Evolve Web site. Information and advocacy are used to promote a comprehensive approach to addressing the multiple needs of the diverse populations served. CHNs seek to learn from the past and to avoid known pitfalls as they search for successful strategies to meet the complex needs of today's populations. As plans for the future are made and as unmet public health challenges are acknowledged, the vision of what nurses in community health can accomplish serves as a sustaining force.

CRITICAL VIEW

1. What changes do you think will occur in the practice of community health nursing during your nursing career?
2. What changes do you think will occur in the practice of community health nursing in reference to nursing informatics?

STUDENT EXPERIENCE

1. What do you know about the history of community health nursing in your province or territory?
2. Add to your knowledge about community health nursing in your province or territory by accessing the University of Ottawa Bibliography: Canadian Nursing History Web site: http://www.health.uottawa.ca/nursinghistory/nhru_biblio.htm.
3. Which aspects of your review of the history of community health nursing have been essential in the development of community health nursing practice in your province or territory? Which experience or situation did you relate to the most? Explain.
4. Who were the community health nursing leaders in your province or territory? Who are currently the leaders in your province or territory? What are some of the commonalities and differences between past and current leaders?

REMEMBER THIS!

- A historical approach can be used to increase understanding of community health nursing in the past, as well as its current and future challenges.
- Community health nursing is a product of social, economic, and political forces and incorporates public health science as well as nursing science and practice.
- Florence Nightingale designed and implemented the first program for training nurses, and her contemporary, William Rathbone, founded the first district nursing association in England.
- Increasing acceptance of public roles for women permitted community health nursing employment for nurses, as well as public leadership roles for their wealthy supporters.
- Lillian Wald, a public health nurse in the United States, played a key role in innovations that shaped public health and community health nursing in its first decades, including school nursing, insurance payments for nursing care, and national organization for public health nurses.
- The Canadian Metropolitan Life Insurance Company, in the 1920s, began a visiting home nursing service for policy holders.
- Eunice Dyke, a public health nursing pioneer in Canada in the early 1900s, played a key role in shaping public health nursing in Canada.
- In the 1920s, the concept of outpost nursing gained momentum, partly due to more PHNs choosing to work in that field.
- The Weir Report of 1932 moved nursing education forward and also addressed several areas related to public health nursing practice.
- In the 1950s and 1960s, public health nursing practice moved from specialized nursing services to generalized nursing services.
- In the late 1960s, Dalhousie University in Nova Scotia offered the first program to educate nurses to work in northern nursing stations as nurse practitioners.
- Industrial nursing practice became known as occupational health nursing practice in 1982. The Canadian Occupational Health Association, in 1984, established the standards of practice for occupational health nurses.
- In 1987, the CHNAC was formed.
- Primary health care nurse practitioner programs were established in most provinces across Canada in the 1990s.
- In 2003, the CHNAC published the *Canadian Community Health Nursing Standards of Practice.*
- In 2004, the Public Health Agency of Canada was developed, and a chief medical officer of health was appointed.
- In 2006, the first community health nursing certification examination was written based on the core competencies for community health nursing.
- In 2006, the core competencies for the public health workforce were launched.
- In 2008, the core competencies for public health nurses in Canada were launched.
- In 2009, the Community Health Nurses Association of Canada changed its name to the Community Health Nurses of Canada.

REFLECTIVE PRAXIS

What Would You Do?

Retrieve the Romanow Report (Romanow, 2002) from the Web site listed in the Weblinks. Complete the following activities and reflect on and respond to the questions below. For many of the questions, you are directed to specific chapters in the report. Record your findings.

1. How does the Romanow Report define *sustainability*?
2. Based on the chapter titled "Primary Health Care and Prevention" (Chapter 5):
   a. What are the opportunities and obstacles related to primary health care?
   b. What are the three recommendations related to prevention?
   c. What is your reflection on these three recommendations in reference to your community? Be sure to consider what exists now and what would be needed to meet these three recommendations.

3. Based on the chapter titled "Rural and Remote Communities" (Chapter 7):
   a. How is *rural* defined?
   b. What are the issues in relation to the disparities between rural and remote communities?
   c. How can rural access to health care be improved?
4. Based on the chapter titled "A New Approach to Aboriginal Health" (Chapter 10):
   a. What federal health programs are available to Aboriginal peoples?
   b. What are the health issues among Aboriginal peoples?
   c. What are the health-related disparities faced by Aboriginal peoples?
5. Select a topic area that is significant to you in the development of community health nursing. Find one refereed article from a nursing journal that further discusses the historical considerations pertaining to your chosen area. Summarize the article and present it to your class.

WEBLINKS

evolve

Direct links to these resources can be found on the text's accompanying Evolve Web site at http://evolve.elsevier.com/Canada/Stanhope/community.

Aboriginal Nurses Association of Canada. *Thirty Years of Community.* This document, available at the ANAC Web site, provides information on the history of the Aboriginal Nurses Association of Canada. This group of professional nurses advocates for capacity building for health for First Nations.

British Columbia History of Nursing Group: Memorial Nursing Portrait Collection. This site provides the reader with the opportunity to experience Canadian nursing in past decades. The use of a variety of costume portrait dolls and personal reflections about these nurses captivate the reader.

Canadian Association for the History of Nursing. This Web site is an affiliate of the CNA Web site to promote and preserve historical nursing materials. Links to other sites that provide historical nursing data are also provided.

Canadian Museum of Civilization. *Symbol of a Profession: One Hundred Years of Nurses' Caps.* This document provides information on symbolism in nursing and why some symbols, such as the nursing cap, have become obsolete. It also provides access to sites that offer an excellent history of nursing in Canada with photographs of various artifacts.

Canadian Nurses Association Position Statement: *The Value of Nursing History Today.* The CNA believes learning from nursing history is critical to advancing the profession in the interests of the Canadian public.

Public Health Agency of Canada. *Building the Public Health Workforce for the 21st Century: A Pan-Canadian Framework for Public Health Human Resources Planning.* This document discusses the collaborative planning needed to improve the public health workforce environment. The framework provided illustrates the building blocks needed to strengthen the public health workforce and includes development of core competencies for public health workers.

Public Health Research, Education & Development (PHRED). *Building Public Health Research, Education & Development in Canada: A Five Site Consultation.* This document provides background into the development of the Ontario PHRED public health program and reviews it as a model to possibly be adopted by other provinces.

Romanow, R. J. *Building on Values: The Future of Health Care in Canada.* This document is the complete Romanow Report in pdf format.

Statistics Canada. *Factors Related to On-the-Job Abuse of Nurses by Patients.* This report provides information about abuse of nurses by patients.

Villeneuve, M., & MacDonald, J. *Toward 2020: Visions for Nursing.* This report, published by the CNA, discusses health care in the year 2020; what the health care system will look like then; and what role nurses and nursing will play in this system to effect positive health care changes.

REFERENCES

Abrams, S. E. (2009). The public health nursing bag as tool and symbol. *Public Health Nursing*, *26*(1), 106–109.

Allemang, M. M. (2000). Development of community health nursing in Canada. In M. J. Stewart (Ed.), *Community nursing: Promoting Canadians' health* (pp. 4–32). Saunders: Toronto, ON.

Buhler-Wilkerson, K. (1993). Public health then and now. Bringing care to the people: Lillian Wald's legacy to public health nursing. *American Journal of Public Health*, *83*(12), 1778–1786.

Cadotte, M. (2006). Epidemic. *The Canadian encyclopedia*. Retrieved from http://www.thecanadianencyclopedia.com/index.cfm?PgNm = TCE&Params = A1ARTA0002629.

Canadian Institute for Health Information (CIHI). (2005). *CIHI update. Home care reporting system*. Retrieved from http://secure.cihi.ca/cihiweb/en/downloads/HOME_CAREupdateNOV05_webENG.pdf.

Canadian Museum of Civilization Corporation. (2004). A brief history of nursing in Canada from the establishment of New France to the present. *Canadian Nursing History Collection Online*. Retrieved from http://www.civilization.ca/tresors/nursing/nchis01e.html.

Canadian Nurses Association. (1968). *The leaf and the lamp*. Ottawa, ON: Author.

Canadian Nurses Association. (1993). *CNA policy statement on Health Information: Nursing Components*. Ottawa, ON: Author.

Canadian Nurses Association. (2006). *CNA awards*. Retrieved from http://cna-aiic.ca/CNA/news/awards/jeannemance/default_e.aspx.

Canadian Occupational Health Nurses Association. (2003). *Occupational health nursing practice standards*. Retrieved from http://www.cohna-aciist.ca/pages/content.asp?CatID = 3&CatSubID = 5.

Canadian Public Health Association. (2009). *About CPHA*. Retrieved from http://www.cpha.ca/en/about.aspx.

Cohen, I. B. (1984). Florence Nightingale. *Scientific American*, *3*, 128–137.

Community Health Nurses Association of Canada. (2003). *Canadian community health nursing standards*. Retrieved from http://www.chnac.ca/index.php?option = com_content&task = view&id = 20&Itemid = 38/.

Dodd, D., Elliott, J., & Rousseau, N. (2005). Outpost nursing in Canada. In C. Bates, D. Dodd, & N. Rousseau (Eds.), *On all frontiers: Four centuries of Canadian nursing* (pp. 139–152). Ottawa, ON: University of Ottawa Press.

Duncan, S. M., Leipert, B. D., & Mill, J. E. (1999). Nurses as health evangelists: The evolution of public health nursing in Canada, 1918–1939. *Advances in Nursing Science*, *22*(1), 40–51.

Epp, J. (1986). *Achieving health for all: A framework for health promotion*. Ottawa, ON: Ministry of Supply & Services.

Frachel, R. R. (1988). A new profession: The evolution of public health nursing. *Public Health Nursing*, *5*(2), 86–90.

Glenbow Museum. (2009). *Archives finding AIDS*. Retrieved from http://www.glenbow.org/collections/search/findingAids/archhtm/colley.cfm.

Green, M. (1984). *Through the years with public health nursing: A history of public health nursing in the provincial government jurisdiction of British Columbia*. Ottawa, ON: Canadian Public Health Association.

Hamilton, D. (1992). Research and reform: Community nursing and the Framingham tuberculosis project, 1914–1923. *Nursing Research*, *41*(1), 8–13.

Hardill, K. (2007). From the Grey Nuns to the streets: A critical history of outreach nursing in Canada. *Public Health Nursing*, *24*(1), 91–97.

Harper-Femson, L. A. (1998). *Nurse practitioners' role satisfaction*. Doctoral thesis, University of Toronto. Retrieved from http://www.collectionscanada.ca/obj/s4/f2/dsk2/tape17/PQDD_0012/NQ35403.pdf.

Health Canada. (2007). *The working conditions of nurses: Confronting the challenges*. Retrieved from http://www.hc-sc.gc.ca/sr-sr/pubs/hpr-rpms/bull/2007-nurses-infirmieres/4_e.html.

Hebert, R., Dubuc, N., Buteau, M., Desrosiers, J., Bravo, G., Trottier, L., & Roy, C. (2001). Resources and costs associated with disabilities of elderly people living at home and in institutions. *Canadian Journal on Aging*, *20*(1), 1–22.

Hollander, M. J. (2001). *Final report of the study on the comparative cost analysis of home care and residential care services. University of Victoria: Centre on Aging*. Retrieved from http://www.homecarestudy.com/reports/full-text/substudy-01-final_report.pdf.

Jan, R. (1996). Rufaida Al-Asalmiya, the first Muslim nurse. *Image*, *28*(3), 267–268.

Kalisch, P. A., & Kalisch, B. J. (1995). *The advance of American nursing* (3rd ed.). Philadelphia, PA: Lippincott.

Keddy, B., & Dodd, D. (2005). The trained nurse: Private duty and VON home nursing (late 1800s to 1940s). In C. Bates, D. Dodd, & N. Rousseau (Eds.), *On all frontiers: Four centuries of Canadian nursing* (pp. 43–56). Ottawa, ON: University of Ottawa Press.

King, M., Harrison, M. J., & Reutter, L. I. (1995). Public health nursing or community health nursing: What's in a name? In M. J. Stewart (Ed.), *Community nursing: Promoting Canadians' health* (pp. 400–412). Toronto, ON: W. B. Saunders.

Lalonde, M. (1974). *New perspective on the health of Canadians*. Ottawa, ON: Government of Canada.

MacDougall, H. (2009). "Truly alarming": Cholera in 1832. *Canadian Journal of Public Health*, *100*(5), 333–336.

MacQueen, J. M. (1997). *Public health nursing in Sudbury, 1920–1956 (Master's thesis)*. Sudbury, ON: Laurentian University.

Mansell, D. (2003). *Forging the future: A history of nursing in Canada*. Ann Arbor, MI: Thomas Press.

McKay, M. (2005). Public health nursing. In C. Bates, D. Dodd, & N. Rousseau (Eds.), *On all frontiers: Four centuries of Canadian nursing*. Ottawa, ON: University of Ottawa Press.

McKay, M. (2008). Community health nursing in Canada. In L. L. Stamler & L. Yiu (Eds.), *Community health nursing: A Canadian perspective* (2nd ed., pp. 1–19). Toronto, ON: Pearson Education Canada.

Mount Saint Vincent University Archives. (2005). *Nursing history digitization project: Nursing education in Nova Scotia*. Retrieved from http://www.msvu.ca/library/archives/nhdp/history/opportunities.htm.

Nightingale, F. (1894). Sick nursing and health nursing. In J. S. Billings & H. M. Hurd (Eds.), *Hospitals, dispensaries, and nursing*. Baltimore, MD: Johns Hopkins Press. (Reprinted New York: Garland Publishing, 1984.)

Nightingale, F. (1946). *Notes on nursing: What it is, and what it is not*. Philadelphia, PA: Lippincott.

Nutting, M. A., & Dock, L. L. (1935). *A history of nursing*. New York, NY: GP Putnam's Sons.

Palmer, I. S. (1983). *Florence Nightingale and the first organized delivery of nursing services*. Washington, DC: American Association of Colleges of Nursing.

Pellegrino, E. D. (1963). Medicine, history, and the idea of man. *Annals of the American Academy of Political and Social Sciences*, *346*, 9–20.

Potter, P. A., Perry, A. G., Ross-Kerr, J. C., & Wood, M. J. (2006). *Canadian fundamentals of nursing* (3rd ed.). Toronto, ON: Elsevier.

Pringle, D. M., & Roe, D. I. (1992). Voluntary community agencies: VON Canada as example. In A. J. Baumgart, & J. Larsen (Eds.), *Canadian nursing faces the future* (2nd ed., pp. 611–626). St. Louis, MO: Mosby.

Public Health Agency of Canada. (2005a). *How healthy are Canadians?* Retrieved from http://www.phac-aspc.gc.ca/ph-sp/phdd/report/toward/back/how.html.

Public Health Agency of Canada. (2005b). *Building the public health workforce for the 21st century: A pan-Canadian framework for public health human resources planning*. Retrieved from http://www.phac-aspc.gc.ca/php-psp/pdf/building_the_public_health_workforce_fo_%20the-21stc_e.pdf.

Public Health Research, Education & Development (PHRED). (2002). *Building public health research, education & development in Canada: A five site consultation*. Retrieved from http://www.phac-aspc.gc.ca/php-psp/pdf/building_public_health_research_eduction_and_development_in_canada_e.pdf.

Romanow, R. J. (2002). *Building on values: The future of health care in Canada*. Retrieved from http://www.collectionscanada.gc.ca/webarchives/20071122004429/http://www.hc-sc.gc.ca/english/pdf/romanow/pdfs/hcc_final_report.pdf.

Rosen, G. (1958). *A history of public health*. New York, NY: MD Publications.

Ross-Kerr, J. C. (2006). The growth of community health nursing in Canada. In J. C. Ross-Kerr & J. MacPhail (Eds.), *An introduction to issues in community health nursing in Canada* (pp. 34–50). Toronto, ON: Mosby.

Ross-Kerr, J. C. (2009). The development of nursing practice in Canada. In P. A. Potter, A. G. Perry, J. C. Ross-Kerr, & M. J. Wood (Eds.), *Canadian fundamentals of nursing* (4th ed., pp. 28–40). Toronto, ON: Mosby Elsevier.

Ross-Kerr, J. C., & Wood, M. J. (2003). *Canadian nursing: Issues and perspectives* (4th ed.). Toronto, ON: Mosby.

Royce, M. (1983). *Eunice Dyke: Health care pioneer*. Toronto, ON: Dundurn Press Limited.

Shah, C. P. (2003). *Public health and preventive medicine in Canada* (5th ed.). Toronto, ON: Saunders.

Spitzer, W. O., Sackett, D. L., Sibley, C., Roberts, R. S., Gent, M., Kergin, D. J., et al. (1974). The Burlington randomized trial of the nurse practitioner. *New England Journal of Medicine*, *290*(5), 251–256.

Stewart, I. (1979). *These were our yesterdays: A history of district nursing in Alberta*. Altona, MN: D. W. Friesen and Sons.

Toth, A., Fackelmann, J., Pigott, W., & Tolomeo, O. (2004). Tuberculosis prevention and treatment: Occupational health, infection control, public health, general duty staff, visiting, parish nursing or working in a physician's office—all nursing roles are key to improving tuberculosis control. *Canadian Nurse*, *100*(9), 27–32.

Underwood, J. M., Mowat, D. L., Meagher-Stewart, D. M., Deber, R. B., Baumann, A. O., MacDonald, M. B., & Munroe, V. (2009). Building community and public health nursing capacity: A synthesis report of the national community health nursing study. *Canadian Journal of Public Health*, *100*(5), I-1–13.

Villeneuve, M., & MacDonald, J. (2006). *Toward 2020: Visions for nursing*. Ottawa, ON: Canadian Nursing Association. Retrieved from http://www.cna-aiic.ca/CNA/documents/pdf/publications/Toward-2020-e.pdf.

Vollman, A. R., Anderson, E. T., & McFarlane, J. (2004). *Canadian community as partner*. Philadelphia, PA: Lippincott Williams & Wilkins.

Weir, G. M. (1932). *Survey of nursing education in Canada*. Toronto, ON: University of Toronto Press.

Worster, A., Sarco, A., Thrasher, C., Fernandes, C., & Chemeria, E. (2005). Understanding the role of nurse practitioners in Canada. *Canadian Journal of Rural Medicine*, *10*(2), 89–94.

CHAPTER 3

Community Health Nursing in Canada: Settings, Functions, and Roles

KEY TERMS

See Glossary on page 593 for definitions.

OBJECTIVES

After reading this chapter, you should be able to:

1. Identify the various types of community health nurses.
2. Describe the various settings in which community health nurses work.
3. Examine the role and scope of practice for community health nurses.
4. Develop an awareness of community health nurses' role in health promotion and disease prevention.
5. Discuss the educational requirements for the various types of community health nurses.
6. Describe examples of work-related illnesses and injuries.
7. Use the epidemiological model to explain work–health interactions.
8. Explain one example each of biological, chemical, environmental or mechanical, physical, and psychosocial workplace hazards.
9. Develop an awareness of other community health nursing specialties.
10. Define *rural* and contrast it with the definition of *urban*.
11. Discuss issues related to delivery of services for rural underserved populations.
12. Define *case management*.
13. Describe a case manager's roles and activities.
14. Explain the principles and steps of the referral process.
15. Explain discharge planning in relation to providing continuity of care.

CHAPTER OUTLINE

The Canadian authors thank Nancy Horan for her contribution of the material regarding sexual assault nurse examiners and Victoria Morley for her contribution to the discussion on public health nursing.

The main types of community health nurses (CHNs) covered in this chapter, presented alphabetically, are home health nurses (HHNs), occupational health nurses (OHNs), parish nurses, and public health nurses (PHNs). Other CHNs include corrections nurses, forensic nurses, nurse entrepreneurs, outpost nurses, primary health care nurse practitioners, street or outreach nurses, and telenurses. The major functions and roles assumed by CHNs in Canada are discussed, as is case management as a method of care delivery in the community. Finally, discharge planning and the referral process are explored.

Underwood et al. (2009) reported on the 2007 demographic profile of Canadian community health nurses. Some of their findings are presented in Table 3-1. These authors reported that, of the total number of nurses working in Canada, approximately 16.3%, or 53,404, were employed as CHNs. These CHNs included registered nurses (RNs), nurse practitioners (NPs), and licensed practical nurses (LPNs). The percentage of community RNs (28%) over 55 years of age was slightly higher than that of all other RNs (22%). The largest number of LPNs working in community health nursing were employed in Alberta and Nova Scotia.

TABLE 3-1 Canadian Community Health Nurses Work Settings Profile for 2007

Settings	Registered Nurses	Licensed Practical Nurses	Total Percentages
Community health centre	27,299	2,331	55.5
Home care agency	7,635	2,288	18.6
Nursing station	1,090	46	2.1
Business/ industry	2,615	333	5.5
Private nursing agency	335	92	0.8
Self-employed	316	120	0.8
Physicians' office	5,150	1,785	13.0
Educational institution	205	13	0.4
Association/ government	749	24	1.4
Other	879	99	1.8
Total	46,273	7,131	100

SOURCE: Underwood J. et al. (2009). *Demographic profile of community health nurses in Canada: 1996–2007* (pp. 19, 31, 32) Hamilton, ON: McMaster University School of Nursing and Nursing Health Services Research Unit. Retrieved from http://www.nhsru.com/documents/Series%2013%20McMaster_Demographic_Profile_of_Community.pdf.

As discussed in Chapter 1, most community health nurses work in primary health care; however, not all CHNs work intensely in the area of community development and planning, and not all use a population-based focus. Some CHNs focus mainly on the individual and family as clients. In community health nursing, the practice settings also vary, but there is some consistency in roles and functions. Currently, the standards of practice for all CHNs are the *Canadian Community Health Nursing Standards of Practice* identified by the Canadian Community Health Nurses Association of Canada (2008). These were initially published in 2003 and updated in 2008 and are presented in Appendix 1. These standards are discussed throughout this text. Prior to the establishment of these standards of practice, the Canadian Public Health Association published *Community Health—Public Health Nursing in Canada: Preparation and Practice* (Canadian Public Health Association, 1990). For many years, this publication defined the activities of public health nurses (PHNs) and outlined their roles, functions, qualifications, and responsibilities. At that time, the emphasis in community health nursing care was on a needs approach, and the umbrella term *community health nurse* was not used. Therefore, there were PHNs and visiting nurses from agencies such as the Victorian Order of Nurses (VON) and Saint Elizabeth Health Care Nurses. Some parts of the current Canadian community health nursing standards of practice are an expansion of the roles and activities outlined in the 1990 Canadian Public Health Association publication, and some community health nursing specialties have developed, or are in the process of developing, their own specific competencies with certification through the Canadian Nurses Association (CNA). Competencies describe the activities that a nurse engages in to meet a standard or set of standards (see the CNA Web site in the Evolve Weblinks listed at the end of this chapter). **Certification** is a mechanism that provides an indication, usually by means of written examination, of professional competence in a specialized area of practice.

THE HOME HEALTH NURSE

Home health care is the most rapidly expanding health care field (Canadian Home Care Association, 2008; Day, Paul, Williams, Smeltzer, & Bare, 2007). Within community health nursing, home health nursing is an important nursing specialty, of which hospice nursing is considered a specialty. Home health providers such as home health nurses (HHNs) and homemakers usually practise in the client's home environment, although this is not always the case, as demonstrated in the "Ethical Considerations" box below. Traditionally, HHNs are RNs who work in the community and who usually provide direct nursing care in the client's home. For more than two centuries, nurses have provided in-home nursing care. In Canada, the VON has provided care to the sick for more than 100 years, often focusing their nursing care and services on teaching, disease prevention, and maternal care (VON, 2006). Refer to the VON Web sites listed in the Weblinks for further information on this traditional Canadian home health nursing agency and home health nursing practice and for stories of how VON volunteers have affected the lives of clients.

Home health nurses function as generalists, incorporating knowledge specialization and skills in areas such as home chemotherapy, enterostomal therapy, mental health, and continence management (VON, 2006). Across Canada, privately operated home health nursing agencies have emerged, and new agencies continue to emerge to meet the demand for home health nursing due to shortened hospital stays. Saint Elizabeth Health Care, a Canadian not-for-profit organization, was established more than 100 years ago and continues to provide home and community health care in settings across Ontario (Saint Elizabeth Health Care, 2009). Bayshore Home Health, established in 1966, identifies itself as Canada's largest provider of home and community health care services, with more than 40 locations across most of the provinces (Bayshore Home Health, 2007). For information about home care in Canada, refer to the Canadian Home Care Association Web site listed in the Weblinks.

Home care offers clients the benefits of familiarity and being surrounded by family, friends, and pets in a setting that is interactional and conducive to expressions of caring and concern. At home, clients have an increased array of choices of food, treatments, medication schedules, and interactions with family and friends, empowering them and leading to a feeling of security and well-being.

When working in a client's home, the CHN is a guest (Fox, Munro, & Brien, 2006) and, to be effective, must earn the trust of the family. In this setting, CHNs have the opportunity to observe family life (a privilege usually reserved for family and friends), including family dynamics, lifestyle choices, communication patterns, coping strategies, responses to health and illness, and the presence of social, cultural, spiritual, and economic issues.

Some of the challenges of home care nursing include meeting the privacy needs of the client and family and adapting as necessary to the family's lifestyle. Some families may view having CHNs, or professional caregivers, in the home as an intrusion of privacy that disrupts the normal daily routine. Families may also have to make spatial adjustments in their home because of durable medical equipment needs. CHNs in the home setting practise autonomously with little structure (Fox, Munro, & Brien, 2006).

ETHICAL CONSIDERATIONS

A home health nurse (HHN) works with Sam, an 11-year-old client, in an elementary school setting, where he requires periodic specialized feeding and monitoring of medication. His teacher asks why he needs all this attention and suggests that Sam be home-schooled or sent to a private institution to avoid disruptions to the class. Sam's mother, a lone parent who works in a low-paying job, is unable to afford such options.

The following ethical principles apply to the above scenario (see Box 6-2 on p. 168 for a more detailed discussion of ethical principles):

- *Respect for autonomy*. This principle requires that individuals be permitted to choose those actions and goals that fulfill their life plans, unless those choices result in harm to another. In this case, Sam and his mother have made the choice for Sam to attend school where he can receive appropriate educational opportunities and some professional health care support without the risk of harm to others.
- *Distributive justice*. This principle requires a fair distribution of the burdens and benefits of society within the limits imposed by its resources. In this case, the family cannot afford to access other options, and to attempt to would cause an undue burden on them and would be an unreasonable expectation when the school option is available.
- *Preserving dignity* (CNA Code of Ethics). Preserving client dignity is a primary ethical value for CHNs. Integrating Sam into the classroom environment, where he has the opportunity for peer interaction, rather than confining him to his home enhances his dignity.

Question to Consider

1. What is the CHN's ethical responsibility in advocating for Sam?

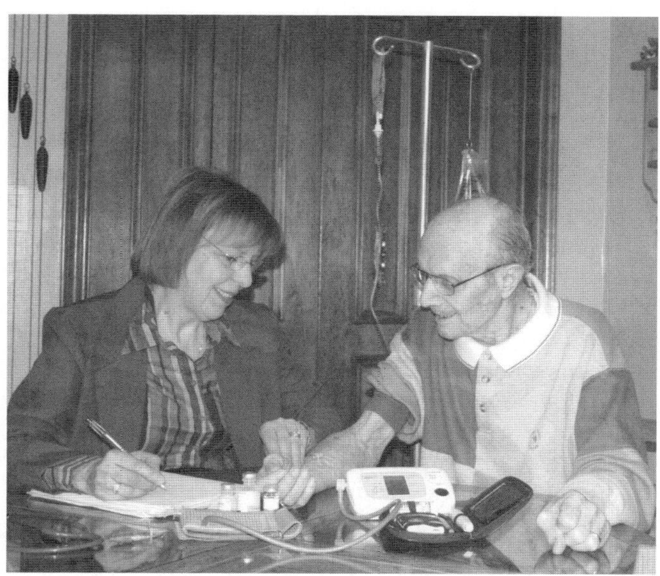

Home health care nurses may provide a variety of services, including assessing a client's response to treatment, reporting their findings to the client's physician, and helping to modify the client's treatment plan as needed.

The home environment lacks many resources typically found in health care institutions, so CHNs need to have good organizational skills, be adaptable to different settings, and demonstrate interpersonal savvy for working with the diverse needs of clients in their homes.

Home health care continues to expand in response to the following:

- Increased demands for cost-effectiveness
- Shorter hospital stays
- Consumer preferences
- Technological advances such as personal-digital-assistant software
- Proven quality of service
- Aging Canadian demographics

Definitions in Home Health Nursing

Home health nursing in today's society cannot be defined simply as "care at home." Home health nursing includes an arrangement of disease prevention, health promotion, and episodic illness-related services provided to people in their places of residence. Home health nurses have the same primary preventive focus of care of aggregates, as all CHNs have. Home health nursing also involves the secondary and tertiary prevention focuses of care of individuals in collaboration with the family and other caregivers.

HHNs usually work with the family in providing care to an individual client. *Family* is defined individually and includes any caregiver or significant person who assists the client in need of care at home. **Family caregiving** by HHNs includes assisting clients to meet their basic needs and providing direct care such as personal hygiene, meal preparation, medication administration, and treatments. The caregiver is essential in providing the needed maintenance care between the skilled visits of the professional health care provider. The in-home care provided today by caregivers was historically offered only in the hospital by a health care provider.

Each client's place of residence has its own uniqueness for providing care and depends on what the person calls home. Home may be a house, apartment, trailer, boarding home, care home, shelter, vehicle, makeshift shelter under a bridge, or cardboard box.

Client goals are always related to the principles of health promotion, maintenance, and restoration. By maximizing a client's level of independence, HHNs help clients function at their highest possible level and prevent their dependence on others. To achieve this, HHNs do the following:

- Provide a combination of direct care and health education
- Enhance self-care skills
- Link the client with community services that provide limited assistance to enable the client to stay at home
- Work to prevent complications in chronically ill persons
- Help to minimize the effects of disability and illness

Practice Settings for Home Health Nursing

The practice setting for home health nursing is usually the client's home, but whenever a client requires direct nursing care, the home health nurse visits the client in his or her current setting, possibly a school, a shelter, a group residence, or the street (Community Health Nurses' Initiatives Group of the Registered Nurses' Association of Ontario, 2004). The client population that home health nurses work with is changing. Formerly, most home care clients were older adults; however, younger clients now also present with myriad health care challenges, often a result of the social determinants of health. Some of the experiences of home health nurses who work with younger clients in Vancouver's Downtown Eastside are captured in a document authored by Giles and Brennan titled *Action-Based Care in Vancouver's DTES* (see the Evolve Weblinks).

Functions and Roles of Home Health Nurses

Home health nurses aim to help prevent the occurrence of illness and to promote the client's well-being. In the home care setting, clients possess more control and determine their own health care needs. The effectiveness of service depends on the client's active involvement in and understanding of plans established jointly by the client and the HHN. The HHN facilitates the development of positive health behaviours for the individual who has had an episode of illness.

A common misconception of home health nursing is that it is a "custodial" type of nursing; however, it is important to remember that home health nursing composes part of community health nursing. Thus, health promotion and disease prevention activities are fundamental components of practice.

Because home health care is often intermittent, a primary objective for the HHN is to facilitate self-care. According to Orem (1995), "*Self-care* is the practice of activities that individuals initiate and perform on their own behalf in maintaining life, health, and well-being" (p. 104). HHNs use this self-care concept for all clients, regardless of the clients' abilities. For example, a client recuperating at home after suffering a cerebrovascular accident (CVA) may be unable to perform activities of daily living without assistance. Such clients can be taught to perform these activities in a modified form. They can thereby regain some control over their life and self-care activities and prevent possible losses in other self-care areas.

Contracting, or establishment of an agreement between two or more parties, is a vital component of all nurse–client relationships. Constantly evolving legislative guidelines, requirements of third-party payers, the high risk of liability, and the level of HHN autonomy make contracts a necessity in the home care environment. Contracting is further discussed in Chapter 12.

LEVELS OF PREVENTION
Related to Home Health Nursing

PRIMARY PREVENTION

The home health nurse visits diabetic clients at home to provide foot care and education on how to care for their feet to prevent infections and foot ulcers.

SECONDARY PREVENTION

The home health nurse provides dietary counselling and education on insulin injections to a newly diagnosed diabetic client and his family.

TERTIARY PREVENTION

The home health nurse provides direct care services to a client who has experienced a cerebrovascular accident to avoid complications.

The process of contracting in-home care involves the client, as individual, and as family, and the home health nurse. **Contracting**, which is the making of a continuously negotiable agreement between two or more parties, involves a shift in responsibility and control toward a shared effort by the client and professional as opposed to an effort by the professional alone. The contract is included in the client's care plan and clinical, notes. Contracting allows the individual, family, and HHN to set mutual goals and facilitates the effectiveness of nursing care and the promotion of self-care.

As an example, during an initial home visit, the HHN gathers data and determines an action plan for care by establishing a contract with the individual and family. Contracts can be formal (written) or informal (verbal), depending on the client's needs. In either case, the HHN records the terms of the contract in the client's chart. The most important aspect of contracting is the client's active participation in developing, implementing, and evaluating the care process within the realm of the contract. To avoid what is often referred to as the "home visit ritual"—visits that have no predetermined goal or outcome—the HHN must establish both short-term and long-term goals with individuals and families. The goals provide for continuity of care and state the criteria for evaluating the client's condition and progress toward an optimum level of self-care.

Home health nursing involves both *direct* and *indirect* functions. In performing these functions, the home health nurse assumes a variety of roles, including that of coordinator of care as part of an interdisciplinary team. *Direct care* refers to the actual physical aspects of nursing care—that is, anything requiring physical contact and face-to-face interaction. By serving as a role model, the HHN facilitates the individual and family development of positive health behaviours.

The HHN needs to be knowledgeable and fully comprehend and apply the agency policies and also be a competent and experienced clinician. *Direct care* activities include the following:

- Observing and evaluating a client's health status and condition
- Administering direct care such as rehabilitative exercises, medications, catheter insertion, colostomy irrigation, and wound care
- Helping the individual and family develop positive coping behaviours
- Educating the individual and family to give treatments and medications how and when indicated
- Educating the individual and family to carry out physicians' orders such as treatments, therapeutic diets, or medication administration

- Reporting to the client's physician changes in the client's condition and arranging for medical follow-up as indicated
- Helping the individual and family identify resources that will help the client attain a state of optimal functioning

Indirect care activities are those that an HHN does on behalf of clients to improve or coordinate care. These activities usually include the following:

- Consulting with other nurses and health care providers
- Organizing and participating in client care conferences
- Advocating for clients within the health care system
- Obtaining results of diagnostic tests
- Documenting care

Home health nursing is interdisciplinary care, and an essential indirect function of the HHN is **care coordination** of an interdisciplinary health care team. The HHN will organize team conferences, which offer an ideal opportunity for increasing coordination and continuity of services for optimal client care and use of resources and services. For example, the HHN will present to the team clients with complex conditions or those with inadequate support in the home; this sharing of information invites joint care planning and problem solving. **Care planning** refers to the HHN, clients, and interdisciplinary team members working together to ensure adequate health care service at home. For example, the HHN and clients may discuss the possible need for resources such as a home care support worker, special equipment to facilitate client mobility, or the involvement of community agencies such as Meals on Wheels, and the HHN, along with the interdisciplinary team, organizes for the delivery of the required resources.

Depending on education and experience, the HHN may engage in the roles of clinician or direct care provider, educator, researcher, manager, referral agent, consultant in home health care, or a combination of any of these. Home health nurses as *clinicians* or *direct care providers* provide direct nursing care to individuals and families. They are *educators* because they educate individuals and families on the "how" and "why" of self-care; they may also provide health education classes to community groups. As well, home health nurses participate in the ongoing education of their colleagues as mentors, both formally, providing in-service education, and informally, as team members. The shortening of hospital stays and the trend toward in-home palliative care have contributed to a growth in importance of the *researcher* role in home health nursing. Potential research areas abound in the home health care setting, and to maintain quality and cost-effectiveness of care, research must remain a priority in the future. As *consultants*, HHNs may provide advice and counsel to clients and others, such as health care providers.

The development of hospice palliative care programs has improved the quality of care for terminally ill persons. **Palliative care** is holistic caring (i.e., physical, psychosocial, and spiritual support), which may include end-of-life care for those facing life-threatening illnesses and for the dying (and their families) so that they experience quality of life through symptom management and supportive care (Canadian Hospice Palliative Care Association [CHPCA], 2002; Harlos, 2009; Public Health Agency of Canada, 2006; World Health Organization [WHO], 2009). Estimates suggest that approximately 62% of the more than 259,000 Canadians who die each year access hospice palliative care services at the end of life (CHPCA, 2007). In Canada, access to hospice palliative care has been challenged because of issues such as health care restructuring and resultant limited service availability; accessibility, especially for those living in remote and rural areas and for persons with severe disabilities; the preference of many Canadians to die at home; inadequate government funding, which places additional burden on family and informal caregivers; inadequate physician education on palliative care pain management; and underfunding for education of other health disciplines such as nursing and social work (CHPCA, 2007). Hospice palliative care can be delivered in-home, in a specially designated palliative care unit in a hospital, or in a hospice facility. **Hospice** is a designated place where hospice care is provided. **Hospice care** refers to the delivery of palliative care of the very ill and dying, offering both respite and comfort. If the individual and family agree, hospice care can be comfortably delivered at home with family involvement under the direction and supervision of health care professionals, especially a home health nurse. The Canadian Hospice Palliative Care Association (CHPCA), in 2006, published *The Pan-Canadian Gold Standards for Palliative and End-of-Life Care at Home*. These standards were developed in partnership with the CHPCA and the Canadian Home Care Association, based on expert input from various health professionals, with the goal of ensuring that all Canadians will have equitable access to the highest possible quality end-of-life care in reference to case management, nursing, palliative-specific pharmaceuticals, and personal care at the end of life (CHPCA, 2006; CHPCA, 2007). Hospice care may be provided in a designated palliative care unit or in a hospice facility when a client experiences severe complications of terminal illness or when the family becomes too exhausted to care for the client in the home.

Canadian Hospice Palliative Care Nursing, or CHPCN(C), is one of the areas of nursing practice that has certification status through the CNA (CNA, 2010). This nursing specialization requires specific cognitive, psychomotor, and affective skills. Box 3-1 lists the hospice palliative care nurse competency categories. Palliative care nursing competencies that

BOX 3-1 The Hospice Palliative Care Nurse Competency Categories

- Care of the Person and Family
- Pain Assessment and Management
- Symptom Assessment and Management
- Last Days/Hours/Imminent Death Care
- Loss, Grief, and Bereavement Support
- Interprofessional/Collaborative Practice
- Education
- Ethics and Legal Issues
- Professional Development and Advocacy

SOURCE: Grantham, D., O'Brien, L. A., Widger, K., Bouvette, M., & McQuinn, P. (2009). *Canadian hospice palliative care nursing competencies case examples*. Retrieved from http://www.carrefourpalliatif.ca/Assets/Canadian%20Hospice%20Palliative%20Care%20Nursing%20Competencies%20Case%20Examples-Revised%20Feb%202010_20100211150854.pdf.

lead to certification can be found on the CNA Web site listed in the Weblinks at the end of this chapter. (See also the *Canadian Hospice Palliative Care Nursing Competencies Case Examples* by Grantham et al., listed in the Evolve Weblinks.)

The CHPCA Web site (see the Weblinks) outlines the "gold standard" optimum nursing care for hospice palliative and end-of-life care at home. This site identifies that the HHN plays an important role within the interdisciplinary team and with the individual and family. Table 3-2 summarizes some of the gold standards for nursing care during hospice palliative care.

Reducing pain and suffering is the goal of hospice palliative care. In both home and hospice settings, HHNs continually do the following:

- Assess the client's response to treatment
- Report their findings to the client's physician
- Collaborate to modify the treatment plan as needed

As the client's level of dependence increases, his or her need for service increases. Agencies that are obligated to maintain quality care and provide for continuity

TABLE 3-2 Gold Standards for Palliative Nursing Care

#	Gold Standard	Community Health Nursing Considerations
1	"Canadians receiving palliative home care have access to skilled, compassionate nursing knowledge and care, 24 hours a day, seven days a week."	• Assessment of individual client needs is essential. • HHNs as members of the interdisciplinary health care team provide support to family and other caregivers. • Clients dying at home and their families can access nursing care whenever they need it either directly (hands-on care) or indirectly through technologies such as telenursing and the Internet.
2	"Home care nurses providing palliative home care have the knowledge, competencies and attitudes to provide high-quality hospice care."	• All HHNs working in hospice palliative care require initial and ongoing education in palliative care management. • Interdisciplinary education in hospice palliative and end-of-life care is essential for all nursing students in Canada. • Employers must offer in-service and continuing education programs on the knowledge and skills of hospice palliative care so generalist and specialist HHNs can access these.
3	"Generalist home care nurses providing palliative home care have timely access to an expert hospice palliative care team."	• Timely access to experts in the field of hospice palliative care as well as appropriate paper and Web-based resources must be provided to all HHNs who have a generalist background and who work with rural, remote, or urban populations. • Employers must assume responsibility for the implementation of innovative technologies to ensure that the HHN has access to experts as outlined above.
4	"Home care nurses are part of a hospice palliative care team that works collaboratively to provide continuity of care for the dying person and his family."	• HHNs function effectively and collaboratively as a member of the interdisciplinary team to ensure continuity of care. • Communication tools such as laptops and common client records are used by all team members in all settings to ensure comprehensive and consistent continuity of care.

SOURCE: Canadian Hospice Palliative Care Association. (2006). *The pan-Canadian gold standards in palliative home care: Toward equitable access to high quality hospice palliative and end-of-life care at home.* Retrieved from http://www.chpca.net/norms-standards/pan-cdn_gold_standards.html.

coordinate health care services, which are tailored to any client health concern. Thus, the range of services provided in home health nursing is extensive. As a result of the hospice movement, persons with terminal diseases now have the option of dying at home with support services available. In addition to prescribed home health nursing services, core services unique to the hospice include the following:

- Volunteers
- Chaplain support
- Respite care
- Financial help with medicines and equipment
- Bereavement support for the family after the family member's death

Palliative (i.e., providing symptom relief) rather than curative care aims to maintain the client's comfort, integrity, and dignity. HHNs contribute to palliative care through actions such as alleviating symptoms and meeting the special needs of dying family members and their families.

Health care providers who work with the dying often experience unique stress. Its presence needs to be identified and appropriately addressed to help ensure quality care and the maintenance of the care provider's integrity. The following are examples of stress experienced by hospice care providers:

- Frustration resulting from clients and caregivers not following the plan of care
- Difficulty deciding how or when to set limits on involvement with clients and families
- Difficulty establishing realistic limitations as to what hospice care can provide

To be effective, the hospice HHN needs the following:

- A firm foundation in nursing skills to meet client physiological needs
- Knowledge of community resources
- The ability to function constructively as a team member
- A level of comfort with death and dying
- The ability to meet the emotional needs of the hospice client and family and their own personal emotional needs

HHNs act as members of palliative interdisciplinary teams with experience in caring for the terminally ill and working with their families. This team may consist of the client's family physician, specialist physicians, social workers, pharmacist, pastoral support workers, personal care workers, volunteers, the client, and his or her family.

Interdisciplinary collaboration, a necessity in home health and hospice settings, is a working agreement in which health care team members carefully analyze their practice roles and work together to determine the best plan for a client's care. Without effective collaboration, the client's home care program would be fragmented, offering decreased or no continuity of care.

The collaborative process for home health nursing directed toward secondary and tertiary prevention activities should begin in the hospital, with the discharge planner and hospital nurse, who identify a client's need for home care and then review their observations and plans with the physician for approval and orders. The discharge planner then contacts the referral intake coordinator of the home care agency and specifies the services requested by the physician. If persons from several disciplines are to be involved, the intake coordinator notifies the appropriate staff and monitors the interdisciplinary collaboration. Either the home health nurse or a physical therapist usually functions as the case manager to ensure the coordination of care. A **case manager** works to enhance continuity and to ensure appropriate care for clients whose health concerns are actually or potentially chronic and complex. Table 3-3 discusses

TABLE 3-3 The Gold Standards for Case Management for Hospice, Palliative, and End-of-Life Care at Home

Standard #	Gold Standard
1	Home care organizations have a timely responsive process for designating clients/patients who need hospice palliative care.
2	Clients/patients and their families have access to timely, knowledgeable, compassionate case management, 24 hours a day, 7 days a week.
3	Home care organizations that provide palliative home care services establish and maintain partnerships with other service providers required for effective case management.
4	Home care providers identify effective case management strategies that reflect the client's/patient's needs and the family's needs and respect diverse cultural beliefs.

(Continued)

TABLE 3-3 The Gold Standards for Case Management for Hospice, Palliative, and End-of-Life Care at Home—Cont'd

Standard #	Gold Standard
5	Case management is provided by professionals who have appropriate knowledge and skills.
6	Members of the care team have the information systems and communication tools to support collaborative practice and effective case management/continuity of care.
7	Canadians are aware of hospice palliative care options available to them, including palliative care.
8	Home care organizations in partnership with other parts of the health system track services available in their communities for people receiving end-of-life care at home, identify gaps, and work collaboratively to meet needs.
9	Jurisdictions monitor the quality and effectiveness of hospice palliative care case management strategies.

SOURCE: Canadian Hospice Palliative Care Association. (2006). *The pan-Canadian gold standards in palliative home care: Toward equitable access to high quality hospice palliative and end-of-life care at home.* Retrieved from http://www.chpca.net/norms-standards/pan-cdn_gold_standards.html.

nine gold standards for case management for hospice, palliative, and end-of-life care at home. Discharge planning and referral considerations are discussed in more detail later in this chapter.

The HHN offering palliative care services will encounter individuals who have not prepared for the possibility of death and so have not completed a living will or considered their end-of-life options such as a do not resuscitate (DNR) order. HHNs need to assess and discuss with their clients (individuals and families) such issues as indicated.

The term *living will* depicts various documents used in the different provinces and territories and includes the *Consent to Treatment Act*, power of attorney for personal care, and the personal directive. The content of such a document varies among the provinces and territories; therefore, the specific act for the applicable province or territory should be consulted.

Evidence-Informed Practice

A qualitative pilot study by Fox, Munro, and Brien (2006) explored the experiences and perceptions of home care nurses who provided diabetes care to homebound clients. The method involved 12 home visits during which the researchers spent time observing nurses working with clients who had diabetes. Also, researchers hosted three focus groups with 17 community health nurses who were involved in providing diabetes care.

The home visits provided the researchers with a deeper understanding of the complexity of managing the medical, social, and emotional needs of clients when caring for them in their homes. The focus groups uncovered the unique role that home care nurses play when delivering care in clients' homes; the challenges and rewards of home care nurses' autonomous practice; and examples of home care nurses' efforts to advocate for their clients within a system of limited resources. The researchers proposed the development of diabetes-specific tools and models for home care clients and the development of diabetes prevention strategies in the community.

Application for CHNs: The findings of this pilot study are important for CHNs because of the need to develop specific tools and models related to diabetes for home care clients in the community. Furthermore, this pilot study emphasized the independent role of home care nurses and the importance of their role as client advocate.

Questions for Reflection & Discussion

1. What health promotion strategies could be used with home care clients who live with diabetes?
2. What programs could a home care nurse provide to clients who live with diabetes?
3. Locate the most recent evidence on diabetes education in home care using the following key words: *home care; advocacy; education; diabetes.*

REFERENCE: Fox, A., Munro, H., & Brien, H. (2006). Exploring diabetes home nursing care: A pilot study. *Canadian Journal of Diabetes, 30*(2), 146–153.

THE OCCUPATIONAL HEALTH NURSE

Most adult Canadians spend a good portion of their day in a workplace setting. All CHNs need to have some basic knowledge about workforce populations, work and related hazards, and methods to control hazards and improve health.

Many substantial workplace changes have occurred, such as the following:

- The nature of work
- Workplace risks
- The work environment
- Workforce composition and demographics
- Health care delivery mechanisms

An analysis of these trends suggests that **work–health interactions** (the influence of work on health) will continue to grow in importance, affecting how work is done, how hazards are controlled or minimized, and how health care is managed and integrated into workplace health delivery strategies. Significant developments are occurring in occupational health and safety programs designed to prevent and control work-related illness and injury and to create environments that foster and support health-promoting activities. In Canada, each of the provinces and territories, as well as the federal government, has its own occupational health and safety legislation outlining the general rights and responsibilities of the employer, the supervisor, and the worker. The Canadian Centre for Occupational Health and Safety (CCOHS) and CanOSH Web sites (listed in the Evolve Weblinks) provide information on such legislation, as well as workers' compensation, regional workplace safety and health acts, and relevant statistics.

An individual with a work-related health problem will often see an occupational health nurse (OHN) before seeing any other health care provider. Consequently, OHNs are in key positions to intervene with working populations at all levels of prevention. They perform critical roles in planning and delivering work-site health and safety services. In addition, the continuing increase in health care costs and concerns about health care quality have prompted the inclusion of primary care and management of non–work-related health concerns through health services programs. Examples of health service programs include smoking cessation programs, cardiac rehabilitation programs, and weight management programs. In some settings, OHNs also provide health service programs for families of workers.

Definitions of Occupational Health Nursing

A nursing specialty within community health nursing, occupational health nursing focuses on workplace health and safety, specifically the delivery of integrated health and safety services and programs to individual employees and employee groups. It encompasses the promotion, maintenance, and restoration of health and the prevention of illness and injury (Canadian Occupational Health Nurses Association Inc., 2009).

Practice Settings for Occupational Health Nurses

Occupational health nurses work in traditional manufacturing, industry, service, health care facility, construction site, and government settings. Their scope of practice is broad and includes the following:

- Worker and workplace assessment and surveillance
- Primary care
- Case management
- Counselling
- Health promotion and protection
- Administration and management
- Research
- Legal and ethical monitoring
- Community orientation

CHNs apply their knowledge in occupational health and safety to the workforce aggregate.

Over the years, a dramatic shift in the types of jobs held by workers has taken place. With the evolution from an agrarian (i.e., agriculture) economy to a manufacturing society and then to a highly technological workplace, the greatest proportion of paid employment is now in the following occupations: service work (e.g., health care, information processing, banking, insurance); professional technical work (e.g., managers, computer specialists); and clerical work (e.g., data entry clerks, secretaries). Along with this change in the nature of work come many new occupational hazards, such as the following:

- Complex chemicals
- Nonergonomic workstation design (i.e., workstation set-ups that do not meet the employee's health and safety needs)
- Job stress
- Burnout
- Exhaustion

Through its services, programs, and legislation for accident and injury prevention, the Canadian government recognizes the importance of a healthy, safe workplace for all employees. For information on workplace

FIGURE 3-1 The Epidemiological Triad

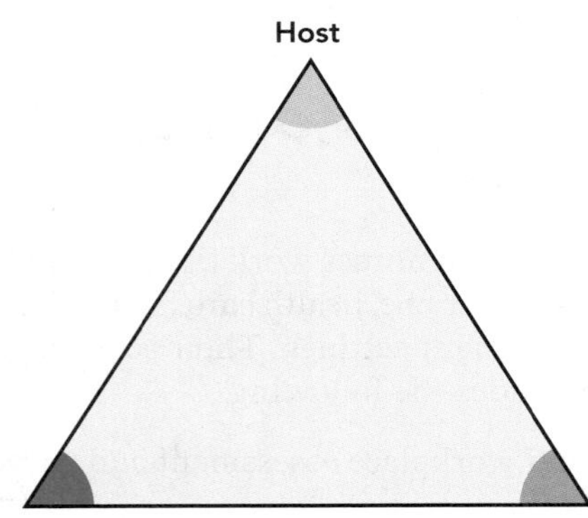

health and safety in Canada, see the Human Resources and Skills Development Canada Evolve Weblink.

The epidemiological triad (see Figure 3-1), discussed more extensively in Chapter 8, can be used to explain the relationship between work and health (Campos-Outcalt, 1994). Using the employed population as an example, the *host* is described as any susceptible human being. Because of the nature of work-related hazards, OHNs must assume that all employed individuals and groups are at risk of exposure to occupational hazards. The *agents*, or factors associated with illness and injury, comprise occupational exposures that are classified as *biological and infectious*, *chemical*, *enviro-mechanical*, *physical*, or *psychosocial* hazards (see Box 3-2). Table 3-4 lists some of the more common workplace exposures, their known health effects, and the types of jobs associated with these hazards.

The third element of the epidemiological triad, the *environment*, includes all external conditions that influence the interaction of the host and agents. The following workplace conditions serve as examples:

- Temperature extremes
- Crowding
- Shift work
- Inflexible management styles

The basic principle of epidemiology is that health interventions for restoring and promoting health result from complex interactions among these three elements. To understand these interactions and to design effective occupational health nursing strategies for dealing with them in a proactive manner, occupational health nurses must look at how each element influences the others.

Occupational health nurses are registered nurses, usually with additional educational preparation and experience, who work in industries and other workplace settings to promote the health and safety of workers. Many OHNs have completed continuing education programs in occupational health and safety at a certificate, diploma, or degree level. Courses taken in these programs help registered nurses to gain further knowledge and skills related to workplace topics such as ergonomics, audiometric testing, and toxicology. The CNA has recognized occupational health nursing as a specialty, and OHNs who have successfully completed the CNA occupational health nursing certification program can place the initials *COHN* after their name. Box 3-3 lists key competency categories for occupational health nurses. Occupational health nursing competencies that lead to certification can be found on the CNA Web site (listed in the Evolve Weblinks at the end of this chapter).

BOX 3-2 Categories of Work-Related Hazards

- Biological and infectious hazards: infectious or biological agents, such as bacteria, viruses, fungi, and parasites, that may be transmitted to others via contact with infected individuals or contaminated body secretions or fluids
- Chemical hazards: various forms of chemicals, including medications, solutions, gases, vapours, aerosols, and particulate matter, that are potentially toxic or irritating to the body system
- Enviro-mechanical hazards: factors encountered in the work environment that cause or potentiate accidents, injuries, strain, or discomfort (e.g., unsafe or inadequate equipment or lifting devices, slippery floors, workstation deficiencies)
- Physical hazards: agents within the work environment, such as radiation, electricity, extreme temperatures, and noise, that can cause tissue trauma
- Psychosocial hazards: factors and situations encountered or associated with one's job or work environment that create or potentiate stress, emotional strain, or interpersonal problems

SOURCE: Rogers, B. (2003). *Occupational health nursing: Concepts and practice* (2nd ed.). St. Louis, MO: Elsevier.

TABLE 3-4 Select Job Categories, Exposures, and Associated Work-Related Diseases and Conditions

Job Categories	Exposures	Work-Related Diseases and Conditions
All workers	Workplace stress	Hypertension, mood disorders, cardiovascular disease
Agricultural workers	Pesticides, infectious agents, gases, sunlight	Pesticide poisoning, "farmer's lung," skin cancer
Anaesthetists	Anaesthetic gases	Reproductive effects, cancer
Automobile workers	Asbestos, plastics, lead, solvents	Asbestosis, dermatitis
Butchers	Vinyl plastic fumes	Meat wrapper's asthma
Caisson workers	Pressurized work environments	Caisson disease, "the bends"
Carpenters	Wood dust, wood preservatives, adhesives	Nasopharyngeal cancer, dermatitis
Cement workers	Cement dust, metals	Dermatitis, bronchitis
Ceramic workers	Talc, clays	Pneumoconiosis
Demolition workers	Asbestos, wood dust	Asbestosis
Drug manufacturers	Hormones, nitroglycerin, etc.	Reproductive effects
Dry cleaners	Solvents	Liver disease, dermatitis
Dye workers	Dyestuffs, metals, solvents	Bladder cancer, dermatitis
Embalmers	Formaldehyde, infectious agents	Dermatitis
Felt makers	Mercury, polycyclic hydrocarbons	Mercury poisoning
Foundry workers	Silica, molten metals	Silicosis
Glass workers	Heat, solvents, metal powders	Cataracts
Hospital workers	Infectious agents, cleansers, radiation	Infections, latex allergies, unintentional injuries
Insulators	Asbestos, fibrous glass	Asbestosis, lung cancer, mesothelioma
Jackhammer operators	Vibration	Raynaud's phenomenon
Lathe operators	Metal dusts, cutting oils	Lung disease, cancer
Office computer workers	Repetitive wrist motion, eye strain	Tendonitis, carpal tunnel syndrome, tenosynovitis

Functions and Roles of Occupational Health Nurses

Optimally, a team of occupational health and safety professionals will provide on-site occupational health and safety services. The usual core members of this team would include the following:

- Occupational health nurse
- Occupational physician
- Industrial hygienist
- Safety professional

Occupational health nurses collaborate with a community physician or occupational medicine physician, who provides consultation and accepts referrals when medical intervention is needed. This collaboration may occur primarily through telephone contact, or the physician may be under contract with the workplace to spend a certain amount of time on-site each week. As workplaces become larger, they are likely to hire the following:

- Ergonomist
- Safety professionals
- Industrial hygienists
- Physicians, part-time or on a consultant basis
- Employee assistance counsellors
- Physiotherapists

BOX 3-3 Occupational Health Nursing Competency Categories

- Provision of Occupational Health, Safety, and Environmental Nursing
- Recognition, Evaluation, and Control of Workplace/Environmental Health and Safety Hazards
- Health Assessment, Planning, Implementation, Monitoring, and Evaluation
- Assessment, Care, and Case Management of Injuries and Illnesses
- Environment, Health, Safety, Wellness Promotion, and Education
- Environment, Health, Safety, and Wellness Management

SOURCE: Canadian Nurses Association. (2008). *Occupational health nursing certification*. Retrieved from http://www.cna-nurses.ca/CNA/documents/pdf/publications/CERT_Occ_Health_e.pdf.

- Health educators
- Physical fitness specialists
- Toxicologists

On-site occupational health programs offer a range of services. Some focus only on work-related health and safety problems; others provide a wide scope of services that includes primary care. Generally, the goals of occupational health nurses are as follows:

- To maintain and promote health and safety in the workplace so that clients maximize their work capacity
- To improve the workplace environment by making it healthy and safe
- To enhance population health through healthy and safe work environments
- To work at the systems level to create a workplace atmosphere that contributes to a productive and comfortable psychosocial work environment

Some specific roles of the occupational health nurse are found in Box 3-4.

In workplaces that have exposures regulated by law, certain programs, such as respiratory protection or hearing conservation, are required. Whether a workplace offers additional programs depends on the employee needs, management's attitudes about and understanding of health and safety, acceptance by the workers, and the employer's economic status. The past few years have seen a significant increase in the number of health promotion and employee assistance programs offered in workplaces. Occupational health promotion programs focus on educating clients about lifestyle choices that cause risks to health. Examples of health promotion programs are: management of job-related stress, strategies to reduce

BOX 3-4 The Role of the Occupational Health Nurse

The occupational health nurse has a diverse role and provides services such as the following:

- Health and safety policy and program development
- Health and safety legislation awareness and interpretation
- Consultation with employees and managers
- Employee attendance-management program development
- Management of occupational and nonoccupational illness and injury
- Preplacement health assessments
- Return-to-work assessments
- Return-to-work coordination
- Rehabilitation and accommodation
- Periodic health monitoring
- Workplace clinic services
- Job demand analysis
- Ergonomic policies and programs
- Chemical monitoring and Workplace Hazardous Materials Information System (WHMIS) education
- Hazard identification, prevention, and surveillance
- Environmental auditing
- Employee assistance programs
- Alcohol and drug programs
- Emergency preparedness and disaster planning
- Pandemic policy and program development
- Overseas travel preparation
- Immunizations
- Customized training
- Healthy lifestyle promotion
- Consultation and support services for Human Resources (HR)

SOURCE: Occupational Health Nurses of British Columbia. (2007). *What is occupational health nursing?* Retrieved from http://www.bcohn.ca/ohnfaq.html. Reprinted by permission of the Occupational Health Nurses' Speciality Association of British Columbia.

obesity, smoking cessation, and promotion of exercise (O'Donnell, 2002). Employee assistance programs are designed to address personal concerns (e.g., marital or family issues, substance abuse, financial difficulties) that affect an employee's productivity. Because such efforts are cost-effective for workplaces, they should continue to increase.

OHNs practise all levels of prevention (Rogers, 2003). They deliver primary prevention services to employees in an effort to avert health issues. Examples of primary prevention measures include offering an immunization program, encouraging use of personal protective equipment such as respirators or gloves, and providing tools for smoking cessation. In the occupational health setting, the purpose of health promotion is to maintain or enhance the well-being of individuals or groups of employees and the workplace in general. To this end, the OHN may implement programs designed to improve coping skills, offer nutrition education and counselling, and provide information to increase knowledge about potential health hazards both in and outside the workplace.

Walk-throughs are carried out in the workplace by the occupational health nurse or other workplace team members to identify workplace hazards so efforts can be aimed at health protection. Health protection efforts seek to eliminate or reduce the immediate risk of disease and to prevent the development of an illness or injury.

Secondary prevention, which occurs after a disease process has already begun, is aimed at early detection, prompt treatment, and prevention of further limitations. For employees, early detection involves health surveillance, periodic health screening to identify an illness at the earliest possible moment in its course, and elimination or modification of the hazard-producing situation. Interventions are intended to prevent further harm or deterioration. Examples of such interventions include referral for counselling in the case of an employee with an emotional or mental health issue whose work performance has been affected and removal from heavy metal exposure for workers who manifest neurological symptoms.

Tertiary prevention is intended to restore health as fully as possible and assist individuals to achieve their maximum level of functioning. Rehabilitation strategies such as return-to-work programs after a heart attack or limited-duty programs after a cumulative trauma injury are examples of tertiary prevention.

The initial step of assessment involves the traditional history and physical assessment but emphasizes exposure to occupational hazards and individual characteristics that may predispose a client in a certain job to an increased health risk. Because work is a part of life for most people, the occupational and environmental health history is an indispensable component of the health assessment of individuals (Rogers, 2003) (see Appendix E-1, "Comprehensive Occupational and Environmental Health History," on the Evolve Web site). An **occupational and environmental health history** contains questions that provide the data necessary to rule out or confirm job-induced conditions and health concerns.

Many workers do not have access to health care services in their workplaces; and it is not unusual to find health care providers in the community who have little or no knowledge about workplaces or expertise in occupation-related illnesses and injuries. Because of the large number of small businesses that do not have the resources for maintaining on-site health care, injured and ill workers are usually first seen in clinics, emergency departments, physicians' offices, and hospitals. Occupational health nurses employed by workplaces are often the first-line assessors of these individuals and perhaps the only contact for education about self-protection from workplace hazards.

LEVELS OF PREVENTION

Related to Occupational Health Nursing

PRIMARY PREVENTION

Occupational health nurses provide education to a group of new employees about safety in the workplace to prevent injury.

SECONDARY PREVENTION

Occupational health nurses provide a mass screening clinic for hearing loss resulting from noise levels in the workplace.

TERTIARY PREVENTION

Occupational health nurses educate a group of workers who have chronic diabetes about appropriate medication use and blood glucose screening to avoid lost workdays.

Identifying workplace exposures as sources of health problems may influence the client's course of illness and rehabilitation and also prevent similar illnesses among others with the potential for exposure (Levy & Wegman, 2000). Including occupational health data in client assessments begins with recognizing the possible relationship between health and occupational factors. The next step is integrating into the nursing history-taking some routine assessment questions that will provide the data necessary to confirm or rule out occupation-induced symptoms. Symptoms of hazardous workplace exposures may be indicated by vague complaints involving any body system. These symptoms often imitate those of common medical problems. Occupational health histories should include the following points:

- A list of current and past jobs the client has held, including specific job titles
- Questions about current and past exposures to specific agents and relationships between the symptoms and activities at work
- Other factors that may enhance the client's susceptibility to occupational agents (e.g., life history including smoking, underlying illness, previous injury, and disability)

Questions about the employee's occupational history can be included in existing short assessment tools such as the one provided in Appendix E-2, "Occupational Health History Form," found on the Evolve Web site. The more complete the data collected, the more likely the OHN is to notice work–health interactions. All employees should be questioned about their employment history. Since not all workers are well informed about the materials with which they work or about potential hazards, the OHN needs to develop basic knowledge about the types of jobs held by clients and the possible hazards associated with them. Because exposures from other environments such as home and yard may interact with workplace exposures, the OHN should extend the questioning to include this information.

Identifying work-related health problems does not require an extensive knowledge of occupational agents and their effects. A systematic approach for evaluating the potential for workplace exposures is the most effective intervention for detecting and preventing occupational health risks. Appendix E-3, "Work-Site Assessment Guide," found on the Evolve Web site, is a brief assessment tool that an OHN can incorporate into a routine history-taking. Similar questions can be included in the assessment of a worker's spouse and dependents, who may have indirect exposure to occupational hazards.

During these health assessments, the OHN has the opportunity to educate clients about workplace hazards and preventive measures. At the same time, the OHN is obtaining information that will be valuable in optimizing the worker–job fit. Such assessments may be done as follows:

- As preplacement examinations before the client begins a job
- On a periodic basis during employment
- With the onset of a work-related health concern or exposure
- When an employee is being transferred to another job with different requirements and exposures
- At termination
- At retirement

These assessments aim to identify agent and host factors that could place the employee at risk and to determine prevention steps that can be taken to eliminate or minimize the exposure and potential health concern.

When the health data from such assessments are considered collectively, the OHN may determine some patterns in risk factors associated with the occurrence of work-related injuries and illnesses in a total population of workers. For example, a nurse practitioner in a clinic noted a dramatic increase in the number of cases of bladder cancer among her clients. When she looked at factors these individuals had in common, she determined that they all worked at a company that used benzidine dyes, which are known bladder carcinogens. She worked with the union and the company to assess the environmental exposure to the employees. This occupational health nursing intervention led to a safer work environment and a decrease in bladder cancer among this population group. Such an approach can be used at the company, industry, and community levels. The initial collection of data and the questioning about workplace exposures are vital steps for any intervention.

The OHN may conduct a similar assessment of the workplace itself. The purpose of this assessment, known as a **work-site walk-through** or survey, is to learn about the following (Rogers, 2003):

- The work processes and the materials
- The requirements of various jobs
- The presence of actual or potential hazards
- The work practices of employees

When the purpose of the work-site walk-through is environmental monitoring or a safety audit, industrial hygienists and safety professionals will conduct more complex surveys. However, most occupational health nurses have developed an expertise in these areas and include such tasks as part of their functions. For any health care provider who assesses workers, this information makes up an important database. For the on-site health care provider, work-site walk-throughs assist the professional in developing rapport and establishing credibility with the employees.

The more information that is collected before the walk-through, the more efficient the process of the survey will be. After the survey is conducted, the OHN can use the information with the aggregate health data to evaluate the effectiveness of the occupational health and safety program and to plan future programs. An environmental scan may be used to assist the occupational health nurse (and other CHNs working in other settings) to complete a more thorough assessment of their work setting to determine the internal and external environmental factors that need to be considered for meeting current and future needs.

CRITICAL VIEW

Both corporate culture and cost-effective programs are key factors in influencing the development of occupational health services.

1. Which determinants of health do occupational health nurses need to consider in work settings?
2. How do the five Community Health Nursing Standards of Practice apply to occupational health nursing?

THE PARISH NURSE

A **parish nurse** is "a registered nurse with specialized knowledge, who is called to ministry and affirmed by a faith community to promote health, healing and wholeness" (Canadian Association for Parish Nursing Ministry [CAPNM], 2004). The parish nurse usually has additional education in pastoral care and social sciences, and uses all the knowledge and skills of this community health nursing specialty to give effective services. The outcome the parish nurse strives for is a truly caring congregation that supports healthy, spiritually fulfilling lives.

Parish nurses address health concerns for individuals, families, and groups of all ages. Members of faith congregations, like other people, experience some or even all life events such as birth, death, acute and chronic illness, stress, dependency concerns, challenges of life transitions, growth and development, and decisions regarding healthy lifestyle choices. Parish nurses work within faith congregations, including communities that serve diverse cultures. Parish nurses also serve faith communities in other countries.

The Canadian Association for Parish Nursing Ministry (CAPNM) (2004) has developed core competencies for parish nursing as guidelines for practice. The practice categories are as follows:

1. Current Standing as a Registered Nurse (Baccalaureate Degree in Nursing Preferred)
2. Orientation to Parish Nursing
3. Spiritual Maturity and Theological Reflection
4. Personal/Interpersonal Skills
5. Teaching/Facilitation
6. Worship

How To... Assess a Worker and the Workplace

Assessing the worker for a work-related problem is a critical practice element. The occupational health nurse should do the following:

- Take a complete general and occupational health history with emphasis on workplace exposure assessment, job hazard analysis, and list of previous jobs.
- Conduct a health assessment to identify agent and host factors that interact to place workers at risk.
- Identify patterns of risk associated with illness or injury.

Assessing the work environment is necessary to determine workplace exposures that create worker health risk. The OHN should do the following:

- Understand the work being done.
- Evaluate the work-related hazards.
- Understand the work process.
- Gather data about the incidence or prevalence of work-related illness or injuries and related hazards.
- Examine the control strategies in place for eliminating exposures.

7. Faith Community Context
8. Collaboration
9. Management
10. Practicum
11. Continuing Education

As of 2010, the CNA does not offer certification status to parish nurses.

Definitions in Parish Nursing

Faith communities are distinct groups of people who acknowledge specific faith traditions and gather in churches, cathedrals, synagogues, or mosques. **Parish nursing** is nursing care provided in the faith community to promote whole-person health among the parishioners (CAPNM, 2004). Parish nurses respond to the health and wellness needs of populations of faith communities and are partners with the church in fulfilling the mission of health ministry.

The faith community includes persons throughout the lifespan, active and less active members, those confined to homes, and those in nursing homes. Often the church's mission includes extending services to individuals and groups in the geographical community who are not part of the congregation. The parish nurse emphasizes the nursing discipline's spiritual dimension and incorporates the physical, emotional, and social aspects of nursing.

Health ministries comprise those activities and programs in faith communities organized around health and healing to promote whole health across the lifespan. Health ministries' services may be specifically planned or more informal and may include visiting the homebound, providing meals for families in crisis or for those returning home after hospitalization, organizing prayer circles, volunteering in community AIDS care groups, serving "heart healthy" church suppers, and holding regular grief support groups.

Parish nurses work closely with other professional health care members, **pastoral care staff** (faith community leaders including clergy, nurses, and educational and youth ministry staff), and lay volunteers who represent various aspects of the life of the congregational community. Along with members of the pastoral team and community partners, the parish nurse assesses, plans, implements, and evaluates health programs. To promote healing, the parish nurse builds on clients' strengths to encourage integrating their inner spiritual knowledge with healthy lifestyle choices for optimal wellness. Providing such holistic care is important with congregation populations. A parish nurse views **holistic care** as the interaction of the body, mind, and spirit in the promotion of holistic wellness (CAPNM, 2004).

Practice Settings for Parish Nursing

In the roots of many faith communities are concerns for justice, mercy, and the need for spiritual and physical healing. Whether participating as individuals or as families, all benefit from their association with a supportive faith community or congregation.

An important aspect of living one's spirituality and religion is being a part of a community of faith from birth to death, throughout wellness and illness. The integration of faith and health within a caring community results in beneficial outcomes. The appeal for caring, the healing of diseases, and the acknowledgement of periods of illness and wellness are universal; however, persons who encounter physical and emotional illness or brokenness and who call upon their faith beliefs and religious traditions may benefit from increased coping skills and realize spiritual growth. These coping skills and spiritual strengths extend beyond the current situation and help with future life challenges and total well-being.

In the late nineteenth and early twentieth centuries, missionaries developed multipurpose activities, which included education and health activities along with religious messages, in their communities. As political and economic forces have changed through the years, health ministries have altered their approaches. Some churches have aligned themselves with community development efforts to help empower people to meet their needs for food, education, clean environments, social support, and primary health care. These efforts have been translated into a variety of positions endorsed by the governing bodies of faith communities, including the position of parish nurse. Parish nursing services were offered as one of the responses to assist with coordinating care and fostering continuity of care.

Parish nursing services emphasize health promotion and disease prevention and provide the benefits of holistic care through the supportive faith community. CHNs functioning as parish nurses need to have skills of leadership; astute and articulate nonverbal and verbal communication; and negotiation and collaboration.

In addition to serving congregations in the community, parish nurses may be employed by older adult living complexes and long-term care facilities that offer a spiritual focus to the nursing practice.

Functions and Roles of Parish Nurses

Parish nursing's goal is to develop and sustain health ministries within faith communities. Health ministries promote wholeness in health and emphasize health promotion and disease prevention within the context of linking healing with the person's faith belief and level of spiritual maturity.

Some of the usual functions of parish nurses include providing personal health counselling and health education, acting as a liaison between the faith community and the local community, facilitating activities, and providing pastoral care. When providing *personal health counselling*, parish nurses explore with clients areas such as health risks, spiritual assessments, and plans for healthier lifestyles as well as provide support and guidance related to acute or chronic actual or potential health problems. Parish nurses may carry out their practice in groups or individually. They make visits to homes, hospitals, and long-term care facilities, and see persons in the faith community's house of worship. Some parish nurses have designated offices; others use space that is most conducive to a particular activity or client need.

Parish nurses participate in *health education* in the following ways:

- Publish information in congregation news bulletins
- Distribute information
- Make available a variety of resources for the physical, mental, and spiritual health of the congregation
- Hold education sessions to address identified health concerns
- Provide individual teaching as needed
- Arrange and host discussions for targeted groups or meetings
- Strive to promote wholeness in health
- Create a fuller understanding of total physical, mental, and spiritual well-being

Acting as a *liaison* between resources in the faith community and the local community, parish nurses accept the following responsibilities:

- Help clients know what resources are available to them for managing their health concerns
- Help individuals and families choose the appropriate resource to deal with their health concerns
- Link clients with the appropriate services to meet their health care needs

Parish nurses are also *facilitators*. They do some or all of the following:

- Link congregational health concerns to the establishment of and referral to support groups
- Facilitate the necessary changes to increase disability access or to extend meals and services to those who are homebound
- Work with a volunteer coordinator to train volunteer caregivers or ensure that interested persons acquire training to function as lay caregivers to meet congregational health concerns

An important function underlying all the previously mentioned functions is that of providing *pastoral care*, which parish nurses fulfill as follows:

- Stress the spiritual dimension of nursing
- Lend support during times of joy and sorrow
- Guide people through health and illness throughout life
- Help faith community members identify the spiritual strengths that assist in coping with particular events

LEVELS OF PREVENTION

Related to Parish Nursing

PRIMARY PREVENTION

Parish nurses encourage faith community leaders to sponsor a safe indoor or outdoor activity area for neighbourhood or at-risk children.

SECONDARY PREVENTION

During home visits, parish nurses conduct family health assessment and counselling as needed—for example, post-hospitalization home visits or postnatal home visits.

TERTIARY PREVENTION

Parish nurses discuss with substance-abusing youth groups and the youths' parents the need for loving, caring friends and parental support during the long-term behaviour modification program.

How To... Intervene in Maternal and Infant Health: Parish Nurses

- Visit the family immediately after the birth of a neonate to assess parenting skills and parent–infant bonding, reinforce a holistic reflection of the life transition, and plan for faith community support as indicated in those areas not addressed by the family or other community agencies.
- Augment community prenatal classes or facilitate classes in a faith community, stressing growth and development of the prenatal and postnatal periods, family transitions, and the health monitoring needed by parents, children, and new family members.
- Facilitate expectant-parent support groups to reinforce positive health during pregnancy; interpret plans negotiated with the health care provider; promote spiritual reflection of the family life transition to encourage connectedness with the Creator and beliefs of the faith community; and provide emotional, social, and community support to the family.

Parish nurses may use hymns, favourite scripture verses, psalms, stories, pictures, church windows, and other images that are important to the individual or group to illustrate the connectedness between faith, health, and well-being.

The parish nurse encourages faith community members to take part in numerous healthy activities and will often work with the congregation to help it stretch beyond its immediate borders to augment community services that promote health and wellness. Congregations are keenly aware that more than half of the members of mainstream churches are part of the growing older adult population of our country. Services offered by parish nurses may include the following:

- Food pantries
- Day care for older adults
- Congregate meals
- Meals on Wheels
- Visits to less mobile members
- Outreach for vulnerable populations

THE PUBLIC HEALTH NURSE

In 2005, the Federal, Provincial, and Territorial Joint Task Group on Public Health Human Resources developed a draft set of core competencies for public health practice in Canada. The task group recommended consultation with the public health community to obtain agreement on a set of core competencies. The Public Health Agency of Canada (PHAC) assumed the lead in this effort, in collaboration with many partners, and discipline-specific public health nursing core competencies became available in 2009 (Community Health Nurses of Canada, 2009). Box 3-5 lists the Canadian public health nursing competency categories. (To read the public health core competencies and a history of their development, see the PHAC Weblink on the Evolve Web site.)

In Canada, public health takes a population health approach to protecting and promoting health and preventing disease for all Canadians. Public health nurses (PHNs) work with many partners, both within the public health

BOX 3-5 Canadian Public Health Nursing Competency Categories

- Public Health and Nursing Sciences
- Assessment and Analysis
- Policy and Program Planning, Implementation, and Evaluation
- Partnerships, Collaboration, and Advocacy
- Diversity and Inclusiveness
- Communication
- Leadership
- Professional Responsibility and Accountability

SOURCE: Community Health Nurses of Canada. (2009). *Public health nursing discipline specific competencies version 1.0.* Retrieved from http://www.chnc.ca/documents/competencies_june_2009_english.pdf.

unit or health authority (e.g., nutritionists, epidemiologists, dental hygienists, health inspectors) and external to the health unit (e.g., community coalitions for heart health, cancer screening, diabetes, and obesity prevention; school and hospital administrators; regional planners; social service and child care workers; lobbyists for health issues such as antismoking legislation and homelessness).

PHNs build partnerships and collaboration among groups and build the capacity of community leaders to address health issues effectively. These are much more powerful strategies in making changes that will have an impact on the health of community members, rather than the PHN working alone or only with individual clients. As an example, a depressed mother having difficulty coping with the activities and responsibilities of daily living and in need of counselling presents a significant public health concern because the mother's, children's, and family's needs are not being met. Frequently, the health concern will not be obvious to the health care professional who sees this woman for the first time. PHNs have the knowledge and skills to identify the strengths of the woman and her family, the health concerns present, and the challenges involved and to consider the impact that all of these things have on the broader community. In this example, consider the following:

- The children may grow to be adults with developmental or mental health concerns.
- The community mental health and social services may not be able to respond to this increased demand on resources.
- The children may become depressed or violent adults, resulting in a need for more health and corrections facilities.
- The mother may need additional mental health and social services.
- The children may be absent from school often and may not be able to complete their education.
- As adults, this mother's children may remain unemployed or be nonproductive in the workplace because their absences from school led to limited or poor job and literacy skills.

The increased burden of care on the health care and other publicly funded systems leads to increased costs and taxes.

Definitions in Public Health Nursing

In public health nursing, the *client* is defined as the population, community, aggregate, group, family, or individual. Public health nursing practice involves primary, secondary, and tertiary preventions. Using population health determinants based on a sound knowledge that includes nursing science, public health science, and social sciences (Community Health Nurses' Initiatives Group, 2004), public health nurses provide services such as health promotion, health protection, disease and injury prevention, and surveillance (Underwood et al., 2009). The minimum educational preparation of PHNs is a baccalaureate degree in nursing with curriculum content in community health nursing, epidemiology, research, management, and leadership.

Practice Settings for Public Health Nursing

PHNs work for an official public health agency referred to as a health department, unit, or regional authority. The official agency is governed by a board of health and funded by provincial or territorial and municipal governments, which develop legislation, such as a public health act, that outlines the requirements for the delivery of programs and services. For example, in Ontario, the *Health Protection and Promotion Act* directs and identifies the roles of public health agencies, and the *Ontario Public Health Standards* (Minister of Health and Long-term Care, 2008) outline the mandate and core functions for public health practice.

The practice settings for PHNs vary and may include home, school, workplace, community health centre, and clinical settings. Historically, PHNs spent a great deal of their time visiting clients in their home and students in schools. In the late 1990s, because of a greater focus on population health, these settings received fewer PHN contact hours. Currently, differences exist across Canada as to the extent of public health nursing involvement in schools. However, there is a movement toward comprehensive school health (see the Communities and Schools Promoting Health Weblink on the Evolve Web site). In schools, PHNs encourage the development of school health committees and promote health through collaboration with principals, teachers, parents, and students. PHNs are very much involved in providing clinic services such as those for influenza prevention, family planning, travel health, immunization, sexual health, breastfeeding and well babies. PHNs work with a variety of groups, including expectant and new parents to promote healthy pregnancy and parenting, smoking cessation and hepatitis C support groups, and other self-help groups dealing with a variety of health issues. PHNs working with the community as client contribute to community and workplace health promotion strategies with a focus on, for example, health issues (e.g., heart health, cancer screening initiatives), childhood obesity, and environmental health issues. More recently, some PHNs have begun working with nontraditional partners such as regional planners, developers, environmentalists, and traffic demand managers to provide consultation and awareness

Evidence-Informed Practice

Female high school students in rural Nova Scotia took part in a pilot study to determine their willingness to participate in a self-test screening program for *Chlamydia trachomatis*. The researchers also wanted to uncover the students' reasons for participating or not participating and to determine whether they would be more inclined to be screened if they practised more risky sexual behaviours. Researchers anticipated that the self-screening approach would lead to screening of an increased number of young women than if they were required to visit a physician or clinic for the testing.

The participants were not required to receive counselling from the school nurse before obtaining test kits from the school's health centre. At the same time as the self-test kits were available to students, a cross-sectional survey was conducted to identify factors related to student participation or nonparticipation. Of the 58% of participants who had had vaginal intercourse at least once, 15% used the self-test kit. The remaining participants who had had vaginal intercourse and who did not use the self-test were aware that females with *Chlamydia* are very often asymptomatic, yet 54% decided not to participate in self-screening because of their lack of symptoms. Forty-nine percent of those not using the kit gave the reason of low probability of infection despite having frequently participated in high-risk sexual activity. Fewer women than anticipated chose to perform the self-test. The researchers attributed the low number to the absence of counselling encouraging the students to participate and connecting knowledge with behaviour. It was recommended that self-testing be further explored to better understand its potential to increase *Chlamydia* screening among Canadian youth.

Application for CHNs: This pilot study suggests that this aggregate is at risk for sexually transmitted infections (STIs). CHNs working with this aggregate need to consider the participants' reasons for not self-testing and to recognize the importance of counselling and education. Youth need to be made aware that their risky behaviour may result in STIs, that being asymptomatic does not ensure an absence of infection, and that if left untreated, they put others at risk for STIs. These study findings suggest important ways for CHNs to assist youth with opportunities to care for themselves.

Questions for Reflection & Discussion

1. What strategies would you choose to promote self-testing for *Chlamydia* in young women who live in rural areas?
2. What determinants of health would be a concern for young women who live in rural Nova Scotia?
3. Locate the latest evidence on STIs in high school populations by using the following key words: *school; self-testing; Chlamydia trachomatis.*

REFERENCE: Langille, D. B., Proudfoot, K., Rigby, J., Aquino-Russell, C., Strang, R., & Forward, K. (2008). A pilot project for *Chlamydia* screening in adolescent females using self-testing: Characteristics of participants and non-participants. *Canadian Journal of Public Health, 99*(2), 117–120.

regarding the health impacts of the built environment in an effort to promote the development of healthy communities. They also work with at-risk populations such as the homeless and immigrants in a variety of settings that may include settlement and outreach centres.

Functions and Roles of PHNs

PHNs have many functions and roles, depending on the needs and resources of an area. Among these roles is advocate. As an advocate, the PHN collects, monitors, and analyzes data and identifies, along with the client (an individual, family, or community), which services and programs best meet the client's needs. The PHN and the client then develop the most effective plan and approach to the health issue. The plan may include activities, alone or in combination, related to education and awareness, personal skills development, the creation of supportive environments, policy development, and community action mobilization. For example, a PHN will work with a client who wants to quit smoking by helping him or her develop the knowledge and skills related to cessation and providing support as the client implements a plan based on stages of change theory. With the PHN's help, the client can increase his or her confidence, take ownership of his or her health, and become more independent in making decisions and obtaining the services necessary to stop smoking.

The PHN may also assume the role of manager with specific aggregate groups and, in this role, assess, plan, implement, and evaluate outcomes to meet clients' needs. As a leader and consultant, the PHN builds and maintains partnerships with community leaders and key stakeholders to identify community needs (e.g., playground safety, access to physical activity opportunities, hand hygiene, pedestrian safety, safer-sex practices), to develop and implement plans to meet these needs, and to identify and implement strategies that promote the adoption of health behaviours over time. As well, communicating complex information clearly is frequently an important component of client management and may involve engaging family members, translators, or religious leaders as the PHN works toward developing the care plan. Other health and social agency participants may not be as familiar as the PHN with the dynamics of family relationships, the family's financial situation, or their living conditions. It is the PHN who has been there, observed the living conditions, and assessed the family's strengths and health concerns, and can support and assist the client to tell his or her story. The PHN as manager assists clients in determining the services they need most and identifies the most effective means of accessing them. For example, a PHN may go into the home to visit a new mother and her baby. Upon assessment, the PHN may find that the mother needs help finding a job, child care, and a pediatrician. The PHN helps the mother in the following ways:

- Assists with prioritizing health concerns
- Reviews research related to how best to address her health concerns and analyzes community data to identify available and accessible resources within the mother's community
- Ensures that resources and services are culturally sensitive and delivered in the appropriate language, literacy level, and environment for the client
- Develops a plan for resolving the health concerns, in partnership with the mother, to identify and work with her strengths
- Supports and encourages the mother to contact other agencies related to employment and child care
- Refers the client to an appropriate community resource or agency as needed
- Follows up with the mother to evaluate her progress and to revise the plan as needed to ensure that her health concerns are being resolved
- Follows up with agencies, such as social services, and shares information with the mother

Being both consultants and specialists, PHNs know how to access and analyze relevant data from a variety of sources. These data often include information related to the social determinants of health (e.g., housing, income, employment, literacy, culture), which provide PHNs with a comprehensive understanding of the health of their community. The PHN then uses this knowledge and skill at community forums and coalitions to facilitate the planning of a variety of health initiatives that may include, for example, mass communication or social marketing campaigns, health fairs for new immigrants, or community mobilization to promote safe routes to schools or increased access to clinical services. PHNs' knowledge of the community also makes them a major referral resource. They maintain or know how to access current information about the health and social needs and the services available within the community. They know what resources a client will find acceptable (e.g., within the social and cultural norms for his or her group). The PHN provides clients education and skill-building opportunities to build their capacity, to enable them to access and use the resources in their community, and to learn self-care. PHNs provide counselling and refer clients to other services in their area, just as other services refer clients to PHNs for care or follow-up. For example, a community agency or hospital may refer a new mother and her baby to a PHN for postnatal care, which would require the PHN to do a postpartum home visit follow-up, or a workplace may contact a PHN for information on how to plan a health fair and flu clinic for its employees, which would require the PHN to provide information on how to access the appropriate community agencies and resources to meet employees' health needs. See the "Evidence-Informed Practice" box on the practice of public health nurses fostering citizen participation and collaborative efforts on the Evolve Web site.

Literacy assessment is a component of public health nursing. Many individuals are limited in their ability to read, write, and communicate clearly; however, being illiterate does not equate to being mentally challenged. A poor literacy level, often a result of restricted educational opportunities or indicative of the length of time an immigrant has been in Canada, may reflect financial limitations. Individuals attending a physician's office, clinic, or hospital who are clean and neatly dressed may be initially assessed as well cared for at home; however, these same people may not be able to read, to answer the assessment questions, or to explain that these are their only clean clothes and do not reflect their true living conditions. It is important that the PHN become culturally sensitive and aware of how cultural and religious norms affect specific or unique health concerns of clients. PHNs need to take a comprehensive and holistic approach in gathering data for their assessment and ensure someone is available to respond accurately to their questions. As well, PHNs must not assume that a client's nod of the head means that he or she understands what has been said. The client may just be anxious to please the health care provider or embarrassed to admit a lack of understanding. It is important for the PHN to follow up on the contacts the individual or family has with medical, social, and legal services to clarify what the client understands and to find answers to questions that have not been asked by the client or answered by the services.

The PHN is also an educator and counsellor. As an **educator**, the PHN identifies the client's learning needs and uses a variety of culturally appropriate and relevant teaching strategies to ensure that information received is information the client can use. The PHN identifies and analyzes the resources available in the community that would best meet the needs of the client. The PHN may have to revise or adapt an existing resource or may have to identify the most appropriate media channel to reach the target population. To this end, the PHN may have to develop skills and experience in video- and teleconferencing, arranging radio or TV presentations, creating online resources, and conducting marketing campaigns. As counsellors, PHNs need to encourage clients, reinforce their positive behaviours, and continually assess their needs in order to develop a relationship of mutual trust and respect and to help clients increase their knowledge and skills and adopt the behaviours necessary to manage their health and self-care.

A PHN uses an evidence-informed approach to practice when identifying the most effective strategies for changing health behaviours. **Evidence-informed practice** (previously known as *evidence-based practice*) is defined as combining the best evidence derived from research with clinical practice, knowledge and expertise, and unique client expectations, preferences, or choices when making clinical decisions (Canadian Nurses Association, 2002; Capital Health, 2010; Straus, Richardson, Glasziou, & Haynes, 2005). Along with education, the PHN plan will include strategies that focus on creating supportive environments, mobilizing the community, developing personal skills, and developing policies. PHNs act as direct primary caregivers in places such as public health clinics and in community activities such as new-baby visits. A **primary caregiver** is the health care provider most responsible for providing for the health care needs of clients. PHNs provide primary care where needed, as determined by community assessment. Such assessments identify gaps to which the private sector is unable to respond and also determine the impact the identified gap in services has on the health of the population. Examples of situations in which a PHN will provide primary care include the following:

- Prenatal services
- Postnatal visits to high-risk mothers
- Breastfeeding clinics
- Immunization services for targeted populations
- Directly observed therapy for clients with active tuberculosis (TB)
- Assessment and treatment for sexually transmitted infections (STIs)

PHNs take on multiple roles in emergency preparedness and planning. At a reception centre, for instance, a PHN may work as part of a team involved in assessing, planning, implementing, and evaluating needs and resources for the different populations being served by the centre. For example, if community members are forced to leave their homes following a tornado or flood, a PHN may be deployed to a reception centre to assess the health status of individuals entering the centre. There, the PHN may have to document clients' personal contact and medical information; develop a communication strategy to keep clients informed of the situation; identify health conditions (e.g., diabetes, heart disease, asthma); assess vital signs; monitor physical, emotional, and mental status; identify medication and diet needs, child or older adult care needs, and clothing and personal needs; and coordinate with community partners and agencies to meet these needs. Whether the disaster is local or national, small or large, natural or caused by humans, PHNs, as skilled professionals, provide services essential to the disaster response effort. As a health care facility, the local public health department has an emergency operations plan, as well as takes a role in the local, regional, and provincial or territorial disaster plans. PHNs' roles in emergency preparedness and relief include the following:

- Providing education that will prepare communities to cope with disasters
- Establishing mass dispensing clinics
- Conducting enhanced communicable disease surveillance
- Working with environmental health specialists to ensure safe food and water for disaster victims and emergency workers
- Serving on the local emergency planning committee

Essential and unique roles for PHNs exist in the area of communicable disease control. Community health nursing skills are necessary for education, prevention, surveillance, and outbreak investigation. PHNs can do the following:

- Find infected individuals
- Notify contacts
- Input findings into regional, territorial, or provincial databases
- Refer clients to other health care providers or agencies for care and treatment as needed
- Educate individuals, families, communities, professionals, and populations
- Act as advocates
- Provide resources to reduce the rate of communicable disease in the community

LEVELS OF PREVENTION

Related to Public Health Nursing

PRIMARY PREVENTION

- PHNs advocate for members of Parliament to address issues such as mandatory seat belt legislation, smoke-free environments, and universal access to health care.
- PHNs conduct ongoing disease surveillance for communicable diseases.

SECONDARY PREVENTION

- PHNs conduct contact tracing for individuals exposed to a client with an active case of TB or an STI. PHNs provide directly observed therapy (DOT) for clients with active TB.
- PHNs participate in screening programs for genetic disorders or metabolic deficiencies in newborns; breast, cervical, and testicular cancers; diabetes; hypertension; and sensory impairments in children, and ensure follow-up services for clients with positive test results.

TERTIARY PREVENTION

- PHNs provide case management services that link clients with chronic illnesses to health care and community support services.

The role of controlling communicable disease is one of the most important for public health nurses during disasters. For example, during the 2003 outbreak of severe acute respiratory syndrome (SARS), PHNs were key in contact tracing and in performing other activities that included, in some communities, screening potential clients at assessment clinics, providing local information and education using dedicated phone centres, and developing resources related to the containment and management of this communicable disease.

The Registered Nurses' Association of Ontario paper *Public Health Nursing: Nursing Practice in a Diverse Environment* (Laforet Fliesser, Schofield, & Yandreski, 2003) provides examples of the roles, functions, and settings of practice of public health nurses (see the Evolve Weblinks). A qualitative research study of PHNs in Nova Scotia titled *Fostering Citizen Participation and Collaborative Practice: Tapping the Wisdom and Voices of Public Health Nurses in Nova Scotia* (Meagher-Stewart et al., 2004) contributes to understanding public health nursing practice as it relates to areas such as primary health care, social justice, population health promotion, collaboration, and partnerships (see the Evolve Weblinks). For an additional resource about PHNs and other CHNs working in school health, see the Communities and Schools Promoting Health Weblink on the Evolve Web site.

OTHER COMMUNITY HEALTH NURSES

The field of community health nursing is expansive and includes many nurses with other designations who practise primary health care, such as forensic nurses, outpost nurses, primary health care nurse practitioners, street or outreach nurses, telenurses, corrections nurses, and nurse entrepreneurs.

The Forensic Nurse

Forensic nursing is an emerging specialty in Canadian community health nursing. Although the CNA does not currently offer certification for this specialty, forensic nurses have had their own interest group within the CNA since 2007 (Forensic Nurses' Society of Canada, 2008).

Forensic nurses work within four subspecialties—as forensic psychiatric nurses, forensic correctional nurses, forensic nurse examiners, or death investigators working with medical examiners (Kagan-Krieger & Rehfeld, 2000; Lynch, 2005). **Forensic nurses** are registered nurses who have additional education in forensic science in order to provide specialized care to persons who have experienced trauma or death from violence, criminal activity, or traumatic accidents (Lynch, 2005). These nurses may provide care in general or psychiatric hospitals, health science centres, correctional institutions, or clinics (Anderson, 2007). Forensic nurses work with victims and perpetrators of violence, especially sexual assault, criminal activity such as physical assault, and traumatic accidents such as suspicious injuries.

In Canada, forensic nurses primarily work as sexual assault nurse examiners (SANEs). The first SANE program began in Winnipeg, Manitoba, in 1993, and similar programs have since opened across Canada. In the absence of national standards of practice for SANEs, provincial and program standards have been developed using templates from the International Association of Forensic Nursing (IAFN) (Lynch, 2005).

Sexual assault nurse examiners are registered nurses who have completed specialized education in forensic science. They assume a wide range of roles and responsibilities in response to the physical, emotional, and psychological needs of persons who have experienced sexual assault, regardless of age or gender. SANEs provide crisis intervention, assess injuries, provide pregnancy prevention by offering the morning-after pill, test for and treat STIs, and collaborate with community partners (Kagan-Krieger & Rehfeld, 2000).

In 2000, Alberta established (in Edmonton) its first sexual assault response team, employing in the emergency department 11 nurses prepared as SANEs, who conduct sexual assault assessments and collect evidence using a sexual assault evidence kit (SAEK) (Kent, 2000). This kit is a standard tool to collect and handle forensic evidence of deoxyribonucleic acid (DNA). Collection must be completed in a timely and nonjudgemental manner, and SANEs must ensure impartial, precise, and credible documentation of personal assault injury for use in court. See the Reflective Praxis section at the end of this chapter for two case studies about forensic nursing, with questions raised for reflection. Additionally, the Antigonish Women's Resource Centre Web site (see Weblinks at the end of this chapter) provides further information about a SANE program.

The Outpost Nurse

Outpost nurses are registered nurses who work in a community health nursing role to provide comprehensive primary health care to clients in remote northern outpost communities (Misener et al., 2008; Tarlier, Johnson, & Whyte, 2003). These nurses usually have experience working in the community and may have additional education, such as a diploma in advanced practice as a primary health care nurse practitioner. Outpost nurses often work with diverse indigenous peoples. Based on data collected from the 2000/2001 Canadian Community Health Survey (CCHS), off-reserve Aboriginals residing in the territories (59%) were less likely to be seen by a doctor than non-Aboriginal people (76%) residing in the territories (Statistics Canada, 2002a). These off-reserve Aboriginals were more likely to contact a nurse (49%) than were the non-Aboriginal population (22%) living in the territories (Statistics Canada, 2002b). These findings indicate the importance of nursing stations to the

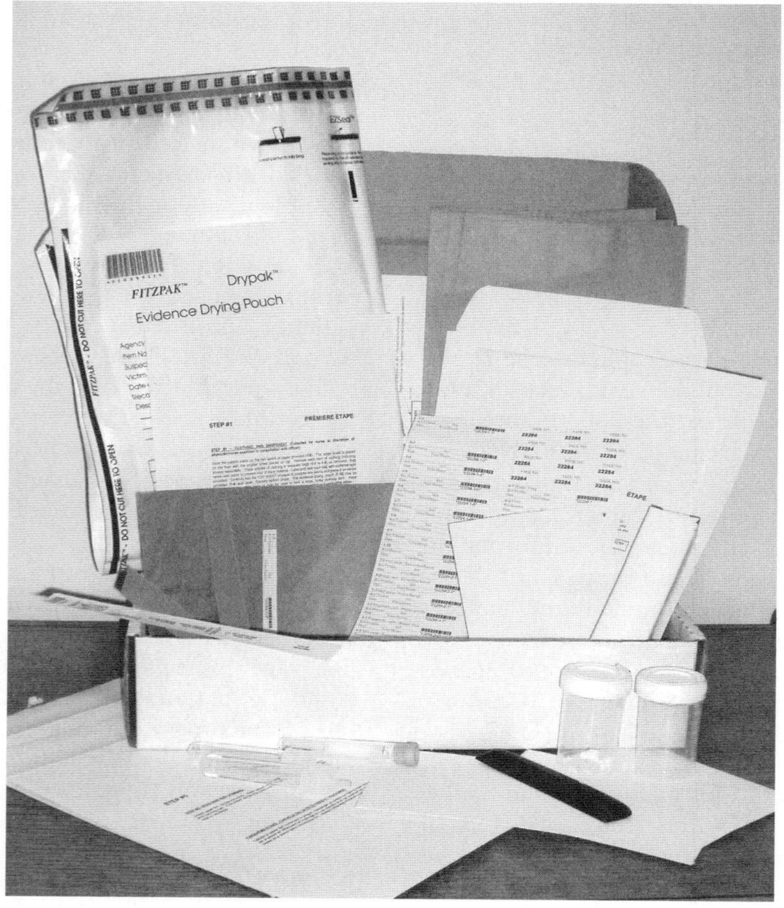

The sexual assault evidence kit includes the following to enable the collection of forensic evidence: bags to collect clothing; oral swabs; envelopes to collect fingernail scrapings or clippings; skin swabs; envelopes and a comb for collecting hair samples; blood and urine collection containers; envelopes for the collection of foreign matter (such as condoms and tampons); a comb and envelopes to collect pubic hair; external, vaginal, and rectal swabs; and a client DNA kit.

health of remote communities (PHAC, 2008). This geographically isolated practice area requires considerable independence and autonomy, with telephone backup available from physicians. Outpost nurses reside in the community where they provide care, and they actively involve community members in the planning and development of community health programs and strategies. Outpost nurses self-reported that they "work with individuals and communities to solve problems collaboratively within a spirit of partnership" (Misener et al., 2008, p. 57). They practise as generalists across the lifespan and have as their main focuses health promotion, disease prevention, medical diagnoses, and treatment of illness and injury (Misener et al., 2008). Additionally, they have on-call responsibilities and accompany clients who require evacuation. In an interpretative study by Tarlier, Johnson, and Whyte (2003), experienced outpost nurses described their community health nursing practice experiences in narrative form. The study findings led to the identification of the following four themes: (1) nurses evolve into the outpost role; (2) experienced outpost nurses build and maintain responsive relationships with the community; (3) primary care competencies are fundamental to outpost practice; and (4) experienced outpost nurses become comfortable with the autonomy and responsibility of practice. Box 3-6 summarizes some of the key study findings for each of the four themes. See the "Evidence-Informed Practice" box on the Evolve Web site discussing the Tarlier, Johnson, and Whyte (2003) research.

The Primary Health Care Nurse Practitioner

Nurse practitioners work collaboratively in health care teams. They are either acute care nurse practitioners (ACNPs) or primary health care nurse practitioners (PHCNPs). **Nurse practitioners** are registered nurses with a minimum of baccalaureate-level academic preparation and, in addition, advanced practice nursing education, usually at a master's degree level. ACNPs specialize in acute care areas, such as cardiology and oncology, and may provide care at the tertiary level of disease prevention in settings such as outpatient clinics.

In Canada, nurse practitioners function in advanced nursing practice roles (CNA, 2008b). In many provinces, in their advanced nursing practice roles, PHCNPs are authorized to independently carry out the following three additional controlled acts: prescribing drugs, ordering specific laboratory tests, and ordering radiographs and ultrasounds. PHCNPs' scope of practice includes assessment, diagnosis, and management of client care for common episodic conditions across the lifespan. These advanced-practice nurses work with families, implement health promotion and disease prevention strategies (primary, secondary, and some tertiary), and participate in community development and planning (Thrasher & Staples, 2005). Also, they manage and monitor clients with chronic illnesses who reside in either their own homes or in institutions such as long-term care facilities. Each province and territory has implemented or

BOX 3-6 Key Findings From Outpost Nurses Working in Northern Canada

1. Nurses evolve into the outpost role:
   - Need to adapt to diverse cultures
   - Need to adapt to geographical, personal, and professional isolation
   - Need to shift focus of care from acute to primary health
   - Need to engage in upstream thinking (i.e., "bigger picture")
2. Experienced outpost nurses build and maintain responsive relationships with the community:
   - Need to develop trust, respect, and acceptance with the community
   - Need to foster responsive relationships in order to effect positive community health outcomes
3. Primary care competencies are fundamental to outpost practice:
   - Need to have advanced assessment and treatment skills
   - Need to address episodic curative situations
   - Need to focus on teaching, supporting, and counselling skills to influence health outcomes
4. Experienced outpost nurses become comfortable with the autonomy and responsibility of practice:
   - Need to recognize and accept the extent of autonomy and responsibility for this practice setting
   - Need to recognize the complex interplay between "autonomy, authority, power, ethics, responsibility and reciprocity of relationships" (p. 183)

Source: Tarlier, D. S., Johnson, J. L. & Whyte, N. B. (2003). Voices from the wilderness: An interpretative study describing the role and practice of outpost nurses. *Canadian Journal of Public Health, 94*(3), 180–184.

is currently working on implementing nurse practitioner legislation and regulations and amendments to the nurses' acts to give these nurses the authority to independently perform additional controlled acts, such as prescribing certain medications and ordering particular diagnostic tests. It is important to note that nurse practitioners complement rather than replace the roles of other health care providers (CNA, 2008b). They work in collaboration with clients and with family physicians but practise autonomously. PHCNPs assume the roles of educator, health promoter, collaborator, researcher, consultant, and leader. Further information on nurse practitioner programs can be found at the Ontario Primary Health Care Nurse Practitioner Program and the College of Registered Nurses of British Columbia Evolve Weblinks. Additional information about nurse practitioners in Canada is found at the NPCanada.ca Evolve Weblink. The CNA report on advanced nursing practice Weblink on Evolve provides more detailed information about the clinical focus and impact of advanced nursing practice, which includes nurse practitioners. Key competency categories for Canadian nurse practitioners are found in Box 3-7.

The Street or Outreach Nurse

Street nurses are registered nurses with community health nursing experience. Often PHNs or nurse practitioners, these CHNs usually work in community health centres or public health units or authorities. Street or outreach nurses usually work with persons in urban centres who have difficulty accessing traditional health care services. These marginalized persons may be homeless, be substance abusers, or have mental illnesses (Self & Peters, 2005).

BOX 3-7 Canadian Nurse Practitioner Core Competency Categories: Family or All Ages Grouping

1. Health Assessment and Diagnosis
2. Health Care Management and Therapeutic Intervention
3. Health Promotion and Prevention of Illness, Injury, and Complication
4. Professional Role and Responsibility

SOURCE: Canadian Nurses Association. (2009). *Canadian nurse practitioner examination program.* Retrieved from http://www.cna-aiic.ca/CNA/nursing/npexam/exam/default_e.aspx.

Street or outreach nurses provide services such as first aid, counselling, referral to community resources such as food banks, testing for STIs, health education and promotion, and advocacy for social issues such as affordable housing, improved social programs to address poverty, and equitable access to health care. Cathy Crowe, a street or outreach nurse, has become well known for her work of more than 20 years in the Greater Toronto Area in Ontario. Her efforts as a social justice activist have earned her several awards, including the Atkinson Charitable Foundations Economic Justice Award, which funds efforts to reduce poverty (CNA, 2007), to further develop initiatives for the homeless in Toronto, and to advocate for national housing policies. The Ontario Ministry of Health and Long-Term Care Nursing Secretariat partnered with the Change Foundation and provided research funding to several researchers co-led by Dyanne Semogas and Ruta Valaitis to develop and evaluate a virtual community of practice for street nursing (McMaster University, 2008). In 2008, 120 members across Canada belonged to this virtual community (see the McMaster University Weblink on the Evolve Web site.) A virtual community of practice provides an opportunity for professionals with similar interests to explore and deal with shared issues or concerns through Web-based communication (Educause Learning Initiative, 2009; Valaitis, 2007). (The specific challenges associated with street nursing are described in the *Forecast Journal* and the Four Pillars Coalition Weblinks on the Evolve Web site. See the Street Health Weblink for a wealth of information about street/outreach nursing, including Cathy Crowe's newsletter.)

The Telenurse

In Canada, telenursing refers to the use of technology for triaging, delivering nursing care, and managing and coordinating health care and services using protocols (College of Nurses of Ontario, 2005; Lapierre, Blackmer, Coutu-Wakulczyk, & Dehoux, 2006). **Telehealth** is the broad term that refers to the use of a variety of technologies to deliver health care services over distance. These technologies include telephones, computers (information systems and the Internet), and teleconferencing using video and audio. **Telenurses** are registered nurses who require specific nursing knowledge and skill that includes enhanced assessment skills and strong clinical knowledge, which are necessary to provide nursing service to clients using only information technology (College of Nurses of Ontario, 2005; Goodwin, 2007).

Proven cost-effective in other countries such as the United States and Japan, telenursing is emerging rapidly in Canada, as it serves to address the accessibility and availability issues in our geographically vast country (Goodwin, 2007). CHNs working in telenursing use evidence-informed protocols and technology-based, standardized responses to address client health concerns. One of the challenges for telenurses is the fact that among their clients are persons travelling outside of their home province or territory, meaning telenurses frequently serve persons who are not in the same province or territory. Since provincial and territorial practice standards vary, possible liability issues arise. This state of cross-jurisdictional health care is being discussed across Canada. The College of Nurses of Ontario (2005) advises telenurses to ensure clear, complete documentation that demonstrates their decision making since they may be required to testify in another jurisdictional community (Goodwin, 2007). In 2003, the National Initiative for Telehealth (NIFTE) developed a framework of guidelines including telehealth policies, procedures, guidelines, and standards for various Canadian health care provider organizations (NIFTE, 2003). The guidelines and principles for telenursing practice standards developed by the College of Registered Nurses of British Columbia and the College of Registered Nurses of Nova Scotia can be found in Weblinks on the Evolve Web site.

The Corrections Nurse

Corrections nurses are registered nurses who work in correctional facilities providing community health nursing interventions that include direct care, health promotion, disease prevention, inmate advocacy, and crisis intervention (Kearley & Steeves, 2010). Their focus of care is on promotion of health. Corrections nurses abide by the *Canadian Community Health Nursing Standards of Practice* and consider the "community" in their case to be the correctional setting. A challenge corrections nurses face is ensuring the safety and security of all clients, including both correctional staff and inmates, at all times prior to health care delivery (Cox, 2008). Some of the other challenges of working with this population include maintaining dignity, confidentiality, and therapeutic relationships; dealing with complex clients because of client vulnerabity due to aging and a lack of awareness of health concerns; and trying to act as a client advocate in a correctional setting (Cox, 2008; Smith, 2005). Corrections nursing requires psychiatric, forensic, occupational health, and communicable and infectious disease interventions. Corrections nurses work autonomously but collaborate with corrections facility employees and other health care providers.

The Nurse Entrepreneur

The **nurse entrepreneur** is a registered nurse who is self-employed in the provision of nursing services to clients in the home or in a variety of settings such as workplaces, government agencies, not-for-profit agencies, and private businesses. Nurse entrepreneurs may be generalists (e.g., a primary health care nurse practitioner working in an independent practice) or specialists (e.g., a nurse offering foot-care clinics).

In 1996, the CNA responded to requests from nurses for direction on being self-employed by releasing a Nursing Now resource titled *On Your Own—The Nurse Entrepreneur* (CNA, 1996). Nurse entrepreneurs were said to work in independent practice and be owners of businesses providing nursing services in areas such as advocacy (e.g., for clients requiring assistive devices), health promotion (e.g., stress management), direct care (e.g., wound therapy), education (e.g., workshops for groups), research (e.g., exploration of the role of lactation consultants in home care), administration (e.g., quality assurance in an agency), and consultation (e.g., workplace health policy) (CNA, 1996). A CHN choosing to work as a nurse entrepreneur is usually precipitated by changing health care needs, often as a result of changing demographics, economic constraints resulting in health care spending cutbacks, and consumer demand for access to alternative health care provider options to replace or supplement available health care resources.

The College of Nurses of Ontario (2009) identifies the following key practice components for nurse entrepreneurs to consider:

- Scope of service
- Conflict of interest
- Endorsement
- Advertising
- Fees
- Informed consent
- Documentation
- Confidentiality
- Other issues and resources (business considerations)

RURAL SETTINGS FOR COMMUNITY HEALTH NURSES

Within the past decade, the health of rural Canadians has captured the attention of researchers, government, and health care advocates, primarily as a result of research demonstrating the specific health needs of this population (Bollman, 2003; DesMeules et al., 2006). Several reports identify and address rural health issues, including *The Federal Role in Rural Health* (Government of Canada, 2000), *Building on Values: The Future of Health Care in Canada* (Romanow, 2002), *How Healthy Are Rural Canadians?* (DesMeules et al., 2006), and *Rural and*

Remote Nursing Practice Parameters: Discussion Document (Canadian Association for Rural & Remote Nursing, 2008). The Nursing Practice in Rural and Remote Canada and the Centre for Rural and Northern Health Research Weblinks on the Evolve Web site provide a more detailed listing of publications and presentations on issues pertaining to rural and remote health care in Canada.

Accessibility to health care in rural areas is related to geographical distance from urban centres (DesMeules et al., 2006; Herbert, 2007). In rural areas of Canada, residents usually live in poorer socioeconomic conditions; attain lower levels of formal education; have less healthy personal health practices (e.g., increased smoking, unhealthy eating, sedentary lifestyle); and suffer increased overall mortality rates than urban Canadians (DesMeules et al., 2006). However, residents in rural areas of Canada experience less stress and perceive a stronger sense of community belonging (DesMeules et al., 2006). Although the many health needs of rural populations are not all unique, they differ from those of **urban** populations. Urban populations live in geographical areas described as nonrural and having a higher population density. The 2000/2001 Statistics Canada *Canadian Community Health Survey* provides data that can be used to compare crucial health indicators between rural and urban areas in Canada (see Box 3-8). Research data suggest that rural people have increased health risks such as being overweight or obese, higher rates of smoking, higher prevalence of heart disease, higher than average likelihood of mental illness (especially depression), and higher than average incidence of hypertension and arthritis (Bollman, 2003; Pitblado, Managhan, Houle, Pong, & Lapalme, 1996).

BOX 3-8 Some Canadian Rural Health Data Compared to Urban Health Data

Rural Canada differs from urban Canada in the following ways:

- Mortality rates due to motor vehicle injuries for all ages are two to three times higher.
- Farmers, fishermen, and loggers have higher levels of occupational hazards.
- Residents under 20 years of age have the highest risk of dying from suicide.
- Incidence of cancer for rural men and women is lower.
- Mortality rates for specific cancers (e.g., breast cancer in women over 45 years of age) are lower.
- Cervical cancer incidence and mortality rates are higher for women in some specific rural areas.
- Mortality rates from lung cancer in men between 45 and 64 years of age are higher.
- Mortality rates from lung cancer in women did not differ between 45 and 64 years of age.
- Mortality rates from circulatory diseases in men are higher.
- Mortality rates from respiratory disease in men are higher.

SOURCE: DesMeules, M., Pong, R., Lagace, C., Heng, D., Manual, D., Pitblado, R., Koren, I. (2006). *How healthy are rural Canadians? An assessment of their health status and health determinants.* Ottawa, ON: Canadian Institute for Health Information. Retrieved from http://secure.cihi.ca/cihiweb/products/summary_rural_canadians_2006_e.pdf.

Historically, care of the sick in small communities was provided by informal social support systems. When self-care and family care did not bring about healing, healing women who lived in the community were called in. For generations, a scarcity of health care providers, poverty, limited access to services, illiteracy, and social isolation have plagued many rural communities and contributed to poor health.

Ninety-five percent of Canada's land mass is considered rural (Ministerial Advisory Council on Rural Health, 2002), and approximately 22% of the total population (about 6.6 million) resides in Canada's rural settings (MacLeod et al., 2004a). Many different definitions of *rural* exist, resulting in an ongoing debate for a universally acceptable definition (Baumann, Hunsberger, Blythe, & Crea, 2006; Herbert, 2007). Generally, **rural** is defined either in terms of the geographical location and population density or the distance from or the time needed (e.g., 40 km or 30 minutes) to commute to an urban centre. Some consider rural to be a state of mind. For the more affluent, *rural* may call to mind images of a recreational, retirement, or resort community located in the mountains or in lake country where one can relax and participate in outdoor activities, such as skiing, fishing, hiking, and hunting. For those with fewer resources, the term can evoke grim scenes.

Travelling time and distance to ambulatory care services affect access to care for both rural and urban residents. For rural people, the difficulty may result from the distance they must travel; for urban people, it may not result from the distance as much as from the travel time due to traffic. Both groups tend to spend the same length of time waiting once they arrive at a clinic or physician's office.

Rural health care providers usually live and practise in a particular community for decades, and they may provide care to people who live in several surrounding districts. A limited number of CHNs such as PHNs or nurse practitioners may offer a full range of services for residents in a specified area, which may span more than 150 km. Consequently, rural physicians and CHNs provide care to individuals and families with all kinds of conditions, in all stages of life, and across several generations.

Within the past decade, research on RNs working in rural and remote Canada has become available. In a national survey exploring nursing practice in rural and remote Canada, questionnaires were sent to nurses residing in rural areas in each of the provinces, nurses working in outpost settings, and nurses working in the Yukon, Northwest Territories, and Nunavut. Their practice areas were divided as follows: acute care (39%), long-term care (17%), community health (14%), home care (8%), primary care (7%), and other (16%), which included areas such as education, administration, research, and government (Stewart et al., 2005). This research study yielded several fact sheets providing statistical information on rural and remote nursing in Canada, including the following: *How Many Registered Nurses Are There in Rural and Remote Canada?*; *What Educational Preparation Do Nurses Need for Practice in Rural and Remote Canada?*; *RNs in Nurse Practitioner Positions in Rural and Remote Canada*; *Aboriginal Nurses in Rural and Remote Canada*; and *Nurses and First Nations and Inuit Community-Managed Primary Health Care Services* (Nursing Practice in Rural and Remote Canada, 2006). These *Nursing Practice in Rural and Remote Canada* fact sheets are found in the Weblinks on the Evolve Web site. It is important to note that until recently there has been a paucity of research available on community health nursing practice in rural and remote settings. Fortunately, this trend is changing.

BOX 3-9 Rural and Remote Settings: Possible Community Health Nursing Challenges

- Autonomous practice with minimal support (MacLeod et. al., 2004a)
- Complex and variable situations (MacLeod et. al., 2004a)
- Limited number of clinical support resources (MacLeod et. al., 2004a)
- Increased demand for functioning in an expanded role (MacLeod et. al., 2004a)
- Difficulty maintaining the nursing workforce (MacLeod et. al., 2004a)
- Difficulty separating personal and professional roles (MacLeod et. al., 2004a)
- Fewer nurses per capita (CNA, 2005)
- Additional recruitment and retention challenges due to isolation or lack of urban amenities (CNA, 2005)
- Limited opportunity for involvement in research (MacLeod, Kulig, Stewart, & Pitblado, 2004b) and more effort required to obtain information about evidenced-informed practice

Community Health Nursing in Rural Settings

In underserved rural areas, gaps usually exist in the continuum of mental health services, which, ideally, should include preventive education, anticipatory guidance, early intervention programs, crisis and acute care services, and follow-up care. As with other aspects of health care, CHNs in rural areas play an important role in community health education, case finding, advocacy, and case management. Although rewarding, the experience of living and working as a CHN in a rural or remote area is complex and presents many challenges (Canadian Association for Rural and Remote Nursing, 2008; Schwartz, 2002). Some of these challenges are outlined in Box 3-9.

Four high-risk industries found primarily in rural areas are forestry, mining, fishing, and agriculture. Rural CHNs need to know the exposures and hazards within their communities and refer to the most recent research evidence in order to advocate and initiate appropriate nursing strategies to maintain and promote health and prevent diseases.

Barriers to health care may include the availability, accessibility, affordability, and acceptability of services and health care providers to rural clients. *Availability* implies that health care services exist and employ the necessary personnel to provide the services. The sparseness of a population limits the number and array of health care services offered in a given geographical region since the cost of providing special services to a few people often is prohibitive. Additionally, where services and personnel are scarce, they must be allocated wisely. *Accessibility* implies that a person has logistical access to, as well as the ability to purchase, needed services. Associated with both availability and accessibility of care, *affordability* implies that services come at a reasonable cost and that a family has sufficient resources to purchase them when needed. *Acceptability* of care means that a particular service is appropriate and offered in a manner that corresponds with the values of a target population. Acceptability can be hampered by both the client's cultural preference and the urban orientation of health professions (see Box 3-10).

Providers' attitudes, insights, and knowledge about rural populations are important to their success in working with those populations. A demeaning attitude, lack of accurate knowledge about rural populations, or insensitivity about the rural lifestyle can diminish a CHN's ability to relate to clients. Moreover, insensitivity generates mistrust, which may cause rural clients to view

BOX 3-10 Barriers to Health Care in Rural Areas

- Need to travel great distances to obtain services
- Lack of personal transportation
- Unavailable public transportation
- Lack of telephone services
- Unavailable outreach services
- Unpredictable weather and travel conditions
- Lack of know-how to procure entitlements and services
- Poor provider attitudes and understanding about rural populations
- Language barriers (caregivers not linguistically competent)
- Lack of culturally appropriate care and services

health care providers as outsiders to the community. On the other hand, some rural health care providers express feelings of being professionally isolated and perceive community nonacceptance. In addressing these rural issues, nursing faculty members can expose students in community health nursing courses to the rural environment by offering rural clinical experiences to help these future health care professionals gain insight about rural community health nursing practice.

CHNs need to have an accurate understanding of rural clients. To design community health programs that are available, accessible, affordable, and appropriate, CHNs need to plan strategies and implement interventions that mesh with clients' belief systems. The implication, then, is that a family and a community actively contribute to the planning and delivery of care for a member who needs it. Although the importance of forming partnerships and ensuring mutual exchange seems obvious, most research about rural communities has been for policy or reimbursement purposes. Currently, minimal empirical data are available about rural family systems in terms of their health beliefs, values, perceptions of illness, health care–seeking behaviours, and beliefs about what constitutes appropriate care. Therefore, CHNs need to assume a more active role in promoting research on the nursing needs of rural populations to expand the profession's theoretical base and subsequently implement empirically based clinical interventions.

Because of the distance, isolation, and sparse resources they encounter, rural residents often develop independent and creative ways to cope. Some prefer to seek help through their informal networks, such as neighbours, extended family, church, and civic clubs, before seeking care from a health care provider. CHNs describe some interesting differences between working in rural areas and urban ones. The boundaries between their home and work roles may blur in that the rural CHN is more likely than the urban CHN to go to the same church, shop at the same stores, and have children in the same schools as their clients. Thus, CHNs personally know many, if not all, clients as neighbours, friends, immediate family members, or part of their extended family. Small towns foster both a social informality and a corresponding lack of anonymity. Some rural CHNs say, "I never really feel like I am off duty because everybody in the area knows me through my work." In part, this may be because community members highly regard CHNs and view them as experts on health and illness. Residents may ask health-related questions when they see the CHN in a grocery store, at a service station, at a basketball game, or at church functions. Rural CHNs may also be expected to know something about everything, and this can be demanding. Some of the challenges of rural nursing practice are professional isolation, difficulty separating personal and professional roles, limited opportunities for continuing education, heavy workloads, having to function well in several clinical areas, and the lack of anonymity (MacLeod et al., 2004a; Tarlier et al., 2003). Many CHNs value the close relationships they develop with clients and co-workers, the diverse clinical experiences that evolve from caring for clients of all ages with a variety of health concerns, the ability to care for clients for long periods (in some cases, across several generations), greater autonomy, and the pleasures of living in a rural area. CHNs can often keep a finger on the pulse of the community by becoming active in the political, social, religious, and employment activities that affect their clients, and they can work toward change, act as community educators, and educate others how to find resources and services.

In summary, considering the unique characteristics of rural communities, strategies such as the following are needed to build rural and remote community health nursing practice capacity:

- Ensuring policymakers and managers of community health nursing organizations appreciate CHNs' practice realities
- Developing and implementing interprofessional practice models that build on the varied assets and community resources
- Involving CHNs working in Aboriginal communities in the development of strategies
- Implementing ways of ensuring continuity of care and culturally appropriate care in Aboriginal communities
- Ensuring undergraduate and postgraduate educational programs prepare nursing students for the realities of community health nursing practice

- Strategically planning continuing education opportunities (e.g., using information technology such as NurseONE)
- Addressing the issue of CHNs leaving rural communities
- Improving identifiers used in databases so that rural and remote settings can be distinguished (MacLeod et al., 2004a; Stewart et al., 2005)

CONCEPTS OF CASE MANAGEMENT

In Canada, case management is a strategy used primarily in community care. Case management settings may include home care (community care access centres [CCACs]), the Workplace Safety and Insurance Board, the Canadian Forces (Canadian Forces Case Management Program), mental health (Mental Health Case Management Association of Ontario), and Veterans Affairs Canada. Case managers may assume roles such as clinician or direct care provider, collaborator, liaison, facilitator, advocate, coordinator, manager, educator, or researcher. In addition, Smith and colleagues (Smith, Smith, Newhook, & Hobson, 2006) identify the roles of negotiator, monitor, and supporter. Various models of case management exist.

Historical Perspective

Canada's case management strategy, influenced by the movement in the United States, where case management was primarily community-based (e.g., home care services), was driven by the need to reduce health care spending while at the same time maintain and improve the quality of client care (Canadian Home Care Association, 2005; Cawthorn, 2006; Daiski, 2000; Petryshen & Petryshen, 1992; Smith et al., 2006). In the 1990s, fiscal constraints, partly due to the decreased transfer payments from the federal to the provincial governments, led to restructuring within the health care system (Daiski, 2000). Other changes to contain health care costs, such as a new emphasis on early hospital discharge to community care and a reduction in the length of time for provision of home care services, led to a need for increased coordination to ensure continuity of care. Many other changes to further control health care costs were also implemented, including a reduction in the number of nurses in the workforce. These factors, along with limited resources, led to the creation of the new strategy referred to as *case management*. CHNs and other health care team members involved in facilitating access to and coordinating care acquired the new title of *case manager*, and the delivery of services became known as *managed care* (Daiski, 2000). Though case management took different forms across Canada, it consistently focused on the advocacy role (Canadian Home Care Association, 2005).

Case management models are being applied in communities across Canada. Home care services serve as an example of a case management model and include community access centres in Ontario and Saskatchewan and continuing care programs in Nova Scotia. In Ontario, for example, CCACs organize access to long-term care, arrange and authorize visiting health care and personal support services in people's homes, authorize services for special needs children in schools, authorize admissions to long-term care homes, and provide information and referrals to the public about other community agencies and services (Ministry of Health and Long-Term Care, 2006). In Saskatchewan, Client/Patient Access Services provides similar community access services to client groups. In Nova Scotia, continuing care programs provide a range of services to people in their homes and in facility care settings. (For information about these programs, see the Weblinks for the Ontario New Community Care Access Centres, Saskatoon Health Region, and Nova Scotia Department of Health Continuing Care Programs on the Evolve Web site.) The case manager advocates for the client, advises the client, coordinates and facilitates access to suitable health care services in a timely manner, and ensures continuity of care for the client.

Definitions of Case Management

The literature uses numerous definitions of *case management*. In this chapter, the definition used for *case management* is that of the Canadian Home Care Association (2005): "a collaborative client-driven strategy for the provision of quality health and support services through the effective and efficient use of available resources in order to support the client's achievement of goals related to healthy life and living in the context of the person and their ability" (p. 13). Smith et al. (2006) further define *case management* as a strategy to improve accessibility and continuity of client care that includes the incorporation of assessment, planning, coordination, delivery, and monitoring of the health care services made available to the client as individual and family. In 2006, the National Case Management Network of Canada was established. The network stated that case management "is a collaborative, client driven process for the provision of quality health and support services through the effective and efficient use of resources" (National Case Management Network of Canada, 2006, p. 1).

Regardless of the definition and implementation of case management, all CHNs using case management strategies will perform the following central activities: targeting, assessment, care planning, implementation, monitoring, and reassessment (Smith et al., 2006) (see Table 3-5). Their clients are usually individuals experiencing complex health challenges that require long-term interventions and various health care services.

The following are examples of the knowledge and skills required in a case management role in the community:

- Knowledge of community resources and ability to identify best resources for the desired outcomes
- Knowledge and skills to apply the referral process
- Written and oral communication skills that facilitate collaboration
- Negotiation and conflict-resolution skills

TABLE 3-5 Case Management Central Activities With Examples

Case Management Central Activities	Description of Activities	Examples of Activities
Targeting	The identification of clients who require case management services	A hospital discharge planner refers the client to a community care access centre case manager, who then contacts the chronic care client and family in the community. An occupational health nurse in industry makes a referral to the Workplace Safety and Insurance Board case manager, who then contacts the client.
Assessment	The process used to gather relevant assessment data appropriate to the client situation in order to establish client health concerns and to prioritize services required; interdisciplinary team assessments are ideal and therefore encouraged	The CHN, physiotherapist, occupational therapist, physician, and social worker conduct physical, cognitive, psychosocial, functional, caregiver support system, and financial assessments in the home to determine the client's health concerns and the community services required. The CHN conducts an assessment focused on how to facilitate a client's return to work based on the client's abilities, disabilities, the client's health concerns, and the available community resources required.
Care planning	The integration of assessment data into an interdisciplinary plan of care so that client health concerns are addressed through the appropriate use of services and resources	Based on individualized client assessment data and knowledge of available services and resources, the case manager develops an interdisciplinary care plan.
Implementation	The carrying out of the care plan through arrangements made with formal and informal support systems to provide the required services to the client; the case manager approves services, assigns resources, and coordinates care	The case manager approves services such as Meals on Wheels and home care and assigns resources such as a home care visiting nurse, homemaker, and physiotherapist. The case manager approves services such as return-to-work programs and assigns resources such as an ergonomist, occupational therapist, and physiotherapist.
Monitoring	The observation of the client situation for changes and the observation of the services provided to ensure that required client outcomes will be met	The case manager monitors the client situation, services, and resources for changes since all systems are dynamic. In this manner, the case manager can respond quickly to changes as needed.
Reassessment	A review of the extent to which goals have been met and of the effectiveness of the plan that has been implemented; also, in consultation with other team members (including the client as a team member), the identification of services still required and of any other changes needed	Keeping resources in mind, case managers review client situations in consultation with the client, family, and service providers. The case manager assesses the client's situation on a regular basis and makes changes to the care plan as needed. For example, if a caregiver becomes ill, additional services and resources may be required. If a new informal support person comes to reside with the client, then certain services and resources may no longer be needed.

SOURCE: Based on Smith, D. L., Smith, J. E., Newhook, C., & Hobson, B. (2006). Continuity of care, service integration, and case management. In J. M. Hibberd and D. L. Smith (Eds.), *Nursing leadership and management in Canada* (3rd ed., pp. 94–95). Toronto, ON: Elsevier.

- Critical-thinking processes to identify and prioritize health concerns from the provider and client views
- Skill in the application of evidence-informed practice in provision of care
- Advocacy skills
- Knowledge and skill in the application of discharge planning
- Knowledge and skill in meeting the legal and professional requirements when documenting and reporting

A CHN seeking a case manager position must develop some additional skills and knowledge through academic programs, orientation, and mentoring experiences.

Case management practice is complex because of the need for *coordinating*, that is, the assembling and directing of the activities of multiple providers and settings throughout a client's continuum of care so that all providers and aspects of care function harmoniously. Care by many (the client, the family, significant others, and community organizations) must be assessed, planned, implemented, adjusted, and based on mutually agreed-upon goals. Although the CHN may be employed and located in one setting, he or she influences the selection and monitoring of care provided in other settings by both formal and informal care providers. When geography presents access challenges, case management activities may be delivered via telephone, e-mail, fax, and video-conferencing in a client's location.

Some examples of case management activities include the application of screening tools to determine eligibility based on agency or program goals and objectives; the organization of and participation in interdisciplinary, individual, and family conferences to identify and monitor client health concerns; negotiation and advocacy on behalf of the client; the coordination of service delivery in the community; and the monitoring of costs of supplies, equipment, and other resources needed for care delivery.

Case management in rural settings is often more complex than in urban settings, partly because of differences in values and beliefs, geographical challenges, differences in social organization, and fewer available community services and resources. Box 3-11 provides examples of the knowledge and skills case managers suggest contribute to their satisfaction and effectiveness when working in rural settings.

Case Manager Tools

Case management has evolved with the introduction of a variety of case management tools that include critical pathways, multidisciplinary action plans, nursing care plans, and care pathways. Care pathways may be referred to as care maps, critical paths, integrated care pathways, and care profiles. It is generally accepted in the literature that *care pathways* are tools that map out the direction of care for clients experiencing specific medical diagnoses (Atwal & Caldwell, 2002; Currie & Harvey, 2000; Grubnic, 2003; Rees, Huby, McDade, & McKechnie, 2004). Care pathways outline the care management steps, with an aim to improve

BOX 3-11 Knowledge and Skills Case Managers Need to Work Effectively with Rural Clients

- Become familiar with the community and its resources including the residents and their health care beliefs and practices.
- Build a rapport with clients and develop strategies to improve communication with the client system (such as family members).
- Demonstrate empathy, respect, genuineness, and commitment in all client interactions, including those with the client system, even if there are conflicting views.
- Promote growth and development of the client as individual and family.
- Coordinate client services to support client autonomy and self-esteem.
- Promote client-to-client support through efforts such as self-help groups and one-to-one client interactions.
- Create channels of client communication that are open and supportive and that respond to changing client situations by involving the client as partner.
- Ensure prompt follow-up of referrals and discharges. Provide extra support to clients who require additional physical and emotional assistance by arranging home visiting and using various channels of communication. The discharge plan should consider transportation and communication challenges.
- Ensure and respect confidentiality with rural clients, who most often know each other well, and involve the clients (individual and family) in exploring creative ways to maintain confidentiality.
- Be a role model by always acting in a caring, professional manner in all work and social encounters. Also, always convey a commitment to and respect for the client as individual, family, and community.

Source: Bushy, A. (2003). Case management: Considerations for working with diverse rural client systems. *Lippincott's Case Management, 8*(5), 214.

CRITICAL VIEW

1. To what extent do the case management programs available in your community meet the needs of the community?
2. a) Which case management tools are used in your community?
   b) What are the advantages and disadvantages of the use of these tools in your community?

efficiency and the outcomes of care and to contribute to a high quality of nursing care (Canadian Hospice Palliative Care Association, 2006; Daiski, 2000).

CONTINUITY OF CARE

The ability to provide a continuum of care has been hindered by the closure of many small hospitals in the past two decades and the possible continuation of this trend. This trend further supports the need for CHNs to build and sustain strong community partnerships that include clients. The roles of the CHN as discharge planner and referral agent facilitate the provision of continuity of care to clients, so it is important for CHNs to become familiar with the principles and steps of the referral process. CHNs need to always consider the resources and client barriers in the referral process and initiate appropriate actions to facilitate a seamless referral to community agencies.

Discharge Planning

Discharge planning is not a new concept; yet, as Pringle stated (as cited in Cawthorn, 2006), models for discharge planning remain scarce, with few currently in development. The integrated model of discharge planning (IMDP) has been developed and is in the early research stages (Cawthorn, 2006; Wells, LeClerc, Craig, Martin, & Marshall, 2002). **Discharge planning** is a process that connects clients and services to ensure continuity of care between hospital and community (Nurses Association of New Brunswick, 2002). Discharge planning, which requires interdisciplinary collaboration, aims to maximize the quality of care so that the transfer of clients from hospital to community is smooth and capitalizes on the available health care resources (Nurses Association of New Brunswick, 2002).

Currently, most hospital clients are discharged early and require a variety of community supports to prevent unnecessary hospital readmission; they benefit from the continuity of care facilitated by discharge planning.

A qualitative research study exploring the perceptions of nurse case managers, social workers, and paraprofessionals about their discharge planning experiences revealed that they frequently assumed the role of advocate for clients and their families affected by shorter lengths of stay in hospital (Corser, 2003). This advocacy role was necessary to support clients' interests when conflict existed between their clients' needs and the expectations of other health care providers or the health care system. Participants identified and viewed as essential to their advocate role the following three major strategies: (1) interacting with clients and families, (2) interacting with other health care providers, and (3) working through the system (Corser, 2003).

Bushy (2003) provides the following insights into considerations that a case manager working in a rural area needs to take into account so that meaningful discharge planning occurs: distance to travel, sufficient time assigned to the CHN to fulfill the role of case manager, weather, and geographical challenges. Bushy (2003) emphasizes the importance of collaboration and increased communication with all relevant multidisciplinary health care providers and the family to facilitate appropriate discharge planning for a rural client and family when a referral is made.

Referral Process

The **referral process** is the process of directing a client to another source of assistance when the client or CHN is unable to address the client's issue (Maurer & Smith, 2009). Hospital discharge planning frequently requires referral to community services; therefore, the discharge planner needs to be familiar both with the referral process, that is, the principles and steps necessary to ensure an efficacious referral, and with the available community resources. Table 3-6 provides a list of the principles and steps in the referral process. The CHN needs to be aware that resource and client barriers may exist that prevent the use of the referral process (see Table 3-7).

The discharge planner often works with a community case manager to facilitate the transition of the client into the community. The client and family as partners need to be included in this process. Regardless of their area of community practice, CHNs most likely use the referral process.

There are many settings, functions, and roles for CHNs. To maintain a holistic focus in their community health nursing practice, CHNs must raise questions when working in and with a community. Following are some questions for CHNs to consider:

- What do I know about this community?
- What do I *not* know about this community but need to know?

TABLE 3-6 The Principles and Steps of the Referral Process

Principles	Steps
There should be merit in the referral.	Establish a working relationship with the client.
The referral should be practical.	Establish the need for a referral.
The referral should be individualized to the client.	Set objectives for the referral.
The referral should be timely.	Explore the availability of resources.
The referral should be coordinated with other activities.	The client decides to use or not to use referral.
The referral should incorporate the client and family into planning and implementing.	Make referral to available resources.
The client should have the right to refuse the referral.	Facilitate the referral. Evaluate client progress. Follow up with the client.

SOURCE: Clemen-Stone, S., McGuire, S. L., & Eigsti, D.G. (1998). *Comprehensive community health nursing: Family, aggregate, and community practice.* St. Louis, MO: Mosby, pp. 271–272, 274–280.

TABLE 3-7 Resource and Client Barriers to the Use of the Referral Process

Resource Barriers	Examples
Attitude of health care provider	The health care provider uses medical terminology without explanation, answers client questions abruptly, or shows an attitude of disrespect and a lack of courtesy in client interactions.
Physical accessibility of resources	The local clinic has limited hours of access (e.g., daytime-only hours); transportation costs to get there are high due to distance.
Cost of resource services	Client perceives a referral to a specialist as prohibitive because of having heard that the recommended treatments (e.g., medications) are extremely costly and not covered by a health plan.
Client Barriers	**Examples**
Priorities	Client values preventive health services (e.g., dental care) less than meeting the basic needs for food, shelter, and clothing.
Motivation	Client is aware of a need for care but is not ready to accept the suggested intervention and take action (e.g., client who has been referred to a dietitian for weight loss acknowledges the need to lose weight but does not follow through with the scheduled appointment).
Previous experience	Client has had a negative experience with a community service or with a resources professional (e.g., for safety reasons, a child has been removed from the home by a community agency).
Lack of knowledge about available resources	Adequate information has not been provided (e.g., services available through genetic counselling).
Lack of understanding regarding need for referral	Client does not realize the importance and the consequences of the suggested referral (e.g., a sexually active teenage female may know that a Papanicolaou test is important and may not understand the possible consequences if this test is not done as recommended; she may therefore not follow through on the referral to her family physician or sexual health clinic).
Client self-image	A client with a low self-image avoids seeking care because of feelings of unworthiness.
Cultural factors	A client who has recently immigrated to Canada has different beliefs and values about health care practices and preventive health activities so resists seeing another health care provider.
Finances	A client does not have the monetary resources necessary to obtain equipment, supplies, or services (e.g., cannot pay for an assistive device such as a motorized wheelchair).
Accessibility	A client cannot access the necessary care because of limited available services or health care professionals—rural settings, in particular, are often underserviced.

SOURCE: Adapted from Clemen-Stone, S., McGuire, S. L., & Eigsti, D. G. (1998). *Comprehensive community health nursing: Family, aggregate, and community practice.* St. Louis, MO: Mosby.

- What determinants of health are relevant to this community?
- What are some possible determinants of health relevant to population health?
- What possible population health issues exist for this community?
- What are the epidemiological considerations and community issues?
- How can I use the available evidence to inform my nursing practice?
- What is the sociopolitical and cultural environment?
- What are the ecological considerations?
- Are there any ethical issues that I need to consider and address?
- Given the setting I work in, what nursing roles might I assume as a community health nurse?
- What health promotion issues need to be addressed in this community and for populations, aggregates, individuals, and families?

CRITICAL VIEW

1. As a community health nurse, what additional questions would you consider that would address social justice issues?
2. What is the rationale for each of the previously stated questions and for your newly developed questions?

Figure 3-2 illustrates the broad range of community health nursing specialty areas, settings, and roles when working with the client and some key concepts used in community health nursing practice. In summary, community health nursing involves working with a variety of clients, fulfilling varying roles, and practising in diverse settings, the extent of which are determined by the area of specialty under the umbrella term *community health nursing*. Community health nursing requires knowledge and skills in concepts such as primary health care and population health; health promotion and levels of prevention; determinants of health; equity and social justice; epidemiology; and evidence-informed practice.

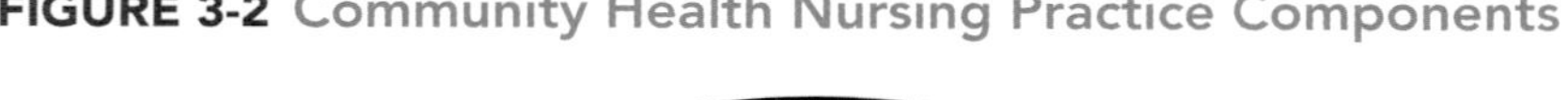

FIGURE 3-2 Community Health Nursing Practice Components

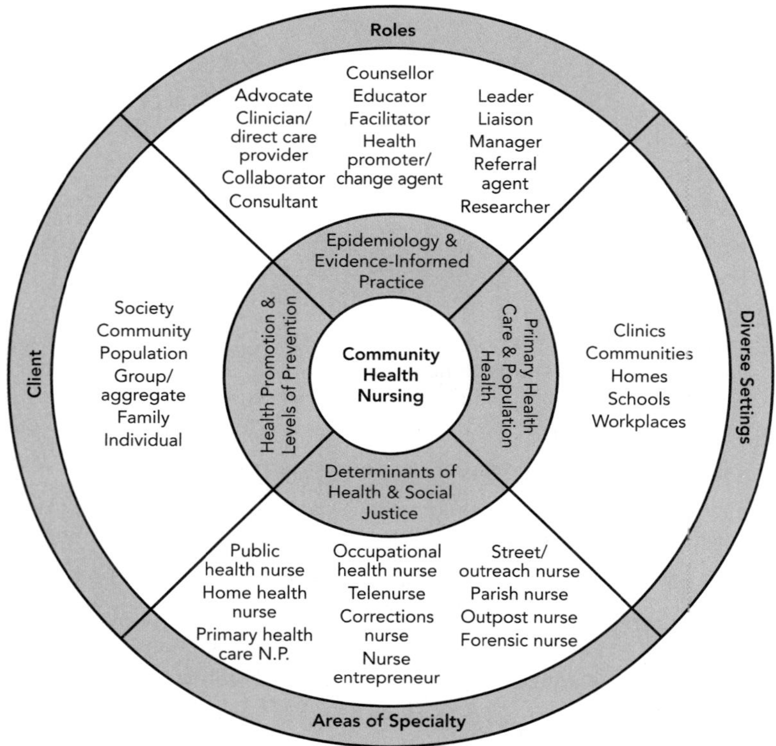

STUDENT EXPERIENCE

A Day in the Life of a Community Health Nurse

The Evolve Web site for this chapter includes blogs* by a variety of community health nurses about their typical day of practice. These community health nurses work in a variety of urban and rural settings, including a public health unit, a home care agency (e.g., Victorian Order of Nurses or Community Care Access), a workplace, and an outpatient clinic. As you read these seven blogs, you will identify and compare their roles, functions, and scope of practice, and relate their experience to your readings from your textbook. Select two of the blogs to use in answering the following questions:

1. Describe the clinical setting of this community health nurse.
2. What are the educational qualifications for this CHN position?
3. What are examples of this CHN's activities that demonstrate the three levels of prevention (if applicable)?
4. What roles does this CHN have?
5. How do this CHN's roles differ from acute-based nursing practice roles?
6. What are the skills required for these CHN roles?
7. What data support this CHN's roles of collaboration and coordination?
8. To what extent does this CHN provide care for the client as individual, family, or group?
9. State one research question pertaining to community health nursing that arose based on the community health nurses' experiences and your readings. For example, a research question might be: Does a mother who breastfeeds bond faster with her new baby than a mother who does not breastfeed? Select one refereed journal article that addresses your research question. Reflect and document the relevance of this article to a community experience that you have had or that you have read about in the blogs.

*The blogs in this exercise were developed for the Laurentian University School of Nursing Distance Education Program.

REMEMBER THIS!

- Home health nurses provide care in the client's environment.
- Family forms an integral part of home health nursing and includes any caregiver or significant person who takes responsibility in assisting a client in need of care at home.
- Health promotion activities form a fundamental component of home health nursing practice.
- Contracting is a vital component of all nurse–client relationships. *Contracting* refers to the development of any working agreement, continuously renegotiable, between the CHN, client, and family.
- Interdisciplinary collaboration is critical in the home health care and hospice settings.
- In home care and hospice care, as in other care settings, health care providers experience stress associated with changing roles and overlapping responsibilities. In collaborating, health care providers should carefully analyze each other's roles to determine whether they overlap and adjust the plan of care as required.
- The scope of occupational health nursing practice is broad, including worker and workplace assessment and surveillance, case management, health promotion, primary care, management or administration, and evidence-informed practice.
- Workplace hazards include exposure to biological and infectious, chemical, enviro-mechanical, physical, and psychosocial hazards.
- The interdisciplinary occupational health team usually consists of the occupational health nurse, occupational medicine physician, industrial hygienist, and safety specialist.
- Parish nurses respond to health, healing, and wholeness within the context of the faith community. Although the emphasis is on health promotion and disease prevention throughout the lifespan, the spiritual dimension of nursing remains central to parish nursing.
- The parish nurse plans programs and considers health-related concerns within faith communities.
- To promote a caring faith community, the parish nurse offers personal health counselling and health teaching, facilitates linkages and referrals to congregation and community resources, advocates for and encourages the development of support resources, and provides pastoral care.
- Parish nurses collaborate to plan, implement, and evaluate health promotion activities while considering the faith community's beliefs and rituals.
- CHNs working in the parish nursing specialty need to attain adequate educational and skill preparation and are held accountable to those served and to those who have entrusted the CHN to serve.
- Other examples of CHNs who practise in primary health care are nurse practitioners, outpost nurses, forensic nurses, telenurses, street or outreach nurses, corrections nurses, and nurse entrepreneurs.
- Public health nurses (PHNs) work with many partners using a population health approach to protect and promote health and prevent disease for populations.
- PHNs work in a variety of settings and have many functions and roles such as those of advocate, manager, educator, consultant, and facilitator.
- PHNs utilize an evidence-informed approach to practice.
- The health status of rural populations depends on genetic, social, environmental, economic, and political factors.
- CHNs must consider the belief systems and lifestyles of a rural population when planning, implementing, and evaluating community services.
- Barriers to rural health care include a lack of availability, affordability, accessibility, and acceptability of services.
- Case management is a strategy that consists of targeting, assessment, care planning, implementation, monitoring, and reassessment.
- Case management is typically an interdisciplinary process in which the client is the focus of the care plan.
- CHNs have within their scope of practice advocacy and case management functions.
- Continuity of care is a goal of community health nursing practice. It requires making linkages with services to improve the client's health status.
- Discharge planning and the referral process promote continuity of care for all clients in the community.
- CHNs need to be aware of the principles, steps, and barriers in the referral process.

REFLECTIVE PRAXIS

Case Study 1*

Jamie and Pat are third-year nursing students who are in the second week of their community health nursing course. Jamie states: "Community nursing is so different from working in the hospital. Learning about community nursing doesn't really matter to me because I plan to work in a coronary care intensive care unit. The population health approach has nothing to do with hospital nursing."

1. a) Do you think that Jamie is correct?
   b) Should all nursing students be required to study community health nursing? Explain.
2. What could Pat say about the population health approach in response to Jamie's statement?

Answers are on the Evolve Web site at http://evolve.elsevier.com/Canada/Stanhope/community.

Case Study 2

During her visit to the regularly scheduled blood pressure clinic in a local apartment complex, Brigit, a 45-year-old woman, complained of feeling dizzy and forgetful. She could not remember which of her six medications she had taken during the past few days. Her blood pressure readings on reclining, sitting, and standing revealed gross elevation. The CHN and Brigit discussed the danger of Brigit's present status and her need to seek medical attention. Brigit called her physician from her apartment and agreed to be transported to the emergency department.

While in the emergency department, Brigit manifested the progressive signs and symptoms of a cerebrovascular accident (i.e., a stroke). During hospitalization, she lost her capacity for expressive language and demonstrated hemiparesis and a loss of bladder control. Her cognitive function became intermittently confused, and she was slow to recognize her physician and neighbours who came to visit. The hospital discharge planning nurse contacted the community case manager to screen and assess for the continuum of care needs as early as possible because Brigit lived alone and family members resided out of town, resulting in family caregiving in the community being intermittent. Brigit had residual functional and cognitive deficits that would demand longer-term care.

1. As the community case manager, place the following actions in sequence to construct a case management plan:
   a) Discuss with the family members their schedule of availability to offer care in the client's home.
   b) Call the client and introduce yourself as a prelude to working with her.
   c) Obtain information on the scope of services covered by your client's benefit plan.
   d) Arrange a community placement facility site visit for the client and family.

Answers are on the Evolve Web site at http://evolve.elsevier.com/Canada/Stanhope/community.

Case Study 3*

Sarah, a 20-year-old female, presents at the emergency department at 5 A.M. She tells the triage nurse that she thinks she was sexually assaulted. The sexual assault nurse examiner (SANE) is notified and arrives within a timely manner. The triage nurse has determined that Sarah does not require emergency medical attention. The SANE escorts Sarah to a private and secure location and obtains the following history. Sarah states, "I was at a dorm party earlier in the evening." She recalls having two beers and denies any use of illegal substances. Sarah states that she remembers feeling "woozy" and then waking up 3 hours later in her room naked and alone. She recalls a thick white substance on her inner right thigh and is complaining of genital "soreness." Sarah is nauseated and appears exceptionally anxious as she is unable to recall a portion of the evening's events. Sarah has a steady boyfriend and is sexually active. She has no known allergies, is not on medication, and has a current immunization status.

1. What are three primary concerns that Sarah may have?
2. What can a forensic nurse (i.e., a SANE) offer Sarah?
3. What might be an advantage of having a forensic nurse care for Sarah?

Answers are on the Evolve Web site at http://evolve.elsevier.com/Canada/Stanhope/community.

Case Study 4*

You are on call as the forensic nurse this evening. You receive a phone call to come to the trauma room of your local emergency department. When you arrive, you are directed to a room where a woman is lying on a stretcher.

* Case Study 1 was contributed by Mary-Louise Batty.

* Case Studies 3 and 4 and answers were created by Nancy Horan.

You observe that she has multiple injuries to her face, neck, and upper arms. The emergency nurse reports to you that the client, Emily, has been given ibuprofen for pain. A series of facial radiographs have revealed no fractures, but Emily will require sutures to a laceration just below her right cheek. You introduce yourself to the client and explain your role as a forensic nurse. Emily reveals that earlier in the evening her boyfriend had repeatedly hit her with his fists; she recalls being "thrown around the apartment." Emily comments that her boyfriend had pushed her over the coffee table last week and that she has a bruise on her left knee as a result. Emily discloses that her boyfriend has been emotionally abusive throughout their 2-year relationship but that this is the first time he has become "so violent."

1. What is your role as a forensic nurse in this case?
2. Emily does not want to return to her apartment. What resources are available in your community that might help Emily?
3. What information and documentation do you think might be important if you were asked to testify in court?

Answers are on the Evolve Web site at http://evolve.elsevier.com/Canada/Stanhope/community.

What Would You Do?

1. You are the home health nurse who has been the direct care provider for Sally in her home. Sally is in the terminal stages of breast cancer and lives on a farm in a small rural community. You have been visiting Sally weekly for the past 6 weeks. Sally is a 30-year-old married mother of a 10-year-old daughter named Brittney.
   a) Reflect on the experiences you have had with death and dying. What values and beliefs do you hold about death and dying?
   b) Based on this situation, what possible family health concerns can you identify?
   c) Review the literature pertaining to women and breast cancer and family stress. What data did you find? How would you use these data to plan your community health nursing interventions with this family?
   d) The following palliative care team members are involved with the family: palliative care volunteers, a homemaker, physiotherapist, chaplain, family physician, pharmacist, dietitian, and social worker. Outline the roles of each of these team members.
2. Initiating, monitoring, and evaluating resources are essential components of nursing case management. Identify the resources available in your community that would facilitate your role as case manager with the following clients:
   a) A client needing cardiac care in the hospital
   b) A hospitalized older adult client who will not return to his or her home and will require long-term care
   c) A young male client who was admitted to an orthopedic clinic due to a work-related accident
3. Initiating, monitoring, and evaluating resources are essential components of community health nursing practice. Identify the resources available in your community that would facilitate your role as discharge planner with the following clients:
   a) A hospitalized client with a cardiac health concern
   b) A hospitalized older adult client who will not return to his or her home and will require long-term care
   c) A young male client who was admitted to an orthopedic clinic due to a work-related accident

TOOL BOX

evolve

The Tool Box contains useful instruments that can be applied in community health nursing practice. These related resources appear either in the appendices at the back of this book or on the Evolve Web site at http://evolve.elsevier.com/Canada/Stanhope/community.

Appendices

- Appendix 1: Canadian Community Health Nursing Standards of Practice
- Appendix E-1: Comprehensive Occupational and Environmental Health History
- Appendix E-2: Occupational Health History Form
- Appendix E-3: Work-Site Assessment Guide

Tools

ActNow BC. *Creating a Healthy Workplace Environment Workbook and Toolkit.*
This Web site provides a resource to assist health care providers in developing activities to improve the health of workers in their workplaces.

Centre to Improve Care of Dying. *Toolkit of Instruments to Measure End-of-Life Care.*
This site provides a variety of tools and information to improve care of the dying. A sample form is available at http://www.chcr.brown.edu/pcoc/TOOLKITRegForm.pdf.

Occupational Health and Safety Council of Ontario. *MSD Tool Kit.*
This site provides information on the prevention and reduction of musculoskeletal disorders (MSD); guidelines for employers are available.

WEBLINKS

evolve

Direct links to these resources appear on the text's accompanying Evolve Web site at http://evolve.elsevier.com/Canada/Stanhope/community.

Antigonish Women's Resource Centre. This Web site provides specific information about one SANE program in Canada.

Canadian Centre for Occupational Health and Safety (CCOHS). This federal government agency's Web site provides a vast array of information on occupational health and safety.

Canadian Home Care Association. This site provides further information on home care in Canada and the various initiatives undertaken by this community organization.

Canadian Hospice Palliative Care Association (CHPCA). The CHPCA is a nonprofit national association that provides leadership in hospice palliative care in Canada. This site provides excellent links about palliative care through its "Other Links" menu option.

Canadian Hospice Palliative Care Association. *The Pan-Canadian Gold Standards in Palliative Home Care: Toward Equitable Access to High Quality Hospice Palliative and End-of-Life Care at Home.* This document outlines the expectations for meeting the four gold standards in case management, nursing, palliative-specific pharmaceuticals, and personal care at the end of life.

Canadian Institute for Health Information and Canadian Nurses Association. *The Regulation and Supply of Nurse Practitioners in Canada: 2006 Update*. This document outlines some of the history in the development of nurse practitioner initiatives in Canada, demographic data for provinces, and legislation and regulations for the provinces and territories.

Canadian Nurses Association. *Advanced Nursing Practice: A National Framework*. This Web site provides valuable information on the national consensus related to the development of advanced practice nursing for nurse practitioners and clinical nurse specialists, their roles, regulations, competencies, and future directions.

Canadian Nurses Association Relevant Position Statements and Competencies:

- Position Statement: "Telehealth: The Role of the Nurse"
- Position Statement: "The Nurse Practitioner"
- Position Statement: "Advanced Nursing Practice"
- Competencies: "Hospice Palliative Care Nursing Competencies"
- Competencies: "Occupational Health Nursing Competencies"

Canadian Occupational Health Nurses Association. This site provides background and historical information on occupational health nursing in Canada and also houses the occupational health nursing practice standards.

CanOSH. Maintained by the Canadian Centre for Occupational Health and Safety, this Web site provides access to the federal, provincial, and territorial occupational health and safety legislation; workers' compensation; workplace safety and health acts for each region; and statistical information relating to occupational health and safety.

Centre for Rural and Northern Health Research (CRaNHR). This site provides direct access to online research reports pertaining to rural health issues and methods of addressing these issues to improve health and access to health care for rural populations.

Centre on Aging, University of Victoria. This site provides several reports on the evaluation of the cost-effectiveness of home care. Substudy 15 provides a literature review and study findings on the barriers in discharge planning from hospitals to home care in Canada.

College of Registered Nurses of British Columbia: *Practice Standard for Registered Nurses and Nurse Practitioners: Telehealth*. This site provides the guidelines and principles for the use of telehealth in nursing practice in British Columbia.

College of Registered Nurses of British Columbia: *A Regulatory Framework for Nurse Practitioners in British Columbia.* This site provides information about the nurse practitioner competencies, roles, and functions in British Columbia.

College of Registered Nurses of Nova Scotia: *Telenursing Practice Guidelines.* This site defines telenursing and provides guidelines, principles, and issues related to the use of telehealth in nursing practice in Nova Scotia.

Communities and Schools Promoting Health. This site provides health care providers and others information pertaining to school health for all provinces and territories.

Community Health Nurses Association of Canada. *Public Health Nursing Discipline-Specific Competencies, Version 1.0.* This site provides information on and access to the newly developed discipline-specific competencies for public health nursing.

Four Pillars Coalition. ***Street Nurse Informs Victoria on Four Pillars Approach.*** This document provides information presented by James Tigchelaar, a street nurse in the Street Nurse Program, Centre for Disease Control, in British Columbia. He describes the changes in the DTES community due to the introduction of various services and programs.

Giles, S., & Brennan, E. *Action-Based Care in Vancouver's DTES.* This document provides two nurses' descriptions of their experiences working as home care nurses in Vancouver's DTES.

Grantham, D., O'Brien, L. A., Widger, K., Bouvette, M., & McQuinn, P. *Canadian Hospice Palliative Care Nursing Competencies Case Examples*. This document provides information on each of the competencies and uses case studies to demonstrate their applications for palliative care nurses.

Herbert, R. *Canada's Health Care Challenge: Recognizing and Addressing the Health Needs of Rural Canadians*. This document discusses rural health definitions, the disparity in health care and health status between urban and rural clients, and the determinants of health specific to rural clients.

Human Resources and Skills Development Canada: Workplace Health & Safety. This site provides information on the various programs, services, and legislation provided by the Government of Canada to protect the rights of Canadian employees.

Laforet Fliesser, Y., Schofield, R., & Yandreski, C. *Public Health Nursing: Nursing Practice in a Diverse Environment*. This Registered Nurses' Association of Ontario paper provides further information on public health nursing, with examples of roles, functions, and settings of practice.

McMaster University. *VCoP: Creating a Virtual Community of Practice for Street Nursing.* This document provides up-to-date information on the progress of a funded research project about a virtual community of practice for street nursing.

Meagher-Stewart, D. *Fostering Citizen Participation and Collaborative Practice: Tapping the Wisdom and Voices of Public Health Nurses in Nova Scotia*. This document provides a report of a qualitative research study conducted in Nova Scotia with public health nurses.

Nova Scotia Department of Health: Continuing Care Programs. This Web site provides information on the various programs and services offered by the Nova Scotia Department of Health.

NPCanada.ca. This site provides information about programs for nurse practitioners and about nurse practitioners in Canada.

Nurse Practitioner Association of Ontario. This site provides information on the standards of practice for PHCNPs in Ontario as well as other information on nurse practitioners in Ontario. "A Day in the Life" provides stories from primary health care nurse practitioners.

Nursing Practice in Rural and Remote Canada: Publications and Presentations. This site provides access to an extensive number of resources on rural and remote health care issues in Canada, including fact sheets.

Ontario Primary Health Care Nurse Practitioner Program. This site provides information about the establishment of the Ontario nursing university consortium and the program educational requirements and preparation.

Ontario's New Community Care Access Centres. This site provides links to the 42 CCACs across the province and the 14 local health integration networks.

Public Health Agency of Canada: Core Competencies for Public Health in Canada. This site explains the core competencies.

Saskatoon Health Region. This site provides information about the services offered by Client/Patient Access Services and provides links to information about programs and services offered by the Saskatoon Health Region. Reports, such as the report on the health status of residents living in Saskatoon, are also available.

Street Health. This site provides links to information on social justice issues, programs, ideas for working with the poor, and discussions on the homeless and other social issues. Cathy Crowe's newsletter can also be accessed via this site.

VON Canada. This site provides access to information on the many services and programs of the Victorian Order of Nurses (VON) of Canada.

VON Canada: *VONetwork*. This site links to VON Canada's newsletter, containing stories about volunteers who have changed the lives of VON clients.

REFERENCES

Anderson, G. S. (2007). *All you ever wanted to know about forensic science in Canada but didn't know who to ask!* Ottawa: Canadian Society of Forensic Science. Retrieved from http://www.csfs.ca/contentadmin/UserFiles/File/Booklet2007.pdf.

Atwal, A., & Caldwell, K. (2002). Do multidisciplinary integrated care pathways improve interprofessional collaboration? *Scandinavian Journal of Caring Science*, *16*(4), 360–367.

Baumann, A., Hunsberger, M., Blythe, J., & Crea, M. (2006). *The new healthcare worker: Implications of changing employment patterns in rural and community hospitals*. Hamilton, ON: Nursing Health Services Research Unit of McMaster University. Retrieved from http://www.nhsru.com/documents/Series%206%20The%20New%20Healthcare%20Worker-Rural.pdf.

Bayshore Home Health. (2007). *Bayshore Home Health named one of Canada's 50 best managed companies*. Retrieved from http://www.bayshore.ca/docs/Bayshore%20Home%20Health%20Named%20One%20of%20Canadas%2050%20Best%20Managed%20Companies.pdf.

Bollman, R. (2003). *Rural and small town Canada: Analysis bulletin*. (Cat. No. 21-006-XIE).Ottawa, ON: Statistics Canada. Retrieved from http://www.statcan.gc.ca/pub/21-006-x/21-006-x2002006-eng.pdf.

Bushy, A. (2003). Case management: Considerations for working with diverse rural client systems. *Lippincott's Case Management*, *8*(5), 214–223.

Campos-Outcalt, D. (1994). Occupational health epidemiology and objectives for the year 2000: Primary care, clinics in office practice. *Occupational Health*, *21*(20), 213.

Canadian Association for Parish Nursing Ministry. (2004). *Guide for parish nursing core competencies for basic parish nurse education programs*. Retrieved from http://www.capnm.ca/core_competencies.htm.

Canadian Association for Rural and Remote Nursing. (2008). *Rural and remote nursing practice parameters: Discussion document*. Retrieved from http://www.carrn.com/files/NursingPracticeParametersJanuary08.pdf.

Canadian Home Care Association. (2005). *Home care case management*. Retrieved from http://www.hc-sc.gc.ca/hcs-sss/alt_formats/hpb-dgps/pdf/pubs/2005-cas-mgmt-gest/2005-cas-mgmt-gest-eng.pdf.

Canadian Home Care Association. (2008). *Home care: Meeting the needs of an aging population*. Retrieved from http://www.cdnhomecare.ca/media.php?mid=1914.

Canadian Hospice Palliative Care Association. (2002). *A model to guide hospice palliative care: Based on national principles and norms of practice*. Retrieved from http://www.cancerboard.ab.ca/maco/pdf/hpcn_chpca_guide_2002_04-12-28.pdf.

Canadian Hospice Palliative Care Association. (2006). *The pan-Canadian gold standards in palliative home care: Toward equitable access to high quality hospice palliative and end-of-life care at home*. (pp. 8–9). Retrieved from http://www.chpca.net/norms-standards/pan-cdn_gold_standards.html.

Canadian Hospice Palliative Care Association. (2007). *Living lessons: Increasing awareness of hospice palliative care in Canada*. Retrieved from http://www.living-lessons.org/main/hospice.asp.

Canadian Nurses Association. (1996). On your own—the nurse entrepreneur. *Nursing Now, 1*(1). Retrieved from http://www.cna-aiic.ca/CNA/documents/pdf/publications/OwnEntrepreneur_Sept1996_e.pdf.

Canadian Nurses Association. (2002). *Policy statement: Evidence-based decision-making and nursing practice*. Retrieved from http://www.cna-nurses.ca/CNA/documents/pdf/publications/PS63_Evidence:based_Decision_making_Nursing_Practice:e.pdf.

Canadian Nurses Association. (2005). *Rural nursing practice in Canada: A discussion paper*. Ottawa: CNA. Retrieved from http://www.carrn.com/files/Rural-Nursing-discussion-paper_Draft3-Sept%2005-1.pdf.

Canadian Nurses Association. (2007). *Street nurse Cathy Crowe and Ottawa nurses tackle health of homeless*. Press release. Retrieved from http://www.cna-aiic.ca/CNA/news/releases/public_release_e.aspx?id=219.

Canadian Nurses Association. (2008a). *Occupational health nursing certification*. Retrieved from http://www.cna-nurses.ca/CNA/documents/pdf/publications/CERT_Occ_Health_e.pdf.

Canadian Nurses Association. (2008b). *Advanced nursing practice: A national framework*. Retrieved from http://www.cna-aiic.ca/CNA/documents/pdf/publications/ANP_National_Framework_e.pdf.

Canadian Nurses Association. (2009). *Canadian nurse practitioner examination program*. Retrieved from http://www.cna-aiic.ca/CNA/nursing/npexam/exam/default_e.aspx.

Canadian Nurses Association. (2010). *CNA certification*. Retrieved from http://www.cna-nurses.ca/CNA/nursing/certification/specialties/default_e.aspx.

Canadian Occupational Health Nurses Association Inc. (2009). *Our scope*. Retrieved from http://www.cohna-aciist.ca/pages/content.asp?CatID=2&CatSubID=8.

Canadian Public Health Association. (1990). *Community health—public health nursing in Canada: Preparation & practice*. Ottawa, ON: Author.

Capital Health. (2010). *Evidence-informed practice*. Retrieved from http://www.cdha.nshealth.ca/default.aspx?page=SubPage¢erContent.Id.0=48427&category.Categories.1=796.

Cawthorn, L. (2006). Discharge planning under the umbrella of advanced nursing practice case manager. *Nursing leadership: On-line exclusive*. Retrieved from http://www.longwoods.com/product.php?productid=19033.

Clemen-Stone, S., McGuire, S. L., & Eigsti, D. G. (1998). *Comprehensive community health nursing: Family, aggregate, and community practice*. St. Louis. MO: Mosby.

College of Nurses of Ontario. (2005). *Practice guideline: Telepractice*. Retrieved from http://www.cno.org/docs/prac/41041_telephone.pdf.

College of Nurses of Ontario. (2009). *Practice guideline: Independent practice*. Retrieved from http://www.cno.org/docs/prac/41011_fsIndepPrac.pdf.

Community Health Nurses Association of Canada. (2008). *Canadian community health nursing standards of practice*. Retrieved from http://www.chnc.ca/documents/standards/chn_standards_of_practice_mar08_english.pdf.

Community Health Nurses of Canada. (2009). *Public health nursing discipline specific competencies version 1.0*. Retrieved from http://www.chnc.ca/documents/competencies_june_2009_english.pdf.

Community Health Nurses' Initiatives Group of the Registered Nurses' Association of Ontario. (2004). *Public health nursing: Position statement*. Retrieved from http://chnig.org/downloads/04.doc.

Corser, W. (2003). A complex sense of advocacy: The challenges of contemporary discharge planning. *The Case Manager, 14*(3), 63–69.

Cox, S. (2008). Nursing on the inside. *Let's Talk, 29*(3). Retrieved from http://www.csc-scc.gc.ca/text/pblct/lt-en/2004/no3/33-eng.shtml.

Currie, V. L., & Harvey, G. (2000). The use of care pathways as tools to support the implementation of evidence-based practice. *Journal of Interprofessional Care, 14*(4), 311–324.

Daiski, J. (2000). The road to professionalism in nursing: Case management or practice based in nursing theory. *Nursing Science Quarterly, 13*(1), 74–79.

Day, R. A., Paul, P., Williams, B., Smeltzer, S. C., & Bare, B. (2007). *Brunner & Suddarth's textbook of medical–surgical nursing* (1st Canadian ed.). Philadelphia, PA: Lippincott, Williams & Wilkins.

DesMeules, M., Pong, R., Lagace, C., Heng, D., Manual, D., Pitblado, R., & Koren, I. (2006). *How healthy are rural Canadians? An assessment of their health status and health determinants*. Ottawa, ON: Canadian Institute for Health Information. Retrieved from http://www.phac-aspc.gc.ca/publicat/rural06/pdf/rural_canadians_2006_report_e.pdf.

Educause Learning Initiative. (2009). *Virtual communities*. Retrieved from http://www.educause.edu/ELI/Archives/VirtualCommunities/576?bhcp=1.

Forensic Nurses' Society of Canada. (2008). *Forensic nurse*. Retrieved from http://www.forensicnurse.ca/.

Fox, A., Munro, H., & Brien, H. (2006). Exploring diabetes home nursing care: A pilot study. *Canadian Journal of Diabetes, 30*(2), 146–153.

Goodwin, S. (2007). Telephone nursing: An emerging practice area. *Nursing Leadership, 20*(4), 38–46.

Government of Canada. (2000). *The federal role in rural health*. Retrieved from http://dsp-psd.tpsgc.gc.ca/Collection-R/LoPBdP/BP/prb0020-e.htm.

Grantham, D., O'Brien, L. A., Widger, K., Bouvette, M., & McQuinn, P. (2009). *Canadian hospice palliative care nursing competencies case examples*. Retrieved from http://www.carrefourpalliatif.ca/Assets/Canadian%20Hospice%20Palliative%20Care%20Nursing%20Competencies%20Case%20Examples-Revised%20Feb%202010_20100211150854.pdf.

Grubnic, S. (2003). Care pathways: Conceptualising and developing a multi-skilling initiative. *International Journal of Health Care Quality Assurance, 16*(6), 286–292.

Harlos, M. (2009). *About palliative care*. Retrieved from http://palliative.info/.

Herbert, R. (2007). Canada's health care challenge: Recognizing and addressing the health needs of rural Canadians. *Lethbridge Undergraduate Research Journal*, *2*(1). Retrieved from http://www.lurj.org/article.php/vol2n1/canada.xml.

Kagan-Krieger, S., & Rehfeld, G. (2000). The sexual assault nurse examiner. *The Canadian Nurse*, *96*(6), 20–25.

Kearley, C., & Steeves, S. (2010). Caring in corrections. *The Canadian Nurse*, *106*(4), 23–27.

Kent, H. (2000). SANE nurses staff Alberta's sexual assault response team. *Canadian Medical Association Journal*, *162*(5), 683–684.

Laforet Fliesser, Y., Schofield, R., & Yandreski, C. (2003). *Public health nursing: Nursing practice in a diverse environment*. Retrieved from http://www.rnao.org/Page.asp?PageID = 122 &ContentID = 1308&SiteNodeID = 405.

Langille, D. B., Proudfoot, K., Rigby, J., Aquino-Russell, C., Strang, R., & Forward, K. (2008). A pilot project for *Chlamydia* screening in adolescent females using self-testing: Characteristics of participants and non-participants. *Canadian Journal of Public Health*, *99*(2), 117–120.

Lapierre, N., Blackmer, J., Coutu-Wakulczyk, G., & Dehoux, E. (2006). Autonomic dysreflexia and telehealth. *Canadian Nurse*, *102*(7), 20–25.

Levy, B. S., & Wegman, D. H. (2000). *Occupational health: Recognizing and preventing occupational disease*. Philadelphia: Lippincott Williams & Wilkins.

Lynch, V. (2005). *Forensic nursing*. St. Louis, MO: Elsevier Mosby.

MacLeod, M., Kulig, J., Stewart, N., Pitblado, J. R., Banks, K., D'Arcy, C., et al. (2004a). The nature of nursing practice in rural and remote Canada. *The Canadian Nurse*, *100*(6), 27–31.

MacLeod, M., Kulig, J., Stewart, N., & Pitblado, R. (2004b). *The nature of nursing practice in rural and remote Canada*. Final Report to Canadian Health Services Foundation. Retrieved from http://www.ruralnursing.unbc.ca/reports/study/RRNFinalReport.pdf.

Maurer, F. A., & Smith, C. M. (2009). *Community/public health nursing practice: Health for families and populations*. (4th ed.). St. Louis, MO: Elsevier.

McMaster University. (2008). *VCoP: Creating a virtual community of practice for street nursing*. Retrieved from http://fhsson.csu.mcmaster.ca/streetnursing/index.php.

Meagher-Stewart, D., Aston, M., Edwards, N., Smith, D., Young, L., & Woodford, E. (2004). *Fostering citizen participation and collaborative practice: Tapping the wisdom and voices of public health nurses in Nova Scotia*. Retrieved from http://www.chnc.ca/documents/phn_study_nov25_2004.pdf.

Minister of Health and Long-Term Care. (2008). *Ontario public health standards*. Retrieved from http://www.health.gov.on.ca/english/providers/program/pubhealth/oph_standards/ophs/progstds/pdfs/ophs_2008.pdf.

Ministerial Advisory Council on Rural Health. Health Canada. (2002). *Rural health in rural hands: Strategic directions for rural, remote, northern and Aboriginal communities*. Retrieved from http://www.srpc.ca/librarydocs/rural_handsbr.pdf.

Ministry of Health and Long-Term Care. (2006). *Ontario's new community care access centres*. Retrieved from http://www.health.gov.on.ca/english/public/contact/ccac/ccac_mn.html.

Misener, R. M., MacLeod, M. L. P., Banks, K., Morton, A. M., Vogt, C., & Bentham, D. (2008). There's rural, and then there's "rural": Advice from nurses providing primary healthcare in northern remote communities. *Nursing Leadership*, *21*(3), 54–63.

National Case Management Network of Canada. (2006). *Connect*. Retrieved from http://ncmn.ca/.

National Initiative for Telehealth. (2003). *National Initiative for Telehealth framework of guidelines*. Retrieved from http://www.ehealthstrategies.com/files/telemed_canada_guide.pdf.

Nurses Association of New Brunswick. (2002). *Position statement: The nurse as discharge planner*. Retrieved from http://www.nanb.nb.ca/PDF/position-statements/NURSE_AS_DISCHARGE_PLANNER_E.pdf.

Nursing Practice in Rural and Remote Canada. (2006). *Factsheets*. Retrieved from http://www.ruralnursing.unbc.ca/factsheets/index.php.

Occupational Health Nurses of British Columbia. (2007). *What is occupational health nursing?*. Retrieved from http://www.bcohn.ca/ohnfaq.html.

O'Donnell, M. (2002). *Health promotion in the workplace*. New York, NY: Delmar.

Orem, D. E. (1995). *Nursing: Concepts of practice*. (3rd ed.). St. Louis, MO: Mosby.

Petryshen, P. R., & Petryshen, P. M. (1992). The case management model: An innovative approach to the delivery of patient care. *Journal of Advanced Nursing*, *17*, 1188–1194.

Pitblado, R. J., Managhan, T., Houle, L., Pong, R. W., & Lapalme, D. (1996). *Mental health status and service utilization in northeastern/northern Ontario*. Sudbury, ON: Northern Health Human Research Unit.

Public Health Agency of Canada. (2006). *Palliative care info-sheet for seniors*. Retrieved from http://www.phac-aspc.gc.ca/seniors-aines/pubs/info_sheets/palliative_care/pall_e.htm.

Public Health Agency of Canada. (2008). *The chief public health officer's report on the state of public health in Canada: Addressing health inequalities*. Retrieved from http://www.phac-aspc.gc.ca/publicat/2008/cphorsphc-respcacsp/index-eng.php.

Rees, G., Huby, G., McDade, L., & McKechnie, L. (2004). Joint working in community mental health teams: Implementation of an integrated care pathway. *Health and Social Care in the Community*, *12*(6), 527–536.

Rogers, B. (2003). *Occupational health nursing: Concepts and practice*. St. Louis, MO: Elsevier.

Romanow, R. (2002). *Building on values: The future of health care in Canada*. Retrieved from http://www.cbc.ca/healthcare/final_report.pdf.

Saint Elizabeth Health Care. (2009). *Join the team*. Retrieved from http://www.saintelizabeth.com/employment-join-our-team.php.

Schwartz, T. (2002). Making it safer down on the farm. *American Journal of Nursing*, *102*(3), 114–115.

Self, B., & Peters, H. (2005). Street outreach with no streets. *The Canadian Nurse*, *100*(1), 21–24.

Smith, D. L., Smith, J. E., Newhook, C., & Hobson, B. (2006). Continuity of care, service integration, and case management. In J. M. Hibberd, & D. L. Smith (Eds.), *Nursing leadership and management in Canada* (3rd ed., pp. 81–112). Toronto, ON: Elsevier Canada.

Smith, S. (2005). Stepping through the looking glass: Professional autonomy in correctional nursing. *Corrections Today*. Retrieved from http://goliath.ecnext.com/coms2/gi_0199-3697147/Stepping-through-the-looking-glass.html.

Statistics Canada. (2002a). *Canadian community health survey (CCHS)—cycle 1.1*. Retrieved from http://www.statcan.gc.ca/concepts/health-sante/index-eng.htm.

Statistics Canada. (2002b). Health of the off-reserve Aboriginal population. *The Daily*, August 27, 2002. Retrieved from http://www.statcan.gc.ca/daily-quotidien/020827/dq020827a-eng.htm.

Stewart, N., D'Arcy, C., Pitblado, R., Forbes, D., Morgan, D., Remus, G., et al. (2005). *Report of the national survey of Nursing Practice in Rural and Remote Canada*. Retrieved from http://www.ruralnursing.unbc.ca/reports/study/SurveyReportEnglish.pdf.

Straus, S. E., Richardson, W. S., Glasziou, P., & Haynes, R. B. (2005). *Evidence-based medicine: How to practice and teach EBM*. London, UK: Elsevier/Churchill Livingstone.

Tarlier, D. S., Johnson, J. L., & Whyte, N. B. (2003). Voices from the wilderness: An interpretative study describing the role and practice of outpost nurses. *Canadian Journal of Public Health*, *94*(3), 180–184.

Thrasher, C., & Staples, E. (2005). Primary health care nurse practitioners. In L. L. Stamler, & L. Yiu (Eds.), *Community health nursing: A Canadian perspective* (pp. 337–340). Toronto, ON: Pearson Prentice Hall.

Underwood, J., Deber, R., Baumann, A., Dragan, A., Laporte, A., Alameddine, M., et al. (2009). *Demographic profile of community health nurses in Canada: 1996–2007*. Hamilton, ON: McMaster University School of Nursing and the Nursing Health Services Research Unit. Retrieved from http://www.nhsru.com/documents/Series%2013%20McMaster_Demographic_Profile_of_Community.pdf.

Valaitis, R. (2007). *What is a virtual community of practice?* Retrieved from http://fhsson.csu.mcmaster.ca/streetnursing/index.php?option=com_content&task=view&id=22&Itemid=25.

Victorian Order of Nurses. (2006). *VON Canada: A century of caring*. Retrieved from http://www.von.ca/en/about/history.aspx.

Wells, D., LeClerc, C., Craig, D., Martin, D., & Marshall, V. (2002). Evaluation of an integrated model of discharge planning: Achieving quality discharges in an efficient and ethical way. *Canadian Journal of Nursing Research*, *34*(3), 103–122.

World Health Organization. (2009). *WHO definition of palliative care*. Retrieved from http://www.who.int/cancer/palliative/definition/en/.

CHAPTER 4

Health Promotion

OBJECTIVES

After reading this chapter, you should be able to:

1. Describe how the various definitions of *health* have influenced the development of health promotion.
2. Compare and contrast health promotion, disease prevention, and harm reduction.
3. Describe the milestones in the development of health promotion.
4. Explain how the determinants of health affect health promotion.
5. Discuss the concepts of literacy and health literacy.
6. Describe how literacy and health literacy relate to the determinants of health.
7. Describe various individual and community health promotion models, theories, and frameworks, and explain their use in community health nursing.
8. Compare the biomedical, behavioural, and socioenvironmental health approaches.
9. Identify health promotion strategies and how, when, and where they would be used.
10. Explain how the *Canadian Community Health Nursing Standards of Practice* are applied in health promotion.
11. Explain the community health nurse's roles and responsibilities in health promotion.

CHAPTER OUTLINE

KEY TERMS

See Glossary on page 593 for definitions.

Over the past four decades, the direction that health has taken in Canada has changed from a medical model to a population health promotion model. Canada has received recognition as a leader in the health promotion movement globally, a process that started with the release of *A New Perspective on the Health of Canadians*, commonly referred to as the Lalonde Report (Lalonde, 1974), followed by the framework by Epp (1986) titled *Achieving Health for All*. Health promotion, as outlined in the Ottawa Charter for Health Promotion, is a strategy to improve health and is defined as "enabling people to increase control over, and to improve, their health" (World Health Organization [WHO], 1986). Recently, "there has been inadequate policy development reflecting what we have learned about population health. In fact, Canada has fallen behind countries such as United Kingdom and Sweden in applying the population health knowledge base that has been largely developed here" (Senate Subcommittee on Population Health, 2009, p. 42). Health promotion applies to the client as individual, family, aggregate or group, population, community, or society. At the time of the Ottawa Charter, use of the term *enabling* marked the beginning of the conceptualization of empowerment (discussed in Chapter 1) as a component of health promotion. **Enabling**, within health promotion, refers to taking action with clients to empower them to gain control over their health and environment with the goal of improving their health.

Optimizing population health and maintaining healthy environments that support the achievement of client health goals require the implementation of health promotion strategies such as strengthening community action, building healthy public policy, creating supportive environments, developing personal skills, and reorienting health services. Health promotion models, frameworks, and activities such as advocacy, health communication and social marketing, and mutual aid are some of the tools CHNs can use to implement these strategies.

This chapter discusses health promotion as a concept and its use by CHNs and introduces select health promotion theories, frameworks, models, strategies, and tools. The topic of health promotion is extensive; for the purposes of this text, only the areas with which CHNs need to be most familiar are discussed. In its efforts toward health promotion, Canada takes a population health approach focusing on the determinants of health, as opposed to placing a more extensive focus on individual health promotion, as is done in some other countries such as the United States.

PROMOTION OF HEALTH

The Canadian Community Health Nursing Practice Model illustrated in Chapter 1 depicts that CHNs promote health in environmental, political, and social contexts. CHNs use the community health nursing process to assess, plan, intervene, and evaluate their practice from a micro level (i.e., individual and family) to a macro level (i.e., systems and society). In their values and beliefs, CHNs incorporate caring, principles of primary health care, multiple ways of knowing, individual and community partnerships, environmental influence, and empowerment. CHNs use the following five standards of practice in all community health nursing practice settings: promoting health, building capacity, building relationships, facilitating access and equity, and demonstrating professional responsibility and accountability. The *Canadian Community Health Nursing Standards of Practice*, presented in Appendix 1, provide detail pertaining to each of the five standards.

Throughout this text, the term *community health nursing process* is used to refer to the processes on which CHNs base their community health nursing decisions. The community health nursing process involves comprehensive community assessment, planning, implementation, and evaluation. Traditional terms such as *nursing process*, *problem solving*, *clinical judgement*, *critical thinking*, and *decision making*, which are used in specific nursing curricula depending upon their underlying philosophy, may be familiar to those who practise nursing. However, reflecting the practice model used in the *Canadian Community Health Nursing Standards of Practice*, this text uses the term *community health nursing process* to describe any of these actions.

Development of the Concept of Health

Understanding health promotion requires looking at the development of the concept of health. The conceptualization of health has taken form over time and with many debates occurring over its definition. In the early to mid-1900s, the medical model ruled, and *health* was therefore defined as the absence of disease. This definition of *health* led to the view of health and illness as two opposing ends on a continuum and to health being measured by indicators of disease, such as morbidity and mortality statistics (Vollman, Anderson, & McFarlane, 2008). As well, this definition had a medical-model perspective because its approach focused primarily on disease in individuals. It also had an individual focus rather than an aggregate or population focus.

In 1947, WHO amended its definition of *health* from "the absence of disease or infirmity" to "health as a state of complete physical, mental, and social well-being, and not merely the absence of disease or infirmity" (WHO, 1947). This expanded definition led to the view of health as a balance between physical, mental, and social well-being which led to a holistic approach to health.

Other *health* definitions followed to include facets such as the environment, predisposing factors such as heredity, family, and community. The influence of epidemiology led to the consideration of aggregates as well

CRITICAL VIEW

1. a) How do you define *health*?
   b) Why do you think you hold this belief about health?
2. How has your definition of *health* influenced your nursing practice?

as individuals in the definition of *health*. Dunn (1959) described health as ever-changing, overlapping levels of wellness (i.e., physical, biological, social, cultural) within the context of the environment. Within the health grid developed by Dunn (1959), high-level wellness can occur only in a favourable environment.

The perspective of health as growth was introduced in the 1960s by Dewey (1963), Erikson (1963), and Piaget (1963), with further development by Havighurst (1972) and Duval in 1985 (as cited in Sheinfeld Gorin & Arnold, 1998). These developmental theorists viewed health as an ongoing process throughout the lifespan influenced by several factors, including lifestyle choices. Other health perspectives include health as functionality, goodness of fit, transcendence, a sense of well-being, wholeness (holistic), and empowerment (Sheinfeld Gorin & Arnold, 1998). The latter three comprise part of the concept of health promotion.

The perspective taken in this Canadian text is based on the Ottawa Charter definition of health: "to reach a state of complete physical, mental and social wellbeing, an individual or group must be able to identify and to realize aspirations, to satisfy needs, and to change or cope with the environment" (WHO, 1986). The WHO thereby identified **health** as a positive resource for everyday living that is holistic—that is, includes physical, social, and personal capabilities. This distinction no longer presents health as an outcome (or a state to be reached); rather, health becomes incorporated into one's activities of daily living. Therefore, a client requires health to live his or her life to its fullest potential. Today, Canada continues to embrace the Ottawa Charter definition of *health*. Viewing health as a resource suggests that communities and individuals can use this resource to manage and even change their surroundings (Health Canada, 2004). Globally, there is no consensus on what constitutes good health; however, consensus on what constitutes poor health is more likely (Maville & Huerta, 2008).

Common Community Health Nursing Foundational Concepts in Health Promotion

Frequently, questions arise about the differences among various concepts such as injury prevention, disease, disease course, illness, illness trajectory, disease prevention, health protection, health promotion, harm reduction, risk avoidance, and risk reduction. These concepts are often referred to in discussions about health and health promotion, and it is important for CHNs to be able to distinguish the differences among them.

Injury prevention refers to the use of strategies to help clients prevent and reduce the risk of injury. Injury prevention occurs at the primary, secondary, and tertiary levels. An example of injury prevention at the primary level is the use of bicycle helmets to prevent head injuries. An example of secondary prevention is the provision of a bicycle safety program for youths who have experienced head injuries. An example of tertiary prevention is the provision of rehabilitation after a head injury resulting from a bicycle accident.

Disease refers to the presence of abnormal alterations in the structure or functioning of the human body that fit within the medical model (Lubkin & Larsen, 2009; Shah, 2003). When an individual experiences a disease, it follows an identifiable progression known as the **disease course**. For example, health practitioners consider the natural history of a disease within the context of signs and symptoms of the disease experienced by the client to identify the disease course.

Illness is an individual's personal experience of, perception of, and reaction to a disease, whereby he or she is unable to function at the desired "usual" level (Lubkin & Larsen, 2009; Shah, 2003). Chronic illness follows a particular trajectory, that is, expected short- and long-term courses over time with a degree of uncertainty about the disease course that requires the affected client, the family, and involved health care providers to adjust to associated changes; this path is referred to as the *illness trajectory* (Lubkin & Larsen, 2009). For example, a client living with rheumatoid arthritis will suffer degenerative physical changes as the disease progresses, possibly requiring assistance from others to adapt and manage activities of daily living such as mobility, bathing, and dressing. Clients adapt differently to chronic illness.

Disease prevention refers to the activities undertaken by the health sector to prevent the occurrence of disease (primary prevention), to detect and stop disease development in those at risk (secondary prevention), and to reduce the negative effects once a disease has established itself (tertiary prevention) (Maville & Huerta, 2008). These activities relate specifically to illness and disease. Disease prevention focuses on individuals and populations that have identifiable risk factors such as genetic predisposition or involvement in risky behaviours such as practising unsafe sex. An example of disease prevention at the primary level is the administration of the H1N1 influenza vaccine to the Canadian population or administration of the seasonal influenza vaccine to the older adult aggregate. An example of disease prevention at the secondary level is the screening for cervical cancer in all sexually active females, using the

Papanicolaou (Pap) smear. An example of the tertiary level of disease prevention is the provision of speech therapy for aphasic clients following a cerebrovascular accident.

Whereas disease prevention focuses on anticipation and avoidance of immediate health risks, **health protection** focuses on health maintenance by dealing with the immediate health risks (Health Canada, 2005a). Health Canada has the responsibility of protecting the Canadian population from current and emerging health threats. With regional offices across Canada (e.g., in British Columbia, Ontario, and New Brunswick), Health Canada safeguards the population's health through surveillance, prevention, legislation, and research in areas such as environmental health, disease outbreaks, drug products, and food safety. In this text, the term *disease prevention* acts as an umbrella term incorporating *illness prevention* and *health protection*.

In 2005, the WHO redefined *health promotion* as the process of enabling people to increase control over the determinants of health and thereby improve their health (Tang, Beaglehole, & O'Byrne, 2005). This definition, developed from that of the Ottawa Charter (WHO, 1986), specifies particular factors that affect health—the determinants of health. These determinants are discussed in Chapter 1 and throughout the text. Health promotion moves beyond health maintenance to incorporate improvements in health resulting in health gains (Health Canada, 2005a). It is critical that clients be actively involved in all aspects of their health to effect improvements. Health promotion embodies a sociopolitical process in which actions are aimed at reducing the effects of social, environmental, and economic conditions on individual, family, aggregate, and community health (Diem & Moyer, 2005).

Using the health issue of adolescent obesity, the following examples show health promotion in action at individual, family, aggregate, and community levels. At an individual level, the adolescent is empowered to make healthy food choices when the school cafeteria offers reasonably priced fresh food and vegetable options. The CHN could advocate on behalf of students to ensure healthier food choices are made available in the school cafeteria and other community eating establishments. The CHN could educate the adolescent's family about meal planning so that family members could plan and implement healthy meals and snacks. The CHN could enable families to purchase healthy foods by providing information on community resources such as community gardens and food banks. At an aggregate level, self-help groups initiated in the school could facilitate adolescents' meeting and sharing ideas on how to promote a healthy weight (the "Ethical Considerations" box below presents an example of health promotion to this same aggregate, but for the issue of smoking). The CHN might advocate for the establishment of life-skill classes that focus on inexpensive healthy food preparation. Within the community, community leaders, adolescents, parents, teachers, and health care providers could work together to establish community recreational opportunities that facilitate physical activity, such as skateboard parks; walking, hiking, and biking trails; and cross-country ski trails and hills. The CHN could advocate for healthy public policy that would support activity promotion through funding opportunities for trail development, lighting for walkways, and tax incentives for enrollment in physical activity programs. **Healthy public policy** is policy developed with the intent of having a positive effect on or promoting health.

ETHICAL CONSIDERATIONS

A PHN assigned to a junior high school has noticed that many of the teenagers smoke. He starts an after-school smoking cessation program targeting the smokers; however, some students just don't want to come. Several students who do want to come can't since they take the bus right after school.

Ethical principles (see Box 6-2 on p. 168 for a more detailed discussion) that apply to the above scenario are as follows:

- *Distributive justice*. The benefits of the program are not equally available to all, since the bused students cannot attend.
- *Respect for autonomy*. The PHN cannot force students to come to the program if they choose not to.
- *Promoting health and well-being* (CNA Code of Ethics). Promoting health and well-being is a primary ethical value for CHNs.

Questions to Consider

1. a) How does a CHN address negative health behaviours while maintaining respect for client autonomy?
   b) What could the CHN in this situation do to maintain respect for client autonomy and address the negative health behaviour of smoking?
2. What is the CHN's responsibility to provide programming for those students who don't yet smoke, that is, to promote client health at a primary level of prevention?

Risk avoidance is a disease prevention strategy used to avoid health problems and to remain at a low-risk level (placing the client at no risk or low risk on the continuum). **Risk reduction** is a disease prevention strategy used to reduce or alter health concerns so that any disease is detected and treated early to prevent moving to a high-risk level (placing the client at low to moderate risk). The risk continuum is often used with clients who have substance use or abuse problems, for example, with alcohol or drugs. **Health enhancement** is a health promotion strategy that is used to increase health and resiliency to promote optimal health and well-being (the client can be at any point on the risk continuum).

Disease prevention and health promotion are foundational to community health nursing practice. Community health nursing interventions aimed at preventing illness or injuries from happening would be primary prevention. Secondary-prevention community health nursing interventions could be to assess and support individuals and populations when risk factors are present so that screening for early detection and treatment occurs. Canadian guidelines, titled *Periodic Health Examination of Adults: Preventive Clinical Practices Guidelines*, provide recommendations for regular adult screening interventions. These recommendations can be found on the Canadian Task Force on Preventative Health Care Weblink on the Evolve Web site. (Focus your reading on the section titled "Recommendations: Motivating Patients to Practice Intervention," pp. 27–33.) In tertiary prevention, community health nursing interventions could involve supporting, educating, monitoring, and referring clients during the rehabilitation stage. The *Canadian Community Health Nursing Standards of Practice* also provide direction for the CHN in dealing with disease prevention. Refer to Appendix 1, specifically "Standard 1: Promoting Health," "Standard 3: Building Relationships," and "Standard 4: Facilitating Access and Equity." See Box 4-1 for Standard 1, Section B, on prevention and health protection and the role of the community health nurse.

While disease prevention measures can contribute to improved population health, individuals may make choices contrary to the interventions proposed by the CHN based on considerations such as culture, religion, or health beliefs. For example, a family in the community might refuse to have their preschool child immunized. In such a situation, the CHN needs to be respectful and nonjudgemental, weigh the risks and benefits to the population, and assess and educate the family appropriately to ensure that the client has made an informed choice.

Community health nursing interventions aimed at health promotion encourage the enhancement of the

BOX 4-1 Canadian Community Health Nursing Standards of Practice

Standard 1, Section B: Prevention and Health Protection

The community health nurse

1. Recognizes the differences between the levels of prevention (primary, secondary, tertiary).
2. Selects the appropriate level of preventive intervention.
3. Helps individuals and communities make informed choices about protective and preventive health measures such as immunization, birth control, breastfeeding, and palliative care.
4. Helps individuals, groups, families, and communities to identify potential risks to health.
5. Uses harm reduction principles to identify, reduce, or remove risk factors in a variety of contexts including the home, neighbourhood, workplace, school, and street.
6. Applies epidemiological principles when using strategies such as screening, surveillance, immunization, communicable disease response and outbreak management, and education.
7. Engages collaborative, interdisciplinary and intersectoral partnerships to address risks to individual, family, community, or population health and to address prevention and protection issues such as communicable disease, injury, and chronic disease.
8. Collaborates on developing and using follow-up systems in the practice setting to ensure that the individual or community receives appropriate and effective service.
9. Practices in accordance with legislation relevant to community health practice (e.g., public health legislation and child protection legislation).
10. Evaluates collaborative practice (personal, team and intersectoral) for achieving individual and community outcomes such as reduced communicable disease, injury, and chronic disease, or impacts of a disease process.

SOURCE: Community Health Nurses Association of Canada. (2008). *Canadian community health nursing standards of practice* (p. 11). Retrieved from http://www.chnc.ca/documents/chn_standards_of_practice_mar08_english.pdf.

well-being of clients. In Canada, many community health nursing strategies are directed to populations and aggregates and emphasize the determinants of health and the use of the health promotion strategies outlined in the Ottawa Charter. Refer to Box 4-2 for Standard 1, Section A, which provides direction for the CHN working in health promotion.

CRITICAL VIEW

1. What do you think distinguishes disease prevention from health promotion?
2. a) Do you think that illness prevention and health protection can be included under the term *disease prevention*?

   b) What supports your decision in answering question 2a?

Different strategies are available to affect the health behaviours of individuals or populations at various levels of risk. Figure 4-1 depicts the health risk continuum and its relationship to health promotion, disease prevention, and treatment. The figure shows the relationship between the three levels of disease prevention and risk. As discussed in Chapter 1, activities and programs at the primary prevention level are initiated when clients are at no risk to low risk and have the goal of risk avoidance. In primary prevention, prevention activities strive to prevent movement toward disability and death. Early treatment and intervention programs at the secondary prevention level are initiated when clients are at moderate risk and have the goal of risk reduction. Treatment programs at the tertiary prevention level (health recovery) are initiated when clients are at high risk and have the goal of rehabilitation. Health promotion activities are intended to move clients toward optimal health. Health enhancement, a health promotion strategy, is used to develop or enhance the health and well-being of clients at any point on the risk continuum.

BOX 4-2 Canadian Community Health Nursing Standards of Practice

Standard 1, Section A: Health Promotion

The community health nurse

1. Collaborates with individual, community, and other stakeholders to do a holistic assessment of assets and needs of the individual or community.
2. Uses a variety of information sources to access data and research findings related to health at the national, provincial, territorial, regional, and local levels.
3. Identifies and seeks to address root causes of illness and disease.
4. Facilitates planned change with the individual, community, or population by applying the Population Health Promotion Model.
   - Identifies the level of intervention necessary to promote health.
   - Identifies which determinants of health require action or change to promote health.
   - Uses a comprehensive range of strategies to address health-related issues.
5. Demonstrates knowledge of and effectively implements health promotion strategies based on the Ottawa Charter for Health Promotion.
   - Incorporates multiple strategies: promoting healthy public policy, strengthening community action, creating supportive environments, developing personal skills, and reorienting the health system.
   - Identifies strategies for change that will make it easier for people to make healthier choices.
6. Collaborates with the individual and community to help them take responsibility for maintaining or improving their health by increasing their knowledge, influence, and control over the determinants of health.
7. Understands and uses social marketing, media, and advocacy strategies to raise awareness of health issues, place issues on the public agenda, shift social norms, and change behaviours if other enabling factors are present.
8. Helps the individual and community to identify their strengths and available resources and take action to address their needs.
9. Recognizes the broad impact of specific issues on health promotion such as political climate and will, values and culture, individual and community readiness, and social and systemic structures.
10. Evaluates and modifies population health promotion programs in partnership with the individual, community, and other stakeholders.

SOURCE: Community Health Nurses Association of Canada. (2008). *Canadian community health nursing standards of practice* (p. 10). Retrieved from http://www.chnc.ca/documents/chn_standards_of_practice_mar08_english.pdf.

FIGURE 4-1 Levels of Disease Prevention on the Risk Continuum

Health concerns are NOT present		Health concerns ARE present	
At no risk	At low risk	At moderate risk	At high risk

→

Primary prevention	Secondary prevention	Tertiary prevention
Risk avoidance	Risk reduction	Rehabilitation

CRITICAL VIEW

1. How would you use the health promotion and disease prevention risk continuum (see Figure 4-1) to explain effective strategies for persons at risk for drug misuse?

Harm reduction is accomplished through strategies such as the implementation of policies or programs (often not requiring abstinence) to decrease the adverse health consequences of substance use (Centre for Addiction and Mental Health, 2006; Davis, 2006; Health Canada, 2005b). Harm reduction strategies focus on the eventual goal of abstinence as opposed to abstinence as a prerequisite for program participation (Davis, 2006).

Examples of harm reduction strategies include needle exchange programs, methadone maintenance programs, and smokeless tobacco programs. Within Canada, although provincial and territorial research findings on the patterns of substance use vary, commonalities exist in its prevalence. For example, alcohol is the most commonly used substance by youth, with binge drinking commonly occurring; cannabis use ranks second and is

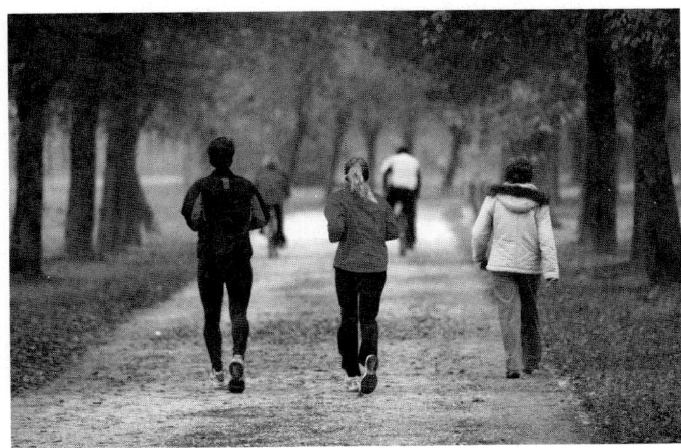

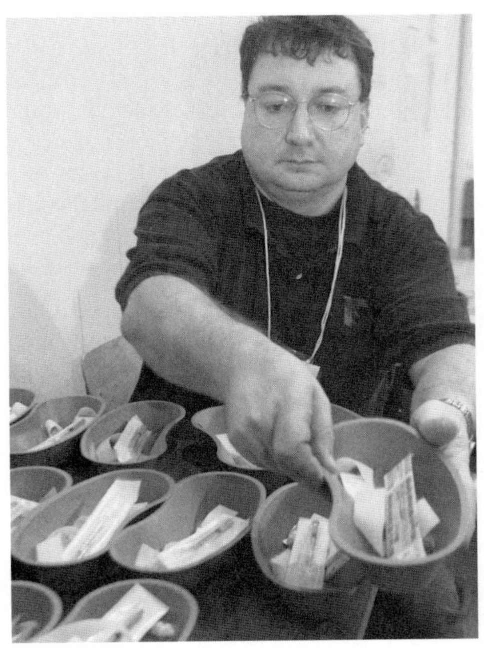

Community nurses may participate in health promotion and harm reduction programs. Health promotion may be aimed at enhancing the well-being of clients, for example, by encouraging participation in exercise programs (as shown at left). On the right, a nurse prepares injection kits for Vancouver's needle-exchange program, an example of a harm reduction program.

more common than cigarette smoking (Canadian Centre on Substance Abuse, 2007). Substance use places youths at high risk for serious harm.

Several strategies to reduce harm from substance use are available. One such strategy targeted junior and senior high-school students in four schools in Nova Scotia with the goal of minimizing harm due to drug (i.e., alcohol, cannabis, tobacco) use. This integrated school- and community-based demonstration intervention project involved a partnership of researchers, school officials, parents, the school board, and the community. A drug education program aimed to minimize the use of these drugs but did not require total abstinence (harm-minimization approach). An evaluation of the harm-minimization approach revealed that the approach was deemed acceptable and effective in the case of the senior high-school students studied; however, there were dangers associated with its use with the junior high-school students in this study (Poulin & Nicholson, 2005). CHNs working with these populations need to consider these study findings when developing educational programs. Harm reduction is discussed further in Chapter 11.

Closely associated with the concept of harm reduction is the concept of resiliency. **Resiliency** is the capacity of clients as individuals, families, groups, and communities to manage effectively when faced with considerable adversity or risk (University of Calgary, 2007). Resiliency develops and changes over time, depending on changes in risk and protective factors. **Risk factors** are variables that create stress and therefore challenge clients' health status. For example, hypertension is a risk factor for a cerebrovascular accident, poverty is a risk factor for certain infectious diseases, and a community disaster is a risk factor for increased community crime rates. **Protective factors** are variables that assist in managing the stressors associated with being at risk. Examples of protective factors include literacy, social support networks, family support systems, and community empowerment through public participation. If stress outweighs one's protective factors, creating an imbalance, a previously resilient client may become incapable of usual functioning. The following are examples of risk factors and associated protective factors:

- Risk factor—inaccessibility to family doctors; protective factor—the provision of local walk-in clinics
- Risk factor—domestic violence; protective factor—extended family support
- Risk factor—gang violence in a community neighbourhood; protective factor—an established community coalition of concerned citizens, the police force, and health care providers

EVOLUTION OF HEALTH PROMOTION

Canada has been at the forefront in the evolution of health promotion. Health promotion extends beyond providing education to individuals, families, aggregates, populations, and communities. A review of the key developments of health promotion in Canada will identify other aspects of health promotion.

The evolution of nursing and health care, presented in Chapter 2, and the discussion earlier in this chapter on the definitions of *health* reveal that when the medical model prevailed, health care's focus was on illness and *health* was defined as the absence of disease. Developmentally and historically, the emphasis was on the control of infectious and communicable diseases. In the mid-1900s, the advent of antibiotics and vaccinations generally brought these diseases under control.

Lalonde Report

It was not until 1974 that Marc Lalonde, then minister of Health and Welfare Canada, introduced the notion of health promotion nationally and internationally with the report titled *A New Perspective on the Health of Canadians: A Working Document*. This report initiated a shift, especially in Canada, from a primarily biomedical view of disease and health to a consideration of certain aspects of health promotion. This document, most commonly known as the Lalonde Report, increased the awareness of human biology, environment, and lifestyle as determinants of health and, therefore, influencers of health (Lalonde, 1974; Vollman et al., 2008). A fourth category of factors affecting the health of Canadians was health care (Lalonde, 1974; Vollman et al., 2008). Lalonde (1974) proposed a need for a more comprehensive approach to health care. He urged improvements to the environment, increased knowledge in human biology, and modifications of self-imposed risks due to individual health choices and related behaviours to increase the population health status of Canadians (Lalonde, 1974; Vollman et al., 2008). These conclusions raised policymakers' awareness of health promotion, not only in Canada but also in the United States and Europe. Consideration of lifestyle factors and their impact on health introduced a focus on individual risk factor behaviours that can negatively affect health, such as smoking, inactivity, unhealthy diet, and substance abuse. A behavioural approach led to a view that individuals were responsible for their own health. Because this individual approach to lifestyle choices did not consider socio-political and economic factors, it led to victim blaming when individuals did not change their behaviours. Box 4-3 lists some of the landmark health promotion movements, and Figure 4-2 presents information on various reports and conferences that illustrate some of the perspectives on health and health policies in Canada.

In response to the Lalonde Report, a focus on lifestyle and personal health occurred, resulting in health promotion research, public policy, and interventions being directed toward lifestyle changes. Health promotion research identified associations between personal risk factors and health status. In public policy, discussions and new legislation at the various government levels focused on areas such as smoking and drinking and driving. Health promotion interventions included the implementation of health education and mass media campaigns to dissuade unhealthy behaviours such as smoking and sedentary lifestyles (Health Canada, 2005c; Health Canada, 2005d).

Alma-Ata Declaration

In 1978, the Alma-Ata Declaration, with its focus on primary health care, was presented at the WHO conference in Alma-Ata, U.S.S.R. (Kazakhstan) to address the unacceptable inequalities in the health status between developed and developing countries. From this conference came an awareness and acknowledgement that to improve health, more had to be done beyond funding health services such as hospitals (Catford, 2004). This shift in thinking brought about primary health care as the chosen strategy for health care delivery to achieve the goal of "health for all by the year 2000." (Refer to Appendix 5 for a copy of the Alma-Ata Declaration.) Primary health care identified social and environmental conditions as determinants of health outside of the health care sector and helped make evident the need for intersectoral cooperation if the population health status was to improve. Unfortunately, however, primary health care did not develop as quickly or as extensively internationally or in Canada as had been envisioned. Power shifted from health care providers to communities and health care consumers (Catford, 2004).

BOX 4-3 Landmark Health Promotion Movements

1974	*A New Perspective on the Health of Canadians* (Lalonde Report)
1978	Alma-Ata Declaration in Alma-Ata, U.S.S.R. (Kazakhstan) (WHO International Conference)
1984	WHO Working Group develops concepts, principles, priorities, and dilemmas of health promotion
1986	Ottawa Charter for Health Promotion in Ottawa, Canada (WHO First International Conference on Health Promotion)
1986	*Achieving Health for All: A Framework for Health Promotion* (Epp Report)
1988	Healthy Public Policy Conference in Adelaide, Australia (WHO Second International Conference on Health Promotion)
1991	Supportive Environments for Health Conference in Sundsvall, Sweden (WHO Third International Conference on Health Promotion)
1996	*Population Health Promotion: An Integrated Model of Population Health and Health Promotion* (Hamilton & Bhatti, 1996)
1997	Jakarta Declaration on Health Promotion Into the Twenty-First Century in Jakarta, Indonesia (WHO Fourth International Conference on Health Promotion)
2000	Bridging the Equity Gap in Mexico City, Mexico (WHO Fifth International Conference on Health Promotion)
2002	Strengthening the Social Determinants of Health: The Toronto Charter for a Healthy Canada in Toronto, Canada
2005	Policy and Partnership for Action: Addressing the Determinants of Health in Bangkok, Thailand (WHO Sixth International Conference on Health Promotion)
2007	World Conference on Health Promotion and Health Education by the International Union for Health Promotion and Education in Vancouver, Canada
2008	World Health Organization Commission on Social Determinants of Health (established in 2005) released final report on the social determinants of health, titled *Closing the Gap in a Generation: Health Equity Through Action on the Social Determinants of Health*
2009	Promoting Health and Development: Closing the Implementation Gap in Nairobi, Kenya (WHO Seventh International Conference on Health Promotion)

FIGURE 4-2 A Conceptual Evolution of "Health": National and International Perspectives on Health and Health Policies From 1974 to the Present

Illness focused

- Provider centred
- Limited community participation
- Public policies based on assumptions that medical technology alone can improve health status

Document	The Lalonde Report: *A New Perspective on the Health of Canadians*	The Alma-Ata Declaration on PHC	The Black Report	The Healthy Communities Initiative: Toronto 2000	The Ottawa Charter: *A Framework for Health Promotion*	Review of PHC and HFA by 2000
Author(s)	(Marc Lalonde) Health and Welfare Canada	WHO and UNICEF	Sir Douglas Black	Dr. Trevor Hancock	(Jake Epp) Health and Welfare Canada	WHO
Place	Ottawa, Ont.	Alma-Ata, Kazakhstan, U.S.S.R.	United Kingdom	Toronto, Ont.	Ottawa, Ont.	Riga, Latvia
Year	1974	1978	1980	1984	1986	1988
Main ideas	Introduction of the "health field concept" (4 domains): • Human biology • Lifestyle • Environment • Health care system as determinant of health Focused on lifestyle modification Approaches seen by some as blaming the victim	5 principles: 1. Accessibility 2. Emphasis on health promotion 3. Intersectoral collaboration 4. Appropriate technology 5. Community participation Plus 8 essential elements	Study of British civil servants—showed that class was associated with mortality outcomes	Began to examine the socioenvironmental determinants of health Multisectoral health policies and health planning emerged Community visioning and empowerment seen as a health-promoting process	Challenges outlined: • Reducing health inequities • Increasing disease prevention Health promotion seen as enabling people to increase control over their health and lives	Renewed commitment to principles of PHC Some disappointment with progress in some areas and locations Health still a highly centralized approach in many parts of the world

Adapted from Ehrlich, A., & Ladouceur, M. G. (2002). *A conceptual evolution of "health": National and international perspectives on health and health policies from 1974 to present.* Hamilton, ON: School of Nursing, McMaster University, with additional information from the Canadian authors.

Health Promotion Principles

In 1984, a working group for the WHO prepared a report on health promotion identifying the concepts, principles, priorities, and dilemmas (Catford, 2004). Table 4-1 presents the health promotion principles with their associated implications. Catford (2004) stated, "The original health promotion principles are alive and well today" (p. 2). It is evident that further support is needed in order that health promotion principles are recognized as one of the basic elements of practitioners' health promotion capacity (McLean, Feather, & Butler-Jones, 2005).

Ottawa Charter

The Ottawa Charter (WHO, 1986) defined and developed the concept and components of health promotion. (Refer to Appendix 6 for the concepts and components found in the Charter.) The Charter increased awareness of and expanded upon the determinants of health in its discussions of the prerequisites for health, such as peace, shelter, education, food, income, a stable ecosystem, sustainable resources, social justice, and equity (Vollman et al., 2008). The Charter identified several health promotion strategies for practice—advocating, enabling, and mediating—as necessary to help communities, groups, and individuals to reach their optimal levels of health. This new perspective on health promotion, included in the Ottawa Charter, contributed to a change in the roles assumed by health care providers (Young & Hayes, 2002), who moved from the expert "in control" role to the roles of advocate, facilitator, supporter, and mediator. The advocacy role is discussed in more detail later in this chapter and in several other chapters throughout the text.

Also at this time, Canada experienced a shift from an individual-based health promotion approach toward a population health promotion (PHP) approach that integrated the Ottawa Charter. The five major action areas (referred to as "action means" in the Charter) for promoting health are as follows:

Improved well-being?

- Better community participation, dialogue, and collaboration

CNA position paper on PHC	RNABC position paper on PHC	ANAC submission to the Royal Commission on Aboriginal Peoples	Community Action Program for Children (CAPC)	Royal Commission on the Future of Health in Canada (the Romanow Report)	The Chief Public Health Officer's Report on the State of Public Health in Canada 2008: *Addressing Health Inequalities*	A Life Course Approach to the Social Determinants of Health for Aboriginal Peoples
CNA	RNABC	ANAC	Health Canada	Roy J. Romanow	Public Health Agency of Canada (Dr. David Butler Jones)	Jeff Reading
Ottawa, Ont.	Vancouver, B.C.	Ottawa, Ont.	Ottawa, Ont.	Saskatoon, Sask.	Ottawa, Ont.	Ottawa, Ont.
1989	1991	1993	1994	2002	2008	2009
		Established a need for dialogue and collaboration and for community-based approaches, including the use of traditional healers	Community-based information gathering for health planning and implementation	Limits of the role of the health care system: • Definition of PHC is reduced to "health care for individuals" and "services to communities" • Intersectoral collaboration is reduced to "inter-disciplinary teamwork" • Prevention is reduced to "early detection and action"	Reports on the health trends in Canada such as the growing prevalence of obesity and diabetes. Includes discussion of the determinants of health and their impact on the health of Canadians and the inequalities that develop because of the determinants of health.	In-depth examination of the social determinants of health, specifically related to the unique context of Aboriginal peoples' health

TABLE 4-1 Health Promotion Principles and Implications

Principles of Health Promotion	Discussion	Implications
1. Health promotion involves the population as a whole in the context of their everyday life, rather than focusing on people at risk for specific diseases.	This principle recognizes the need to enable persons to take charge of and responsibility for their health. It identifies population health as a major part of health promotion.	• Health professionals need to empower and promote self-care with clients. • Populations require access to information about health. • Health professionals need to use a variety of dissemination methods.
2. Health promotion is directed toward action on the determinants or causes of health.	The intersectoral aspects of health promotion are evident. Intergovernmental responsibility exists for the "total" environment, which is outside of individual and group influence.	• All levels of government are responsible for ensuring that all environments support and promote health by implementing appropriate and timely interventions. • Health professionals should assume an advocacy role and be involved in intersectoral collaboration to influence the development of healthy public policy.

(Continued)

TABLE 4-1 Health Promotion Principles and Implications—Cont'd

Principles of Health Promotion	Discussion	Implications
3. Health promotion combines diverse but complementary methods or approaches.	Diverse strategies and approaches could include communication, education, legislation, organizational change, community development, and health hazard management.	• Health professionals need to carefully plan and be selective in choosing appropriate and mixed strategies and approaches.
4. Health promotion aims particularly at effective and concrete public participation.	Public participation collectively and individually requires further development of problem definition and decision-making life skills.	• Health professionals need to be flexible, innovative, and transparent to facilitate individual, group, and community involvement in decision making. • Health professionals need to build on and support individual, group, and community strengths.
5. Health professionals—particularly in primary health care—have an important role in nurturing and enabling health promotion.	Health promotion is not a medical service; it is an activity mainly used in the health and social fields.	• Health professionals need to develop skills in health promotion, such as empowerment, health education, and advocacy.

SOURCE: Adapted from Catford, J. (2004). Health promotion's record card: How principled are we 20 years on? *Health Promotion International, 19*(1), 2.

- Building healthy public policy (e.g., mandatory seat belt use in automobiles)
- Creating supportive environments (e.g., smoke-free workplaces)
- Strengthening community action (e.g., funding for heart health initiatives such as healthy food choices in restaurants)
- Developing personal skills (e.g., through community literacy programs)
- Reorienting health services (e.g., interdisciplinary community health centres)

These five action areas shifted the health promotion emphasis to include communities and shifted responsibilities for health primarily to the governments, communities, and individuals (Shah, 2003; Young & Hayes, 2002). Note that these five "action means" are referred to as "health promotion strategies" in this textbook; recent Canadian literature has also called them "health promotion strategies" (Canadian Public Health Association, 1996; Community Health Nurses Association of Canada, 2008; Health Canada, 2005a; Ministry of Health Promotion, 2008; Reutter & Eastlick Kushner, 2009; University of Ottawa, 2008). Strategies make up the "how" component of a plan to meet specified goals. Therefore, the population health promotion model (see Figure 1-4 on p. 16) considers the question "*How* should we take action?" in light of the five Charter action means.

Canadian Framework for Health Promotion

Jake Epp, as the minister of Health and Welfare Canada, proposed a national framework for health promotion as a strategy to achieve the goal of "health for all." In his framework, the following three identified national health challenges were highlighted as requiring particular focus: (1) reducing health inequities between low- and high-income groups; (2) increasing prevention efforts by reducing or eliminating risks to decrease injuries, diseases, chronic illnesses, and related disabilities; and (3) enhancing coping abilities, especially helping people to manage chronic conditions, mental health problems, and disabilities (Epp, 1986).

The Epp framework (Epp, 1986) identified the following mechanisms as necessary for health promotion and for meeting the identified health challenges:

CRITICAL VIEW

1. What differences do you think exist between equity and equality?
2. What are the relationships between social justice, equity, and equality?

- Self-care as related to healthy personal decisions and actions regarding an individual's own health (e.g., an individual deciding to become physically active)
- Mutual aid associated with individuals helping and supporting other individuals to deal with health concerns (e.g., bereavement groups)
- The creation of healthy environments to enhance health (e.g., smoke-free spaces)

Epp's framework further supported a community and policy focus in health promotion through the actions of fostering public participation (e.g., encouraging physical activity for heart health), strengthening community health services (e.g., increasing community mental health services), and coordinating healthy public policy (e.g., banning the sale and use of baby walkers).

A socioenvironmental approach is evident in the Ottawa Charter and the Epp Report since in these documents "health is seen as more than just the absence of disease and engaging in healthy behaviours; rather, this approach emphasizes connectedness, self-efficacy, and capacity to engage in meaningful activities" (Reutter & Eastlick Kushner, 2009, p. 4).

Other Developments in Health Promotion

Importantly, the Canadian identification of the determinants of health within the framework of health promotion introduced by Lalonde (1974), Epp (1986), and the Ottawa Charter (WHO, 1986) demonstrated very progressive thinking. As noted in Chapter 1, the research to date has provided evidence that many of the 12 determinants, specifically economic and social inequities, influence the health status of Canadians. Also of note is the influence of poverty on health; poverty increases the risk for health problems especially during childhood, which continue throughout the lifespan, diminishing individuals' full potential and their contributions to Canadian society (Raphael, 2004). For further discussion of each of the determinants of health, including policy implications, refer to the Mikkonen and Raphael Web site "Social Determinants of Health: The Canadian Facts," listed in the Weblinks on the Evolve Web site. This timely, succinct document reviews the determinants of health from the Canadian perspective.

The WHO hosted the second international conference on health promotion in Adelaide, Australia, in 1988. It focused on the importance of healthy public policy and the re-establishment of commitment to the Ottawa Charter (Wass, 2000). Industrial countries were urged to establish policies to reduce inequities between rich and poor countries. Other priorities identified for action included the health of women, the elimination of malnutrition and hunger, a decreased availability of alcohol and tobacco, and the provision of increased supportive environments through alliance formations (Vollman et al., 2008).

The third international conference on health promotion, held in Sundsvall, Sweden, had as its main focus the provision of supportive environments to promote health at a community level. The four key actions to promote the creation of these supportive environments were as follows:

> *(1) strengthening advocacy through community action, particularly through groups organized by women; (2) enabling communities and individuals to take control over their health and environment through education and empowerment; (3) building alliances for health and supportive environments in order to strengthen the co-operation between health and environmental campaigns and strategies; and (4) mediating between conflicting interests in society in order to ensure equitable access to supportive environments for health.* (WHO, 1991, pp. 3–4)

Population Health Promotion Model Revisited

In 1994, a document titled *Strategies for Population Health: Investing in the Health of Canadians*, prepared by a federal, provincial, and territorial advisory committee, endorsed a population health approach (as cited in Public Health Agency of Canada [PHAC], 1994). This population health approach had originally been introduced in 1989 by the Canadian Institute of Advanced Research (CIAR). The CIAR had started the discussion on population health as a new concept to aid in understanding the determinants of health and the interplay among them (Evans, Barer, & Marmor, 1994). This population health approach created much debate about how it related to or was different from health promotion, especially since it also focused on the determinants of health (Young & Hayes, 2002). Many health promotion leaders in Canada expressed concerns about the population health approach and its possible negative influence on the integration of health promotion into public health practice in Canada (Bhatti, 1996; Labonte, 1995; Raphael & Bryant, 2002; Robertson, 1998).

A few years later, Hamilton and Bhatti (1996) introduced a population health promotion (PHP) model. This model builds on the Ottawa Charter as it considers and adds to the determinants of health and health promotion strategies. It integrates the challenge of reducing inequities in the population as outlined by both the Epp Report (Health Canada, 2005a; Shah, 2003) and the CIAR population health model (Young & Hayes, 2002). This PHP model clarifies the relationship between health promotion and population health. In support of the model, the Health Canada (2005a) document *Health Promotion: Does It Work?* clearly identifies the two theories as "synergistic" rather than contrasting concepts, and PHAC (2001, p. 1) describes the PHP model as showing "how a population health approach can be implemented through action on the full range of health determinants by means of health promotion strategies."

Figure 1-4 in Chapter 1 presents the three-dimensional diagram of the PHP model. The interrelating parts of the model that guide actions to improve health are (1) "what" (referring to the determinants of health); (2) "who" (referring to the top of the cube); and (3) "how" (referring to the health promotion strategies from the Ottawa Charter). The foundations of the model are evidence-informed decision making; sources for evidence-informed decision making, which include research, experiential learning, and evaluation; and values and assumptions. With this model, any of the five health promotion strategies can be developed and implemented at various levels, from societal to individual. The choice of health promotion strategy depends upon factors such as the values and assumptions held about the determinants of health, desired outcomes, and available evidence. The model can be used from a variety of entrance points (PHAC, 2001). For example, the determinants of health to be influenced or a health issue for a particular aggregate can serve as starting points, and, as well, one or more of the determinants can be addressed. Figure 4-3 demonstrates the application of the PHP model to an at-risk aggregate—girls and young women (9 to 26 years of age) at risk for a sexually transmitted infection. This infection is caused by exposure to the human papillomavirus (HPV) and can be prevented by the administration of an HPV vaccine.

The PHAC has identified eight key elements that need to be addressed in the population health approach model (see the Weblinks on the Evolve Web site). These elements, presented in Figure 4-4, are as follows (PHAC, 2008a):

1. Focus on the health of populations. A population health approach assesses health status and disparities in health status through the lifespan at the population level.

2. Address the determinants of health and their interactions. A population health approach appraises the determinants of health and their interrelationships.

FIGURE 4-3 The Population Health Promotion Model Applied to a Female Aggregate

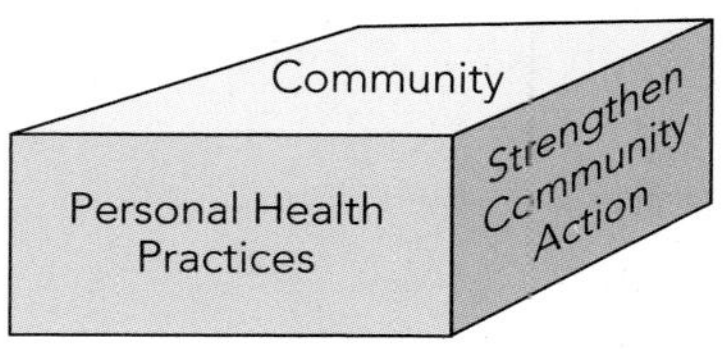

e.g.: Support community action to obtain available HPV vaccine and establish an HPV program.

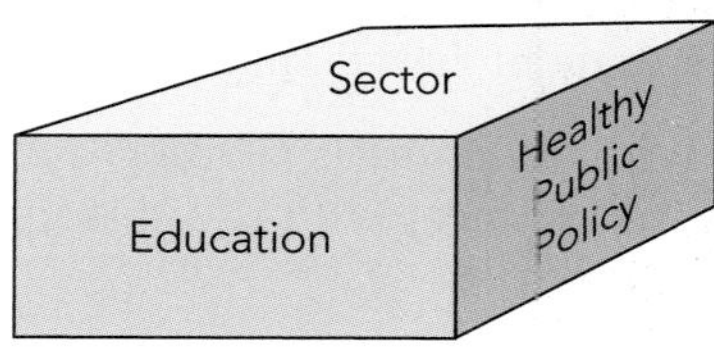

e.g.: Boards of Education can ensure that HPV vaccine information is included in the school curriculum.

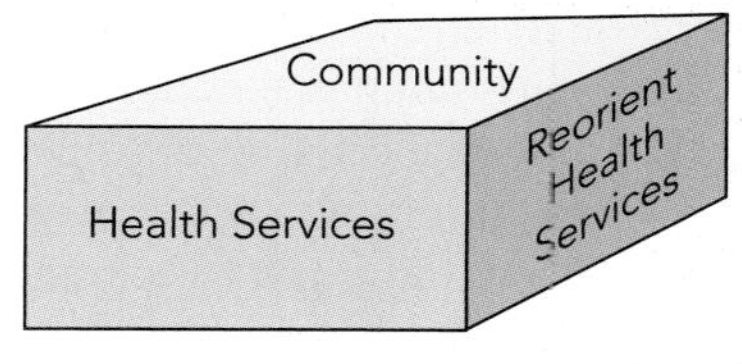

e.g.: Communities can provide opportunities for HPV testing, HPV counselling, and administration of the HPV vaccine and ensure that all opportunities are available and accessible.

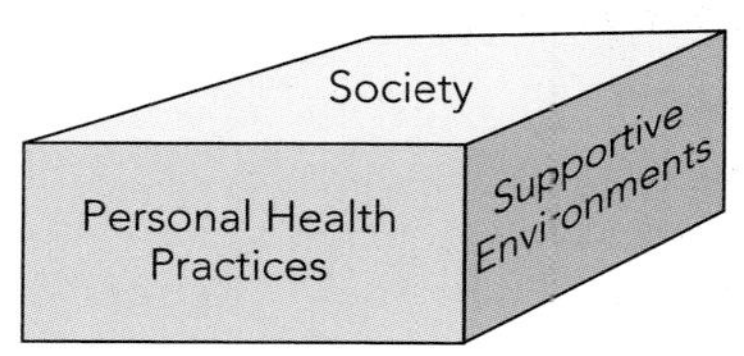

e.g.: Social marketing campaigns can heighten public awareness of the importance and availability of the HPV vaccine.

Adapted from Public Health Agency of Canada. (2001). *Population health promotion: An integrated model of population health and health promotion.* Retrieved from http://www.phac-aspc.gc.ca/ph-sp/php-psp/index-eng.php.

3. Base decisions on evidence. A population health approach uses evidence in assessment, planning, and development of interventions in health promotion.

4. Increase upstream investments. A population health approach capitalizes on its potential by focusing its energy and interventions to deal with foundational contributors to health and wellness.

5. Apply multiple interventions and strategies. A population health approach uses a variety of interventions and strategies to address the health concerns of client as individual, family, group or aggregate, community, population, or society.

6. Collaborate across sectors and levels. A population health approach includes horizontal and vertical intersectoral collaboration to affect health.

FIGURE 4-4 Population Health Approach: The Organizing Framework

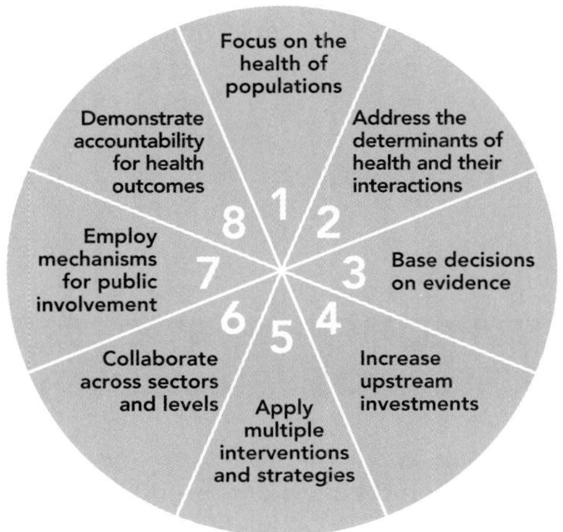

Public Health Agency of Canada. (2008). *Population health approach: The organizing framework*. Retrieved from http://cbpp-pcpe.phac-aspc.gc.ca/population_health/index-eng.html.

7. Employ mechanisms for public involvement. A population health approach partners with the community for planning, implementation, and evaluation of health promotion programs.
8. Demonstrate accountability for health outcomes. A population health approach focuses on the extent of change that can be a result of interventions in relation to health outcomes.

It bears repeating that CHNs need to note that in health promotion, Canada has primarily adopted the PHP approach, whereas other countries such as the United States have focused on an individual approach. The PHP approach integrates the determinants of health.

Although CHNs may work in health promotion with individuals and families, many work with populations and aggregates in their communities. CHNs need to always assess the determinants of health; consider social and economic inequalities; consider interventions needed to affect the determinants of health, such as empowering communities; advocate for healthy public policy; and establish and promote partnerships that contribute to the highest level of health for the client. This integration of the determinants of health is complex. To assist CHNs with the development of health promotion activities to effect change in population health determinants, Labonte (2003) prepared for Health Canada *How Our Programs Affect Population Health Determinants: A Workbook for Better Planning and Accountability* (see the Weblinks on the Evolve Web site).

Other International Health Promotion Conferences

The fourth international conference on health promotion took place in Jakarta, Indonesia, in 1997. The conference produced *The Jakarta Declaration on Leading Health Promotion into the 21st Century* (WHO, 2001). This was the first health promotion conference held in a developing country and the first to involve the private sector. To the prerequisites for health introduced in the Ottawa Charter, the Jakarta conference added social security, social relations, empowerment of women, and respect for human rights. Poverty (income) was identified as the social determinant influencing health the most. In addition, the declaration expanded on the Ottawa Charter strategies. The five priorities identified for the twenty-first century were (1) to promote social responsibility for health; (2) to increase investments for health development; (3) to consolidate and expand partnerships for health; (4) to increase community capacity and empower the individual; and (5) to secure an infrastructure for health promotion. The WHO site listed in the Weblinks on the Evolve Web site offers further information.

The fifth international conference on health promotion, Health Promotion: Bridging the Equity Gap, was held in Mexico City, Mexico, in 2000. Its primary emphasis was on dealing with the equity gap by focusing on the social determinants of health relating to those populations experiencing poverty and social challenges (Shah, 2003). The conference confirmed the importance of the provision of health services and of making health promotion a key component of public policies and programs globally to promote equity and health for all (WHO, 2000). The formation of international networks was recognized as one action for health promotion (WHO, 2000).

The sixth international conference on health promotion, titled Policy and Partnership for Action: Addressing the Determinants of Health, took place in Bangkok, Thailand, in 2005 and produced *The Bangkok Charter for Health Promotion in a Globalized World* (WHO, 2005). This charter addresses the need for global governance of health as affected by all the determinants of health, especially the health gaps between the rich and the poor. Four new global health promotion commitments included in the Bangkok Charter are as follows: "central to the global development agenda; a core responsibility for all of government; a key focus of communities and civil society; a requirement for good corporate practice" (WHO, 2005). The following five action areas were identified for all sectors and settings to narrow the inequalities in the social determinants that affect health: (1) advocacy for health for all; (2) policies, actions, and infrastructures in place to maintain sustainability; (3) capacity building in areas of policy development, leadership, health promotion practice, knowledge transfer and research, and health literacy; (4) an optimal level of security from harm to provide opportunity for health and well-being for all that is equal, based on regulation and legislation; and (5) the establishment of partnerships and alliances to create sustainable measures between nongovernmental and international organizations including public, private, and civil society (WHO, 2006).

The seventh international conference on health promotion, held in Nairobi, Kenya, in 2009, followed up on the work done at the Bangkok conference. Member states were encouraged to work toward meeting the four global health promotion commitments established in the Bangkok Charter. Support was provided to member states to develop and implement pilot projects to address the social determinants of health to reduce the gap between the rich and the poor (WHO, 2010). (See the WHO Overview Weblink listed at the end of this chapter.)

Summary

Catford (2004) captures the development of health promotion during the past several decades by categorizing health promotion dimensions related to its main focuses. According to Catford, in the 1970s, the first dimension of health promotion focused on managing preventable diseases and risk behaviours (e.g., heart disease, tobacco use). The health promotion strategy most countries adopted was providing health information and "simple" education. In the 1980s, the emphasis shifted to the importance of complementary intervention approaches as outlined in the Ottawa Charter, such as building healthy public policy and strengthening community action. In the 1990s, the focus was on providing health promotion to individuals and groups in their communities (e.g., cities, neighbourhoods, workplaces, schools, health care settings).

Catford (2004) suggests that in the 2000s, a fourth dimension of health promotion is evident in the inclusion of the social determinants of health, which provide a much broader focus than disease control and prevention. To ensure continued growth in health promotion, leadership development, one of the challenges for the current decade, is necessary (Catford, 2004); therefore, CHNs actively promoting health in their nursing practice need to continue demonstrating their leadership role by influencing healthy public policy, creating supportive environments, and strengthening community action. In addition, CHNs need to take action on the determinants of health, especially the social determinants of health, rather than focusing on disease prevention such as risk avoidance and risk reduction. Canadian community health nursing practice incorporates strategies from primary health care, the Ottawa Charter, the Epp framework, the population health model, and the determinants of health. For a synopsis of the reports and initiatives that contributed to the shift from an illness-focused perspective to a population- and health-promotion focus in primary health care in Canada, refer to Ehrlich and Ladouceur (2002). Figure 4-2 outlines this evolution in health care up to the present.

HEALTH PROMOTION MODELS, THEORIES, AND FRAMEWORKS

Models, theories, and frameworks provide different ways to look at health and health promotion. Several theories and models have been developed in an attempt to explain health behaviour and health behavioural change (Clark, 2008; Heiss, 2009). Some of these theories and models are directed toward behavioural change in individuals, while others focus on health changes in communities and organizations, and a few on healthy public policy. Only the models and theories most widely associated with health promotion and used in community health are discussed here. The Theories of Reasoned Action and of Planned Behaviour and the Transtheoretical (Stages of Change) Model focus on explaining an individual's behavioural health change. These theories and model serve to explain and facilitate personal health practices, one of the determinants of health. Theories, frameworks, and models that attempt to explain changes in communities include the Diffusion of Innovation Theory, Community Organization Models of Practice, Theories and Models of Community Development, and Community Mobilization Framework. The healthy public policy frameworks and models comprise Milio's framework, Weiss's framework, and the health impact assessment (HIA).

Theories of Reasoned Action and of Planned Change

In 1980, Ajzen and Fishbein developed the Theory of Reasoned Action to explain an individual changing his or her health behaviour (Clark, 2008). The theory assumes a relationship among attitudes, beliefs, intention, and behaviour (McKenzie, Neiger, & Thackeray, 2009). Another underlying assumption of this theory is that the most influencing factor in behavioural change is the intent to act. The theory postulates that beliefs, attitudes, and perceived behavioural control influence individual, group, and aggregate behavioural intention and thus their action and behaviour (McKenzie, Neiger, & Thackeray, 2009). Therefore, to develop interventions

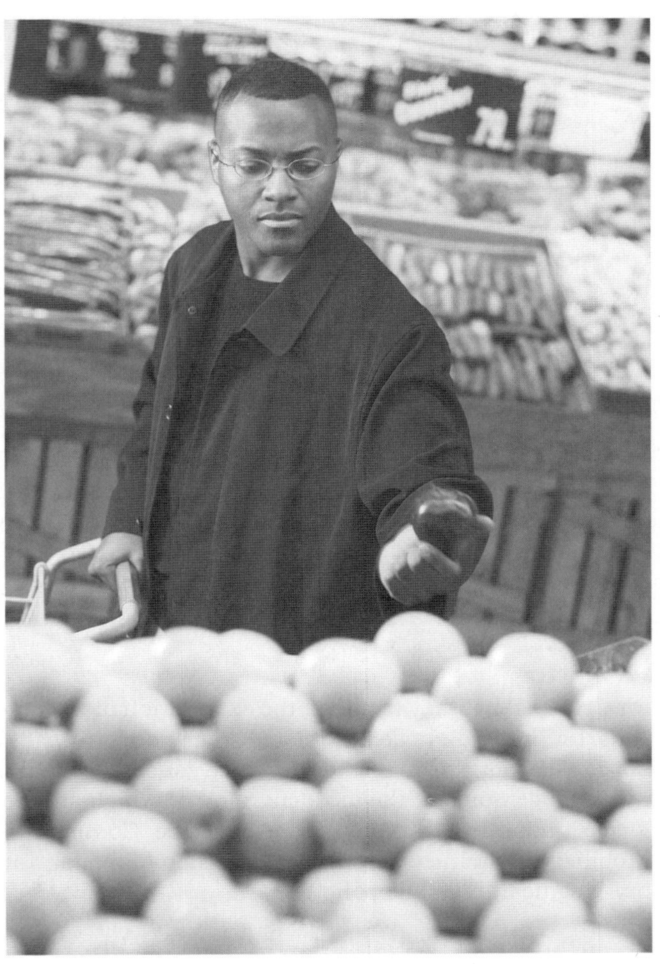

Making healthy choices when grocery shopping is one way in which a person practises self-efficacy.

and programs that will meet client needs, the CHN needs to assess these three influences in all client situations. In addition, the CHN needs to identify the client's intent for behavioural change. For further information on these theories, see the Ontario Health Promotion Resource System Weblink on the Evolve Web site.

Transtheoretical (Stages of Change) Model

The Transtheoretical Model, often referred to as the Stages of Change Model, was introduced in the early 1980s by Prochaska and DiClemente (1983). It proposes that the process of intentional change, that is, health behavioural actions and changes, usually proceeds through five stages. A sixth stage, termination, has been identified most often in association with changing addictive behaviours such as substance use (see Table 4-2).

The Transtheoretical Model includes the stages (i.e., precontemplation, contemplation, etc.) and processes (i.e., consciousness raising, recognition of the benefits of change, etc.) of change and the constructs, such as situational self-efficacy and temptations (e.g., coping with a situation with confidence without reverting to previous unhealthy behaviours), and decisional balance (e.g., consideration of the pros and cons of changing behaviour) (Cancer Prevention Research Center, n.d.). For a more comprehensive discussion of this model (and other models), refer to the *Theory at a Glance: A Guide for Health Promotion Practice* and the Cancer Prevention Research Center Weblinks on the Evolve Web site.

Many research studies have used this model with aggregates such as smokers in smoking cessation

TABLE 4-2 Application of the Transtheoretical Model to Promote Smoking Cessation

Stages of Change	Client Behaviour	Challenge	Suggested Actions for the Community Health Nurse
Precontemplation	Client has no intention to change behaviour within the next 6 months (no readiness for change)	Consciousness raising	• Assess client interest in quitting smoking • Provide information to the client on the health risks associated with smoking • Explore with the client the feasibility of smoking cessation
Contemplation	Client thinking of changing behaviour within the next 6 months	Recognition of the benefits of change	• Discuss information on the potential benefits of quitting smoking
Preparation	Client has serious intention to change behaviour within the next 30 days (readiness for change)	Support to overcome barriers to quitting smoking	• Assist client to identify potential barriers • Explore with the client how to overcome the barriers

(Continued)

TABLE 4-2 Application of the Transtheoretical Model to Promote Smoking Cessation—Cont'd

Stages of Change	Client Behaviour	Challenge	Suggested Actions for the Community Health Nurse
Action	Client has initiated behaviour change within past 6 months (behaviour change)	Program of change	• Develop a smoking cessation plan with the client • Monitor client progress
Maintenance	Client has changed behaviour for longer than 6 months (behaviour change)	Follow-up with continued support	• Plan routine follow-up contacts with the client • Prepare a plan to prevent relapse
Termination	Client is no longer tempted to re-establish the unhealthy behaviour (permanent behaviour change)	No need for follow-up	• Capacity building by identifying strengths • Supporting changed behaviour

SOURCE: Adapted from Nutbeam, D., & Harris, E. (2004). *Theory in a nutshell: A practical guide to health promotion theories.* Sydney, Australia: McGraw Hill, based on Prochaska, J. O., & DiClemente, C. C. (1983). Stages and processes of self-change of smoking: Toward an integrative model of change. *Journal of Consulting and Clinical Psychology, 51*(3), 390–395.

programs (Callaghan & Herzog, 2006; Spencer, Pagell, Hallion, & Adams, 2002); obese individuals in weight loss programs (Beresford, Curry, Kristal, Lazovich, & Bhatti, 1996; Glanz et al., 1998); and persons and aggregates with sedentary lifestyles trying to increase their physical activity behaviours (Riebe et al., 2005; Spencer, Adams, Malone, Roy, & Yost, 2006).

Recently, debate has arisen to create some division in support of the use of the Transtheoretical Model (Herzog, 2005; Prochaska, 2006; West, 2005). Critics have raised several issues including challenges of the scientific merit of the model, despite the finding that more than 500 published studies used this model for change for smoking cessation (see Herzog [2005] and West [2005] for specifics on the debate).

For a CHN working with clients or developing programs, this model of change provides direction regarding what to assess, which processes to use, and what nursing actions to take when clients are at different stages of change. The CHN needs to be familiar with community resources that would benefit clients going through the stages of change for their specific behaviour.

Summary

The previously discussed models focus mainly on health promotion interventions that shape individuals' or groups' health behaviours (Sallis et al., 2006; Young & Hayes, 2002). These individual-focused models tend to encourage victim blaming because they view individuals as being responsible for their health and therefore when people do not change their health behaviour, poor health is viewed as their fault. The advantage of these models for CHNs is that they facilitate the exploration of the reasons for individual health-related behaviours (Meade, 2007). We now turn to theories that concern community change, some of the most common of which are the Diffusion of Innovation Theory and the Community Mobilization Framework, and a discussion of models for building healthy public policy.

Diffusion of Innovation Theory

The Diffusion of Innovation Theory provides guidance on effective ways to encourage clients to adopt ideas, practices, programs, or products that are considered "new" and are adopted in a community or society. *Innovation* is any new idea, practice, or product, and *diffusion* is the process for gaining acceptance in the community or throughout society (Nutbeam & Harris, 2004). This theory shows that individuals adopt innovations at different rates. Clients exposed to an innovation are classified in one of the following five categories: innovators (quick adopters), early adopters (keeners), early majority, late majority, and laggards. Nutbeam and Harris indicate that early-majority clients usually comprise 30% to 35% of the general population and they are open to change and recognize the benefits of it. Late-majority clients usually comprise 30% to 35% of the general population and are doubtful about adopting the innovation. The laggards are resistant to adopting the innovation. The early adopters are willing to change and have the resources to adopt the innovation. Although the innovators hastily adopt the innovation, these people are often viewed as impulsive and not trustworthy (Nutbeam & Harris, 2004). Clients are more likely to adopt health-related practices if the following conditions exist: compatibility, flexibility, reversibility, simplicity, advantageousness, and cost-efficiency. (For further information, see the Ontario Health Promotion Resource System Weblink listed on the Evolve Web site.) Dearing (2009) describes the potential adopter's perception of the attributes of the innovation as follows:

- Perception of advantage on the basis of effectiveness and cost-efficiency in relation to the alternatives
- Complexity, that is, how easy it is to understand the innovation
- Compatibility, that is, similarity to past ways for the same goal
- Observability, that is, the degree to which the impact can be observed
- Trialability, that is, the degree of commitment for full adoption

To be effective, CHNs involved in the development and implementation of new health promotion ideas and practices need to consider the types of responders to innovation and the six conditions influencing adoption of the innovation. Social marketing strategies, which are discussed later, assist with dissemination and acceptance of the innovation. The theory components need to be considered to make programs sustainable. With the introduction of innovations in a community, diffusion can include implementing new initiatives, advancing policies, and using mass media (National Cancer Institute, 2005). With the introduction of innovations in an organization, diffusion can include initiating programs, modifying regulations, and adjusting worker roles. With the introduction of innovations to individuals, diffusion includes adopting a health behaviour and requires changes in lifestyle.

CHNs must know the community they work with and be able to anticipate what would most likely influence the community's response to new health promotion ideas, practices, and programs. Also, CHNs can identify community leaders as role models for change, which can speed up the adoption of the innovation. See Table 4-3 for the Top 10 Dissemination Mistakes That Can Happen in Practice to Work Against Diffusion. CHNs need to be aware of these mistakes to avoid a misapplication of the theory.

TABLE 4-3 Top 10 Mistakes That Can Happen in Practice That Can Work against Diffusion

1. We assume that evidence matters in the decision making of potential adopters.

Interventions of unknown effectiveness and of known ineffectiveness often spread while effective interventions do not. Evidence is most important to only a subset of early adopters and is most often used by them to reject interventions.
Solution: Emphasize other variables in the communication of innovations such as compatibility, cost, and simplicity.

2. We substitute our perceptions for those of potential adopters.

Inadequate and poorly performed formative evaluation is common as experts in the intervention topical domain engage in dissemination.
Solution: Seek out and listen to representative potential adopters to learn wants, information sources, advice-seeking behaviors, and reactions to prototype interventions.

3. We use intervention creators as intervention communicators.

While the creators of interventions are sometimes effective communicators, the opposite condition is much more common.
Solution: Enable access to the experts, but rely on others whom we know will elicit attention and information-seeking by potential adopters.

4. We introduce interventions before they are ready.

Interventions are often shown as they are created and tested. Viewers often perceive uncertainty and complexity as a result.
Solution: Publicize interventions only after clear results and the preparation of messages that elicit positive reactions from potential adopters.

5. We assume that information will influence decision making.

Information is necessary and can be sufficient for adoption decisions about inconsequential innovations, but for consequential interventions that imply changes in organizational routines or individual behaviours, influence is typically required.

Solution: Pair information resources with social influence in an overall dissemination strategy.

(Continued)

TABLE 4-3 Top 10 Mistakes That Can Happen in Practice That Can Work against Diffusion—Cont'd

6. We confuse authority with influence.
Persons high in positional or formal authority as influential, but often this is not the case. Solution: Gather data about who among potential adopters is sought out for advice and intervene with them to propel dissemination.
7. We allow the first to adopt (innovators) to self-select into our dissemination efforts.
The first to adopt often do so for counter-normative reasons and their low social status can become associated with an intervention.
Solution: Learn the relational structure that ties together potential adopters so that influential members can be identified and recruited.
8. We fail to distinguish among change agents, authority figures, opinion leaders, and innovation champions.
It is unusual for the same persons to effectively play multiple roles in dissemination into and within communities and complex organizations. Solution: Use formative evaluation to determine the functions that different persons are able to fulfill.
9. We select demonstration sites on criteria of motivation and capacity.
Criteria of interest and ability make sense when effective implementation is the only objective. But spread relies on the perceptions by others of initial adopters. Solution: Consider which sites will positively influence other sites when selecting demonstration sites.
10. We advocate single interventions as the solution to a problem.
Potential adopters differ by clientele, setting, resources, etc., so one intervention is unlikely to fit all. Solution: Communicate a cluster of evidence-informed practices so that potential adopters can get closer to a best fit of intervention to organization prior to adaptation.

SOURCE: Dearing, J. W. (2009). Applying diffusion of innovation theory to intervention development. *Research on Social Work Practice, 19*(5), 503–518.

Community Mobilization Framework

Health promotion involves working with communities that can be defined as a geographic community (e.g., neighbourhood, town) or a community of interest (e.g., older adults, disabled group with diabetes, obese children, transgendered persons). Rothman's Community Mobilization Framework identifies the following three health promotion community mobilization approaches to bring about community change: (1) social planning (i.e., problem solving at the community level to deal with community physical, mental, and social health concerns), which is described as a task-oriented strategy with a health care provider as expert "leader"; (2) locality development (i.e., community participation and cooperation to deal with community health concerns with a focus on process, consensus, and community self-help with a health care provider as facilitator); and (3) social action (i.e., a process with the focus on shifting power relationships and resources so that change occurs to the benefit of the disadvantaged in the community) (Nutbeam & Harris, 2004). (See the Ontario Health Promotion Resource System Weblink for further elaboration.)

The distinction between "working with," "working for," and "working on" communities is important as one examines the perspective of community-level work (Wass, 2000). When "working with" the community, health care providers form partnerships with community members as community development and capacity building occur. Thereby, communities incorporate health promotion approaches to bring about needed changes. When "working for" the community, health care providers are recognized as the experts who lead the planning and implementation of health promotion approaches, with some involvement of community members as required to bring about the needed changes. When "working on" the community, health care providers, using health promotion approaches, are viewed as the experts and assume complete planning and decision making responsibilities with little or no input from the community to bring about the needed changes. "Working with" the community is the approach CHNs prefer for fostering community engagement and mobilization.

BUILDING HEALTHY PUBLIC POLICY MODELS

CHNs practise in a sociopolitical environment (Community Health Nurses Association of Canada [CHNAC], 2008), guided and influenced by municipal (local), provincial or territorial, and federal health policies. Health is considered in its broadest sense, for example, including physical, psychosocial, economic, and cultural perspectives. Therefore, CHNs need to be familiar with and knowledgeable about the available models for healthy public policy development, the policies and legislation that mandate their professional practice roles and responsibilities, and the healthy public policies mandated within their community programs and service delivery. It is also important for CHNs to recognize the need for intersectoral coordination in relation to healthy public policy development. Within a population health focus with an emphasis on the determinants of health, policy development is broader than just health care. Therefore, depending upon the issue, other societal sectors may need to be involved (e.g., agriculture, justice, and transportation) in the building of healthy public policy.

Nutbeam and Harris (2004) indicate that models for building healthy public policy in health promotion are in their early stages of development. At present, the following three frameworks are available to help in understanding healthy public policy: Milio's framework for the development of healthy public policy, Weiss's framework on the relationships between evidence and policy, and the health impact assessment (HIA) on policy development and implementation.

Milio, in 1987, coined the term *healthy public policy* and identified that policy development proceeds through initiation, action, implementation, evaluation, and reformulation stages (as cited in Nutbeam & Harris, 2004). These stages are cyclical and dynamic rather than linear as policy moves through the social and political processes. In Milio's framework, *policyholders* (i.e., politicians, bureaucrats), *policy influencers* (i.e., aggregates inside and outside of governments), the *public* (i.e., individuals who influence policy adoption, such as taxpayers and voters), and the *media* (i.e., print and electronic, affecting policymakers and public knowledge and perceptions about the issue) are foundational to healthy policy development. Milio maintains that the community or organization must become a key stakeholder, even though most policy development is initiated by only a few individuals. The four elements that affect policy development as identified by Milio are *social climate* (i.e., social, economical, and political context when the policy is introduced), *influence* (best if the policy is associated with committed groups who have the most power on the issue), *interests* (i.e., what could be gained, lost, or compromised), and *capacity* (i.e., ability to affect the issue). Social climate is the most powerful of these elements.

The CHN's roles as an advocate in creating public policy, as a support for community action to influence public policy, and as an advocate for societal change are identified in the *Canadian Community Health Nursing Standards of Practice*. In community health nursing, with its health promotion focus, development of healthy public policy is often directed at particular aggregate groups based on age, health challenges, lifestyle, and healthy choice issues. Examples include crib safety for infants and young children, restraint use in long-term care institutions, seat belt use for populations, and a tobacco ban in communities. An understanding of Milio's framework would, for example, help the CHN identify the main players and key elements to consider in strategy development when proposing a health issue for healthy policy development.

Weiss developed knowledge-driven, problem-solving, interactive, political, and tactical models to provide clarification of the different ways that evidence has guided healthy policy development (as cited in Nutbeam & Harris, 2004). Box 4-4 provides a synopsis of each of these models Weiss developed.

HIA models are used to inform decision making in relation to policy development and practice. They are also used to examine the impact on the health of populations (Nutbeam & Harris, 2004).

BOX 4-4 Weiss's Models of Policy Development

Model	Key Considerations
Knowledge-driven	• New research knowledge immediately influences healthy public policy. • New knowledge is rapidly accepted into policy development.
Problem-solving	• Mechanisms during the decision-making process related to policy development include collection and consideration of the evidence. • The evidence is collected from a variety of sources.
Interactive	• During policy development, knowledge from research is one consideration. • Other considerations include social pressures, experience, and political situation.
Political	• "Evidence is used to justify a predetermined position" (Nutbeam & Harris, 2004, p. 65). • Preferable data are used.
Tactical	• Evidence is used to support an unpopular decision or to explain and avoid an unpopular decision. • Unsubstantiated research findings are used to delay decision making.

SOURCE: Adapted from Nutbeam, D., & Harris, E. (2004). *Theory in a nutshell: A practical guide to health promotion theories.* Sydney, Australia: McGraw Hill.

Other Models

Ecological models in health promotion address broad contextual factors that influence health (Green & Kreuter, 1999; Lyons & Langille, 2000). These models have a system-level focus and explore the relationships between individuals and communities and between sociocultural and environmental factors that influence health (McLaren & Hawe, 2005). Therefore, when using an ecological perspective, the health promotion strategies target multiple levels, such as healthy public policy, community, organization, and intrapersonal and interpersonal factors that affect health (Green & Kreuter, 1999; McLaren & Hawe, 2005; Sallis et al., 2006). One example of an ecological model is the PRECEDE–PROCEED Model developed by Green and Kreuter (1999). Sallis et al. (2006) describe a more recent example of the application of the ecological model to change population health in communities through improving physical activity. The researchers explored the ecological model and its influence on the four domains of active living: recreation, transport, occupation, and household. (See the article by Sallis et al. [2006] for further details on the approach used.) The PRECEDE–PROCEED Model is discussed in depth in Chapter 10.

In recent literature, existential and humanistic theoretical perspectives have emerged as orientations that inform nursing practice. Within these orientations, the classic and evolving theoretical work of Watson (1979, 1999) emphasizes caring for humankind as foundational to nursing as a profession and, more specifically, the therapeutic interpersonal relationship between the nurse and the client. Watson's description of caring as the moral imperative to act justly and ethically to effect a positive change in the welfare of others aligns well with health promotion initiatives for community clients. Watson's emphasis on holistic health identifies that all human beings have "carative" needs that can be met through individualized nursing interventions focused on a human care process involving mutual participation of both the nurse and the client (Watson, 1999). Although not widely acknowledged as a health promotion model, Watson's Theory of Human Caring, when applied in health promotion initiatives within the community context, provides a holistic and progressive client-inclusive approach.

CRITICAL VIEW

1. How does community health nursing practice differ when using the humanistic approach for health promotion rather than the behaviourist approach?
2. Which health promotion programs are available in your community?

HEALTH PROMOTION APPROACHES

The following three approaches provide different ways of viewing health and of promoting optimal health and well-being: (1) biomedical, (2) behavioural, and (3) socioenvironmental. These approaches were originally referred to as *models*. Table 4-4 describes the components of each of these approaches.

Biomedical Approach

The biomedical approach was introduced in the eighteenth century with the discovery of disease pathogens and has continued to develop to the present. "Health promotion began with a medical approach focusing on immunization and screening for existing diseases, then shifted to a focus on changing individual risk behaviours" (Clark, 2008). This approach focuses on the treatment and prevention of disease, especially on the biological and physiological risk factors associated with disease and ill health. The prevention of disease includes the three levels of prevention. For example, hypertension is a risk factor for cardiovascular events such as cerebrovascular accidents. Finding hypertension in clients early and counselling about dietary changes, especially fat and salt intake, are important preventive strategies.

Behavioural Approach

The behavioural approach was first introduced with the Lalonde Report (1974) and has further developed to the present. This approach focuses on using lifestyle changes, especially behavioural risk factors, to promote health. For example, obesity is a risk factor for hypertension, and obesity and smoking are risk factors for cardiovascular disease. Health communication activities in this example would focus on quit-smoking campaigns and physical activity and nutritional messages for weight loss. Social marketing, the use of mass media, or both could be used to support the adoption of a healthy lifestyle.

Socioenvironmental Approach

The socioenvironmental approach started with the Alma-Ata Conference on Primary Health Care in 1978, when community participation and intersectoral collaboration were identified as necessary for dealing with social and environmental determinants of health. This approach focuses on health as a resource and considers the psychosocial and environmental risk factors related to the determinants of health in relation to health and health promotion. For example, the risk condition associated with the social determinant of health of poverty in the community affects people's ability to purchase healthy foods and, thereby, affects their cardiovascular

TABLE 4-4 Three Approaches Used in Health Promotion

Approach	Perception of Health	Examples of Leading Health Problems	Examples of Strategies to Manage Health Problems
Biomedical	Health is the absence of diseases, conditions, and disorders.	• Hypertension • Cardiovascular diseases • Diabetes • Obesity • Human immunodeficiency virus/acquired immunodeficiency syndrome	• Medical and pharmacological treatments specific to health problem • Primary prevention, e.g., immunization • Secondary prevention, e.g., early case finding through screening programs • Tertiary prevention, e.g., cardiovascular rehabilitation programs
Behavioural	Health is the result of lifestyle choices, specifically healthy ones.	• Poor stress management • Smoking • Sedentary lifestyle • Poor eating habits • Substance abuse	• Health communication • Health education • Self-help or mutual aid • Advocacy for healthy public policies to change behaviours and promote healthy lifestyle choices (e.g., smoking bans)
Socioenvironmental	Health is the result of the determinants of health, specifically social, economical, and environmental, that provide benefits and barriers to individual and community health.	• Unemployment • Poverty • Lack of social support and isolation • Environmental pollution	• Building healthy public policy • Creating supportive environments • Strengthening community action • Developing personal skills • Reorienting health services

SOURCE: Adapted from Ontario Health Promotion Resource System. (n.d.). *HP-101: Health promotion on-line course*. Retrieved from http://www.ohprs.ca/hp101/mod3/module3c1.htm.

health. Community policy development pertaining to "food security" would address this social determinant of health. This health promotion approach uses the five strategies for health promotion outlined in the Ottawa Charter. Lending support for the importance of the socio-environmental approach in health promotion, the WHO (2008) summarizes this approach to health as follows:

> *Lack of health care is not the cause of the huge global burden of illness; water-borne diseases are not caused by lack of antibiotics but by dirty water, and by political, social and economic forces that fail to make clean water available to all; heart disease is not caused by a lack of coronary care units but by the lives people lead; which are shaped by the environments in which they live; obesity is not caused by moral failure on the part of individuals but by the excess availability of high-fat and high-sugar foods. The main action on the social determinants of health must come from outside the health sector.* (p. 43)

The Senate Subcommittee on Population Health (2009) recommends a focus on the determinants of health and the population health framework as an investment in Canada's future in the twenty-first century. It recommends that priority be given to the following determinants of health: clean water; food security; parenting and early childhood learning; violence against Aboriginal women, children, and elders; education; housing; economic development; and health care. The report also addresses health disparities, promotes the well-being of all Canadians, and recommends a whole-government approach to address health issues of Canadians.

Health care providers usually subscribe to one or all of these approaches, influencing their view of health and health promotion, their definitions of *health*, and their decisions about which health promotion strategies and activities to use to deal with client health challenges. CHNs often subscribe to all three approaches, but depending on the setting in which they work, they usually place greater emphasis on the socioenvironmental approach.

HEALTH PROMOTION STRATEGIES

Several strategies are used to promote population, community, group, family, and individual health. As noted earlier, the Ottawa Charter identified five areas requiring action in health promotion practice: strengthening community action, building healthy public policy, creating supportive environments, developing personal skills, and reorienting health services. Because of the complexity of health issues, addressing them is best done using a combination of strategies to achieve an identified goal or goals. The Ottawa Charter shifted the health promotion approach from an individual level with a focus on behavioural and disease orientation to a population health level with a focus on the determinants of health and a health orientation (Tang, Beaglehole, & O'Byrne, 2005). Each of the Ottawa Charter strategies is discussed below.

Strengthening Community Action

The strategy of strengthening community action, as outlined in the Ottawa Charter, refers to empowering communities. It involves engaging communities from the grassroots, or "bottom up" (referred to as locality development as outlined by Rothman), so as to involve community members in identifying health issues and planning and initiating interventions specific to their communities. Thereby, communities take ownership and have control over health issues affecting them and the health of their members. The term most frequently used for this in Canada (as well as Australia and the United Kingdom) is *community development*; in the United States, the strategy is most often referred to as *community organizing* or *community building* (Labonte, 1997). **Community development**, therefore, is a process whereby community members identify health concerns or issues affecting their community that require the development of capacity building skills to bring about a needed change (Shah, 2003). Partnerships are essential in community development. The goal is a secure and healthy community with buy-in from all community members.

The resources or assets and possible contributions of the partners are identified and "mapped" to build a capacity list rather than a deficiency list. *Asset mapping* with a capacity building focus serves as the starting point for determining the resources and assets available in the community, identifying further community resources to be developed. The asset mapping approach sees the glass half full rather than half empty and usually shows the connections between and among community assets because communities are built on these types of connections and supports. A community with a limited view (i.e., that sees the glass as half empty) would focus on the high numbers of homeless, high numbers of illegal drug users, and inadequate numbers of health care providers. A community working on capacity building (i.e., that sees the glass as half full) would focus on establishing green space, sponsoring numerous support groups, and working toward low crime rates.

The information gained from asset mapping should be used to promote community development. Often, a coalition of community partners is engaged with this goal of effecting positive community change. The Canadian Heart Health Initiative serves as an example of a capacity-building project using partnerships. This multilevel-strategy project links local, provincial, and national health departments by producing widespread partnerships as a way of developing and distributing knowledge about the major preventable risk factors for heart disease (Canadian Heart Health Database Centre, 2009).

The Canadian Healthy Communities project, developed and launched by Health Canada in 1987, is an example of community development. (WHO established its Healthy Communities program shortly afterward.) Currently, provincial Healthy Communities networks are found primarily in Quebec and Ontario. The Healthy Communities process includes an intersectoral approach with health being the major focus for policymaking and citizen engagement at the municipal level. The project includes the following components: wide community participation (communities identify their own health issues), involvement of all sectors of the community, local government commitment, and creation of healthy public policies (Ontario Healthy Communities Coalition, n.d.). These components relate directly to the Ottawa Charter health promotion strategies.

The significance of the Healthy Communities process to CHNs is that it deals with many of the determinants of health that fall outside the scope of the health care system. For example, implementing policies to provide better access to nutritious food would have a significant positive impact on clients' health status. CHNs in several Canadian communities have contributed to building healthy communities by identifying health issues in the community, assisting community members to explore health issues, advocating for identified issues, and establishing coalitions with other organizations and sectors such as education and housing (Canadian Nurses Association [CNA], 2005). The CNA backgrounder titled *Healthy Communities and Nursing: A Summary of the Issues* provides information on why the issue of healthy communities is important to nurses and offers some suggestions as to what nurses can do about this issue, for example, becoming informed about community health issues and working with others in the community to advocate for healthier communities (CNA, 2005).

The PHAC has a Healthy Communities Division within the Centre for Health Promotion, which addresses the issues of family violence, rural health, mental health, injury prevention, and physical activity and also provides consultation with regard to community capacity building with the goal of improving Canadians' health (PHAC, 2008b). The use of community capacity to bring about change through an action plan, usually developed and implemented with community partners, is known as **community mobilization**. *Community mobilization* refers to individuals in a community working together as a group to influence healthy public policy and to bring about change regarding a health issue. Reductions in tobacco use provide an example of community mobilization. The healthy public policy around this issue developed from the grassroots, meaning it was initiated by individuals in the community who felt a concern about the effects of smoking and formed community groups, which partnered with community agencies and organizations to advocate for policy changes at the municipal, provincial, and federal levels. Usually, these groups included CHNs, either as representatives of their local health agency or as fellow concerned citizens. As a result of the community mobilization around tobacco use, municipal, provincial, and federal governments in Canada have developed and implemented policies to restrict tobacco use.

A distinction has been made between community-based strategies and community development strategies (Boutilier, Cleverly, & Labonte, 2000; Labonte, 1997; Ontario Health Promotion Resource System, n.d.). Usually defined by an outside organization or professional, *community-based strategies* connect programs and services to community groups. The decision-making power is most often with the sponsoring organization or professional and not with the community participants. *Community development strategies*, on the other hand, involve a health concern or issue defined by community residents, rather than by a sponsoring organization or professional. When community development strategies are used, the decision-making power rests primarily with the community residents. In community development strategies, the CHN may fulfill a liaison role.

Having gained recognition in the 1990s (Ontario Prevention Clearinghouse, 2002), the term **capacity building** refers to the specific services, resources, and programs that can assist communities, individuals, or organizations to deal with their health issues by focusing on community strengths but also acknowledges deficits. Capacity building requires a strong foundation that can support and sustain what the community needs to address its health concerns or issues, often through the establishment and maintenance of partnerships. A project led by the Canadian Public Health Association serves as an example of capacity building. Voluntary Organizations Involved in Collaborative Engagement (VOICE) in Health Policy was a national project with the goal of enhancing the policy capacity of volunteer health organizations. The project was divided into three phases to reach the goals and objectives and concluded in 2004 with an action plan to continue enhancing policy collaboration (PHAC, 2005). Health Canada's Community Action Program for Children (CAPC) and Canada Prenatal Nutrition Program (CPNP) provide two other examples of capacity building.

Community capacity includes the identification of resources, commitment, and time required to ensure the success of the health project or program. As well, capacity building at the community level involves community members' taking action to deal with their needs as well as the social and political support required for successful implementation of programs (Smith, Tang, & Nutbeam, 2006).

To build community capacity, CHNs needs to work collaboratively with the community. When working with the community, the CHN begins with an assessment to (1) determine what stage the community is at, (2) assist the community to identify health concerns and strengths, (3) assist the community to identify how to use its strengths to deal with the identified health challenges, and (4) explore how the community feels it can best manage its health challenges. Following assessment and planning, the CHN works with the community to develop strategies. The *Canadian Community Health Nursing Standards of Practice* Standard 2, "Building Individual/Community Capacity," provides specific community health nursing responsibilities (see Appendix 1).

Empowerment, a key concept in health promotion, refers to an active process whereby individuals, groups, and communities are able to state their health requirements and be involved in and take charge of the strategies required to achieve improved health. Community empowerment results from collective individual efforts to influence and manage the effects of the determinants of health. Currently, client empowerment is a key component of health promotion (Uys, Majumdar, & Gwele, 2004).

CRITICAL VIEW

On the Evolve Web site, go to the WHO Weblink entitled *7th Global Conference on Health Promotion* and read the following tracks: Community Empowerment (track 1); Partnerships and Intersectoral Action (track 4); and Building Capacity for Health Promotion (track 5).

1. How is community empowerment different from individual empowerment?
2. How has globalization affected your community's development?
3. How can capacity building specifically the establishment of partnerships for health promotion be developed in your community?

Community inclusion and engagement are aspects of health promotion and part of the dialogue within the field of population health. People need to experience a sense of belonging if they are to feel comfortable actively participating in decisions that will affect the health of their community. Social networks and supports contribute to the development of this sense of belonging. There needs to also be social and political actions that influence policy to ensure equity, social justice, and addressing the determinants of health. For further information about inclusion, see Health Canada's *An Inclusion Lens* (a workbook developed in Atlantic Canada) and Health Nexus (previously known as the Ontario Prevention Clearinghouse) in the Evolve Weblinks. Table 4-5 provides examples of inclusion and exclusion in relation to eight dimensions of inclusion identified in *An Inclusion Lens*.

The Community Health Action Model, a new model currently in development, considers many of the concepts that have been discussed in this section. The model does the following:

- Serves as a model for community health promotion
- Incorporates community development and community health assessment
- Incorporates a population health approach
- Empowers the community
- Views health care providers as resources for the community versus experts
- Considers community assets and strengths
- Considers community resiliency and community capacity (Racher & Annis, 2007)

CHNs value and believe in the concepts of partnerships and empowerment, which are supported in the *Canadian Community Health Nursing Standards of Practice*. They build partnerships derived from the concepts of primary health care, caring, and empowerment (CHNAC, 2008). In the standards of practice, the two primary health care principles directly related to partnerships and empowerment are that individuals and communities should actively participate in decisions affecting their health and life and that partnerships should be established between disciplines, communities, and all health sectors (CHNAC, 2008).

Building Healthy Public Policy

Building healthy public policy, an Ottawa Charter strategy, refers to creating environments that support health

TABLE 4-5 Examples of Inclusion and Exclusion in Relation to the Eight Dimensions of the Inclusion Lens

Dimension	Examples of Inclusion	Examples of Exclusion
Cultural	• Valuing of contributions • Acknowledgement of differences and diversity	• Intolerance • Gender stereotyping
Economic	• Fewer disparities • Personal security	• Unemployment • Stigma • Inequality
Functional	• Ability to be involved • Valuing of social roles	• Inability to function • Overextended
Participatory	• Ability to make choices • Accessibility of programs	• Lack of encouragement to participate in decision making • Blockage of communication
Physical	• Friendly environment • Access to community services	• Unfriendly environment • Unsustainable environments
Political	• Social protection of vulnerable groups • Active participation by citizens in the community	• Victim blaming • Restrictive policies
Relational	• Belonging • Supportive family	• Isolation • Family violence
Structural	• Community capacity building • Two-way communication	• Withholding of information • Restrictive boundaries

SOURCE: Adapted from Health Canada. (2002). *An inclusion lens: Workbook for looking at social and economic exclusion and inclusion.* Retrieved from http://www.phac-aspc.gc.ca/canada/regions/atlantic/pdf/inclusion_lens-E.pdf.

and reduce inequities in health and social policies. It requires coordinated action by federal, provincial, and municipal government levels, and specific areas of governments such as agriculture and health, to identify and develop public policies that affect health. An example of healthy public policy is the ban in several provinces on the use of hand-held cellphones and other hand-held devices while driving is a policy developed to reduce the risk of motor vehicle–related injuries. Various community groups advocated for this healthy public policy. Another example is the law banning smoking in vehicles carrying children, implemented in some provinces to decrease the health risks from second-hand smoke. CHNs have advocated at the community and provincial levels to develop the aforementioned healthy public policies.

A focus on the concept of health, rather than illness, has engaged policy discussions over the past two decades regarding the relationship between health and social and economic conditions such as education, housing, employment, and the environment. A shift from institution-based care to community-based care has presented the opportunity for individuals to participate in health decisions with health care providers. This empowerment of individuals and communities has resulted in the development of healthy public policy such as bylaws that restrict smoking in public places, environmental protection legislation prohibiting the use of leaded gasoline in motor vehicles, and laws requiring seat-belt use. Policies can be developed from the top down (i.e., originating from the government) or from the bottom up (i.e., originating from the community).

Having established that the setting of health goals or strategies is critical, the 1974 Lalonde Report put an emphasis on health care organization, particularly the provision of services, as one of several components affecting health (Lalonde, 1974). This view was restated in the 1986 Epp Report, which emphasized that all public policy sectors (e.g., income security, employment, education, housing, agriculture) have an impact on health (Epp, 1986). In 1994, a federal, provincial, and territorial advisory committee identified five categories of factors that determine the health of Canadians: (1) social and economic environment, (2) physical environment, (3) personal health practices, (4) individual capacity and coping skills, and (5) health services. These factors provided the basis for the development of *Strategies for Population Health: Investing in the Health of Canadians*; pursuing these strategies would improve the health status of the Canadian population and provide a more integrated approach to health (Health Canada, 1994).

The current health policy development challenge pertains to the constraints of changing social, economic, and political climates. The final report of the 2002 Commission on the Future of Health Care in Canada, referred to as the Romanow Report, recommended policies that would ensure longstanding sustainability of a universally accessible, publicly funded health care system with quality health services within constraints such as fiscal (Romanow, 2002). However, very few recommendations from the Romanow Report have been implemented (Walkom, 2008). One recommendation that has been gradually addressed in recent years is the need for a national policy on mental health. Davis (2006) proposed that the Government of Canada had not addressed mental health in Canada at a policy level. He indicated that the Romanow Report identified "mental health … as one of the orphan children of medicare" with the need to "bring mental health into the mainstream of public health care" (p. 91). In 2007, the Government of Canada established the Mental Health Commission, a national mental health strategy for Canada. In 2009, this commission released a document titled *Toward Recovery and Wellbeing: A Framework for Mental Health Strategy for Canada*, developed from input from a variety of sectors across Canada. This strategy is discussed further in Chapter 11.

Canada's first ministers, in 2004, committed to a collaborative process to set health goals and targets for Canada (PHAC, 2009a). In 2005, provincial, territorial, and federal ministers of health outlined health goals for Canada based on the following four areas: basic needs (social and physical environments); belonging and engagement; healthy living; and a system for health (PHAC, 2009b). These health goals were developed using an extensive consultation, confirmation, and approval process involving experts and grassroots representatives from all provinces and territories. For further reading on the historical efforts of the federal, provincial, and territorial governments to develop and implement population health policy in Canada, refer to the Senate of Canada report *Population Health Policy: Federal, Provincial, and Territorial Perspectives* (see the Evolve Weblinks). The Senate Subcommittee on Population Health (2009) has recommended that the 2005 Health Goals for Canada be updated and that the Population Health Promotion Expert Group develop a national set of indicators of health disparities that correspond with the revised Health Goals of Canada. Advocacy, at a policy level, is an activity for this strategy within the Ottawa Charter.

Creating Supportive Environments

Creating supportive environments, an Ottawa Charter strategy, refers to providing environments in all settings such as home, work, and play that are safe, satisfying, stimulating, and enjoyable. Health equality and the social determinants of health contribute to the creation of supportive environments for health promotion. Environment is a determinant of health and is, therefore, interconnected with health. This interconnectedness leads to improved population health if improvements have been made in the environment. Butler-Jones (2009) stated that "people's actions are very much shaped by the social and environmental conditions in which they live and work" (p. 47). For example, poor communities often experience population health disparities. These populations live in environments that lack material and social supports and tend to experience poorer health as compared to the general Canadian population. A large body of evidence links poverty to poor health (Auger & Alix, 2009). The physical environment influences health outcomes by approximately 10%, and socioeconomic factors give explanation to approximately 50% of the health of populations (Senate Subcommittee on Population Health, 2009). The environment as a determinant of health is discussed in Chapter 15. Despite Canada's reputation as a leader in health promotion and population health, disparities continue to exist (Raphael, 2009). Child poverty has persisted as a major Canadian issue, with income disparity among families with children continuing to create a bigger gap (Ungerleider & Burns, 2004).

As an example of the CHN role in creating a supportive environment, consider the case of a CHN working in a rural agricultural community. This CHN works with this community to plan and implement a program pertaining to farm safety. In the words of the PHAC, "a farm is more than an industrial worksite, it's a home" (PHAC, 2008c). The CHN uses strategies such as providing education about farm safety by working with parent–school councils, local youth groups such as 4-H clubs, school staff, and organizations such as the Canadian Agricultural Safety Association (CASA), an association that works to improve farm safety practices and decrease the chances of injury in Canada.

Another example of the creation of a supportive environment is the Baby-Friendly Hospital Initiative (BFHI). This initiative was developed by the World Health Organization (WHO) and UNICEF in 1991 (UNICEF, 2009). This program, known in Canada as the Baby Friendly Initiative (BFI) and available at six designated sites across the country (Alberta Breastfeeding Committee, 2009), integrates both hospital and community care for breastfeeding mothers and infants. Breastfeeding protects the health of babies, mothers, and families and supports the environment (Horta, Bahl, Martines, & Cesar, 2007). Quebec and New Brunswick have mandated the implementation of BFI (Alberta Breastfeeding Committee, 2009). Refer to the Alberta Breastfeeding Committee and UNICEF Weblinks on the Evolve Web site for further information.

Creating a supportive environment, within the Ottawa Charter, includes the activities of social marketing, advocacy, health communication, and mutual aid, which are discussed later in this chapter. Refer to the WHO Weblink on Evolve for the WHO's report on addressing health inequalities. For further information on how to address the multiple determinants of health, refer to the Senate of Canada Report Weblink on Evolve.

CRITICAL VIEW*

1. Refer to the Web sites listed below for the corresponding behaviours. List at least two health risks for mother and infant associated with choosing the following behaviours:
   a) Smoking tobacco (http://www.cps.ca/caringforkids/pregnancy&babies/SafeSleepForBaby.htm)
   b) Not using an infant car seat (http://www.cps.ca/caringforkids/keepkidssafe/CarSeatSafety.htm)
   c) Not immunizing an infant (http://www.cps.ca/caringforkids/immunization/index.htm)
   d) Not breastfeeding an infant (http://www.breastfeedingalberta.ca/baby-friendly_initiative.htm)
2. How can CHNs support the BFI initiative?

*This box and the section on the Baby-Friendly Initiative were contributed by Mary-Louise Batty.

Literacy and Health Literacy

In Canada, *literacy* refers to having nine skills essential to achieving success and safety in work, learning, and life (Human Resources and Skills Development Canada, 2009). These essential skills are reading, writing, oral communication, numeracy, thinking, document use, working with others, computer use, and continuous learning (Human Resources and Skills Development Canada, 2009). Literacy has also been linked to empowerment (Vollman et al., 2008). Empowerment implies clients' having the ability to take control of and manage their own health. For example, clients would be able to read and understand information provided by health care providers.

Health literacy is defined as "the ability to access, understand, evaluate, and communicate information as a way to promote, maintain, and improve health in a variety of settings across the lifespan" (Rootman & Gordon-El-Bihbety, 2008, p. 11). In ethnocultural communities, illiteracy can prove a barrier to accessing health services because of limited language abilities and therefore a lack of information on health service availability (Zanchetta & Poureslami, 2006). Persons with lower levels of literacy are inclined to live and work in less healthy environments (Ronson & Rootman, 2009).

Health literacy has been an issue in health promotion for many years. In 1986, literacy was identified as a national priority; in 1994, the Canadian Public Health Association (CPHA) initiated a national literacy and health program; in 2000, Ottawa hosted the first Canadian conference on literacy and health; in 2005, a Health and Learning Knowledge Centre, focused on research, was created in British Columbia; in 2007, the results of the International Adult Literacy and Skills Survey (IALSS), which included thousands of Canadians and resulted in the development of a health literacy measurement tool, were published; and in 2008, a report titled *A Vision for a Health Literate Canada: Report of the Expert Panel on Health Literacy* was released by CPHA, providing information on the extent of the literacy problem in Canada and proposing a national strategy for health literacy (see the Evolve Weblinks). This report includes definitions, concepts, an assessment of the scope of the problem, a discussion of the barriers to literacy and the effectiveness of interventions, and the panel's recommendations.

Ronson and Rootman (2009) suggest that literacy is related to the following:

- Overall health status
- Co-morbidity burden
- Life expectancy
- Lifestyle practices
- Culture
- Income and socioeconomic status
- Living and working conditions
- Educational attainment
- Gender
- Early life

Literacy, therefore, is linked to some of the determinants of health (e.g., income and education). In addition, the data suggest that literacy is associated with health status, community involvement, and health literacy. The CHN needs to be constantly aware of the challenges that health literacy presents in many client situations. The CHN works with clients to develop personal skills and partners with others to create supportive environments, strengthen community action on literacy, and build healthy public policy to address health literacy issues.

Developing Personal Skills

Developing personal skills, an Ottawa Charter strategy, builds individual capacity so that persons will make lifestyle choices that promote health. One aspect of this strategy is the provision of health education to empower clients as individuals and to promote client involvement in health care decisions. This strategy also includes the adoption of healthier behaviours, such as stress management, healthy eating, and physical activity. Moving toward the adoption of healthier lifestyles through behavioural change is difficult even for motivated clients. The theories, models, and frameworks previously discussed in this chapter assist the CHN to plan interventions suitable to a client's need and situation; however, many social and economic factors included in the social determinants of health hinder behavioural change (Shah, 2003).

An intervention commonly used by CHNs, health education is the provision of learning opportunities that

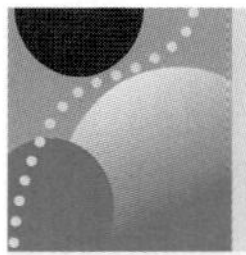

Determinants of Health
Literacy

- Low literacy and low health literacy contribute to lower incomes and decreased community engagement, which are related to poorer health.
- Approximately 55% of working-aged Canadian adults have less than adequate health literacy skills.
- Approximately 88% of older adults (65 years of age and older) have less than adequate health literacy skills.
- Approximately 10% of Canadians live with a learning disability, approximately 80% of whom experience difficulty learning to read.
- Canadians with the lowest health literacy scores are 2½ times more likely than Canadians with high health literacy scores to report their health status as "fair" to "poor."

SOURCE: Rootman, I., & Gordon-El-Bihbety, D. (2008). *A vision for a health literate Canada: Report of the Expert Panel on Health Literacy.* Ottawa, ON: Canadian Public Health Association. Retrieved from http://www.ccl-cca.ca/NR/rdonlyres/3865A9D0-F2FE-4A95-A8C0-8FFF6BE466A9/0/20080225VisionforHealthLiterateCanReportEN.pdf.

improve health knowledge, perceptions, and actions to enhance clients' decision-making and other skills (Bhatti & Hamilton, 2002). CHNs provide health teaching with populations, groups, and individuals in a variety of settings. Health education with populations can occur, for example, in public places or through social marketing strategies such as mass media announcements for issues such as sun safety or safer sex. Health education with community groups may occur in schools, workplaces, churches, and health departments on a range of issues, such as alcohol use or ergonomics. CHNs also educate groups of learners who then become educators for other groups in the community. This activity is usually referred to as "train the trainer" sessions. One example is a CHN who educates a select community group to teach about healthy food choices to promote a healthy lifestyle. These trainees then individually teach nutrition information to community groups in various settings. Health teaching with individuals may occur in homes, clinics, or older adult centres, for example, for a variety of issues, such as nutrition, child care, and safety.

Several teaching methods are available for health education, including lectures, demonstrations, small groups, and health fairs. Health fairs are commonly used with populations to disseminate information and to determine population interest and further learning needs. One example of a program for developing personal skills is Aboriginal Head Start (AHS), a national program provided in urban and northern settings to Aboriginal preschool children and their families. AHS aims to promote the development of a positive sense of self to encourage learning. CHNs in their communities could facilitate community development through the administration of this type of program for children and their parents. (See the Tool Box on the Evolve Web site for links to resources for planning general and workplace health fairs.)

Shah (2003) proposes that for population behaviour change to occur, attention to the "4 E's: education, environmental supports, economic levers, and enforcement of regulation and legislation" (p. 27) is necessary. CHNs develop interventions that address each of these areas as they work toward promoting health in communities.

Low literacy produces a barrier to understanding health information (Ronson & Rootman, 2009; Rootman & Gordon-El-Bihbety, 2008); creates stress (Literacy B.C., 2005); and may prevent people from seeking health care.

The most common activities used to further the Ottawa Charter strategy of developing personal skills include health communication, social marketing, mutual aid, and advocacy directed at the individual. These activities are discussed later in this chapter.

LEVELS OF PREVENTION

Related to Community Health Education

PRIMARY PREVENTION

Community health nurses provide education at a health fair regarding healthy eating using *Eating Well With Canada's Food Guide*.

SECONDARY PREVENTION

Community health nurses provide education at a health fair about the need for blood pressure screening for early diagnosis and treatment of hypertension.

TERTIARY PREVENTION

A community health nurse provides education to a community group of individuals and their families coping with the effects of brain injury.

Reorienting Health Services

The strategy of reorienting health services, as outlined in the Ottawa Charter, refers to reforming health services and the health sector so that they include a health promotion focus. This change requires movement beyond the focus on cure and clinical services. Health care reform would need to consider areas such as the link between the determinants of health and population health; social justice; the individual as a holistic being; community-based care that is accessible, affordable, acceptable, and appropriate for the clients; a greater focus on population health and on health research; and modifications to professional education (Vollman et al., 2008). In contributing toward achieving this goal, a CHN may, for example, work with community partners to reorient mental health services from a hospital to a community location that is accessible, available, and appropriate to meet specific community mental health promotion needs. The most common activities used to further the Ottawa Charter strategy of reorienting health services include health communication and social marketing. These activities are discussed later in this chapter.

Activities to Facilitate Health Promotion Strategies

Health Communication and Social Marketing Activities

Used in the delivery of health promotion messages to various targeted populations, health communication and social marketing activities are designed to inform individuals so that they can make decisions related to maintaining and improving their health and well-being and those of their families and communities. In 1971, ParticipACTION became the first Canadian government program that incorporated health communication and social marketing strategies with a mandate to improve the health of Canadians (Bauman, Madil, Craig, & Salmon, 2004; Health Canada, 2005d). Extremely successful, this program spanned a 30-year period ending in January 2001. ParticipACTION was directed at positively influencing attitudes, beliefs, values, and behaviours to increase physical activity in the general population and at the same time targeting specific aggregates such as youth, older adults, and workers. In February 2007, ParticipACTION was officially renewed, with funding from sources such as government, labour, education, and business (ParticipACTION, 2010).

Health communication involves disseminating information to promote knowledge, distributing health risk information, demonstrating how to access health care programs, and creating awareness of health issues using various forms of mass media. Examples of mass media are television, radio, flyers, newspapers, magazines, and Internet-based messages. ParticipACTION used mass media such as television and radio and, at a national level, a print-based monograph called *Canada's Physical Activity Guide to Active Living.* The CHN needs to plan health communication messages that are inclusive and considerate of the client's ability to access health information. For example, not all clients use the Internet, and some have lower literacy levels. The CHN also needs to develop and use appropriate activities to ensure equity and accessibility in the planning, implementation, and evaluation stages of the activity.

Focusing on populations, social marketing uses structured messages to effect positive behaviour change in lifestyle areas such as diet and substance use to improve health and decrease health inequalities (French, Blair-Stevens, McVey, & Merritt, 2009). It is extremely important to be aware that social marketing is a process that includes more than promotion (Thackeray & McCormack Brown, 2005). The four *P*s of social marketing, also known as the marketing mix, form the key elements of social marketing: *product* (benefits), *price* (costs such as physical, psychological, social, and financial for the target audience related to the benefits), *place* (convenient access), and *promotion* (utilizing the most appropriate media form to convey the messages to the target audience) (Grier & Bryant, 2005). ParticipACTION demonstrated use of the four Ps of social marketing in the following ways:

- Product—Canadians saw benefits such as improved health and well-being
- Price—physical activity was inexpensive, easy to do, and readily available
- Place—physical activity could be carried out in the home, school, or workplace or outdoors in the community
- Promotion—various communication approaches were used (e.g., inclusion of physical activity in school curricula and encouragement by health professionals such as CHNs and community dietitians)

Weinreich (2006) has added the following four additional *P*s to social marketing: *publics*, *partnership*, *policy*, and *purse strings*. "Publics" includes the external groups, such as policymakers and the target audience, and the internal groups, such as organizational managers. "Partnership" includes teaming up with relevant agencies and organizations in the community with similar goals. "Policy" includes creating a supportive environment by introducing and supporting policies that fit with the social marketing program for sustainability. "Purse strings" includes the identification of and utilization of funding from sources such as grants or donations that will assist with creating and operating the program.

Campaigns that use communication forms such as mass media only are not social marketing strategies. In fact, according to Andreasen (2002) all of the following benchmarks must be present to identify an approach as a social marketing strategy: (1) interventions are designed and evaluated based on behaviour change; (2) audience research is used, along with pretesting and monitoring of interventions for each project; (3) specific audiences are targeted; (4) the main component is building attractive and motivational interactions with target audiences; (5) the approach uses the four *P*s (product, price, place, promotion); and (6) benefits and barriers associated with the desired behaviour are identified.

In 1974, the Lalonde Report contributed strongly to influencing broader approaches to health in Canada and internationally and led to an assortment of social marketing campaigns, including "Dialogue on Drinking" (alcohol moderation focus in 1976), "Operation Lifestyle" (healthy lifestyle focus in 1976), and "Generation of Non-Smokers" (nonsmoking focus for teens in 1981) (Mintz, 2005). In 1978, the Health Promotion Directorate was established, and, in 1981, this directorate established the Social Marketing Unit with the role of developing social marketing campaigns to positively change the health behaviours of Canadians (Mintz, 2005). Advances in communication technology and marketing skills contributed to the development of numerous campaigns in the 1980s and beyond, including initiatives for antismoking and antidrug use, physical activity, healthy eating, diabetes prevention, healthy pregnancy, healthy children (Brighter Futures), older adults' issues, injury prevention, prevention of sexually transmitted infections, prevention of human immunodeficiency virus/acquired immune deficiency syndrome (HIV/AIDS), healthy environment, education (e.g., literacy, stay in school), and a number of Aboriginal campaigns directed at tobacco, diabetes, and healthy pregnancy (Mintz, 2005).

In January 2003, two very familiar social marketing campaigns were launched in Canada. One, a national television advertisement, featured "Bob," an average Canadian man who was trying to quit smoking. This campaign used the Prochaska model of change and was targeted to 40- to 55-year-old Canadians who wanted to quit smoking. The target audience could order print information and access information through an Internet site. You may also remember Heather, a 40-year-old Canadian waitress who had never smoked but who had developed lung cancer as a result of second-hand smoke. Heather's story was promoted through national television advertisements, print media, and posters displayed on buses and other public areas, and through public appearances across Canada by Heather herself (Mintz, 2005).

2ND HAND SMOKE
CAN KILL YOU.
JUST ASK HEATHER.
Heather never smoked, but she worked in smoke-filled restaurants.
Now she's dying from lung cancer. Some tobacco companies say that
2nd hand smoke bothers people. Health Canada says it kills.
Refuse to be a target. Call 1 800 O-Canada (1 800 622-6232) TTY: 1 800 465-7735
www.GoSmokefree.ca
LA FUMÉE SECONDAIRE
PEUT VOUS TUER.
DEMANDEZ À HEATHER.
HEATHER CROWE, NEVER SMOKED, DYING OF LUNG CANCER
HEATHER CROWE, N'A JAMAIS FUMÉ, SE MEURT DU CANCER DU POUMON
Health Canada Santé Canada
Canada

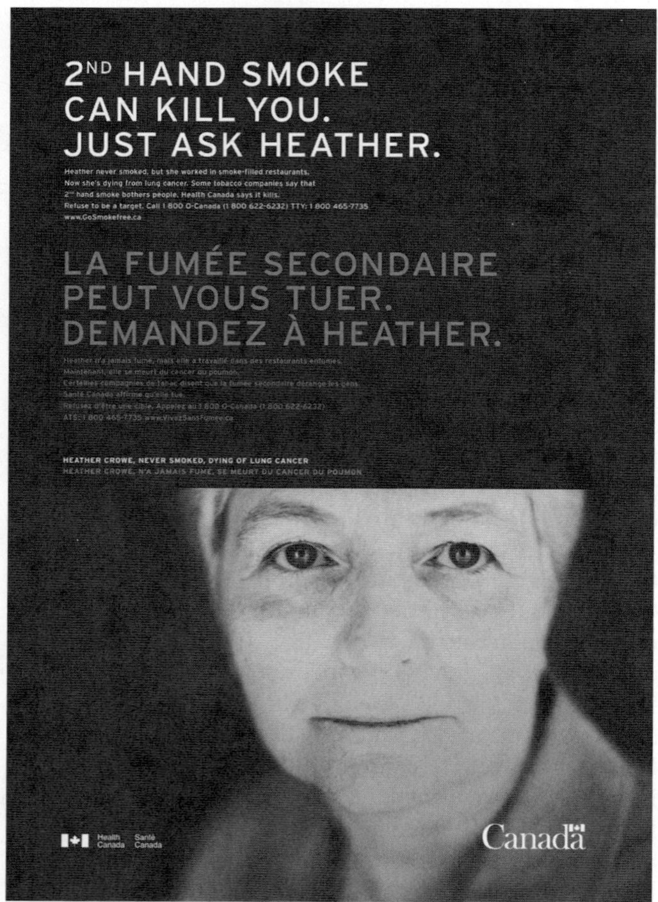

Heather Crowe developed lung cancer after years of exposure to second-hand smoke in her work environment. The antismoking campaign based on her experience provides an example of a social marketing strategy aimed at educating the public about the risks of tobacco use.

Mutual Aid

In *A Framework for Health Promotion*, Jake Epp identified mutual aid as a health promotion mechanism (Epp, 1986). *Mutual aid*, most commonly referred to as self-help, is defined as a process whereby persons share common experiences, situations, or problems with others and view each other as equals (Shah, 2003; Self-Help Resource Centre, n.d.; Young & Hayes, 2002). Self-help groups are used for individual support usually when professional support (e.g., after office hours) or family support is not readily available, and access to persons who have gone through a similar problem is viewed as helpful. Self-help groups provide persons experiencing a certain type of issue with emotional and practical support, information exchange, and, often, assistance with problem solving (Self-Help Resource Centre, n.d.). Some self-help groups, such as breast cancer groups, Alcoholics Anonymous, and the Anxiety and Mood Disorders Support Group, also engage in community education and advocacy. Self-help groups serve as a social support network, one of the social determinants of health.

A Canadian mental health promotion program with a slightly different "helping" slant is the Canadian Community Helpers Program. This program works with existing community strengths, finding community members to act as "natural helpers" to work with youth with mental health problems. In contrast to traditional models of help, these natural helpers already have a youth connection and are persons whom youth have related to in the past when they have encountered problems (PHAC, 2004).

CHNs can support the use of self-help groups by discussing with clients (individuals and families) appropriate self-help group availability and the assistance provided; referring clients to self-help groups as appropriate; and assisting in the establishment of self-help groups as needed in and identified by the community. Self-help groups use available technologies such as the Internet, telephone, and teleconferencing.

Advocacy

Advocacy is defined as "interventions such as speaking, writing or acting in favour of a particular issue or cause, policy or group of people" (PHAC, 2008d). Advocacy enhances the power of clients by involving them in the identification of their health concerns or issues and encouraging them to participate in developing solutions, including policy development and policy promotion. Advocacy is action taken to influence decision makers in communities and governments to support a policy or cause that promotes health. Advocacy for health includes looking after those who are helpless or have been discriminated against and empowering clients to raise awareness of their health issues, such as concerns about traffic patterns in a school area. Regardless of the need for advocacy, CHNs need to work *with* the client rather than do *for* the client. Advocacy is discussed throughout the text.

HEALTH PROMOTION SKILLS

CHNs practising health promotion strategies need to be familiar with resources that are available to facilitate and enhance their health promotion interventions. Often, CHNs have the theoretical knowledge of *what* needs to happen to effect change to improve client health; the also necessary "how to" information on facilitating change is available through many resources (many of them Web-based). Working in focus groups and preparing funding proposal applications—two techniques or skills that CHNs use in their health promotion practice—are briefly introduced here.

Evidence-Informed Practice

To deal with rising health care costs, the lengths of hospital stays for women who had just delivered babies were decreased in the 1990s. Early postpartum discharge (EPD) involves discharging patients within 48 hours post–vaginal delivery and 96 hours post–non-complicated Caesarean delivery. Sustaining this early discharge strategy has required the involvement of public health nurses (PHNs). A qualitative study using focus groups of PHNs explored perceptions of EPD and its effects on public health nurses' practice in Winnipeg, Manitoba. The study identified three main themes: passion for the PHN role, the influence of EPD on practice, and building a PHN future. The following 10 subthemes also came to light: valuing public health nursing, building capacity and developing relationships, changes in practice, erosion of health promotion, a new role, proper tools, continuity of care, relationships with community partners, and resources to support public health programs. The PHNs perceived that the introduction of EPD reduced their role in community-level interventions and health promotion activities, thus altering their practice. Although the PHNs in this study valued their new role in EPD, they identified a need for resources and funding to be directed to the public health system to support PHNs' increased scope of practice and to continue support of their traditional health promotion roles with all clients.

Application for CHNs: It is important to understand the impact new programs such as the EPD have on the roles of public health nurses. The introduction of EPD added new responsibilities for PHNs, but additional resources and staffing were not provided, putting at risk PHNs' other program commitments. PHNs perceived that they were being forced to give up their established community commitments and involvements. Time normally allocated for population health approach activities, including health promotion activities, was now directed to individual and family care in the community. Organizations need to consider and plan for the introduction of new programs for health care delivery, and CHNs such as PHNs need to be involved in this planning process to ensure the availability of sufficient resources and staffing. CHNs' involvement would contribute to making sure that the established population health programs would not be compromised with the introduction of new program delivery modes.

Questions for Reflection & Discussion

1. What health promotion activities could a PHN implement with early discharge clients (mother, neonate, and family) in their homes?
2. What questions would be important to ask PHNs when a new program of delivery is being considered?

Reference: Cusack, C., Hall, W., Scruby, L., & Wong, S. (2008). Public health nurses' (PHNs) perceptions of their role in early postpartum discharge. *Canadian Journal of Public Health, 99*(3), 206–211.

Focus Groups

Focus groups in health promotion are informal sessions using an interactive strategy to gain insight into the perceptions, beliefs, and opinions of generally 6 to 12 representatives. Focus groups are used in assessment, particularly social assessment, and serve as "pretests" in health promotion program development and evaluation. In most cases, focus groups are led by skilled moderators who create supportive environments so that group members can speak liberally and instinctively about the issues, programs, or services. The leader usually follows a structured interview format in a 60- to 90-minute facilitated and taped discussion. Several Web resources elaborate on the "how to" of this skill (see the Tool Box on the Evolve Web site).

Funding Applications

Health program survival may be challenged due to fiscal constraints and therefore is dependent on government funding. This funding involves the submission of an application for funding to various government organizations. Stiff competition for available funds often exists; therefore, succinct and skilled completion of funding proposals is critical. CHNs need to become familiar with how to write funding proposals so that they can apply directly or assist a program in the community to successfully apply. Several Web-based tools guide CHNs in writing a funding proposal (see the Health Communication Unit online proposal writing course and the Health Promotion Clearinghouse found in the Weblinks on the Evolve Web site).

Health Promotion Capacity

In summary, health promotion practice has undergone a shift from a primary focus on the individual to a primary focus on populations. However, health promotion areas continue to be addressed with individuals as clients. CHNs need to develop many skills applicable to working with clients. Table 4-6 summarizes the knowledge, skills, commitment, and resources health care providers, including CHNs, require. Table 4-7 presents the organizational elements necessary to support CHNs as they function within their health promotion practice.

STUDENT EXPERIENCE

Working alone or with a student study group, identify a health promotion program or policy relevant to your community. Create your own inclusion and exclusion lens by responding to the questions and using the template found on the Health Canada Web site titled *An Inclusion Lens: Workbook for Looking at Social and Economic Exclusion and Inclusion* (listed in the Evolve Weblinks for this chapter).

Bring your completed work to class for discussion.

TABLE 4-6 The Basic Elements of Practitioners' Health Promotion Capacity

Category	Basic Elements of Capacity
Knowledge	• A holistic understanding of health and its determinants • An awareness of population health promotion principles • An understanding of a variety of strategies and processes through which effective health promotion interventions can be undertaken • A recognition of the contextual specificity of the strengths and weaknesses of different health promotion strategies and processes • A familiarity with the conditions, aspirations, and culture of the population(s) with which one works

(Continued)

TABLE 4-6 The Basic Elements of Practitioners' Health Promotion Capacity—Cont'd

Category	Basic Elements of Capacity
Skills	• Program planning (needs assessment, design, implementation, and evaluation) • Communication across sectors, disciplines, and socioeconomic or community boundaries • Working with others (e.g., nurturing relationships, participation, and intersectoral partnerships; facilitation; conflict mediation) • Integrating research and practice (both in the program planning cycle and as a means of critically reflective practice) • Capacity building (both within one's own organization and with the external communities and organizations with which one works) • Being strategic and selective in making decisions about what to do and how to do it
Commitment	• Personal energy, enthusiasm, patience, and persistence • Values of population health promotion • Willingness to be flexible, to innovate, and to take thoughtful risks • Learning from experience of oneself and others • Self-confidence and credibility • Believing in and advocating for health promotion
Resources	• Time to engage in health promotion practice and in personal and professional development that enhances such practice • Tools for more efficient and effective practice, including resource inventories and repertoires of good ideas and best practices • Infrastructure, including office space, capital equipment, and effective means of communication • Supportive managers, colleagues, and allies with whom to work and learn • Access to adequate funding for health promotion activities

Source: Reprinted with permission of the Publisher from *Building health promotion capacity: Action for learning, learning from action*, by McLean, S., et al.

TABLE 4-7 The Basic Elements of Organizational Health Promotion Capacity

Category	Basic Elements of Capacity
Commitment	• Health promotion is valued at all levels of the organization. • There are a shared vision, a mission, and strategies for engaging in population health promotion to address the determinants of health. • Policies, programs, and practices are consistent with the organization's vision, mission, and strategies ("walking the talk"). • Partnerships are valued and nurtured both across the organization and with diverse external organizations and communities.
Culture	• Styles of leadership and management empower health promotion practice, foster lifelong learning, and support healthy working environments. • Positive and nurturing relationships are fostered among employees. • Communication is open and timely, enabling employees to solve problems, learn from mistakes, and share successes. • Critical reflection, innovation, and learning are fostered.

(Continued)

TABLE 4-7 The Basic Elements of Organizational Health Promotion Capacity—Cont'd

Category	Basic Elements of Capacity
Structures	• Health promotion is a shared responsibility, being an integral part of job titles, job descriptions, and performance evaluations among at least several employees. • There are effective policies and practices of human resource recruitment, retention, and professional development. • There are participatory, empowering, and evidence-informed practices for strategic planning, needs assessment, program planning, and evaluation. • Employees are organized into work teams that promote intra-institutional collaboration.
Resources	• A significant number of employees in key positions and units have high levels of individual capacity for health promotion. • Adequate funding is provided for the programmatic and infrastructural costs of engaging in health promotion activities. • Appropriate infrastructure exists, including office space, capital equipment, technology, and effective means of communication. • Active engagement with communities brings additional resources.

SOURCE: Reprinted with permission of the Publisher from *Building health promotion capacity: Action for learning, learning from action*, by McLean, S., et al.

REMEMBER THIS!

- Many definitions of *health* have developed over time and have influenced the development of health promotion.
- Differences exist between the concepts of injury prevention, disease, disease course, illness, illness trajectory, disease prevention, health protection, health enhancement, health promotion, risk avoidance, risk reduction, harm reduction, and resiliency.
- Many reports and national and international conferences have contributed to the development of health promotion in Canada.
- In Canada, the Ottawa Charter strategies of strengthening community action, building healthy public policy, creating supportive environments, developing personal skills, and reorienting health services are fundamental to community health nursing practice.
- The community health nursing practice model and the *Canadian Community Health Nursing Standards of Practice* define the scope of community health nursing practice.
- The population health promotion (PHP) model, a shift away from an individualized lifestyle health promotion focus, is currently used by many CHNs in their practice.
- CHNs consider the determinants of health, which are key factors that influence health.
- Literacy and health literacy influence client access to health care.
- The three health promotion approaches are biomedical, behavioural, and socioenvironmental; CHNs place greater focus on the socioenvironmental approach.
- Many theories, models, and frameworks have contributed to the development of health promotion in community health nursing.
- Many CHNs use socioenvironmental multilevel approaches in their practice.
- Health communication, social marketing, mutual aid, and advocacy are activities used to facilitate the Ottawa Charter health promotion strategies.
- CHNs use a variety of health promotion skills during interactions with clients.

REFLECTIVE PRAXIS

Case Study

Tim, a CHN, lives and works in a large urban centre. He has been teaching prenatal classes to high-school students in his assigned district for a couple of years; however, this is his first time teaching at a particular high school. The students at this high school comprise a multicultural population consisting mainly of second-generation immigrants from Asia and Africa. There are 10 pregnant girls in the prenatal class, eight of whom are from ethnocultural communities. Tim usually incorporates various teaching methods such as lecture, the use of videos, and the dissemination of print materials.

1. If you were Tim, what you would include in your assessment as you prepared to teach this particular aggregate?
2. Locate a pamphlet (from the Internet, a pharmacy, or a local health unit) on a topic related to pregnancy and prenatal care. Using a tool to assess readability (see the resources on plain language and readability in the Tool Box on the Evolve Web site), evaluate the pamphlet for readability and usability for this aggregate. Identify whether you would use this pamphlet and provide a rationale. Bring your pamphlet and results to class.

Answers are on the Evolve Web site at http://evolve.elsevier.com/Canada/Stanhope/community/.

What Would You Do?

1. Locate one peer-reviewed article for each of the following: primary level of prevention; secondary level of prevention; tertiary level of prevention; health promotion with an individual; health promotion with an aggregate group; and health promotion with the community. Describe briefly (i.e., in no more than 200 words per article) the client being studied, the settings, and examples of levels of prevention or health promotion, and identify the role of the CHN.
2. Observe your community and identify one relevant health promotion issue. Collect observational data, for example, many overweight adults, few recreational facilities, and many fast-food restaurants. Review subjective data, for example, media coverage of recreational facilities closing or high poverty levels in the community due to industry closures and the resultant high unemployment rates. Find two evidence-informed peer-reviewed articles that identify possible interventions to address

your selected health promotion issue. For example, interventions might include self-help groups, health fairs, policy changes, and mass education through media sources. From your two articles, choose one intervention and reflect on and record the following:

a) Who is (are) the aggregate(s) related to the issue in your community? Provide supporting data.

b) What would be involved in implementing your chosen intervention in your community?

c) What barriers and facilitators need to be considered in order to implement your chosen intervention?

3. Identify one personal health and health promotion behaviour that you wish to change, for example, weight reduction, smoking cessation, or increased physical activity. Reflect and document the change you would like to make. For example, "I would like to increase my weekly physical activity to 30 minutes of walking three times a week." Locate at least one research article on Prochaska and DiClemente's change theory. Address in writing the following questions:

a) What health behaviour have you identified as needing to be changed? Provide your rationale.

b) What have you done in the past in regard to this behaviour? State your goal(s).

c) At what stage in the Transtheoretical Model of change would you place yourself? Provide a rationale.

d) What are your health strengths? What are your health weaknesses or challenges?

e) What health promotion activities will you use to work toward reaching your goal(s)? Implement your health promotion activities for 1 week. Record the health promotion activities you used, your behaviours, thoughts, health strengths, areas needing improvement, and changes you identify that will be needed to reach your goal(s).

f) Based on your 1-week experience, what have you learned about yourself and the process of changing behaviour? Record your reflections.

g) What family and community supports or barriers have you identified that affected your ability to reach your goal(s)? Record your findings.

h) What did you learn from this experience that you could transfer to future client interactions?

4. Attend one municipal council meeting in your community. Identify the issues observed. Describe one public policy issue addressed during this council meeting. For example, should smoking in public places such as outdoor sporting events be banned? If no issue was discussed, identify one issue that could have arisen based on the topics discussed at the council meeting. Address in writing the following questions:

a) Who initiated discussion of the issue (e.g., councillor, mayor, concerned citizen, or municipal employee), and what was his or her rationale?

b) Why is it a policy issue?

c) What actions were discussed?

d) What impact could this policy change have on the community and on individuals residing in the community?

e) What was not discussed that could have been considered in reference to this issue? Provide a rationale.

TOOL BOX evolve

The Tool Box contains useful resources that can be applied in community health nursing practice. These related resources are found either in the appendices at the back of this book or on the book's Web site at http://evolve.elsevier.com/Canada/Stanhope/community/.

Appendices

- Appendix 1: Canadian Community Health Nursing Standards of Practice
- Appendix 5: Declaration of Alma-Ata
- Appendix 6: Ottawa Charter for Health Promotion

Tools

Basics of Conducting Focus Groups.
This is an excellent resource for anyone planning to conduct or learn about focus groups. It provides a step-by-step guide for the novice.

Community Tool Box.
This resource acts as a support for nurses in the community who strive to promote health. The resource is organized as a tool box and provides practical skill-building information on more than 250 topics as well as examples, checklists, and resources relating to community health.

How to Organize a Workplace Health Fair.
This step-by-step guide includes the phases from planning to evaluation of a workplace health fair.

How to Plan a Health Fair.
This guide for the development of health fairs in the community provides a step-by-step process.

Literacy and Essential Skills Toolkit.
This Human Resources and Skills Development Canada tool kit is a series of user-friendly tools that offer support in the following areas: assessment, learning, and training applicable to employees and learners; community groups; and employers and practitioners. The tool kit also offers many tip sheets and resources on how to take action on literacy.

Mental Health Promotion Toolkit: *A Practical Resource for Community Initiatives.*
This excellent resource provides information to facilitate the understanding of mental health in the community.

Neighbour to Neighbour Toolkit: Media Tool Kit.
This guide for using the media in community advocacy provides information on how to write a press release.

Plain Language.
This Web site provides a guide for the use and evaluation of plain language and how to write using plain language. Other links about literacy and language are also provided at this site.

Plain Language Handbook.
This site provides the reader with information and tools to assist in the preparation of plain-language documents.

Readability Tests.
This site provides an explanation of readability and provides tools on how to measure written materials for readability such as the Gunning, Fog index and the Flesch-Kincaid grade index.

Rural Communities Impacting Policy. *Rural Tackle Box.*
This site provides tools on how to influence policy to maintain healthy communities.

10 Tips for Running Successful Focus Groups.
This site provides tips that can help CHNs conduct more effective focus groups.

WEBLINKS

evolve

Direct links to these resources can be found on the text's accompanying Evolve Web site at http://evolve.elsevier.com/Canada/Stanhope/community.

Alberta Breastfeeding Committee. *BFI in Canada*. This Web site provides the evolution and the steps for successful breastfeeding and the plan for the protection, promotion, and support of breastfeeding in community health care. This BFI example also links the relationship between hospital and community health nursing practice and therefore contributes to continuity of care for families with newborns.

Canadian Public Health Association. *A Vision for a Health Literate Canada: Report of the Expert Panel on Health Literacy*. This Web site provides a definition and statistics on health literacy and discusses the relationship between literacy and health literacy, the scope of the problem in Canada, barriers to health literacy, and interventions and recommendations to improve health literacy.

Canadian Task Force on Preventive Health Care, United States Preventive Services Task Force, Quebec and Canadian Guidelines. *Periodic Health Examination of Adults: Preventive Clinical Practices Guidelines*. This site provides evidence-informed information for preventive clinical practices such as cardiovascular and respiratory diseases, cancer, infectious diseases, trauma and sensory deficits, psychosocial issues, and dental problems and a tracking tool for the periodic examination of adults.

Cancer Prevention Research Center. *Transtheoretical Model: Detailed Overview of the Transtheoretical Model*. This site provides material that has been adapted from Velicer, Prochaska, Fava, et al. (1998) on the Transtheoretical Model, a model of intentional change.

Community Health Nurses of Canada. This Web site contains a great deal of information on community health nursing, including Standards of Practice.

Health Canada: *How Our Programs Affect Population Health Determinants: A Workbook for Better Planning and Accountability*. A document to assist CHNs with developing health promotion activities to effect change in population health determinants.

Health Canada. ***An Inclusion Lens: Workbook for Looking at Social and Economic Exclusion and Inclusion.*** This workbook developed in Atlantic Canada contains information on the issues of social and economic exclusion and inclusion.

The Health Communication Unit. ***Online Proposal Writing Course.*** This online course uses six modules to help learners with the planning and preparation of proposals.

Health Promotion Clearinghouse. ***Proposal and Grant Writing.*** This site provides additional e-links to many resources on grant writing.

Mikkonen, J. and Raphael, D. ***Social Determinants of Health: The Canadian Facts.*** This timely succinct document reviews the determinants of health from the Canadian perspective.

National Cancer Institute. ***Theory at a Glance: A Guide for Health Promotion Practice.*** This Web-based book defines and explains many of the theories for health promotion and behaviour change. Examples are provided. Click the View button to access the book.

Ontario Health Promotion Resource System. ***Health Promotion (HP) 101.*** This free Web-based course for health care providers offers modules about health promotion information and resources.

Ontario Prevention Clearinghouse. ***Inclusion: Societies That Foster Belonging Improve Health.*** This document resulted from a project titled *Inclusion and Engagement: Health Promotion's Way Forward.* It reports on the "Count me in!" forums convened by the Ontario Prevention Clearinghouse to focus on inclusion and health.

Public Health Agency of Canada. ***Population Health Approach: The Organizing Framework.*** This Web site provides extensive information and additional links for the eight identified key elements that need to be addressed in the population health approach model. Click on each of the elements to access the information.

Senate of Canada Report. ***Population Health Policy: Federal, Provincial, and Territorial Perspectives.*** This site provides further historical information on the federal, provincial, and territorial government efforts to develop and implement population health policies in Canada.

UNICEF. ***The Baby-Friendly Hospital Initiative.*** This Web site provides information on the development of the baby friendly initiative. It lists the 10 steps to promote successful breastfeeding and links to other sites that provide information on nutrition and health plus educational material pertaining to breastfeeding for professionals.

World Health Organization. ***Overview: 7th Global Conference on Health Promotion.*** This Web site provides a discussion of the 2009 Nairobi, Kenya, conference and community empowerment; health literacy and health behaviour; strengthening health systems; partnerships and intersectoral action; and building capacity for health promotion.

World Health Organization. ***Closing the Gap in a Generation: Health Equity Through Action on the Social Determinants of Health.*** This Web site provides an extensive report commissioned by WHO to examine the inequities so that action might be taken to improve health and the lives of the citizens of the world.

REFERENCES

Alberta Breastfeeding Committee. (2009). *BFI in Canada.* Retrieved from http://www.breastfeedingalberta.ca/bfi_in_canada.htm.

Andreasen, A. R. (2002). Marketing social marketing in the social change marketplace. *Journal of Public Policy and Marketing, 21*(1), 3–13.

Auger, N., & Alix, A. (2009). Income, income distribution, and health in Canada. In D. Raphael (Ed.), *Social determinants of health* (2nd ed., pp. 61–74). Toronto, ON: Canadian Scholars' Press.

Bauman, A., Madil, J., Craig, C. L., & Salmon, A. (2004). Particip ACTION: This mouse roared, but did it get the cheese? *Canadian Journal of Public Health, 96*(Suppl. 2), S14–S19.

Beresford, S. A., Curry, S. J., Kristal, A. R., Lazovich, D., & Bhatti, T. (1996). *Report of the roundtable on population health and health promotion.* Ottawa, ON: Health Canada, Health Promotion Development Division.

Bhatti, T. (1996). *Report of the roundtable on population health and health promotion.* Ottawa, ON: Health Canada, Health Promotion Development Division.

Bhatti, T., & Hamilton, N. (2002). Health promotion: What is it? *Health Policy Research Bulletin, 1*(3), 5–7.

Boutilier, M., Cleverly, S., & Labonte, R. (2000). Community as a setting for health promotion. In B. D. Poland, L. W. Green, & I. Rootman (Eds.), *Settings for health promotion: Linking theory and practice* (pp. 250–307). Thousand Oaks, CA: Sage.

Butler-Jones, D. (2009). The role of public health in the health of Canada's children. *Chronic Diseases in Canada, 29*(2), 47.

Callaghan, R. C., & Herzog, T. A. (2006). The relation between processes-of-change and stage-transition in smoking behavior: A two-year longitudinal test of the transtheoretical model. *Addictive Behaviors, 31*(8), 1331–1345.

Canadian Centre on Substance Abuse. (2007). *Substance abuse in Canada: Youth in focus*. Retrieved from http://www.ccsa.ca/2007%20CCSA%20Documents/ccsa-011521-2007-e.pdf.

Canadian Heart Health Database Centre. (2009). *Canadian heart health initiative*. Retrieved from http://www.med.mun.ca/chhdbc/chhimore.htm.

Canadian Nurses Association. (2005). *Healthy communities and nursing: A summary of the issues*. Retrieved from http://www.cna-nurses.ca/CNA/documents/pdf/publications/BG5_Healthy_Communities_e.pdf.

Canadian Public Health Association. (1996). *Action statement for health promotion in Canada*. Retrieved from http://www.cpha.ca/en/programs/policy/action.aspx.

Cancer Prevention Research Center. (n.d.). *Transtheoretical model: Detailed overview of the transtheoretical model*. Retrieved from http://www.uri.edu/research/cprc/TTM/detailedoverview.htm.

Catford, J. (2004). Health promotion's record card: How principled are we 20 years on? *Health Promotion International*, *19*(1), 1–4.

Centre for Addiction and Mental Health. (2006). *Health promotion resources*. Retrieved from http://www.camh.net/Health_Promotion/Health_Promotion_Resources/healthpromo_resources_index_pr.html.

Clark, M. J. (2008). *Community health nursing: Advocacy for population health* (5th ed.). Upper Saddle River, NJ: Pearson Prentice Hall.

Community Health Nurses Association of Canada. (2008). *Canadian community health nursing standards of practice*. Retrieved from http://www.chnc.ca/documents/chn_standards_of_practice_mar08_english.pdf.

Cusack, C., Hall, W., Scruby, L., & Wong, S. (2008). Public health nurses' (PHNs) perceptions of their role in early postpartum discharge. *Canadian Journal of Public Health*, *99*(3), 206–211.

Davis, S. (2006). *Community mental health in Canada: Theory, policy, and practice*. Vancouver, BC: UBC Press.

Dearing, J. W. (2009). Applying diffusion of innovation theory to intervention development. *Research on Social Work Practice*, *19*(5), 503–518.

Diem, E., & Moyer, A. (2005). *Community health nursing projects: Making a difference*. Philadelphia, PA: Lippincott Williams & Wilkins.

Dunn, H. L. (1959). High-level wellness for man and society. *American Journal of Public Health*, *49*(6), 786–792. Retrieved from http://www.pubmedcentral.nih.gov/picrender.fcgi?artid=1372807&blobtype=pdf.

Ehrlich, A., & Ladouceur, M. G. (2002). *A conceptual evolution of "health": National and international perspectives on health and health policies from 1974 to present*. Hamilton, ON: School of Nursing, McMaster University.

Epp, J. (1986). *Achieving health for all: A framework for health promotion*. Ottawa, ON: Minister of Supply & Services.

Evans, R. G., Barer, M. L., & Marmor, T. R. (Eds.). (1994). *Why are some people healthy and some people not?* New York, NY: Aldine de Gruyter.

French, J., Blair-Stevens, C., McVey, D., & Merritt, R. (2009). *Social marketing and public health: Theory & practice*. Oxford, UK: Elsevier.

Glanz, K., Patterson, R. E., Kristal, A. R., Feng, Z., Linnan, L., Heimendinger, J., & Hebert, J. (1998). Impact of worksite health promotion on stages of dietary change: The Working Well Trial. *Health Education and Behavior*, *25*(4), 448–463.

Green, L. W., & Kreuter, M. W. (1999). *Health promotion planning: An educational and ecological approach* (3rd ed.). Mountain View, CA: Mayfield.

Grier, S., & Bryant, C. (2005). Social marketing in public health. *Annual Review of Public Health*, *26*, 319–339.

Hamilton, N., & Bhatti, T. (1996). *Population health promotion: An integrated model of population health and health promotion*. Ottawa, ON: Health Promotion Development Division, Health Canada.

Health Canada. (1994). *Strategies for population health: Investing in the health of Canadians*. Retrieved from http://www.phac-aspc.gc.ca/ph-sp/pdf/strateg-eng.pdf.

Health Canada. (2002). *An inclusion lens: Workbook for looking at social and economic exclusion and inclusion*. Retrieved from http://www.phac-aspc.gc.ca/canada/regions/atlantic/pdf/inclusion_lens-E.pdf.

Health Canada. (2004). *Canadian addiction survey: A national survey of Canadians' use of alcohol and other drugs*. Retrieved from http://www.ccsa.ca/2005%20CCSA%20Documents/ccsa-004028-2005.pdf.

Health Canada. (2005a). *Health promotion: Does it work?*. Retrieved from http://www.hc-sc.gc.ca/sr-sr/pubs/hpr-rpms/bull/2002-3-promotion/method-eng.php.

Health Canada. (2005b). *National framework for action to reduce the harms associated with alcohol and other drugs and substances in Canada*. Retrieved from http://www.nationalframework-cadrenational.ca/uploads/files/HOME/NatFRA1steditionEN.pdf.

Health Canada. (2005c). *Social marketing*. Retrieved from http://www.hc-sc.gc.ca/ahc-asc/activit/marketsoc/index_e.html.

Health Canada. (2005d). *Social marketing in health promotion: The Canadian experience*. Retrieved from http://www.hc-sc.gc.ca/ahc-asc/activit/marketsoc/socmar-hcsc/experience_e.html.

Heiss, G. L. (2009). Health promotion and risk reduction in the community. In F. A. Maurer, & C. M. Smith (Eds.), *Community/public health nursing practice: Health for families and populations* (4th ed., pp. 472–490). St. Louis, MO: Saunders Elsevier.

Herzog, T. A. (2005). When popularity outstrips the evidence: Comment on West. *Addiction*, *100*(8), 1040–1041.

Horta, B., Bahl, R., Martines, J., & Cesar, G. (2007). *Evidence on the long-term effects of breastfeeding*. Geneva, Switzerland: World Health Organization.

Human Resources and Skills Development Canada. (2009). *Taking action: An introduction*. Retrieved from http://www.hrsdc.gc.ca/eng/workplaceskills/essential_skills/taking_action_introduction.shtml.

Labonte, R. (1995). Population health and health promotion: What do they have to say to each other? *Canadian Journal of Public Health*, *86*(3), 165–168.

Labonte, R. (1997). Community, community development, and the forming of authentic partnerships: Some critical reflections. In M. Minkler (Ed.), *Community organizing and community building for health* (pp. 88–102). New Brunswick, NJ: Rutgers University Press.

Labonte, R. (2003). *How our programs affect population health determinants: A workbook for better planning and accountability*. Retrieved from http://www.phac-aspc.gc.ca/ph-sp/progphd-progdsp/pdf/progphd_work_e.pdf.

Lalonde, M. (1974). *A new perspective on the health of Canadians: A working document*. Ottawa, ON: Government of Canada.

Literacy, B. C. (2005). *Literacy and health*. Retrieved from http://www2.literacy.bc.ca/facts/health.htm.

Lubkin, I. M., & Larsen, P. D. (2009). *Chronic illness: Impact and interventions* (7th ed.). Sudbury, MA: Jones & Bartlett.

Lyons, R., & Langille, L. (2000). *Healthy lifestyle: Strengthening the effectiveness of lifestyle approaches to improve health*. Retrieved from http://www.ahprc.dal.ca/lifestylefinal.pdf.

Maville, J. A., & Huerta, C. G. (2008). *Health promotion in nursing* (2nd ed.). Clifton Park, NY: Delmar, Cengage Learning.

McKenzie, J. F., Neiger, B. L., & Thackeray, R. (2009). *Planning, implementing, and evaluating health promotion programs: A primer* (5th ed.). Upper Saddle River, NJ: Pearson Education.

McLaren, L., & Hawe, P. (2005). Ecological perspectives in health research. *Journal of Epidemiology and Community Health*, *59*, 6–14.

McLean, S., Feather, J., & Butler-Jones, D. (2005). *Building health promotion capacity: Action for learning, learning from action*. Vancouver, BC: UBC Press.

Meade, C. D. (2007). Community health education. In M. A. Nies & M. McEwan (Eds.), *Community/public health nursing: Promoting the health of populations* (4th ed., pp. 104–134). St. Louis, MO: Saunders Elsevier.

Ministry of Health Promotion (2008). *Ontario public health standards*. Retrieved from http://www.health.gov.on.ca/english/providers/program/pubhealth/oph_standards/ophs/progstds/workshops/chronic_diseases_injuries_family_health_walsh_gertler.pdf.

Mintz, J. (2005). *Social marketing in health promotion … the Canadian experience*. Retrieved from http://www.hc-sc.gc.ca/ahc-asc/activit/marketsoc/socmar-hcsc/experience-eng.php.

National Cancer Institute. (2005). *Theory at a glance: A guide for health promotion practice* (2nd ed.). Retrieved from http://www.cancer.gov/PDF/481f5d53-63df-41bc-bfaf-5aa48ee1da4d/TAAG3.pdf.

Nutbeam, D., & Harris, E. (2004). *Theory in a nutshell: A practical guide to health promotion theories*. Sydney, Australia: McGraw Hill.

Ontario Health Promotion Resource System. (n.d.). *HP-101: Health promotion on-line course, module 4*. Retrieved from http://www.ohprs.ca/hp101/mod4/module4c6.htm.

Ontario Healthy Communities Coalition. (n.d.). *About us: What makes a community healthy?* Retrieved from http://www.ohcc-ccso.ca/en/what-makes-a-healthy-community.

Ontario Prevention Clearinghouse (2002). *Capacity building for health promotion: More than bricks and mortar*. Retrieved from http://www.healthnexus.ca/our_programs/hprc/resources/capacity_building.pdf.

ParticipACTION (2010). *About ParticipACTION*. Retrieved from http://www.participaction.com/en-us/AboutParticipaction/AboutParticipaction.aspx.

Poulin, C., & Nicholson, J. (2005). Should harm minimization as an approach to adolescent substance use be embraced by junior and senior high schools? Empirical evidence from an integrated school and community-based demonstration intervention addressing drug use among adolescents. *International Journal of Drug Policy*, *16*(6), 403–414.

Prochaska, J. O. (2006). Further commentaries on West (2005): Moving beyond the transtheoretical model. *Addiction*, *101*(6), 768–774.

Prochaska, J. O., & DiClemente, C. C. (1983). Stages and processes of self-change of smoking: Toward an integrative model of change. *Journal of Consulting and Clinical Psychology*, *51*(3), 390–395.

Public Health Agency of Canada. (1994). *Strategies for population health: Investing in the health of Canadians*. Retrieved from http://www.phac-aspc.gc.ca/ph-sp/pdf/strateg-eng.pdf.

Public Health Agency of Canada. (2001). *What is the population health approach?* Retrieved from http://www.phac-aspc.gc.ca/ph-sp/php-psp/php3-eng.php#Developing.

Public Health Agency of Canada. (2004). *Discovering assets—the Community Helpers program*. Retrieved from http://www.phac-aspc.gc.ca/mh-sm/mhp-psm/pub/community-communautaires/ccbm_3_e.html.

Public Health Agency of Canada (2005). *The VOICE in health policy project*. Retrieved from http://www.phac-aspc.gc.ca/vs-sb/voice_e.html.

Public Health Agency of Canada. (2008a). *Population health approach: The organizing framework*. Retrieved from http://cbpp-pcpe.phac-aspc.gc.ca/population_health/index-eng.html.

Public Health Agency of Canada. (2008b). *Centre for Health Promotion: Healthy Communities Division*. Retrieved from http://www.phac-aspc.gc.ca/chhd-sdsh/index-eng.php.

Public Health Agency of Canada. (2008c). *Home: Is your child safe?* Retrieved from http://www.phac-aspc.gc.ca/dca-dea/allchildren_touslesenfants/she_security-eng.php#safehome.

Public Health Agency of Canada. (2008d). *Glossary of terms relevant to the core competencies for public health, A–D*. Retrieved from http://www.phac-aspc.gc.ca/ccph-cesp/glos-a-d-eng.php.

Public Health Agency of Canada. (2009a). *Health goals for Canada: A federal, provincial and territorial commitment to Canadians*. Retrieved from http://www.phac-aspc.gc.ca/hgc-osc/home.html.

Public Health Agency of Canada. (2009b). *Health goals for Canada: A federal, provincial and territorial commitment to Canadians*. Retrieved from http://www.phac-aspc.gc.ca/hgc-osc/new-1-eng.html.

Racher, F. E., & Annis, R. C. (2007). *The community health action model: Health promotion by the community*. Retrieved from http://www2.brandonu.ca/organizations/rdi/Publications/Health/CHA_ModeWorkingPaper.pdf.

Raphael, D. (2004). *Social determinants of health: Canadian perspectives*. Toronto, ON: Canadian Scholars' Press.

Raphael, D. (2009). *Social determinants of health: Canadian perspectives* (2nd ed.). Toronto, ON: Canadian Scholars' Press.

Raphael, D., & Bryant, T. (2002). The limitations of population health as a model for a new public health. *Health Promotion International*, *17*(2), 189–199.

Reutter, L., & Eastlick Kushner, K. (2009). Health and wellness. In P. A. Potter, A. G. Perry, J. C. Ross-Kerr, & M. J. Wood. (2009). *Canadian fundamentals of nursing* (4th ed., pp. 1–13). Toronto, ON: Mosby Elsevier.

Riebe, D., Blissmer, B., Greene, G., Caldwell, M., Ruggiero, L., Stillwell, K. M., & Nigg, C. (2005). Long-term maintenance of exercise and healthy eating behaviors in overweight adults. *Preventive Medicine*, *40*(6), 769–778.

Robertson, A. (1998). Shifting discourses on health in Canada. From health promotion to population health. *Health Promotion International*, *13*(2), 155–166.

Romanow, R. (2002). *Building on values: The future of health care in Canada. Final report.* Retrieved from http://publications.gc.ca/pub?id = 237274&sl = 0.

Ronson, B., & Rootman, I. (2009). Literacy and health literacy: New understandings about their impact on health. In D. Raphael (Ed.), *Social determinants of health* (2nd ed., pp. 171–185). Toronto, ON: Canadian Scholars' Press.

Rootman, I., & Gordon-El-Bihbety, D. (2008). *A vision for a health literate Canada*. Canadian Public Health Association. Retrieved from http://www.ccl-cca.ca/NR/rdonlyres/3865A9D0-F2FE-4A95-A8C0-8FFF6BE466A9/0/20080225VisionforHealthLiterateCanReportEN.pdf.

Sallis, J. F., Cervero, R. B., Ascher, W., Henderson, K. A., Kraft, M. K., & Kerr, J. (2006). An ecological approach to creating active living communities. *Annual Review of Public Health*, *27*, 297–322.

Self-Help Resource Centre. (n.d.). *Self-help and health promotion.* Retrieved from http://www.selfhelp.on.ca/resource/health_promo_factsheet.pdf.

Senate Subcommittee on Population Health. (2009). *A healthy productive Canada: A determinant of health approach*. Retrieved from http://www.parl.gc.ca/40/2/parlbus/commbus/senate/com-e/popu-e/rep-e/rephealth1jun09-e.pdf.

Shah, C. (2003). *Public health and preventive medicine in Canada*. Toronto, ON: Elsevier.

Sheinfeld Gorin, S., & Arnold, J. (1998). *Health promotion handbook*. St. Louis, MO: Mosby.

Smith, B. J., Tang, K. C., & Nutbeam, D. (2006). WHO health promotion glossary: New terms. *Health Promotion International*, *21*(4), 340–345.

Spencer, L., Adams, T. B., Malone, S., Roy, L., & Yost, E. (2006). Applying the transtheoretical model to exercise: A systematic and comprehensive review of the literature. *Health Promotion Practice*, *7*(4), 428–443.

Spencer, L. S., Pagell, F., Hallion, M. E., & Adams, T. B. (2002). Applying the transtheoretical model to tobacco cessation: A review of the literature. *American Journal of Health Promotion*, *17*(1), 7–71.

Tang, K., Beaglehole, R., & O'Byrne, D. (2005). Policy and partnership for health promotion: Addressing the determinants of health. *Bulletin of the World Health Organization*, *83*(12), 884–885.

Thackeray, R., & McCormack Brown, K. (2005). Social marketing's unique contributions to health promotion practice. *Health Promotion Practice*, *6*(4), 365–368.

Ungerleider, C., & Burns, T. (2004). The state and quality of Canadian public education. In D. Raphael (Ed.), *Social determinants of health: Canadian perspectives* (pp. 139–153). Toronto, ON: Canadian Scholars' Press.

UNICEF. (2009). *The baby-friendly hospital initiative*. Retrieved from http://www.unicef.org/nutrition/index_24806.html.

University of Calgary. (2007). *Introduction to children's mental health*. Retrieved from http://fsw.ucalgary.ca/cmhp/introduction.

University of Ottawa. (2008). *Individual and population health*. Retrieved from http://www.med.uottawa.ca/Curriculum/IPH/data/Health_Promotion_e.htm.

Uys, L. R., Majumdar, B., & Gwele, N. (2004). The Kwazulu-Natal health promotion model. *Journal of Nursing Scholarship*, *36*(3), 192–196.

Vollman, A. R., Anderson, E. T., & McFarlane, J. (2008). *Canadian community as partner: Theory & multidisciplinary practice*. (2nd ed.) Philadelphia, PA: Lippincott Williams & Wilkins.

Walkom, T. (2008). Post mortem on Romanow. *Toronto Star*. Retrieved from http://www.emerginghealthleaders.ca/resources/Post-mortem-on-Romanow.pdf.

Wass, A. (2000). *Promoting health: The primary health care approach*. (2nd ed.). Sydney, Australia: Harcourt Saunders.

Watson, J. (1979). *Nursing: The philosophy and science of caring*. Boston, MA: Little, Brown and Company.

Watson, J. (1999). *Human science and human care: A theory of nursing*. Sudbury, MA: Jones & Bartlett.

Weinreich, N. K. (2006). *What is social marketing?* Retrieved from http://www.social-marketing.com/Whatis.html.

West, R. (2005). Time for a change: Putting the transtheoretical (stages of change) model to rest. *Addiction*, *100*(8), 1036–1039.

World Health Organization. (1947). *World Health Organization Act 1947. Constitution of the World Health Organization, section 3.* Retrieved from http://www.austlii.edu.au/au/legis/cth/consol_act/whoa1947273/sch1.html.

World Health Organization. (1986). *Ottawa charter for health promotion*. Retrieved from http://www.who.int/hpr/NPH/docs/ottawa_charter_hp.pdf.

World Health Organization. (1991). *Third international conference on health promotion, Sundsvall, Sweden*. Retrieved from http://www.who.int/hpr/NPH/docs/sundsvall_statement.pdf.

World Health Organization. (2000). *Health promotion: Bridging the equity gap*. Retrieved from http://www.who.int/hpr/NPH/docs/mxconf_report_en.pdf.

World Health Organization. (2001). *The Jakarta declaration on leading health promotion into the 21st century*. Retrieved from http://www.who.int/hpr/NPH/docs/jakarta_declaration_en.pdf.

World Health Organization. (2005). *The Bangkok charter for health promotion in a globalized world*. Retrieved from http://www.who.int/healthpromotion/conferences/6gchp/hpr_050829_%20BCHP.pdf.

World Health Organization. (2006). *Health promotion in a globalized world*. Retrieved from http://apps.who.int/gb/ebwha/pdf_files/WHA59/A59_21-en.pdf.

World Health Organization. (2008). *Closing the gap in a generation: Health equity through action on the social determinants of health*. Retrieved from http://whqlibdoc.who.int/publications/2008/9789241563703_eng.pdf.

World Health Organization. (2010). *Overview: 7th global conference on health promotion*. Retrieved from http://www.who.int/healthpromotion/conferences/7gchp/overview/en/index.html.

Young, L. E., & Hayes, V. E. (2002). *Transforming health promotion practice: Concepts, issues, and applications*. Philadelphia, PA: F. A. Davis.

Zanchetta, M. S., & Poureslami, I. M. (2006). Health literacy within the reality of immigrants' culture and language. *Canadian Journal of Public Health, 97*(Suppl. 2), 526–530.

Evidence-Informed Practice in Community Health Nursing

CHAPTER 5

OBJECTIVES

After reading this chapter, you should be able to:

1. Explain evidence-informed practice.
2. Provide examples of evidence-informed practice in community health nursing.
3. Apply evidence-informed practice in the context of community health nursing practice.

CHAPTER OUTLINE

KEY TERMS

See Glossary on page 593 for definitions.

EVIDENCE-INFORMED PRACTICE

In this chapter, the basic principles of evidence-informed practice are described as they apply to nursing in general and more specifically to the practice of community health nursing. The dynamics of the practice setting are described as they relate to implementing evidence-informed practice in the current health care system. Also included is a discussion and reinforcement of the importance of the integration of evidence-informed practice into community health nursing practice. Additional resources are provided for access to more information on evidence-informed practice.

Evidence-informed practice has become central to daily nursing practice (DiCenso, Guyatt, & Ciliska, 2005) and it provides nurses with guidance in current nursing practice to help make the most relevant and individualized nursing care decisions in their practice (DiCenso et al., 2005; Melnyk & Fineout-Overholt, 2005). Consequently, CHNs need to acquire skills for evidence-informed practice, to develop clinical questions, to access available evidence to answer these questions, to interpret the information appropriately, and to apply the evidence appropriately in their nursing practice in order to deliver the highest quality of care to clients (Canadian Nurses Association [CNA], 2002; Community Health Nurses Association of Canada, 2008; Sanzero Eller, Kleber, & Wang, 2003). In addition, CHNs need to stay up to date in the knowledge related to their area of practice and to appropriately apply this knowledge to client situations to be competent practitioners and to be able to validate decisions made in their daily nursing practice.

In Canada, the National Forum on Health recommended that the health care sector focus on the development of an evidence-informed health system (DiCenso et al., 2005). The underlying principle of evidence-informed practice is that high-quality care is based on evidence rather than on tradition or intuition (DiCenso et al., 2005; Melnyk & Fineout-Overholt, 2005). The application of scientific evidence in nursing is not new. For example, infection control measures, such as hand washing, were based on sound scientific knowledge. However, it is important to note that evidence-informed practice includes more than the use of research, as will be discussed in this chapter. As well, this chapter provides an overview of research aspects but students will need to review the research process using additional resources.

Evidence-informed practice is defined as combining the best evidence derived from research with clinical practice, knowledge, and expertise, and unique client expectations, preferences, or choices when making clinical decisions (CNA, 2002; Straus, Richardson, Glasziou, & Haynes, 2005). It is critical to utilize evidence-informed practice within the caring context in community health nursing. Sources of evidence, such as professional knowledge, client preferences, scientific evidence, and community milieu, need to be considered by CHNs in evidence-informed practice. The CNA describes evidence-informed decision making as an ongoing interactive process that involves thorough and carefully reviewed evidence to provide the best possible nursing care for clients (CNA, 2002). The CNA position statement on evidence-informed decision making and nursing practice (see the Weblinks at the end of this chapter) outlines the responsibilities for nurses, nursing regulatory and specialty associations, researchers, educators and educational institutions, employers of registered nurses and governments, and national and provincial health information institutions (CNA, 2002). The Sigma Theta Tau International Honour Society of Nursing (2005) in its position statement defines evidence-informed nursing as "an integration of the best evidence available, nursing expertise, and the values and preferences of the individuals, families and communities who are served" (p. 1). **Best practices** are recommendations pertaining to specific health issues or practice areas based on the most recent research evidence and key expert experiences and judgments (Health Canada, 2007). Refer to the Weblinks for the Institute for Clinical Evaluative Sciences and the Public Health Agency of Canada on the Evolve Web site for access to several sources on best practices.

CRITICAL VIEW

1. a) What are the differences between research application and evidence-informed practice?
   b) How has your provincial or territorial professional nursing association supported evidence-informed nursing practice?
2. What, if any, changes do you think will promote the use of evidence-informed practice by community health nurses?

EVIDENCE-INFORMED PRACTICE PROCESS

The sources of evidence-informed practice as applied to community health nursing practice are these:

- Identification of a clinical question based on client health status and client situation
- Use of the CHN's professional knowledge and clinical experience
- Scientific knowledge of all types
- Client experiences, values, preferences, and choices
- Consideration of community milieu, resources, accessibility, and availability

In community health nursing practice, assumptions are made every day about the client health situations. These assumptions need to be challenged and the most appropriate evidence accessed, interpreted, and appropriately applied. Also, CHNs need to use the best available evidence to make policy recommendations.

Historically, nurses have used multiple sources of knowledge in their practice. Unsystematic clinical observations by a CHN can lead to the development of hypotheses (hunches) of what might be happening. Upon reflection, the CHN would develop the clinical/community question. This reflection would include consideration of the components of the model identified in Figure 5-1.

See the evidence-informed practice puzzle in Figure 5-2 that depicts the evidence-informed practice process and the related challenges to CHNs as they make community health nursing practice decisions to provide the highest-quality care to their clients. As previously mentioned, the term *client* is used in the broadest sense, that is, client as individual, family, group, aggregate, population, and community. To some extent, the client will be determined by the area of community health nursing practice. Refer again to Figure 5-2 for areas where the CHN can apply evidence-informed practice. This puzzle presents the different parts of the evidence-informed practice process that need to be considered for each client situation. Every piece of the puzzle calls for reflection and decision making in each unique client situation.

FIGURE 5-1 Model for Evidence-Informed Practice and Decision Making in Community Health Nursing

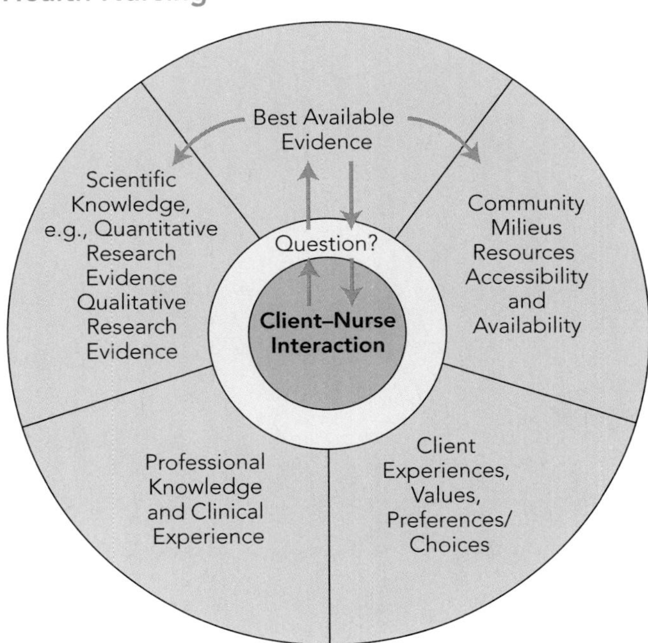

The formulation of a searchable question, which involves defining and refining the question, is an important first step in the evidence-informed practice process. To effectively answer the formulated clinical questions, CHNs have access to a variety of sources, such as the client, the community, and research such as systematic reviews, experimental and nonexperimental research studies, and clinical practice guidelines. Clinical nursing practice guidelines are systematically developed recommendations that facilitate nursing decision making and provide the most suitable clinical interventions for particular clients (CNA, 2002). The most rigorous research available is used in the development of clinical practice guidelines. However, when research evidence is found to be weak, these guidelines are developed using expert opinion and consensus (CNA, 2002; DiCenso et al., 2005). Examples of nursing clinical practice guidelines—such as *Crisis Intervention, Screening for Delirium, Dementia and Depression in the Older Adult*, and *Caregiving Strategies for Older Adults with Delirium, Dementia, and Depression*—are available through the Registered Nurses' Association of Ontario clinical practice guidelines found in the Evolve Weblinks. The "Ethical Considerations" box on page 154 relates to researching guidelines during emergencies.

The question directs the search for research evidence in the literature. A well-formulated question provides the key words to search the literature in order to retrieve relevant research evidence. At first glance, this may seem easy; however, the CHN needs to formulate the question in such a way that it is answerable and searchable if the literature searches are to be effective and provide relevant information. DiCenso et al. (2005) describe different types of questions and the corresponding types of studies that would be most appropriate for them. For example, they indicate that quantitative studies answer "how many" and "how much" questions, whereas qualitative studies answer questions related to how people feel about or how people experience situations and conditions. Also, these authors identify the different parts of the question for each type of study. For example, the parts of questions for quantitative studies include the populations, the interventions or exposures, and the outcomes, whereas questions related to qualitative studies include the population and the situation. Box 5-1 provides two examples of how to formulate a question. Further information on formulating questions and other examples can be found in DiCenso et al. (2005). Remember, the key words used in your search will determine how successful you are in extracting the relevant information from the available literature related to your question. Information on how to acquire the skills

ETHICAL CONSIDERATIONS

Public health emergencies present ethical challenges. An example is the H1N1 influenza; it can cause disproportionate damage or harm to vulnerable populations. When this happens, the CHN needs to identify and address ethical issues and evidence-informed guidelines to deliver the highest quality care to these clients.

Ethical principles that apply to the above situation (see Box 6-2 on page 168 for more detail):

- *Nonmaleficence*. The CHN acts according to the standards of due care, always seeking to produce the least amount of harm possible.
- *Beneficience*. This principle is complementary to nonmaleficence and requires that CHNs do good. The CHNs are limited by time, place, and talents in the amount of good they can do. CHNs have obligations to perform actions that maintain or enhance dignity of the clients whenever those actions do not place an undue burden on health care providers.

Questions to Consider

Outcomes of vulnerability may be negative, such as a lower health status. You are the CHN working with a vulnerable population.

1. Identify barriers to implementing evidence-informed guidelines in minimizing the spread of H1N1 among the vulnerable population.
2. a) How do the ethical principles of nonmaleficence and beneficience specifically apply to this situation?
   b) How would these principles guide your practice as the CHN?

FIGURE 5-2 Evidence-informed practice puzzle: The steps in evidence-informed practice

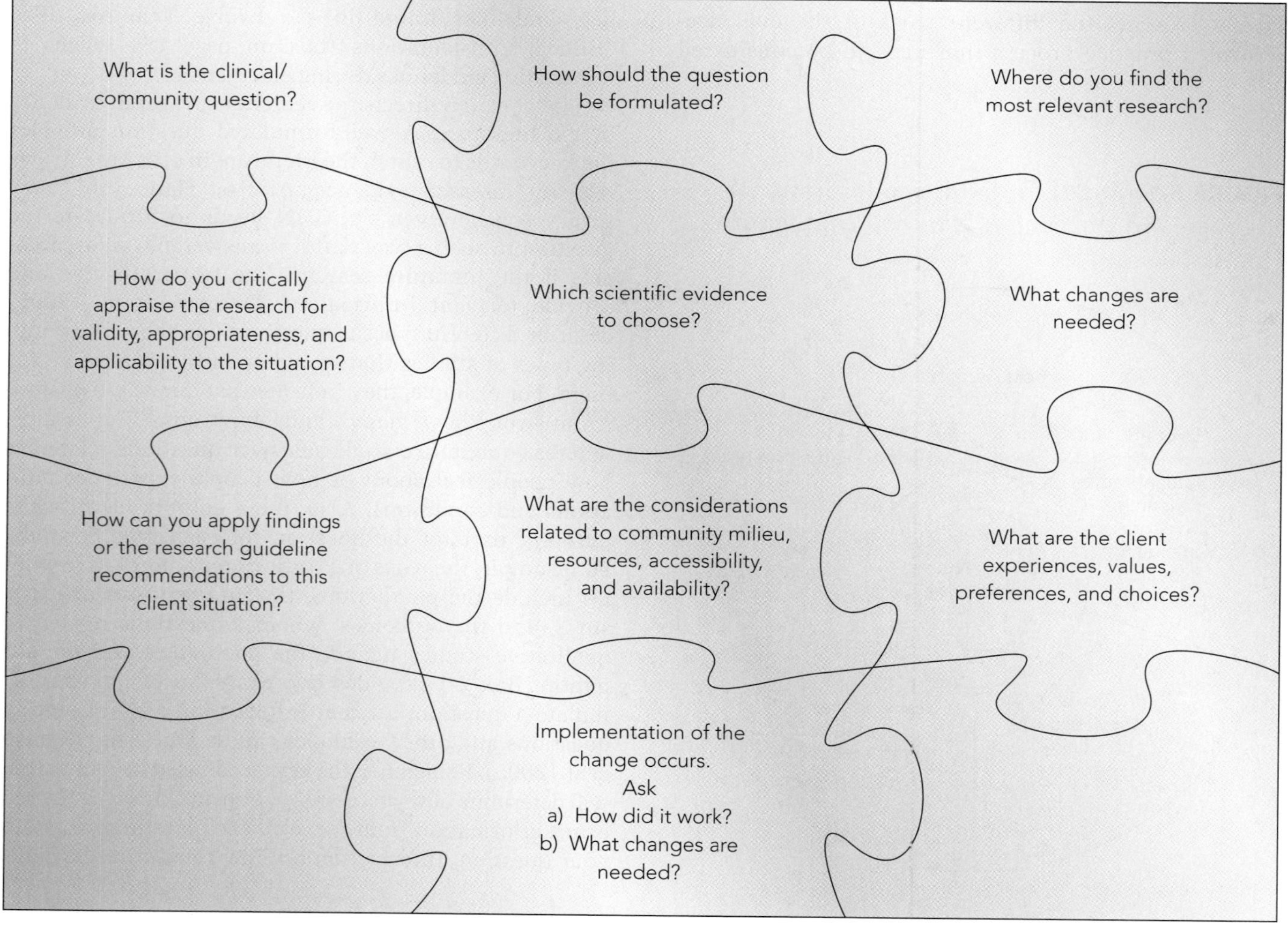

BOX 5-1 Examples of Transforming Unstructured Clinical Questions Into Structured Clinical Questions

Example 1: Smoking Cessation

You are a school nurse at a large high school in your community. You have just completed a day of information sessions with students on the harmful effects of smoking and have offered to meet with whoever is interested in quitting smoking. The next day, an 18-year-old girl, who has been smoking half a pack of cigarettes a day for the past year, drops in at your office. She has tried to quit smoking a number of times but with no success. She asks you whether "the patch" is an effective aid to quit smoking.

Type of Study: Quantitative Initial

Question: Is the nicotine patch effective?

Digging Deeper: One limitation of this type of question is that it does not specify the population. The effectiveness of the nicotine patch may differ in adolescents versus adults, in women versus men, in heavy smokers versus light smokers, as well as in those who have smoked for many years versus those who have smoked only for a few years. Another limitation of this question is that it does not include an outcome, which we know is smoking cessation.

Improved (Searchable) Question: A searchable question would specify the relevant patient population, the management strategy, and the patient-relevant consequences of that intervention, as follows:

Population: Young women who are moderate smokers

Intervention: Nicotine replacement therapy

Outcome: Smoking cessation

Formulated Question: Among young women who are moderate smokers, does nicotine replacement therapy increase the probability of smoking cessation?

Example 2: Caregiver Stress

You are a public health nurse making home visits to an elderly man with Alzheimer's disease. His daughter is his primary caregiver. As his condition deteriorates, she is increasingly worried about his safety and finds the situation physically and emotionally draining. She is experiencing anguish and guilt as she realizes that her father will soon need to be placed in a special care unit. She asks you whether others in this situation have similar feelings and what she can expect to feel once he is placed in the special care unit.

Type of Study: Qualitative

Initial Question: What feelings does one experience when placing a relative in special care?

Digging Deeper: The limitations of this question include failure to specify the population and insufficient details about the situation.

Improved (Searchable) Question: A searchable question would specify the relevant patient population and situation, as follows:

Population: Caregivers

Situation: Placing a relative with Alzheimer's disease in a special care unit

Formulated Question: How do caregivers describe their experiences of deciding to place a relative with Alzheimer's disease in a special care unit?

SOURCE: DiCenso, A., Guyatt, G., & Ciliska, D. (2005). *Evidence-based nursing: A guide to clinical practice* (pp. 24–27). St. Louis, MO: Mosby. Reprinted with permission.

of question formulation and key word searches can be obtained through attending evidence-informed practice workshops and reading relevant texts (e.g., DiCenso et al., 2005). Librarians are also excellent sources of help in library searches, but the information needed for the questions must be clearly stated. Some available Internet sources are outlined and discussed in Box 5-2. Depending on your community health nursing practice setting, as well as your roles and responsibilities, some Internet resources will be more helpful than others. Caution needs to be exercised while using information on Web sites that claim to contain data on evidence-informed practice.

Some examples of client clinical questions are these:

1. For new parents, does providing free smoke detector alarms to homes help reduce injuries from fires?
2. What type of guidance should be provided to a group of new mothers regarding infant car seats?
3. Which community programs are most effective in reducing obesity among school-age children?
4. Should a policy be instituted requiring vaccination for hepatitis A and B for all adults travelling out of Canada?

EVIDENCE-INFORMED PRACTICE IN COMMUNITY HEALTH NURSING

As discussed earlier, the first step in the evidence-informed practice process is formulating the question, which includes defining and refining the question.

BOX 5-2 Resources for Implementing Evidence-Informed Practice

Listed below are some of the available resources that community health nurses can utilize in developing their evidence-informed nursing practice.

1. The Cochrane Database of Systematic Reviews is an extensive collection of systematic reviews on health care issues. These reviews can be accessed at http://www.thecochranelibrary.com. A nursing segment of this group, the Cochrane Nursing Care Network, established in 2009, can be accessed at http://www.joannabriggs.edu.au/cncn/.
2. Health-evidence.ca: Promoting Evidence-Informed Decision Making is a Canadian Web site that consists of a collection of systematic reviews that are relevant to public health practice. They can be accessed at http://health-evidence.ca.
3. National Collaborating Centre for Methods and Tools is a Canadian resource that provides evidence-informed practice for public health and can be accessed at http://www.nccmt.ca.
4. The University of Sheffield, in the United Kingdom, provides evidence-informed practice sites and can be accessed at http://www.shef.ac.uk.
5. The University of Iowa Hospitals and Clinics and College of Nursing under the direction of Dr. Marita Titler provides evidence-informed practice resources to improve health care as well as help with understanding the evidence-informed practice process and can be accessed at http://www.nursing.uiowa.edu/sites/users/Gardery/ebp/Index.htm.
6. The *Evidence-Based Nursing Journal* provides reports on select articles that include the research question, methods, results, and evidence-informed conclusions and is accessed at http://ebn.bmj.com/.
7. Clinical Practice Guidelines based on the best available evidence to aid in clinical decision making are available at the following sites: http://www.rnao.org and http://www.bcguidelines.ca/gpac/.
8. *Clinical Evidence,* published by the *British Medical Journal,* is an online resource that provides a summary of the available scientific evidence on prevention and treatment and is available at http://www.clinicalevidence.bmj.com.
9. PubMed provides information on clinical questions and can be accessed at http://www.pubmed.gov.
10. The Institute for Clinical Evaluative Studies (ICES) provides scientific insights based on the latest evidence-informed research to guide health care practitioners and can be accessed at http://www.ices.on.ca.
11. CINAHL is a library database that provides references to individual journal articles and is available at http://www.ebscohost.com/cinahl/.
12. *Worldviews on Evidence-Based Nursing* is a journal that provides research information for nurses on clinical issues and can be accessed at http://onlinelibrary.wiley.com/journal/10.1111/(ISSN)1741-6787.

SOURCE: Adapted from: DiCenso, A., Guyatt, G., & Cileska, D. (2005). *Evidence-based nursing: A guide to clinical practice.* St. Louis, MO: Elsevier Mosby.

To answer the client clinical question that has been formulated, the sources of evidence-informed practice related to community health nursing include the best available evidence, that is, CHNs' professional knowledge and clinical experience; scientific knowledge of all types; client experiences, values, preferences, and choices; and consideration of community milieu, resources, accessibility, and availability.

The first source in the evidence-informed practice process is consideration of the CHNs' professional knowledge and clinical experience. The CHNs' background experiences in the community and their use of clinical reasoning skills will help in (1) identifying client issues for study and anticipating possible client responses to proposed strategies; (2) integrating all available evidence into nursing practice decisions; and (3) evaluating the community health nursing practice decisions. When CHNs access scientific knowledge of all types, they need to choose the most relevant information for each client's clinical situation. Asking relevant questions will help determine what acceptable evidence is. As well, CHNs need to have the skills to critically appraise the available evidence, including both quantitative and qualitative research evidence. The choice of research methodology is dependent on the nature of the client health concern.

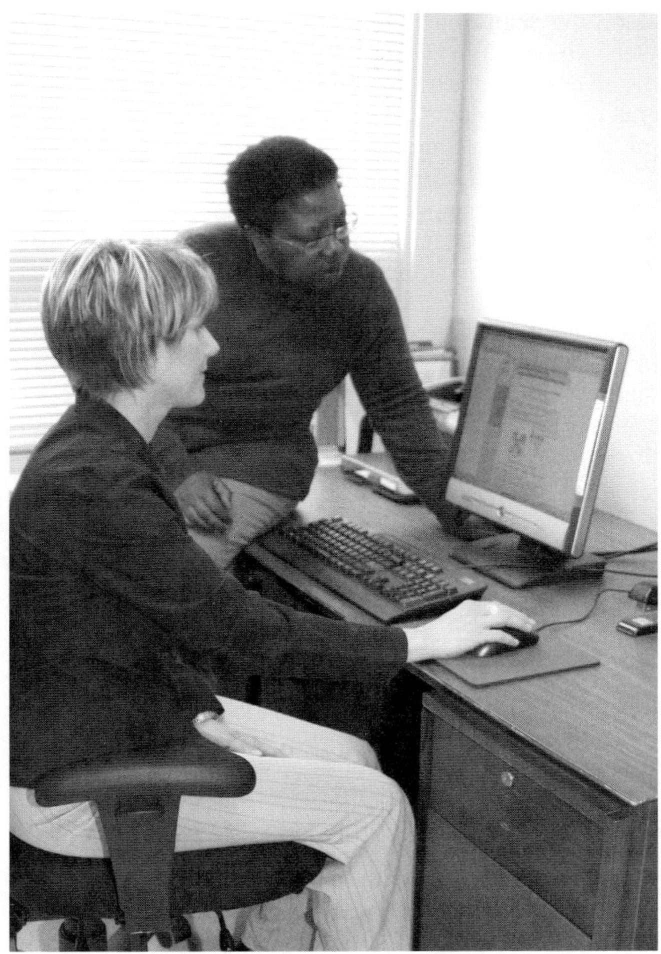

Although it might sometimes be easier to rely on past experience and knowledge, community health nurses strive to use the most recent evidence-informed data as one of their primary sources of decision making. Community health nurses use e-technology to acquire new knowledge.

As studies are reviewed, CHNs need to ask the following questions in order to determine their acceptability:

1. Is the study sufficiently well conducted in order to use the study findings?
2. What is the fit between the clinical/community question and the study design?
3. Can this research evidence be used in this client situation?
4. How can this research evidence be used in this client situation?
5. What are the implications for the client?

You may refer to resources listed or research textbooks to review study designs and the research process in depth. Also, some guidelines and Web sites are provided later in the chapter.

A **systematic review**, often called an overview, is a summary or synthesis of the research evidence that relates to a specific question and to the effects of an intervention. The "Evidence-Informed Practice" box provides one example of a systematic review found in the Cochrane Library. Systematic reviews can involve a rigorous process with several steps and several evaluators to evaluate a group of randomized controlled trials that relate to the same question.

Using specific criteria for systematic reviews, a grade is assigned, and the grade indicates the strength of the evidence; the higher the grade, the greater is the strength of the study. The abundance of research information that is available to CHNs can be overwhelming. Systematic reviews assist CHNs to manage this information overload and provide a grading of the quality of the available information. In addition, systematic reviews are useful knowledge sources, providing quick and easy access to large amounts of available research information that has been reviewed and summarized. In systematic reviews, meta-analysis is sometimes used. **Meta-analysis** is a technique that results in a summary statistic of the results when studies are comparable (Ciliska, Cullum, & Marks, 2001; Stumbo, 2003). Past and current systematic reviews that are of relevance to CHNs in their nursing practice are available from the Effective Public Health Practice Project (EPHPP) Web site (see the Tool Box on the Evolve website).

Ciliska, Cullum, and Marks (2001) identify the following three critical questions to consider when evaluating systematic reviews:

1. *Are the results of this systematic review valid?* Areas to consider in answering this critical appraisal question are these:
   a. Is this a systematic review of randomized controlled trials?
   b. Does the systematic review include a description of the strategies used to find all relevant trials?
   c. Does the systematic review include a description of how the validity of the individual studies was assessed?
   d. Were the results consistent from study to study?
   e. Were individual or aggregate data used in the analysis?
2. *What were the results?* Areas to consider in answering this critical appraisal question are these:
   a. How large was the treatment effect?
   b. How precise is the estimate of treatment effect?

3. *Will the results help me in caring for my clients?* Areas to consider in answering this critical appraisal question are these:
   a. Are my clients so different from those in the study that the results do not apply?
   b. Is the intervention/treatment feasible in my setting?
   c. Were all clinically important outcomes (harms as well as benefits) considered?

An overview of appraising a systematic review is provided by Stumbo (2003) (see the Evolve Weblinks). This Web site, in a two-part series, provides information on the conducting and appraisal of systematic reviews for evidence-informed practice.

One of the considerations with systematic reviews is the possible problem of bias, particularly publication bias. The reviewer(s) developing the systematic review may select only published studies that have significant results. However, other, unpublished studies may confirm or contradict the reported results (DiCenso et al., 2005; Melnyk & Fineout-Overholt, 2005). Systematic reviews can overestimate the effectiveness of the intervention, especially if unpublished studies are not included in the review. In the systematic review, the reviewer needs to be transparent about the efforts made to access unpublished studies as well as the process used for obtaining published studies. The Cochrane Collaboration Web sites listed in the Evolve Weblinks address many of the areas that have been discussed previously and provide guidance on conducting a systematic review and searching the health promotion and public health literature. The quality of the primary research studies included in systematic reviews will, in turn, influence the quality of the systematic reviews themselves. Guidelines for the reporting of primary empirical research studies in education have been developed by the Evidence for Policy and Practice Information Coordinating Centre (EPPI-Centre) (see the Tool Box on the Evolve Web site). This site provides questions to consider when appraising a process evaluation—for example, health promotion interventions. The City of Hamilton, Ontario: Effective Public Health Practice Project Weblink (see Evolve Web site) also provides systematic reviews and summary statements of relevance to CHNs.

Randomized controlled trials (RCTs) are considered by many as the gold standard of evidence gathering in evidence-informed practice. RCTs are considered one of the best sources for clinical effectiveness, interventions, and drug efficacy (DiCenso et al., 2005; Melnyk & Fineout-Overholt, 2005). RCTs are often considered the strongest evidence because of random assignment to either the control group or the experimental group, which controls for biases and differences that can occur due to the intervention. You may refer to research textbooks

Evidence-Informed Practice

One health promotion activity implemented by nurses and other health care professionals is advising or counselling clients regarding smoking cessation. A practising nurse might question whether this is an effective activity. Rice and Stead (2006) conducted a systematic review to determine the effectiveness of nursing interventions in smoking cessation. The authors, using an evidence-informed approach, conducted their search using the resources of CINAHL and the Cochrane Tobacco Addiction Group to identify the randomized trials exploring nursing interventions for smoking cessation. Twenty of the 29 studies identified that smoking cessation interventions significantly increased the odds of the client quitting smoking, particularly when the activity was provided during hospitalization. Smoking cessation interventions in nonhospitalized clients also indicated some benefit from the advice and support provided by the nurses. Overall, the systematic review indicated reasonable evidence that smoking cessation interventions by nurses could be effective.

Application for CHNs: The review of the trials indicated that the health promotion activity of advising and counselling smokers had some benefit and therefore should be utilized as a community health nursing intervention for encouraging smoking cessation. As well, community health nurses need to provide follow-up care for the clients discharged from hospital who require continued support and counselling for smoking cessation.

Questions for Reflection & Discussion

1. State one clinical question raised by the systematic review described above.
2. What evidence-informed practice sources would you use to obtain answers to this clinical question? Elaborate on why you have chosen these evidence-informed practice sources.

REFERENCE: Rice, V. H., & Stead, L. F. (2006). *Nursing interventions for smoking cessation.* Cochrane Database of Systematic Reviews. ISSN: 1464-780X. Retrieved from www.cochrane.org.

to review random allocation, blinding, and loss to follow-up, which are used to control for bias. Frequently in community health, RCTs are not feasible or ethical.

Community health nursing has had minimal involvement in RCTs; however, all types of evidence may be as applicable to nursing practice in communities as to other areas of health care. The reason for the limited participation of community health nursing in RCTs is related to ethical issues. It is often unethical to withhold an intervention or program—for example, withholding administration of the human papillomavirus (HPV) vaccine from a group of teens to determine the psychological effects of HPV infection. It would also be unethical to assign persons to an experimental group when harm could occur—for example, assigning pregnant women to a smoking group (experimental group) to determine the effects of smoking on the fetus.

CHNs need to consider and use available evidence, but this needs to be done taking into consideration individual client beliefs, perceptions, and concerns. Since the goal in nursing is to deliver the best possible care to clients and to have the best possible client outcomes, evidence can also be based on "unsystematic observations" by the nurse, discussions with the clients, and qualitative research findings (DiCenso et al., 2005).

Regardless of the type of study design, the quality of a study must always be established before a decision is made to use the study's findings. There are several tools available to evaluate the quality of quantitative study designs. Refer to the Effective Public Health Practice Project quality assessment tool listed in the Tool Box on the Evolve Web site. This tool can help CHNs determine whether the findings of a study can be used in their community health nursing practice.

Qualitative research, a research methodology that explores human experiences and uses words, text, and themes, rather than numbers, to describe the experiences, has gained importance because of the exploration of the "meaning" of certain situations to clients and the contribution of this methodology to the development of theories relevant to nursing practice. The qualitative evidence hierarchy of strength has yet to be developed; however, meta-synthesis—summarizing qualitative study results—has been initiated and is likely to lead to the development of a hierarchy. It is important to be aware that qualitative research evidence is also valuable. Qualitative research, with its interpretive perspective, assigns meaning to experiences. The types of qualitative approaches most familiar to CHNs are **phenomenology** (to understand the meaning of the lived experience); **grounded theory** (for theory development); **ethnography** (to understand a culture from the emic [insider] perspective), and **action research** (a systematic study of practice interventions) (Melnyk & Fineout-Overholt, 2005). You may refer to research textbooks for in-depth discussions on qualitative research.

Participatory action research (PAR), widely used in community health nursing practice (Stringer & Genat, 2004), is action-oriented research that helps CHNs develop client-centred interventions and services and influence policy. For example, researchers and CHNs may partner with community stakeholders to initiate, design, implement, and evaluate an action research study. The partnership also involves determining how the findings will be used. PAR is often conducted to (1) resolve health service delivery issues and problems and (2) empower individuals, populations, and communities with the motivation for promoting social action (Melnyk & Fineout-Overholt, 2005; Stringer & Genat, 2004).

It is critical that CHNs recognize that both quantitative and qualitative study designs contribute to nursing knowledge. DiCenso et al. (2005) describe these two paradigms as complementary to each other. In the qualitative paradigm, meanings of phenomena are explored, theories are generated, and "relationships between identified concepts" are identified. In the quantitative paradigm, hypotheses are tested and numbers are used in data analysis and in presenting study findings in order to make generalizations about aggregates and populations and for making predictions. In addition, this paradigm tests the theories developed in qualitative studies (DiCenso et al., 2005). Fade (2003) also posited the need for both types of study designs to achieve complete understanding of issues.

After CHNs have determined the validity, appropriateness, and applicability of the available research, they need to evaluate client openness and readiness to implement the change recommended by the research (DiCenso et al., 2005). In this process, it is important to assess client experiences, values, preferences, and choices. These client experiences, values, preferences, and choices will influence client willingness to implement the change or intervention. Also, at times, clients may request a particular intervention, but the CHN may have determined, on the basis of the critical appraisal of the available evidence, that this would not be a wise choice. The CHN would then need to explain to the client the evidence presented by the research and help the client make an informed decision. Refer to Box 5-3 for questions to consider regarding appropriateness and applicability for evidence-informed practice.

In partnership with the client, the CHN would consider the community milieu to determine which interventions would most likely be of benefit to the client. Community milieu includes such factors as expertise available in the community, urban or rural setting, social and physical environments, and resource availability and

BOX 5-3 Questions to Consider Regarding Appropriateness and Applicability for Evidence-Informed Practice

1. How will the results direct my client care practice?
   a. What is the fit between the study participants and my client and can the study results be applied?
   b. What is the feasibility of applying the treatment in our setting?
   c. How were the clinically relevant outcomes—that is, harms and benefits—considered?
   d. What are my client experiences, values, preferences, or choices for prevention of the outcome and the potential side effects?
   e. What community milieu, resources, accessibility, and availability need to be considered?
2. How can the study findings be applied to the care of my client?
   a. What is the meaning and relevance of the study to my practice?
   b. How does the study facilitate my understanding of the context of my practice?
   c. How does the study enhance my knowledge about my practice?

SOURCE: Adapted from Ciliska, D., & Thomas, H. (2008). Research. In J. L. Leeseberg Stamler & L. Yiu, *Community health nursing: A Canadian perspective* (2nd ed., pp. 227–244). Toronto, ON: Pearson Education Canada.

accessibility. For example, fiscal and human resources should be available in the community to support selected programs, and interventions have to be based on the best available evidence for the clinical and community question.

Mowinski Jennings and Loan (2001), when applying evidence-informed practice to clients, identify the importance of assisting the client with decision making, ensuring that the evidence is an appropriate literacy level for each client, advising the client of the benefits and risks of an intervention, and considering client preferences and values in practice decisions. In community health nursing practice, evidence would be applied with input from the client as partner. CHNs can use evidence-informed practice as a process to improve practice and client outcomes and to influence policies that will improve the health of communities (DiCenso et al., 2005).

Knowledge exchange refers to researchers and decision makers solving problems collaboratively so that research is planned, developed, disseminated, and applied (Canadian Health Services Research Foundation, 2007). Through knowledge exchange, CHNs, in their roles as researchers and in working collaboratively with other researchers and health care decision makers, can influence health care policy, and the ensuing health care policy changes and application of research evidence will positively affect community health. Access and utilization of evidence-informed practice encourage CHNs to be professional, to provide care in a safe manner, and to be accountable for their community health nursing practice. The evidence-informed content in this chapter provides information necessary for the community health nurse to meet this practice challenge.

CHNs are often confronted with situations "filled with uncertainty" (Melynk & Fineout-Overholt, 2005, p. 3). Evidence-informed practice skills can help CHNs deal with these uncertainties as they occur in daily nursing practice. Application of evidence-informed practice also assists CHNs to explain and justify the decisions they make on a daily basis in their community health nursing practice.

CRITICAL VIEW

Many believe that "an ounce of prevention buys a pound of cure." Others believe that "early detection is good for everyone."

1. What do you think about these two statements? Do you agree? Why or why not? After you have reflected on these two statements, go to the Web site http://www.chsrf.ca/mythbusters/index_e.php and select the link for each of these statements.
2. How has the evidence found on these links changed your thinking about these two statements?

Refer to the CNA position statement, *Evidence-Based Decision-Making and Nursing Practice* (listed in the Evolve Weblinks), which outlines the responsibilities at various levels and by various bodies to facilitate evidence-informed practice in nursing.

STUDENT EXPERIENCE

Choose one of the following client situations to demonstrate the use of evidence-informed practice.

Client 1: Many local schools have vending machines that contain high-fat, high-carbohydrate foods. As the CHN, you are suggesting that these vending machines be removed because of the increasing numbers of overweight and obese children within the community and the school. Does the removal of vending machines contribute to improved children's nutritional status?

Client 2: A 24-year-old paraplegic client who is bedridden has developed a reddened broken skin area in the coccyx area. This client became paraplegic due to a motorcycle accident and has just been discharged home where he will be living with his recently separated mother. What is the best treatment for a pressure sore in early development?

Client 3: Identify a client situation from your own community clinical practice. State a question in relation to that clinical practice situation.

Activity:

1. Choose one of the above client situations.
2. a. Improve the question so that it is searchable.
   b. Formulate the question.
3. Search the literature (quantitative and qualitative research evidence that includes systematic reviews and meta-analyses).
4. Critically appraise the research for validity, appropriateness, and applicability to the client situation.
5. Decide on the scientific evidence that works best for the client's situation.
6. Outline how you would apply the findings to the client situation.
7. Outline the considerations related to the community milieu, resources, accessibility, and availability.
8. Identify questions that you would ask in relation to client experiences, values, preferences, and choices.
9. Evaluate by raising questions that would address how it worked and what changes would be needed.

Questions:

1. What have you learned from this evidence-informed practice exercise?
2. How has this exercise changed your thoughts and feelings about evidence-informed practice?

REMEMBER THIS!

- Evidence-informed practice combines the best evidence from research, clinical practice, knowledge and expertise, and unique client expectations, preferences, or choices when making clinical decisions.
- Sources of evidence for CHNs include professional knowledge and clinical experience, scientific knowledge, client experiences, values, preferences and choices, community milieu, resources, accessibility, and availability.
- CHNs need to learn to follow the evidence-informed practice process in order to deliver the highest-quality care to clients in their nursing practice.
- Formulation of a searchable problem is an important first step in the evidence-informed practice process.
- Quantitative and qualitative studies contribute to research knowledge in evidence-informed practice.
- The quality of research studies needs to be assessed before study findings are applied in community health nursing practice.
- Client experiences, values, preferences, and choices need to be explored and considered.
- Consideration of community milieu, resources, accessibility, and availability are part of the assessment.
- Evaluation of the outcome related to the decision is essential.
- Knowledge exchange affects community health.

REFLECTIVE PRAXIS

Case Study

The director of a part-time, nurse-managed community health clinic is in the process of determining how best to expand services to operate as a full-time clinic in the most cost-effective as well as clinically effective manner. The nurse, who is the director, gathers evidence on nurse-managed community clinics in other rural settings to evaluate cost-effectiveness and clinical effectiveness of various models. The nurse also considers evidence from the following sources in the decision-making process: client satisfaction research data, knowledge of clinic staff, expert opinion of community advisory board members, evidence from community partners, and data on service needs in the province. Having examined the evidence, the nurse decides that incremental (step-by-step) growth toward full-time status is warranted. Evidence of needs in the community and analysis of statistical data indicate that adding services for children is a priority. As the first step, a community health nurse (CHN) with a pediatric clinical background is hired, while planning for full-time status continues.

1. Which of the following is demonstrated by the evaluation of the evidence gathered?
   a. Effectiveness of the intervention in communities
   b. Application of the data to populations and communities
   c. Economic consequences of the intervention
   d. Barriers to implementation of the interventions in communities
2. Explain how this example applies principles of evidence-informed practice.

Answers are on the Evolve Web site at http://evolve.elsevier.com/Canada/Stanhope/community/.

What Would You Do?

1. You are a CHN working with adolescents diagnosed with diabetes mellitus. Mary, newly diagnosed with diabetes, tells you that she injects insulin through her clothes because it is faster and easier for her. Also, she tells you that her best friend was told that sterile technique is no longer needed. The clinical question is, can clients with diabetes mellitus safely inject insulin through clothing? How would you obtain the answer to this question? Refer to the sources for evidence-informed practice provided in this chapter and find the answer to your clinical question. Bring your findings to class for discussion.

Adapted from Lock, S.E. (2010). Evidence-based practice. In M. Stanhope & J. Lancaster, *Foundations of nursing in the community: Community-oriented practice* (3rd ed., pp. 178–187). St. Louis, MO: Mosby Elsevier.

TOOL BOX

evolve

The Tool Box contains useful instruments that can be applied in community health nursing practice. These related resources are found either in the appendices at the back of this book or on the Evolve Web site at http://evolve.elsevier.com/Canada/Stanhope/community/.

Tools

The Cochrane Collaboration. *Cochrane Reviews.*
This Web site provides reviews from A–Z on such topics as cardiovascular health, drugs and alcohol, infectious diseases, sexual health, human immunodeficiency virus/acquired immunodeficiency syndrome (HIV/AIDS), various types of injuries, mental and social health, nutrition, overweight and obesity, physical activity, occupational health and safety, population screening and population group, and tobacco control.

Effective Public Health Practice Project. *The Quality Assessment Tool.*
This site provides links to the tool and a dictionary for tool use. Also, there is a link that provides access to public health literature reviews.

Evidence for Policy and Practice Information and Coordinating Centre (EPPI-Centre).
Guidelines for the reporting of primary empirical research studies in education (The REPOSE Guidelines). This site provides a tool for evaluating primary research studies.

WEBLINKS

evolve

Direct links to these resources can be found on the text's accompanying Evolve Web site at http://evolve.elsevier.com/Canada/Stanhope/community.

Canadian Nurses Association Position Statement. *Evidence-Based Decision-Making and Nursing Practice*. This CNA position statement on evidence-informed decision making and nursing practice outlines the responsibilities for nurses, nursing regulatory and specialty associations, researchers, educators and educational institutions, employers of registered nurses and governments, and national and provincial health information institutions. Choose Position Statements under Quick Links and then select Research.

City of Hamilton, Ontario. *Effective Public Health Practice Project*. This Web site is a result of a partnership between the Public Health Research Education and Development Program (PHRED), funded by the Ministry of Health and Long-Term Care, and the City of Hamilton Public Health Services. The Web site provides systematic reviews and summary statements of relevance to CHNs.

The Cochrane Collaboration. *Cochrane Handbook for Systematic Reviews of Interventions.* Version 5.0.2. This site explains systematic reviews, the need for a systematic review, and how to prepare a Cochrane review, etc.

The Cochrane Collaboration. *What's New?* This Web site explains the latest handbook updates and discusses systematic reviews.

Cochrane Public Health Group. The Web site reviews the protocols relevant to health promotion and public health on the Cochrane Library. It provides links to health promotion and public health literature.

Institute for Clinical Evaluative Sciences (ICES). *Informed*. This Web site provides access to peer-reviewed publications of value to primary care providers. From the ICES homepage, choose Publications, scroll down, and click on "informed."

Public Health Agency of Canada. *Canadian Best Practices Portal for Health Promotion and Chronic Disease Prevention*. This Web site provides access to many sources on best practices in chronic disease prevention and control interventions and on health promotion initiatives. The information provided will also assist in policy development, and access to best practice interventions is available for many areas.

Registered Nurses' Association of Ontario. *Clinical Practice Guidelines*. Several best-practice guidelines for nurses are available at this Web site. Some examples include best-practice guidelines on abuse of women, breastfeeding, client-centred care, crisis interventions, establishing therapeutic relationships, primary prevention of childhood obesity, and enhancing healthy adolescent development. Select the Nursing Best Practice Guidelines link and from there choose Clinical Practice Guidelines.

REFERENCES

Canadian Health Services Research Foundation. (CHSRF). (2007). *Glossary of knowledge exchange terms as used by the foundation*. Retrieved from http://www.chsrf.ca/keys/glossary_e.php.

Canadian Nurses Association. (2002). *Evidence-based decision-making and nursing practice*. Retrieved from http://www.cna-nurses.ca/CNA/documents/pdf/publications/PS63_Evidence_based_Decision_making_Nursing_Practice_e.pdf.

Ciliska, D., Cullum, N., & Marks, S. (2001). Evaluation of systematic reviews of treatment of prevention interventions. *Evidence-Based Nursing*, *4*(4), 100–105.

Ciliska, D., & Thomas, H. (2008). Research. In J. L. Leeseberg Stamler & L. Yiu (Eds.), *Community health nursing: A Canadian perspective* (2nd ed., pp. 227–244). Toronto, ON: Pearson Education Canada.

Community Health Nurses Association of Canada. (2008). *Canadian Community Health Nursing Standards of Practice*. Retrieved from http://www.chnc.ca/documents/chn_standards_of_practice_mar08_english.pdf.

DiCenso, A., Guyatt, G., & Ciliska, D. (2005). *Evidence-based nursing: A guide to clinical practice*. St. Louis, MO: Mosby.

Fade, S. A. (2003). Communicating and judging the quality of qualitative research: The need for a new language. *Journal of Human Nutrition and Dietetics*, *16*(3), 139–149.

Health Canada. (2007). *Best practices: Treatment and rehabilitation for seniors with substance use problems*. Retrieved from http://www.hc-sc.gc.ca/hc-ps/pubs/adp-apd/treat_senior-trait_ainee/background-contexte-eng.php.

Lock, S. E. (2010). Evidence-based practice. In M. Stanhope, & J. Lancaster (Eds.), *Foundations of nursing in the community: Community-oriented practice* (3rd ed., pp. 178–187). St. Louis, MO: Mosby Elsevier.

Melnyk, B. M., & Fineout-Overholt, E. (2005). *Evidence-based practice in nursing and healthcare: A guide to best practice*. Philadelphia, PA: Lippincott, Williams & Wilkins.

Mowinski Jennings, B., & Loan, L. A. (2001). Misconceptions among nurses about evidence-based practice. *Journal of Nursing Scholarship*, *33*(2), 121–127.

Rice, V. H., & Stead, L. F. (2006). *Nursing interventions for smoking cessation*. Cochrane Database of Systematic Reviews. ISSN: 1464–780X. Retrieved from www.cochrane.org.

Sanzero Eller, L., Kleber, E., & Wang, S. L. (2003). Research knowledge, attitudes, and practices of health professionals. *Nursing Outlook*, *51*(4), 165–170.

Sigma Theta Tau International Honour Society of Nursing. (2005). *Evidence Based Nursing Position Statement*. Retrieved from http://www.nursingsociety.org/aboutus/PositionPapers/Pages/EBN_positionpaper.aspx.

Straus, S. E., Richardson, W. S., Glasziou, P., & Haynes, R. B. (2005). *Evidence-based medicine: How to practice and teach EBM*. London, UK: Elsevier/Churchill Livingstone.

Stringer, E., & Genat, W. J. (2004). *Action research in health*. Upper Saddle River, NJ: Merrill Prentice Hall.

Stumbo, N. J. (2003). Systematic Reviews Part I: How to conduct systematic reviews for evidence-based practice and Systematic Reviews Part II: How to appraise systematic reviews for evidence-based practice. *Annual in Therapeutic Recreation*, *12*, 29–55. Retrieved from http://www.atra-tr.org/members/annual/2003/volume12.pdf.

CHAPTER

6

Ethics in Community Health Nursing Practice

OBJECTIVES

After reading this chapter, you should be able to:

1. Describe a brief history of the ethics of community health nursing.
2. Discuss ethical decision-making processes.
3. Compare and contrast ethical theories and principles, virtue ethics, ethic of care, and feminist ethics.
4. Explain how ethics is part of the core functions of community health nursing.
5. Analyze codes of ethics for nursing and community health nursing.
6. Apply the ethics of advocacy to community health nursing.
7. Apply principles of ethical decision making in community health nursing practice.

CHAPTER OUTLINE

KEY TERMS

See Glossary on page 593 for definitions.

The Canadian authors gratefully acknowledge the contribution of Manon Lemonde.

The work of community health nurses (CHNs) involves ethical activities. CHNs who practise in this area focus on protecting, promoting, preserving, and maintaining health while preventing disease. These goals reflect the ethical principles of promoting good and preventing harm. CHNs also struggle with the rights of individuals and families versus the rights of local groups within a community. These struggles reflect the tensions between respect for autonomy, rights-based ethical theory, and community-based ethical theory.

In addition, CHNs deal with consequence-based ethical theory and obligation-based ethical theory. They also deal with the ethical components of advocacy, justice, health policy, caring, women's moral experiences, and the moral character of health care practitioners. They are guided by codes of ethics and ethical decision-making frameworks. Ethics is a body of knowledge and, as such, is more than "being a good person." Ethics is a part of clinical decision making and practice (Bernheim & Melnick, 2008). This chapter applies the core knowledge of ethics to community health nursing.

BOX 6-1 The Nightingale Pledge

The Nightingale Pledge was written by Lystra Gretter in 1893. It states:

I solemnly pledge myself before God and in the presence of this assembly, to pass my life in purity and to practice my profession faithfully. I will abstain from whatever is deleterious and mischievous, and will not take or knowingly administer any harmful drug. I will do all in my power to maintain and elevate the standard of my profession, and will hold in confidence all personal matters committed to my keeping and all family affairs coming to my knowledge in the practice of my calling. With loyalty will I endeavor to aid the physician, in his work, and devote myself to the welfare of those committed to my care. (Registered-nurse-canada.com, 2009)

HISTORY OF NURSING AND ETHICS

Modern nursing has a rich heritage of ethics and morality, beginning with Florence Nightingale (1820–1910). The morals and values she gave to nursing have endured. **Morals** are shared and generational societal norms about what constitutes right or wrong conduct; **values** are beliefs about the shared worth or importance of what is desired or esteemed within a society. Florence Nightingale saw nursing as a call to service, and she thought that those who became nurses should be people of good moral character. She was passionate about the need to provide care to poor people and also about the importance of a sanitary environment, as seen in her work with soldiers in the Crimean War (1854–56). Because of her commitment to poor individuals in communities, her championing of primary prevention, and the work she did to show that healthy environments save soldiers' lives, she is seen as nursing's first moral leader and the first community health nurse.

Nurses' codes of ethics are important in the history of nursing practice in the community. A nursing **code of ethics** is a framework that nurses use to guide their ethical obligations and actions within the profession. Nurses' codes of ethics clarify the values and guidelines of ethical conduct in nursing practice. The Nightingale Pledge (see Box 6-1) is generally considered to be nursing's first code of ethics (American Nurses Association [ANA], 2001). After the Nightingale Pledge, a suggested code and a tentative code were published in the *American Journal of Nursing* but were not formally adopted. The *Code for Professional Nurses* was formally adopted by the ANA House of Delegates in 1950. It was amended and revised five more times until, in 2001, after 5 years' work, the ANA House of Delegates adopted the *Code of Ethics for Nurses with Interpretive Statements.*

Shortly after the first ANA code was adopted in the United States, the first known international code of ethics for nursing was developed by the International Council of Nurses (ICN) and was adopted in Canada in 1954 (Canadian Nurses Association [CNA], 2008). Since that time, the *ICN Code of Ethics for Nurses* has undergone various reviews with the most recent revisions made in 2006 (ICN, 2010).

In 1980, the CNA developed the *CNA Code of Ethics: An Ethical Basis for Nursing in Canada.* This code of ethics was adopted in 1985 as the *Code of Ethics for Nursing.* It was revised and updated four more times by 2008 and was retitled *Code of Ethics for Registered Nurses* (CNA, 2008).

ETHICAL DECISION MAKING

Ethical decision making is that component of ethics that focuses on the process of how ethical decisions are made. It involves making decisions in an orderly process that considers ethical principles, client values and abilities, and professional obligations, and it occurs when health care professionals must make decisions about ethical issues and ethical dilemmas. **Ethical issues** are moral challenges facing the nursing profession. In community health nursing, one such challenge is how to prepare an adequate and competent workforce for the future. In contrast, **ethical dilemmas** are puzzling moral problems in which a person, group, or community can envision morally justified reasons for both taking and not taking a certain course of action. In community health nursing, an example of an ethical dilemma is how to allocate resources to two equally needy populations when the resources are sufficient to serve only one. Ethical decision-making frameworks help nurses think through these issues and dilemmas.

Ethical decision-making frameworks use problem-solving processes. They serve as guides to making sound ethical decisions that can be morally justified. Some of these many frameworks are discussed in this chapter.

A generic ethical decision-making framework is presented in Table 6-1, along with rationales. The steps of a generic ethics framework are often nonlinear, and, with one exception, they do not change substantially. Step 5 (the one exception) lists six approaches (utilitarianism, deontology, principlism, virtue ethics, ethic of care, feminist ethics) to the ethical decision-making process. These approaches are outlined throughout the chapter in the "How To" boxes.

ETHICS

Definition, Theories, and Principles

Ethics is a branch of philosophy that includes both a body of knowledge about the moral life and a process of reflection for determining what persons ought to do or be regarding this life. It addresses such questions as the following: How should I behave? What actions should I perform? What kind of person should I be? What are my obligations to myself and to fellow humans? Some of the general obligations that humans have as members of society follow:

- To not harm others
- To respect others
- To tell the truth
- To keep promises

Veracity is telling the truth, and it is a CHN's duty to tell the truth. Veracity promotes trust in the nurse–client therapeutic relationship. Sometimes, however, a situation arises in which it is necessary to tell a lie or break a promise since the consequences of telling the truth or keeping the promise may bring about more harm than good. For example, a CHN has promised a family that he or she will visit them at a certain time, but the CHN is delayed because of unexpected circumstances—one of the other families in the CHN's caseload is in a state of crisis, their adolescent child is suicidal, and community health nursing interventions are needed immediately. Most CHNs would agree that this is not a good time to keep the original promise. In this example, the CHN is morally justified in breaking a promise because more harm than good would be done if the promise were kept.

TABLE 6-1 Rationale for Steps of Ethical Decision-Making Framework

Steps	Rationale
1. Identify the ethical issues and dilemmas.	Persons cannot make sound ethical decisions if they cannot identify the ethical issues and dilemmas.
2. Place them within a meaningful context.	The historical, sociological, cultural, psychological, economic, political, communal, environmental, and demographic contexts affect the way ethical issues and dilemmas are formulated and justified.
3. Obtain all relevant facts.	Facts affect the way ethical issues and dilemmas are formulated and justified.
4. Reformulate ethical issues and dilemmas, if needed.	The initial ethical issues and dilemmas may need to be modified or changed on the basis of context and facts.
5. Consider appropriate approaches to actions or options (utilitarianism, deontology, principlism, virtue ethics, ethic of care, feminist ethics).	The nature of the ethical issues and dilemmas determines the specific ethical approaches used.
6. Make decisions and take action.	Professional persons cannot avoid choice and action in applied ethics.
7. Evaluate decisions and action.	Evaluation determines whether the ethical decision-making framework used resulted in morally justified actions related to the ethical issues and dilemmas.

The aforementioned example illustrates the following about ethical thinking:

- Ethical judgements are concerned with values. The goal of an ethical judgement is to choose that action or state of affairs that is good or right in the circumstances.
- Ethical judgements generally do not have the certainty of scientific judgements. For example, in community health nursing, CHNs initially assess a situation on the basis of the best available information and then choose the course of action that seems to provide the best ethical resolution to the issue.
- At times, the decision is based on outcomes or consequences. In this approach, called **consequentialism**, the right action is the one that produces the greatest amount of good or the least amount of harm in a given situation. **Utilitarianism** is a well-known consequentialist theory that appeals exclusively to outcomes or consequences in determining which choice to make. In utilitarianism, "the moral value of an action is determined by its overall benefit" (Chaloner, 2007, p. 43). It involves weighing morally significant outcomes or consequences regarding the overall maximizing of good and minimizing of harm for the greatest number of people.

In other scenarios, CHNs are faced with options that challenge fundamental beliefs. In such circumstances, the CHNs may conclude that the action is right or wrong in itself, regardless of the amount of good that might come from it. This is the position known as **deontology.** It is based on the premise that persons should always be treated as ends in themselves and never as mere means to the ends of others.

Health professionals have specific obligations that exist because of the practices and goals of the profession. These health care obligations can be interpreted in terms of a set of principles in bioethics, an approach called **principlism.** The *primary principles* are respect for autonomy, nonmaleficence, beneficence, and distributive justice, as shown in Box 6-2. These principles have dominated the development of the field of **bioethics,** "a general term for the kind of principled reasoning used by health care providers in making ethical decisions" (Oberle & Bouchal, 2009, p. 299). One of the best descriptions and fullest articulations of principlism is in the sixth edition of Beauchamp and Childress's *Principles of Biomedical Ethics* (2008). The principlism approach to ethical decision making in health care arose in response to life-and-death decision making in acute care settings, where the question to be resolved tended to concern a single localized issue such as the withdrawing or withholding of treatment (Holstein, 2001). In these circumstances, preserving and respecting a client's autonomy became the dominant issue.

Despite its success as a basis for analysis in bioethics, principlism has come under attack from a variety of quarters (e.g., Boylan, 2000; Callahan, 2000; Clouser & Gert, 1990; Walker, 2009), and there are grounds for the criticism. First, some people say the principles are too abstract to serve as guides for action. Second, the principles themselves can conflict in a given situation, and there is no independent basis for resolving the conflict. Third, some persons claim that effective ethical problem solving must be rooted in concrete, individual experiences. Fourth, ethical judgements are alleged to depend more on the judgement of sensitive persons than on the application of abstract principles. Fifth, principlists should explain why morality is so narrowly constrained.

BOX 6-2 Ethical Principles

Respect for autonomy. Based on human dignity and respect for individuals, autonomy requires that individuals be permitted to choose those actions and goals that fulfill their life plans unless those choices result in harm to another.

Nonmaleficence. According to ancient writings from Hippocrates, nonmaleficence requires that we do no harm. It is impossible to avoid harm entirely, but this principle requires that health care professionals act according to the standards of due care, always seeking to produce the least amount of harm possible.

Beneficence. This principle is complementary to nonmaleficence and requires that we do good. We are limited by time, place, and talents in the amount of good we can do. We have general obligations to perform those actions that maintain or enhance the dignity of other persons whenever those actions do not place an undue burden on health care providers. Health care professionals have special obligations of beneficence to clients.

Distributive justice. Distributive justice requires that there be a fair distribution of the benefits and burdens in society based on the needs and contributions of its members. This principle requires that, consistent with the dignity and worth of its members and within the limits imposed by its resources, a society must determine a minimal level of goods and services to be available to its members. For community and public health professionals, this principle takes on considerable importance.

How To... Apply the Utilitarian Ethics Decision Process*

1. Determine moral rules that are important to society and that are derived from the principle of utility.†
2. Identify the communities or populations that are affected or most affected by the moral rules.
3. Analyze viable alternatives for each proposed action based on the moral rules.
4. Determine the consequences or outcomes of each viable alternative on the communities or populations most affected by the decision.
5. Select the actions on the basis of the rules that produce the greatest amount of good or the least amount of harm for the communities or populations that are affected by the action.

*Note that the utilitarian ethics decision process is one of the approaches in step 5 of the generic ethical decision-making framework (see Table 6-1).

†Moral rules of action that produce the greatest good for the greatest number of communities or populations affected by or most affected by the rules.

How To... Apply the Deontological Ethics Decision Process*

1. Determine the moral rules (e.g., tell the truth) that serve as standards by which individuals can perform their moral obligations.
2. Examine personal motives for proposed actions to ensure that they are based on good intentions in accord with moral rules.
3. Determine whether the proposed actions can be generalized so that all persons in like situations are treated similarly.
4. Select the action that treats persons as ends in themselves and never as mere means to the ends of others.

*Note that the deontological ethics decision process is one of the approaches in step 5 of the generic ethical decision-making framework (see Table 6-1).

Autonomy is often emphasized in acute care settings, whereas beneficence and distributive justice are emphasized more in community health. For this reason, it is useful to consider other models for ethical decision making. Utilitarianism and deontology were developed from the Enlightenment's focus on universals, rationality, and isolated individuals. Each theory maintains that there is a universal first principle, the principle of utility for utilitarianism and the categorical imperative for deontology, that serves as a rational norm for our behaviour and allows us to calculate the rightness or wrongness of each individual action. According to both utilitarianism and deontology, as in classic liberalism, the individual is the special centre of moral concern (Steinbock, London, & Arras, 2008). Giving priority to individual rights and needs means that the "rights and dignity of the individual should never (or rarely) be sacrificed to the interests of the larger society" (Steinbock et al., 2008). The focus on individual rights leads to complications in the interpretation of distributive or social justice.

Distributive or *social justice* refers to the allocation of benefits and burdens to members of society. Benefit refers to basic needs, including material and social goods, liberties, rights, and entitlements. Some benefits of society are wealth, education, and public services. Among the burdens to be shared are such things as taxes, military service, and the location of incinerators and power plants. Justice requires that the distribution of benefits and burdens in a society be fair or equal. It is widely agreed that the distribution should be based on what one needs and deserves, but there is considerable disagreement as to what these terms mean. Three primary theories of distributive justice are defended today. They are the egalitarian, libertarian, and liberal democratic theories.

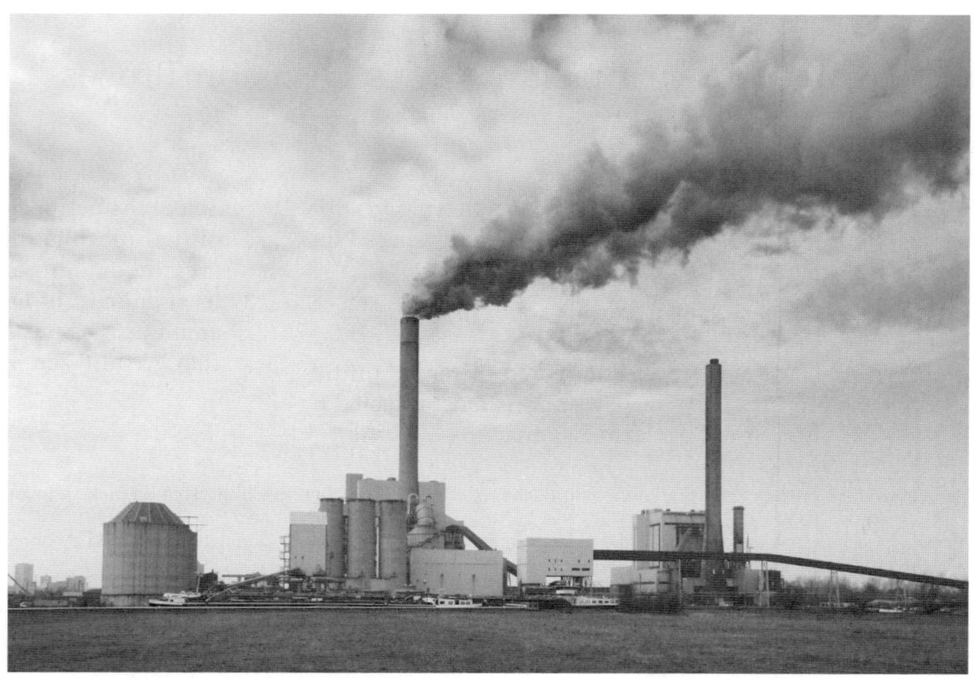

Distributive justice means that as a society, we share both benefits and burdens. Some shared benefits are wealth, education, and public services. Among the burdens to be shared, however, are such things as taxes, military service, and the location of incinerators and power plants.

How is it possible to apply the distributive justice principle to prenatal services? A CHN can face this interesting question when the target group is women with low educational levels who cannot afford health care visits or the time to attend them. This is a challenging issue considering that quality prenatal care can potentially reduce the rates of incidence of maternal mortality and morbidity (US Department of Health and Social Services and Centers for Disease Control and Prevention, 2008). Phillippi (2009) identified societal, maternal, and structural barriers to access to prenatal care. Suggestions for the reduction of structural barriers include the creation of child-friendly waiting and examining rooms. Maternal and societal barriers can be addressed through community education. The CHN could seize the opportunity to minimize the impact and ensure justice to this population.

Egalitarianism is the view that everyone is entitled to equal rights and equal treatment in society. Ideally, each individual has an equal share of the goods of society, and it is the role of government to ensure that this happens. The government has the authority to redistribute wealth if necessary to ensure equal treatment. Thus, egalitarians are supportive of *welfare rights*—that is, the right to receive certain social goods necessary to satisfy basic needs. These include adequate food, housing, education, police and fire protection (Anderson, Reimer-Kirkham, Khan, & Lynam, 2009), and the opportunity to acquire these things (Kayman & Ablorh-Odjidja, 2006). There are practical and theoretical weaknesses in egalitarianism. For example, it would be almost impossible to ensure the equal distribution of goods and services in any moderately complex society. But the distribution of material resources must be sufficient to ensure participants' independence and "voice" (Kirkham & Browne, 2006). Also, egalitarianism cannot provide an incentive for each of us to do our best because there is no promise of our merit being rewarded.

The *libertarian* view of justice says that the right to private property is the most important right. Libertarians recognize only *liberty rights,* the right to be left alone to accomplish our goals. Stubager (2008) notes that "libertarians . . . loathe social hierarchies and value instead the free and equal interaction of people without regard to social positions of any kind" (p. 329). Libertarians see a limited role for government, namely the protection of property rights of individual citizens through providing police and fire protection. Although they also agree that there is a need for jointly shared, publicly owned facilities such as roads, they reject the idea of welfare rights and view taxes to support the needs of others as coercive taking of their property. In addition, the libertarian position entails a basic respect for and tolerance of other people—including those who deviate from one's own norms or the norms of the society (Stubager, 2008).

Rawls (2001), discussing the *liberal democratic* theory, attempts to develop a theory that values both liberty and

How To... Apply the Principlism Ethics Decision Process*

1. Determine the ethical principles (respect for autonomy, nonmaleficence, beneficence, distributive justice) that are relevant to an ethical issue or dilemma.
2. Analyze the relevant principles within a meaningful context of accurate facts and other pertinent circumstances.
3. Act on the principle that provides, within the meaningful context, the strongest guide to action that can be morally justified by the tenets foundational to the principle.

*Note that the principlism ethics decision process is one of the approaches in step 5 of the general ethical decision-making framework (see Table 6-1).

equality. He acknowledges that inequities are inevitable in society, but he tries to justify them by establishing a system in which everyone benefits, especially the least advantaged. This is an attempt to address the inequalities that result from birth, natural endowments, and historical circumstances. Imagining what he calls a "veil of ignorance" (Rawls, 2001, p. 15) to keep us unaware of our actual advantages and disadvantages, Rawls would have us choose the basic principles of justice. Once impartiality is guaranteed, Rawls (2001) maintains that all rational people will choose a system of justice containing the following two basic principles:

> *Each person has the same indefeasible claim to a fully adequate scheme of equal basic liberties, which scheme is compatible with the same scheme of liberties for all; and social and economic inequalities are to satisfy two conditions: first, they are to be attached to offices and positions open to all under conditions of fair equality of opportunity; and second, they are to be to the greatest benefit of the least advantaged members of society (the difference principle).* (p. 42)

As the veil-of-ignorance device and the justice principles indicate, Rawls and other justice theorists all assume the Enlightenment concept of isolated selves in competition for scarce resources. The significance of justice, then, becomes the assurance of fairness to individuals. In justice as fairness, the original position of equality corresponds to the state of nature in the traditional theory of the social contract (Rawls, 1999, p. 11). Violating the dictates of distributive justice is an offence to the dignity of the collective preferences of autonomous, rational moral agents. The interests of the community may be in conflict with the interests of individuals; yet, confined to the Enlightenment ideal, the needs of society are not directly addressed, nor is society given any priority. This Enlightenment assumption has been challenged recently by a number of ethical theories loosely grouped together under the heading *communitarianism.* **Communitarianism** maintains that abstract, universal principles are not an adequate basis for moral decision making; instead, these theorists argue, history, tradition, and concrete moral communities should be the basis of moral thinking and action (Solomon, 1993). Among the theories with a communitarian focus are virtue ethics, the ethic of care, and feminist ethics.

Justice considerations play prominent roles in community health work. According to the CNA (2008), "justice includes respecting the rights of others, distributing resources fairly, and preserving and promoting the common good (the good of the community)" (p. 26). Kass (2005), while describing principles of public health, highlights the importance of fairness in decision procedures and in balancing benefits and burdens. Stone and Parham (2007) describe the principle of justice as building on and functioning with the principle of equal and substantial respect. "Justice informs how to show such respect and how to respond when people are disrespected" (Stone & Parham, 2007, p. 356). For example, justice arises regarding equitable or fair dealing or treatment or equitable opportunity for participation and input.

To effect equity, which refers to fairness or justice, CHNs need to assure equity in access to health care and equity in health outcomes (Pauly, MacKinnon, & Varcoe, 2009). For example, people who are street-involved, either homeless or drug users, often delay or do not access health care for a variety of complex and multifaceted reasons, including concerns about stigma related to drug use and homelessness. In this case, attention is required in addressing the stigma and discrimination experienced by those who are disadvantaged.

There should be some emphasis on terminology used to describe concepts that can be misleading. The definition of **equity** in health care refers to "the fulfillment of each individual's needs as well as the individual's opportunity to reach full potential as a human being" (CNA, 2006, p.14). **Equality** is also an important concept and refers to equal rights under the law, such as security, voting rights, freedom of speech and assembly, and the extent of property rights. However, it also includes access to education, health care, and other social goods such as economic good and fundamental political rights (Easley & Allen, 2007). It includes equal opportunities and obligations and involves the whole society. *Egalitarianism* is closely related to the concept of equality, that all people ought to be treated equally. In order to respect these elements, it becomes important for the CHN to ensure that the assessment leads to the fair distribution of resources without compromising the access and opportunities for the targeted group to benefit from it.

Social justice refers to "the fair distribution of society's benefits and responsibilities and their consequences. It focuses on the relative position of one social group in relation to others in society as well as on the root causes of disparities and what can be done to eliminate them" (CNA, 2006, p. 7). The issue of social justice is a concern for public health. A social justice framework can be useful in addressing the vulnerabilities of people; this framework has the potential to engage all community players. The Canadian Strategy on HIV/AIDS is based on the belief that social justice should guide the development of all Canadian public policy across all jurisdictions—equity, fairness, and inclusion of all Canadians—reflecting broad determinants of health and the broadest definition of health. The guiding principles for a social justice approach are (1) an integrative approach, (2) an approach that operates across the determinants of health, (3) a rights-based approach that respects, promotes, and fulfills rights, and (4) an approach that presents a lens of social inclusion for policy design, program development, and evaluation (Public Health Agency of Canada, 2006).

Virtue Ethics

Virtue ethics, one of the oldest ethical theories, dates back to the ancient Greek philosophers Plato and Aristotle. It is not concerned with actions, as utilitarianism and deontology are, but instead asks, What kind of person should I be? The goal of virtue ethics is to enable persons to flourish as human beings. According to Aristotle, **virtues** are acquired, excellent traits of character that dispose humans to act in accord with their natural good. During the seventeenth and eighteenth centuries, the Greek concept of the good as a principle of explanation went out of favour. Because virtue ethics was closely tied to the concept of the good, interest in virtues as an element of normative ethics also declined. Examples of virtues include benevolence, compassion, discernment, trustworthiness, integrity, and conscientiousness (Beauchamp & Childress, 2008). The appeal to virtues results in a significantly different approach to moral decision making in health care (Fletcher, 1999). In contrast to moral justification via theories or principles, the emphasis is on practical reasoning applied to character development.

Caring and the Ethic of Care

Another ethical theory, referred to as caring or the ethic of care, is based on feminist theory. Caring in nursing, the ethic of care, and feminist ethics are all interrelated, and, historically, all converged between the mid-1980s and early 1990s. Nurses have written about caring as the essence of or the moral ideal of nursing (Leininger, 1984; Watson, 1985). This view was a response to the technological advances in health care science and to the desire of nurses to differentiate nursing practice from medical practice. The ethic of care is a core value of community health nursing.

Carol Gilligan and Nel Noddings are considered to be among the developers of the ethic of care (Volbrecht, 2002). Gilligan's moral orientation toward care and responsibility distinguishes the moral agency of women from men (Storch, Rodney, & Starmzomski, 2004). Her work can easily be used in community health nursing. In fact, Gilligan (1982) describes a personal journey where, by listening and talking to people, she began to notice two distinct voices about morality and two ways of describing the interpersonal relationships between self and others. Contrary to what has been written about Gilligan and the two distinct voices (i.e., male and female) related to moral judgement, here is what she actually wrote (Gilligan, 1982):

> *The different voice I describe is characterized* not by gender *[emphasis added] but theme. Its association with women is an empirical observation, and it is primarily through women's voices that I trace its development. But this association is not absolute, and the contrasts between male and female voices are presented here to highlight a distinction between two modes of thought and to focus [on] a problem of interpretation rather than to represent a generalization about either sex.* (p. 2)

Her 1982 book is based on three qualitative studies about conceptions of morality and self and about experiences of conflict and choice. From these studies, she formulated her basic premises about responsibility, care, and relationships.

These premises, in Gilligan's (1982) own voice, are as follows:

1. "Sensitivity to the needs of others and the assumption of responsibility for taking care lead women to attend to voices other than their own." (p. 16)
2. "Women not only define themselves in a context of human relationships but also judge themselves in terms of their ability to care." (p. 17)
3. "The truths of relationship, however, return in the rediscovery of connection, in the realization that self and other are interdependent and that life, however valuable in itself, can only be sustained by care in relationships." (p. 127)

Noddings's (1984) personal journey started at a point different from that of Gilligan. Noddings noticed that ethics was described in the literature primarily using principles and logic. The goal for Noddings's book, therefore, was to express a feminine view that could be accepted or rejected by women *and* men.

How To... Apply the Virtue Ethics Decision Process*

1. Identify communities that are relevant to the ethical dilemmas or issues.
2. Identify moral considerations that arise from a communal perspective and apply the considerations to specific communities.
3. Identify and apply virtues that facilitate a communal perspective.
4. Modify moral considerations as needed to apply to the specific ethical dilemmas or issues.
5. Seek ethical community support to enhance character development.
6. Evaluate and modify the individual or community character traits that impede communal living.

*Note that the virtue ethics decision process is one of the approaches in step 5 of the generic ethical decision-making framework (see Table 6-1).
SOURCE: Modified from Volbrecht, R. M. (2002). *Nursing ethics: Communities in dialogue*. Upper Saddle River, NJ: Prentice Hall, p. 138.

How To... Apply the Ethic of Care Decision Process*

1. Recognize that caring is a moral imperative.
2. Identify personally lived caring experiences as a basis for relating to self and others.
3. Assume responsibility and obligation to promote and enhance caring in relationships.

*Note that the ethic of care decision process is one of the approaches in step 5 of the generic ethical decision-making framework (see Table 6-1).

The basic premises of Noddings's book (1984), in her own voice, are as follows:

1. "The essential elements of caring are located in the relation between the one caring and the cared-for." (p. 9)
2. "Caring requires me to respond . . . with an act of commitment: I commit myself either to overt action on behalf of the cared-for or I commit myself to thinking about what I might do." (p. 81)
3. "We are not 'justified'—we are *obligated*—to do what is required to maintain and enhance caring." (p. 95)
4. "Caring itself and the ethical ideal that strives to maintain and enhance it guide us in moral decisions and conduct." (p. 105)

What both Gilligan and Noddings have in common has been called a **feminine ethic**—a belief in the morality of responsibility in relationships that emphasize connection and caring. To them, caring is not a mere nicety but a moral imperative. Nevertheless, a long-term healthy debate has surrounded their premises.

Feminist Ethics

Recently, the beliefs of feminist ethics have begun to be seen as relevant to CHNs. Leipert (2001) notes that a feminist perspective supports critical thinking and a focus on such issues as gender, power, and socioeconomic status. Clearly, these issues affect health and the work of CHNs. Defining the terms *feminists* and *feminist ethics* is helpful. **Feminists** are women *and* men who hold a world view advocating economic, social, and political statuses for women that are equivalent to those of men. Consequently, feminists reject the devaluing of women and their experiences through systematic oppression based on gender. According to Volbrecht (2002), "a feminist is also someone who works to bring about the social changes necessary to promote more just relationships among women and men" (p. 160). Feminists also can support the ethic of care. They think that the oppression of women is morally wrong.

The study of **feminist ethics** entails knowledge about and critique of classical ethical theories developed by men as well as ethical theories developed by women. The study also entails knowledge about the social, cultural, political, economic, environmental, and professional contexts that insidiously and overtly oppress women as individuals or within a family, group, community, or society.

The idea of feminist bioethics exposes the fact that the tradition does not view women's rights as human rights; thus, a "feminist ethic would always be only a partial ethics" (Rawlinson, 2001, p. 406). Rawlinson (2001) recommends that a feminist bioethics pay attention to sexual difference—the body and material forms of life—and advances a political and ethical program that focuses not on the equality of rights, but on women's rights. This approach will consider women's experience (Mackenzie, 2007) and women's bodies to articulate those civil rights identified through access to universality. In fact, it is a way to approach human rights, for the CHN needs to identify structural injustices that are masked by dominating (even paternalistic) approaches; reorganize social conditions to promote the autonomy, health, and well-being of peoples across diverse cultures and traditions; and ultimately remove barriers that interfere with women's

How To... Apply the Feminist Ethics Decision Process*

1. Identify the social, cultural, political, economic, environmental, and professional contexts that contribute to the identified problem (e.g., under-representation of women in clinical trials).
2. Evaluate how the preceding contexts contribute to the oppression of women.
3. Consider how women's lives are defined by their status in subordinate social groups.
4. Analyze how social practices marginalize women.
5. Plan ways to restructure those social practices that oppress women.
6. Implement the plan.
7. Evaluate the plan and restructure it as needed.

* Note that the feminist ethics decision process is one of the approaches in step 5 of the generic ethical decision-making framework (see Table 6-1).

Source: Modified from Volbrecht, R. M. (2002). *Nursing ethics: Communities in dialogue*. Upper Saddle River, NJ: Prentice Hall, p. 219.

CRITICAL VIEW

1. What are some ethical issues in reference to the determinants of health?
2. a) What ethical issues need to be considered when working with local community-based groups?

   b) What ethical issues need to be considered when working with populations?

full participation in their local network. This work should always consider the preservation of the universal dimension of human rights without neglecting the contribution local groups or networks can make to overcoming oppressive conditions (Donchin, 2003).

Community health nursing uses a broader, population-focused approach to concentrate on specific groups of people regardless of geographical locations instead of focusing mainly on providing care to individuals and families. This approach requires skill in interpreting epidemiological data, in partnering with groups to resolve problems, and in being aware of the environment's effect on health (Meagher-Stewart, Aston, Edwards, Young, & Smith, 2007).

It is important to understand that this approach could cause challenges for the CHN, particularly when the care of the individual is still highly valued but the individual's active participation is being influenced by factors that are not under the CHN's control. The focus of the broader population approach will certainly change the CHN role by recognizing the fact that this approach uses predisposing enabling and reinforcing factors within a given population to develop strategies designed to minimize behaviours associated with health risk and prevent the re-emergence of these behaviours (Radzyminski, 2007).

An example of this approach using a broader population health model could be one that follows the assessment of children with repeated bronchitis, considers why the children contract the disease in spite of treatment, and asks what contributes to the large number of children who contract the disease repeatedly. The ethical decision-making frameworks could certainly provide a relevant framework to understand not only the challenges but the approach in focusing on the population rather than the individual.

NURSING CODE OF ETHICS

As noted earlier in this chapter under "History of Nursing and Ethics," Canadian nurses have adopted the CNA *Code of Ethics for Registered Nurses* (CNA, 2008). The CNA, a national nursing body, links with all provincial and territorial associations representing nurses. This national organization works with these affiliated associations in developing standards of nursing practice, education, and ethical conduct (Keatings & Smith, 2010). The CNA code "can assist nurses in practising ethically and working through ethical challenges that arise in their practice with individuals, families, communities and public health systems" (p. 1). Specific purposes of the *Code of Ethics for Registered Nurses* are listed as follows (CNA, 2008):

- Provides guidance for ethical relationships, responsibilities, behaviours, and decision making
- Serves as a means for self-evaluation and self-reflection for ethical nursing practice
- Provides a basis for peer feedback and review
- Serves as an ethical basis from which nurses can advocate for quality work environments that support the delivery of safe, compassionate, competent, and ethical care
- Informs other health care professionals and members of the public about the ethical commitments of nurses
- Upholds the responsibilities nurses accept as being part of a self-regulating profession

- Concerns the social responsibility of the professionals who are accountable to society and to communities and implies an understanding of these foundations (Slomka, Quill, DesVignes-Kendrick, & Lloyd, 2008).

These purposes are reflected in the seven primary values of the code. Refer to the CNA Weblink to access the *Code of Ethics for Registered Nurses* listed in the Evolve Weblinks. For each of the primary values, the CNA has identified responsibility statements for nurses pertaining to ethical considerations.

NURSING CODE OF ETHICS AND COMMUNITY HEALTH NURSING

In nursing practice, CHNs are required to uphold the values identified in the CNA *Code of Ethics for Registered Nurses.* For CHNs, the client includes the individual, group or family, aggregates, community, populations, or society. CHNs are often faced with unique situations of ethical conflict that challenge such nursing values as choice; **confidentiality,** which means that nurses are obligated to not disclose specific client information; and **accountability,** which means nurses act in a manner consistent with their professional responsibilities and standards of practice (CNA, 2008). Oberle and Tenove (2000) explored ethical issues in public health nursing with a group of Canadian public health nurses working in rural and urban settings and identified some strategies to support ethical nursing practice. See the "Evidence-Informed Practice" box on this page for further information.

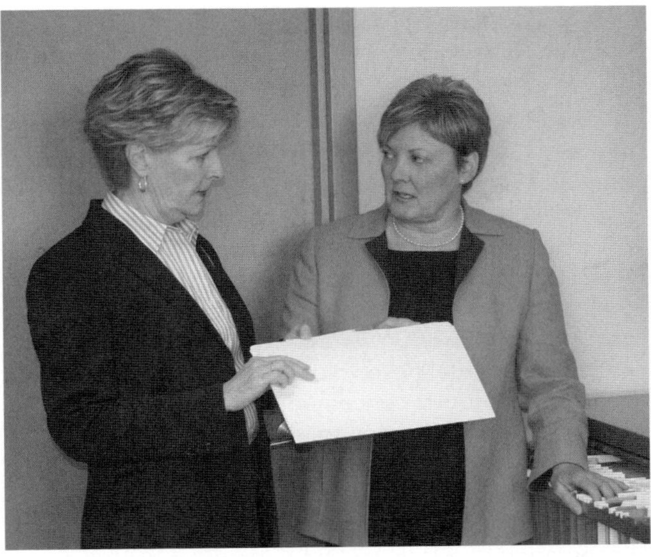

Confidentiality is one of the primary nursing values listed in the CNA code of ethics.

The *Canadian Community Health Nursing Standards of Practice,* discussed in Chapter 1 and found in Appendix 1, must also be followed in ethical, legal, and professional

Evidence-Informed Practice

The purpose of this Canadian study was to identify recurring ethical problems faced by community health nurses (CHNs), specifically public health nurses. The design was an exploratory qualitative study in which 22 nurses who were deemed by supervisors to be reflective and articulate regarding ethical problems were interviewed. The CHNs worked in public health nursing centres in both urban (n=11) and rural (n=11) settings. The interviews, which were basically unstructured, were tape-recorded and lasted from 30 minutes to 2 hours. The tape recordings were transcribed and then analyzed.

The analyses resulted in five interrelated themes: "relationships with health care professionals; systems issues; character of relationships; respect for persons; and putting self at risk" (Oberle & Tenove, 2000, p. 425). Each of the five themes had two or three subthemes related to ethical problems in public health nursing. Examples of subtheme ethical problems were perceived inequities in power, unacceptable practice, inequitable resource allocation, conflict between ethics and law, inadequate systems support for nursing, conflicts between individual and community rights, conflicts between nurses' and clients' values, and conflicts between service to clients and physical danger to self.

Application for CHNs: This study concluded that ethics permeated every aspect of public health nursing.

Questions for Reflection & Discussion

1. Are more ethical concerns likely to arise for CHNs working in rural versus urban communities? Support your thinking with an example.
2. Have you observed or experienced ethical problems as listed in the subthemes outlined in the study findings? Explain.

Reference: Oberle, K., & Tenove, S. (2000). Ethical issues in public health nursing. *Nursing Ethics, 7*(5), 425.

Evidence-Informed Practice

A case study analysis was used in this Toronto, Ontario, teen survey* to explore ethical issues related to conducting adolescent sexual health research in identifying access barriers and facilitators to their use of community services health resources. One of the ethical issues was regarding parental consent. In fact, the authors had the following concerns about parental consent: that it was unwarranted, unjust, and confusing and could silence those voices that most need to be heard. Other topics concerned safeguarding youth by paying more attention to issues of confidentiality and anonymity and ensuring youth-friendly processes, protocols, and consent procedures. In addition to suggesting that institutional review boards should be encouraged to adopt context-dependent strategies that address unique vulnerabilities of the adolescent, the authors state that "attention to flexibility, vulnerability, and community-specific needs is necessary to ensure appropriate ethical research practices that attend to the health and well-being of young people" (Flicker & Guta, 2008, p. 3).

Application for CHNs: CHNs need to be sensitive to ethical issues related to adolescent health research to avoid inadvertent harm. This case study analysis provides some strategies for CHNs to use to encourage adolescent participation in sexual research. It also highlights legal and ethical areas in public health that CHNs may find useful in evidence-informed clinical practice.

Questions for Reflection & Discussion

1. What are some examples of specific ethical situations with which CHNs, specifically involved with the research team, might be confronted?
2. Refer to the CNA Weblink *Code of Ethics for Registered Nurses* listed in the Evolve Weblinks. With regard to the primary nursing values, outline the CHN's specific responsibilities in relation to the conducting of research projects with adolescents.

REFERENCE: Flicker, S., & Guta, A. (2008). Ethical approaches to adolescent participation in sexual health research. *Journal of Adolescent Health, 42*, 3–10.

*Further information on the Toronto teen survey can be found at the Canadian Institute of Health Research Weblink on the Evolve Web site.

LEVELS OF PREVENTION

Related to Ethics

PRIMARY PREVENTION

Community health nurses (CHNs) use the CNA *Code of Ethics for Registered Nurses* to guide their nursing practice.

SECONDARY PREVENTION

If CHNs do not behave in accordance with *the Code of Ethics for Registered Nurses* (e.g., a CHN speaks in a way that does not communicate respect for a client), then the CHN needs to take steps to correct his or her behaviour. The CHN could explain the error to the client and apologize. It is important to reflect on ways to change this unethical behaviour.

TERTIARY PREVENTION

If a CHN has treated a client or staff member in a way that is inconsistent with ethics practices, reflection on this praxis and seeking guidance on other choices that could be made are the actions that need to be taken.

nursing practice situations. These standards outline the expectations for CHNs about the knowledge, skills, values, and decision making required for community health nursing practice. Additionally, CHNs need to consider factors that affect the health status of clients such as the determinants of health. These factors are outlined in Chapter 1 of this book.

The code of ethics and the community health nursing standards provide guidance to the CHN; assist the CHN in identifying ethical problems, issues, and dilemmas; and contribute to professional conduct. Should the code and standards not be followed, ethical distress, professional misconduct, or legal ramifications would be likely to result.

ADVOCACY AND ETHICS

Definitions, Codes, and Standards

Advocacy is a powerful ethical concept in community health nursing. But what does *advocacy* mean? Christoffel (2000) offers two definitions that are useful since they seem to differentiate between nursing in community health and public health nursing. The following definition related to community health nursing seems appropriate: "*Advocacy* is the application of information and resources (including finances, effort, and votes) to effect systemic changes that shape the way people in a community live" (p. 722). In contrast, "*public health advocacy* is advocacy that is intended to reduce death or disability in groups of people. . . . Such advocacy involves the use of information and resources to reduce the occurrence or severity of public health problems" (pp. 722–723). The former definition is intended to address the quality of life of individuals in a community, whereas the latter is intended to address the quality of life for aggregates or populations. Thus, both definitions have an ethical basis grounded in quality of life. Advocacy is addressed in the CNA *Code of Ethics for Registered Nurses* (CNA, 2008) as well as in the *Canadian Community Health Nursing Standards of Practice* (Community Health Nurses Association of Canada [CHNAC], 2003 [Revised 2008]).

According to the CNA code of ethics, advocacy is a nursing responsibility, and according to Hogan (2008), a new body of literature emphasizes the importance of advocacy ethics in informing public health nursing practice (Cohen & Reutter, 2007). This notion is reflected in the responsibility statements for the primary values of health and well-being, informed decision making, dignity, privacy and confidentiality, and justice (see the Canadian Nurses Association Weblink in the Evolve Weblinks). For example, under the nursing value of preserving dignity, the code states, "When a person receiving care is terminally ill or dying, nurses foster comfort, alleviate suffering, advocate for adequate relief of discomfort and pain and support a dignified and peaceful death" (CNA, 2008, p. 14). For the nursing value of privacy and confidentiality, the code maintains that nurses advocate for persons in their care to receive access to their own health care records through a timely and affordable process when such access is requested. In addition, nurses respect policies that protect and preserve people's privacy, including safeguards in information technology. Under the nursing value of justice, the code states that nurses should "advocate for fair treatment and for fair distribution of resources for those in their care" (CNA, 2008, p. 17). Encompassed in the nursing value of health and well-being is the notion that nurses use and advocate for the use of the least restrictive measure possible for those in their care when a community health intervention interferes with the individual rights of persons receiving care.

Finally, for the nursing value of informed decision making, "nurses advocate for persons in their care if they believe that the health of those persons is being compromised by factors beyond their control, including the decision-making of others" (CNA, 2008, p. 11).

Similarly, the *Community Health Nursing Standards of Practice* lists advocacy as part of the CHN's role. This document states that CHNs need to "use supportive and empowering strategies to move individuals and communities toward maximum autonomy" (CHNAC, 2003 [Revised 2008], p. 12); that they need to support individuals, families, communities, and populations to develop

NT SINAI HOSPITAL
MEDICIN
HOSPITAL EMERGENCY
Staff shortages put your health at risk

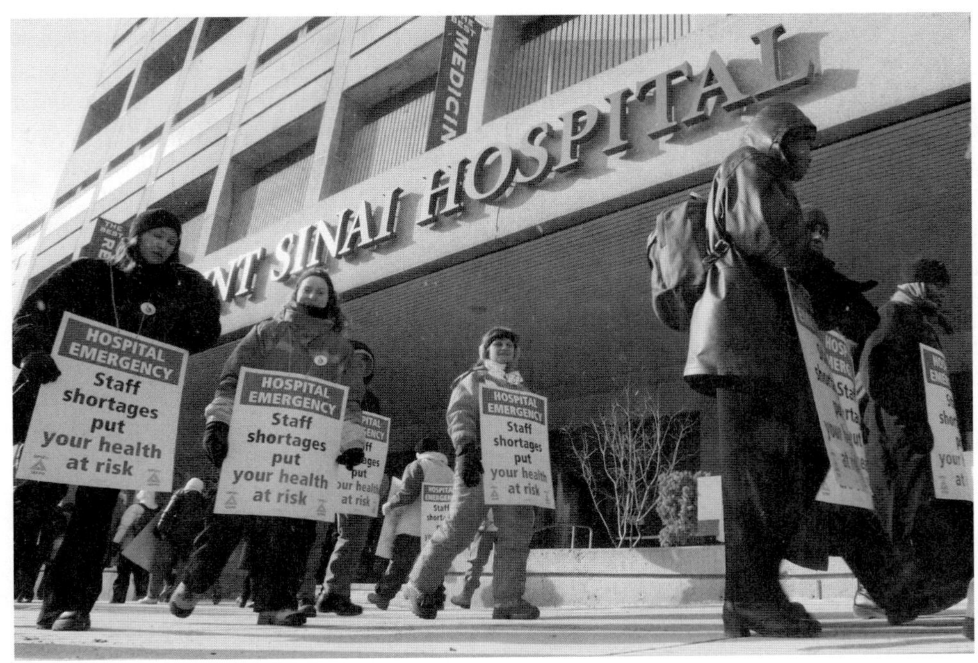

Advocacy is a responsibility of all nurses. Ontario nurses are shown here, protesting against staff shortages that they fear will put patient health and safety at risk.

the skills necessary to advocate for themselves; and that they need to support communities' efforts to change policies to improve health. Furthermore, it states that the CHN also "advocates for healthy public policy by participating in legislative and policymaking activities that influence health determinants and access to services" (CHNAC, 2003 [Revised 2008], p. 14). (See the Canadian Nurses Association and International Council of Nurses Weblinks on the Evolve Web site for further information on codes of ethics, and the Community Health Nurses of Canada site for incorporation of the codes into community health nursing practice. For an example of a code of ethics developed by a health care agency, refer to the VON Canada Weblink on the Evolve Web site).

Conceptual Framework for Advocacy

Hogan (2008), in addressing the public health nurses' needs, puts forward the fact that these nurses should be aware of their ethical responsibilities related to advocacy. "Advocacy ethics is perhaps an area of public health nursing training and education including familiarity with frameworks for advocacy" (p. 36) such as the conceptual framework identified by Christoffel (2000) or the practical approach to advocacy suggested by Bateman (2000).

Christoffel (2000) identifies the following three stages of her conceptual framework for advocacy:

1. *Information stage,* which focuses on gathering data about public health problems, including such factors as extent of the problem, patterns of frequency, and effectiveness of and barriers to public health programs
2. *Strategy stage,* which focuses on such tactics as disseminating the gathered information and policy statements to lay and professional audiences, identifying objectives, building and funding coalitions, and working with legislators
3. *Action stage,* which focuses on implementing the strategies through such tactics as lobbying, testifying, issuing press releases, passing laws, and voting

Some of the principles that underlie this framework include scientific integrity in data gathering and dissemination, respect for persons (i.e., lay and professional audiences), honesty regarding fundraising, truthfulness in lobbying and testifying, and justice in passing laws.

Practical Framework for Advocacy

Bateman (2000) takes a practical approach to advocacy. He places the advocate's core skills (i.e., interviewing, assertiveness and force, negotiation, self-management, legal knowledge and research, and litigation) within the context of six ethical principles for effective advocacy, as shown in Box 6-3. Although his focus is on the individual, it can also apply to groups and communities.

BOX 6-3 Ethical Principles for Effective Advocacy

1. Act in the client's (group's, community's) best interests.
2. Act in accordance with the client's (group's, community's) wishes and instructions.
3. Keep the client (group, community) properly informed.
4. Carry out instructions with diligence and competence.
5. Act impartially and offer frank, independent advice.
6. Maintain client confidentiality.

SOURCE: Adapted from Bateman, N. (2000). *Advocacy skills for health and social care professionals.* Philadelphia, PA: Jessica Kingsley, p. 63.

Regarding the first ethical principle, Bateman (2000) is sensitive to the ethical conflict between clients' best interests and the best interests of groups, communities, and societies but does not elaborate on this conflict. The second ethical principle works in tandem with the first principle and puts the client in charge. For example, the CHN might state, "This is what I think we can do. What do you want me to do?" (Bateman, 2000, p. 51). Of course, the advocate can refuse the request if self or others may be harmed. By following the third ethical principle, the client is empowered to make knowledgeable decisions. The fourth ethical principle addresses standards of practice. The fifth addresses fairness and respect for persons (nursing in community health is more collaborative in nature than independent). The last ethical principle, confidentiality, ensures that information will be shared only on a need-to-know basis.

PRINCIPLES FOR THE JUSTIFICATION OF PUBLIC HEALTH INTERVENTION

According to Upshur (2002), the following principles are relevant to ethical deliberation in public health: the Harm Principle, the Principle of Least Restrictive Means, the Reciprocity Principle, and the Transparency Principle.

The Harm Principle is a foundational principle for ethics. It sets out the justification to take action to restrict the liberty of an individual or a group in order to prevent harm to others. The Principle of Least Restrictive Means recognizes that a variety of means exist to achieve public health needs, but the full authority and power should be used for exceptional circumstances; education, facilitation, and discussion should precede any restriction or coercive measures. The Reciprocity Principle holds that society must be prepared to facilitate individuals and communities in their efforts to discharge their duties. The Transparency Principle refers to the manner and context in which decisions are made (Upshur, 2002).

CRITICAL VIEW

The following case from Upshur (2002) encompasses mainly the Harm Principle.

The health department is called to investigate community concerns regarding chemicals leaching into the water table. An epidemiological investigation fails to show any linkage of the exposure to health outcomes, but the community persists in its belief of adverse health effects.

1. As a CHN, how would you address the harm principle and respect the need for transparency and reciprocity in order to facilitate health promotion and competent care values?

STUDENT EXPERIENCE

1. To access the CNA *Code of Ethics and Social Justice* (2008), go to the CNA Weblink listed in the Evolve Weblinks.
2. Read through the documents and familiarize yourself with the attributes and framework of social justice in addition to the nursing values and ethical responsibilities.
3. Answer the following questions using this scenario:

   Mr. Smith is an 85-year-old man who resides on the eighth floor in an older adults' apartment building. His spouse passed away 4 months ago and he has no other family. He has had many falls over the last 3 weeks, resulting in severe leg and hip pain that has prevented him from attending church or socializing with his friends. He is experiencing urinary incontinence and is having difficulty managing his own personal care. He is unable to complete household tasks and has lost 12 pounds since his wife died. He has a diagnosis of chronic obstructive pulmonary disease (COPD) and hypertension and is having difficulty taking his medications on schedule. You are the CHN assigned to Mr. Smith.

   a) How would you apply an ethical model of your choice for reflection and decision making in this situation for Mr. Smith?

   b) How would you apply the social justice decision tree model in the Smith situation?

REMEMBER THIS!

- Nursing has a rich heritage of ethics and morality, beginning with Florence Nightingale.
- During the late 1960s, the field of bioethics began to emerge and influence nursing.
- Ethical decision making is the component of ethics that focuses on the process of how ethical decisions are made.
- Many different ethical decision-making frameworks exist; however, underlying each is the problem-solving process.
- Ethical decision making applies to all approaches to ethics: utilitarianism, deontology, principlism, virtue ethics, the ethic of care, and feminist ethics.
- Classic ethical theories are utilitarianism and deontology.
- Principlism consists of respect for autonomy, nonmaleficence, beneficence, and distributive justice.
- Other approaches to ethics include virtue ethics, the ethic of care, and feminist ethics.
- CHNs in Canada are required to uphold the values identified in the CNA *Code of Ethics for Registered Nurses.*
- Advocacy is the application of information and resources to effect systemic changes that shape the way people in a community live (Christoffel, 2000).
- The *Code of Ethics for Registered Nurses* and *the Canadian Community Health Nursing Standards of Practice* both address advocacy as a nursing responsibility.

REFLECTIVE PRAXIS

Case Study 1

Jeff, a community health nurse, was preparing to visit Chris, a 59-year-old client recently diagnosed as having emphysema. Chris, who was unemployed because of a farming accident several years earlier, was well known to the community care agency. Hypertensive and overweight, he was also a heavy, long-term cigarette smoker despite his decreased lung function. Jeff visited Chris to find out why the client had missed his latest chest clinic appointment. He also wanted to determine if the client was continuing his medications as ordered.

As Jeff parked his car in front of his client's house, he could see Chris sitting on the front porch smoking a cigarette. A flash of anger made him wonder why he continued trying to teach Chris reasons for not smoking and why he took the time from his busy home care schedule to follow up on Chris's missed clinic appointments. This client certainly did not seem to care enough about his own health to give up smoking.

During the home visit, Jeff determined that Chris had discontinued the use of his prophylactic antibiotic and was not taking his expectorant and bronchodilator medication on a regular basis. Chris's blood pressure was 210/114 mm Hg, and he coughed almost continuously. Although he listened politely to Jeff's concerns about his respiratory function and the continued use of his medications, Chris simply made no effort to take responsibility for his health care. Even so, another clinic appointment was made, and Jeff encouraged the client to attend.

As he drove to his next home visit, Jeff wondered to what extent he was obligated as a nurse to spend time with clients who took no personal responsibility for their health. He also wondered if there was a limit to the amount of nursing care a noncooperative client could expect from a service provided in the community.

1. What are Jeff's professional responsibilities for Chris's rights to health care?
2. What authority defines the moral requirements and moral limits of nursing care to clients?

Adapted from Fry, S. T., & Veatch, R. M. (2006). *Case studies in nursing ethics* (3rd ed.). Toronto, ON: Jones and Bartlett.

Answers are on the Evolve Web site at http://evolve.elsevier.com/Canada/Stanhope/community/.

Case Study 2*

Because finding affordable housing was difficult, 26-year-old Terri lived with her 6-month-old son, Tommy, and her common-law husband, Billy, in one room of her landlord's own house. Terri was morbidly obese and diagnosed with bipolar disease; Billy had served time for drug dealing and was out on parole and staying straight. Neither had finished high school. Billy's past drug use

*Written by Deborah C. Conway and adapted by the Canadian authors.

had rendered him unable to do much manual labour because of heart damage, but on occasion he would work at construction to support the family.

Jim, a CHN, had received a referral on Tommy when he was diagnosed with failure to thrive 2 months earlier. Terri, who had had two children removed from her custody by family services (child protective services) in the past, and Billy seemed to adore their baby, so much so that Terri would hold the baby all day long. In the past 2 months, the CHN had taught Terri about infant nutrition and encouraged her to attend the Healthy Babies program in her community, and now Tommy had increased his rate of physical growth and was above 5% of the growth percentile. Yet, he was not meeting his gross motor milestones per the Nipissing District Developmental Screen tool. Jim thought that Tommy was not allowed to play on the floor enough to progress in sitting, pushing his shoulders up, and crawling. Most of their small room was taken up with the bed and the boxes that stored their belongings. There was not really space for "tummy time" or play. When not in the room, the family would take the bus to a discount store and spend the day walking around to get a change of scene.

One week, Terri told Jim she was not taking her medications for bipolar disease any more because they caused her to gain weight. The next week, she confided that Billy had had a "dirty" urine specimen check and would have to return to prison in the near future. The following week, Jim found the family living in a rundown motel since they had been evicted by their landlord after a disagreement. Terri was very agitated. She confided to Jim that they had $100 left, Billy was going to have to return to prison that week, and the motel bill was already $240. Terri knew she would be homeless soon without the support of Billy but refused to talk with her social worker about her needs. She asked Jim not to tell anyone about her situation because she was afraid that family services would take Tommy from her, as they had her other children. It was clear to Jim that he might not know where Tommy was after the family left this motel.

1. What are some of the ethical dilemmas with which the CHN is confronted in this case?
2. How would you apply the four primary ethical principles to this case?

Answers are on the Evolve Web site at http://evolve.elsevier.com/Canada/Stanhope/community/.

Case Study 3

Ralph, a recently widowed man in his mid-60s, was discharged from the hospital after exploratory surgery that disclosed colon cancer with metastases to the lymph nodes. His physician referred him to a home health agency for nursing care follow-up. In reading the referral, the CHN learned that Ralph had been living with a married daughter and her family since his wife's death. An unmarried daughter apparently lived nearby, visiting him regularly and helping with his daily care. The referral did not explain what, if anything, the client had been told by his physician concerning his condition.

During the first home visit, it became apparent that Ralph did not know that the tumour removed from his body had been diagnosed as cancerous or that it had metastasized to the lymph nodes. He did not realize the seriousness of his condition, but he did express concern about his health. He complained of vague pain in the abdomen, asked for information about the results of the tests performed before discharge from the hospital, and wanted to know how soon he would be able to return to his work as a cabinetmaker. When the CHN avoided a direct answer to these questions, Ralph asked directly, "Is everything all right?" The married daughter, who was present when her father asked these questions, assured him that everything was all right and that he would soon be up and around.

Walking the CHN to her car when the visit was over, the married daughter confided that it was the family's wish that their father not be told of the seriousness of his condition. She said that her mother's recent death had been very difficult for him to accept. They did not want him to be further burdened with the knowledge of his condition. The CHN listened, acknowledging the difficulties posed by the wife's recent death and the father's serious condition. She told the daughter, however, that it would be difficult, if not impossible, for anyone from her agency to continue to provide nursing care to Ralph without his knowledge of his condition.

When she returned to her office, the CHN discussed Ralph's situation with her supervisor. The CHN did not want to continue visiting the client, knowing he was being deceived by the physician and family. The supervisor suggested that she consult with the attending physician as soon as possible and explain that Ralph was asking questions about his condition. Luckily, the CHN was able to reach the physician before it was time to make the next home visit. She asked the physician what the client had been told about his condition. The physician said that, at the family's request, Ralph had not been told that he had cancer. He said he agreed with the family that Ralph could probably not withstand the anxiety of knowing he had a terminal illness so soon after his wife's death. The physician also expressed concern about Ralph's daughters, who, as he put it, "need a little time to accept the mother's death, as well as the impending death of the old man." The physician said that he would consider any act of disclosure on the CHN's part at this time to be inappropriate to her role as a visiting nurse and inconsistent with the well-being of the client and his family.

1. What is the professional duty of veracity?
2. What reasons might the CHN give for telling Ralph the truth?
3. Which of the values from the *Code of Ethics for Registered Nurses* would apply to this case? Provide your rationale for the identified values.

Adapted from Fry, S. T., & Veatch, R. M. (2006). *Case studies in nursing ethics.* Philadelphia, PA: Lippincott.

Answers are on the Evolve Web site at http://evolve.elsevier.com/Canada/Stanhope/community/.

Case Study 4

In October 2005, the news media in Canada focused on the evacuation of Aboriginal people from the community of Kashechewan, a Cree First Nations community of about 1,900 people located near the western shore of James Bay on the Albany River in Northern Ontario. The measure was essential because the community's water supply was tainted and had become a serious health threat. Prior to the evacuation, high levels of *Escherichia coli* were found in the reserve's drinking water, requiring that chlorine levels be increased to "shock" levels, which, in turn, caused an increase in common skin problems such as scabies and impetigo. Part of the problem was that an intake pipe for the community's water treatment plant was downstream from the sewage lagoon. This resulted in many boil-water orders and eventually the evacuation.

This community was not just facing problems with water quality, however. The tainted water drew attention to the living conditions on the reserve: deteriorating and inadequate housing and community services, as well as repeated spring flooding requiring multiple evacuations since 2004 at the public's expense. The conditions inspired public debate over the quality of life for the members of the Kashechewan First Nations community and the need to relocate to a safer location.

An Ontario agency organizing the October 2005 evacuation from the Cree reserve searched for communities to take in the displaced people. Many were taken to surrounding northern communities such as Sudbury, Cochrane, and Timmins. Another 250 were flown to Ottawa. The Kashechewan people remained away for a month while the Canadian military installed water purification systems that supplied up to 50,000 L of clean water per day; also, building materials were shipped in for housing reconstruction. However, spring flooding in April 2006 necessitated yet another evacuation. As part of a longer-term solution, the federal government offered to move the community to a better area a short distance from its current location. However, the Kashechewan people wished to relocate within their traditional lands. The government signed an agreement with the First Nation on July 30, 2007, giving the reserve $200 million to improve and repair the infrastructure of the existing community, including housing and flood control services.

This scenario is an example of a situation that CHNs might face while working in remote communities.

1. Identify two ethical dilemmas presented by this population health crisis and describe the potential involvement of CHNs in this situation.
2. What do you think of the quality of life of residents who were evacuated and relocated in different communities? (Reflect on the residents' beliefs and values that make up their personal value system.)
3. How should the Aboriginal culture have been considered in relocating the residents from the community of Kashechewan?
4. Which aspects of the CNA code of ethics might apply to this situation, especially considering the health concerns of the Aboriginal population (e.g., diseases of the respiratory system, which accounted for 18.8% and 11.6% of all hospital separations for First Nations males and females, respectively, in 1997, and injuries and poisonings, which accounted for 17.7% and 9.3% of all hospital separations for First Nations males and females, respectively, in 1997 [Health Canada, 2005])?
5. Which of the CHNC standards could be employed to help empower the community of Kashechewan to deal with this crisis?

Answers are on the Evolve Web site at http://evolve.elsevier.com/Canada/Stanhope/community/.

What Would You Do?

1. A 90-year-old Caucasian woman refuses to have her community health nursing care provided by an African Canadian CHN. Should the community agency assign a CHN from another racial group to care for the client, or should the client be transferred to another community health agency? What is the most ethical approach to take?

SOURCES: Brennan, R. (2007). Ottawa to rebuild troubled reserve. *The Toronto Star,* July 30. Retrieved from http://www.thestar.com/News/article/241308; Government of Canada. (2005). *Progress on Kashechewan action plan.* Retrieved from http://www.ainc-inac.gc.ca/ai/mr/nr/s-d2005/2-02730-eng.asp; McGuire, A. (2006, April 24). Flooding forces evacuation of Kashechewan First Nation. *Ottawa Citizen,* p. A1; CBC News.(2006). *Kashechewan: Water crisis in Northern Ontario.* Retrieved from http://www.cbc.ca/news/background/aboriginals/kashechewan.html; and Health Canada. (2005). *Statistical profile on the health of First Nations in Canada.* Retrieved from http://www.hc-sc.gc.ca/fniah-spnia/intro-eng.php.

2. Suppose public-opinion surveys about professional aid in dying suggested that 50 to 75% of adults favour allowing health care professionals to assist the suicide of those who are terminally ill. Nurses, however, are ethically and legally prohibited from assisting the suicide of anyone and from participating in acts of euthanasia. What should a CHN do when a terminally ill and suffering client asks the CHN to help him die? Provide your rationale based on the CNA code of ethics.

TOOL BOX evolve

The Tool Box contains useful instruments that can be applied in community health nursing practice. These related resources are found either in the appendices at the back of this book or on the Evolve Web site at http://evolve.elsevier.com/Canada/Stanhope/community/.

Appendices

- Appendix 1: Canadian Community Health Nursing Standards of Practice

Tools

University of Toronto Joint Centre for Bioethics. *Community Ethics Toolkit.*

The *Community Ethics Toolkit* was created to facilitate the broader implementation of a common approach for ethical decision making across the community health and support sector. The toolkit consists of a code of ethics for the community health and support sector; a decision-making worksheet; guidelines for using the decision-making worksheet; guidelines for conducting case reviews; and additional resources.

WEBLINKS evolve

Direct links to these resources can be found on the text's accompanying Evolve Web site at http://evolve.elsevier.com/Canada/Stanhope/community.

Canadian Institute of Health Research. *From Research to Action: KTE and the Toronto Teen Survey.* This Web site describes the findings about youth sexual issues and discusses the plans for future community strategies to improve adolescent health outcomes.

Canadian Nurses Association. This comprehensive Web site contains a wealth of material relevant to Canadian nursing, including the CNA code of ethics. Click on "Nursing Practice" and go to "Nursing Ethics" to find the 2008 *Code of Ethics for Registered Nurses.* To access information on social justice, at the CNA homepage, search social justice. Choose Social Justice . . . A Means to an End, an End in Itself.

Canadian Nurses Protective Society (CNPS). The CNPS offers legal liability protection related to nursing practice to eligible registered nurses, by providing information, education, and financial and legal assistance.

Community Health Nurses of Canada. This Web site contains a great deal of information on community health nursing.

International Council of Nurses. The ICN represents nurses through their national health professional associations; this site provides information on global nursing issues. When you go to the site, enter the term "code of ethics" in the search box.

NursingEthics.ca. This Web site—administered by Chris MacDonald, PhD, president of the Canadian Society for the Study of Practical Ethics—contains links to books and Web-based ethics resources.

The Provincial Health Ethics Network (PHEN) of Alberta. PHEN is a nonprofit organization that provides resources on addressing ethical issues related to health. PHEN does not advocate for or take positions on particular ethical issues; its role is to facilitate thoughtful, informed, and reasoned ethical decision making from all perspectives.

Victorian Order of Nurses. This is a general Web site for this not-for-profit, national health care organization. Click on "About VON" and select "Code of Ethics" in the menu.

REFERENCES

American Nurses Association. (2001). *Code of ethics for nurses with interpretive statements.* Washington, DC: American Nurses Publishing.

Anderson, J. M., Rodney, P., Reimer-Kirkham, S., Browne, A., Khan, K., & Lynam, J. (2009, October/December). Inequities in health and healthcare viewed through the ethical lens of critical social justice: Contextual knowledge for the global priorities ahead. *Advances in Nursing Science, 32*(4), 282–294.

Bateman, N. (2000). *Advocacy skills for health and social care professionals.* Philadelphia, PA: Jessica Kingsley.

Beauchamp, T. L., & Childress, J. F. (2008). *Principles of biomedical ethics* (6th ed.). New York, NY: Oxford University Press.

Bernheim, R. G., & Melnick, A. (2008). Principled leadership in public health: Integrating ethics into practice and management. *Journal of Public Health Management, 14*(4), 348–366.

Boylan, M. (2000). Interview with Edmund D. Pellegrino. In M. Boylan (Ed.), *Medical ethics: Basic ethics in action.* Upper Saddle River, NJ: Prentice Hall.

Brennan, R. (2007). Ottawa to rebuild troubled reserve. *The Toronto Star*, July 30. Retrieved from http://www.thestar.com/News/article/241308.

Callahan, D. (2000). Universalism and particularism fighting to a draw. *Hastings Center Report, 30*(1), 37.

Canadian Nurses Association. (2006). *Social justice.* Retrieved from http://www.cna-aiic.ca/CNA/documents/pdf/publications/Social_Justice_e.pdf.

Canadian Nurses Association. (2008). *Code of ethics for registered nurses.* Retrieved from http://www.cna-aiic.ca/CNA/documents/pdf/publications/Code_of_Ethics_2008_e.pdf.

CBC News. (2006). *Kashechewan: Water crisis in Northern Ontario.* Retrieved from http://www.cbc.ca/news/background/aboriginals/kashechewan.html.

Chaloner, C. (2007). An introduction to ethics in nursing. *Nursing Standard, 21*(32), 42–45.

Christoffel, K. K. (2000). Public health advocacy: Process and product. *American Journal of Public Health, 90*(5), 722–723.

Clouser, K. D., & Gert, B. (1990). A critique of principlism. *Journal of Medicine and Philosophy, 15*, 219.

Cohen, B. E., & Reutter, L. (2007). Development of the role of public health nurses in addressing child and family poverty: A framework for action. *Journal of Advanced Nursing, 60*(1), 96–107.

Community Health Nurses Association of Canada. (2003). *Canadian community health nursing standards of practice.* [Revised 2008]. Retrieved from http://www.chnc.ca/documents/chn_standards_of_practice:mar08_english.pdf.

Donchin, A. (2003). Converging concerns: Feminist bioethics, development theory, and human rights. *Journal of Women in Culture and Society, 29*(2), 299–324.

Easley, C. E., & Allen, C. A. (2007). A critical intersection: Human rights, public health nursing, and nursing ethics. *Advances in Nursing Practice, 30*(4), 367–382.

Fletcher, J. J. (1999). Virtues, moral decisions, and healthcare. *Nursing Connections, 12*(4), 26–32.

Flicker, S., & Guta, A. (2008). Ethical approaches to adolescent participation in sexual health research. *Journal of Adolescent Health, 42*, 3–10.

Fry, S. T., & Veatch, R. M. (2006). *Case studies in nursing ethics.* (3rd ed.). Toronto, ON: Jones and Bartlett.

Gilligan, C. (1982). *In a different voice: Psychological theory and women's development.* Cambridge, MA: Harvard University Press.

Government of Canada. (2005). *Progress on Kashechewan action plan.* Retrieved from http://www.ainc-inac.gc.ca/ai/mr/nr/s-d2005/2-02730-eng.asp.

Health Canada. (2005). *Statistical profile on the health of First Nations in Canada.* Retrieved from http://www.hc-sc.gc.ca/fniah-spnia/intro-eng.php.

Hogan, M. (2008). *Public health practice in Canada: A review of the literature.* Retrieved from http://www.chnc.ca/documents/Final_PHN_Lit_Review_May_26_2008.pdf.

Holstein, M. B. (2001). Bringing ethics home: A new look at ethics in the home and the community. In M. B. Holstein, & P. B. Mitzen (Eds.), *Ethics in community-based elder care.* New York, NY: Springer.

International Council of Nurses. (2010). *ICN code of ethics for nurses.* Retrieved from http://www.icn.ch/about-icn/code-of-ethics-for-nurses/.

Kass, N. E. (2005). An ethics framework for public health and avian influenza pandemic preparedness. *Yale Journal of Biology and Medicine, 78*, 235–250.

Kayman, H., & Ablorth-Odjidja, A. (2006). Revisiting public health preparedness: Incorporating social justice principles into pandemic preparedness planning for influenza. *Journal of Public Health and Management Practice, 12*(4), 373–380.

Keatings, M., & Smith, O. B. (2010). *Ethical and legal issues in Canadian nursing.* (3rd ed.). Toronto, ON: Mosby.

Kirkham, S. R., & Browne, A. (2006). Toward a critical theoretical interpretation of social justice discourses in nursing. *Advances in Nursing Science, 29*(4), 324–339.

Leininger, M. (Ed.), (1984). *Care: The essence of nursing and health.* Thorofare, NJ: Slack.

Leipert, B. D. (2001). Feminism and public health nursing: Partners for health. *Scholarly Inquiry for Nursing Practice, 15*(1), 49–61.

Mackenzie, C. (2007). Feminist bioethics and genetic termination. *Bioethics, 21*(9), 515–516.

McGuire, A. (2006, April 24). Flooding forces evacuation of Kashechewan First Nation. *Ottawa Citizen*, A1.

Meagher-Stewart, D., Aston, M. L., Edwards, N. C., Young, L., & Smith, D. (2007). Managements' perspective on Canadian public health nurses' primary health care practice. *Primary Health Care Research & Development, 8*, 170–182.

Noddings, N. (1984). *Caring: A feminine approach to ethics and moral education.* Berkeley, CA: University of California Press.

Oberle, K., & Bouchal, S. R. (2009). *Ethics in Canadian nursing practice: Navigating the journey.* Toronto, ON: Pearson-Prentice Hall.

Oberle, K., & Tenove, S. (2000). Ethical issues in public health nursing. *Nursing Ethics*, *7*(5), 425–439.

Pauly, B. M., MacKinnon, K., & Varcoe, C. (2009). Revisiting "who gets care?" Health equity as an arena for nursing action. *Advances in Nursing Practice*, *32*(2), 118–127.

Phillippi, J. C. (2009). Women's perceptions of access to prenatal care in the United States: A literature review. *Journal of Midwifery & Women's Health*, *54*(3), 219–225.

Public Health Agency of Canada. (2006). *Direction # 9: Move to a social justice framework*. Retrieved from http://www.phac-aspc.gc.ca/aids-sida/fi-if/direct/csha/29-eng.php.

Radzyminski, S. (2007). The concept of population health within the nursing profession. *Journal of Professional Nursing*, *23*(1), 37–46.

Rawlinson, M. C. (2001). The concept of a feminist bioethics. *Journal of Medicine and Philosophy*, *26*(4), 405–416.

Rawls, J. (1999). *A theory of justice (revised edition)*. Cambridge, MA: Harvard University Press.

Rawls, J. (2001). *Justice as fairness: A restatement* (E. Kelly, Ed.). Cambridge, MA: Harvard University Press.

Registered-nurse-canada. (2009). *The Nightingale Pledge*. Retrieved from http://www.registered-nurse-canada.com/nightingale_pledge.html.

Slomka, J., Quill, B., DesVignes-Kendrick, M., & Lloyd, L. (2008). Professionalism and ethics in the public health curriculum. *Public Health Reports*, *123*(Suppl. 2), 27–35.

Solomon, R. C. (1993). *Ethics: A short introduction*. Dubuque, IA: Brown & Benchmark.

Steinbock, B., London, J., & Arras, A. J. (2008). *Ethical issues in modern medicine*. Toronto, ON: McGraw-Hill.

Stone, J. R., & Parham, G. P. (2007). An ethical framework for community health workers and related institutions. *Family Community Health*, *30*(4), 351–363.

Storch, J. L., Rodney, P., & Starzomski, R. (2004). *Toward a moral horizon: Nursing ethics for leadership and practice*. Toronto, ON: Pearson Prentice-Hall.

Stubager, R. (2008). Education effects on authoritarian-libertarian values: A question of socialization. *British Journal of Sociology*, *59*(2), 327–350.

Upshur, R. E. G. (2002). Principles of the justification of public health intervention. *Canadian Journal of Public Health*, *93*(2), 101–103.

U.S. Department of Health and Social Services and Centers for Disease Control and Prevention. (2008). *Safe motherhood: Promoting health for women before, during, and after pregnancy*. Retrieved from http://www.cdc.gov/NCCDPHP/publications/aag/pdf/drh.pdf.

Volbrecht, R. M. (2002). *Nursing ethics: Communities in dialogue*. Upper Saddle River, NJ: Prentice Hall.

Walker, T. (2009). What principlism misses. *Journal of Medical Ethics*, *35*, 229–231.

Watson, J. (1985). *Nursing: Human science and human care*. Norwalk, CT: Appleton-Century-Crofts.

CHAPTER

7 Diversity

KEY TERMS

allophones 191
cultural awareness 202
cultural blindness 204
cultural competence 199
cultural interpretation 211
cultural knowledge 202
cultural nursing assessment 207
cultural safety 206
cultural skill 203
culture 187
culture shock 205
diversity 187
ethnicity 192
ethnocentrism 204
immigrant 210
interpretation 211
linguistic interpretation 211
multiculturalism 188
newcomer 210
person in need of protection 210
prejudice 205
race 192
racially visible 187
racism 205
refugee 210
stereotyping 205
translation 211
visible minority 187

See the Glossary on page 593 for definitions.

OBJECTIVES

After reading this chapter, you should be able to:

1. Describe demographic trends and immigration and refugee patterns that will affect future community health nursing in Canada.
2. Identify the ethnic composition of Canada.
3. Discuss the effect of diversity on community health nursing practice in Canada.
4. Identify how gender, culture, income, and social status as determinants affect health.
5. Explain how the concepts of macroscopic (upstream), microscopic (downstream), and the Ottawa Charter health promotion strategies related to diversity can be applied to community health nursing practice.
6. Describe some of the cultural group variations in Canada.
7. Explain cultural competence and its application to community health nursing.
8. Explain the concept of cultural safety and its application to community health nursing.
9. Evaluate the effects of cultural organizational factors on health and illness.
10. Conduct a cultural assessment of a person from a cultural group other than one's own.
11. Explain the difference between interpretation and translation and describe how to select and use an interpreter.
12. Within a cultural context, apply community health nursing interventions to promote positive health outcomes for community clients.

CHAPTER OUTLINE

The Canadian authors gratefully acknowledge the contribution of Catherine Aquino-Russell and Lisa Perley-Dutcher in this chapter pertaining to the Aboriginal peoples in Canada and Catherine Aquino-Russell for her contribution on Deaf culture and hard-of-hearing persons in Canada.

Canada is considered to be a multicultural nation and a nation of diversity. Increasingly, community health nurses (CHNs) in Canada care for culturally diverse groups, and more CHNs come from culturally diverse groups themselves. There are significant differences in beliefs about health and illness among various cultural groups, and CHNs want to practise in a manner that is respectful of their clients' beliefs when intervening to promote and maintain wellness. This chapter discusses Canada's ethnic mix, multiculturalism, culture, diversity, and strategies to enable CHNs to provide culturally competent and culturally safe care to clients. Within this chapter, Srivastava's (2007) definition of **culture** is used, that is, "a term that applies to all groups of people where there are common values and ways of thinking and acting that differ from those of another group" (p. 15). Within this broad definition of culture, examples of cultural groups are based on gender, sexual orientation, geographic location, physical and mental health challenges, religion, age, race, and ethnicity. Some of these groups are discussed in other chapters in this text and some are discussed in this chapter. For more extensive discussion on culture and diversity in health care, refer to additional resources.

The Canadian Nurses Association (CNA) position statement on promoting culturally competent care says that nurses require "knowledge, skill, attitudes and personal attributes" to provide culturally competent care and services to their clients (CNA, 2004, p. 1) (refer to the CNA Weblinks at the end of this chapter). In its broad definition of culture, "ethnicity, language, religion, and spiritual beliefs, gender, socio-economic class, age, sexual orientation, geographic origin, group history, education, upbringing and life experiences" are identified (CNA, 2004, p. 2). Appendix 1 presents the Community Health Nurses Association of Canada (CHNAC) Standards of Practice 1 through 5. In CHNAC Standard 1A, Health Promotion, various actions by CHNs are identified under the determinants of health, of which culture is one determinant, and in Standard 1C, Health Maintenance, Restoration, and Palliation, respect for client diversity and uniqueness is identified as part of providing culturally competent care. (Diversity and culturally competent care will be discussed later in this chapter.) CHNAC Standard 3, Building Relationships, states that CHNs in culturally relevant interactions need to be aware of and use culturally appropriate verbal, nonverbal, and written communication. And CHNAC Standard 4, Facilitating Access and Equity, outlines that the CHN, by providing culturally competent care, of which cultural sensitivity is a part, facilitates equitable access to services in the community (CHNAC, 2008).

Statistics Canada and the federal government of Canada use the term **visible minority** to describe people of colour, that is, people who are neither Aboriginal nor Caucasian. However, the term **racially visible** is becoming more popular since population projections indicate that "people of colour" will eventually make up the majority of the population in Canadian cities. Racially visible often includes Aboriginals (Canadian Policy Research Network [CPRN], 2006), although for statistical discussions the groups are sometimes separated. Srivastava (2007) identifies a limitation that occurs when the terms *visible minority* or *people of colour* are used: heterogeneous groups of non-Caucasian people are slotted into one category, which results in class and ethnic differences being concealed.

In this text, diversity in the broadest sense refers to the uniqueness of the client within the cultural context. Diversity focuses on client assets that build capacity. The two types of diversity are visible and invisible (Clair, Beatty, & MacLean, 2005). Visible diversity includes aspects such as age, physical appearance, and gender (Clair et al., 2005). With visible diversity, there is an increased risk of discrimination, stereotyping, and marginalization (Srivastava, 2007). Consideration needs to be given to groups that are regarded as invisibly diverse because differences such as religion, national origin, occupation, sexual orientation, and illness are not visible and therefore are not overt (Srivastava, 2007). Throughout this chapter, the two terms *visible minority* and *racially visible* will be used, as they are the terms used by Statistics Canada under the *Employment Equity Act*. **Diversity** in the cultural context includes consideration of similarities and differences. Therefore, in this text culture and diversity consider the similarities and differences of the client as part of a society, population, community, aggregate/group, and family and as an individual.

CRITICAL VIEW

1. a) What is the value of upstream thinking for CHNs?
   b) What is the relationship between using a macroscopic approach in community health nursing and upstream thinking?
2. What are some examples of interventions in community health nursing that are appropriate to culture as a determinant of health for the Ottawa Charter health promotion strategies of
   a) building healthy public policy,
   b) creating supportive environments,
   c) strengthening community action,
   d) developing personal skills, and
   e) reorienting health services?

IMMIGRATION TO CANADA 1900 TO PRESENT

Historically, patterns of immigration to Canada have varied throughout the years, with a mix of places of origin represented. Many immigrants have come from Europe, Asia, the United States, Africa, and the Caribbean. Frequently, reasons for leaving the country of origin have included persecution and war. Given Canada's diverse historical immigration background, it is not surprising that Canada has moved in the direction of **multiculturalism,** a belief that promotes the recognition of diversity of citizens with respect to their ancestry and supports acceptance and belonging (Government of Canada, 2006).

The varied ethnocultural composition of the country has often been compared to a rich tapestry or mosaic. Over time, the pattern of this tapestry has changed; there has been a shift from mainly European immigrants to an increasing number of visible minority groups, such as Chinese, South Asians, and Blacks (Astle & Pacquiao, 2006; Statistics Canada, 2010). (Refer to Figure 7-1.) Also, where immigrants choose to live is changing. Immigrants are showing a preference for metropolitan areas such as Toronto, Vancouver, and Montreal (Statistics Canada, 2010). These three cities are the most racially and culturally diverse in Canada. Canada has a history of admitting large numbers of immigrants of various ethnic origins. In 2009, Canada's immigration numbers were one of the highest for Canada since the early 1990s, with approximately 240,000 to 265,000 immigrants admitted as new permanent residents (Citizenship and Immigration Canada, 2008). For further information about immigration to Canada, see the Statistics Canada *Portraits of Immigrants in Canada* Weblink.

During the nineteenth century, as immigration to Canada progressed and the country became a federation, the need arose for a system that would provide the federal and provincial governments with an organized approach to immigration in this geographically vast nation. At the time of Confederation, under the *Constitution Act* of 1867, the federal and provincial governments agreed to share jurisdiction over immigration; however, if a conflict arose, federal law was to take precedence over provincial law.

The *Immigration Act* of 1906 provided criteria, such as insanity and crime-related behaviour, for the deportation of immigrants from Canada, should the need arise. The 1910 *Immigration Act* gave the government legal authority to prevent the landing of immigrants if they belonged to any race not desired in Canada. In 1950, the first Department of Canadian Citizenship and Immigration was created, and within 3 years a very extensive and new *Immigration Act* was passed in parliament, which identified people who would not be allowed into Canada and who could be deported. At this time, the Immigration Appeals Board was established, with the *Immigration Appeal Board Act* being passed in the House of Commons in 1967. The new *Immigration Act* of 1978 required consultation between the provinces and the government in planning immigration policies. In 1985, the Immigration Appeal Board membership increased due, in part, to the assumed role of hearing claims from refugees, which were increasing in numbers.

The *Constitution Act* of 1867 remained in place until 1991, when the province of Quebec, under the Canada–Quebec Accord of 1991, was granted sole decision-making authority about immigration to that province. Currently, Manitoba and British Columbia have negotiated similar agreements, and other provinces and territories are at various stages of negotiating immigration agreements with the federal government.

FIGURE 7-1 Percentage of Canada's Visible Minority Population in 2006 (including Canadian born*)

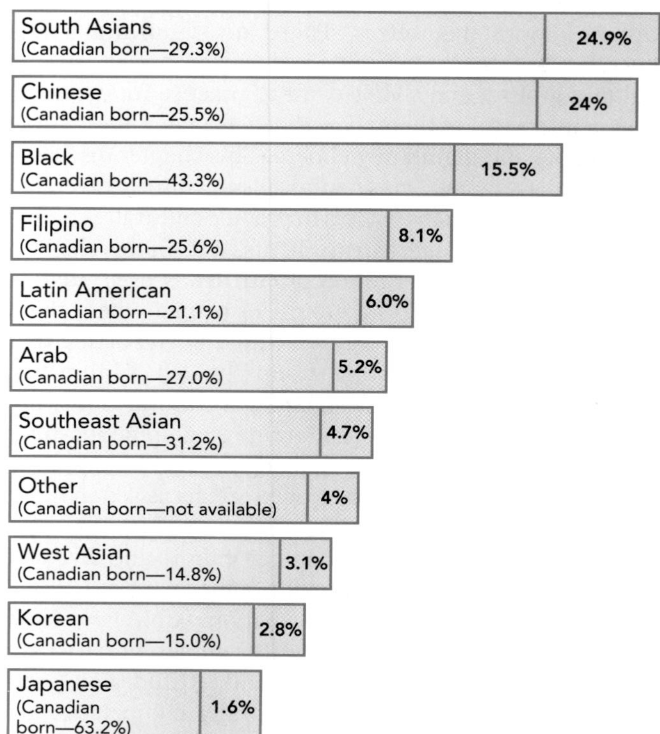

*"Canadian born" refers to the percentage of these population groups who were born in Canada, which can be explained by earlier immigration patterns.

Adapted from Statistics Canada. (2010). *Canada's ethnocultural mosaic, 2006 Census: National picture.* Retrieved from http://www12.statcan.ca/census-recensement/2006/as-sa/97-562/p6-eng.cfm.

CURRENT AND FUTURE CULTURAL PATTERNS IN CANADA

The Aboriginal peoples include North American Indian (68%), Métis (27%), and Inuit (5%), with the Inuit being the fastest-growing group (CPRN, 2006). The distribution of the most prominent cultural groups for Canada, provinces, and territories is outlined in Table 7-1.

In addition to knowledge of current cultural patterns, an awareness of population projections for the future is important for CHNs in order to plan for relevant programs that will meet the needs of the Canadian population. Such projections might be used, for example, to lend support for the continuation or expansion of existing programs or the development of new programs to improve the quality of nursing and client services. The face of Canada is changing rapidly, particularly in urban areas, mainly because of increased rates of non-European immigration in recent decades. Immigrants are making up an increasingly large proportion of the general population. This means that there are growing numbers of Canadians who do not speak English or French and whose religion is non-Christian. These facts affect how health care is delivered to large segments of the community and their ability to access health care.

Population projections are estimates of how the population will grow and change in the future. Based on Statistics Canada data, Belanger and Malenfant (2005) anticipate some important trends in Canadian demographics by the year 2017:

- One in five Canadians could be a visible minority person (i.e., belonging to the Chinese, South Asian, Black, Filipino, Latin American, Southeast Asian, Arab, West Asian, Japanese, or Korean groups).
- The visible minority population will have grown by 56 to 111% (depending on the projection scenario used) compared with only 1 to 7% for the rest of the population.
- Visible minorities will continue to gravitate to urban centres. Almost 95% of the racially visible population will live in census metropolitan areas—75% in Toronto, Montreal, and Vancouver alone.

Currently in Canada, South Asians and Chinese form the two largest racially visible groups, with each group having a population of over 1 million (Statistics Canada, 2010). In 2006, for the first time South Asians were the largest visible minority group (Statistics Canada, 2010). In 2017, they are expected to remain so and to make up nearly half of the total racially visible population in Canada. By 2017, Blacks and Filipinos are expected to be the third- and fourth-largest visible minority groups (Belanger & Malenfant, 2005). In fact, based on the 2006 census data, Blacks had already reached the third-largest group, and Filipinos had already reached the fourth-largest visible minority position (Statistics Canada, 2007a). Of all Canada's racially visible groups,

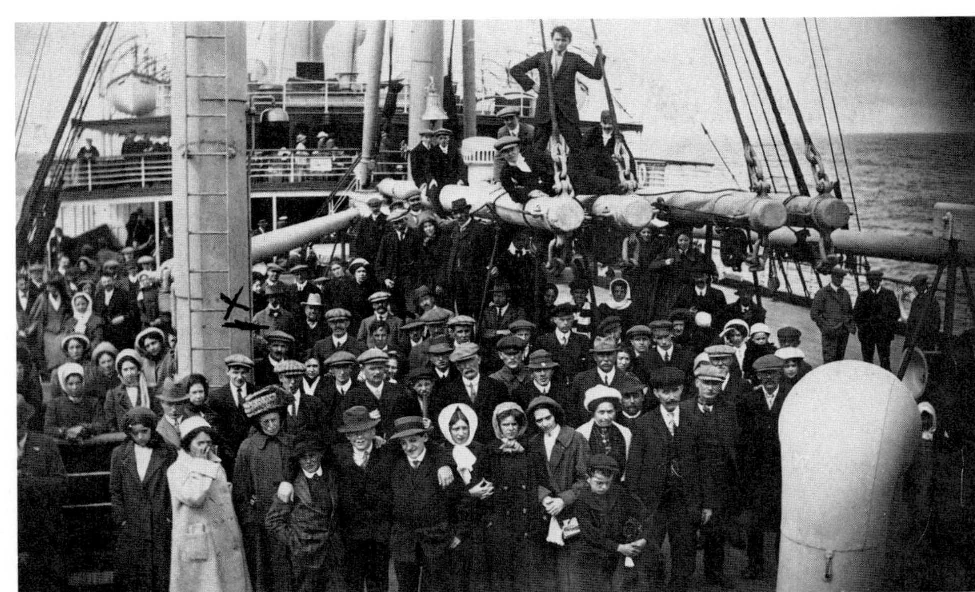

In the early 1900s, immigrants to Canada were mainly European in origin, as with the group shown here setting sail on the Empress of Ireland *in 1910. Today, however, most immigrants coming to Canada are from other parts of the world, especially Asia and Africa.*

TABLE 7-1 Population of Selected Prominent Cultural Groups, by Province and Territory

Group	Canada	BC	Alta.	Sask.	Man.	Ont.	Que.	Nfld.	PEI	NS	NB	YT	NWT	Nvt.
Canadian*	11,682,680	939,460	813,485	240,535	252,330	3,350,275	4,897,475	271,345	60,000	425,880	415,810	7655	7255	1175
French*	4,668,410	331,535	332,675	109,800	139,145	1,235,765	2,111,570	27,785	28,410	149,785	193,470	3815	3860	805
North American Indian	1,000,890	175,085	144,040	102,285	109,515	248,940	130,165	16,030	2360	28,560	23,815	6370	13,375	350
Métis	307,845	45,445	63,620	40,110	57,075	60,535	21,755	6120	245	4395	4955	570	2955	70
Inuit	—	—	—	—	—	—	—	7445	120	—	—	215	4140	22,625
Chinese	1,029,395	365,485	99,095	8,085	11,930	481,505	56,830	925	205	3290	1530	225	255	35
Black	662,210	25,465	31,390	4165	12,820	411,095	152,195	840	370	19,670	3850	115	170	65
Total visible minority population†	3,983,845	836,440	329,925	27,580	87,110	2,153,045	497,975	3850	1180	34,525	9425	1025	1545	210
Total population	29,639,035	3,868,870	2,941,150	963,150	1,103,695	11,285,550	7,125,580	508,075	133,385	897,570	719,710	28,520	37,105	26,665

*Not considered a "visible minority."

†Not all visible minorities are shown in this table. Although visible minority groups are heterogeneous, the data presented here are as available from Statistics Canada.

SOURCE: Adapted from Statistics Canada. (2009). *Population by selected ethnic origins, by province and territory (2006 census)*. Retrieved from http://www.40.statcan.ca/l01/cst01/demo26a.htm; Statistics Canada. (2009). *Visible minority population, by province and territory (2006 census)*. Retrieved from http://www.40.statcan.ca/l01/cst01/demo52a.htm.

CRITICAL VIEW

1. What are the implications of these population projections for community health nursing practice?

the West Asian, Korean, and Arab groups are increasing at the fastest rates, although their overall numbers are smaller than those of the Chinese or South Asians (CPRN, 2006). Due to high birth rates, the Aboriginal group is expected to increase at twice the rate of the rest of the population. Of the Aboriginal peoples, the Inuit are increasing fastest (CPRN, 2006), although, again, their numbers are comparatively small. See Table 7-2 for population projections for 2017. The projections provided in this table have implications for policy development and health care service delivery. CHNs need to be cognizant of changing patterns in their communities so that they can be proactive in their program planning. For example, if the community's growth reflects an increase in a cultural group that is susceptible to certain diseases, then the CHN would assess current services offered and work with the community to identify and fulfill program and service needs.

With regard to the provincial distribution of Canada's visible minority population, by 2017 the racially visible population is expected to make up 20% of the total population of British Columbia, 57% of Ontario, 8% of Alberta, and 11% of Quebec (Statistics Canada, 2005a). At that time, 77% of Canada's racially visible inhabitants will be located in Ontario and British Columbia. Aboriginal peoples are concentrated in the Prairie Provinces and the North. Currently, nearly 53% of Aboriginal peoples live in British Columbia, Alberta, and Ontario. By 2017, a slight shift is expected away from British Columbia and toward Alberta so that 51% will be living in Alberta, Ontario, and Manitoba, as well as a slight shift away from urban centres (27% in 2001 compared with 25% in 2017) and toward Indian reserves (48% in 2001 versus 57% in 2017) (Statistics Canada, 2005b). For further information on the profile of visible minorities in Canada, see the Statistics Canada Weblink on Canada's ethnocultural mosaic.

All these statistical projections have implications that will affect health care and CHNs. For example, racially visible people and Aboriginals will be, on average, much younger than the rest of the population in 2017 (see Table 7-3). The future composition of the population will also have an impact on cultural factors such as language and religion. For example, in 2001, 17% of Canadians were **allophones,** or people whose native language is other than French or English. By 2017, that is expected to rise to between 21 and 25% (CPRN, 2006). Similarly, 6.3% of Canadians belonged to a non-Christian religion in 2001, and that number is projected to rise to between 9.2 and 11.2% by 2017 (CPRN, 2006) (see Figures 7-2 and 7-3). CHNs who are aware of these trends will be better able to prepare themselves to deliver the best care possible to the clients in their community. Based on the identified trends, part of the CHNs' preparation would be to learn about and obtain the needed skills required to address the health care needs for the identified cultural groups.

CULTURE AS A DETERMINANT OF HEALTH

Health is influenced by the 12 determinants of health. According to the Public Health Agency of Canada (PHAC) and World Health Organization (WHO), culture is one of the determinants of health (PHAC, 2003; WHO, 2009). The "Determinants of Health" box on page 193 suggests that culture and other forms of diversity, including age, race, ethnicity, and access to health care,

TABLE 7-2 Racially Visible, Aboriginal, and Immigrant Populations as a Percentage of the Total Canadian Population

Group	2001 Census Data (% of general population)	Projections for 2017 (% of general population)	Increase (%)
Racially visible*	13	19–23	6–10
Aboriginals	3.4	4.1	0.7
Immigrants	18	22.2	4.2

*Refers to Chinese, South Asian, Black, Filipino, Latin American, Southeast Asian, Arab, West Asian, Japanese, and Korean groups and excludes Aboriginals.

SOURCE: Statistics Canada. (2005). *Population projections of visible minority groups, Canada, provinces and regions 2001-2017.* Retrieved from http://www.statcan.ca/english/freepub/91-541-XIE/91-541-XIE2005001.pdf; and Statistics Canada. (2005). *Projections of the Aboriginal populations, Canada, provinces and territories 2001 to 2017.* Retrieved from http://www.statcan.ca/english/freepub/91-547-XIE/91-547-XIE2005001.pdf.

TABLE 7-3 Projections for 2017: Median Age of Racially Visible and Aboriginal Groups and the Rest of Canada

Group	2017 Projections (median age in years)
Racially visible*	35.5
Canadian born	16.6
Born outside Canada	44.3
Rest of Canada†	43.3
Aboriginals	27.8
Rest of Canada‡	41.3

*Refers to Chinese, South Asian, Black, Filipino, Latin American, Southeast Asian, Arab, West Asian, Japanese, and Korean groups and excludes Aboriginals.
†Refers to all persons, including Aboriginals, but not persons included under racially visible.
‡Refers to all persons, including racially visible, but not Aboriginals.

SOURCE: Statistics Canada. (2005). *Population projections of visible minority groups, Canada, provinces and regions 2001–2017.* Retrieved from http://www.statcan.ca/english/freepub/91-541-XIE/91-541-XIE2005001.pdf; Statistics Canada. (2005). *Projections of the Aboriginal populations, Canada, provinces and territories 2001 to 2017.* Retrieved from http://www.statcan.ca/english/freepub/91-547-XIE/91-547-XIE2005001.pdf.

FIGURE 7-2 Canadians Who Speak a Language Other Than French or English (allophones), 2006 Census Data and Projections for 2017

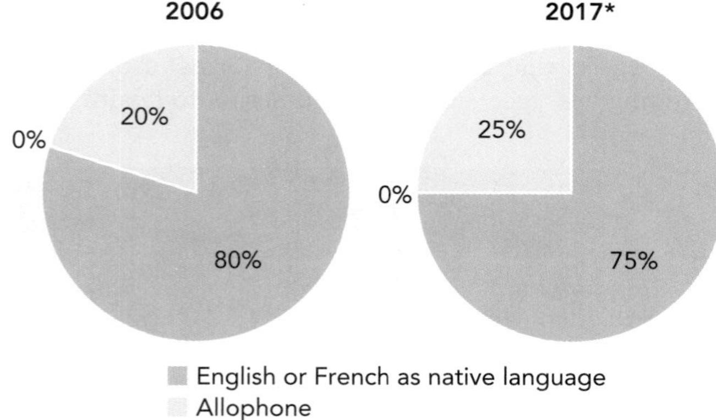

*Projected range is 21 to 25%.

Statistics Canada. (2005). *Population projections of visible minority groups, Canada, provinces and regions 2001–2017.* Retrieved from http://www.statcan.ca/english/freepub/91-541-XIE/91-541-XIE2005001.pdf; Statistics Canada. (2009). *2006 census: The evolving linguistic portrait, 2006 census: Sharp increase in population with a mother tongue other than English or French.* Retrieved from http://www.12.statcan.ca/census-recensement/2006/as-sa/97-555/p2-eng.cfm.

FIGURE 7-3 People Whose Religion is Non-Christian, 2001 Census Data and Projections for 2017

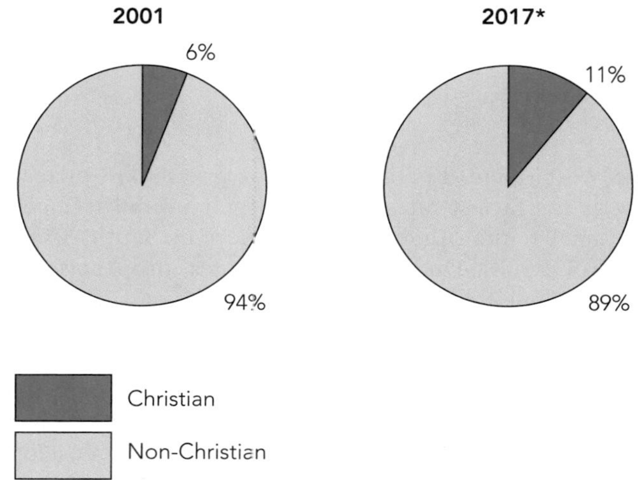

*Projected range is 9.2–11.2%.
Adapted from Statistics Canada. (2005). *Population projections of visible minority groups, Canada, provinces and regions 2001–2017.* Retrieved from http://www.statcan.ca/english/freepub/91-541-XIE/91-541-XIE2005001.pdf.

have an impact on the health of Canadians. These examples suggest some of the contributors to health disparities among diverse groups. CHNs need to recognize the importance of improving the determinants of health and therefore in their advocacy role to pressure governments to institute policies to reduce health inequities.

CULTURE AND CULTURAL GROUPS' VARIATIONS

The concepts of culture, race, and ethnicity influence our understanding of human behaviour. Culture provides direction as to the appropriate behaviours for situations in everyday life (Allender & Spradley, 2005). Race and ethnicity lead to the identification of distinguishable groups within cultures (Jarvis, 2004). However, these three terms are often used inaccurately.

Race is primarily a social classification that relies on physical characteristics such as skin colour to identify group membership (Maville & Huerta, 2008). Individuals may be of the same race but of different cultures. For example, Blacks—who may have been born in Africa, the Caribbean, North America, or elsewhere—are a heterogeneous group, but they are often (wrongly) viewed as culturally and racially homogeneous.

Ethnicity refers to cultural membership and is based on individuals sharing similar cultural patterns (e.g., beliefs, values, customs, behaviours, traditions) that, over time, create a common history that is resistant to change.

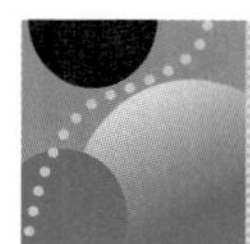

Determinants of Health
Culture and Diversity

- One in six Canadian adults has experienced racism (Ipsos-Reid, 2005). Racism is a form of social exclusion, one of the determinants of health (Hyman, 2009; Raphael, [in press]), and also contributes to lower socioeconomic status (WHO, 2007), another determinant of health.
- Visible minorities, when compared with Caucasians, are less likely to use preventive screening services such as mammogram, PAP tests, and PSA tests and are less likely to be admitted to hospital (Quan et al., 2006.)
- The use of health services among visible minorities varies. For example, Japanese and Korean people tend to visit family physicians less often than South Asians (Quan, et al., 2006).
- Children and families in Aboriginal communities have high rates of unintentional injuries and accidents, including deaths from drowning (Vollman, Anderson, & McFarlane, 2008).
- In 2005, recent-immigrant men earned 63 cents for every dollar earned by Canadian-born men, and recent-immigrant women earned 56 cents for every dollar earned by Canadian-born women (Statistics Canada, 2009a), thereby contributing to lower socioeconomic status.
- Almost 66% of Aboriginal children take part in sports regularly (about the same as Canadian children in general), with Métis and Inuit children being most involved (Statistics Canada, 2007b). First Nations children living off-reserve have higher rates of sports participation than those living on reserves, and parents of Aboriginal children participating in sports generally have higher levels of education and income than parents of nonparticipating children (Statistics Canada, 2007b).
- In 2006, 7.3% of the visible minority population in Canada was over 65 years of age, compared with 13.0% of the total population (Statistics Canada, 2009e), indicating that as a whole, the visible minority population is younger than the overall Canadian population.

Ethnicity represents the identifying characteristics of culture (e.g., race, religion, national origin). It is influenced by education, income level, geographical location, and association with individuals from ethnic groups other than one's own. Therefore, a reciprocal relationship exists between the individual and society. Some examples of ethnicity are African, Chinese, Greek, Irish, Italian, Ukrainian, and Vietnamese. Ethnicity has replaced the term *race* when assigning identity and describing culture (Srivastava, 2007).

CHNs who work with people from a variety of backgrounds would benefit from an understanding of and use of the concepts of culture, race, and ethnicity in their nursing practice. Awareness and understanding of these concepts assist the CHN to be more culturally sensitive about the variations and implications related to the terms used. CHNs also need to consider aspects of cultural safety, which will be discussed later in this chapter.

Srivastava (2007) states that the term *culture* is difficult and ambiguous. Although there are many definitions, Srivastava's definition of culture being "a term that applies to all groups of people where there are common values and ways of thinking and acting that differ from those of another group" (2007, p. 15) is a broad and inclusive definition. Srivastava describes culture using the acronym CULTURE, that is, C = commonly, U = understood, L = learned, T = traditions, U = unconscious, R = rules of, E = engagement.

According to Srivastava (2007), there are six characteristics shared by all cultures:

1. Culture is learned based on the events and experiences that we internalize as we grow and develop from infancy onward. We are not born with culture:
2. Culture is adaptive in that persons adjust to the environmental and technological changes occurring over time.
3. Culture is dynamic in that persons respond to changes. Culture is not static.
4. Culture is invisible and is evident only by rituals, language, celebrations, and attire. Culture is not visible.
5. Culture is shared in that persons from the same culture identify with the same values, beliefs, and patterns of behaviour, yet maintain individuality. Everyone is unique.
6. Culture is selective in that boundaries are identified for desirable, acceptable, or unacceptable behaviours; it also influences how people view and respond to situations and issues. Culture differentiates between outsiders and insiders.

CRITICAL VIEW

Reflect on the information provided in the "Determinants of Health" box and consider the following:

1. a) What other determinants of health might have relevance to culture?
   b) What are some of the cultural implications in reference to equity, social justice, inclusion and exclusion, health disparities, and empowerment?
2. As a CHN working with culturally diverse groups, how would you implement the health promotion strategies of strengthening community action, building healthy public policy, creating supportive environments, developing personal skills, and reorienting health services?

CHNs need to be aware of the possible cultural variations and acquire the skills to work comfortably and effectively with persons from diverse cultural groups. This awareness is a recognition of the uniqueness of various cultures and not a focus on cultural differences. When CHNs approach clients equitably, they are practising nursing with awareness and an underlying belief that respects the uniqueness and variations based on culture. To enhance CHNs' awareness, information on some of the prevalent cultural groups in Canada, that is, the Chinese, First Nations, and South Asians, is briefly discussed. Further information on Chinese and South Asian cultural groups can be found at the Statistics Canada *Canada's Ethnocultural Mosaic, 2006 Census: Findings* Weblink. The Government of Canada Weblink *Aboriginal Canada Portal* provides online resources and information on government programs and services about First Nations, Métis, and Inuit. See also Box 7-1, which discusses another type of cultural diversity.

BOX 7-1 Enhancing Understanding of Deaf Culture and of Hard-of-Hearing Persons in Canada

One population of persons that is often *not* thought of when considering cultural diversity is the Deaf. Many people with deafness (living with no sound) may consider themselves belonging to a Deaf culture, sharing unique values, norms, and sign language (McCreary Stebnicki & Coeling, 1999; Padden, 2000). In addition to persons from the Deaf culture, many others experience hearing loss of varying degrees, affecting their ability to communicate with others, including health care providers. Community health nurses (CHNs) need to be aware of this cultural diversity as they would for any other form of diversity, in order to provide the best possible care to their clients.

Hearing loss, affecting approximately 10% of the world's population, is a silent and often overlooked condition, which deprives people of one of the most basic of human needs—the ability to communicate effectively with others. "In 2005, about 278 million people had moderate to profound hearing impairment, 80% of them live in low-and middle-income countries" (WHO, 2010). There are over 310,000 culturally Deaf Canadians and over 3,000,000 hard-of-hearing Canadians (Canadian Association of the Deaf, 2007; Canadian Hard of Hearing Association, 2010). As well, 50% of persons over the age of 60 live with loss of hearing. Given these figures, one can see that hearing loss is a lived experience of many people around the world, and given predictions of population statistics, these numbers will increase.

The labels *deaf* and *hard of hearing* are generally used interchangeably in our society. There is a movement to try to change this, however, because some people who are Deaf (with a capital D) prefer to have their deafness brought into the open and made visible to others, describing themselves as having their own culture (Padden & Humphries, 2005). "Deaf people are typically identified early in life, living with no sound and the majority usually benefit from special education programs and resources" (Getty & Hetu, 1994, p. 267). They share a common language (sign language) and culture (Padden, 2000; Padden & Humphries, 2005). On the other hand, "most hard of hearing people … develop hearing loss during adulthood which generally progresses insidiously, and unless they wear a noticeable hearing aid, their loss of hearing may be invisible to others" (Getty & Hetu, 1994, p. 267). Stigmatization and misunderstanding surface because "the public uses the word *deafness* as an umbrella term to cover all forms of hearing loss" (Ashley, 1985, p. 61). Labels and names may or may not be welcomed by individuals in the Deaf community or those living with hearing loss depending on the person's perspective or world view.

Aquino-Russell (2003) noted that there is a lack of understanding on the part of society, family, and

BOX 7-1 Enhancing Understanding of Deaf Culture and of Hard-of-Hearing Persons in Canada—Cont'd

friends of what it is like to live with a different sense of hearing. For example, one study participant stated:

> *I think of my father and how lonely it must have been for him to live out his last year in a world of his own in almost complete silence. This sometimes leaves me to wonder if and when my hearing reaches that point if I too will be living alone in my own world because family and friends do not understand.* (p. 210)

In addition, people tend not to realize that the value of amplification with the assistance of hearing aids varies according to a person's residual hearing and the ability to make sense of what is heard, and that amplification or a hearing aid is not a substitute for normal hearing (Bess & Humes, 1995). The benefits of hearing aids depend on the person and environment (Gatehouse, Naylor, & Elberling, 2003).

It has been argued that because hearing loss is invisible (i.e., people do not see it), hard-of-hearing and Deaf persons receive less understanding or sympathy than people with more visible differences. According to Vernon (1989), the public is inclined to blame them for their problems rather than expressing concern and compassion (p. 152). Comments such as "He can hear when he wants to," "She doesn't pay attention," or "Grandfather is just stubborn" show the tendency to stigmatize and blame the hard-of-hearing person, with no consideration of the hearing loss for difficulties that may arise. Typically, with blame come feelings of anger and hostility on the part of both the person living with hearing loss and the person with normal hearing (Vernon, 1989). Concurrently, "the problem for Deaf people is as always, how to articulate their views … in a world that finds it easier *not* to understand them" (Padden & Humphries, 2005, pp. 179–180).

CHNs need to be sensitive to the existence of stigma and individuals' preferences. Each person is unique and will have a unique experience of hearing loss or being deaf. CHNs have the responsibility to listen to people with hearing loss if they wish to describe their experience. CHNs must also enable interpreters to work with persons from the Deaf culture within the health care system in a language of their choice. Equally important is to respect those who do not wish to tell of their experiences. "Parse proposes that speaking about something is a way of being with it and thus silence may, for some [people] be a strategy for continuing on" (cited in Carson & Mitchell, 1998, p. 1247). Rather than considering themselves experts concerning people's health, CHNs need to learn from the people living the experience by listening to them describe their experiences and by assisting them with the needs they identify, rather than focusing on the needs the CHN feels are important.

CHNs need to respect the views and choices of persons with a different sense of hearing. Those living with hearing loss may not only choose to reveal or conceal their experience to others, they may also choose to connect with or separate from sounds and others' words. People have described removing hearing aids because the sounds were indiscernible, too loud, or too muffled, or when they just wished to enjoy their own sound of silence (Aquino-Russell, 2003). It is interesting to note that persons do know that with every choice there are opportunities and limitations, consequences that will open some doors and close others. For example, by choosing to remove hearing aids to enjoy one's sound of silence, these people know there may be sounds that will be missed, while at the same time the choice to keep their hearing aids in place to hear sounds can create unbearable noise. Persons who come from the Deaf community need to have their care in conjunction with sign language interpreters. It is vital for CHNs to appreciate that individuals live their own value priorities—they live what is important to them for their own quality of life—and that understanding personal meaning is important to people. "To feel understood is to experience the fact that one's personal meaning is shared by another" (Howell, 1998, p. 15).

Practice Strategies

Aquino-Russell (2003) found that, in general, health care professionals do not know or practise strategies to enhance interpersonal communication and quality of life. However, an enhanced understanding of what it is like to live with hearing loss can be lived in professional practice through the choices the CHN makes about how to be *with* others. When exploring the meaning of living with hearing loss with persons who actually live the experience, the CHN might ask: "Please help me to understand what it is like for you." The explanations to this simple question can guide CHN practice in unbounded ways.

There are other helpful strategies for working with persons who live with loss of hearing, such as the use of technology in the form of personal communication devices (one type is called a Pocket-Talker). As well, CHNs should

(Continued)

BOX 7-1 Enhancing Understanding of Deaf Culture and of Hard-of-Hearing Persons in Canada—Cont'd

- face the person who has loss of hearing directly,
- keep one's face in the light with no light behind one's head,
- speak clearly, never covering one's mouth or turning one's head away (Aquino-Russell, 2005).

For those who come from the Deaf community, sign language interpreters are legislated to provide interpretation of health care activities. The *Canadian Human Rights Act* recognizes that persons with disabilities have a right to full integration and participation in society (Deaf and Hard of Hearing Society, 2010). CHNs have a responsibility to learn how individuals wish to be helped, if they do, and what is important to those living the experience. All individuals should be invited to share their personal realities and strategies. People who live with hearing loss and those who come from the Deaf community know the simple and intricate ways that help or hinder. They know what they want and when it would be best to try (or not to try) new or different strategies. CHNs might ask, for example: "What strategies might we try to make our communication better for you?" "The linguistic and social lives of Deaf persons [and those who live with hearing loss] provide us with unique and valuable ways of exploring the vast potential for human language and culture" (Padden & Humphries, 2005, p. 180).

Immigrant Population in Canada

Based on the 2006 census data, the largest number of visible minorities were in Toronto (42.9%), Vancouver (17.3%), and Montreal (11.6%) and other larger Canadian centres such as Halifax, Winnipeg, and Calgary (Statistics Canada, 2010). In 2006, 9.6% of Canada's Chinese lived in Toronto and 18.2% of Vancouver's total population was Chinese, making it the largest visible minority group in that city (Statistics Canada, 2010). Many early Chinese immigrants arrived in Canada as manual labourers; recent Chinese immigrants arrive with education and monetary resources and enter Canada as skilled workers (Chui, Tran, & Flanders, 2005). In Canada, the Chinese language (made up of many dialects) is the third most common mother tongue, following those of English and French (Statistics Canada, 2007a). The Chinese culture values family, and aging parents often reside with their children. Generally, in the 2001 Canadian census, 60% of the Chinese population reported no religious affiliation (Christian and non-Christian) compared with 16% of the general population (Chui et al., 2005).

In 2006, the largest Canadian South Asian population resided in Toronto (54.6%) with Abbotsford, British Columbia, having the highest proportion to its total population (16.3% versus 13.5% in Toronto) (Statistics Canada, 2010). South Asians are usually referred to in Canada as "East Indian," with some countries of origin being India, Sri Lanka, Pakistan, and Nepal. The South Asian culture values family, and aging parents usually reside with a family member. Most South Asians value their ethnocultural community and frequently work and socialize together and marry within their own group. Not surprisingly, they value maintaining their ethnic customs and traditions such as food, holiday celebrations, and clothing. Their religion is important to them. They tend to actively participate in religious activities, local group activities, and organizations (Tran, Kaddatz, & Allard, 2005). According to the 2001 census data, most South Asians reported a strong sense of belonging to Canada, their province, and their municipality (Tran et al., 2005).

In Montreal, according to the 2006 census data, the largest visible minority group was Black (169,100) while the Arab population in Montreal was approximately 100,000 and was the fastest growing visible minority group in that large urban centre (Statistics Canada, 2010). According to the 2006 census data, in Montreal compared to the rest of Canada, the percentage of visible minorities (16.5%) was slightly above the national average 16.2%) (Statistics Canada, 2010).

Aboriginal Peoples in Canada

Aboriginal refers to the original inhabitants of a country who identify with a particular heritage based on their linguistics and culture. In Canada, it is generally known that the term *Aboriginal peoples* or *First Peoples* of Canada refers to the Indian, Inuit, and Métis peoples of Canada. In section 35(2) of the *Constitution Act,* 1982, the term *Inuit* replaced the term *Eskimo* and the term *First Nations* replaced the term *Indian* (Inuit Tapiriit Kanatami, 2007, p. 13).

Inuit Peoples

The Inuit people of the Arctic and subarctic regions (north of 60° latitude) mainly reside in northern Canada. The majority of Inuit (over 80%) live in 53 communities spread across two provinces and two territories (Inuit Tapiriit Kanatami, 2009). Over 90% of these communities are accessible by air only. Inuit communities are located in four land-claim regions: Nunatsiavut (Labrador), Nunavik (Northern Quebec), Nunavut Territory, and Inuvialuit Settlement Region (Northwest Territories), and Inuit live as well in southern Canada (Inuit Tapiriit Kanatami, 2009).

Métis Peoples

The Métis National Council (2009) defines a Métis person as "a person who self-identifies as Métis, is of historic Métis Nation Ancestry, is distinct from other Aboriginal Peoples and is accepted by the Métis Nation" (p. 1). The "Historic Métis Nation" refers to the Aboriginal people historically known as Métis or mixed blood (with parents of Aboriginal and European ancestry) who resided in the "Historic Métis Nation Homeland," which refers to the area of land in west central North America used and occupied as the traditional territory of the Métis. "Métis Nation" refers to the Aboriginal people descended from the Historic Métis Nation, which is now made up of all Métis Nation citizens and who are considered members of one of the Aboriginal peoples of Canada within section 35 of the *Constitution Act* of 1982. They have their own distinct dialect, referred to as the Michif language, but the Métis people are diverse linguistically depending on the combination of ancestry (e.g., Cree, Dene, English, and French). The Métis had the greatest population gain of all Aboriginal groups between 1996 and 2001. The Métis population grew by 43% during this period (Statistics Canada, 2003).

First Nation Peoples

The most important means of Canadian control over First Nations communities was, and still is, the *Indian Act,* which consolidated the various laws relating to Indians that had been passed by the Canadian government in the years since Confederation and by the British colonial authorities before them. The *Indian Act* exists to this day and is used to set out certain federal governmental obligations and to continue to exert power and complete control of all aspects of Indian life, such as reserve lands, Indian moneys, and other resources. "Amendments in the early years of the *Indian Act* enabled the Canadian government to outlaw traditional Aboriginal ceremonies such as the potlatch and sacred dancing including the Sun Dance" (Helin, 2006, p. 95). The *Indian Act* also defines who has Indian status and who does not. Until 1985, the *Indian Act* discriminated against Indian women who married non-Indian men; these women were not considered to have Indian status, but Indian men did not lose their status if they married a non-Indian. In fact, their non-Aboriginal wives gained status. Women are considered the carriers of the culture, and so when Indian woman were excluded from living in their communities and non-Indian woman who married Indian men were welcomed into the community, this created another means for assimilation to seep into the very fibre of the community (Dutcher, 2008). The *Indian Act* was amended in 1985 to allow those who had lost status to regain it, as well as their children. However, this change in the Act created a new form of discrimination in that the grandchildren of the women who had originally lost their status would continue to lose their status if they married a nonstatus person. The case of Sharon McIvor in British Columbia contested this further discrimination to future generations and was successful in the B.C. Court of Appeal. She appealed the amended *Indian Act* section that discriminated against the children of Aboriginal women who married a non-Aboriginal, resulting in their loss of Indian status (Court of Appeal for British Columbia, 2009). Efforts by Aboriginal and non-Aboriginal leaders have, in recent years, focused on the self-government and self-determination for all Aboriginal peoples in Canada (Auer & Andersson, 2001). There are ongoing governmental and nongovernmental efforts focusing on the self-government and self-determination for all Aboriginal peoples in Canada. For information on the Government of Canada's approach to implementation of the inherent right and the negotiation of Aboriginal self-government, refer to the Indian and Northern Affairs Canada Web site titled "Government of Canada's Approach to Implementation of the Inherent Right and the Negotiation of Aboriginal Self-Government" found in the Weblinks. This Web site contains information on existing policies pertaining to self-governance, approaches to self-government, and process issues.

The health transfer process, which started in 1989 throughout Canada, was an effort of the federal government to relinquish some of its authority and control to First Nation and Inuit communities regarding the managing of health programs. Aboriginal peoples have long asserted their rights as the First (Indigenous) Peoples of North America. This has been particularly true since the 1970s, with the rise of Aboriginal self-determination, which was fuelled by many successful court challenges by various Aboriginal peoples, including the following three widely considered as the most significant milestone cases in advancing Aboriginal rights in Canada. In the 1973 *Calder* decision, the Nisga'a people in Pacific Northwest lost on a technicality but a majority of the Supreme Court of Canada justices recognized for the first time that Aboriginal rights did indeed exist in Canadian law. In the 1991 *Delgamuukw* decision, two other peoples in the Pacific Northwest—the Gitksan and Wet'swet'en peoples—succeeded in getting the Supreme Court to recognize for the first time that oral evidence by Aboriginal elders was "a repository of historical knowledge for a culture" and would be considered on par with other types of evidence (Dickason & McNab, 2009, p. 330). As well, in the 1999 *Marshall* decision, the Supreme Court held that the Mi'kmaq had, based on eighteenth-century treaties of peace and friendship, the Aboriginal right to fish. The Supreme Court later clarified that this right was subject to conservation regulations and restricted to earning a moderate livelihood (Dickason & McNab, 2009). Aboriginal peoples continue to maintain their rights and identity as indigenous people in Canadian society, while also trying to address the vast complexities of health and social issues.

Historical Context

The historical context of all Aboriginal people in Canada has had a profound impact on the present-day realities as well as the current health status of Aboriginal people. Prior to European contact, more than 500 years ago, it is well established historically that the Aboriginal people lived in harmony and in balance with the environment that they inhabited. Harmony and balance was embedded in every aspect of life, including the cultural practices and teachings passed on by the elders. Maintaining the balance of the spiritual, psychological, emotional, and physical well-being of the person with the environment was the basis for Aboriginal philosophy. This philosophy of being in the world was vastly different from European immigrants' philosophy to have dominion over the earth. Initial contact with Europeans and the conflicting world views caused a massive disruption to the way of life and also caused a decline in the population (from the sixteenth to the twentieth centuries). It is estimated that prior to European contact, 500,000 Aboriginal or Indigenous persons lived in what is now known as Canada, and that this was reduced to 102,000 persons as a result of infectious diseases, such as influenza, smallpox, measles, and tuberculosis, to which the Aboriginal peoples had no immunity (Indian and Northern Affairs Canada, 1996). European immigrants forced some Aboriginal communities to relocate while claiming the land and resources as their own. Aboriginal people were resistant to the governmental agenda to control and monopolize Canadian resources, and so an assimilation policy was developed (Indian and Northern Affairs Canada, 1996b).

Residential School Legacy

Attempts to intentionally assimilate and colonize Aboriginal people included the suppression of language, ceremonies, and culture and a destruction of family, often done through residential schools. In 1920, residential schools were made compulsory by the Deputy Superintendent General of Indian Affairs Duncan Campbell Scott. Residential schools, in particular, had a damaging impact on Aboriginal peoples as children were often seized by force and sent away to live in impersonal and oppressive institutions run by the churches and financed by the federal government. The children were often subject to physical, emotional, and even sexual abuse in the residential schools (Chansonneuve, 2005). The schools also had a multigenerational effect as children did not grow up learning about their traditional roles as children and eventually as parents: "Instead, they grew up in an environment where adults frequently exerted 'power and control' through abuse" (Dion Stout & Kipling, 2003, p. 52). Many children who attended these schools learned that their culture and language were of no value within a new European-dominated society (Dutcher, 2008). Many Aboriginal people who attended these schools still carry the psychological baggage, which they pass on to the following generations. This process of passing historical trauma on to the following generations has created intragenerational grief that affects the mental, physical, emotional, and spiritual well-being of individuals, families, and communities (Wesley-Esquimaux & Smolewski, 2004). The Aboriginal Healing Foundation was established to help survivors of the residential schools and their families deal with the impacts of their experiences. It was not until 1996 that the last government-run residential school closed (Wesley-Esquimaux & Smolewski, 2004). However, the traumatic experiences that many generations of Aboriginal people had to endure in these institutions are only one example of the attempts to assimilate and colonize the indigenous people of North America. People throughout the world who have experienced colonization also display patterns of poor health, including high rates of infectious disease, high mortality rates, and increased chronic and degenerative illnesses (Smylie, 2000).

Aboriginal Population Statistics

This brief introduction to First Nations, Inuit, and Métis peoples living in Canada, and the specific statistics for each group of peoples will help provide a greater understanding of the diversity among the various groups of Aboriginal peoples in Canada. Statistics gathered for each distinct group are variable and in some cases not collected at all. This is true especially for the Métis population, since the two federal departments, the First Nations and Inuit Health and the Department of Indian Affairs, have not included Métis with the First Nations and Inuit populations' statistics. However, Statistics Canada gathers information on all three Aboriginal groups (Health Council of Canada, 2005). According to the 2006 census data, the Aboriginal population constitutes 4% of the Canadian population, with the First Nations (698,025) being the largest group, the Métis (389,785) being the

TABLE 7-4 Comparison of Non-Aboriginal, First Nations, Inuit, and Métis Populations in Canada

Criteria	Non-Aboriginal	First Nations	Inuit	Métis
Age	Median age: 40 18% <15 years	Median age 25 yrs 33% <15 yrs 5% seniors >65	Median age 22 yrs 35% <15 yrs	Median age 25 yrs
Fertility rates	Low	High	High	High
Employment rate	81.6%	51.9% on reserve 66.3% off reserve	61.2%	74.6%
Median income (2005)	$25,955	$14,517	$16,955	Not available
Report crowded homes and needing major repairs	3%	More likely for those living on reserves	33% more likely	69% live off reserves; 3% and more likely to live in homes needing repairs
Suicide rate	29%	33%	40%	Not available
Percentage deaths per 100,000 population				

SOURCE: Statistics Canada. (2009). *2006 Census: Aboriginal Peoples in Canada in 2006: Inuit, Métis and First Nations, 2006 Census: Highlights.* Retrieved from http://www12.statcan.ca/census-recensement/2006/as-sa/97-558/index-eng.cfm.

next largest, and the Inuit (50,485) being the smallest (Statistics Canada, 2009c). Aboriginal people are the fastest-growing population in Canada, and the Aboriginal population is considered a young population, as indicated by the fact that 50 to 56% of First Nations and Inuit persons are under the age of 25 (Human Resources and Skills Development, 2010). See Box 7-2 for statistics on Aboriginal peoples in Canada. There are 606 First Nations communities and 53 Inuit communities in Canada (Health Canada, 2008). See Table 7-4 for a comparison of the statistics of the non-Aboriginal, First Nations, Inuit, and Métis populations based on 2006 Statistics Canada data.

CULTURAL COMPETENCE

In today's climate of multiculturalism, there is an increasing demand for CHNs to provide high-quality, effective, and "culturally competent" care. Many definitions of cultural competence exist. In this text, **cultural competence** refers to an ongoing process, rather than an outcome, whereby the health care professional respects, accepts, and applies knowledge and skill appropriate to the client interactions without allowing one's personal beliefs to influence the clients' differing views (Giger et al., 2007; Srivastava, 2007). Cultural competence includes CHNs acknowledging the fundamental variations in the ways clients respond to health care challenges. This can include paying attention to health promotion activities, coping with pain and death and dying, and understanding culturally specific beliefs, values, and practices such as modesty, eye contact, closeness, and how one touches others.

In Nova Scotia, primary health care professionals, led by Sharon Davis-Murdoch, have developed a document, *A Cultural Competence Guide for Primary Health Care Professionals* (see the Weblinks on the Evolve Web site), which addresses the diverse communities of First Nations, African Canadians, immigrant Canadians, Acadians, and Francophone Canadians (Nova Scotia Department of Health, 2005). For example, this document includes a discussion on eight steps in developing cultural competence (see Box 7-3), consideration of the determinants of health such as equity and access, and inclusion of primary health care.

One example of cultural competence with a community-level focus was the establishment of a coalition between two Saskatchewan Aboriginal communities, a health region and three tertiary educational institutions. The objective was to determine cultural elements that demonstrated respect in the delivery of direct health care and ways to deliver health education programs for Aboriginal peoples that were respectful of their cultural diversity, resulting in the establishment of relationships among coalition members that led to an enhanced understanding of Aboriginal culture, specifically healing and ways of knowing (Canadian Institutes of Health Research, 2006).

BOX 7-2 Aboriginal Peoples of Canada Based on the 2006 Census Data

- There are over 1 million Aboriginal people in Canada.
- Aboriginal people make up 3.8% of the Canadian population.
- The percentage of Métis people has increased the most within the Aboriginal population.
- More than 50% of the population who resided in the territories identified as being of Aboriginal ancestry.
- The largest populations of Aboriginal peoples are in Ontario, Nunavut, Northwest Territories, Manitoba, and Saskatchewan.
- Aboriginal peoples' population growth is faster than Canada's non-Aboriginal population growth.
- Many Aboriginal people (54%) live in urban areas.
- Eighty percent of Aboriginal people live either in Ontario or in Manitoba, Saskatchewan, Alberta, and British Columbia.
- The First Nations population was the largest, followed by Métis, then Inuit population.
- In 2006, the average age of the Aboriginal population was 13 years lower than the average age of the non-Aboriginal population.

SOURCE: Human Resources and Skill Development Canada. (2010). *Canadians in context–Aboriginal population*. Retrieved from http://www.4.hrsdc.gc.ca/.3ndic.1t.4r@-eng.jsp?iid=36.

BOX 7-3 Eight Steps for CHNs to Develop Cultural Competence

- Know yourself by analyzing your principles, behaviours, views, and assumptions.
- Be aware of racism and the systems or behaviours that foster racism.
- Reframe your thinking by engaging in activities that encourage others' views and perspectives.
- Become familiar with the core cultural aspects of your community.
- Partner with clients to facilitate a comparison of their perceptions and your findings of the core cultural aspects of the community.
- Familiarize yourself with different cultures and their perceptions and practices for health and illness, and explore with clients their cultural uniqueness (diversity) regarding health and illness.
- Establish rapport, respect, and trust with clients and co-workers by being open, understanding, and willing to accept varying perceptions.
- Establish an environment that is welcoming for the diverse cultures within your community.

SOURCE: Adapted from Government of Nova Scotia. (2005). *A cultural competence guide for primary health care professionals in Nova Scotia* (p.18, Section 2). Retrieved from http://www.gov.ns.ca/health/primaryhealthcare/diversity.asp.

The approach used by these communities demonstrates cultural competence because it was collaborative, was respectful, and promoted trust.

A second example of cultural competence at a community level is a project involving a team of seven community partners from the Windsor, Ontario, area who worked together in conducting an extensive literature review of research pertaining to breast screening practices of North American ethnocultural women from continental Africa and Asia who have cultural and language challenges. The team surveyed the Windsor/Essex community to determine its capacity for providing culturally competent breast health care and interviewed 80 ethnocultural women to discover their knowledge of and beliefs about breast cancer, their views of health, and their breast screening practices. The results of the surveys informed the development and delivery of health promotion workshops on breast cancer prevention for newcomer women, resulting in knowledge translation and community programs that are culturally competent (Centre for Urban Health Initiatives, 2008).

An example of cultural competence focused at an individual level is that of a woman, a recent Chinese immigrant, who speaks little English and goes to an urban community health centre because of a urinary tract infection. The culturally competent CHN understands the need to use strategies that allow the CHN to communicate effectively with the client. The CHN also understands that the client has the right to effective care, to judge whether she has received the care she wants, and to follow up with appropriate action if she does not receive the expected care. In this interaction, the CHN demonstrates cultural competence by being sensitive to the client's modesty by using a female interpreter to explain the physical examination procedures. The CHN also explores with this client the use of traditional medicines and practices for pain and infections.

As well, CHNs working with Aboriginal Canadians need to understand that this group has specific health

ETHICAL CONSIDERATIONS

In Canada, a multicultural country, the CHN needs to work within the system to improve the health of many different culturally diverse groups; therefore, cultural competence is essential. CHNs work with some cultural groups whose cultural values and beliefs about health and illness differ from theirs.

A CHN is working with a cultural group that believes prayer along with advice and permission from their Church leaders is necessary prior to receiving any medical treatment. This group also uses folk and alternative medicine to cure illnesses because of their belief system, and it is less expensive and more accessible in their community. The CHN identifies the need for a community immunization clinic, but suspects that clients will not want to come.

Ethical principles that apply to this scenario:

- *Beneficence:* The CHN is bound by this principle to do good. Immunization has been proven to reduce the incidence of vaccine-preventable communicable diseases.
- *Respect for autonomy:* Some clients do not wish to be immunized, and CHNs respect client autonomy.
- *Promoting and respecting informed decision making (CNA Code of Ethics):* This primary ethical value requires respect for informed decision making. CHNs have an ethical responsibility to provide essential health care information so that clients can make informed decisions.

Question to Consider

1. Given the above ethical principles, the importance of cultural competence, and the necessity for cultural safety, how can the CHN provide the best care for these clients?

care beliefs and care practices. They have healers, often called medicine healers or shamans, who provide service to people in their communities. Some of the traditions found in Aboriginal communities are burning sweet grass and smoking tobacco; using sweat lodges, which are associated with spirituality; using the medicine wheel for spiritual balance; and connecting with the circle of life to reach balance and harmony (Srivastava, 2007). CHNs need to be aware of their own values, beliefs, and biases toward healing and alternative health care practices. The "Ethical Considerations" box, on this page, deals with a similar theme.

Developing Cultural Competence

Culturally competent care is provided not only to individuals of racial or ethnic minority groups but also to individuals belonging to groups held together by factors such as age, religion, sexual orientation, and socioeconomic status. Nurses need to be culturally competent to provide nursing care that meets the needs of these persons. Culture has been widely studied, and many theories, frameworks, and cultural assessment guides are available to assist the CHN to provide culturally competent care (Astle & Pacquiao, 2006; Giger & Davidhizar, 2008; Kulig, 2000; Leininger, 2002). Cultural nursing assessment is discussed later in this chapter. "Cultural competence can work to reduce disparities in health services, address inequitable access to primary health care and respectfully respond to diversity" (Government of Nova Scotia, 2005b).

Developing cultural competence is an ongoing life process that involves every aspect of client care. It is challenging and at times painful as nurses struggle to adopt new ways of thinking and performing. Leininger (2002) suggests the following two principles that are useful in developing cultural competence:

1. Maintain a broad, objective, and open attitude toward individuals and their cultures.
2. Avoid seeing all individuals as alike.

Nurses develop cultural competence in different ways, but the key elements are experiences with clients of other cultures, an awareness of these experiences, and the promotion of mutual respect for differences. Because degrees of cultural competence vary, not all nurses may reach the same level of development.

Burchum (2002) used the method of concept analysis to identify the key attributes of cultural competence. She found the following six attributes most often in her review of the concept of cultural competence: (1) cultural awareness, (2) cultural knowledge, (3) cultural understanding, (4) cultural sensitivity, (5) cultural interaction, and (6) cultural skill. Table 7-5 presents a modification of Burchum's (2002) attributes and dimensions of cultural competence.

TABLE 7-5 Attributes and Dimensions of Cultural Competence

Attributes and Definitions	Dimensions	Nursing Considerations
Cultural awareness is self-examination and in-depth exploration of one's own beliefs and values as they influence behaviour (Campinha-Bacote, 2002; Misener, Sowell, Phillips, & Harris, 1997).	• Understand your own culture • Know your ethnocentric views, biases, and prejudices • Be aware of similarities and differences between and among cultures	Nurses who have developed cultural awareness are • receptive to learning about the cultural dimensions of the client. • able to understand their own cultural beliefs and behaviour and how these can influence the delivery of competent care to persons from cultures other than their own (Pottinger, Perivolaris, & Howes, 2007). • able to recognize that health is expressed differently across cultures and that culture influences an individual's responses to health, illness, disease, and death.
Cultural knowledge is information about organizational elements of diverse cultures and ethnic groups. Emphasis is on learning about the client's world view from an emic (native) perspective. An understanding of the client's culture decreases misinterpretations and the misapplication of scientific knowledge and facilitates the client's cooperation with the health care regimen (Campinha-Bacote, 2002; Leininger, 2002).	• Know about cultures other than your own • Be able to recognize differences in communication styles and etiquette between and within cultures • Acquire familiarity with conceptual and theoretical frameworks	Cultural competence is knowledge-based care (Srivastava, 2007). Leininger (2002) points out that nurses who lack cultural knowledge may develop feelings of inadequacy and helplessness because they are often unable to effectively help their clients. Eliason's (1998) research shows that there is a significant positive relationship between students' comfort level and the amount of experience they have had in caring for culturally diverse clients. Although it is unrealistic to expect that nurses will have knowledge of all cultures, they need to be aware of and know how to obtain the knowledge of cultural influences that affect groups with whom they most frequently interact.
Cultural understanding refers to continuous reflections on the effects of culture (values, beliefs, and behaviours) for diverse clients (Burchum, 2002).	• Understand that "Western medicine" does not have all the answers • Recognize how culture shapes your beliefs, values, and behaviours • To avoid stereotyping, be aware that there are racial, ethnic, and cultural variations • Understand the concerns and issues that occur when your values, beliefs, and practices differ from those of the dominant culture • Know that marginalization influences patterns of seeking care	Nurses who achieve cultural understanding practise with clients in a manner that demonstrates recognition of a variety of ways of knowing. The nurses also recognize and accept that clients from various cultures use alternative and complementary therapies. The nurses also deal with problems such as marginalization that result from differing beliefs and values.
Culture sensitivity is "knowing how" (Srivastava, 2007). Cultural sensitivity refers to being able to appreciate, "respect, and value cultural diversity" (Burchum, 2002, p. 7). Therefore, it involves a realization about the influence of one's own personal and professional identity on practice.	• Appreciate and respect your individual client's beliefs and values • Appreciate and value diversity • Appreciate and genuinely care about those of other cultures • Recognize how your own cultural background may influence professional practice	In all client interactions, the nurses are aware and respect client cultural diversity. The nurses also consider how personal and professional identity influence nursing practice. Nurses' verbal and nonverbal behaviours are polite and respective (Giger et al., 2007).

TABLE 7-5 Attributes and Dimensions of Cultural Competence—Cont'd

Attributes and Definitions	Dimensions	Nursing Considerations
Cultural interaction refers to the verbal and nonverbal communication between persons of different cultures.	• Interact with those of other cultures • Engage in practice with those of other cultures	Nurses engage in effective communication, use the appropriate language and literacy level, and learn directly from clients about their life experiences and the significance of these experiences for health (Leininger, 2002).
Cultural skill refers to the effective integration of cultural awareness and cultural knowledge to obtain relevant cultural data and meet the needs of culturally diverse clients (Stanhope & Lancaster, 2010).	• Perform cultural assessments that consider beliefs and values, family roles, health practices, and the meanings of health and illness • Perform physical assessments that incorporate knowledge of racial variations • Be sure to communicate, either personally or through appropriate use of interpreters and other resources, in a manner that is understood and that effectively responds to those who speak other languages • Make sure your nonverbal communication techniques take into consideration the client's use of eye contact, facial expressions, body language, touch, and space • Know how to provide care that incorporates the development of a respectful and therapeutic alliance with the client • Provide care that overcomes biases and is modified to respect and accommodate the values, beliefs, and practices of the client without compromising your own values • Provide care that is beneficial, safe, and satisfying to your client • Know how to provide care that elicits a feeling by the client of being welcome, understood, important, and comfortable • Provide care that addresses disadvantages arising from the client's position in relation to networks • Use self-empowerment strategies in your client care	Culturally skillful nurses use appropriate touch during conversation, modify the physical distance between themselves and others, and use strategies to avoid cultural misunderstandings while meeting mutually agreed-upon goals (Stanhope & Lancaster, 2010).
Cultural proficiency refers to the demonstration of new knowledge and cultural skills, including the communication of this information.	• Add new knowledge by conducting research, by developing new culturally sensitive therapeutic approaches, and by delivering this information to others • Evidence a commitment to change	The nurses participate in and use research in nursing practice with culturally diverse clients.

Source: Adapted from Burchum, J. L. (2002). Cultural competence: An evolutionary perspective. *Nursing Forum, 37*(4), 5–15.

CHNs can help clients who come from different cultures in relation to their health care practices. Through educational groups facilitated by the CHN or others, such as self-help groups, clients from these different cultures can learn new adaptation strategies from each other and a variety of ways to relate to families, community, and workplace. One very important role of the CHN working with the community is that of advocate to support and ensure that there are appropriate and accessible health care services. CHNs also advocate at the local, provincial, and federal levels for policies that support adaptation of culturally diverse groups to their new or unfamiliar environment. For example, one of the policy changes initiated to assist the culturally diverse group of physically disabled persons in wheelchairs was the requirement that all public buildings have ramps to accommodate wheelchairs. This change resulted in all such physically challenged persons having access to all public buildings in their communities. Therefore, CHNs need to assess communities through the use of environment health scans to ensure that issues affecting culturally diverse group are addressed.

To provide culturally competent care, CHNs need to appreciate and understand the cultural backgrounds of their clients. Although certain health beliefs and practices have been identified within Aboriginal, Inuit, Francophone, Black, and Chinese cultures, the CHN needs to remember that the beliefs and practices differ among regions and localities of the country and among individuals. Box 7-4 presents some attributes and nursing considerations when dealing with Aboriginal people. For further information on developing cultural competence, refer to the Registered Nurses Association of Ontario (RNAO) Weblink on developing cultural competence.

Inhibitors to Developing Cultural Competence

When CHNs fail to provide culturally competent nursing care, it may be because they do not understand transcultural nursing, they are pressured by supervisors to improve productivity by increasing their caseloads, or they are pressured by colleagues who are not knowledgeable about other cultures and who are offended when others use these concepts. These and similar issues inhibit delivery of culturally competent care and may result in some of the following CHN behaviours:

- **Ethnocentrism.** Ethnocentrism is a type of cultural prejudice in which one believes that his or her "own cultural values, beliefs, and behaviours are the best, preferred, and the most superior ways" (Srivastava, 2007, p. 5). CHNs who assume that their way of providing nursing care is the only right way are ethnocentric.
- **Cultural blindness.** Cultural blindness is a denial of diversity and the inability to recognize the uniqueness of individual clients. An example is CHNs who, attempting to be culturally unbiased, treat all clients in the same manner by conducting their nursing assessments using the same questions, do not actively listen to the responses, and fail to modify their questioning to gain an understanding of client culture and diversity.

BOX 7-4 Attributes and Dimensions of Aboriginal Culture and Nursing Considerations

Some important cultural and community health nursing considerations when working with Canadian Aboriginal clients are these:

- Know the history and culture within the community of practice.
- Know the Aboriginal cultural behaviours that demonstrate respect.
- Have an awareness of one's own cultural beliefs, values, and attitudes to interact in a nonjudgemental manner.
- Distinguish the similarities and differences among Aboriginal cultures; have an awareness that health care for Aboriginal people is a "treaty right and not a privilege."
- Participate in traditions, such as attending powwows and other activities in the community.
- Know the community health resources, particularly the community elders.

SOURCE: Foster, C.H. (2006). What nurses should know when working in Aboriginal communities. *Canadian Nurse, 102*(4), 28–31.

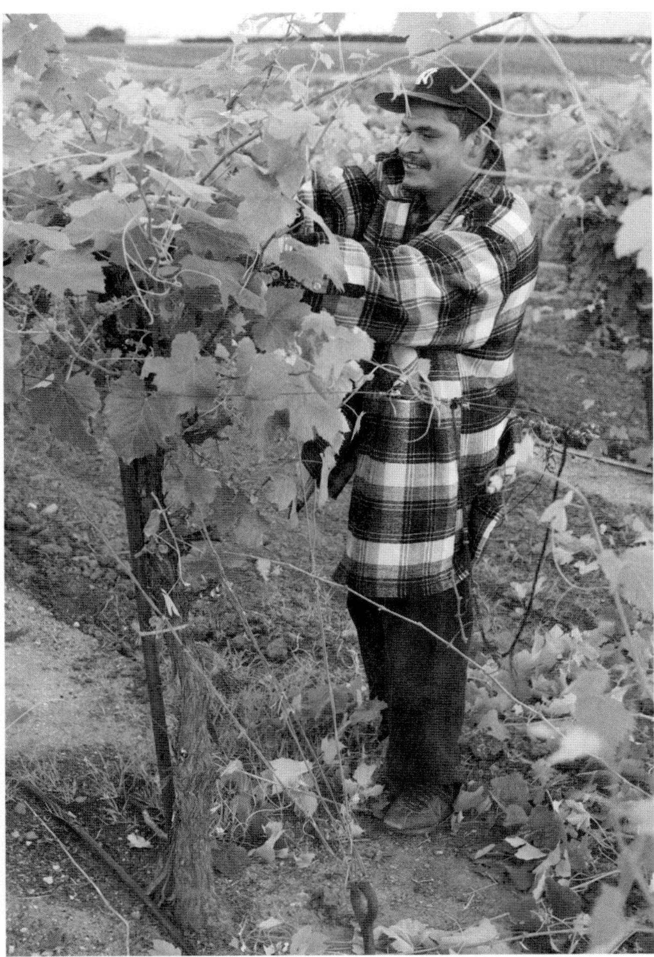

CHNs work with clients from a diverse cultural and economic background. One such group is migrant workers, who often have high occupational mobility and who may seek health care only when they are too ill to work. It is important for a community health nurse to teach these clients about disease prevention, health maintenance, health protection, and health promotion activities before the client moves.

- **Culture shock.** Culture shock is a condition that involves feelings of anxiety because of exposure to unfamiliar environments and culture. The person feels threatened and helpless while trying to adapt to the unfamiliar culture with its different practices, values, and beliefs. For example, a newcomer from Somalia arrives in Canada and finds the unfamiliar environment and culture overwhelming.
- **Stereotyping.** Stereotyping occurs when generalizations are applied to an individual without exploring individual values, beliefs, and behaviours. For example, a CHN decides that an Italian client with diabetes eats too much pasta and therefore cannot control blood sugar levels. The CHN does not ask the client about this.
- **Prejudice.** A prejudice is a negative attitude about a person or group without factual data (Srivastava, 2007), e.g., "older adults do not have sex."
- **Racism.** Racism is a prejudice in which members of one cultural group perceive themselves to be superior to another cultural group (Ontario Human Rights Commission, 2008), e.g., "the white race in Canada is superior to all newcomers."

Being aware of clients' cultural beliefs and knowing about other cultures may help CHNs to be less judgemental, more accepting of cultural variations, and less likely to engage in the behaviours previously listed, which inhibit cultural competence.

Racism

Racism is most frequently thought of in terms of responding to skin colour, ethnic origin, or religion; however, it can occur based on other aspects of culture such as cultural celebrations, traditional dress, and traditional food. The most commonly found types of racism in the literature are overt and systemic. *Overt racism* is an open demonstration by attitudes, actions, policies, and practices of a feeling of superiority over individuals or groups with the intent of harming or damaging (Government of Canada, 2003b). Hate crimes, for example, are considered as one example of overt racism. *Systemic racism,* also known as institutional racism, involves policies within organizations, corporations, and institutions that are not equally applied to all individuals and groups (RNAO, 2007), such as when a job position is available only to persons who are Canadian-born. The Ethnic Diversity Survey revealed that visible minority groups, especially Black Canadians, reported perceptions of discrimination and unfair treatment "often" or "sometimes" (32%) and "rarely" (17%) (Government of Canada, 2003a). However, this survey also found that Canadians (50%) have a strong sense of belonging to their ethnic background and that the majority (86%) of the population, including visible minorities, perceived they had not been discriminated against or unfairly treated (Government of Canada, 2003a).

Racism may be encountered in nursing practice (RNAO, 2007). The CHN may experience racism in client interactions, collegial nursing interactions, workplace organizational systems, and community systems. Racism in community health nursing practice needs to be labelled and addressed when it occurs or it can lead to oppression. It may also be detrimental to client health and access to health care services. The CHN needs to consider the culture of the clients and their associated lifestyles, health beliefs, and behaviours, as well as the power imbalance and possible oppression that might occur in each client–nurse interaction.

CRITICAL VIEW

1. To what extent do you think race influences health and health care for Aboriginal people?
2. Read "Racism as a Determinant of Immigrant Health" (Hyman, 2009) found at http://canada.metropolis.net/pdfs/racism_policy_brief_e.pdf.
    a) For CHNs, what are some of the equity issues related to health?
    b) What are some equity issues related to access to health care?

CULTURAL SAFETY

Cultural competence is defined by the health care provider, whereas cultural *safety* is defined by the client. Cultural safety recognizes the diversity, that is, the uniqueness of the client. **Cultural safety** refers to gaining an understanding of others' health beliefs and practices so that one's actions demonstrate working toward equity and the avoidance of discrimination by recognition and respect for cultural identity so that a power balance exists between the health care provider and client (Anderson et al., 2003; Srivastava, 2007). Gray and Thomas (2006) support the view of culture as relational, and as a sociopolitical construct it involves power relationships in health professional and client interactions. Therefore, when CHNs use a cultural safety lens, they involve the client to address health inequities and to strive for social justice.

De and Richardson (2008) maintain that cultural safety is based on the following three premises:

- Analysis by the health professional of their cultural self and its influence on client interactions
- Acknowledgement of the power imbalance favouring the health professional and addressing this so that the client cultural environment is safe
- Learning and applying new foundational skills by the health professional

These authors identify cultural awareness and cultural sensitivity as the steps to reaching cultural safety (De & Richardson, 2008). Cultural awareness is the initial understanding that variations exist, and cultural sensitivity is showing respect and valuing cultural diversity in CHN behaviours (Giger et al., 2007). Refer to Table 7-5 on pp. 202–203 for a further discussion of these two concepts. De and Richardson (2008) state, "Cultural safety is a way to work in highly diverse communities in a way that helps remove the barriers of 'power' and 'authority' and promotes equality. Working in this way places the responsibility for appropriateness firmly with the nurse while giving the service user the right to declare when care does not feel culturally sensitive or safe" (p. 330). For the CHN to work effectively with clients from varying cultural backgrounds and to provide culturally responsive health care, cultural safety and cultural competence need to be addressed and implemented in client interactions (De & Richardson, 2008; Dion Stout & Downey, 2006).

The concept of cultural safety was developed by Maori nurse leaders in New Zealand to gain an understanding of the health care interactions between indigenous Maori people and white European-descended health care providers (Anderson et al., 2003; Srivastava, 2007). The National Aboriginal Health Organization (NAHO) (2008) identified Aboriginal peoples as one group requiring cultural safety. The experiences of colonialism on non-European cultures have shaped the social systems and policies used in postcolonial times (Anderson et al., 2003; Boyer, 2006). In a discussion paper, the NAHO (2006) argues that colonization affected the traditional values and social structures of Aboriginals and also contributed to many of the inequalities in the health status of Aboriginal women in Canada. The sociopolitical context of colonialism encouraged the development of dominant systems of care, resulting in feelings of discrimination and disempowerment. Some of the historical colonial influences have carried over to the postcolonial times and warrant study, especially with regard to cultural safety. See the NAHO Weblink on cultural competency and safety.

Anderson and colleagues (2003) reported on two ethnographic studies exploring cultural safety within a postcolonial context. The study participants included Canadians of South Asian and Chinese ancestry who immigrated to Canada, Canadians of European ancestry who had been born in Canada, and health care providers. Their study findings and reflections in reference to cultural safety included the following:

- Participant accounts (both health care providers and clients) often identified issues of communication.
- Health care providers reported feeling distressed when unable to communicate with the clients, and clients who could not speak English were also distressed.
- Some non–English-speaking participants felt safe because they felt respected and observed health care provider behaviours that suggested the provision of appropriate care.
- Some clients who could communicate in English with health care providers reported feeling vulnerable.
- Some health care providers reported that they were too busy to seek out resources such as interpreters, and other health care providers decided that interpreter services were not needed.
- Language is critical if relationships are likely to be developed.

CRITICAL VIEW

Respond to the following questions:

1. a) To what extent might race, culture, gender, and social status influence CHNs' decisions to seek interpreter services?

   b) What can CHNs do if there are no interpreter services available in their community?
2. Should clients have the right to refuse care from a CHN (with a different cultural background) on the basis of cultural variations? Explain.
3. How would you communicate with clients to ensure feelings of cultural safety?

- People must be able to communicate with each other if they are to feel culturally safe.
- There is a need to identify what the meaning of communication is within culturally safe care.
- Nurses who were "women of colour" reported instances where they were discriminated against by white clients who refused care by these nurses.
- An older adult couple from the dominant culture reported possible discrimination based on age when assumptions were made by the health care providers that the couple did not require access to home care based on their social status and network.

CULTURAL NURSING ASSESSMENT

Culturally competent care requires culturally congruent attitudes, knowledge, and skills, which are developed and enhanced through cultural assessment. A **cultural nursing assessment** is a systematic way to identify the beliefs, values, meanings, and behaviours of people while considering their history, life experiences, and the social and physical environments in which they live.

CHNs need to conduct a cultural assessment for all clients when they first come in contact with them. It is important that CHNs be aware that some clients might be reluctant to acknowledge cultural identity openly, such as racial background, religion, age, and sexual orientation. This reluctance to disclose information may be due to a fear of prejudice, a commitment to assimilation as a Canadian, a fear of identification as an illegal immigrant, or discomfort with direct questioning or other forms of nonverbal communication such as direct eye contact. CHNs need to seek information from sources such as family members, interpreters, traditional cultural health practitioners, and educational resources on how to integrate cultural concepts into other aspects of client care to meet their clients' total health care needs. In addition, they need to be able to distinguish between cultural and socioeconomic class issues and not misinterpret behaviour as having a cultural origin when, in fact, it should be attributed to socioeconomic class. Giger and Davidhizar (2008) have identified many factors to be considered when conducting a cultural assessment, such as communication, space, social organization, time, environmental control, and biological variations. A synopsis of Giger and Davidhizar's Transcultural Assessment Model is provided in Appendix 7. CHNs need to know the following when completing a cultural assessment: population demographic changes in their practice area; general information about the various cultural groups; how and when to use a focused assessment; how to use an interpreter; and how to assess and consider the social, political, and economic factors in the community (Astle & Barton, 2009).

Evidence-Informed Practice

This article, focusing on nursing practice possibilities, was based on qualitative human science research completed to uncover the meaning of the lived experience of persons who have a different sense of hearing (Aquino-Russell, 2003, cited in Aquino-Russell, 2005). The meaning is this:

> *Living with a different sense of hearing is experiencing the joy-sorrow of hearing-not hearing unfolding through discovering gained-lost communication surfacing all-at-once with diminished-enhanced feelings of self while choosing the rhythm of revealing-concealing amid potential regard-disregard of others (Aquino-Russell, 2003, p. ii, cited in Aquino-Russell, 2005, p. 33).*

Examples of how persons wished to be treated were the following:

- I wish to be treated with respect and for others to stop labelling, stigmatizing, and treating me like I'm stupid.
- I wish health care professionals would just listen.

Evidence-Informed Practice—Cont'd

- I wish I only had to ask *once* for others to change their pattern of speaking to me, for example: to face me, to speak clearly and articulately, with no hands covering their faces or mouths.
- I wish for patience, understanding, and for others to keep trying to communicate with me rather than just giving up and saying "never mind" (Aquino-Russell, 2005, p. 34).

Enhanced understanding of lived experiences prepares CHNs to discover how individuals define and live with experiences in their own ways. Although research informs CHNs about lived experiences, it does not define them for others. Rather, it opens the way for others to be considered in the same and different ways. Each unique person will have an inimitable lived experience. Others can never truly understand what it is like to have a different sense of hearing, but clearly CHNs have the responsibility to listen to clients if they wish to describe what it is like and change their way of being, if needed.

Application for CHNs: When working with clients with a different sense of hearing, CHNs need to understand the importance of using a caring approach and enhanced communication skills to maximize their partnerships with each client and with this cultural group. CHNs need to demonstrate cultural competence and cultural safety in a l client interactions.

Questions for Reflection & Discussion

1. You are going to dc a home visit with a person who lives with a different sense of hearing. What might you consider related to communication strategies and practice possibilities prior to the visit? What questions might you ask during the visit?
2. You are going to be presenting a paper of an important health topic at the local chapter of the Canadian Hard of Hearing Association. What do you need to consider wnen doing this presentation? How might you prepare for the presentation?
3. Which of the components from the evidence-informed practice model discussed in Chapter 5 would be applicable to this research evidence?

REFERENCE: Aquino-Russell, C. (2005). Practice possibilities for nurses choosing true presence with persons who live with a different sense of hearing, *Nursing Science Quarterly, 18*(1), 32–36.

Giger and Davidhizar's (2008) cultural assessment model includes the following categories: culturally unique individual, communication, space, social organization, time, and biological variations. Under each category, the model provides items to consider in your assessment:

1. Culturally Unique Individual. CHNs need to elicit client cultural data as outlined in the "Culturally Unique Individual" section (see Appendix 7).
2. Communication. An understanding by the CHN of differences in communication patterns can help overcome communication barriers due to culture; therefore, the quality of client care will be improved. Some clients from diverse cultural backgrounds may be reluctant to speak to a traditional CHN about nontraditional health care beliefs and practices. The use of therapeutic communication skills such as conveying respect, warmth, and genuineness is necessary. The CHN should assess the client's need for an interpreter and, based on this need, make health care decisions based on the client's health concerns rather than based on interpreter accessibility and availability, and nursing time constraints.
3. Space. The physical distance between the client and the CHN is an important consideration in promoting the comfort level of the client during interactions. For example, Asians usually are more guarded about their personal space and prefer at least a space of 150 to 180 cm (5 to 6 feet) of distance in interactions; this is viewed as a sign of respect.
4. Social Organization. There are various types of family forms, such as traditional nuclear family, one-parent family, reconstructed or blended family, gay family, and communal family. CHNs need to incorporate the family cultural beliefs and concerns into a client care plan. For example, the CHN may arrange to meet with a group of clients to discuss child care within the context of their family cultural beliefs and practices.
5. Time. It is important for the CHN to recognize that clients from variant cultures may view time differently. The CHN may become quite frustrated when many members arrive approximately 30 minutes past the scheduled start time of the group meeting. A culturally sensitive CHN will be aware that this lateness is not an avoidance of the topic but rather reflects the group's cultural view of time.
6. Biological Variations. To provide culturally competent and safe nursing care, CHNs need to be familiar

CRITICAL VIEW

1. What should be included in completing a cultural assessment on the client (individual, family, and community)? Provide a rationale based on cultural considerations.
2. What are the specific questions that a CHN would need to ask for each area identified in question 1?

with the biological variations associated with racial groups and to consider the uniqueness of cultural groups and individuals. This awareness also needs to incorporate the fact that biological parameters are usually based on Caucasian standards and that these norms may not be applicable to non-Caucasian clients.

Skills such as listening, explaining, acknowledging, recommending, understanding, and negotiating help the CHN to be nonjudgemental. It is vital that CHNs listen to clients' perceptions of their health concerns and, in turn, that CHNs explain to clients their perceptions of their concerns. To develop recommendations for managing health concerns, CHNs and clients need to acknowledge and discuss similarities and variations between their perceptions. CHNs also negotiate with clients on nursing care actions to meet clients' needs.

LEVELS OF PREVENTION

Related to Culture and Literacy

PRIMARY PREVENTION

CHNs determine that the health information on immunization requirements is culturally appropriate and is at an appropriate health literacy level for each client.

SECONDARY PREVENTION

CHNs screen clients to determine literacy level so that programs are developed and provided at the appropriate health literacy level.

TERTIARY PREVENTION

CHNs, through intersectoral partnerships, establish literacy community programs and services to meet the needs of clients requiring culturally appropriate teaching about health during cardiac rehabilitation.

APPLICATION TO COMMUNITY HEALTH NURSING

Culture is a key determinant of health. All CHNs work with clients from a variety of cultural backgrounds. Therefore, when CHNs come in contact with clients who are culturally different from themselves, they need to adapt general cultural concepts to the situation until they are able to learn directly from the clients about their culture. CHNs can further develop cultural competence by reading about, taking courses on, and discussing various cultures within multicultural settings.

CHNs need to know if there are specific risk factors for a given cultural population. For example, Southeast Asians are often at risk for hepatitis B (with its attendant effects on the liver), tuberculosis, intestinal parasites, and visual, hearing, and dental problems; the incidence of hypertension in Blacks is higher and more severe and occurs earlier in life than in Caucasians (Arcangelo & Peterson, 2006); and the incidence of type 2 diabetes in Aboriginal peoples (First Nations, Inuit, and Métis) is considerably higher than in the general population. However, it is important to note that some health concerns that appear to be linked to culture may in fact be more closely linked to other social determinants of health. For example, the higher incidence of type 2 diabetes among Aboriginal peoples is linked to determinants of health such as low income, unemployment, lower educational levels, poor social conditions, and difficulty accessing health care (Statistics Canada, 2007b). Therefore, it is important for the CHN to consider that "it is these socioeconomic factors such as poverty, employment, housing, and violence, that have a great influence on health, not race and ethnicity" (Beckmann Murray, Proctor Zentner, Pangman, & Pangman, 2009, p. 9). The Ottawa Charter health promotion strategy of strengthening community action is evident in a variety of community-based projects in British Columbia related to diabetes (see the Health Canada *Making Change Happen* Weblink for examples).

CHNs need to understand the nontraditional healing practices that their clients use. Many of these treatments have proved effective and can be blended with traditional Western medicine. The key is to know which practices are being used so that the blending can be done knowledgeably. For example, Chinese clients may use traditional practices such as acupuncture or massage therapy, and Aboriginal peoples may wish to consult community elders, sometimes called shamans (Srivastava, 2007).

An awareness of cultural values, beliefs, and practices will guide the nurse in planning and delivering culturally appropriate, holistic care (Giger & Davidhizar, 2008). Different cultural groups have varying values and beliefs that are transmitted in different ways. The cultural values and beliefs need to be considered and respected by the CHN when planning health care for the client. For example, Aboriginal and Inuit peoples value harmony with the environment, spirituality, and family (Arnold & Bruce, 2005); most older Chinese Canadians believe that soup is good for their health (Lai & Surood, 2009); and some First Nations people use verbal stories to transmit cultural beliefs about life and reality (Arnold & Bruce, 2005). In order to plan appropriate nursing interventions with clients, CHNs need to be cognizant of the ways various cultures may transmit their cultural beliefs. CHNs need to explore clients' cultural values, beliefs, and behaviours rather than memorizing facts about each culture.

Working with Newcomer Populations

A **newcomer** is a person who arrives in a new country to settle there for a variety of reasons and with a variety of background experiences. Newcomers come from all parts of the world and bring with them unique cultural, health care, and religious backgrounds. In Statistics Canada information, the term most frequently applied to a newcomer is *immigrant.* However, newcomers include immigrants, refugees, and persons in need of protection, which are defined as follows: an **immigrant** is a person who has chosen to live in Canada and has been accepted by the Government of Canada and who may apply for permanent residency; a **refugee** is a person who has come to Canada, without choice, having had to leave his or her country because of persecution or war, or who lives in a refugee camp; and "a **person in need of protection** is a person who cannot return to his or her country because of a danger of torture, a risk of cruel and unusual treatment or punishment or a risk to his or her life and has been given protection by the Government of Canada" (Immigration and Refugee Board of Canada, 2009, p. 6).

Access to health care may be limited if newcomers lack health benefits, resources, language ability, and transportation. CHNs need to be astute in considering the cultural backgrounds of their newcomer clients and populations. Often, the community, and family if available, must be relied on to provide information, support, and other aid. Also, CHNs need to know the major health concerns and risk factors within each cultural group, such as vulnerability to specific diseases, and consider the social determinants of health. For further information on newcomers and stories of their experiences, see the Government of Canada *Going Places: Success Stories* and the United Nations Development Program Weblinks.

The complex issues surrounding newcomers and their health are beyond the scope of this discussion, but several issues are particularly relevant for CHNs as they may affect the health care of newcomers:

- Language barriers
- Low literacy levels
- Financial constraints
- Differences in social, religious, and cultural backgrounds between the newcomer and the health care provider
- Providers' lack of knowledge about high-risk diseases in the specific newcomer groups for whom they care
- The fact that many newcomers rely on traditional healing or folk health care practices that may be unfamiliar to their Canadian health care providers
- Refugees experience more physical and mental health problems, and tend to be poorer compared to immigrants (Beckmann Murray et al., 2009).

When working with newcomer populations, CHNs need to take into account that their own background, beliefs, and knowledge may be significantly different from those of the people receiving their care. CHNs can assess their cultural beliefs and practices by using cultural competence checklists.

CHNs need to be aware of the importance of the family to newcomer clients. Often, children and adolescents adjust to the new culture more easily than their elders do. This can lead to family conflict and, at times, violence that usually has warning signs of family stress and tension. On the other hand, family members can help translate their culture, religion, beliefs, practices, support systems, and risk factors for the health care provider. They also can assist with decision making and provide support to enable the person or group seeking care to change behaviours to become more health conscious. CHNs need to strive to understand the role of the family for newcomer populations and to treat individuals in the context of their families.

Similarly, the role of the community in the care of newcomers is important. Communities can help clients with communication, explanation, crisis intervention, emotional and other forms of support, and housing. CHNs need to assess the community carefully and learn what strengths, resources, and talents are available. For further information about newcomers, see the Ontario Council of Agencies Serving Immigrants (OCASI) Weblink.

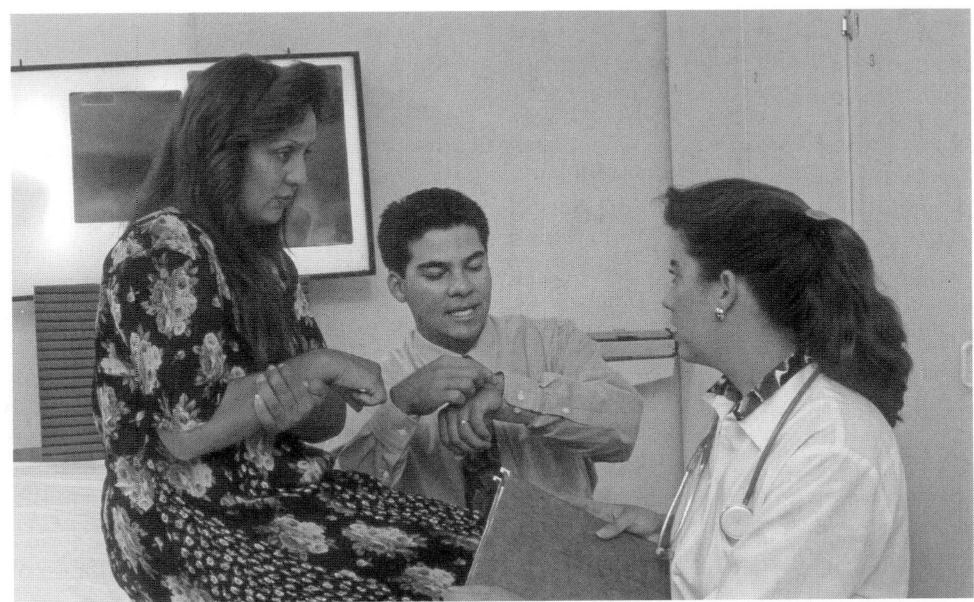

Community health nurses who come in contact with clients who are culturally different from themselves need to adapt general cultural concepts to the situation until they are able to learn directly from the clients about their culture. Here, a community health nurse is seen communicating with a client using an interpreter.

USING AN INTERPRETER

Clear communication between nurses and clients and their families is obviously of vital importance. Language barriers may interfere with CHNs' efforts to provide assistance or to obtain cultural assessments. When CHNs do not speak or understand the client's language, they need to obtain an interpreter (Ku & Flores, 2005). **Interpretation** is the process by which a spoken or signed message in one language is relayed, with the same meaning, in another language. Srivastava (2007) distinguishes **linguistic interpretation** as interpretation of spoken word only from **cultural interpretation,** being the interpretation of the spoken word but with additional information about the culture. **Translation** is the written conversion of one language into another (Health Canada, 2006). It is best not to use community members as interpreters; however, a lack of available interpreters residing outside the client community may warrant using community members. Regardless of the place of residence of the interpreter, the need for confidentiality must be addressed with the interpreter. Strategies to help CHNs select and use an interpreter effectively are listed in the "How To" box. In areas where interpreters are not available, the CHN could use interpreters at a distance by telephone or videoconferencing and provide paper-based information in a variety of languages that would meet the needs of the diverse populations in that community. Sometimes it may be necessary to use a health professional within the community to function as an interpreter.

How To... Select and Use an Interpreter

1. When feasible, select an interpreter who has knowledge of health-related terminology.
2. Use family members with caution because of the client's need for privacy when discussing intimate matters; family members may lack the ability to communicate effectively in both languages, and family members may

How To... Select and Use an Interpreter—Cont'd

exhibit a bias that influences the client's decisions.

3. The sex of the interpreter may be of concern; in some cultures, women may prefer a female interpreter and men may prefer a male.
4. The age of the interpreter may also be of concern. For example, older clients may want a more mature interpreter. Children tend to have limited understanding and language skills, and when used as interpreters, they may have difficulty interpreting the information.
5. Differences in socioeconomic status, religious affiliation, and educational level between the client and the interpreter may lead to problems in interpreting of information.
6. Identify the client's origin of birth and language or dialect spoken before selecting the interpreter. For example, Chinese clients speak different dialects depending on the region in which they were born.
7. Avoid using an interpreter from the same community as the client to avoid a possible breach of confidentiality.
8. Avoid using professional jargon, colloquialisms, abstractions, idiomatic expressions, slang, similes, and metaphors (Randall-David, 1994). Speak slowly and use words that are common in the client's culture.
9. Clarify roles with the interpreter.
10. Introduce the interpreter to the client and explain to the client what the interpreter will be doing.
11. Observe the client for nonverbal messages, such as facial expressions, gestures, and other forms of body language (Giger & Davidhizar, 1999). If the client's responses do not fit with the question, the nurse needs to check to be sure that the interpreter understood the question.
12. Increase accuracy in transmission of information by asking the interpreter to translate the client's own words and ask the client to repeat the information that the interpreter communicated.
13. At the end of the interview, review the material with the client to ensure that nothing has been missed or misunderstood.

SOURCES: Giger, J. N., & Davidhizar, R. (2004). *Transcultural nursing: Assessment and intervention* (4th ed.). St. Louis, MO: Mosby; Randall-David, E. (1994). *Culturally competent HIV counseling and education.* McLean, VA: Maternal and Child Health Clearinghouse.

Be aware that interpreters may not understand medical language, and this can influence the accuracy of the interpretation. Interpreters may emphasize their personal preferences by influencing both the nurse's and the client's decisions to select and participate in treatment modalities. CHNs may minimize this risk by learning basic words and sentences of the most commonly spoken languages in the community and by having key written materials translated into the language of sizable client populations. Five steps CHNs need to consider in order to work effectively with interpreters are these:

- Identify when the need for an interpreter exists.
- Use an appropriate interpreter.
- Explain the role of the interpreter and the health professional.
- Verbally engage the client in conversation.
- Monitor for interpretation errors (Srivastava, 2007).

See Box 7-5 for points that the CHN can use when working with clients requiring interpreters.

As in all areas of health care, resources for interpretation are finite and choices must be made about how best to serve the needs of the whole community. The degree of accommodation depends on the proportion of clients in the community who speak a language other than French or English. If there is a large volume of a particular cultural or linguistic group, agencies may be required to provide translations of all their written materials and to use interpreters regularly. If the volume of clients is not sufficiently large, perhaps only portions of the written materials will be translated and no interpreter provided. Health care agencies have a responsibility to communicate effectively with their clients. Literacy levels need to

BOX 7-5 Working with Interpreters: The Interpretation Session

- Face the client directly.
- Always speak in the first person as if talking directly to the client.
- Introduce yourself (and the interpreter) to the client(s).
- Describe your role and the purpose of the session.
- Speak slowly, clearly, and directly to the client, not the interpreter.
- While the interpreter is speaking, observe the client's nonverbal communication.
- Verify interpretations of any nonverbal behaviour ("I notice you are tapping your foot—is this something you do when you are nervous, or is there something else...?").
- Use simple language and short, straightforward sentences.
- Be patient; remember that the interpreter may require much more time to interpret something than you needed when you spoke in English.
- Ask open-ended questions as needed, to clarify what the client says or to hear what the client may wish to convey.
- Observe and evaluate what is going on before interrupting the interpreter.
- Always ask that the client repeat instructions.
- Provide written information (preferably in the client's language) for instructions, appointments, and contact information.
- Provide information as to how the client may access an interpreter (preferably the same interpreter) in the future.

SOURCE: Srivastava, R. H. (2007). *The health care professional's guide to clinical cultural competence*. Toronto, ON: Elsevier Canada, p. 140. Reprinted with permission.

be considered in any written and oral communication with clients. Communication needs to be in plain language—that is, language that is direct, clear, and simple, using common words.

It is important for CHNs when caring for clients to understand and respect culturally diverse populations by being comfortable with the aspects of cultural assessment with individuals, family, and community. Culturally competent CHNs need to reflect on their personal values, attitudes, and beliefs about health and culture and be open to change so that they can provide effective culturally competent care to clients in their practice. It is imperative that CHNs consider culture in its broadest sense as including groups based on age, socioeconomic status, and physical and mental abilities, and not just groups of newcomers.

STUDENT EXPERIENCE

Storytelling, for professional practice, can assist learners to develop ways of knowing and to explore issues (Lordly, 2007). Based on your past experiences and through storytelling, you will recognize similarities in your experiences and enhance your knowledge on culturally competent care.

1. Reflect and journal on one experience that you have had with one specific cultural group such as an ethnic group, a group of older adults, members of a homeless culture, the Deaf, or members of a drug culture.
2. Choose a culture that you are unfamiliar with and write, using storytelling, about
   a) Your attitudes, beliefs, values, and experiences as a member of that culture; and
   b) Your difficulties in accessing health care services.

REMEMBER THIS!

- The population of Canada is increasingly diverse. Changes in immigration laws and policies have increased migration, contributed to changes in community demographics, and heightened the need to recognize the impact of culture on health care and the need for nurses, particularly CHNs, to learn about the culture of the individuals for whom they provide care.
- Culture is a learned set of behaviours that are widely shared among a group of people; a people's culture helps guide individuals in problem solving and decision making. Culture is learned, adaptive, dynamic, invisible, shared, and selective.
- CHNs need to consider in assessment and planning, implementing, and evaluating nursing care that all cultures are not the same.
- Culturally competent community health nursing care incorporates the client's beliefs, values, attitudes, and behaviours and is provided with sensitivity. Such community health nursing care helps improve health outcomes and reduce health care costs.
- A culturally competent CHN uses cultural knowledge as well as specific skills, such as intracultural communication and cultural assessment, in assessing and selecting interventions for client care.
- Barriers to providing culturally competent care are stereotyping, prejudice and racism, ethnocentrism, and cultural shock.
- Cultural safety addresses the imbalance in power between CHNs and clients and is defined by the client.
- When CHNs use a cultural safety lens, they involve the client to address health inequities and to strive for achievement of social justice.
- CHNs need to perform a cultural assessment on every client with whom they interact. Cultural assessments help CHNs understand clients' perspectives of health and illness and thereby guide them in discussing culturally appropriate interventions. The needs of clients vary with their age, education, religion, and socioeconomic status.
- When CHNs do not speak or understand the client's language, they need to use an interpreter. In selecting an interpreter, CHNs need to consider clients' cultural needs and respect their right to privacy.

REFLECTIVE PRAXIS

Case Study

Shu Ping was concerned about her father's deteriorating health and contacted her friend, Sally Wong, a grade-school teacher, for advice. Mr. Ping recently immigrated to Canada from China to live with his only child, Shu. Mary, the CHN, had been visiting Mr. Ping since his recent discharge from the hospital, and he had asked her not to discuss his diagnosis with his family. After several contacts with Mr. Ping, Sally was able to establish a close enough relationship with Mr. Ping to engage him in a private discussion about his health. He confided to Sally that he had been diagnosed with cancer of the small intestine, and he feared he was dying. Mr. Ping did not want his family to know the "bad news." He refused treatment because he believed that people never got better after they were diagnosed with cancer; they always died.

1. What actions should Mary take that would demonstrate her ability to provide culturally competent care to the Ping family?
2. If Sally volunteered to be an interpreter for Mr. Ping, what are some of the possible limitations of this interaction that Mary would need to consider?
3. Identify how Mary would apply Giger and Davidhizar's Transcultural Assessment Model to the Ping family situation.

Answers are on the Evolve Web site at http://evolve.elsevier.com/Canada/Stanhope/community/.

What Would You Do?

1. Select a culture from your community that you would like to learn more about. Go to an appropriate Web site and gather information about the cultural group. Identify the group's health-seeking behaviours. Validate this information with a member of the group in your community. List differences between the two sources of data. How do you explain these findings? Explain how you can use this information in your clinical practice. Which major ethnic and religious groups

are represented in the community where you live? What resources are available to service their needs? What mechanisms are in place to facilitate access to these services by these groups?

2. Recall a first meeting with a client whose culture differed from yours. Did you form an immediate impression about the reason for the individual's contact with the health care system? Discuss your assumptions about this client. What led you to make them? How did your assumptions influence your interaction with the client or family member? Give specific examples.

3. Interview an older person. What would you do to prepare for this interview? Discuss the individual's perspective of health and illness. Explore the use of Western and alternative health practices and determine the individual's decision-making process in seeking out these health services. Prepare a list of alternative health care practitioners who practise in your community.

TOOL BOX

evolve

The Tool Box contains useful instruments that can be applied in community health nursing practice. These related resources are found either in the appendices at the back of this book or on the book's Web site at http://evolve.elsevier.com/Canada/Stanhope/community/.

Appendices

- Appendix 1: Canadian Community Health Nursing Standards of Practice
- Appendix 7: Giger and Davidhizar's Transcultural Assessment Model

Tools

Better Communication, Better Care: Provider Tools to Care for Diverse Populations.
This tool kit was prepared for health care professionals and contains information on how to interact and communicate with clients from diverse cultures.

Cultural Competence Checklist: Personal Reflection.
This Web-based tool is a one-page cultural competence checklist to increase awareness of how clients from different cultures are viewed.

Cultural Competence Checklist: Service Delivery.
This Web-based tool is a one-page cultural competence checklist to assess how to improve service delivery to culturally diverse clients.

WEBLINKS

evolve

Direct links to these resources can be found on the text's accompanying Evolve Web site at http://evolve.elsevier.com/Canada/Stanhope/community.

Canadian Nurses Association Position Statement. ***Promoting Culturally Competent Care.*** "The CNA believes that to provide the best possible patient outcomes, nurses must provide culturally competent care." At the home page, click on "CNA on the Issues" and select "Position Statements," then choose "Practice" in the legend on the left.

Government of Canada. ***Aboriginal Canada Portal.*** This Web site provides online resources and government programs and services about First Nations, Métis, and Inuit. Information can be found in many categories, including education, employment, research, and statistics. Selecting the "Research, Statistics and Maps" link takes the reader to a variety of choices on data on these cultural groups obtained from the 2006 census survey.

Government of Canada. ***Going Places: Success Stories.*** This Web site provides stories of newcomers living in various places across Canada and their experiences of moving to Canada.

Government of Nova Scotia. ***Cultural Competence Guide for Primary Health Care Professionals in Nova Scotia.*** This guide, prepared for Nova Scotia primary health care professionals, addresses the diverse communities of First Nations, African Canadians, immigrant Canadians, Acadians, and Francophone Canadians. The guide provides information on cultural competence that will be of value to primary health care professionals. It contains several excellent tools relevant to community health nursing practice.

Health Canada. ***Making Change Happen: Stories from British Columbia Diabetes Projects.*** This Web site includes stories of projects related to diabetes. For example, reducing barriers particularly related to culture is evident in projects titled "Stepping Their Way to Health" and "More Than Translating Pamphlets." These projects provide excellent examples of establishing community partnerships and sustainability.

Indian and Northern Affairs Canada. ***Government of Canada's Approach to Implementation of the Inherent Right and the Negotiation of Aboriginal Self-Government.*** This Web site contains information on existing policies pertaining to self-governance, approaches to self-government, and process issues.

National Aboriginal Health Organization (NAHO). ***Cultural Competency and Safety: A Guide for Healthcare Administrators, Providers, and Educators.*** This site provides a discussion on the historical development of cultural competency and cultural safety and an examination of the application of culturally safe environments in health care and education for First Nations, Inuit, and Métis.

National Aboriginal Health Organization (NAHO). ***Social Determinants of Métis Health.*** This resource provides information on the determinants of health for Canada's Aboriginal people and specifically speaks to Métis social determinants of well-being.

Ontario Council of Agencies Serving Immigrants (OCASI). ***Health Care Debate—The Impact on Newcomers.*** Go to this site for a discussion on the Supreme Court decision on access to private health care and its effect on the marginalized such as recent immigrants and refugees to Canada. It discusses the health care challenges for these aggregates.

Qulliit Nunavut Status of Women Council. ***The Little Voices of Nunavut: A Study of Women's Homelessness North of 60 Territorial Report.*** This research report provides qualitative study findings on Nunavut women's homelessness north of 60 degrees latitude, as well as the determinants of homelessness for this study population. Recommendations for change are also provided in this extensive report.

Registered Nurses' Association of Ontario. ***Embracing Cultural Diversity in Health Care: Developing Cultural Competence.*** This Web site provides extensive information on the background of cultural diversity and how to develop cultural competence for nurses.

Statistics Canada. ***Canada's Ethnocultural Mosaic, 2006 Census: Findings.*** A vast amount of information on the national profile of visible minorities in Canada, based on census 2006 data, can be found through this site. It also provides information on visible minorities in each province and the territories, including information such as ancestry and distribution of visible minorities, as well as information on visible minorities in various cities across Canada.

Statistics Canada. ***Canadian Social Trends: Asian Culture.*** This site provides the results of a Canadian survey and census data on the ethnic and cultural backgrounds of Canadians. The focus of this site is South Asians residing in Canada, and it provides historical background, statistics, and some of the beliefs and values held in South Asian culture.

Statistics Canada. ***Chinese Canadians: Enriching the Cultural Mosaic.*** The results of a Canadian survey and census data give information on the ethnic and cultural backgrounds of Chinese Canadians. The Web site provides historical background, statistics, and some of the beliefs and values held in the Chinese culture.

Statistics Canada. ***Portrait of Immigrants in Canada.*** This Web site provides information on immigrants numbers to Canada and supplies information on demographic variables such as age and marital status.

United Nations Development Programme. ***Human Development Report 2009.*** This report discusses how to foster understanding of mobility and human development and looks at the who, when, and why people move and how those who migrate manage in areas such as socioeconomic status, health, and education and explores policies relevant to migrants.

REFERENCES

Allender, J. A., & Spradley, B. W. (2005). *Community health nursing: Promoting and protecting the public's health* (6th ed.). Philadelphia, PA: Lippincott, Williams & Wilkins.

Anderson, J., Perry, J., Blue, C., Browne, A., Henderson, A., Khan, K., Smye, V. (2003). Rewriting cultural safety within the postcolonial and postnational feminist project: Towards new epistemologies of healing. *Advances in Nursing Science, 26*(3), 196–214.

Aquino-Russell, C. (2003). *Understanding the lived experience of persons who have a different sense of hearing.* Perth, Australia: Curtin University of Technology. Retrieved from http://adt.curtin.edu.au/theses/available/adt-WCU20040219.113721/.

Aquino-Russell, C. (2005). Practice possibilities for nurses choosing true presence with persons who live with a different sense of hearing. *Nursing Science Quarterly, 18*(1), 32–35.

Arcangelo, V., & Peterson, A. M. (2006). *Pharmacotherapeutics for advanced practice: A practical approach* (2nd ed.). Philadelphia, PA: Lippincott, Williams & Wilkins.

Arnold, O., & Bruce, A. (2005). Nursing practice with Aboriginal communities: Expanding worldviews. *Nursing Science Quarterly, 18*(3), 259–263.

Ashley, J. (1985). A personal account. In H. Orlans (Ed.), *Adjustment to adult hearing loss* (pp. 59–70). San Diego, CA: College Hill Press.

Astle, B. J., & Barton, S. (2009). Culture and ethnicity. In P. A. Potter, A. G. Perry, J. C. Ross-Kerr, & M. J. Wood (Eds.), *Canadian fundamentals of nursing* (4th ed., pp. 114–131). Toronto, ON: Elsevier Canada.

Astle, B. J., & Pacquiao, D. (2006). Culture and ethnicity. In P. A. Potter, A. G. Perry, J. C. Ross-Kerr, & M. J. Wood (Eds.), *Canadian fundamentals of nursing* (3rd ed., pp. 128–147). Toronto, ON: Elsevier Canada.

Auer, A. M., & Andersson, R. (2001). Canadian Aboriginal communities: A framework for injury surveillance. *Health Promotion International*, *16*(2), 169–177.

Beckmann Murray, R., Proctor Zentner, J., Pangman, V., & Pangman, C. (2009). *Health promotion strategies through the lifespan* (2nd Canadian ed.). Toronto, ON: Pearson Prentice Hall.

Belanger, A., & Malenfant, E. (2005). Ethnocultural diversity in Canada: Prospects for 2017. *Canadian Social Trends*, *79*, 18–21.

Bess, F. H., & Humes, L. E. (1995). *Audiology: The fundamentals* (2nd ed.). Baltimore, MD: Williams & Wilkins.

Boyer, Y. (2006). *Discussion paper series in Aboriginal health. Legal issues: First Nations, Métis, and Inuit Women's health.* Retrieved from http://www.naho.ca/english/documents/NAHOPaperNo.4.pdf.

Burchum, J. L. (2002). Cultural competence: An evolutionary perspective. *Nursing Forum*, *37*(4), 5–15.

Campinha-Bacote, J. (2002). The process of cultural competence in the delivery of healthcare services: A model of care. *Journal of Transcultural Nursing*, *13*(3), 181–184.

Canadian Association of the Deaf. (2007). *Statistics on Deaf Canadians.* Retrieved from http://www.cad.ca/en/issues/statistics_on_deaf_canadians.asp.

Canadian Hard of Hearing Association. (2010). *Broadcasting Notice of Consultation CRTC 2009-661 Review of community television policy framework.* Retrieved from http://chha.ca/documents/chha_submission032910.pdf.

Canadian Institutes of Health Research. (2006). *Evidence in action, acting on evidence: Exploring culturally respectful care in Aboriginal communities.* Retrieved from http://www.cihr-irsc.gc.ca/e/30680.html.

Canadian Nurses Association. (2004). *Promoting culturally competent care.* Retrieved from http://www.cna-nurses.ca/can/documents/pdf/publications/PS73_Promoting_Culturally_Competent_Care_March_2004_e.pdf.

Canadian Policy Research Network (2006). *Population projections for 2017.* Retrieved from http://www.cprn.com/en/diversity-2017.cfm?print = true.

Carson, M. G., & Mitchell, G. J. (1998). The experience of living with persistent pain. *Journal of Advanced Nursing*, *28*(6), 1242–1248.

Centre for Urban Health Initiatives. (2008). *Community based research.* Retrieved from http://www.utoronto.ca/cuhi/awards/merit.html.

Chansonneuve, D. (2005). *Reclaiming connections: Understanding residential school trauma among Aboriginal People.* A report prepared for the Aboriginal Healing Foundation. Ottawa: Aboriginal Healing Foundation.

Chui, T., Tran, K., & Flanders, J. (2005). *Chinese Canadians: Enriching the cultural mosaic.* Retrieved from http://estat.statcan.ca/contenglishish/articles/cst/cst-pop20.pdf.

Citizenship and Immigration Canada. (2008). *Minister Kenney announces immigration levels for 2009; Issues instructions on processing federal skilled workers.* Retrieved from http://www.cic.gc.ca/english/DEPARTMENT/MEDIA/releases/2008/2008-11-28.asp.

Clair, J., Beatty, J., & MacLean, T. (2005). Out of sight but not out of mind: Managing invisible social identities in the workplace. *Academy of Management Review*, *30*(1), 78–95.

Community Health Nurses Association of Canada. (2008). *Canadian community health nursing standards of practice.* Retrieved from http://chnc.ca/documents/chn_standards_of_practice_mar08_english.pdf.

Court of Appeal for British Columbia. (2009). *McIvor versus Canada (Registrar of Indian and Northern Affairs)*. BCCA 153. Retrieved from http://www.kahnawake.com/org/docs/McIvorDecision.pdf.

De, D., & Richardson, J. (2008). Cultural safety: An introduction. *Pediatric Nursing*, *20*(2), 39–43.

Deaf and Hard of Hearing Society. (2010). *Rights and responsibilities.* Retrieved from http://www.dhhs.ca/programs-services/interpreting-services/right-responsibilities/.

Dickason, O. P., & McNab, D. (2009). *Canada's First Nations: A history of founding peoples from earliest times* (4th ed., pp. 315–335). Toronto: Oxford University Press.

Dion Stout, M., & Downey, B. (2006). Nursing, Indigenous peoples and cultural safety: So what? Now what? *Contemporary Nurse*, *22*, 327–332.

Dion Stout, M., & Kipling, G. (2003). *Aboriginal people, resilience and the residential school legacy.* Ottawa: The Aboriginal Healing Foundation.

Dutcher, L. (2008). *Colonization and the health impacts on Aboriginal people in Canada.* Unpublished course paper for History 3374. University of New Brunswick.

Eliason, J. (1998). Correlates of prejudice in nursing students. *Journal of Nursing Education*, *37*(1), 27–29.

Foster, C. H. (2006). What nurses should know when working in Aboriginal communities. *Canadian Nurse*, *102*(4), 28–31.

Gatehouse, S., Naylor, G., & Elberling, C. (2003). Benefits of hearing aids in relation to the interaction between user and the environment. *International Journal of Audiology*, *42*, S77–S85. Retrieved from http://213.129.10.63/eprise/main/SiteGen/Uploads/Public/Downloads_Oticon/GSRC/Benefits_of_Hearing_Aids.pdf.

Getty, L., & Hetu, R. (1994). Is there a culture of hard-of-hearing workers? *Journal of Speech-Language Pathology & Audiology*, *18*(4), 267–270.

Giger, J. N., & Davidhizar, R. (1999). *Transcultural nursing: Assessment and intervention* (3rd ed.). St. Louis, MO: Elsevier Science.

Giger, J. N., & Davidhizar, R. (2004). *Transcultural nursing: Assessment and intervention* (4th ed.). St. Louis, MO: Mosby.

Giger, J. N., & Davidhizar, R. E. (2008). *Transcultural nursing: Assessment and intervention* (5th ed.). St. Louis, MO: Mosby Elsevier.

Giger, J., Davidhizar, R., Purnell, L., Harden, J., Phillips, J., & Strickland, O. (2007). American Academy of nursing expert panel report: Developing cultural competence to eliminate health disparities in ethnic minorities and other visible populations. *Journal of Transcultural Nursing*, *18*(2), 95–102.

Government of Canada. (2003a). *Government of Canada survey reveals diversity trends in Canadian society*. Retrieved from http://www.pch.gc.ca/newsroom/index_e.cfm?fuseaction=displayDocument&DocIDCd=3N0292.

Government of Canada. (2003b). *Views on racism*. Retrieved from http://www.pch.gc.ca/progs/em-cr/eval/archive/2002_15/5_e.cfm.

Government of Canada. (2006). *What is multiculturalism?*. Retrieved from http://www.canadianheritage.gc.ca/progs/multi/what-multi_e.cfm.

Government of Nova Scotia. (2005a). *A cultural competence guide for primary health care professionals in Nova Scotia*. Retrieved from http://healthteamnovascotia.ca/cultural_competence/Cultural_Competence:guide_for_Primary_Health_Care_Professionals.pdf.

Government of Nova Scotia. (2005b). *Cultural competence guidelines for the delivery of primary health care in Nova Scotia*. Retrieved from http://www.healthteamnovascotia.ca/cultural_competence/CulturalCompetenceGuidelines_Summer08.pdf.

Gray, P. D., & Thomas, D. J. (2006). Critical reflections on culture in nursing. *Journal of Cultural Diversity*, *13*(2), 76–82.

Health Canada. (2006). *Language barriers in access to health care*. Retrieved from http://www.hc-sc.gc.ca/hcs-sss/pubs/acces/2001-lang-acces/index-eng.php.

Health Canada. (2008). *Fact Sheet: First Nations and Inuit Health Branch*. Retrieved from http://www.hc-sc.gc.ca/ahc-asc/branch-dirgen/fnihb-dgspni/fact-fiche-eng.php.

Health Council of Canada. (2005). *The health status of Canada's First Nations, Métis and Inuit Peoples*. Retrieved from http://healthcouncilcanada.ca.c9.previewyoursite.com/docs/papers/2005/BkgrdHealthyCdnsENG.pdf.

Helin, C. (2006). *Dances with dependency: Indigenous success through self-reliance*. Vancouver, BC: Orca Spirit Publishing and Communications.

Howell, D. (1998). Reaching to the depths of the soul: Understanding and exploring meaning in illness. *Canadian Oncology Nursing Journal*, *8*(1), 12–23.

Human Resources and Skill Development Canada. (2010). *Canadians in context—Aboriginal population*. Retrieved from http://www.4.hrsdc.gc.ca/.3ndic.1t.4r@-eng.jsp?iid=36.

Hyman, I. (2009). *Racism as a determinant of immigrant health*. Ottawa, ON: Public Health Agency of Canada. Retrieved from http://canada.metropolis.net/pdfs/racism_policy_brief_e.pdf.

Immigration and Refugee Board of Canada. (2009). *An overview*. Retrieved from http://www.cisr-irb.gc.ca/eng/brdcom/publications/oveape/Pages/index.aspx.

Indian and Northern Affairs Canada. (1996a). *The burden of ill health: From the past to the present*. Retrieved from http://www.collectionscanada.gc.ca/webarchives/20071115053257/http://www.ainc-inac.gc.ca/ch/rcap/sg/sgmm_e.html.

Indian and Northern Affairs Canada. (1996b). *Report of the Royal Commission on Aboriginal Peoples (RCAP)*. Retrieved from http://www.collectionscanada.gc.ca/webarchives/20071115053257/http://www.ainc-inac.gc.ca/ch/rcap/sg/sgmm_e.html.

Inuit Tapiriit Kanatami. (2007). *Inuit in Canada: A statistical profile, 2007*. Retrieved from http://www.itk.ca/system/files/Inuit-Statistical-Profile.pdf.

Inuit Tapiriit Kanatami. (2009). *Inuit in Canada*. Retrieved from http://www.itk.ca/Inuit-Approaches-to-Suicide-Prevention.

Ipsos-Reid. (2005). *March 21st, international day for the elimination of racial discrimination: One in six Canadians say they have been the victim of racism*. Retrieved from http://www.dominion.ca/Downloads/IRracismSurvey.pdf.

Jarvis, C. (2004). *Physical examination and health assessment* (4th ed.). St. Louis, MO: Elsevier Science.

Ku, L., & Flores, G. (2005). Pay now or pay later: Providing interpreter services in health care. *Health Affairs*, *24*(2), 435–444.

Kulig, J. C. (2000). Culturally diverse communities: The impact on the role of community health nurses. In M. J. Stewart (Ed.), *Community nursing promoting Canadians' health* (2nd ed., pp. 194–210). Toronto, ON: Harcourt Canada.

Lai, D. W. L., & Surood, S. (2009). Chinese health beliefs of older Chinese in Canada. *Journal of Aging and Health*, *21*(1), 38–62.

Leininger, M. (2002). Essential transcultural nursing care concepts, principles, examples, and policy statements. In M. M. Leininger, & M. McFarland (Eds.), *Transcultural nursing: Concepts, theories, research, and practices* (3rd ed., pp. 45–69). New York: McGraw-Hill.

Lordly, D. (2007). Once upon a time.... Storytelling to enhance teaching and learning. *Canadian Journal of Dietetic Practice and Research*, *68*(1), 30–35.

Maville, J. A., & Huerta, C. G. (2008). *Health promotion in nursing*. Clifton Park, NY: Thomson Delmar Learning.

McCreary Stebnicki, J. A., & Coeling, H. V. (1999). The culture of the Deaf. *Journal of Transcultural Nursing*, *10*(4), 350–357. Retrieved from http://tcn.sagepub.com/cgi/content/short/10/4/350 DOI: 10.1177/104365969901000413.

Métis National Council. (2009). Métis definition. Retrieved from http://www.metisnation.ca/who/definition.html.

Misener, T. R., Sowell, R. L., Phillips, K. D., & Harris, C. (1997). Sexual orientation: A cultural diversity issue for nursing. *Nursing Outlook*, *45*(4), 178–181.

National Aboriginal Health Organization. (2006). *Discussion paper series in Aboriginal health: Legal issues: First Nations, Métis, and Inuit women's health*. Retrieved from http://www.naho.ca/english/documents/NAHOPaperNo.4.pdf.

National Aboriginal Health Organization. (2008). *Cultural competency and safety: A guide for health administrators, providers, and educators*. Retrieved from http://www.naho.ca/publications/culturalCompetency.pdf.

Nova Scotia Department of Health. (2005). *A cultural competence guide for primary health care professionals in Nova Scotia*. Retrieved from http://www.healthteamnovascotia.ca/cultural_competence/Cultural_Competence:guide_for_Primary_Health_Care_Professionals.pdf.

Ontario Human Rights Commission. (2008). *Racism and racial discrimination: Your rights and responsibilities*. Retrieved from http://www.ohrc.on.ca/en/issues/racism.

Padden, C. (2000). The Deaf community and the culture of Deaf people. In M. Adams (Ed.), *Readings for diversity and social justice* (pp. 343–352). New York: Routledge.

Padden, C., & Humphries, T. (2005). *Inside Deaf culture*. Cambridge, MA: Harvard University Press.

Pottinger, A., Perivolaris, A., & Howes, D. (2007). The end of life. In R. H. Srivastava (Ed.), *The health care professional's guide to clinical cultural competence* (pp. 227–246). Toronto, ON: Mosby Elsevier.

Public Health Agency of Canada. (2003). *What makes Canadians healthy or unhealthy?*. Retrieved from http://www.phac-aspc.gc.ca/ph-sp/determinants/determinants-eng.php.

Quan, H., Fong, A., DeCoster, C., Wang, J., Musto, R., Noseworthy, T. W., et al. (2006). Variation in health services utilization among ethnic populations. *Canadian Medical Association Journal, 174*(6), 787–791.

Randall-David, E. (1994). *Culturally competent HIV counseling and education*. McLean, VA: Maternal and Child Health Clearinghouse.

Raphael, D. (in press). Critical perspectives on the social determinants of health. In E. McGibbon (Ed.), *Oppression as a determinant of health*. Halifax, NS: Fernwood Publishers.

Registered Nurses' Association of Ontario. (2007). *Embracing cultural diversity in health care: Developing cultural competence*. Retrieved from http://www.rnao.org/Storage/29/2336_BPG_Embracing_Cultural_Diversity.pdf.

Smylie, J. (2000). A guide for health professionals working with Aboriginal Peoples: The sociocultural context of Aboriginal Peoples in Canada. *Journal of SOGC, 100*, 1–12.

Srivastava, R. H. (2007). *The health care professional's guide to clinical cultural competence*. Toronto, ON: Elsevier Canada.

Stanhope, M., & Lancaster, J. (2010). *Foundations of nursing in the community: Community-oriented practice* (3rd ed.). St. Louis, MO: Mosby Elsevier.

Statistics Canada. (2003). *2001 Census: analysis series. Aboriginal peoples of Canada: A demographic profile* (Catalogue no. 96F0030XIE2001007). Ottawa: Author.

Statistics Canada. (2005a). *Population projections of visible minority groups, Canada, provinces and regions 2001–2017*. Retrieved from http://www.statcan.ca/english/freepub/91-541-XIE/91-541-XIE2005001.pdf.

Statistics Canada. (2005b). *Projections of the Aboriginal populations, Canada, provinces and territories 2001 to 2017*. Retrieved from http://www.statcan.ca/english/freepub/91-547-XIE/91-547-XIE2005001.pdf.

Statistics Canada. (2007a). *2006 Census: Immigration, citizenship, language, mobility and migration*. Retrieved from http://www.statcan.gc.ca/daily-quotidien/071204/dq071204a-eng.htm.

Statistics Canada. (2007b). *Study: Sports participation among Aboriginal children*. Retrieved from http://www.statcan.gc.ca/daily-quotidien/070710/dq070710b-eng.htm.

Statistics Canada. (2009a). *Earnings and incomes of Canadians over the past quarter century, 2006 Census*. (Cat. No. 97-563-XIE2006001). Ottawa: Author. Retrieved from http://www.12.statcan.ca/census-recensement/2006/as-sa/97-563/p13-eng.cfm.

Statistics Canada. (2009b). *Population by selected ethnic origins, by province and territory (2006 census)*. Retrieved from http://www.40.statcan.ca/l01/cst01/demo26a.htm.

Statistics Canada. (2009c). *2006 Census: Aboriginal Peoples in Canada in 2006: Inuit, Métis and First Nations, 2006 Census: Highlights*. Retrieved from http://www.12.statcan.ca/census-recensement/2006/as-sa/97-558/p1-eng.cfm.

Statistics Canada. (2009d). *2006 census: The evolving linguistic portrait, 2006 census: Sharp increase in population with a mother tongue other than English or French*. Retrieved from http://www.12.statcan.ca/census-recensement/2006/as-sa/97-555/p2-eng.cfm.

Statistics Canada. (2009e). *Visible minority population, by province and territory (2006 census)*. Retrieved from http://www.40.statcan.ca/l01/cst01/demo52a.htm.

Statistics Canada. (2010). *Canada's ethnocultural mosaic, 2006 census: National picture*. Retrieved from http://www.12.statcan.ca/census-recensement/2006/as-sa/97-562/p6-eng.cfm.

Tran, K., Kaddatz, J., & Allard, P. (2005). *South Asians in Canada: Unity through diversity*. Retrieved from http://www.cansim.org/english/kits/pdf/social/asian.pdf.

Vernon, M. (1989). Assessment of persons with hearing disabilities. In T. Hunt, & C. J. Lindley (Eds.), *Testing older adults: A reference guide for geopsychological assessments* (pp. 150–162). Austin, TX: Pro-Ed, Inc.

Vollman, A. R., Anderson, E. T., & McFarlane, J. (2008). *Canadian community as partner: Theory and multidisciplinary practice* (2nd ed.). Philadelphia, PA: Lippincott, Williams & Wilkins.

Wesley-Esquimaux, C., & Smolewski, M. (2004). *Historical trauma and Aboriginal healing: A report prepared for the Aboriginal Healing Foundation*. Ottawa, ON: Aboriginal Healing Foundation.

World Health Organization. (2007). *A conceptual framework for action on the social determinants of Health*. Discussion paper for the Commission on Social Determinants of Health. Geneva: Author.

World Health Organization. (2009). *The determinants of health*. Retrieved from http://www.who.int/hia/evidence/doh/e.

World Health Organization. (2010). *Fact sheet No. 300—Deafness and hearing impairment*. Retrieved from http://www.who.int/mediacentre/factsheets/fs300/en/index.html.

CHAPTER

8

Epidemiological Applications

KEY TERMS

See Glossary on page 593 for definitions.

OBJECTIVES

After reading this chapter, you should be able to:

1. Define epidemiology and describe how it has developed over time.
2. Describe the essential concepts of epidemiology and an epidemiological approach.
3. Discuss the steps in the epidemiological process.
4. Describe the basic methods used in epidemiology.
5. Analyze critically the concept of screening and screening tests used in epidemiology.
6. Explain the basic epidemiological concepts of population at risk, natural history of disease, levels of prevention, host–agent–environment relationships, and the web-of-causation model.
7. Differentiate among descriptive, analytical, ecological, and experimental or intervention epidemiological studies.
8. Explain how community health nurses use epidemiology in their nursing practice.

CHAPTER OUTLINE

Epidemiology is the study of the distribution and factors that determine the health, related states, or events in a population, as well as the use of this information to control health problems. The term originally referred to infectious epidemics, such as cholera or tuberculosis (TB). It now includes infectious diseases; chronic diseases, such as cancer and cardiovascular disease; mental health–related and other health-related events, including accidents, injuries, and violence; occupational and environmental exposures and their effects; and even positive health states. The public health science of epidemiology has made major contributions to (1) understanding the factors that contribute to health and disease, (2) the development of health promotion and disease prevention measures, (3) the detection and characterization of emerging infectious agents, (4) the evaluation of health services and policies, and (5) the practice of nursing in community health. This chapter presents a review of the key epidemiological concepts and processes. CHNs need to have knowledge of epidemiological data and to have the skill of using these data. Readers are encouraged to consult epidemiological resources that provide detailed information.

DEFINITIONS

Epidemiology investigates the **distribution,** or the patterns, of health events in populations and the determinants or the factors that influence those patterns. When using the term **descriptive epidemiology,** one looks at health outcomes in terms of what, who, where, and when. What is the disease? Who is affected? Where are they? When do these events occur? Thus, descriptive epidemiology discusses a disease in terms of person, place, and time. On the other hand, **analytical epidemiology** looks at the etiology (origins or causes) of the disease and deals with determinants of health and disease, which, as discussed in Chapter 1, are the factors, exposures, characteristics, and behaviours that determine (or influence) the patterns. How does it occur? Why are some people affected more than others? Determinants may be individual, relational, social, communal, or environmental.

Epidemiology, like both the research process and community health nursing process, consists of a set of steps. The first step is to define the outcome. The health outcome can be a disease, or it can refer to injuries, accidents, or even wellness. Using epidemiological methods, a CHN describes the distribution—who, where, and when—of a disease, event, or injury and searches for factors that explain the pattern or risk of occurrence. The CHN asks what influences the occurrence of a particular disease or injury or why and how events occurred as they did.

Like nursing, epidemiology builds on and draws from other disciplines and methods, including clinical medicine, laboratory sciences, social sciences, quantitative methods (especially biostatistics), and public health policy and goals, among others. Important distinctions are that epidemiology focuses on *populations,* whereas clinical medicine focuses on the diagnosis and treatment of disease in *individuals.* As well, epidemiology studies populations to determine the causes of health and disease in communities and to investigate and evaluate interventions that will prevent disease and maintain health.

Epidemiology differs from clinical medicine in that it studies populations to (1) monitor the health of the population, (2) identify the determinants of health and disease in communities, and (3) investigate and evaluate interventions to prevent disease and maintain health. Effective community health nursing practice connects the disciplines of epidemiology, medicine, and nursing. CHNs focus on clients as populations, groups/aggregates, and as individuals, and on the health care provided for the identified client. Focus by CHNs is also on the broader context in which clients live and the complex interplay of social and environmental factors that affect their well-being. This task involves CHNs using epidemiological methods and findings in identifying and developing community health programs and in implementing preventive measures.

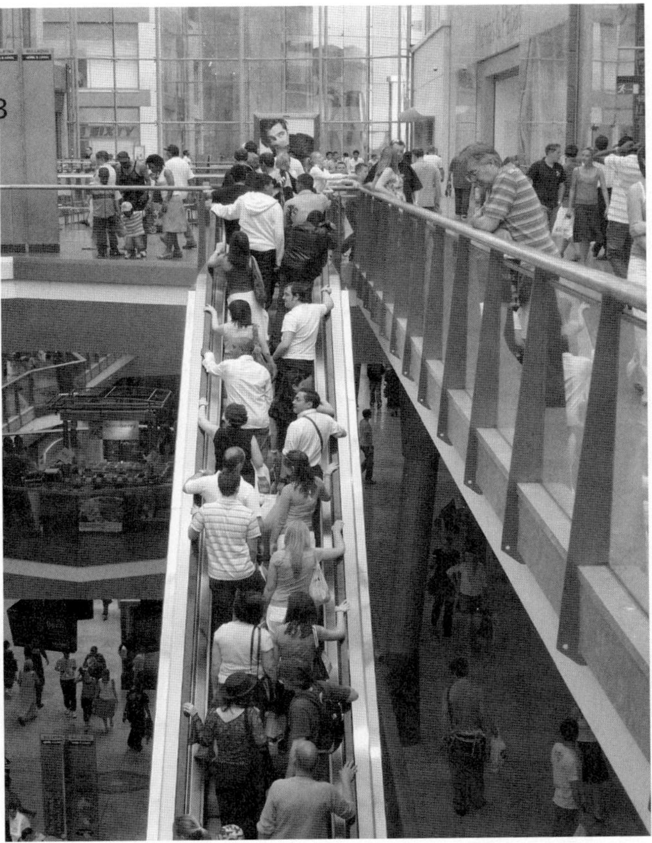

Epidemiology is the study of the health of populations.

HISTORY

Hippocrates was the first to use the ideas that are now part of epidemiology as early as in the fourth century BC (Merril & Timmreck, 2006). He examined health and disease in a community by looking at geography, climate, the seasons of the year, the food and water consumed, and the habits and behaviours of the people. His approach, like descriptive epidemiology, looked at how health is influenced by personal characteristics, place, and time. During the nineteenth century, Louis Pasteur developed the germ theory as well as pasteurization. Pasteur also recognized the role of personal factors, such as immunity and host resistance, when he saw that only certain people were susceptible to disease (Vandenbroucke, 1990). Other major discoveries during this century were made by Joseph Lister, a British surgeon, who developed antiseptic surgery, and Robert Koch, a German scientist, who developed pure culture and identified the organisms that cause such diseases as TB, anthrax, and cholera. In the eighteenth and nineteenth centuries, the comparison of groups began to be used to measure change in or the effects of some action or treatment on an experimental group. Also at this time, quantitative methods (numerical measurements or counts) came into use. One of the most famous studies using a comparison group is the mid-nineteenth-century investigation of cholera by John Snow, whom some call the "father of epidemiology" (Merril & Timmreck, 2006). Snow drew a map of the areas of cholera occurrence and found that the cases were clustered around a single public water pump. He was thus able to show that the contaminated water supply was related to the outbreak of cholera. He later observed that cholera rates were higher among households supplied with water obtained from downstream than among households whose water came from farther upstream, where there was less contamination. However, when households in the same area had different sources of water, differences observed in rates of cholera could not be attributed to location or economic status. Snow showed that households receiving water from the Lambeth Company, which moved its water intake away from sewage contamination, had cholera rates considerably lower than those supplied by Southwark and Vauxhall, a company that still drew water from a contaminated section of the river. Snow conducted a "natural experiment" (see Table 8-1) and was able to document that foul water was the vehicle of transmission of the agent that caused cholera (Rothman, 2002).

In the field of nursing, Florence Nightingale made a major contribution to the development of epidemiology in her work with British soldiers during the Crimean War (1854–1856). At this time, sick and injured soldiers were cared for in cramped quarters that had poor sanitation, were infested by lice and rats, and had insufficient food and medical supplies. She looked at the relationship between the environmental conditions and the recovery of the soldiers. Using simple epidemiological measures, such as rate of illness per 1,000 soldiers, she was able to show that improving environmental conditions and additional nursing care decreased the mortality rates among the soldiers (Cohen, 1984; Palmer, 1983).

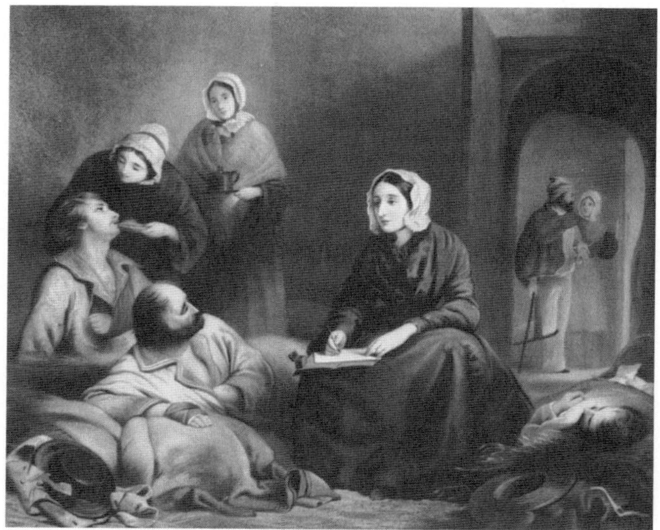

Florence Nightingale, a skilled statistician for her time, had a significant influence on the study of epidemiology.

TABLE 8-1 Cholera Death Rates per Household by Source of Water Supply in John Snow's 1853 Investigation

Company	Number of Houses	Death from Cholera	Deaths per 10,000 Households
Southwark and Vauxhall	40,046	1263	315
Lambeth	26,107	98	37
Rest of London	256,423	1422	59

Source: Snow, J. (1855). On the mode of communication of cholera. In *Snow on cholera*. New York, NY: The Commonwealth Fund.

Several changes followed and influenced the development of epidemiology. Before the twentieth century, the epidemiological focus was on the elimination of infectious diseases, such as cholera and bubonic plague (Naidoo & Wills, 2005). Improvements in sanitation, water, and housing were considered most essential to improve health. During the twentieth century, prevention and treatment of many infectious and communicable diseases were made possible, and the study of the causes of death shifted to chronic conditions, such as heart disease and cancer. Negative lifestyle factors have been found to contribute to many of the chronic conditions that lead to death. Highly effective vaccinations, immunizations, and mass screening programs contributed to the downward shift in disease (morbidity) and death (mortality) statistics.

Table 8-2 shows the leading causes of death in Canada for the years 2003 to 2006 (Statistics Canada, 2010a). Many of these deaths were due to chronic illnesses. Within a biomedical approach, cardiovascular diseases are often associated with negative lifestyle behaviours, such as smoking, unhealthy diets, and physical inactivity (Spenceley, 2007). Raphael (2009) reports that the social determinants of health, specifically those that affect socio-economic conditions for the client, contribute to chronic disease and other negative health outcomes. The Health Nexus and the Ontario Chronic Disease Prevention Alliance document titled *Primer to Action: Social Determinants of Health* (see the Weblinks on the Evolve Web site) provides the reader with information on the relationship of the social determinants of health and chronic disease and suggests actions to be taken.

In addition, the development of genetic and molecular techniques increased the epidemiologist's ability to classify persons in terms of exposures or inherent susceptibility to disease. Examples included the identification of genetic traits that indicated an increased risk for breast cancer and markers that identified exposures to environmental toxins, such as lead or pesticides. These developments are of particular interest to CHNs who deal with people in their living and work environments and

TABLE 8-2 Age-Standardized Mortality Rates in Canada by Selected Causes (Both Sexes), 2003 and 2005

	Rates per 100,000 Population		
	2003	2005	2006
All causes of death	586.9	563.7	540.5
Septicemia	4.0	4.1	4.3
Viral hepatitis	1.0	1.0	1.1
HIV/AIDS	1.3	1.3	1.2
Malignant neoplasms (colon, rectum, anus, pancreas, trachea, bronchus, lung, breast)	175.6	170.3	166.5
Diabetes mellitus	20.5	19.1	17.1
Alzheimer's disease	13.1	12.7	12.0
Cardiovascular disease (ischemic and other)	133.3	121.5	113.5
Cerebrovascular diseases	37.7	32.5	30.7
Influenza and pneumonia	12.0	13.2	11.2
Chronic lower respiratory diseases	25.8	25.1	22.7
Chronic liver disease and cirrhosis	6.4	6.1	6.0
Renal failure	8.5	8.3	8.1
Certain conditions originating in the perinatal period	4.2	4.4	4.1
Congenital malformations, deformations, and chromosomal abnormalities	3.3	3.2	3.0
Accidents (unintentional injuries)	25.5	25.6	25.3
Intentional self-harm (suicide)	11.3	10.9	10.0
Assault (homicide)	1.5	1.9	1.6

Note: Age-standardized mortality rates are calculated using the 1991 population of Canada as standard population.

Source: Adapted from Statistics Canada. (2010). *Summary tables, latest indicator tables.* CANSIM, Table 102-0552. Last modified May 13, 2009. Retrieved from http://www40.statcan.gc.ca/l01/cst01/health30a-eng.htm.

have to understand the interaction of environment(s) on health and well-being. CHNs are then enabled to assess a broad range of health outcomes as well as factors that contribute to wellness and illness.

Unfortunately, in recent years, new infectious diseases (e.g., Lyme disease, legionnaires' disease, hantavirus, Ebola virus, severe acute respiratory syndrome [SARS], HIV/AIDS, avian influenza), as well as new forms of old diseases (e.g., drug-resistant strains of TB, new forms of *Escherichia coli* [*E. coli*]), have emphasized the potential dangers to community health. Also, possible threats from terrorist attacks with infectious agents (e.g., anthrax, smallpox) have once again brought infectious disease epidemiology to the spotlight. There is an urgency to use epidemiological tools to safeguard the community and to improve health care management. As mentioned earlier, epidemiological methods are applied to a broader spectrum of health-related outcomes, including accidents, injuries, and violence; occupational and environmental exposures; psychiatric and sociological phenomena; health-related behaviours; and health services research.

In the United States, following the terrorist attacks of September 11, 2001, and the apparently unrelated appearances of "anthrax letters," public health acquired a broader significance and heightened public awareness. In Canada, in 2004, the Public Health Agency of Canada (PHAC) was established in response to the SARS outbreak, with additional responsibilities for chronic disease prevention, injury prevention, and emergency preparedness (Issa, 2008; PHAC, 2006). In the United States and especially in Canada, there is renewed awareness of the importance of a sound public health infrastructure, particularly with regard to disease surveillance and outbreak investigations. This infrastructure can carry on critical day-to-day public health functions while also monitoring, anticipating, and responding to events. Epidemiologists were among the first to respond to events such as the 9/11 terrorist attacks, anthrax letters, and SARS. Subsequently, numerous epidemiological studies were designed and initiated to understand the impact of a range of exposures related to those events. Epidemiological methods and epidemiologists play a key role in public health planning and emergency preparedness.

HEALTH SURVEILLANCE

The Government of Canada provided funding in 2004 to support the start-up of the pan-Canadian Health Surveillance System as an electronic information system to collect health data that would guide public health actions in areas such as communicable diseases and population health issues, as well as the management of infectious diseases (KPMG, 2009). One resulting initiative is the Centre for Surveillance Coordination, which offers internet-based training called "Skills Enhancement for Health Surveillance." This initiative, through self-study modules, provides health professionals across Canada opportunities for skills enhancement in epidemiology, surveillance, and information management (PHAC, 2007). **Health surveillance** is defined by the Network for Health Surveillance in Canada as "the tracking and forecasting of any health event or health determinant through the collection of data, and its integration, analysis and interpretation into surveillance products, and the dissemination of those surveillance products to those who need to know" (cited in Shah, 2003, p. 89). Health surveillance is an important aspect of public health and will be discussed later.

DETERMINANTS OF HEALTH

The "Determinants of Health" box on p. 225 provides examples of populations and their determinants of health. Socioeconomic status has been identified as one of the most influential determinants of health. The term *socioeconomic status* includes income and social position, education, employment, and working conditions. Gender is also a determinant of health, and research findings often demonstrate differences between men and women in areas such as disease processes and access to care (Gender & Health Collaborative Curriculum, 2009). Income influences food choices based on purchasing power. Low income puts people at risk for food insecurity (inconsistent access to sufficient food to achieve health) (Shah, 2003).

BASIC CONCEPTS IN EPIDEMIOLOGY

Epidemiology looks at the distribution of health states and events in the community. Individuals differ in their probability or risk of disease, so the primary concern is to identify how they differ. Mapping cases of a disease in an area—as John Snow mapped cholera cases in one area of London, and as many epidemiologists currently map various health-related events—can be instructive, even though it is limited in what it can reveal. A current example of mapping social determinants of health in one province in Canada is available at the National Collaborating Centre for Determinants of Health (see the Evolve Weblinks). A higher number of cases may simply be the result of a larger population with more potential cases or the result of a longer period of observation. Any description of disease patterns should take into account the size of the population at risk for the disease. That is, we should look not only at the numerator (the number of cases) but also at the denominator (the number of people in the population at risk) and at the amount of time each was observed. For example, 50 cases of influenza might

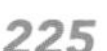

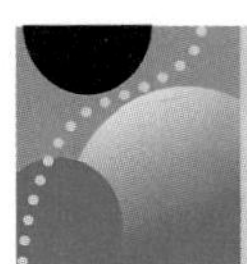

Determinants of Health

Gender, Income, Social Status, Education, Employment, and Working Conditions

- The appropriate treatments for alcohol and drug addictions differ in the cases of men and women (Palm, 2007).
- Men and women vary in their health-seeking behaviours for mental health (Oliver, Pearson, Coe, & Gunnell, 2005).
- Men earn significantly more than women do within 5 years following graduation (Finnie & Wannell, 2004). Some possible explanations for the gender wage gap are associated with more women working part-time (Clark, 2010; Finnie & Wannell, 2004; Maritime Provinces Higher Education Commission, 2004); or women working full time but working shorter work week hours (Finnie & Wannell, 2004; Maritime Provinces Higher Education Commission, 2004); fewer women are self-employed (Finnie & Wannell, 2004); and the fields of study chosen by women often do not lead to full-time employment opportunities (Maritime Provinces Higher Education Commission, 2004) or women often work in low-paying occupations (Clark, 2010).
- Canadians view homelessness, street crime, motor vehicle accidents, and unemployment as serious health hazards that are related to the social environment (Krewski et al., 2006; Lemyre, Lee, Mercier, Bouchard, & Krewski, 2006).
- Groups experiencing food insecurity in Canada: 9.2% of Canadian households experienced moderate or severe food insecurity; 33.3% of Aboriginal households experienced food insecurity; 8.8% of non-Aboriginal households experienced food insecurity; 10.4% of households with children compared to 8.6% of households without children experienced food insecurity; 7% of female lone-parent households experienced severe food insecurity compared to 1.4% of couple-led households (Health Canada, 2007).
- The unemployment rate among core working-age immigrants was 6.6%, compared to 4.6% among the Canadian-born (Statistics Canada, 2008a). Some reasons for higher unemployment rate in immigrants is that they may not have the necessary language skills, their credentials may not be acknowledged, and they may lack similar work experiences in Canada (Canadian Chamber of Commerce, 2009). The longer immigrants have been in Canada, the more the gap narrows between their unemployment rate and that of people born in Canada (Canadian Chamber of Commerce, 2009).
- Lower education and literacy skills increase the risk for health problems related to unhealthy eating, obesity, sedentary lifestyle, and smoking (Heart & Stroke Foundation of Canada, 2003).
- The income gap between the very rich and the very poor has increased between 1980 and 2005 as the median income for the top 20% earners in Canada increased by 16.4% compared to median income for the poorest, which fell 20.6% (Statistics Canada, 2008d).
- In 2007, 37% of immigrants between the ages of 25 and 54 years held a university degree compared to 22% of people in the same age group born in Canada (Statistics Canada, 2008c).
- Among immigrants, women are more likely to be living on low incomes compared with their male counterparts and those born in Canada (Statistics Canada, 2010c).

be seen as a serious epidemic (outbreak of influenza) in a population of 250 but would be a low rate in a population of 250,000. Using proportions (ratio) and rates (measure of frequency) instead of simple counts of cases correctly identifies population at risk.

Commonly Encountered Epidemiological Measures in Community Health Nursing

There are many epidemiological measures that a CHN needs to be familiar with when working with populations. **Morbidity** refers to the occurrence of disease in a population—for example, the number of reported cases of coronary artery disease in males between the ages of 40 and 60 years. Measures for morbidity include incidence and prevalence rate. In contrast, **mortality** refers to the number of deaths in a population—for example, the number of deaths from coronary artery disease among men between the ages of 40 and 60 years. Mortality rates include case fatality rate, infant mortality rate, and proportionate mortality rate.

Table 8-3 presents definitions, examples, and formulas for the epidemiological measures that CHNs need to be familiar with. These measures help them identify and understand health issues present in the communities they serve, diseases in the community, populations most at

TABLE 8-3 Basic Epidemiology Measurements, Definitions, and Examples

Measurement	Definition	Example or Formula
Proportion	**Proportion** is a type of ratio that shows the relationship between the total number and the frequency of occurrence in the case of a particular health event.	In 2000, there were 2,404,624 deaths recorded in Country X, of which 709,894 were reported as caused by cardiovascular diseases. Therefore, the proportion of deaths caused by heart disease in 2000 was 709,894/2,404,624 = 0.295, or 29.5%.
Rate	**Rate** is a measure of the frequency of a health event in a specific population in a defined time period.	The formula for calculating rate is Events × 1000 (10,000 or 100,000) Population at risk For example, in Country X, the birth rate for a given year would be calculated as follows: # of births in (year) Total population in (year) 37,850 (2005) 3,970,000 (2005) = 0.0095 × 1000 = 9.5 Therefore, in Country X, 9.5 births per 1,000 population occurred in the year 2005.
Risk	Refer to Table 8-4	Refer to Table 8-4
Ratio	Refer to Table 8-4	Refer to Table 8-4
Incidence rate	**Incidence rate** is measure of the number of new cases of a disease or an event in a population at risk over a defined period.	The formula for calculating incidence rate is # of new cases in a specified period # of population at risk
Prevalence rate	**Prevalence rate** identifies the number of persons in a population who have a disease or experienced an event at a specific period (old and new cases included).	The formula for calculating prevalence rate is # of population with the disease # of population at risk For example, 8,000 women are screened for breast cancer, and 35 of them have previously been diagnosed with a cancer event and 20 are newly diagnosed with a cancer event; the prevalence rate in this group is as follows: 55/8000 = 0.006875 Or 687.5 per 100,000
Epidemic	An **epidemic** is an outbreak of a disease, injury, or other condition that exceeds the usual (endemic) level of that condition. Therefore, the incidence of the disease has increased (new cases).	For example, by this definition, with the global eradication of smallpox, any occurrence of smallpox anywhere might be considered an epidemic.
Endemic	The **endemic** rate of a disease, injury, or other condition is the rate of occurrence that is usual in a population.	For example, community-acquired pneumonia that is usually present in a particular population within a region.
Pandemic	The **pandemic** rate of a disease, injury, or other condition is the rate of its occurrence in geographically widespread populations.	For example, the bubonic plague of the 1300s.

= number.

Note: Country X could be Canada; note, however, that these numbers are fictitious.

Source: The above definitions are adapted from Greenberg, R. S., Daniels, S. R., Flanders, W. D., Eley, J. W., & Boring, J. R. (2005). *Medical epidemiology* (4th ed.). New York, NY: The McGraw-Hill Companies.

risk, or health services needed in the community. A more detailed discussion of the measurement of proportion, rate, risk, incidence rate, and prevalence rate and the concepts of epidemic, endemic, and pandemic follows.

A proportion is a type of ratio in which the denominator must include the numerator. Because of this, proportions can range from 0 to 1. Proportions are often multiplied by 100 and expressed as a percent, literally meaning per 100. In public health statistics, however, if the proportion is very small, a larger multiplier is used in order to avoid small fractions, so the proportion may be expressed as a number per 1,000 or per 100,000.

A rate is a ratio, but it is not a proportion because the denominator is a function of both the population size and the dimension of time and reflects the total population that experienced the event, whereas the numerator is the number of events. Furthermore, depending on the units of time and the frequency of events, a rate may exceed 1. As its name suggests, a rate is a measure of how quickly something is happening—how rapidly a disease is developing in a population or how rapidly people are dying. Rates deal with change, that is, moving from one state of being to another—from well to ill, from alive to dead, or from ill to cured. Because they deal with events (moving from one state of being to another), time is involved. A population must be monitored over time to observe the changes in state, and typically, those persons who have already experienced the event are excluded from the population that is monitored.

A *population at risk* comprises those for whom there is some finite probability (even if small) of experiencing that event. For example, although the risk of breast cancer in men is small, a few men do develop breast cancer and therefore are part of the population at risk. There are some outcomes for which certain people would never be at risk (e.g., men can never be at risk for ovarian cancer, nor can women be at risk for testicular cancer). A high-risk population, on the other hand, would include those persons who, because of exposure, lifestyle, family history, or other factors, are at greater risk for a disease than the population at large. It seems that all persons are susceptible to HIV infection, although the degree of susceptibility may vary. Persons who have multiple sexual partners without adequate protection or intravenous drug users are in the high-risk population for HIV infection. However, others who do not fit these categories may unknowingly be at high risk—for example, women who are in monogamous relationships but are unaware that their partners have multiple sexual relationships. Similar to proportions, risk estimates also have no dimensions, but they are a function of the length of time of observation. Given a continuous rate, increasing exposure time will mean that a larger proportion of the population will eventually become ill.

A *ratio* can be used to calculate an approximation of a risk. For example, the infant mortality "rate" is the number of infant deaths (i.e., infants are defined as being younger than 1 year) in a given year divided by the number of live births in that same year. It approximates the risk of death in the first year of life for infants born in a specific year. It is important to note that in a particular year, some of the infants who die before their first birthday would have been born in the previous year, and some of the infants born that year may die in the following year. However, because about two-thirds of infant deaths occur within the first 28 days of life, the number of infants in the numerator (deaths in a given year) but not in the denominator (live births in that same year) will be small. It can be assumed that the current-year deaths among the previous year's cohort (group of individuals with similar characteristics) will approximately equal the following-year deaths among the current year's cohort. Although technically a ratio, this is an approximation to the true proportion and, therefore, an estimate of the risk. Infant mortality rate is calculated using the following formula:

$$\frac{\text{number of infant deaths under 1 year of age during a given year}}{\text{number of live infant births under 1 year during the same year}} \times 1000$$

For example, in City X in Canada, which has a population of 200,000, there have been 200 infant deaths and 20,000 live births in 2006. Therefore, the infant mortality rate for 2006 would be

$$\frac{200}{20{,}000} \times 1000 = 10$$

Therefore, there have been 10 infant deaths per 1,000 live births during 2006 in City X.

Measures of *incidence* reflect the number of new cases or events. The population at risk is considered to be individuals who have not experienced the event or outcome of interest but who are at risk of experiencing it. Note that for this calculation, existing (or prevalent) cases are excluded from the population at risk because they already have the condition and are no longer at risk of developing it.

The prevalence rate is a measure of existing disease in a population at a particular time (i.e., the number of existing cases divided by the current population). The prevalence of a specific risk factor or exposure can also be calculated. For example, if a breast cancer screening program reveals that 35 of the 8,000 women screened have a previous diagnosis of breast cancer and 20 with no previous history of breast cancer are diagnosed as having breast cancer, then the prevalence rate would be calculated as shown in Table 8-3.

In community health nursing practice, the CHN needs to be familiar with the concepts of epidemics, endemics, and pandemics because diseases tend to occur at specific times in specific geographical locations and affect specific populations (see Table 8-3). People who are exposed to specific agents or pathogens are more likely to develop a disease or a condition that may spread to others in their community. In some situations, the disease or condition may also spread to other communities and geographical locations, as in the case of the global spread of SARS, which will be discussed in a later chapter.

Point epidemic is a time-and-space–related pattern that is particularly important in infectious disease investigations. It is also a significant indicator for toxic exposures in environmental epidemiology. A point epidemic is most clearly seen when the frequency of cases is graphed against time. The sharp peak that is characteristic of such graphs indicates a concentration of cases over a short interval of time. The peak often indicates a population's response to a simultaneous exposure to a common source of infection or contamination. Knowledge of the incubation or latency period (the time between exposure and development of signs and symptoms) for the specific disease entity can help determine the probable time of exposure. A common point epidemic is an outbreak of gastrointestinal illness caused by a food-borne pathogen. CHNs need to be alert for a sudden increase in the number of cases of a disease and then need to chart the outbreak, determine the probable time of exposure, and, by careful investigation, isolate the probable source of the agent.

Table 8-4 provides examples of commonly used mortality rates. *Mortality rates* reflect both the incidence and prevalence of death rates. Many commonly used mortality rates are not true rates but proportions. Although measures of mortality reflect serious health problems and changing patterns of disease, they have limited usefulness. They provide information only about fatal diseases and do not provide direct information about either the level of an existing disease in the population or the risk of getting a particular disease. Also, a person may have one disease (e.g., prostate cancer) and yet die from a different cause (e.g., cerebrovascular accident). A clinical epidemiology glossary is provided on the Web site (see the Tool Box on the Evolve Web site). This glossary provides common terms used in epidemiology and their definitions. For some of the terms, such as odds ratio, relative risk, and specificity calculation, links are also provided on this site.

Because of population changes during the course of a year, the usual practice is to estimate the population at mid-year as the denominator for annual rates. The *crude annual mortality rate* is an estimate of the risk of death for a person in a given population for that year. These rates are multiplied by a scaling factor, usually 100,000, to avoid small fractions. The result is then expressed as the number of deaths per 100,000 persons. Although the crude mortality rate is calculated easily and represents the actual death rate for the total population, it has certain limitations. It does not reveal specific causes of death, which change in relative importance over time. Also, the mortality rate is affected by the population's age distribution since older people are at much greater risk of death than are younger people.

Mortality rates also are calculated for specific groups (e.g., age-specific, gender-specific, or race-specific mortality rates). In *age-specific mortality rates*, the number of deaths occurring in the specified group is divided by the population at risk at a specific time. This rate is then considered the risk of death for persons in the specified group during the period of observation. Differences in the age distribution between two populations can lead to bias. *Standardized mortality rates* (SMR) build on age-specific mortality rates and correct for age distribution differences and therefore control for bias.

How To... Determine If a Health Concern Exists in the Community

Planning for resources and personnel often requires quantifying the level of a health concern in a community. For example, to know how different districts compare in the rates of very-low-birth-weight infants, one would calculate the number of very-low-birth-weight infants in each district:

1. Determine the number of live births in each district from birth certificate data obtained from the vital records division of the health department.
2. Use the birth-weight information from the birth certificate data to determine the number of infants born weighing less than 1,500 grams in each district.
3. Calculate the number of very-low-birth-weight infants by district: the number of infants weighing less than 1,500 grams at birth divided by the total number of live births.
4. If the number of very-low-birth-weight infants in each district is small, use several recent years of data to obtain a more stable estimate.

TABLE 8-4 Common Mortality Rates

Rate/Ratio	Definition/Description and Example*
Crude mortality rate	An estimate of the risk of death for a person in a given population at a specified time **Example:** In year X, there were 2,304,500 deaths in a total population of 295,364,888, or 780.2 per 100,000.
Age-specific rate	Number of deaths among persons of a given age group/the total number of deaths in the population of that age group at a specified time. **Example:** In year X, the age-specific mortality rate for 40- to 60-year-olds was 240 per 100,000.
Cause-specific rate	Number of deaths from a specific cause in a population at a specified time **Example:** In year X, the cause-specific rate for accidents was 42.6 per 100,000.
Case fatality rate	The proportion of persons diagnosed with a particular disease (i.e., cases) who die within a specified period **Example:** If 15 of every 100 males diagnosed with prostate cancer dies within 5 years, the 5-year case fatality rate is 15%. The 5-year survival rate is 85%.
Proportionate mortality ratio	The proportion of all deaths that are the result of a specific cause who die within a specified period **Example:** In year X, there were 650,670 deaths from cardiovascular diseases and 2,506,451 deaths from all causes, or 26% of all deaths were due to heart disease.
Infant mortality rate	Number of infant deaths before 1 year of age in a year/number of live births in the same year **Example:** In year X, there were 29,200 infant deaths and 3,068,715 live births, or.9.5 per 1000 live births.
Neonatal mortality rate	Number of infant deaths under 28 days of age in a year/number of live births in the same year **Example:** In year X, there were 17,886 neonatal deaths and 4,068,914 live births, or 4.4 per 1,000 live births.
Postneonatal mortality rate	Number of infant deaths from 28 days to 1 year of age in a year/number of live births in the same year **Example:** In year X, there were 8489 postneonatal deaths and 4,068,914 live births, or 2.1 per 1,000 live births.

*Examples are not based on actual data. Refer to chapter discussion for calculation formulas.

The *cause-specific mortality rate* is an estimate of the risk of death from a specific disease in a population. It is the number of deaths from a specific cause divided by the total population at risk, usually multiplied by 100,000. Two related measures should be distinguished from the cause-specific mortality rate. **Case fatality rate** (CFR) is the proportion of persons diagnosed with a particular disease (i.e., cases) who die within a specified period. The CFR is considered an estimate of the risk of death within that period for a person newly diagnosed with the disease (e.g., the proportion of persons globally with cases of avian influenza A/(H5N1) who die within 5 years). Since the CFR is the proportion of diagnosed individuals who die within the period, 100 minus the CFR yields the survival rate. For example, if 433 cases of H5N1 were diagnosed over a 5-year period and 262 deaths occurred, the CFR would be 60.5%, and the 5-year survival rate would be 39.5% (Proteus, 2009). To review further information on case fatality rates and on the avian influenza, see the Proteus Weblink on the Evolve Web site. Persons diagnosed with a particular disease often want to know the probability of their survival. Case fatality rates provide that information.

The second measure to be distinguished from the cause-specific mortality rate is the **proportionate mortality ratio** (PMR), the proportion of all deaths that are the result of a specific cause. The denominator is not the population at risk of death but the total number of deaths in the population; therefore, the PMR is not a rate, nor does it estimate the risk of death. The magnitude of the PMR is a function of both the number of deaths from the cause of interest and the number of deaths from other causes. The formula for calculating the PMR, usually expressed as a percentage, is as follows:

$$\frac{\text{Total number of deaths due to a specific cause}}{\text{Total number of deaths from all causes}} \times 100$$

If rates of death from certain causes decline over time, rates of death from other causes that remain fairly constant may have increasing PMRs. For example, in Canada in 2003, motor vehicle accidents (MVAs) accounted for 16 deaths per 100,000 persons 15 to 19 years of age, with the total number of deaths from all causes in this age group reported as 46.4 per 100,000 persons (Statistics Canada, 2003). This was 34.5% of all deaths in the age group 15 to 19 years (PMR). By comparison, MVAs accounted for 1.8 deaths per 100,000 persons 5 to 9 years of age, with the total number of deaths from all causes in this age group reported as 10.4 per 100,000 persons (Statistics Canada, 2003). This was 17.3% of all deaths in the age group 5 to 9 years (PMR). This example demonstrates that the risk of death from an MVA in the age group 15 to 19 years was more than twice that of the age group of 5 to 9 years (based on the rates) and that such accidents accounted for a far greater proportion of all deaths in this older age group (based on the PMR).

The infant mortality rate (the number of deaths to infants in the first year of life divided by the total number of live births) is used all over the world as an indicator of overall health and availability of health care services. The risk of death declines considerably during the first year of life, so neonatal (i.e., newborn) and postneonatal mortality rates are of significance. In Canada, in 2003, infant mortality rates were 5.3 per 1,000 live births, compared with 5.1 per 1,000 live births in 2007 (Statistics Canada, 2010b). Refer to Table 8-5 for a comparison of Canadian infant mortality rates for the years 2003 to 2007. Some provinces and territories (New Brunswick, Newfoundland and Labrador, Prince Edward Island, Quebec, and the Yukon), however, reported an increase in infant mortality rates per 1,000 live births.

The most frequently used analytical measures of association in epidemiology are displayed in Table 8-6. These

CRITICAL VIEW

Since the 1900s, in Canada, there have been remarkable improvements in the health of Canadians. Table 8-5 indicates a reduction in infant mortality rates in Canada.

1. What do you think are the contributing factors to this reduction?
2. a) What epidemiological data exist to explain the increase in the infant mortality rates for the provinces and territories listed in the table?

   b) What empirical evidence exists to support your answers?

TABLE 8-5 Comparison of Canadian Infant Mortality Rates for Both Sexes 2003–2007

	2003	2004	2005	2006	2007
Canada	5.3	5.3	5.4	5.0	5.1
Newfoundland and Labrador	5.0	5.1	6.2	5.3	7.5
Prince Edward Island	4.9	4.3	2.2	2.1	5.0
Nova Scotia	5.7	4.6	4.0	4.0	3.3
New Brunswick	4.1	4.3	4.1	4.0	4.3
Quebec	4.4	4.6	4.6	5.1	4.5
Ontario	5.3	5.5	5.6	5.0	5.2
Manitoba	8.0	7.0	6.6	6.0	7.3
Saskatchewan	6.3	6.2	8.3	6.1	5.8
Alberta	6.6	5.8	6.8	5.3	6.0
British Columbia	4.2	4.3	4.5	4.1	4.0
Yukon	6.0	11.0	0.0	8.2	8.5
Northwest Territories	5.7	0.0	4.2	10.2	4.1
Nunavut	19.8	16.1	10.0	13.4	15.1

Note: The infant mortality rate is calculated as the number of deaths of children less than 1 year of age per 1,000 live births.

Source: Statistics Canada. (2010). *Infant mortality rates.* Retrieved from http://www40.statcan.ca/l01/cst01/health21a-eng.htm.

TABLE 8-6 Analytical Measurements of Association

Measurement	Description	Example of Formula
Risk	*Risk* refers to the probability that an event will occur within a specified period.	There are different measures of risk, such as absolute risk, attributable risk, and relative risk, which are considered in determining morbidity and mortality of a disease. These specific calculations can be found in various epidemiological texts.
Relative risk (RR)	A measure that identifies the probability of the occurrence of a negative event for persons exposed and those not exposed.	$\frac{\text{Incidence in exposed group}}{\text{Incidence in non-exposed group}}$
Attributable risk (AR)	A measure of the incidence of disease in individuals who have been exposed to the risk (risk factors) and expressed in percentages.	$\frac{\text{Incidence in exposed group–incidence in non-exposed group}}{\text{Incidence in exposed group}}$
Ratio	A measure of the relationship between 2 numbers expressed as the quotient of one divided by the other.	$\frac{\text{Number X}}{\text{Number Y}}$
Odds ratio (OR)	A measure of the odds/probability that an event is the same for two groups. Used when incidence rates are not available.	$\frac{\text{Odds of exposure for cases}}{\text{Odds of exposure for controls}}$ Calculated by using contingency tables (refer to epidemiology text for specifics)

frequently used measures include relative risk, attributable risk, odds ratio, risk, and ratio. Of note, attributable risk and relative risk are used by epidemiologists to compare rates of exposure between those exposed to a risk and those not exposed to a risk.

Epidemiological concepts and data are used in ongoing assessments of client health concerns. As will be discussed in Chapter 9, an initial component of a community health assessment is the collection of vital statistics such as incidence, prevalence, morbidity, and mortality rates for specific diseases and other data such as patterns of the use of health services and immunization rates.

Epidemiological Triangle: Agent, Host, and Environment

Epidemiologists understand that disease results from complex relationships among causal agents, susceptible persons, and environmental factors. These three elements—agent, host, and environment—are called the **epidemiological triangle** (see Figure 8-1A). Changes in any one of the elements of the triangle can influence the occurrence of disease by increasing or decreasing a client's risk for disease. Frequently, the client is an individual; however, a client can be a group. For example, a group of miners (host) were diagnosed with pneumoconiosis, as a result of their working conditions in an underground mine (environment) and their exposure to coal dust (agent). Figure 8-1B shows that the agent and the host, as well as their interaction, are influenced by the environment in which they exist. Alternatively, the agent and the host may also influence the environment. Specifically, these elements, or variables, are defined as follows:

- **Agent:** an animate or inanimate factor that must be present or lacking for a disease or condition to develop
- **Host:** a living species (human or animal) capable of being infected or affected by an agent
- **Environment:** all that is internal or external to a given host or agent and that is influenced by and influences the host and the agent. Environment also includes social and physical factors.

Some examples of these three components are listed in Box 8-1. Figure 8-2 provides examples of client situations using the epidemiological triangle for the events of TB, MVA, family violence, and homelessness. In the tuberculosis example, the host is a new immigrant with poor nutritional status; the agent is the mycobacterium tuberculosis organism; and the environment is the crowded housing in which the host lives, and the fact that the host has poor hygiene and has been in contact with a person infected with tuberculosis.

The epidemiological triangle and the web of causation are models that help CHNs identify and explore connections among various factors and causes affecting specific health challenges. Causal relationships (one

FIGURE 8-1 A & B Two Models of the Agent–Host–Environment Interaction (the Epidemiological Triangle)

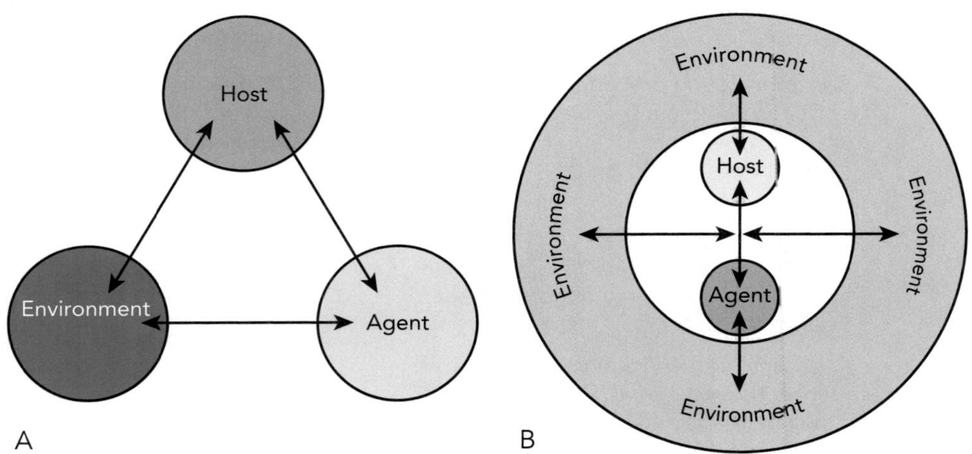

BOX 8-1 Examples of Agent, Host, and Environmental Factors in the Epidemiological Triangle

Agent
- Infectious agents (bacteria, viruses, fungi, parasites)
- Chemical agents (heavy metals, toxic chemicals, pesticides)
- Physical agents (radiation, heat, cold, machinery)

Host
- Genetic susceptibility
- Immutable characteristics (age, sex)
- Acquired characteristics (immunological status)
- Lifestyle factors (diet, exercise)

Environment
- Climate (temperature, rainfall)
- Plant and animal life (agents or reservoirs or habitats for agents)
- Human population distribution (crowding, social support)
- Socioeconomic factors (education, resources, access to care)
- Working conditions (levels of stress, noise, satisfaction)

thing or event causing another) are often more complex than the epidemiological triangle conveys. The term **web of causation,** also referred to as web of causality, recognizes the complex interrelationships of many factors, sometimes interacting in subtle ways to increase (or decrease) the risk of disease. Also, associations are sometimes mutual, with lines of causality going in both directions. Refer to Figure 8-3 for an example of the application of the web of causation for the causal variables for cardiovascular disease, a medical event. In this web diagram, the contributing factor identified as "social pressures" would include the social and economic determinants of health. There is a growing body of evidence that poverty, social exclusion, and unavailability of health and social services are major factors contributing to the incidence of cardiovascular disease in populations (Raphael, 2004). As well, gender, especially being female, contributes to differences in causes, risk factors, processes, and treatment of cardiovascular disease (Armstrong, 2010).

In this web of causality, the linked factors illustrate relationships among the data. For example, such factors as heredity, diet, and exercise can contribute to prevention or development of myocardial infarction. To explore the relationships in the web of causality, Edwards and Moyer (2000) suggest asking the following two questions: (1) "What factors are contributing to the problem?" (2) "What issues does each problem cause?" (p. 432). The CHN can use the web of causation for assessment purposes and to identify prevention intervention strategies.

Refer to Figure 8-4 for another example of the application of the web of causation applied to homelessness, a social event. In reference to this figure, it is evident that homelessness is a complex social event and multiple factors do not act in isolation but involve many complex interactions. Some of the key interrelated factors contributing to homelessness are income, social support networks, education, physical and social environments, employment and working conditions, health services, and culture. Conditions such as lack of affordable housing and lack of community supports and services can lead to an inability to manage other aspects of living, such as maintenance of relationships with family and friends and

FIGURE 8-2 Examples of Client Situations Using the Epidemiological Triangle

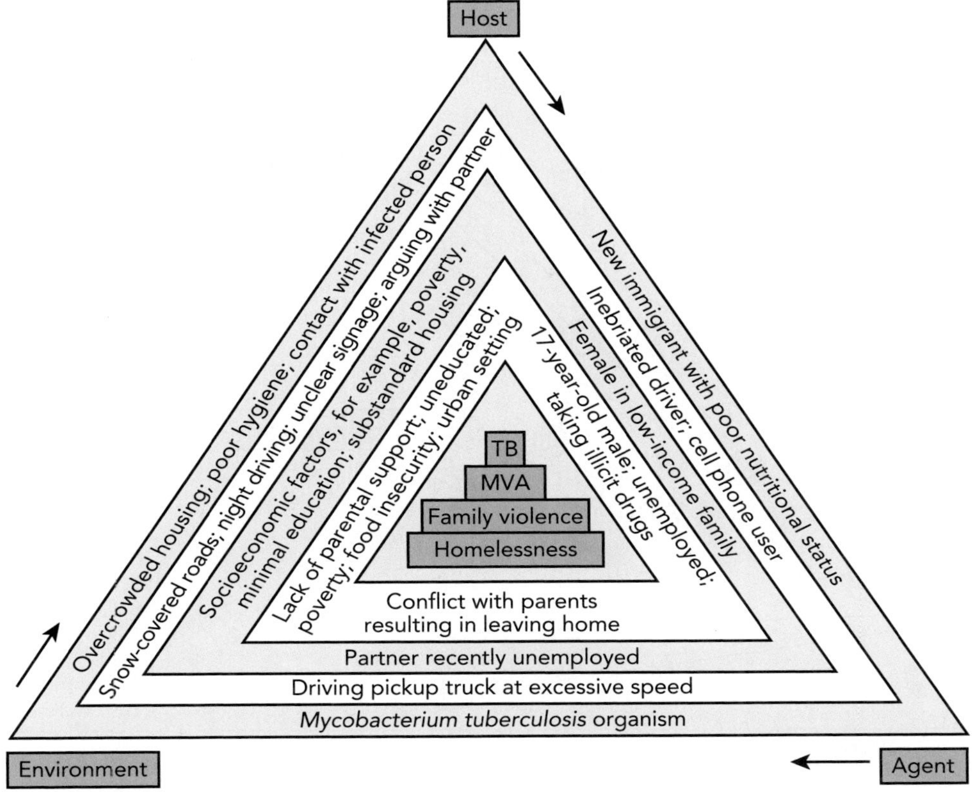

TB, Tuberculosis; *MVA*, motor vehicle accident

FIGURE 8-3 The Web of Causation for Myocardial Infarction

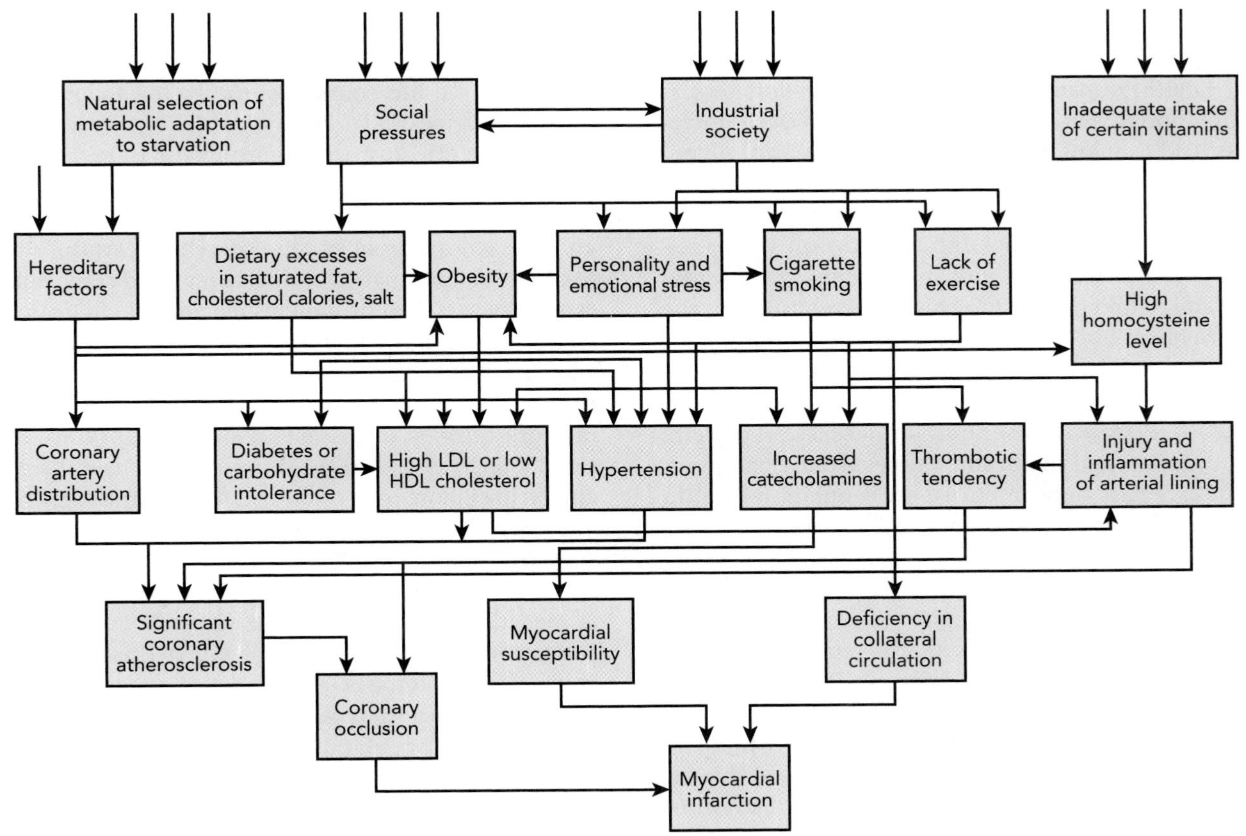

Friedman, G. D. (2004). *Primer of epidemiology* (5th ed., p. 4). New York, NY: McGraw-Hill.

FIGURE 8-4 The Web of Causation Applied to Homelessness

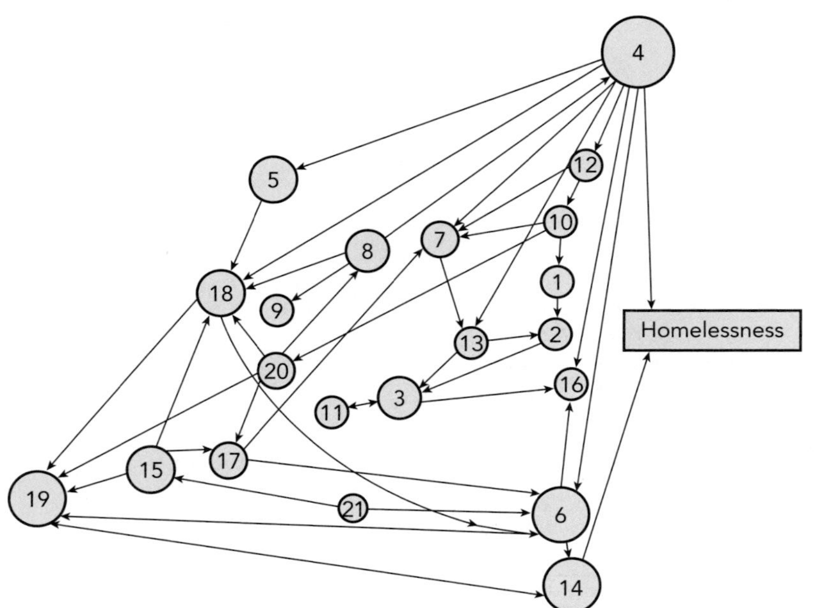

1. Changed economic factors
2. Decreased job market
3. Loss of employment
4. Poverty
5. Decreased food security
6. Lack of affordable housing
7. Access to health care
8. Cuts to social programs
9. Domestic violence
10. Physical chronic diseases
11. Educational level
12. Stress
13. Occupation
14. Poor hygiene
15. Loss of friends
16. Loss of family support
17. Addiction problems
18. Criminalization
19. Mental illness
20. Lack of available community services
21. Culture (e.g., Aboriginal)

Note: These are some possibilities and are not to be considered all-inclusive.

maintaining employment status, and these conditions may also enhance health risks such as malnutrition.

It needs to be noted that the relationship between mental health, substance abuse, and homelessness is multidirectional. The questions raised are "Does homelessness lead to mental illness and abuse of alcohol and drugs?" "Does having mental illness lead to homelessness?" and "Does being a substance abuser lead to homelessness?" For further information on homelessness, see the British Columbia Partners for Mental Health and Addictions Information Weblink on the Evolve Web site.

In recent years, with the introduction of life course approaches, there has been a paradigm shift in the understanding of disease; prevention of disease, especially chronic illnesses; and health and wellness (Ben-Schlomo & Kuh, 2002; Senate Subcommittee on Population Health, 2009). The life course epidemiological approach includes biological, psychosocial, and behavioural data collected from longitudinal studies starting from childhood and through to adulthood. This approach attempts to link early life factors with diseases that occur in adulthood (Kuh, Ben-Shlomo, Lynch, Hallqvist, & Power, 2003)—that is, how factors such as early childhood influence disease outcomes. Adopting a life course approach also involves exploring how the social determinants of health influence development across the lifespan in relation to immediate as well as long-term health and illness status (Ben-Shlomo & Kuh, 2002; Hertzman, Power, Matthews, & Manor, 2001; Raphael, 2009; Senate Subcommittee on Population Health, 2009).

Within the life course approach, the following three possible courses have been identified by researchers to explain the effect of the environment in early life on a person's health in adulthood: latent effects (early environment affects fetal and infancy stages, and these effects are masked until later in life when certain diseases become evident); pathway effects (early life environment, especially social environment, may direct children to different life courses that influence their childhood and adult health); and cumulative effects (the environmental risks experienced at different ages accumulate and increase the risk of disease in adulthood) (Hertzman et al., 2001; PHAC, 2009). Many studies have been conducted to explore each of these effects to link early life factors and diseases in adulthood (Ben-Schlomo & Kuh, 2002; Hertzman et al., 2001; PHAC, 2009). The life course approach is in its early development, and further research is needed. However, life course research studies are difficult to conduct due to the complexity of this type of cohort study (Ben-Schlomo & Kuh, 2002). Canadian researcher Clyde Hertzman was influential in creating a framework that "connects population health to human development, highlighting the unique role of early childhood development as a determinant of health" (WHO, 2006). The conference titled "Measuring Early Child Development"

Evidence-Informed Practice

The findings in this population-based preliminary study are the result of a 3-year national surveillance coordinated by the Canadian Pediatric Surveillance Program (CPSP), in which physicians provided, on a monthly basis, information on clients with specific conditions. The study population comprised clients with select conditions grouped as syndrome CHARGE (coloboma, heart defects, atresia choanae, retarded growth and development, genital hypoplasia, and ear abnormalities). The birth prevalence of CHARGE was calculated on the basis of national and provincial birth rates obtained from Statistics Canada.

The main objective of the study was to estimate the prevalence of CHARGE syndrome. The average Canadian birth rate of those with CHARGE syndrome was 3.5 per 100,000 live births. There were no reported cases of this syndrome in Alberta. The incidence of CHARGE in Newfoundland and Labrador was 10.66 per 100,000, and in the Maritime provinces, the incidence was 12.84 per 100,000. The occurrence in the Atlantic provinces was found to be 1 in every 8,500 live births. Provincial and regional variations in the birth rate of those with this syndrome were identified to be higher than previously reported in the literature. The findings of this study are consistent with previous reports, in that newborns and infants who survive these time frames are more likely to survive into childhood.

Application for CHNs: Consideration of epidemiological measures, such as prevalence and incidence of disease, is important for the CHN when planning community health nursing care for aggregates in their geographical area.

Questions for Reflection & Discussion

1. Explain the difference between the terms *prevalence* and *incidence.*
2. How would knowledge of change in the occurrence of CHARGE syndrome over time contribute to the assessment and planning role of a community health nurse?
3. Visit the Web site listed at the end of the chapter for current research and epidemiological information about CHARGE syndrome and the prevalence of this syndrome across Canada.
4. There is a higher incidence of CHARGE in the Maritime provinces and Newfoundland and Labrador. What could community health nurses explore about client experiences, values, preferences or choices when conducting home visits with families?

REFERENCE: Karina, A., Issekutz, K. A., Graham, J. M., Prasad, C., Smith, I. M., & Blake, K. D. (2005). An epidemiological analysis of CHARGE syndrome: Preliminary results from a Canadian study. *American Journal of Medical Genetics, 133A,* 309–317.

(chaired by Fraser Mustard and Richard Tremblay) that took place in April 2006 in Vaudreil, Quebec, addressed life course research and the development of the linkage of population health to human development, especially early child development as a determinant of health. The PHAC has funded the establishment of the Centres of Excellence for Children's Well-Being in partnership with several community groups, such as Canadian universities, First Nations communities, and professional associations. These Centres make available the latest research on social and emotional development of young children through the *Encyclopedia on Early Childhood Development* (see Evolve Weblinks), thus providing a valuable resource for CHNs.

Natural History of Disease Related to Levels of Prevention

The goal of epidemiology is to identify and understand the causal factors and mechanisms of disease, disability, and injuries so that effective interventions can be implemented to prevent the occurrence of these adverse processes before they begin or before they progress. The **natural history of disease** refers to the progression of the disease process from onset to recovery. Leavell and Clark (1965) provide a classic description of two clear periods in the natural history of the disease process that includes the prepathogenesis (susceptibility to disease) period and the period of pathogenesis (from the preclinical stage to death, disability, or recovery). These two periods in the natural history of a disease are related to the three levels of prevention commonly used in community health nursing practice: primary, secondary, and tertiary prevention of communicable and noncommunicable diseases. Leavell and Clark also depicted the natural history of disease in a figure (see Figure 8-5). This figure illustrates the relationship between the natural history of disease and the three levels of prevention.

FIGURE 8-5 The Natural History of a Disease

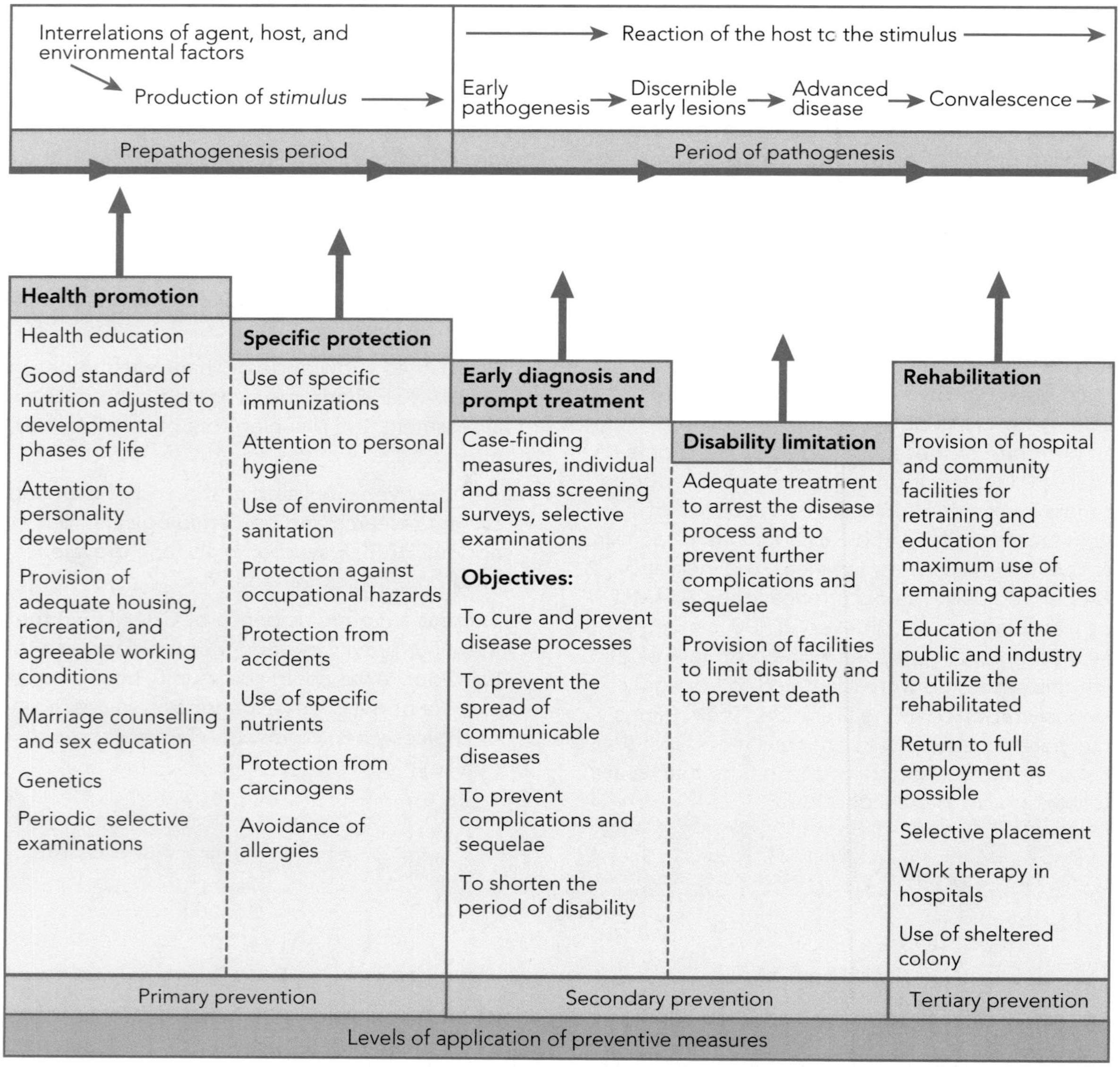
Interrelations of agent, host, and environmental factors
Production of *stimulus*
Reaction of the host tc the stimulus
Early pathogenesis
Discernible early lesions
Advanced disease
Convalescence
Prepathogenesis period
Period of pathogenesis
Health promotion
Health education
Good standard of nutrition adjusted to developmental phases of life
Attention to personality development
Provision of adequate housing, recreation, and agreeable working conditions
Marriage counselling and sex education
Genetics
Periodic selective examinations
Specific protection
Use of specific immunizations
Attention to personal hygiene
Use of environmental sanitation
Protection against occupational hazards
Protection from accidents
Use of specific nutrients
Protection from carcinogens
Avoidance of allergies
Early diagnosis and prompt treatment
Case-finding measures, individual and mass screening surveys, selective examinations
Objectives:
To cure and prevent disease processes
To prevent the spread of communicable diseases
To prevent complications and sequelae
To shorten the period of disability
Disability limitation
Adequate treatment to arrest the disease process and to prevent further complications and sequelae
Provision of facilities to limit disability and to prevent death
Rehabilitation
Provision of hospital and community facilities for retraining and education for maximum use of remaining capacities
Education of the public and industry to utilize the rehabilitated
Return to full employment as possible
Selective placement
Work therapy in hospitals
Use of sheltered colony
Primary prevention
Secondary prevention
Tertiary prevention
Levels of application of preventive measures

Source: Leavell, H. R., & Clark, I. G. (1965). *Preventive medicine for the doctor in his community: An epidemiological approach.* New York, NY: McGraw-Hill (p. 21).

LEVELS OF PREVENTION

In their daily practice, CHNs are often involved in activities related to all three levels of prevention. For example, in the natural history of disease during the prepathogenesis period, CHNs use primary prevention in health promotion programs with both the general population and specific vulnerable groups (e.g., the homeless, HIV-positive persons, certain vulnerable immigrant groups) to improve general health status and to reduce the incidence of specific diseases, such as TB. In the early period of pathogenesis, secondary prevention activities include, for example, routine Mantoux testing of specific groups (e.g., health care providers, child care workers) and identification and screening of persons who have had contact with a client with known active TB. The use of directly observed therapy (DOT) for clients with TB and teaching range-of-motion exercises for clients in the community fall within the realm of tertiary prevention. Given the emergence of new drug-resistant strains of TB, CHNs are now facing the challenge of designing and implementing programs to increase long-term compliance and provide aftercare for clients in a variety of community settings.

Primary Prevention

Primary prevention refers to interventions to prevent the occurrence of disease, injury, or disability. Interventions at this level of prevention are aimed at individuals, groups, and populations who are susceptible to disease but have no discernible pathology (i.e., they are in a state of prepathogenesis). This first level of prevention includes broad efforts, such as the following:

- *Environmental protection,* from basic sanitation and food safety to home and workplace safety plans and air quality control. An example is a CHN working proactively to develop and advocate for policies and legislation that lead to prevention of environmental hazards. Another example is a CHN consulting with industries, local governments, and groups of concerned citizens and public educators about preventable environmental health problems.
- *Specific protection* against disease or injury, which includes immunizations, proper use of seat belts and infants' car seats, preconception folic acid supplementation to prevent neural tube defects, fluoridation of the water supply to prevent dental caries, and actions taken to reduce exposure to cancer-causing agents.

Many CHNs are actively involved in primary prevention implemented in homes, in community settings, and at the primary level of health care (e.g., in public health clinics, physicians' offices, community health centres, and rural health clinics).

Secondary Prevention

Secondary prevention (early detection of disease during the preclinical period) refers to interventions designed to increase the probability of an early diagnosis so that treatment is likely to result in cure. Health screenings are the mainstay of secondary prevention. Early and periodic screenings are critical for diseases, such as breast cancer, for which there are few specific primary prevention strategies.

Interventions at the secondary level of prevention may occur in community settings as well as at primary and secondary levels of health care. In developing countries, wherever safe water can be made available, oral rehydration therapy (ORT) is an inexpensive and effective way to treat infant diarrheal disease. An example is CHNs teaching mothers to recognize the early signs of infant dehydration and administer a homemade ORT solution made with water, sugar, and salt. Again, in secondary prevention, the CHN obtains a family history of cancer, heart disease, diabetes, or mental illness as part of a client's health history and then follows up with education about appropriate screening procedures. Other secondary prevention interventions include mammography to detect breast cancer, a Papanicolaou (Pap) test to detect cervical cancer, colonoscopy for early detection of colon cancer, and screening of pregnant women for gestational diabetes.

Tertiary Prevention

During the middle and later periods of pathogenesis, **tertiary prevention** includes interventions aimed at minimizing disability and rehabilitation from disease, injury, or disability. Tertiary prevention interventions occur most often at secondary and tertiary levels of care (e.g., in specialized clinics, hospitals, rehabilitation centres) but may also occur in community and primary care settings. Examples of tertiary prevention are medical treatment, physical and occupational therapy, and rehabilitation.

SCREENING

Screening, a key component of many secondary prevention interventions, involves the testing of groups of individuals who are at risk for a certain condition but do not manifest any symptoms. The goal is to determine the likelihood that these individuals will develop the disease. From a clinical perspective, the aim of screening is early detection and treatment when these are likely to result in a more favourable prognosis. From a public health perspective, the objective is to sort out, efficiently and effectively, those who probably have the disease from those who probably do not, again to detect early cases for treatment or begin prevention and control programs. A screening test is *not* a diagnostic test. Effective screening programs must include referrals for diagnostic evaluation for those who have positive results for the disease to confirm if they do have the disease and need treatment.

CHNs need to stay current on screening guidelines, since they are regularly reviewed and revised on the basis of epidemiological research results. In Canada, these screening guidelines are referred to as Clinical Practice Guidelines, which recommend routine screening for such conditions as dyslipidemia, diabetes mellitus, hypertension, women's health, and men's health. As community health advocates, CHNs are responsible for planning and implementing screening and prevention programs aimed at high-risk populations. Box 8-2 outlines criteria for a successful screening program. Box 8-3 provides the World Health Organization classic screening criteria that were developed by Wilson and Jungner as commissioned by the WHO and first released in 1965 (cited in Andermann, Blancquaert, Beauchamp, & Dery, 2008). Box 8-3 also includes a synthesis of the screening criteria up to the present time. Andermann et al. (2008) report that the Wilson and Jungner screening criteria are still the "gold standard of screening assessment" (p. 18).

Reliability and Validity

Reliability

The reliability, accuracy, and validity of a measure are important considerations to keep in mind. The **reliability** of a measure refers to its consistency or repeatability. For example, while blood pressure screening is being carried out in a community, a large number of people are screened, and follow-up or repeat measurements are taken for some individuals with higher pressures. If the sphygmomanometer used for the screening shows extremely varying measures on two consecutive readings for the same person, then the sphygmomanometer lacks reliability. The instrument would be unreliable even if the overall mean of repeated measurements was

BOX 8-2 Characteristics of a Successful Screening Program

1. Valid (accurate): A high probability of correct classification of persons tested
2. Reliable (precise): Results are consistent from place to place, time to time, and person to person
3. Facility for large group administration: (a) fast both in administration of the test and in obtaining results; (b) inexpensive in both personnel required and the materials and procedures used
4. Innocuous: Few, if any, side effects, and the test is minimally invasive
5. High yield: Can detect enough new cases to justify the effort and expense (*yield* defined as the amount of previously unrecognized disease that is diagnosed and treated as a result of screening)

BOX 8-3 WHO Screening Criteria

Wilson and Jungner's classic screening criteria:

1. The condition sought should be an important health problem.
2. There should be an accepted treatment for patients with recognized disease.
3. Facilities for diagnosis and treatment should be available.
4. There should be a recognizable latent or early symptomatic stage.
5. There should be a suitable test or examination.
6. The test should be acceptable to the population.
7. The natural history of the condition, including development from latent to declared disease, should be adequately understood.
8. There should be an agreed policy on whom to treat as patients.
9. The cost of case-finding (including diagnosis and treatment of patients diagnosed) should be economically balanced in relation to possible expenditure on medical care as a whole.
10. Case-finding should be a continuing process and not a "once and for all" project.

Synthesis of emerging screening criteria proposed over the past 40 years:

1. The screening program should respond to a recognized need.
2. The objectives of screening should be defined at the outset.
3. There should be a defined target population.
4. There should be scientific evidence of screening programmed effectiveness.
5. The program should integrate education, testing, clinical services, and program management.
6. There should be quality assurance, with mechanisms to minimize potential risks of screening.
7. The program should ensure informed choice, confidentiality, and respect for autonomy.
8. The program should promote equity and access to screening for the entire target population.
9. Program evaluation should be planned from the outset.
10. The overall benefits of screening should outweigh the harm.

SOURCE: Wilson, J. M. G., & Jungner, G. (1968). *Principles and practice of screening for disease*. Geneva: WHO. Available from: http://whqlibdoc.who.int/php/WHO_PHP_34.pdf; Andermann, A., Blancquaert, I., Beauchamp, S., & Dery, V. (2008). Revisiting Wilson & Jungner in the genomic age: A review of the screening criteria over the past 40 years. *Bulletin of the World Health Organization, 86*(4), 317–319. Retrieved from http://www.who.int/bulletin/volumes/86/4/07-050112.pdf.

close to the true overall mean for the persons measured. The problem would be that the readings would not be reliable for any individual, and reliability is what a screening program requires.

On the other hand, suppose the readings on a particular sphygmomanometer are reliably reproducible but tend to be about 10 mm Hg too high. This instrument is producing consistent readings, but the uncorrected (or uncalibrated) instrument lacks accuracy. In short, a measure can be consistent without producing valid results.

The following three major sources of error can affect the reliability of tests:

1. Variation inherent in the trait being measured (e.g., blood pressure changes with time of day, activity, level of stress, and other factors)
2. Observer variation, which can be divided into intraobserver reliability (consistency by the same observer) and interobserver reliability (consistency from one observer to another)
3. Inconsistency in the instrument, which includes the internal consistency of the instrument (e.g., whether all items in a questionnaire measure the same thing) and the stability (or test–retest reliability) of the instrument over time

Validity: Sensitivity, Specificity, and Predictive Values

Validity refers to whether a measure is really measuring what we think it is, and how exactly. Validity in a screening test is measured by sensitivity and specificity. **Sensitivity** quantifies how accurately the test identifies those with the condition or trait and represents the proportion of persons with the disease whom the test correctly identifies as positive (true positives). High sensitivity is needed when early treatment is crucial and when identification of all cases is important.

Specificity indicates how accurately the test identifies those without the condition or trait (i.e., the proportion of persons whom the test correctly identifies as negative for the disease [true negatives]). High specificity is needed when rescreening is impractical and when reducing false positives is important. The sensitivity and specificity of a test are determined by comparing the results from a particular test with results from a definitive diagnostic procedure (sometimes called the *gold standard*). For example, the Pap test is used frequently to screen for cervical dysplasia and carcinoma. The definitive diagnosis of cervical cancer requires a biopsy and histological confirmation of malignant cells.

The ideal for a screening test is 100% sensitivity and 100% specificity. That is, the test is positive for 100% of those who actually have the disease and is negative for all those who do not have the disease. In practice, sensitivity and specificity are often inversely related. That is, if the test results are such that one can choose a particular point beyond which a person is considered positive (a "cutpoint")—as in a blood pressure reading to screen for hypertension or a serum glucose reading to screen for diabetes—then moving that critical point to improve the sensitivity of the test will result in a decrease in specificity; in other words, an improvement in specificity can be made only at the expense of sensitivity.

A third measure associated with sensitivity and specificity is the predictive value of the test. The **positive predictive value** (also called *predictive value positive*) is the proportion of persons with a positive test who actually have the disease, interpreted as the probability that an individual with a positive test has the disease. The **negative predictive value** (or *predictive value negative*) is the proportion of persons with a negative test who are actually disease-free. Although sensitivity and specificity are relatively independent of the prevalence of disease, predictive values are affected by the level of disease in the screened population and by the sensitivity and specificity of the test. When the prevalence is very low, the positive predictive value will be low, even with tests that are sensitive and specific. In addition, lower specificity produces lower positive predictive values because of the increase in the proportion of false-positive results. Refer to Table 8-7 for a description of each of these measurement terms with an accompanying formula. Screening tests are related to the period of pathogenesis in the natural history of disease as part of secondary prevention during early diagnosis, specifically early case-finding. Refer again to Figure 8-5 for an illustration of the natural history of disease to see this relationship between screening and secondary prevention.

Two or more tests can be combined, in a series or in parallel, to enhance sensitivity or specificity. In *series testing,* the final result is considered positive only if *all* the tests in the series were positive, and it is considered negative if *any* test was negative. For example, if a blood sample were screened for HIV, a positive enzyme-linked immunosorbent assay (ELISA) might be followed up with a Western blot, and the sample would be considered positive only if both tests were positive. Series testing enhances specificity, producing fewer false positives, but sensitivity will be lower. In series testing, sequence is important; a very sensitive test is often used first to pick up all cases, including false positives, and then a second, very specific test is used to eliminate the false positives. In *parallel testing,* the final result is considered positive if *any* test was positive and is considered negative only if *all* tests were negative. To return to the example of a blood sample being tested for HIV, a blood bank might consider a sample positive

TABLE 8-7 Screening Tests: Sensitivity, Specificity, and Predictive Values

Measurement	Description	Formula
Sensitivity	A measure in percent that identifies a test's ability to identify those persons with the disease.	$\frac{\text{Number of persons with a positive test}}{\text{Total number of persons with the disease}} \times 100$
Specificity	A measure in percent that identifies a test's ability to identify those persons who do not have the disease.	$\frac{\text{Number of persons with a negative test}}{\text{Total number of persons without the disease}} \times 100$
Positive predictive value	A measure in percent that identifies the probability that a person with a positive test has the disease.	$\frac{\text{Number of persons with a positive test and who have the disease}}{\text{Total number of persons with a positive test}} \times 100$
Negative predictive value	A measure in percent that identifies the probability that a person with a negative test does *not* have the identified disease.	$\frac{\text{Number of persons with a negative test and who do } \textit{not} \text{ have the disease}}{\text{Total number of persons with a negative test}} \times 100$

SOURCE: Adapted from Fletcher, R. W., & Fletcher, S. W. (2004). *Clinical epidemiology: The essentials*. Philadelphia, PA: Lippincott, Williams & Wilkins; and Gordis, L. (2008). *Epidemiology* (4th ed.). Philadelphia, PA: Elsevier/Saunders.

if a positive result was found on either the ELISA or the Western blot. Parallel testing enhances sensitivity, resulting in fewer false negatives, but specificity will be lower. Genetic testing is becoming more common, but most tests indicate only susceptibility to disease, not certainty of the presence of disease. Screening tests are never perfect, so there is always some probability of misclassification of screened subjects.

CRITICAL VIEW

In a surveillance cohort study with 529 asymptomatic women with a high familial risk for breast cancer, researchers identified the mammogram as a screening tool for breast cancer with a sensitivity of 33% overall and a specificity of 96.8% (Kuhl et al., 2005). The mammography screening test had a positive predictive value ranging from 21.4 to 28.6.

1. **a)** How would you interpret specificity and sensitivity results?

   b) How would you use the results of this test?

2. How would you interpret this positive predictive value?

BASIC METHODS IN EPIDEMIOLOGY

Sources of Data

It is important to know early in any epidemiological study how data will be obtained (Gordis, 2008). The following three major categories of data sources are commonly used in epidemiological investigations:

1. Routinely collected data: census data, collected by Statistics Canada; vital records (birth and death certificates) collected by provincial government offices; and **surveillance** data (systematic collection of data about disease occurrence) as carried out by the PHAC Centre for Infectious Disease and Emergency Preparedness branch (IDEP)
2. Data collected for other purposes but useful for epidemiological research: medical, health department, and insurance records
3. Original data collected for specific epidemiological studies

Routinely Collected Data

The Canadian census is conducted every 5 years and collects population data, including demographic distribution (age, race, and sex), geographical distribution, and additional information about economic status, housing, and education. These data provide denominators for various rates, such as CFR, infant mortality rate, and maternal mortality rate.

Vital records are the primary source of birth and mortality statistics. Registration of births and deaths, mandated in most countries, serves as one of the most complete sources of health-related data. However, the quality of specific information varies. For example, on birth information forms, sex and date of birth are fairly reliable, whereas such information as gestational age, level of prenatal care, and the mother's smoking during pregnancy is less reliable. On death certificates, the quality of the cause-of-death information varies between differing history forms used and varies from place to place, depending on diagnostic capabilities and local practice. Vital records are readily available in most parts of the world; they are an inexpensive and convenient resource and allow the study of long-term trends. Mortality data, however, are informative only in the case of fatal diseases.

Data Collected for Other Purposes

Hospital, physician, health department, and insurance records provide information on morbidity, as do surveillance systems, such as cancer registries and health-department reporting systems, which solicit reports of all cases of a particular disease within a geographical region. Other information, such as occupational exposures, may be available from employer records.

Epidemiological Data

Statistics Canada and the Canadian Institute for Health Information (CIHI) support and carry out surveys that provide information on the health of Canadians, such as lifestyle behaviours of the Canadian population. For example, the 1978 Canada Health Survey (CHS) provided lifestyle information, and the 2001 Canadian Community Health Survey (CCHS) explored health status, risk factors, and health care access. Surveys are also carried out by provincial governments to collect statistical information on the health of the population in the province. Since 1999, various health units in the province of Ontario have been conducting an ongoing monthly telephone provincial survey as part of program planning. In this study, a random sample of 100 adults 18 years and older are interviewed about risky behaviours that have an impact on public health—for example, excessive sun exposure, failure to use a seat belt, and smoking. This survey conducted on behalf of the participating health units, in partnership with the Institute for Social Research (ISR) at York University, is called the Rapid Risk Factor Surveillance System (RRFSS, 2009).

Rate Adjustment

Rates, which are key to epidemiological studies, can be misleading when compared across different populations. For example, the risk of death increases considerably after 40 years of age, so a higher crude death rate is expected in a population of older people compared with a population of younger people (Gordis, 2008). Comparing the overall mortality rate of an area having a large population of older adults with that of an area having a younger population would be misleading. Methods that adjust for differences in populations can be used to compare death rates.

Age adjustment is based on the assumption that a population's overall mortality rate is a function of the age distribution of the population and age-specific mortality rates. Age adjustment, or standardization of rates, reduces bias when the populations to be compared comprise different age groups (Cassells, 2007). Age adjustment can be performed by direct or indirect methods. Both methods require *a standard population,* which can be an external population, such as the Canadian population in a given year; a combined population of the groups under study; or some other standard chosen for relevance or convenience.

A direct age-adjusted method applies the age-specific death rates from the study population to the age distribution of the standard population. The result is the (hypothetical) death rate of the study population if it had the same age distribution as the standard population. The CHN can then compare the two populations, which are now similar in age distribution. The indirect age-adjusted method, as the name suggests, is more complicated. The age-specific death rates of the standard population when applied to the study population's age distribution produce an index rate that is used with the crude rates of both the study population and the standard population to produce the final indirect adjusted rate, which is also hypothetical.

The indirect method may be required when the age-specific death rates for the study population are unknown or unstable (e.g., when based on relatively small numbers). Often, instead of an indirect adjusted rate, a standardized mortality ratio (SMR) is calculated. That is, the number of observed deaths in the study population is divided by the number of deaths expected on the basis of the age-specific rates in the standard population and the age distribution of the study population (Gordis, 2008; Greenberg, Daniels, & Flanders, 2005).

CHNs incorporate epidemiology into their daily practice and function in a variety of ways. In many settings, CHNs collect, report, analyze, interpret, and communicate epidemiological data. CHNs involved in the care of individuals with communicable diseases, such as TB, gonorrhea, and gastroenteritis, are practising epidemiology as they identify, report, treat, and provide follow-up on cases and contacts. Those working in schools collect data on the incidence and prevalence of accidents, injuries, and illnesses in the school population. CHNs are also key players in the detection and control of local epidemics, such as outbreaks of mumps. CHNs practise in a variety of settings and are actively involved in primary, secondary, and tertiary prevention (see "Natural History of Disease Related to Levels of Prevention," page 235, and the "Levels of Prevention" box below).

Comparison Groups

Comparison groups are often used in epidemiology. To determine the rate of disease based on a suspected risk factor, the exposed group should be compared with a group of unexposed persons. For example, to investigate the effect of smoking during pregnancy on the rate of low birth weight, calculate the rate of low-birth-weight infants born to women who smoked during their pregnancy and the (lower) rate of low-birth-weight infants born to nonsmoking women. Ideally, you want to compare one group of people who all have a certain characteristic, exposure, or behaviour with a group of people who are like them in all ways except that characteristic, exposure, or behaviour. In the absence of that ideal, you can either randomize people to exposure or treatment groups in experimental studies or select comparison groups that are comparable in observational studies.

LEVELS OF PREVENTION

RELATED TO CARDIOVASCULAR DISEASE

Primary Prevention

At a large competitive industrial facility, the occupational health nurse (OHN) discusses strategies to manage various psychosocial stresses with a group of high-level management personnel who have no diagnosed medical conditions.

Secondary Prevention

The OHN implements blood pressure screening for all workers at the worksite in an industrial facility.

Tertiary Prevention

In an industrial facility, the OHN holds monthly group meetings with personnel diagnosed with back conditions related to injury to discuss back care and prevention of further back injuries.

CRITICAL VIEW

Refer to the following Web site to answer the questions below:
http://www.phac-aspc.gc.ca/cpip-pclcpi/vf/panvac-eng.php

1. a) What is pandemic epidemiology?
   b) What are some advantages of using a pandemic epidemiological approach?
   c) What are some considerations in using a pandemic prioritization framework?
2. What are some suggested actions that can be taken to provide equitable access globally to the pandemic vaccines?

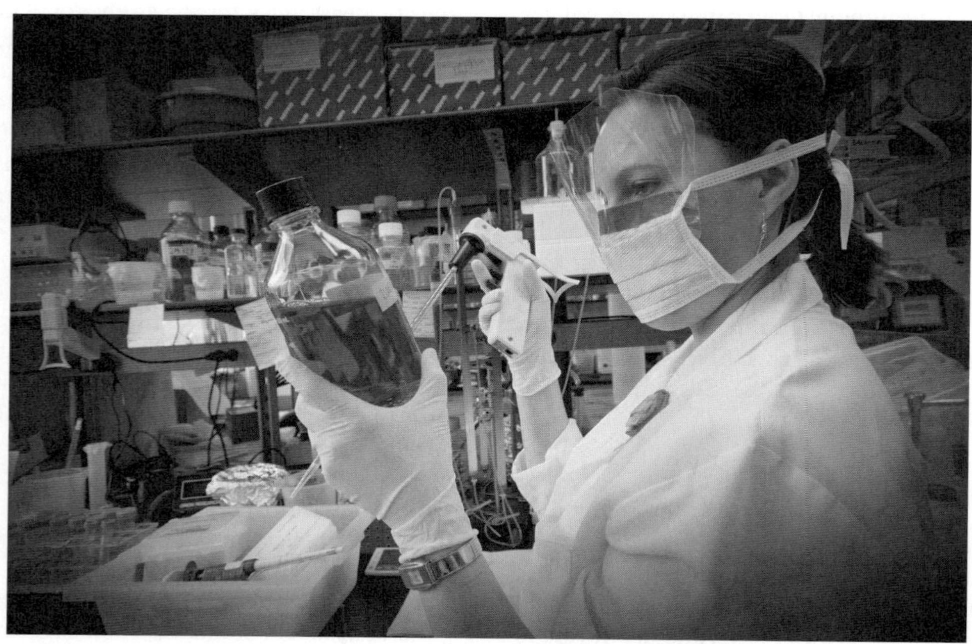

Epidemiological methods and epidemiologists are at the very centre of public health planning and response to terrorist threats.

Types of Epidemiological Studies

Four types of studies that are used by epidemiologists to explore health and illness in populations are (1) descriptive, (2) analytical, (3) ecological, and (4) experimental or intervention studies. Descriptive and analytical studies are observational. In these studies, the investigator observes events as they are or have been and does not intervene to change anything or to introduce a new factor. An **ecological study** bridges descriptive and analytical epidemiology. **Experimental or intervention studies** include interventions to test preventive or treatment measures, techniques, materials, policies, or drugs.

Descriptive epidemiology describes the distribution of disease, death, and other health outcomes in a population according to person, place, and time. This type of epidemiology provides a picture of how things are or have been—the who, where, and when of disease patterns. In this type of study, common measures of disease occurrence are frequency, incidence rates, morbidity and mortality rates, and prevalence that describe the disease patterns. Populations based on certain factors, such as age, socioeconomic status, and gender, that are at high or low risk for diseases can be identified using descriptive measures. Also, in descriptive epidemiology, trends for specific diseases can be observed over time. Descriptive epidemiology generates hypotheses, and analytical epidemiology tests the hypotheses (Cassells, 2007). One Canadian example of a descriptive epidemiology study was conducted using the CCHS (national survey) data to describe the epidemiology of major depression in Canadians (Patten et al., 2006). The study participants were 15 years of age or older and lived in family homes. Households were randomly selected, and one study participant 15 years of age or older from the household was interviewed (based on willingness to participate). The Statistics Canada national survey data that were reviewed had been collected between May and December 2002. As expected in descriptive epidemiology, the findings included annual and lifetime prevalence rates based on characteristics such as gender, age group, marital status, socioeconomic status, urban and rural status, and presence or absence of one or more chronic medical conditions. One of the rationales for conducting this descriptive epidemiology was to generate etiological hypotheses.

Analytical epidemiology searches for the determinants of the patterns observed—the how and why. That is, epidemiological concepts and methods are used to identify what factors, characteristics, exposures, or behaviours might account for differences in the observed patterns of disease occurrence. Analytical epidemiology includes study designs such as cross-sectional (correlational or prevalence), case control (retrospective, case comparison), prospective cohort (concurrent cohort, longitudinal, follow-up), and retrospective cohort (nonconcurrent cohort). Surveys and polls are examples of cross-sectional studies. Two well-known and influential longitudinal studies conducted in the United States on heart disease and other common health conditions were the Framingham Heart Study and the Nurses Health Study. A recent Canadian cohort study example is the National Longitudinal Survey of Children and Youth in Canada. The study, started in 1994, collected data on child development and related issues every 2 years until 2002 (Statistics Canada, 2008b). This study was primarily developed to obtain child development and risk factor databases that could be used to direct program and policy in Canada. Cohorts of study participants were monitored from birth to early adulthood, and data were collected at specific intervals throughout the study (Statistics Canada, 2008b). Some of the findings were as follows: (1) children were more aggressive in their behaviour when parenting practices were more punitive; (2) children experienced higher levels of anxiety when parental practices were punitive; (3) children became less aggressive in their behaviour over an 8-year span of time when parental practices had changed from punitive to nonpunitive practices; (4) children became less anxious when parental practices had changed from punitive to nonpunitive practices; and (5) children from low-income homes, when tested 8 years later, had higher scores in aggressive behaviour than children from higher-income homes (Statistics Canada, 2008b).

The identifying characteristic of ecological studies is that only aggregate data, such as population rates, are used rather than data on individuals' exposures, characteristics, and outcomes. In ecological studies, the descriptive component considers variations in disease rates by person, place, or time. The analytical component in ecological studies tries to determine if there is a relationship between disease rates and variations in rates for possible risk (or protective) factors or characteristics.

Experimental or intervention studies, such as clinical trials and community trials, have particular significance for CHNs. The goal of a clinical trial is generally to evaluate the effectiveness of an intervention, such as a medical treatment for disease, a new drug or an existing drug used in a new or different way, a surgical technique, or other treatment. Randomized clinical trials are used to test hypotheses about specific interventions. In clinical trials, the sample should be randomly assigned to two treatments, that is, the new treatment or the currently used treatment. In randomization, treatments are assigned to patients (subjects) so that all possible treatment assignments have a predetermined probability; however, neither the subject nor the investigator determines the actual assignment of any participant. Randomization avoids the bias that may result if subjects choose to be in one group or the other or if the investigator or clinician chooses particular subjects for each group.

Masking or "blinding" treatment assignments is a second kind of treatment allocation. Generally, it is best to use the double-blinded study method, in which neither the subject nor the investigator knows who is getting which treatment. Clinical trials usually are the best way to show causality because of the objective way in which subjects are assigned and the greater control over other factors that could influence outcome. Like cohort studies, they are prospective and provide the clearest evidence of using a time sequence.

Clinical trials tend to be conducted in a contrived (versus natural) situation, under controlled conditions, and with specific client populations. That means that treatment may not be as effective when applied in more realistic clinical or community conditions in a more diverse patient population. There are also more ethical considerations in experimental studies than in observational studies. For example, the question arises as to whether it is fair to withhold a treatment if the treatment truly appears to have the potential to cure a disease or alleviate suffering in order to systematically evaluate the treatment using experimental and control groups. Finally, clinical trials are expensive with regard to time, personnel, facilities, and, in some cases, supplies.

Community trials are similar to clinical trials in that an investigator determines what the exposure or intervention will be. However, community trials often deal with health promotion and disease prevention rather than treatment of an existing disease. The intervention is usually undertaken on a large scale, and the unit of treatment is a community, region, or group rather than individuals. Although a pharmaceutical process, such as fluoridation of water or mass immunizations, may be involved in a community trial, these trials often involve educational, programmatic, or policy interventions. Examples of community interventions would be measuring the rate of diabetes or cardiovascular disease in a community after increasing the availability of exercise programs and facilities or where a much larger supply of healthful fresh foods has been made available.

Although community trials provide the best means of testing whether changes in knowledge or behaviour, policy, programs, or other mass interventions are effective, they do present some problems. For many interventions, it may take years for the effectiveness to become evident—for example, the effect of exercise programs and healthful food on the rates of either diabetes or heart disease. While the study is being carried out over time, other factors can influence the outcome either positively (making the intervention look more effective than it really is) or negatively (making the intervention look less effective than it really is). Comparable community populations without similar interventions for comparative analysis are often difficult to find. Even when comparable communities are available—especially when the intervention is improved knowledge or changed behaviour—it is difficult and unethical to prevent the control communities from making use of generally available information, thereby making them less different from the intervention communities. Finally, because community trials are often undertaken on a large scale and over long periods, they can be expensive, require a large staff, have complicated logistics, and need extensive communication about the study.

The advantages and disadvantages of major epidemiological study designs are summarized in Table 8-8. Descriptive and analytical epidemiological studies have not been included in the table. However, note that ecological studies encompass descriptive and analytical epidemiology with aggregate data.

CRITICAL VIEW

1. Find one example of a clinical trial applicable to community health nursing in Canada. How was the clinical trial controlled for ensuring validity?
2. Identify a Canadian community trial study and describe the relevance of the study findings to community health nursing practice.

HOW COMMUNITY HEALTH NURSES USE EPIDEMIOLOGY

CHNs use the epidemiological results of various databases such as morbidity and mortality rates when planning and conducting a community health assessment. In their community practice, CHNs use epidemiology to identify the extent of the health concern, identify health threats or unhealthy behaviours occurring in their practice community, and to identify populations at risk in their practice community (case-finding).

CHNs frequently are members of interdisciplinary teams, consisting of epidemiologists, researchers, policy makers, and others, that are analyzing health and disease causation in the community in order to develop and initiate appropriate prevention programs using the most relevant and up-to-date evidence-informed community interventions. CHNs may identify client health concerns and work with nurse researchers and other discipline-specific researchers to explore options that would improve clients' quality of life. Based on the available epidemiological data, policy makers at the various

TABLE 8-8 Comparison of Major Epidemiological Study Designs

Study Design	Advantages	Disadvantages
Ecological	Is a quick, easy, and inexpensive first study Uses readily available existing data May prompt further investigation or suggest other/new hypotheses May provide information about contextual factors not accounted for by individual characteristics	Ecological fallacy: the associations observed may not hold true for individuals Problems in interpreting temporal sequence (cause and effect) More difficult to control for confounding and "mixed" models (ecological and individual data); more complex statistically
Cross-sectional (prevalence survey)	Gives general description of scope of problem; provides prevalence estimates Is often based on a population (or community) sample, not just those who sought care Is useful in health care evaluation and planning Data obtained at once; less expensive and quicker than cohort because there is no follow-up Baseline for prospective study or to identify cases and controls for case-control study Correlational cross-sectional studies identify relationships (associations)	No calculation of risk; prevalence, not incidence Temporal sequence unclear Not good for rare diseases or rare exposures unless large sample size or stratified sampling Selective survival can be major source of selection bias; surviving subjects may differ from those who are not included (e.g., death, institutionalization) Selective recall or lack of past exposure information can create bias
Case-control (retrospective, case comparison)	Less expensive than cohort; smaller sample required Quicker than cohort; no follow-up Can investigate more than one exposure Best design for rare diseases If well designed, can be important tool for etiological investigation Best suited to disease with relatively clear onset (timing of onset can be established so that incident cases can be included)	Greater susceptibility than cohort studies to various types of bias (selective survival, recall bias, selection bias in choice of both cases and controls) Information on other risk factors may not be available, resulting in confounding Antecedent consequence (temporal sequence) not as certain as in cohort; not well suited to rare exposures Gives only an indirect estimate of risk Limited to a single outcome because of sampling effect on disease status
Prospective cohort (concurrent cohort, longitudinal, follow-up)	Best estimate of disease incidence Best estimate of risk Fewer problems with selective survival and selective recall Temporal sequence more clearly established Broader range of option for exposure assessment	Expensive in time and money More difficult to organize Not good for rare diseases Attrition of participants can bias estimate Latency period may be very long; may miss cases May be difficult to examine several exposures
Retrospective cohort (noncurrent cohort)	Combines advantages of both prospective cohort and case-control Shorter time (even if follow-up into future) than prospective cohort Less expensive than prospective cohort because relies on existing data Temporal sequence may be clearer than case-control	Shares some disadvantages with both prospective cohort and case-control Subject to attrition (less to follow-up) Relies on existing records that may result in misclassification of both exposure and outcome May have to rely on surrogate measure of exposure (e.g., job title) and vital records information on cause of death

levels of government often make health care spending decisions, such as the amount and type of financial support (e.g., grants) and the allocation of resources such as the availability of various health care providers, community programs, and material resources.

CHNs are a key part of interdisciplinary teams that analyze the causes of health and disease in the community and are responsible for both preventing and treating illnesses. CHNs often use epidemiological principles and techniques to deal with the factors that affect individuals, families, and population groups that cannot be as easily controlled in the community as might be the case in acute care settings. For example, it is difficult to control water and food supplies; air quality conditions, including pollutants; disposal of garbage and trash; and ensuring the use of lead-free paint.

CHNs are involved in the surveillance and monitoring of disease trends. Those working in homes, clinics, schools, occupational health, and public health often can identify patterns of disease in a group. For example, if several children in a school experience abdominal problems within a short period (e.g., a 24-hour period), the CHN would try to trace the common source of contamination. Did they eat the same food, drink water from the same source, or swim in the same pool? Similarly, if workers in a factory all displayed similar symptoms, the CHN would look for causative factors in the workplace.

Nursing documentation on client records is an important source of data for epidemiological reviews. For example, client demographics and health histories are often collected or verified by nurses. As nurses collect and document client information, they might not be thinking about the epidemiological connection. However, the reliability and validity of such data can be key factors in the quality of future epidemiological studies.

CHNs need to apply findings from epidemiological studies, particularly population studies, in their community health nursing practice. Inclusion of population study findings can be used to plan for prevention programs for populations at risk and community programs (Cassells, 2007). In a descriptive epidemiology study of Aboriginal Canadians, the researchers studied the influence of ethnicity on the incidence of severe trauma (Karmali et al., 2005). In addition, the purpose of the study was to identify the characteristics associated with severe trauma in this population group in Alberta. When the Aboriginal study group was compared with an Alberta reference population, some of the study findings were as follows: (1) a four-fold higher risk for experiencing severe trauma; (2) a five-times higher risk for trauma from MVAs; (3) a ten-fold higher risk for trauma from assault; (4) a three-fold higher risk for traumatic suicide; and (5) a "post-traumatic survival advantage" (Karmali et al., 2005, p. 1010). More research is needed about severe trauma in Aboriginal Canadians before appropriate community interventions can be developed. However, CHNs need to be aware that this population is at greatly increased risk for these various types of trauma. The CHN needs to discuss with the community elders the relevance of these study findings to their Aboriginal population. The CHN works with the elders to identify and develop a community action plan that would involve the establishment of community partnerships to address community needs and develop appropriate interventions. In summary, CHNs need to understand that epidemiology assists in explaining the

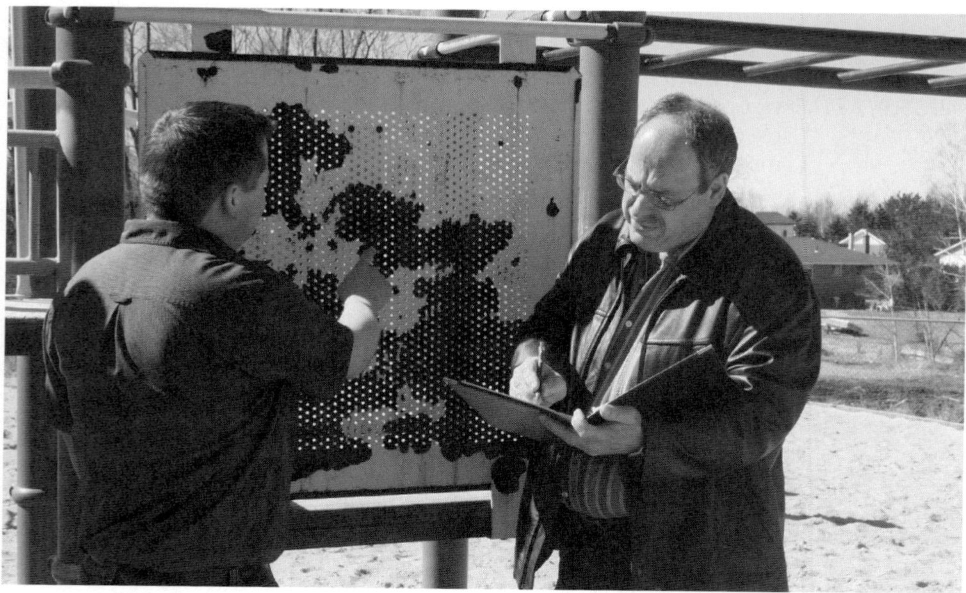

Community health nurses working in schools, for example, collect data on the incidence and prevalence of accidents, injuries, and illnesses in the school population.

multiplicity of factors influencing population health and illness (Clark, 2008).

Epidemiologists continue to struggle with the best approaches needed to gain an understanding of causation (Barreto, 2005). In the late 1990s, chronic disease epidemiology was an area of research focus by epidemiologists (Susser & Susser, 1996), and this focus continues into the twenty-first century. Debate has arisen around the risk factor approach used in epidemiology. This approach looks at relationships between risk factors and disease in populations as client. Supporters argue that identifying risk factors is crucial in public health research and that risk factor studies need to continue with a greater focus on validity and precision (McMichael, 1999; Susser, 2004). An issue raised in the use of the risk factor epidemiological approach, focusing primarily on identifying risk factors, is that it takes a narrow view and limits findings by studying individuals, rather than the environment and societal influences, where risks often begin (Stanley, 2002). McMichael (1999) maintained that a social-ecological systems perspective was needed with a focus on population health and upstream thinking in order to gain an understanding of the determinants of health and disease causation and well-being. Up to the present time, epidemiologists have taken different approaches in their study of causation, such as individual health, population health, and the life course approach (Krieger, 2001; McMichael, 1999; Susser, 2004). Susser and Susser (1996) proposed a paradigm shift referred to as *eco-epidemiology*, which takes a multidimensional focus that integrates molecular, societal, individual, and population levels. Susser (2004) proposes that "an integrated approach to investigating disease and its prevention will necessarily subsume levels of causation, life course trajectories, kinds of causes, and types of disease" and challenges epidemiologists to unite and adapt the eco-epidemiology framework (p. 520). The life course approaches challenge the traditional view of young adults and those needing to adopt healthy lifestyles to prevent chronic diseases, such as cardiovascular disease and diabetes (Raphael, 2004; PHAC, 2009; Senate Subcommittee on Population Health, 2009). The life course approach proposes that risks accumulate over time, starting in the prenatal period and childhood, and increase the risk of later adult onset of chronic diseases. The debate continues about the best approaches to use in epidemiology as we progress into the twenty-first century.

CRITICAL VIEW

1. How do you think the determinants of health would be studied when an integrated approach is used in epidemiology?
2. What are the implications for community health nursing practice?

Evidence-Informed Practice

This quantitative study analyzed the incidence of all-cause injury and specific injury categories reported for 2004 in Ontario Aboriginal communities (N = 28,816). The research study was a comparison of rate and categories of injuries that led to hospitalization for First Nations peoples in comparison with residents living in smaller northern and southern Ontario communities (N = 211,834). Hospital discharge data were used to determine the incidence rate for all-cause injury and specific injury type. In the First Nations communities, the relative risk for injury was 3.0 relative to southern communities and 2.5 relative to northern communities. The study findings indicated that the most likely reasons for hospitalization of residents in First Nations communities compared to those in non-Aboriginal communities was accidental poisoning, assault, and intentional self-harm, with females in First Nations communities being the most vulnerable to these injuries.

Injuries that required a hospital admission were higher in northern Ontario First Nations communities relative to those non-Aboriginal residents in northern and southern Ontario. This interesting finding underscores the importance of using a geographic comparison group when doing research.

Application for CHNs: Geographical information is a useful way for CHNs to identify populations priorities. By knowing which aggregates or populations have the greatest risk of disease or injury, CHNs can focus on programs that will more effectively fit the needs of the communities they serve.

Questions for Reflection & Discussion

1. Which determinants of health are evident in this study?
2. Explain the relevance of each of the identified determinants of health.
3. What primary care interventions could the community health nurse implement that would address injury prevention?

REFERENCE: Fantus, D., Shah, B. R., Qiu, F., Hux, J., & Rochon, P. (2009). Injury in First Nations communities in Ontario. *Canadian Journal of Public Health, 100*(4), 258–262.

STUDENT EXPERIENCE

Complete the following chart, providing as many examples as you can by exploring Web sites such as the Public Health Agency of Canada Infectious Diseases site: http://www.phac-aspc.gc.ca/id-mi/index-eng.php.

Infectious diseases currently prevalent in Canada	Infectious diseases that were prevalent in Canada in the early 1900s	Infectious diseases currently prevalent in developing countries

Identify reasons for the different prevalence rates listed above.

REMEMBER THIS!

- Epidemiology is the study of the distribution and determinants of health-related events in human populations and the application of this knowledge to improving the health of communities.
- Epidemiology is a multidisciplinary science that recognizes the complex interrelationships of factors that influence disease and health at both the individual level and the community level; it provides the basic tools for the study of health and disease in communities.
- Epidemiological methods are used to describe health and disease and to investigate the factors that promote health or influence the risk or distribution of disease. This knowledge can be useful in planning and evaluating programs, policies, and services and in clinical decision making.
- Basic epidemiological concepts are the interrelationships between agent, host, and environment (the epidemiological triangle); the interactions of factors, exposures, and characteristics in a causal web affecting risk of disease; and the levels of prevention corresponding to stages in the natural history of disease.
- Primary prevention involves interventions to reduce the incidence of disease by preventing disease processes from developing.
- Secondary prevention includes programs (e.g., screening) designed to detect disease in the early stages, before signs and symptoms are clinically evident, to intervene with early diagnosis and treatment.
- Tertiary prevention provides treatments and other interventions directed toward persons with clinically apparent disease, with the aim of lessening the course of disease, reducing disability, or rehabilitating.
- Epidemiological methods are also used in the planning and design of screening (secondary prevention) and community health intervention (primary prevention) strategies and in the evaluation of their effectiveness.
- Basic epidemiological methods include the use of existing data sources to study health outcomes and related factors and the use of comparison groups to assess the association between exposures or characteristics and health outcomes.
- Epidemiologists use rates and proportions to quantify levels of morbidity and mortality.
- Prevalence gives a picture of the level of existing diseases or events in a population at a given time.
- Incidence rates and proportions measure the rate of new case development in a population and provide an estimate of the risk of disease.
- Incidence gives a picture of the new diseases or events in a population at a given time.
- By accessing various sources of epidemiological data, CHNs will be prepared to care for populations in their communities.
- Descriptive epidemiological studies provide information on the distribution of disease and health states according to personal characteristics, geographical region, and time. This knowledge enables practitioners to target programs and allocate resources more effectively and provides a basis for further study.
- Analytical epidemiological studies investigate associations between exposures or characteristics and health or disease outcomes, with a goal of understanding the etiology of disease. Analytical studies provide the foundation for understanding disease causality and for developing effective intervention strategies aimed at primary, secondary, and tertiary prevention.
- Depending on the work setting, CHNs may be involved in clinical and community trials. As well, information gained from these intervention studies may be of value to CHNs.
- Screening tests are not diagnostic tests.
- CHNs are responsible for organizing screening programs.
- Sensitivity, specificity, and predictive values are measurements that CHNs need to understand and consider when using screening tests.

REFLECTIVE PRAXIS

Case Study

Marnie, a public health nurse (PHN) employed by the Warren Public Health Unit, was contacted by a local church after several church members became sick following its annual picnic. Of the 200 people who attended the picnic, 100 were ill with diarrhea, nausea, and vomiting. Ten people required emergency medical treatment or hospitalization. Incubation periods ranged from 1½ to 30 hours, with a mean of 6 hours and a median of 3½ hours. The duration of the illness ranged from 1 to 80 hours, with a mean of 30 hours and a median of 15 hours.

The annual church picnic was a potluck lunch buffet. The menu included macaroni casserole (brought by the Carusos), turkey with gravy and stuffing (brought by the Smiths), potato salad (brought by the Changs), green bean casserole (brought by the Champs), chili (brought by the Turners), homemade bread (brought by Grand-Maman Rivest), chocolate cake (brought by the Bushes), and cookies (brought by the Beckmans). Marnie interviewed the church members who were ill and discovered that three specific food items were clearly associated with the illness: turkey, gravy, and stuffing.

Marnie interviewed the Smiths, who brought the turkey, gravy, and stuffing to the picnic. Review of their food-handling procedures showed that after it had been cooked, the turkey had been left out for 4 hours to come to room temperature—a time and temperature sufficient for bacterial growth and toxin production. Furthermore, the same dishes were used for cooking the turkey and the other foods.

Marnie educated the Smiths on proper food-handling practices, emphasizing handwashing, proper cooling and preserving methods, and better sanitation of dishes. Marnie also offered a similar educational session to the entire church congregation.

1. Apply the data in this situation to the epidemiological triangle.

Answers are on the Evolve Web site at http://evolve.elsevier.com/Canada/Stanhope/community/.

What Would You Do?

1. Identify a health issue, such as obesity, smoking, or coronary artery disease, that affects your community. Using government records, determine the rate, risk, incidence, prevalence, and mortality rate for the health issue identified.
2. Locate one evidence-informed article pertaining to your identified health issue. On the basis of this article, indicate the possible interventions for the health issue identified.

TOOL BOX

evolve

The Tool Box contains useful instruments that can be applied in community health nursing practice. These related resources are found either in the appendices at the back of this book or on the Evolve Web site at http://evolve.elsevier.com/Canada/Stanhope/community.

Tools

Clinical Epidemiology Glossary. This site provides commcn terms used in epidemiology and their definitions. For some of the terms, such as odds ratio, relative risk, and specificity calculation, links are also provided.

WEBLINKS

evolve

Direct links to these resources can be found on the text's accompanying Evolve Web site at http://evolve.elsevier.com/Canada/Stanhope/community.

British Columbia Partners for Mental Health and Addictions Information. This resource provides information on homelessness.

Canadian Institute for Health Information (CIHI). This nongovernmental organization provides information for health agencies, health professionals, health associations, researchers, and the general public on the health of Canadians by reporting on health spending, health care services, human resources in health care, and population health. Click on your desired language and select Top Links of your choice.

Centre of Excellence for Early Childhood Development. This site contains information and articles on a variety of topics pertaining to child health from conception to 5 years of age.

CHARGE Syndrome Canada. This site provides epidemiological information about CHARGE syndrome, including the prevalence of this syndrome across Canada and current research.

Encyclopedia on Early Childhood Development. This site provides the latest research on the social and emotional development of young children.

Haydon, E., Raerecke, M., Giesbrecht, N., Rehm, J., and Kover-Matthews, K. *Chronic Disease in Ontario and Canada: Determinants, Risk Factors and Prevention Priorities.* This Web site provides examples of the epidemiology of selected chronic conditions such as cancer and cardiovascular disease.

Health Canada. Health Canada is a federal department that provides statistical data about diseases affecting Canadians. Click on your preferred language and select your area of interest from the menu.

Health Nexus and the Ontario Chronic Disease Prevention Alliance. *Primer to Action: Social Determinants of Health.* This document provides the reader with information on the relationship between the social determinants of health and chronic disease and actions to be taken.

National Collaborating Centre for Determinants of Health. *Mapping Social Determinants of Health.* This PowerPoint presentation demonstrates the technique of mapping and provides examples of the distribution of the social determinants of health for Nova Scotia using some of the census 2006 data.

Proteus: Avian Influenza Information Page. The Proteus site is part of a service for health professionals and the public that is provided by Ryerson's School of Occupational and Public Health. Included on this site are updates on the swine flu (H1N1) as well as information about influenza pandemics.

Public Health Agency of Canada. This recently formed federal agency was established to renew the public health system in Canada and support a sustainable health care system by focusing efforts on preventing chronic diseases, preventing injuries, and dealing with disease outbreaks and public health emergencies.

Statistics Canada. Click on your preferred language, select Health and Subject, and choose "Subject of Interest." To access the *Canadian Community Health Survey* that provides information on health status, risk factors, and health care use by Canadians, select the search feature and type in "Canadian Community Health Survey." Scroll down to find the health issue of interest. To access the report on the results of the National Population Health Survey titled *Statistical Report on the Health of Canadians* (1999), select the search feature and type in the title.

REFERENCES

Andermann, A., Blancquaert, I., Beauchamp, S., & Dery, V. (2008). Revisiting Wilson & Jungner in the genomic age: A review of the screening criteria over the past 40 years. *Bulletin of the World Health Organization, 86*(4), 317–319. Retrieved from http://www.who.int/bulletin/volumes/86/4/07-050112.pdf.

Armstrong, E. (2010). Gender, health, and care. In T. Bryant, D. Raphael, & M. Rioux (Eds.), *Staying alive: Critical perspectives on health, illness, and health care* (pp. 331–346). Toronto, ON: Canadian Scholars' Press.

Barreto, M. L. (2005). Commentary: Epidemiologists and causation in an intricate world. *Emerging Themes in Epidemiology, 2*(3), 1–2.

Ben-Schlomo, Y., & Kuh, D. (2002). A life course approach to chronic disease epidemiology: Conceptual models, empirical challenges and interdisciplinary perspectives. *International Epidemiological Association, 31*, 285–293.

Canadian Chamber of Commerce. (2009). *Immigration: The changing face of Canada*. Policy Brief: Economic Policy Series, February 2009. Retrieved from http://www.chamber.ca/images/uploads/Reports/economic-immigration-0209.pdf.

Cassells, H. (2007). Epidemiology. In M. A. Nies & M. McEwen (Eds.), *Community/public health nursing: Promoting the health of populations* (4th ed., pp. 50–73). St. Louis, MO: Saunders.

Clark, M. J. (2008). *Community health nursing: Advocacy for population health* (5th ed.). Upper Saddle River, NJ: Pearson Prentice Hall.

Clark, W. (2010). Economic gender equality indicators. In D. Raphael (Ed.), *Health promotion and quality of life in Canada: Essential readings* (pp. 234–247). Toronto, ON: Canadian Scholars' Press.

Cohen, I. B. (1984). Florence Nightingale. *Scientific American, 250*(3), 128–137.

Edwards, N. C., & Moyer, A. (2000). Community needs and capacity assessment: Critical component of program planning. In M. J. Stewart (Ed.), *Community nursing: Promoting Canadians' health* (pp. 420–442). Toronto, ON: Harcourt Canada.

Fantus, D., Shah, B. R., Qiu, F., Hux, J., & Rochon, P. (2009). Injury in First Nations communities in Ontario. *Canadian Journal of Public Health, 100*(4), 258–262.

Finnie, R., & Wannell, T. (2004). *The evolution of the gender earnings gap amongst Canadian university graduates.* (Cat. No. 11F0019MIE2004235). Ottawa, ON: Statistics Canada.

Fletcher, R. W., & Fletcher, S. W. (2004). *Clinical epidemiology: The essentials.* Philadelphia, PA: Lippincott, Williams & Wilkins.

Friedman, G. D. (2004). *Primer of epidemiology* (5th ed.). New York: McGraw-Hill.

Gender & Health Collaborative Curriculum. (2009). *Introduction to gender and health.* Retrieved from http://www.genderandhealth.ca/.

Gordis, L. (2008). *Epidemiology* (4th ed.). Philadelphia, PA: Elsevier/Saunders.

Greenberg, R. S., Daniels, S. R., Flanders, W. D., Eley, J. W., & Boring, J. R. (2005). *Medical epidemiology* (4th ed.). New York, NY: McGraw-Hill.

Health Canada. (2007). *Canadian community health survey cycle 2.2, nutrition 2004: Income-related household food security in Canada.* Retrieved from http://www.hc-sc.gc.ca/fn-an/surveill/nutrition/commun/income_food_sec-sec_alim-eng.php.

Heart & Stroke Foundation of Canada. (2003). *The growing burden of heart disease and stroke in Canada.* Retrieved from http://www.cvdinfobase.ca/cvdbook/CVD_En03.pdf.

Hertzman, C., Power, C., Matthews, S., & Manor, O. (2001). Using an interactive framework of society and life course to explain self-rated health in early adulthood. *Social Science & Medicine, 53*(12), 1575–1585.

Issa, J. (2008). Revisiting SARS, five years later: Public health chief David Butler-Jones on warding off the next one. *National Review of Medicine, 5*(4). Retrieved from http://www.nationalreviewofmedicine.com/issue/2008/04/5_policy_politics04_4.html.

Karina, A., Issekutz, K. A., Graham, J. M., Prasad, C., Smith, I. M., & Blake, K. D. (2005). An epidemiological analysis of CHARGE syndrome: Preliminary results from a Canadian study. *American Journal of Medical Genetics, 133A*, 309–317.

Karmali, S., Laupland, K., Harrop, A. R., Findlay, C., Kirkpatrick, A. W., Winston, B., Hameed, M. (2005). Epidemiology of severe trauma among status Aboriginal Canadians: A population-based study. *Journal of Canadian Medical Association, 172*(8), 1007–1011.

KPMG. (2009). *2009 performance evaluation of the Canada Health Infoway public health surveillance program.* Retrieved from http://www2.infoway-inforoute.ca/documents/Infoway-PHS%20Evaluation-Final-March%202009%20-%20EN.pdf.

Krewski, D., Lemyre, L., Turner, M. C., Lee, J. E. C., Dallaire, C., Bouchard, L., Mercier, P. (2006). Public perception of population health risks in Canada: Health hazards and sources of information. *Human & Ecological Risk Assessment, 12*(4), 626–644.

Krieger, N. (2001). Theories of social epidemiology in the 21st century: An ecosocial perspective. *The International Journal of Epidemiology, 30*(4), 668–677.

Kuh, D., Ben-Shlomo, J., Lynch, J., Hallqvist, J., & Power, C. (2003). Life course epidemiology. *Journal of Epidemiology and Community Health, 57*, 778–783.

Kuhl, C. K., Schrading, S., Leutener, C. C., Molrakkabati-Spitz, N., Wardelmann, E., Schild, H. (2005). Mammography, breast ultrasound, and magnetic resonance imaging for surveillance of women at high familial risk for breast cancer. *Journal of Clinical Oncology, 23*(33), 8469–8476.

Leavell, H. R., & Clark, I. G. (1965). *Preventive medicine for the doctor in his community: An epidemiological approach.* New York: McGraw-Hill.

Lemyre, L., Lee, J. E. C., Mercier, P., Bouchard, L., & Krewski, D. (2006). The structure of Canadians' health risk perceptions: Environmental, therapeutic and social health risks. *Health, Risk & Society, 8*(2), 185–195.

Maritime Provinces Higher Education Commission. (2004). The gender gap in employment outcomes of university graduates. *Trends in Maritime Higher Education, 3*(1), 1–11. Retrieved from http://www.mphec.ca/resources/TrendsV32004E.pdf.

McMichael, A. J. (1999). Prisoners of the proximate: Loosening the constraints on epidemiology in an age of change. *American Journal of Epidemiology, 149*(10), 887–897.

Merril, R., & Timmreck, T. C. (2006). *Introduction to epidemiology* (4th ed.). Boston, MA: Jones and Bartlett Publishers.

Naidoo, J., & Wills, J. (2005). *Public health and health promotion: Developing practice* (2nd ed.). Toronto, ON: Baillière Tindall.

Oliver, M., Pearson, N., Coe, N., & Gunnell, D. (2005). Health-seeking behavior in men and women with common mental health problems: Cross-sectional study. *The British Journal of Psychiatry, 186*(4), 297–301.

Palm, J. (2007). Women and men—same problems, different treatment. *International Journal of Social Welfare, 16*(1), 18–31.

Palmer, I. S. (1983). *Florence Nightingale and the first organized delivery of nursing services.* Washington, DC: American Association of Colleges of Nursing.

Patten, S. B., Wang, J. L., Williams, J. V. A., Currie, S., Beck, C. A., Maxwell, C. J., & El-Guebaly, N. (2006). Descriptive epidemiology of major depression in Canada. *Canadian Journal of Psychiatry, 51*(2), 84–90.

Proteus. (2009). *Avian influenza information page.* Retrieved from http://www.ryerson.ca/~tsly/avian_flu_page.htm.

Public Health Agency of Canada. (2006). *Centre for Infectious Disease and Emergency Preparedness Branch (IDEP).* Retrieved from http://www.phac-aspc.gc.ca/about_apropos/pdf/idep-eng.pdf.

Public Health Agency of Canada. (2007). *Skills enhancement for public health.* Retrieved from http://www.phac-aspc.gc.ca/sehs-acss/index-eng.php.

Public Health Agency of Canada. (2009). *The Chief Public Health Officer's Report on the state of public health in Canada 2009: Growing up well—Priorities for a healthy future.* Retrieved from http://www.phac-aspc.gc.ca/publicat/2009/cphorsphc-respcacsp/pdf/cphorsphc-respcacsp-eng.pdf.

Raphael, D. (2004). *Social determinants of health: Canadian perspectives.* Toronto, ON: Canadian Scholars' Press.

Raphael, D. (2009). *Social determinants of health* (2nd ed.). Toronto, ON: Canadian Scholars' Press.

Rapid Risk Factor Surveillance System (RRFSS). (2009). *History*. Retrieved from http://www.rrfss.ca/index.php?pid=3#History.

Rothman, K. J. (2002). *Epidemiology: An introduction*. New York, NY: Oxford University Press.

Senate Subcommittee on Population Health. (2009). *A healthy, productive Canada: A determinant of health approach*. Retrieved from http://senate-senat.ca/health-e.asp.

Shah, C. P. (2003). *Public health and preventive medicine in Canada* (5th ed.). Toronto, ON: Saunders.

Snow, J. (1855). On the model of communication of cholera. In *Snow on cholera*. New York: The Commonwealth Fund.

Spenceley, S. (2007). Chronic illness. In R. Day, P. Paul, B. Williams, S. C. Smeltzer, & B. Bare (Eds.), *Brunner and Suddarth's textbook of medical-surgical nursing* (1st Canadian ed., pp. 148–159). Philadelphia, PA: Lippincott, Williams & Wilkins.

Stanley, F. (2002). From Susser's causal paradigms to social justice in Australia. *International Journal of Epidemiology*, *31*(1), 40–45.

Statistics Canada. (2003). *Mortality, summary list of causes*. (Cat. No. 84F0209XIE). Retrieved from http://www.statcan.gc.ca/bsolc/olc-cel/olc-cel?catno=84F0209X&lang=eng.

Statistics Canada. (2008a). *Canada's immigrant labour market*. Retrieved from http://www.statcan.gc.ca/daily-quotidien/080513/dq080513a-eng.htm.

Statistics Canada. (2008b). *National longitudinal survey of children and youth (NLSCY)*. Retrieved from http://www.statcan.gc.ca/cgi-bin/imdb/p2SV.pl?Function=getSurvey&SDDS=4450&lang=en&db=imdb&adm=8&dis=2.

Statistics Canada. (2008c). *Study: Canadian immigrant labour market: Analysis by region of highest postsecondary education*. Retrieved from http://www.statcan.gc.ca/daily-quotidien/080718/dq080718b-eng.htm.

Statistics Canada. (2008d). *2006 census: Earnings, income and shelter costs*. Retrieved from http://www.statcan.gc.ca/daily-quotidien/080501/dq080501a-eng.htm.

Statistics Canada. (2010a). *Age-standardized mortality rates by selected causes, by sex (both sexes)*. Retrieved from http://www40.statcan.ca/101/cst01/health30a-eng.htm.

Statistics Canada. (2010b). *Infant mortality rates*. Retrieved from http://www40.statcan.ca/l01/cst01/health21a-eng.htm.

Statistics Canada. (2010c). *Women in Canada: A gender based statistical report*. Ottawa, ON: Statistics Canada. (Cat. No. 89-503-XWE). Retrieved from http://www.statcan.gc.ca/bsolc/olc-cel/olc-cel?catno=89-503-x&lang=eng.

Susser, E. (2004). Eco-epidemiology: Thinking outside the black box. *Epidemiology*, *15*(5), 519–520.

Susser, M., & Susser, E. (1996). Choosing a future for epidemiology: II. From black box to Chinese boxes and ecoepidemiology. *American Journal of Public Health*, *86*(5), 674–677.

Vandenbroucke, J. P. (1990). Epidemiology in transition: A historical hypothesis. *Epidemiology*, *1*(2), 164.

Wilson, J. M. G., & Jungner, G. (1968). *Principles and practice of screening for disease*. Geneva: WHO. Available from http://whqlibdoc.who.int/php/WHO_PHP_34.pdf.

World Health Organization. (2006). *Socio-economic determinants of health*. Retrieved from http://www.euro.who.int/socialdeterminants.

CHAPTER 9

Working with Community

KEY TERMS

asset mapping 264
change agent 278
change partner 278
coalition 264
community capacity 264
community competence 266
community forums 271
community health 261
community health assessment 266
community health concerns 268
community health strengths 268
community partnerships 263
data collection 267
data gathering 267
data generation 268
database 268
evaluation 279
focus groups 268
goals 275
healthy community 262
implementation 278
informant interviews 268
interdependent 257
intervention activities 277
objectives 275
participant observation 269
partnership 263
secondary analysis 272
surveys 272
sustainability 266
windshield survey 258

See Glossary on page 593 for definitions.

OBJECTIVES

After reading this chapter, you should be able to:

1. Define community as partner.
2. Explain selected concepts basic to community health nursing practice: community, community as partner, community health, partnership for health, community development, capacity building, community competence, community engagement, community mobilization, coalition building, sustainability, and healthy communities.
3. Identify the relationship of community and the determinants of health.
4. Apply the community health nursing process to community health nursing practice.
5. Explain the role of the community health nurse when working with the community as partner.
6. Describe which methods of assessment, intervention, and evaluation are most appropriate in selected situations.

CHAPTER OUTLINE

Florence Nightingale defined her community as war-torn Africa and discovered that the lack of fresh air, sanitation, and hygiene was contributing to the illnesses of the soldiers. Lillian Wald found that the New York neighbourhoods in her practice were impoverished, with poor housing conditions and sanitation, improper nutrition, and crowding contributing to the problems of new mothers and children. Both women became political activists, worked with the leaders in their communities, and even solicited help from their respective governments to help change the conditions for the individuals and families in their communities. Community health nurses (CHNs) need to know how to assess a community and work with the community as a partner in order to maximize community health.

Conceptualizing community as client is different from conceptualizing community as partner. A CHN who conceptualizes the community as client provides prevention and early intervention programs for the total population, such as offering mass screening and immunization programs in the community; the CHN is often viewed as the expert. In the community-as-client approach, a community assessment emphasizes the use of epidemiological data and disease occurrences with a focus that is needs defined. The interventions used by the CHN are often directed by government policy and legislation or regulations with an expectation of client compliance.

In contrast, when the CHN approaches the community as partner, the emphasis is on community strengths or assets in order to deal with community-identified health concerns and to further develop community capacity in a collaborative milieu that is supportive to and meaningful for community members (the "Ethical Considerations" box, below, deals with this type of partnership). The CHN partners with community groups such as other health care professionals, community stakeholders, and nonprofit agencies. The CHN blends professional knowledge with knowledge of the specific community to use and work with community resources for planning and implementation purposes. During this partnership, epidemiological data and disease and injury prevention data are also considered by the CHN but are not the key elements in the community assessment process.

CRITICAL VIEW

1. What is meant by the term *community as the unit of care*?
2. What are the differences between community as client and community as partner?

Ethical Considerations

Working with a CHN, a group of women residents of a low-income neighbourhood have identified food security as a major issue for many of the children in their community. They proposed to the local government that programs could be developed by the community members, such as a breakfast program for school children, food banks for individuals and families, a community kitchen program, and the establishment of a community garden if start-up funding and support by the local government could be provided. This is the first time that this community has worked together to address some of its community health concerns. The response of the local government was to zone for a grocery store chain in the neighbourhood that provides bulk discount food, a change that would also provide increased tax revenue for the city.

Ethical principles that apply to the above case:

- *Beneficence:* Clients are most empowered and their dignity most respected if their own input is recognized. In this case, the community members' suggestions were ignored.
- *Distributive justice:* The bulk discount store does not solve all of the community's food security problems. Many people may still not be able to afford or access the food there.
- *Respect for autonomy:* CHNs recognize the importance of client autonomy when working with the community as partner. The community members were trying to achieve autonomy by having their own garden so that they did not have to depend on external sources.
- *Promoting justice:* (CNA *Code of Ethics*). This primary CHN ethical value states that CHNs have a responsibility to promote social justice.

Questions to Consider

1. What are the CHN's responsibilities in promoting social justice in this situation?
2. What are some actions the CHN could take to promote social justice in this situation?

This chapter clarifies community concepts and provides a guideline for community health nursing practice with the community as the unit of care. The *Canadian Community Health Nursing Standards of Practice* (Community Health Nurses Association of Canada [CHNAC], 2008) includes expectations for assessment, planning, intervention, and evaluation when working with the community. Some of these expectations are listed in Box 9-1. For the complete *Standards of Practice,* refer to Appendix 1.

Working with the community as the unit of care and as partner may be a new experience for some CHNs, as many are accustomed to working with individuals and families as clients. The term *community health nursing process,* coined in the *Canadian Community Health Nursing Standards of Practice* (CHNAC, 2008), is used in this chapter to refer to the process by which CHNs make their community health nursing practice decisions. This process involves comprehensive health community assessment, planning, implementation, and evaluation. It involves working with the community to collect data and to draw conclusions about the community's strengths and assets, resources, and health concerns (assessment) and includes further decision making during planning, implementation, and evaluation. This

BOX 9-1 The *Canadian Community Health Nursing Standards of Practice* Examples for Working with the Community as the Unit of Care

The standards for CHNs provide direction in working with the community. Some examples from these five standards are presented below:

Standard 1: Promoting Health

- Collaborates with the individual or community and other stakeholders in conducting a holistic assessment of the assets and needs of the individual or community
- Collaborates with the individual or community to assist members in taking responsibility for maintaining or improving their health by increasing their knowledge, influence, and control over the determinants of health
- Assists the individual or community in identifying strengths and available resources and taking action to address needs
- Assists individuals, groups, families, and communities in identifying potential risks to health
- Engages collaborative, interdisciplinary, and intersectoral partnerships to address risks to individual, family, community, or population health and to address prevention and protection issues such as communicable disease, injury, and chronic disease
- Evaluates collaborative practice (personal, team, or intersectoral) in achieving individual or community outcomes

Standard 2: Building Individual or Community Capacity

- Uses community development principles
- Uses a comprehensive mix of community- or population-based strategies such as coalition building, intersectoral partnerships, and networking to address issues of concern to groups or populations
- Supports the individual, family, community, or population in developing skills for self-advocacy
- Supports community action to influence policy change in support of health

Standard 3: Building Relationships

- Respects and trusts the family's or community's ability to know the issue members are addressing and solve their own problems
- Involves the individual or community as an active partner in identifying relevant needs, perspectives, and expectations

Standard 4: Facilitating Access and Equity

- Assesses and understands individual and community capacities, including norms, values, beliefs, knowledge, resources, and power structure
- Takes action with and for individuals or communities at the organizational, municipal, provincial or territorial, and federal levels to address service gaps and accessibility issues
- Monitors and evaluates changes and progress in access to the determinants of health and appropriate community services

Standard 5: Demonstrating Professional Responsibility and Accountability

- Takes preventive or corrective action individually or in partnership with others to protect the individual or community from unsafe or unethical circumstances

SOURCE: Modified from Community Health Nurses Association of Canada (CHNAC). (2008). *Canadian community health nursing standards of practice* (pp. 10–17). Retrieved from http://www.chnac.ca/images/downloads/standards/chn_standards_of_practice_mar08_english.pdf.

chapter provides the CHN with the knowledge necessary to conduct a community health assessment and to complete the community health nursing process with the community as the unit of care and as partner. CHNs are interested in knowing how the community's health affects their client(s) (individual, family, group, aggregate, population, and society). Completing a community health assessment will assist the CHN in identifying community strengths and assets and community health concerns (actual, possible, and potential).

WHAT IS COMMUNITY?

The concept of *community* is broad, but generally refers to persons who interact and have similar goals or interests and share common social supports and may or may not come from within the same geographic boundaries. When community agencies such as schools, social services, and government interact, solutions to health concerns are more probable. CHNs quickly learn that society consists of many different kinds of communities, such as a community of interest (e.g., a group of individuals who want to cut hiking and walking trails in their community or a group of older adults meeting to support affordable healthy food options); community of concern (e.g., communities concerned about low literacy levels in their communities or a group of older adults who perceive a need for enhanced lighting of city sidewalks); neighbourhood community (e.g., neighbours in a specific geographic area who meet to set up a neighbourhood watch program); and communities of practice (e.g., practitioners sharing knowledge and learning). CHNs also may work in partnership with political communities, such as school districts, municipalities, or counties, to develop a health promotion policy pertaining to bullying. Because each community is unique, and its defining characteristics will affect the nature of the partnership, CHNs planning an intervention with a community must take into account its specific characteristics.

In most definitions, *community* includes three dimensions—*people, place,* and *function:*

1. The *people* are the community residents.
2. *Place* refers both to geographical and time dimensions.
3. *Function* refers to the aims and activities of the community.

CHNs regularly need to examine how the personal, geographical, and functional dimensions of community shape their nursing practice with individuals, families, and groups. They can use both a conceptual definition and a set of indicators for the concept of community in their practice.

In this chapter, the following definitions are used: *community* is a locality-based entity composed of systems of formal organizations reflecting society's institutions, informal groups, and aggregates (groups within a population). The components of community are **interdependent**—they are mutually reliant upon each other—and their function is to meet a wide variety of collective needs. This definition of community includes personal, geographical, and functional dimensions and recognizes the interaction among the systems within a community. The three community dimensions—place, people or person—and function are listed in Table 9-1 with indicators of their measure and examples of data sources included.

THE COMMUNITY AS PARTNER

The community is primarily the setting for practice for the CHN providing health promotion and disease prevention interventions with clients using a population health approach model. Community health nursing has often been considered unique because the focus of care is the community. The idea of health-related care being provided within the community is not new. In the early twentieth century, most persons who were ill stayed at home. As a result, the practice environment for most nurses was the home rather than the hospital.

As the range of community health nursing services expanded, many different kinds of agencies were started and their services often overlapped. For instance, voluntary agency home visiting nurses such as Victorian Order of Nurses and official government health agency nurses such as public health nurses visited mothers with newborn babies or clients with tuberculosis. These CHNs practised in clients' homes, not in the hospital. Early textbooks on public health nursing included lengthy descriptions of the home environment and tools for assessing the extent to which that environment promoted the health of family members. Health education about the domestic environment was often a major part of home nursing care.

By the 1950s, schools, prisons, industries, and neighbourhood health centres, as well as homes, had all become areas of practice for nurses in community health. CHNs in these settings focused on the individual client or family seeking care and were referred to as providing community-based nursing (Kushner, 2006; Zotti, Brown, & Stotts, 1996). These nurses practising in the community (*location of practice*) and caring for the individual, family, or group living in the community (*unit of care*) were not necessarily focusing on the community itself as the unit of care.

Viewing the community as the unit of care and as a partner means embracing the two key concepts of

TABLE 9-1 Concept of Community Specified

Dimensions	Measures	Examples of Data Sources
Place	Geopolitical boundaries Local or folk name for area Size in kilometres, acres, blocks, or census tracts Transportation avenues, such as rivers, highways, railroads, and sidewalks History Physical environment such as land-use patterns and condition of housing	Maps Local newspaper Census data Chamber of Commerce Municipal offices Library archives and local histories Local housing office
People or person	Population: number and density Demographic structure of population, such as age, sex, socioeconomic and racial distributions, rural and urban character, and dependency ratio Informal groups such as block clubs, service clubs, and friendship networks Formal groups such as schools, churches, businesses, industries, governmental bodies, unions, and health and welfare agencies Linking structures (intercommunity and intracommunity contacts among organizations)	Census data Churches, seniors' centres Civic groups Local newspaper Telephone directory United Way Social service agencies Chamber of Commerce District health units/health authority Tourist bureau Local and government offices Chamber of Commerce
Function	Production, distribution, and consumption of goods and services Socialization of new members Maintenance of social control Adaptation to ongoing and expected change Provision of mutual aid	Provincial or territorial offices Business and labour Local library Social and local research reports Police station Social and local research reports Churches and religious organizations

community—health and partnership for community health. Together, these form not only the goal but also the means of community practice.

Vollman, Anderson, and McFarlane (2008) present a community model that entails a community-as-partner focus. A partnership conveys an egalitarian relationship between the CHN and the community (Ervin, 2002). This egalitarian relationship encourages community involvement, autonomy, and empowerment. Vollman et al. (2008) suggest that the people in your community are your partners and the partners need to be included during the entire community health nursing process. To facilitate the community partnership, the CHN may work with a community agency, perhaps directly with someone in that agency with ties to the particular community health issue (Jessup-Falcioni & Viverais-Dresler, 2005).

Community partners can facilitate the development of community rapport and trust that are necessary for the CHN to gain access to and information from the community. Consideration for gaining access to aggregates or the entire community is the same as for dealing with the client as individual or family. For example, the community must perceive that a health concern exists, believe that the CHN can assist in addressing this health concern, perceive that its contributions are valued, be assured of confidentiality for nonpublic information, and be involved from the beginning in this partnership. Role negotiation (who will do what) and role separation (CHN as data collector and CHN as facilitator) are other important aspects of partnership and trust. For example, a school principal speaks to a CHN regarding concerns about the number of overweight and obese children in the school and requests assistance to deal with this health concern. The community of interest in this situation is the schoolchildren. The CHN examines the pediatric literature to determine the incidence and prevalence of childhood obesity and reviews the literature for strategies and their effectiveness pertaining to this issue in the school population. The CHN partners with the school principal and school community to conduct a community health assessment, which includes a "windshield survey" of the school and the surrounding school catchment area to determine factors such as nutrition policies and practices, food costs, and food security, with the focus of the assessment being the school environment. A **windshield survey** is an observational method used as part of a community assessment that scans the community's physical environment. A windshield survey is discussed in more detail later in this chapter. The CHN decides to interview certain members individually and conduct focus groups with students, teachers, parents, lunch monitors, and physical activity coordinators. School community strengths and assets are identified and strategies for implementation determined by all stakeholders.

The Community-as-Partner Model diagram and a brief description are found in Appendix 8. The Community-as-Partner Model, based on Betty Neuman's system model, is a nursing framework for community health assessment that incorporates two central components—that is, the nursing process and the community as partner. The community in this community-as-partner model is composed of a central population and eight subsystems depicted diagrammatically as a wheel with population as the hub surrounded by the subsystems. Working as partners, the CHN and the community plan, implement, and evaluate strategies to reduce stressors, restore stability, and avert future health concerns. (A comprehensive discussion of the Community-as-Partner Model is presented in Vollman et al. [2008].)

Other community health assessment models that are sometimes used in community health are the general systems model for community and population assessment, comprehensive health assessment (looks for all relevant community health information), familiarization assessment (windshield survey), problem-oriented assessment (assesses the community with regard to one problem), subsystem or population-oriented assessment (assessment of one single aspect of community such as schools or resources for older adults), and assets assessment (focuses on strengths and capacities rather than only health concerns) (Maurer & Smith, 2009).

COMMUNITY AND THE DETERMINANTS OF HEALTH

The "Determinants of Health: Community and Determinants of Health" box below provides examples of some determinants of health that relate to community and that influence the health of populations. Health status variations exist between populations residing in urban and rural communities, which suggests that the determinants of health need to be addressed especially to deal with the health disparities that exist in rural communities. CHNs need to consider other determinants of health that might exist in their community, such as social and physical environments.

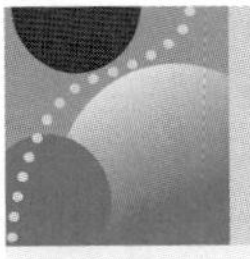

Determinants of Health
Community and Determinants of Health

- Rural Canadians, compared with their urban counterparts, have completed a lower level of education; live in poorer socioeconomic conditions; demonstrate less healthy behaviours; and have more chronic diseases, lower life expectancy, higher mortality rates, and a stronger sense of community belonging (Canadian Institute for Health Information, 2006). Dunn (2002) stated that "social and economic factors strongly influence the health of Canadians and such factors can be modified by social and economic policy" (p. ii). Low income and unemployment contribute to rural Canadians facing greater economic difficulties than their urban counterparts (Pong, 2007). Some of the differing health behaviours by rural residents are higher smoking rates (especially in men), greater exposure to second-hand smoke, and lower likelihood of eating the recommended five servings of fruit and vegetables (especially males) (Health Canada, 2010). The most common causes of mortality due to injury in rural communities are due to motor-vehicle and farm accidents and injuries (Health Canada, 2010).
- Poverty is on the rise in Canadian cities (Khosla, 2005).
- Many (approximately 49%) of Aboriginal children living off the reserve are living in poverty (Campaign 2000, 2009).
- In 1970, of 905 neighbourhoods 86% were middle class, but in 2005 the number had dropped to 61% (*Toronto Star,* February 8, 2009). In Canada, the gap between the poor and rich families is widening (Campaign 2000, 2009). Neighbourhood quality is one part of the social environment (Clark, 2008), another determinant of health.
- From March 2007 to March 2008, there was an increase of 17.6%, or almost 120,000 people, in need of food assistance from food banks across Canada, with increases noted in every region (Society and Culture, 2009). This increase in persons unable to afford food supports the widening gap in socioeconomic status and therefore the increase in poverty experienced by Canadians.

CRITICAL VIEW

1. How do the socioeconomic features of a community (e.g., employment, income, and cultural diversity) promote health or cause ill health?
2. What are the effects of inequalities in socioeconomic features in your community?

CHARACTERISTICS OF COMMUNITY HEALTH NURSING PRACTICE

The most effective means of completing healthy changes in the community is through collaborative partnership of the CHN with various partners. Their common goal of community health involves an ongoing series of health promoting changes.

Community Health

Like the concept of community, community health has three common characteristics. These characteristics or dimensions are status, structure, and process. Each dimension has a unique effect on a community's health.

Status

Community health is often measured by traditional morbidity and mortality rates, life expectancy indices, and risk-factor profiles. This information for all regions in Canada is available through the Statistics Canada Web site (see the Weblinks on the Evolve Web site). It is a Government of Canada site that provides an accurate source of data such as profiles of individual communities, a profile of Canada, and detailed data for small groups (such as one-parent families, ethnic groups, occupational groups, and immigrants). The 2006 census findings are available at the Statistics Canada Web site. The Canadian census is collected every 5 years and aims to include every Canadian in Canada on "census day" plus any Canadians who are living outside of Canada. Individuals without an address, such as the homeless, are not likely to be included and therefore are invisible aggregates. The census also includes those who are residing in Canada and who have a permit to do so, such as a study, work, or temporary resident permit, and their dependants (Statistics Canada, 2009b). The questions used every 5 years are similar, so similarity comparisons can be made to determine changes that have occurred in Canada's population over time. The release of the 2006 census data began in March 2007, and data reports are released as they become available. The Government of Canada's decision in the summer of 2010 to make voluntary the previously mandatory long-form census has research and evaluation implications. According to Collier (2010), "The population data obtained from a voluntary survey will be biased, researchers say, and will inhibit research into the social determinants of health" (p. E563). It will be difficult to monitor for changes in population health patterns. The proposed changes are being challenged and may be reversed prior to the 2011 census due to pressure on the government to maintain the census status quo.

The Canadian Institute for Health Information (CIHI) is a not-for-profit autonomous organization that provides data and analysis on the health of Canadians and Canada's health system. The CIHI, along with Statistics Canada, reports on the health indicators that reflect and affect the health of Canadians and the performance of the Canadian health care system. The Canadian Community Health Survey (CCHS), initiated in 2000, closely examines health determinants and is a 2-year cycle survey that is the data source for many of the health indicators. The CCHS is "conducted by Statistics Canada to provide cross-sectional estimates of health determinants, health status and health system utilization for 133 health regions across Canada, plus the territories" (Statistics Canada, 2009a). Health indicators provide information on the health of the population, health services, and community characteristics.

Some of the health surveys that have been conducted in Canada over the years are the Canada Health Survey (1978), Health Promotion Surveys (1985, 1990), the National Population Health Survey (1994 and every 2 years thereafter, which now includes the CCHS), Canadian Heart Health Surveys (1986, 1990), and the National Longitudinal Survey of Children and Youth (1994) (Shah, 2003). These surveys, and others, generally provide prevalence rates for risk factors, disease, disability, and use of health services and are used to look at associations among the risk factors (Shah, 2003). (For a brief history of Canadian health surveys, see the Public Health Agency of Canada Weblink on the Evolve Web site.) In 2006, Health Canada published *Healthy Canadians: A Federal Report on Comparable Health Indicators, 2006* (see the Weblinks on the Evolve Web site). This site provides the executive summary of highlights of the report, which includes statistics on findings such as that smoking among teenagers continued to decline and that more than half of Canadians over age 12 were active or moderately physically active (Health Canada, 2006).

Structure

Community health, when viewed from the structure of the community, is usually defined in terms of community characteristics, as well as *services* and *resources*. Indicators used to measure community health services and resources include service-use patterns, treatment data from various health agencies, and provider-to-client ratios. These data provide information such as the number of available hospital beds or the number of emergency room visits to a particular hospital.

Characteristics of the community structure are commonly identified as social indicators, or correlates, of health. Characteristics of community structure include demographic characteristics such as age, gender, socioeconomic and racial distributions, and educational levels. Their relationships to health status have been thoroughly documented (Shah, 2003).

Recent evidence identifies key factors that influence the health of populations. These are referred to as the *social determinants of health* (Raphael, 2009) (see Chapter 1) and include such factors as gender, housing, income and income distribution, and educational levels (Mikkonen & Raphael, 2010). Some studies have found that certain social determinants of health have more impact on health and the incidence of illness than traditional biomedical and behavioural risk factors (Raphael, 2009).

Process

The view of community health as the process of effective community functioning or problem solving is well established. However, it is especially appropriate to community health nursing because it directs the study of community health to promote effective community action for health promotion, which is an important aim of CHNs.

A broad, commonly accepted definition of **community health** is the process of involving the community in maintaining, improving, promoting, and protecting its own health and well-being. This definition emphasizes the process dimension but also includes the dimensions of status and structure. Indicators for the dimensions of community health (status, structure, and process) are listed with measures and examples of data sources in Table 9-2. The use of status, structure, and process

TABLE 9-2 Concept of Community Health Specified

Dimension	Measures	Examples of Data Sources
Status	Vital statistics (live births, neonatal deaths, infant deaths, maternal deaths)	Census data District health unit annual vital statistics
	Incidence and prevalence of leading causes of mortality and morbidity	Census data District health unit/health authority
	Health-risk profiles of selected aggregates	District health unit Support groups Local nonprofit organizations
	Functional ability levels	Census data
Structure	Health facilities such as hospitals, long-term care facilities, industrial and school health services, health units, voluntary health associations	Local Chamber of Commerce United Way
	Health-related planning groups	Local newspapers Local magazines Local government
	Health personnel resources, such as physicians, dentists, and nurses	Telephone directory Provincial and labour statistics Professional licensing boards
	Health-resource use patterns, such as bed-occupancy days and client or provider visits	Statistics Canada District health units and hospital annual reports
Process	Commitment to community health	Local government
	Awareness of self and others and clarity of situational definitions	Local history Neighbourhood help organizations Local or neighbourhood newspapers and radio programs Local government
	Conflict containment and accommodation	Social services department
	Participation	Existence of and participation in local organizations
	Management of relationships with society	Windshield survey—observation of interactions
	Machinery for facilitating participant interaction and decision making	Notices for community organizations and meetings in public places (supermarkets, newspapers, radio)

dimensions to define community health is an effort to develop a broad definition of community health, involving indicators that often are not included when discussions focus only on individual and family risk factors as the basis for community health.

Strategies to Improve Community Health

There are several different approaches to community disease prevention and health promotion, but regardless of which approach is taken, specific strategies to improve community health often depend on whether the status, structure, or process dimension of community health is being emphasized, as follows:

- If the emphasis is on the *status dimension,* activities from primary or secondary prevention at the community level are usually the best strategies because the objective is either to prevent a disease or to treat it in its early stages. Immunization programs are an example of a community health nursing intervention at the primary prevention level when contracting the disease will likely occur if the immunization is not received.
- Community health nursing intervention strategies focused on the *structural dimension* are directed at either health services or population demographic characteristics. Intervention aimed at altering health services might include developing a new program in occupational health nursing because of the illnesses and injuries identified through an assessment at a certain workplace. Interventions aimed at affecting demographic characteristics may include community development. A group of community leaders may come together because they have recognized that school-age children do not have easy access to recreational opportunities after school hours. The leaders, in partnership with the health units or authorities and the school board, may be able to plan for after-school recreational activities.
- When the emphasis is on the *process dimension*—usually the level of intervention of the CHN—the best strategy is usually health promotion. For example, if family-life education is lacking in a community because of ineffective communication among families, children, school board members, religious leaders, and health professionals, the most effective CHN strategy may be to open discussion among these groups and help community members develop education programs and advocate for programs.

Healthy Communities

In the mid-1980s, an international movement promoting healthy communities was developed in Europe by the World Health Organization (WHO). The term "Healthy Cities movement" is used interchangeably with "Healthy Communities movement." This movement, also discussed in Chapter 4, incorporates the primary health care principles of health promotion to achieve "health for all." "A '**healthy community**' is one where people, organizations and local institutions work together to improve the social, economic and environmental conditions that make people healthy—the determinants of health" (Rural Communities Impacting Policy, 2006, p. 1).

The health of a community includes the health care system and involves policies that affect social, economic, and environmental life, and the activities of individuals, groups, and corporations (Capital Regional District, 2008). Characteristics of a healthy community are the following:

- "Clean and safe physical environments
- Peace, equity and social justice
- Adequate access to food, clean water, shelter, income, safety, work and recreation for all
- Strong, mutually-supportive relationships and networks
- Wide participation of residents in decision-making
- Strong cultural and spiritual heritage
- Diverse and robust economy
- Opportunities for learning and skill development
- Access to health services, including public health and preventive programs" (Vancouver Coastal Health, 2009)

There is an emphasis on the determinants of health, which include social determinants (e.g., healthy public policy), environmental determinants (e.g., green space), economic determinants (e.g., stable employment), physical determinants (e.g., physical activity), psychological and spiritual determinants (e.g., sense of belonging), and cultural determinants (e.g., community identity) (British Columbia Healthy Communities, 2009). (Further information about healthy communities can be found at the Healthy Cities/Healthy Communities Weblink on the Evolve Web site.) Communities in many provinces have adopted the movement, such as Victoria in British Columbia, Buffalo Narrows in Saskatchewan, Brandon in Manitoba, Waterloo in Ontario, Trois-Rivières in Quebec, and Bathurst in New Brunswick. The *Directory of the Networks of Healthy Communities and Cities in Canada* Evolve Weblink provides a history of the Healthy Cities/Healthy Communities movement and direct connections to the many cities and communities across Canada that have joined this Canadian network. For additional information on other Canadian communities engaged in the Healthy Communities movement, see pp. 32–38 of the document found at the *Senate Subcommittee on Population Health* Weblink on the Evolve Web site.

The Canadian Nurses Association (CNA) provides a summary of the issues pertaining to Healthy Communities and nursing (see the Weblinks on the Evolve Web site). This issue is important to nurses as it deals with several of the determinants of health. Some of the ways that CHNs have been involved in the Healthy Communities movement have been to identify community health issues; support community members in the research, organization, and presentation of the issues; and establish coalitions with other partners such as the educational sector. The backgrounder provides information on the Healthy Communities process and, in particular, the range of policies at the community level that can affect health—for example, a policy for sidewalk snow removal that should result in fewer falls and injuries. The process of Healthy Communities development is important to CHNs as it deals with several of the determinants of health and policy development to improve on these determinants, which is one strategy that CHNs can support. Additionally, CHNs can apply for funding where available for community projects that support healthy community initiatives (British Columbia Healthy Communities, 2009; Ontario Ministry of Health Promotion, 2009).

Community Partnerships and Coalitions

A **partnership** is a relationship between individuals, groups, organizations, or governments, in which the parties are actively working together in all stages of assessment planning, implementation, and evaluation. In the community context, it is often used synonymously with *coalitions* and *alliances,* ideally with power shared among all participants in the processes of change for improved community health. **Community partnerships** involve collaborative decision-making efforts in health planning with the goal of reducing health inequalities and improving community health. Consequently, successful strategies for improving community health must include collaborative partnerships in the community for greater health impact. Vollman et al. (2008) use the Community-as-Partner Model to emphasize the fundamental thinking of interdisciplinary primary health care and the developing reverence for public involvement in health decision making.

Partnership is a concept that is essential for CHNs to know and use, as are the concepts of community, community as partner, and community health. Experienced CHNs know that partnership is important because health is generated through new and increasingly effective means of lay and professional collaboration at the individual, family, group, or community level. For example, polluted air is an issue for many urban neighbourhoods. An example of an informal partnership is one that developed among parents of asthmatic children, local politicians, and other citizens to create a policy about leaf burning in the township. Another is the spring cleanup organized in several communities, whereby citizens volunteer to pick up garbage along roadways on a selected activity day, sponsored by a local business such as Tim Hortons in partnership with the local government, with the intention of promoting exercise and cleaner neighbourhoods. An example of a formal partnership is the PeaceWorks Community Partnership Project, which took place in the late 1990s in the eastern part of Prince Edward Island. Partnerships were established between families, youth groups, schools, police, and local businesses to address the issue of increased community violence, with the goal of more peaceful schools and communities. Effective partnerships usually have the following characteristics:

- Equality in decision making
- A shared vision
- Integrity
- Agreement on specific goals
- A plan of action to meet the goals

The significance and effectiveness of partnership in improving community health are supported by a growing body of literature. Some Government of Canada partnership initiatives that have an impact on the determinants of health are the National Homelessness Initiative, which assists governments and community organizations in 61 communities across Canada to address homelessness (physical environment as the determinant of health) (Human Resources and Skills Development Canada, 2009b); the Workplace Partners Panel (Human Resources and Skills Development Canada, 2006), which brings business and labour leaders together to centre on labour market and skills issues currently facing Canada (employment and working conditions as the determinant of health); and the Community Development and Partnerships Directorate (Human Resources and Skills Development Canada, 2009a), which is working toward addressing the social concerns of the Government of Canada in reference to children and their families by working with the voluntary sector (social environment as the determinant of health).

In international health, partnership models generally are viewed as empowering people, through their lay leaders, to control their own health destinies and lives. Partnerships can also be established between nurses. The CNA believes that nurses and the nursing profession in Canada must contribute to the advancement of global health and equity and that one way this can be achieved is by establishing partnerships with nurses and nursing associations around the world, especially in developing countries. The CNA's position statement "International Health Partnerships" (see the Weblinks on the Evolve Web site) shows that CNA has been establishing partnerships with national nursing associations in developing countries for more than 30 years with the goal of increasing the ability of these nursing associations to fortify the nursing profession as well as the quality of nursing and health services provided to their populations (CNA, 2005).

Another example of a different type of partnership is the Healthy Cities/Healthy Communities movement previously discussed. The Healthy Communities movement promotes the creation of multisectoral partnerships among the various community groups, such as individual community members, voluntary and nonvoluntary agencies, businesses, local government, and citizens, to address issues of health and quality of life that have been identified as priorities (Vollman et al., 2008). To improve and promote the health and well-being of the community, existing community resources are used to identify and prioritize community health needs and concerns. Existing resources are also used in the planning, implementation, and evaluation of the chosen strategies and programs (Vollman et al., 2008).

Many of the activities pertaining to the Healthy Communities movements or projects are conducted by coalitions. A **coalition** refers to two or more groups that share a mutual issue or concern and join forces, thereby increasing their influence in achieving a common goal. The groups can vary but most often are representative of organizations and agencies that have an assigned interest (mandate) in the issue and citizens who have come together to form a "community of interest." These community coalitions are one type of partnership that usually extends over a long period of time. Members come to a coalition as representatives of their own organization or as a community member; however, there is an expectation that members will advocate on behalf of the coalition to advance their shared interests in health promotion and not their own self-interest (Moyer, 2005; Nies & McEwen, 2007). Coalitions can have many purposes, and many coalitions are not just locally based but have provincial and national affiliates. For example, Heart Health coalitions have been established in at least 10 provinces and territories and in more than 50 Canadian communities (Health Canada, 2004), and Healthy Communities coalitions are located in several provinces, such as British Columbia, Saskatchewan, Manitoba, Ontario, Quebec, and New Brunswick. Coalitions often add credibility to the health community because they have broad community support and present a united front with a coordinated, consistent message. However, conflict may be evident at times due to the variety of groups in a coalition, their varying strengths and weaknesses, and the personalities that they bring to the coalition. The management of conflict and group building skills are necessary to deal with issues that arise in coalitions. These group management processes are discussed in Chapter 14.

COMMUNITY CONCEPTS

Kretzmann and McKnight (1993) identify community development as "building communities from the inside out." (See the Kretzman and McKnight Weblink on the Evolve Web site for introductory information on community development.) Community development occurs when a community is engaged in a dynamic continuous process of social change that can lead to permanent enhancements in people's lives; this can include a broad range of strategies such as capacity building and empowerment (Winnipeg Regional Health Authority, 2007). The process also includes working with the community as the unit of care and implies partnering with the community so that the CHN and other health professionals work with community members to identify their health concerns and work toward community change. Table 9-3 outlines the steps in the community development process. **Community capacity** identifies and works with existing community strengths to promote a positive view of the community; it therefore helps communities to become stronger based on these strengths rather than focus on their weaknesses (McKnight & Kretzmann, 2005; Shields & Lindsey, 2002). The process of capacity building relies strongly on collaboration and partnerships. Building capacity ensures that partners develop the skills and resources required to hold programs together, thereby increasing their chances for long-term success. Table 9-4 describes nine features of community capacity (Public Health Agency of Canada, 2008).

As a result of this shift in thinking about community approaches, a tool called "mapping community capacity" was introduced by McKnight and Kretzmann (2005). Asset mapping is one of the skills required of CHNs when working in community development. **Asset mapping** refers to identifying community-based initiatives such as community development, strategic planning, and organizational development. There are three approaches to asset mapping: the whole-assets approach (which is comprehensive and provides a complete map of the community and its support system), the storytelling approach (a social history that reveals assets in the community), and the heritage approach (a picture, map, or list of anything that is part of a community's heritage) (Government of Canada, 2009). Some examples of asset mapping are found at the following Weblinks on the Evolve Web site: (1) the Canadian Community Economic Development Network, which provides detail on socioeconomic indicators and mapping, and links to related resources, (2) the Strong Neighbourhoods Task Force Web site, which provides examples of the application of asset mapping, and (3) the Human Resources and Social Development Canada site, which provides extensive guidelines on and examples for using mapping as a tool.

TABLE 9-3 Steps in the Community Development Process

Defining the issue	Articulate the issue; what is known about it, and who is affected
Initiating the process	Research the veracity of the issue and perspectives, identify the full range of stakeholders, and gather people together to create commitment for action
Planning community conversations	Invite all stakeholders to participate; develop both informal and formal processes of consultation that allow all viewpoints to be properly aired
Talking, discovering, and connecting	Prepare handouts that outline the issue and why you are gathering information and mobilizing the community; connect with key people and community members; share information and gather support
Creating an asset map	Develop lists as you talk to people and initiate relationships, communicate regularly and widely, attract resources
Mobilizing the community	Bring people together in central locations to discuss options, share experiences, create a common vision, and plan activities
Taking action	Involve and educate community members, help to shape opinion, and galvanize commitment
Planning and implementing	Have a vision in mind of what must change so community-driven initiatives improve the situation, organize people and work, and sustain efforts

SOURCE: Vollman, A. R., Anderson, E. T., & McFarlane, J. (2008). *Canadian community as partner* (2nd ed., p. 118). Philadelphia, PA: Lippincott, Williams & Wilkins.

TABLE 9-4 Features and Descriptions of Community Capacity

Feature	Description
Participation	Is the active involvement of people in improving their own and their community's health and well-being. Participating in a project means the target population, community members, and other stakeholders are involved in project activities, such as making decisions and evaluation.
Leadership	Includes developing and nurturing both formal and informal local leaders during a project. Effective leaders support, direct, deal with conflict, acknowledge and encourage community members' voices, share leadership, and facilitate networks to build on community resources. Leaders bring people with diverse skill sets together and may have both interpersonal and technical skills. Finally, an effective leader has a strategic vision for the future.
Community structures	Refers to smaller or less formal community groups and committees that foster belonging and give the community a chance to express views and exchange information. Examples of community structures are church groups, youth groups, and self-help groups.
External supports	Refers to (funding bodies) such as government departments, foundations, and regional health authorities that can link communities and external resources. At the beginning of a project, early external support may nurture community momentum.
Asking why	Refers to a community process that uncovers the root causes of community health issues and promotes solutions. The community comes together to critically assess the social, political, and economic influences that result in differing health standards and conditions. Exploration through "asking why" helps refine a project to reflect the community needs.
Obtaining resources	Includes finding time, money (other than from funding bodies), leadership, volunteers, information, and facilities both from inside and outside the community.
Skills, knowledge, and learning	Refers to the qualities in the project team, the target population, and the community that the project team uses and develops.
Linking with others	Refers to linking your project with individuals and organizations. These project links help the community deal with its issues. Examples include creating partnerships or linking with networks and coalitions.
Sense of community	Is fostered through building trust with others. Community projects can strengthen a sense of community when people come together to work on shared community problems.
	Collaborations give community members confidence to act and courage to feel hopeful about change.

SOURCE: Public Health Agency of Canada. (2008). *The community capacity building tool* (pp. 1–14). Retrieved from http://www.phac-aspc.gc.ca/canada/regions/ab-nwt-tno/downloads-eng.php.

The use of community capacity to bring about change through an action plan, usually developed and implemented with community partners, is known as community mobilization. It refers to influencing healthy public policy and may include individuals residing in the community joining together to bring about change in reference to a health issue. Some examples of community mobilization are "Fighting for a Supervised Injection Site in Vancouver," which is a group of citizens who mobilized over the issue of safe drug use in downtown eastside Vancouver, and "Building a gay, lesbian, bisexual and transgendered (GLBT) community organization in Nova Scotia," which is a group of concerned citizens who mobilized to create a safe community for its GLBT community members. For further information on these examples of community mobilization and others, refer to the Canadian HIV/AIDS Legal Network Weblink on the Evolve Web site.

As the community and its members are involved as partners in community development, outcomes such as empowerment, sustainability, and community competence are most likely to occur. By using partnership in the community development process, members and the community should gain control over the issues that affect them and thereby become empowered. Participation that encourages empowerment of a community is crucial in promoting community health and sustainability (Diem, 2005). **Sustainability** refers to the maintenance and continuation of established community programs and is more likely to occur when members of the community are involved as partners in the community development process. **Community competence** has been linked to community empowerment (Minkler & Wallerstein, 2005); a competent community is able to use its problem-solving abilities to identify and deal with community health issues (Minkler & Wallerstein, 2005). Through the identification and management of their own issues, communities are more likely to experience feelings of empowerment. CHNs are in an ideal position to be involved in community development as they possess both the knowledge required to work with the community and the nursing practice skills in community development. As mentioned in Chapter 1, CHNs take the approach of *working with* as opposed to *doing for* the community, which demonstrates the forward thinking needed in community development. They have established rapport with members in their communities and can therefore mobilize the community in meeting its health needs through utilization of the community health nursing process. Additional resources that CHNs could employ to help guide community development, capacity building, and asset mapping are found on the Community Building Resources Web site, the Human Resources and Social Development Canada Web site, and the Strong Neighbourhoods Task Force Web site found in the Weblinks on the Evolve Web site.

COMMUNITY ASSESSMENT TO EVALUATION

As mentioned earlier, the community health nursing process is used in community health assessment. The phases of this process that directly involve the community as partner begin at the start of the contract or partnership; these phases are assessment, planning, implementation, and evaluation.

Assessing Community Health

There are many approaches to assessing a community. According to Maurer and Smith (2009), some of these are a comprehensive needs assessment that tries to determine what the particular problems or needs are within a community using an extensive systematic process to assess all community aspects; a problem-oriented approach that assesses a community based on a specific health concern; a single-population approach that is an assessment of one population group in a community such as older adults or men; and the familiarization approach that uses existing data on a community such as census data, surveys, or health reports. One current and widely used comprehensive community assessment model in Canada is the Vollman, Anderson, and McFarlane Community-as-Partner Model (Vollman et al., 2008). Another model used in Canada that provides thorough community health assessment is the *Community Health Assessment Guidelines, 2009,* which are endorsed by the Community Health Assessment Network of Manitoba and also incorporate the determinants of health. These guidelines are listed in the Weblinks on the Evolve Web site under the Manitoba Health and Healthy Living Accountability Support Branch.

Community health assessment is the process of thinking critically about the community and involves getting to know and understand the community client as partner. This helps the CHN to understand the client health concerns and to know what community strengths and resources are available for the CHN to work as a partner with the client to address the client's concerns. The community health assessment phase involves a logical, systematic approach to the initial phase of the community health nursing process. Community health assessment helps to (1) identify community strengths, resources, assets, capacities, and opportunities; (2) clarify health concerns; (3) identify community constraints; (4) identify the economic, political, and social factors affecting the community; and (5) identify the determinants of health affecting community health.

Community health assessments can be extensive, such as the comprehensive community assessment, or shorter, such as the single-population approach. Either way, the necessary initial assessment phase of the community health nursing process with the community client as partner is applied. CHNs undertake a community health assessment for many reasons that direct the type of data collected, the emphasis on different clusters of data, the sources of data, and the data collection methods. One reason to conduct a community health assessment could be as a response to a suspected or identified health concern in order to validate the existence and determine the extent of the health concern and generate some possible resolutions. A second reason is to identify community assets and gaps in resources so that alternative solutions can be developed to address the identified gaps. Finally, the CHN undertakes a community health assessment to determine the actual health status of the community. The CHN may focus on a particular population group (aggregate) within the community or may assess the entire community.

Some examples will help to clarify these differing purposes. For instance, a CHN concerned about an apparent increase in the incidence of rubella in a community might conduct a community health assessment to verify the existence and extent of the health concern within a susceptible population, such as females of child-bearing years, and their level of immunity. This action might enable the CHN to prevent fetal deformities either by increasing immunization levels among the target group or by promoting contraceptive use by those who are not immune. Another example is a CHN who has been recently assigned to a new or rapidly expanding town. A comprehensive community health assessment is conducted to establish baseline information on the health status of a community and the capacity of the community to meet its health concerns. Before a community health assessment is started, certain planning considerations must be addressed. See the *Manitoba Community Health Assessment Guide* (specifically pp. 6–22) in the Weblinks on the Evolve Web site, for a discussion on planning considerations.

Assessing community health requires the following three steps:

1. Gathering relevant existing data and generating missing data
2. Developing a composite database
3. Interpreting the composite database to identify community strengths and health concerns

Data Collection and Interpretation

Data collection is the process of acquiring existing, readily available information or developing new information about the community and its health. The systematic collection of data about community health requires the following:

- Gathering or compiling existing data
- Generating missing data
- Interpreting data
- Identifying community abilities and health concerns

See the Weblink for the *Manitoba Community Health Assessment Guide* (pp. 23–26) for key considerations on data gathering and analysis for community health assessments.

There is a multitude of data to be collected to complete a comprehensive health assessment of a community as client. An assessment model or framework identifies the various categories of data to be collected and assists in organizing the data collected. There is no sole instrument that provides all the information needed; therefore, CHNs often select parts of various assessment instruments that meet their needs and that address concerns of relevance to the community. Even though an assessment model or framework assists with data gathering and generation, in a comprehensive assessment of a community, the amount of community information can become overwhelming. Therefore, the CHN needs to make decisions about what information is most important to collect, the data sources most appropriate to use, and the data-collection methods deemed most effective. Most frequently, CHNs will conduct smaller and more focused assessments. These condensed community assessments could be done using the windshield survey method to gain beginning insights about the community or using a small-scale community assessment (Escoffery, Miner, & Trowbridge, 2004). Depending on factors such as health concern, purpose, and resource availability, the CHN may conduct either a comprehensive community health assessment or a condensed community health assessment.

Data Gathering

Data gathering is the process of obtaining existing, readily available data. The following data usually describe the demography of a community:

- Age of residents
- Gender distribution of residents
- Socioeconomic characteristics
- Racial distributions
- Vital statistics, including selected mortality and morbidity data
- Community institutions, including health care organizations and the services they provide
- Health personnel characteristics

Often these data have been collected by others via structured interviews, questionnaires, or surveys and are available in published reports at the library or local public health department. These data give the CHN a snapshot of how the clients receiving services fit into the community.

The CHN also needs to be aware that some statistics may not be easily accessed for the community being examined. A primary source survey may sometimes need to be repeated, as in the need for accurate data for smaller geographical areas. This type of survey requires close partnership to facilitate complete community response and cooperation. This partnership helps to ensure the accuracy and validity of community health nursing assessment.

Data Generation

Data generation is the process of developing data that do not already exist, through interaction with community members. This type of information is more difficult to obtain and is generally not statistical in nature. Data that often must be generated include information about the following:

- Knowledge and beliefs
- Values and sentiments
- Goals and perceived concerns
- Norms
- Problem-solving processes
- Power
- Leadership
- Influence structures

These data are more likely to be collected by interviews and observation.

Composite Database Analysis

The gathered and generated data are combined to create a composite **database.** Data analysis, with the community, seeks to make sense of the data, as follows:

1. Data are analyzed and synthesized, and themes are noted.
2. **Community health concerns**—actual, possible, or potential community health challenges with identifiable contributing factors in the environment—are determined.
3. **Community health strengths**—resources available to meet community health concerns—are identified.
4. Community health strengths, which are the resources available, are implemented to meet the health concerns that have been identified.

Data collection and interpretation (diagnostic reasoning) are critical aspects of the community health nursing process.

Data-Collection Methods

Several methods to collect data are needed. Methods that encourage the CHN to consider the community's perception of its health concerns and abilities are as important as those methods structured to identify knowledge that the CHN considers essential. Six useful methods of collecting data follow:

1. Informant interviews
2. Focus groups
3. Participant observation
4. Windshield surveys
5. Community forums
6. Secondary analysis of existing data
7. Surveys

These methods can be grouped into the following two distinct but complementary categories: methods that rely on what is directly observed by the data collector and methods that rely on what is reported to the data collector.

Collection of Direct Data

Informant interviews, focus groups, participant observation, windshield surveys, and community forums are five methods of directly collecting data. All five methods require sensitivity; openness; curiosity; the ability to listen, taste, touch, and smell; and the ability to see life as it is lived in a community.

Informant interviews, which consist of directed talks with selected members of a community about community members or groups and events, are basic to effective data collection. Talking to key informants is a critical part of the community assessment. Key informants are not always people who have a formal title or position—they often have an informal role within the community. Examples are a member of a minority group who is listened to by other members of the group, a church deacon, or a parent who is active and vocal about the school health curriculum. What is critical in using key informants is to acquire those whose views represent those of the community.

Focus groups consist of talking with a group of individuals residing in the community who share their beliefs, opinions, and experiences about a selected discussion topic. In focus groups, the members are able to interact and share and build on each other's ideas. During a community health assessment, focus groups are usually used throughout the assessment phase. For example, a focus

How To... Identify a Key Informant for Interviews

The following may be key informants:

- Health care providers such as public health nurses
- Church leaders
- Many community members whom CHNs know and who can identify other key informants
- A president of the school council organization
- The mayor or other local politicians
- Informal leader, such as a mother who organized the local chapter of Mothers Against Drunk Driving (informal leader)

group may be conducted to explore high-risk behaviour in specific aggregate groups; in this case, they might try to determine factors contributing to smoking behaviour in youth. Also, a focus group may be conducted to explore possible alternative interventions for identified health concerns in youth who smoke to determine youth perceptions of actions to promote smoking cessation. Another example of the use of a focus group could be to evaluate the effectiveness of a smoking program that has been implemented among youth.

Also basic is **participant observation,** the deliberate sharing, if conditions permit, in the life of a community. For example, if the CHN lives in the community, participating in activities such as clinical organizations and church life and reading the newspaper provides the CHN with "observations" of the community's life. Informant interviews and participant observation are good ways to generate information about community beliefs, norms, values, power and influence structures, and problem-solving processes. Such data can seldom be reported in numbers, so often they are not collected. Even worse, conclusions that are based on intuition and are unchecked are sometimes used to replace this type of data. Conclusions from direct data-collection methods should be confirmed by those people providing the information.

Informant interviews with social workers and religious leaders can provide data that describe a community that has well-defined clusters of individuals with similar concerns, such as persons of low income, those with concerns about adolescent pregnancy, and those with worries about the health of babies. These data could be difficult to acquire without personal interviews.

A windshield survey or walking survey can be conducted by walking or driving through a community. It involves the CHN looking through the car windshield while performing a quick collection of data that facilitates an understanding of the geographical features of the community and "the location of agencies, services, businesses, and industries and location of possible areas of environmental concern through "sight, sense, and sound" (Cassells, 2007, p. 77). Observational data may also be collected by conducting a walking survey (Vollman et al., 2008).

While walking, driving a car, or riding public transportation, the CHN can observe many dimensions of a community's life and environment through the windshield, such as these:

- Common characteristics of people on the street
- Accessibility, such as access to buildings and sidewalk design
- Neighbourhood gathering places
- The rhythm of community life
- Housing quality and alternatives
- Recreational opportunities
- Geographical boundaries

Windshield surveys can be used by themselves for short and rapid community health assessments. See the "How To..." on p. 271. A CHN doing such a survey as part of a community health assessment should go out twice: once during the day when people are at work and children are at school, and a second time in the evening after work is done and school is out. This survey can be completed on foot to provide the opportunity for interaction and a "feel" for the community, or by driving slowly through the community if it covers a large geographical area. An example of a walking or windshield survey is found in Figure 9-1.

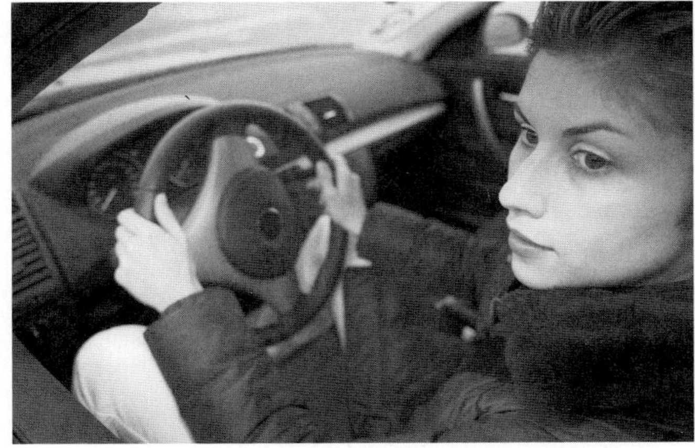

A windshield/walking survey is an observational technique used in community health assessment that offers the community health nurse some early insights about the community in which he or she is working.

FIGURE 9-1 Windshield/Walking Survey

I. Community Core (Elements)	Observations	Data
1. *History.* What can you glean by looking (e.g., old, established neighbourhoods; new subdivision)? Ask people willing to talk: How long have you lived here? Has the area changed? As you talk, ask if there is an "old-timer" who knows the history of the area.		
2. *Demographics.* What sorts of people do you see? Young? Old? Homeless? Alone? Families? Is the population homogeneous?		
3. *Ethnicity.* Do you note indicators of different ethnic groups (e.g., restaurants, festivals)? What signs do you see of different cultural groups?		
4. *Values and beliefs.* Are there churches, mosques, temples? Does it appear homogeneous? Are the lawns cared for? With flowers? Gardens? Signs of art? Culture? Heritage? Historical markers?		
II. Subsystems	**Observations**	**Data**
1. *Physical environment.* How does the community look? What do you note about air quality, flora, housing, zoning, space, green areas, animals, people, human-made structures, natural beauty, water, climate? Can you find or develop a map of the area? What is the size (e.g., kilometres, blocks)?		
2. *Health and social services.* Is there evidence of acute or chronic conditions? Shelters? Alternative therapists or healers? Are there clinics, hospitals, practitioners' offices, public health services, home health agencies, emergency centres, nursing homes, social service facilities, mental health services? Are there resources outside the community but readily accessible to residents?		
3. *Economy.* Is it a "thriving" community, or does it feel "seedy"? Are there industries, stores, places of employment? Where do people shop? Are there signs that people can find employment (e.g., Help Wanted signs, classified ads)? Are there signs of thrift stores, pawn shops, and other services for people with money issues? How active is the food bank?		
4. *Transportation and safety.* How do people get around? What types of private and public transportation are available? Do you see buses, bicycles, taxis? Are there sidewalks, bike trails? Is getting around in the community possible for people with disabilities? What types of protective services are there (e.g., fire, police, sanitation)? Is air quality monitored? What types of crimes are committed? Do people feel safe? Are there signs of racism or intolerance?		
5. *Politics and government.* Are there signs of political activity (e.g., posters, meetings)? What party affiliation predominates? What is the governmental jurisdiction of the community (e.g., elected mayor, city council with single-member districts)? Are people involved in decision making in their local governmental unit?		
6. *Communication.* Are there "common areas" where people gather? What newspapers do you see in the stands? Do people have TVs, mobile music devices, cell phones? What do they watch and listen to? What are the formal and informal means of communication?		

FIGURE 9-1 Windshield/Walking Survey—Cont'd

7. *Education.* Are there schools in the area? How do they look? How does it function? What is the reputation of the school(s)? What are major educational issues? What are the dropout rates? Are extracurricular activities available? Are they used? Is there a school health service? A school nurse? Are there adult education and second-language programs readily available?		
8. *Recreation.* Where do children play? What are the major forms of recreation? Who participates? What facilities for recreation do you see? Are they in good order or disrepair? Are there signs that pets are welcome? What about the performing arts and social and other leisure activities (e.g., festivals, zoo, museum, sports teams)?		
III. Perceptions	**Observations**	**Data**
1. *The residents.* How do people feel about the community? What do they identify as its strengths? Problems? Ask several people from different groups (e.g., old, young, unskilled/skilled workers, service worker, professional, clergy, stay-at-home parent, lone parent) and keep track of who gives what answer.		
2. *Your perceptions.* What are your general statements about the "health" of this community? What are its strengths? What concerns or potential concerns can you identify? Who are the gatekeepers to the community and/or population of interest? Who are the champions that might support your work? Who in the community might become a partner in the process? Where will resistance be found?		

Vollman, A. R., Anderson, E. T., & McFarlane, J. M. (2008). *Canadian community as partner: Theory and multidisciplinary practice in nursing* (2nd ed., pp. 248–249). Philadelphia: Lippincott, Williams & Wilkins. Adapted from Anderson, E. T., & McFarlane, J. M. (2006). *Community as partner: Theory and practice in nursing* (5th ed., pp. 220–221). Philadelphia, PA: Lippincott, Williams & Wilkins. Reproduced with permission.

Community forums provide an opportunity for involved parties to gain an understanding of a particular issue of concern to them. For community forums to be effective, it is important to build a trusting, open relationship. Community forums do not include decision making. Some examples of community forums are town hall meetings where the public meet face to face in a community centre to discuss a community issue; community-to-community forums where the members from neighbouring communities such as a First Nations reserve and a local community meet face to face to discuss mutual issues; and an Internet forum that provides the opportunity for a discussion to occur using online technology. For an example of a community forum, see the *Guide to Community Forums in British Columbia* Weblink on the Evolve Web site.

How To... Obtain a Quick Assessment of a Community

- One way of getting a quick, initial sense of the community is to do a windshield assessment using a format like the one provided in Figure 9-1.
- CHNs interested in doing a windshield assessment need to take public transportation, have someone else drive while they take notes, or stop frequently to write down what they see.
- The windshield survey example is organized into 14 elements with specific questions to answer that are related to each element. Some of the questions need to be answered by visiting the library to get secondary data.
- CHNs who use this approach will have an initial descriptive assessment of the community when they are finished.
- Interventions are planned based on the windshield survey findings.

Evidence-Informed Practice

The authors describe the findings of a qualitative study using interpretive descriptive analysis to uncover the experience of capacity building among health education workers in the Yukon. Individual and small group interviews were held with 21 study participants. Themes that emerged included ways in which the participants build on their own and the community members' strengths; the ways they focus on achieving outcomes that are immediately important and relevant to the members of the community; and how these health education workers lived and worked in their communities, which helped them to identify assets that promoted capacity building. The health educators asked for personal, relevant community experiences and used these in their teaching. This strategy engaged the learners. It is very important to understand that health education workers who live in their communities can make a difference in capacity building. Policies and organizational practices can support communities to enhance capacity building.

Application for CHNs: The findings support the importance of the experiences of community members being recognized and the importance of their involvement in capacity building. CHNs need to work with community strengths and assets and build on these to promote capacity building. Engaging a community is often a result of CHNs also being engaged with a community at a relationship level ("living in relationship with the community"), as well as at a working level ("working in interactive relationships with community members") (Horton & MacLeod, 2008, p. 71). *Relationship level* refers to the personal level of residing in a community, whereas the *working level* refers to the professional aspect of working with the community while residing in that community.

Questions for Reflection & Discussion

1. Why is it important to promote community capacity building?
2. Do you think that living in and knowing the community would be a disadvantage to a CHN who also works in that community? Support your viewpoint.
3. Based on the study findings, what is one clinical question (also referred to as a structured question) that you would ask in order to search the literature?

REFERENCE: Horton, J., & MacLeod, M. (2008). The experience of capacity building among health education workers in the Yukon. *Canadian Journal of Public Health, 99*(1), 69–72.

Collection of Reported Data

Secondary analysis and surveys are two methods of collecting reported data. In **secondary analysis,** the CHN uses previously gathered data, such as minutes from community meetings and use of available epidemiological data. This type of analysis is extremely valuable because it saves time and effort. Many sources of data are readily available and useful for secondary analysis, including the following:

- Public documents
- Census data
- Health surveys
- Health surveillance
- Minutes from meetings
- Statistical data
- Internet sites and informatics
- Health records

Surveys report data from a sample of persons. A health survey can be cross-sectional (provided to participants once only) or longitudinal (provided to the same participants at different times) (Shah, 2003). Surveys can be conducted by interview, telephone, mail, or the Internet. The use of computers for linking databases and for conducting surveys has created ethical and social issues (Shah, 2003). Health surveys most often are used for surveillance of health behaviour, illness levels, and health consequences (Shah, 2003). They are as useful as observational methods and secondary analyses but require time-consuming and costly data collection as the reliability and validity of the questions need to be determined. Thus, the CHN does not often use the survey method. There are many population health surveys conducted in Canada, such as the Canadian Community Health Survey (CCHS), Canadian Health Measures Survey (CHMS), National Population Health Survey (NPHS), and Participation Activity Limitation Survey (PALS) (Statistics Canada, 2009c).

Assessment Issues

Gaining entry or acceptance into the community is perhaps the biggest challenge in assessment. If the CHN does not live in the community, he or she is most likely to be considered an outsider. The CHN is often seen to represent an established health care system that is neither known nor trusted by community members, who may therefore react with indifference or even active hostility to the CHN. In addition, CHNs may feel insecure about their skills as a community worker, and the community may refuse to acknowledge its need for those skills. Because the CHN's success depends largely on the way he or she is viewed, entry into the community is critical. It takes time to establish trust and rapport. It is crucial that ethical principles such as autonomy, beneficence, justice, and nonmaleficence are followed and that the possibility for bias is minimized by upholding professional standards and being aware of the influence on one's own values and beliefs and how these may affect the establishment of trust with community clients. Often the CHN can gain trust and entry into the community in the following ways:

- Taking part in community events
- Looking and listening with interest
- Visiting people in formal leadership positions
- Using an assessment guide
- Using a peer group for support
- Keeping appointments
- Clarifying community members' perceptions of health needs
- Respecting an individual's right to choose whether he or she will work with the CHN

If the CHN lives in the community, the establishment and maintenance of professional boundaries may be problematic. In small communities, the clients may also be very familiar to the CHN in that they could be relatives or friends. CHNs may have to set boundaries between their personal and professional lives in order to find a balance that is respected by the client and the CHN. For example, if the CHN is well known in the community, some community members may solicit, in a public place, the CHN's advice, or the CHN may inadvertently ask a client about his or her progress in a public place.

Maintaining *confidentiality* is important. CHNs need to protect the identity of community members who provide sensitive or controversial data. In some cases, the CHN may consider withholding data; in other situations, the CHN may be legally required to disclose data. For example, CHNs are required by law to report child abuse.

Identifying Community Health Concerns

Based on the data collected from the various sources and the creation of a composite database will result in a list of community strengths and health concerns. Each health concern needs to be identified and clearly stated. The health risk to the community is stated, the persons affected are identified, and the community factors that led to the health concern(s) are defined. This assessment process is an important first step for planning. In the planning phase, priorities are established and interventions are identified.

Each community has its own unique characteristics. Some of these characteristics are strengths that the CHN can build upon, but other characteristics contribute to the health concern identified. An example of a community health concern is infant malnutrition. Based on community health assessment data, the community health concern for infant malnutrition using this format would be described as follows:

1. Infant malnutrition health concern—children younger than 1 year
2. Risk to community—because of children in poor health, may need to provide new services
3. Persons affected—some families in Stanfield Township
4. Community factors:
    - Lack of regular developmental screening for infants in the community
    - No outreach program to identify at-risk infants
    - Families' lack of knowledge about the community nutrition program
    - Confusion among community families about criteria for enrolment in nutrition health program
    - Community families' lack of infant-related nutritional knowledge
    - Community expectations

(See the *Manitoba Health and Healthy Living Accountability Support Branch* Weblink on the Evolve Web site for the Community Health Assessment Guidelines, specifically pp. 23–24.)

Planning for Community Health

The planning phase includes analyzing the community health data to identify the community health concerns, establishing priorities among them, establishing goals and objectives, and identifying intervention activities that will accomplish the objectives. (See the *Community Health Assessment Guidelines* Weblink on the Evolve Web site, specifically pp. 25–26, for key considerations in analyzing and planning community health assessment data.)

Analyzing Health Concerns

Analyzing health concerns seeks to clarify the nature of the concern. The CHN identifies the origins and effects of the health concern, the points at which intervention might be undertaken, and the parties that have an interest in the health concern and its solution. Analysis often requires identifying the following:

- The direct and indirect factors that contribute to the health concern
- The outcomes of the health concern
- Relationships among health concerns (whether one health concern contributes to or is affected by other health concerns)

This analysis is important because the CHN can anticipate that several of the factors that contribute to a health concern and affect its outcomes also contribute to many other health concerns.

Analysis should be undertaken for each identified health concern. It often requires organizing a special group composed of the CHN and persons whose areas of expertise relate to the health concern, individuals whose organizations are capable of intervening, and representatives of the community experiencing the health concern—the client. Together, they can identify the contributing factors and explain the relationships between each factor and the health concern.

This process is seen in Table 9-5, an example of a health concern analysis for infant malnutrition. All the tables pertaining to the health concern for Stanfield Township are based on fictitious data. Factors that contribute to the health concern of infant malnutrition and its outcomes are listed in the first column. These factors are from all areas of community life. Social and environmental factors are as appropriate as those oriented to the individual. For example, teenage pregnancy is a social factor, and high unemployment is an environmental factor; both are related to infant malnutrition. In the second column of Table 9-5, the relationships between each factor and the health concern are noted. The third column contains data from the community and the literature that support the relationship, using the example of suspected infant malnutrition. From the best evidence available, infant malnutrition is thought to be related to inadequate diet, community norms, poverty, disturbed mother–child relationships, and teenage pregnancy. This is an example of how some of the determinants of health can affect a client situation.

Health Concern Priorities

Infant malnutrition represents only one of several community health concerns identified by the community assessment (see Table 9-6). In reality, several community health concerns may be identified. They may include a lack of clinics, poor housing conditions, a mortality rate from cardiovascular disease that is higher than the national norm, and—as expressed by many residents—a desire to quit smoking.

Each health concern identified as part of the assessment process must be put through a ranking process to determine its importance. This is known as *prioritizing*. See the *Community Health Assessment Guidelines* Weblink

TABLE 9-5 Health Concern Analysis: Infant Malnutrition

Name of community: Stanfield Township

Health concern statement: Infant malnutrition in Stanfield Township

Factors Contributing to the Health Concern and Outcomes	Relationship of Factors	Data Supportive to Relationships
1. Inadequate diet	Diets lacking in required nutrients contribute to malnutrition.	All township infants and their mothers seen by public health nurses in 2004 were referred to dietitians because of poor diets.
2. Community norms	Bottle-fed babies are less apt to receive adequate amounts of safe milk containing necessary nutrients.	Area general practitioners and CHNs agree that 90% of mothers in township bottle-feed.
3. Poverty	Infant formulas are expensive.	Of new mothers in township, 60% are receiving social assistance.
4. Disturbed mother–child relationship	Poor mother–child relationship may result in infant's failure to thrive.	Data from charts of 43 nursing mothers show infants diagnosed with failure to thrive.
5. Teenage pregnancy	Teenage mothers are most apt to have inadequate diets prenatally, to bottle-feed, to be poor, to lack parenting skills, and to have low literacy skills.	Of births in 2004, 90% were to women19 years of age or younger.

TABLE 9-6 Health Concern Priority: Infant Malnutrition in Stanfield Township

Criteria	Rationale for Rating	Problem Priority
1. Community awareness of the health concern	Health service providers, teachers, and a variety of leaders have mentioned health concern.	2
2. Community motivation to resolve the health concern	Most believe that this health concern is not solvable because most of those affected are poor.	4
3. CHN's ability to influence health concern resolution	CHNs are skilled at raising consciousness and mobilizing support.	3
4. Ready availability of expertise relevant to health concern resolution	Public health unit/regional health authority nutrition program and nutritionists or dietitians are available.	1
5. Severity of outcomes if health concern is left unresolved	Effects of marginal health services are not well documented.	5
6. Quickness with which health concern resolution can be achieved	The time taken to mobilize a rural community with no history of social action is lengthy.	6

on the Evolve Web site, specifically pp. 27–29, for selecting priorities.

Community Health Concern Priority Criteria

Answers to the following questions have been helpful in ranking an identified health concern:

1. How aware is the community of the health concern?
2. Is the community motivated to resolve or better manage the health concern?
3. Is the CHN able to influence a solution for the health concern?
4. Are experts available to solve the health concern?
5. How severe are the outcomes if the health concern is unresolved?
6. How quickly can the health concern be solved?

Using the example of infant malnutrition again, the criteria are listed in the first column of Table 9-6. Note that this one health concern is only an example to show how to evaluate each health concern using the six criteria.

The members of the partnership answer questions related to their ability to influence or change the situation, and the CHN and the community agree on the ability to resolve the health concern. One example of the difference between the perceptions of the CHN and community members is smoking in public buildings; the CHN might identify smoking as a public health concern, but community members might view smoking as an issue of individual choice and personal freedom. For example, recently, a mid-size community, through the local municipal government and the health unit, passed a regulation to forbid smoking in all public places, including restaurants and bars. The outcry from the community residents has been loud. Many of the residents believe their individual rights and freedoms have been taken away by government regulations. It does not matter to them that lung cancer rates are high.

This process is repeated separately for each identified health concern, and all the health concerns are compared. Priorities among the identified health concerns are established. The health concerns with the highest priority are the ones selected as the focus for interventions. Table 9-7 shows how all health concerns in Stanfield Township community example were prioritized after each one was separately evaluated.

Establishing Goals and Objectives

Once high-priority health concerns are identified, relevant goals and objectives are developed. **Goals** are generally broad statements of desired outcomes. **Objectives** are the precise statements indicating the means of achieving the desired outcomes. Table 9-8 provides an example of one of the goals and the specific objectives associated with it for the infant malnutrition health concern in Stanfield Township. The goal is to reduce the incidence and prevalence of infant malnutrition. Using a humanistic caring model, the broadly stated goal is used to measure the desired client outcomes. However, when using behavioural models, the objectives are *precise, behaviourally stated,* and *measurable* and can be reached in a series of steps implemented over time rather than all at once. In this Stanfield Township example, the specific objectives pertain to (1) assessing infant developmental levels, (2) determining nutrition program eligibility, (3) implementing an outreach program, (4) enrolling infants in the nutrition program, and (5) providing supplemental foods in existing diets. See the *Creating S.M.A.R.T. Goals* and the Province of British Columbia *S.M.A.R.T. Goal Setting* Weblinks

TABLE 9-7 Community Health Concern Priority: All Identified Community Health Concerns in Stanfield Township

Criteria	Health Concern	Rationale for Rating	Concern Priority
1. Community awareness of the health concern	Community's desire to be smoke-free	Health service providers, teachers, and a variety of leaders have mentioned health concern.	2
2. Community motivation to resolve the health concern	Poor housing standards	Most believe that this health concern is not solvable because most of those affected are extremely poor.	4
3. CHN's ability to influence health concern resolution	Mortality rate from cardiovascular disease	CHNs are skilled at raising consciousness and mobilizing support.	3
4. Ready availability of expertise relevant to health concern resolution	Infant malnutrition in Stanfield Township	Public health unit/regional health authority nutrition program and nutritionists and dietitians are available.	1
5. Severity of outcomes if health concern is left unresolved	Lack of primary health care clinics	Effects of marginal health services are not well documented.	5
6. Quickness with which health concern resolution can be achieved	Teen pregnancy	The time to mobilize a rural community with no history of social action is lengthy.	6

TABLE 9-8 Goals and Objectives: Infant Malnutrition in Stanfield Township

Name of community, Health concern: Stanfield Township, Infant malnutrition

Goal statement: To reduce the incidence and prevalence of infant malnutrition

Present Date	Objectives	Completion Date
2009	1. Developmental levels will be assessed for 80% of the infants seen by the health unit, neighbourhood health centre, and private physicians.	2012
2009	2. Nutrition program eligibility will be determined for 80% of infants seen by the health unit, neighbourhood health centre, and private physicians.	2012
2009	3. An outreach program will be implemented to identify at-risk infants not now known to health care providers.	2012
2009	4. Nutrition program eligibility will be determined for 25% of at-risk infants.	2013
2009	5. Of all infants eligible for nutrition program food supplements, 75% will be enrolled in the program.	2012
2009	6. Of the mothers of infants enrolled in the nutrition program, 50% will demonstrate three ways of incorporating nutrition program supplements into their infants' diets.	2013

for help developing skill in writing objectives using the acronym S.M.A.R.T. (Specific, Measurable, Attainable, Realistic, Timely). Writing goals and objectives will be covered in more detail in Chapter 10.

As noted, establishing goals and objectives involves collaboration between the CHN and representatives of the community groups affected by both the health concern and the proposed intervention. This often requires a great deal of negotiation among everyone taking part in the planning process. One important advantage offered by the continuous active involvement of people affected by the outcomes is that they have a vested interest in those outcomes and are therefore supportive of and committed to the success of the intervention. Once goals and objectives are chosen, intervention activities to accomplish the objectives can be identified.

Identifying Intervention Activities

Intervention activities are the strategies used to meet the objectives, the ways change will be effected, and the ways the health concern cycle will be broken. Because alternative intervention activities do exist, they must be identified and evaluated. An example of how intervention activities are identified then prioritized for infant developmental levels for Stanfield Township is illustrated in Table 9-9.

To achieve the objective related to the assessment of infant developmental levels for Stanfield Township (see Table 9-8, objective 1), five intervention activities are listed in the second column of Table 9-9. Each is relevant to the first objective. The first two activities involve nutrition program personnel as the principal change agents. The last three involve the CHN, nutrition program personnel, and the staff of the health unit, neighbourhood health centre, and private physicians' offices as the change partners.

The expected effect of each of the activities is considered in the second column of Table 9-9. The value, or the likelihood that the activity will help meet the objective and finally resolve the health concern, is noted in the third column. It is more valuable in the long term to educate others on how to assess infant development (activity 4) than to do it for them (activity 1). It is also necessary to analyze the change process needed to complete the objective (activity 5). Activity 5 must be done before any other interventions can be considered.

As a result, activities 4 and 5 have higher value scores than activity 1, in which the professional staff alone carries out the intervention. How does one decide the priority value? Answer the questions on page 275. Read the literature to find evidence about what works best. If five interventions are possible, assign a score between 1 and 5 based on the answers to the questions and what the literature says is the best approach.

TABLE 9-9 Plan: Intervention Activities to Assess Infants' Developmental Levels in Stanfield Township

Name of community: Stanfield Township

Objective 1: Developmental levels will be assessed for 80% of infants seen by health unit, neighbourhood health centre, and private physicians

Current Date	Possible Interventions	Intervention Health Concern and Resources	Priority Intervention for Best Outcome
2011	1. The nutrition program supplies personnel to assess infant developmental levels.	Personnel and time are insufficient; existing community resources (potential) are ignored.	5
2011	2. The nutrition program provides in-service education to staff on the assessment of infant development.	Antipathy between the nutrition personnel health workers and other workers is high. The need for education must be assessed first, and enthusiasm for objectives must be created.	4
2011	3. The CHN provides in-service education to staff in assessment of infant development.	The CHN cannot do it alone.	3
2011	4. The CHN helps the nutrition program personnel identify in-service educational needs of area health care providers regarding the assessment of infant development.	This is most likely to build on existing community strengths; a CHN skilled in needs assessment and interpersonal techniques is needed to decrease antipathy.	2
2011	5. The CHN helps the nutrition program personnel identify driving and restraining forces relative to implementation of objective.	Without this, change effort is likely to fail.	1

Implementation for Community Health

Implementation, the third phase of the community health nursing process, involves the work and activities aimed at achieving the goals and objectives. Implementation efforts may be made by the person or group that established the goals and objectives, or they may be shared with or even delegated to others.

Factors Influencing Implementation

Implementation is shaped by the CHN's chosen roles, the type of health concern selected as the focus for intervention, the community's readiness to take part in solving the health concern, and the characteristics of the social change process. The CHN taking part in community intervention has knowledge and skills that the other interveners do not have; the question for the CHN is how to use the position, knowledge, and skills.

The CHN's Role

CHNs can act as content experts, helping communities select and attain task-related goals. In the Stanfield Township example of infant malnutrition, the CHN can use epidemiological skills to determine the incidence and prevalence of malnutrition. The CHN can serve as a process expert by increasing the community's ability to document the health concern rather than only by providing help as an expert in the area.

Content-focused roles often are considered change agent roles, whereas process roles are called *change partner roles*. The roles of the **change agent** stress gathering and analyzing facts and implementing programs, whereas the roles of the **change partner** include those of enabler-catalyst, teacher of problem-solving skills to address health concern, and activist advocate.

The Community Health Concern and the CHN's Role

The role the CHN chooses depends on the nature of the health concern, the community's decision-making ability, and professional and personal choices. Some health concerns clearly require certain intervention roles:

- If a community lacks democratic problem-solving abilities, the CHN may select educator, facilitator, and advocate roles. Problem-solving skills must be explained, and the CHN becomes a role model.
- A difficulty with determining the health status of the community, on the other hand, usually requires fact-gatherer and analyst roles.
- Some health concerns require multiple roles. Managing conflict among the involved health care providers demands process skills.
- Collecting and interpreting the data necessary to document a health concern require both interpersonal and analytical skills.
- The community's history of taking part in decision making is a critical factor. In a community skilled in identifying and successfully managing its health concerns, the CHN may best serve as technical expert or advisor.

Different roles may be required if the community lacks problem-solving skills or has a history of unsuccessful change efforts. The CHN may need to focus on developing problem-solving capabilities or on making one successful change so that the community becomes empowered to take on the job of promoting change on its own behalf.

Social Change Process and the CHN's Role

The CHN's role also depends on the social change process. Not all communities are open to change. Ability to change is often related to the extent to which a community focuses on traditional norms. The more traditional the community, the less likely it is to change. Other barriers such as lack of human and fiscal resources and accessibility to health services in the community may also hinder change; the CHN needs to determine what these are so that appropriate interventions can be initiated.

The CHN, as a change agent, in applying the community health assessment process needs to be familiar with the principles of change and the types of community organizations that support change (Maurer & Smith, 2009). The Rothman Model of Community Organization is most commonly used to initiate community change. Rothman identified three models of community organization: locality development, social planning, and social action (Maurer & Smith, 2009). In practice, Rothman's three models are often used in combination. For further information on Rothman's models, see the City of Calgary Weblink on the Evolve Web site. 

CRITICAL VIEW

Refer to the key strategies for health promotion as outlined in the Ottawa Charter for Health Promotion.

1. a) How do the environmental features of your community contribute to health promotion and disease prevention?
   b) What physical characteristics in your community might contribute to inequalities? Explain.
2. Which community programs exist in your community to address each of the Ottawa Charter strategies?

Evaluating the Intervention for Community Health

Simply defined, **evaluation** is the appraisal of the effects of some organized activity or program. Evaluation may involve the design and conduct of evaluation research or the more elementary process of assessing progress by contrasting the objectives and the results. For key considerations on the evaluation of a community health assessment, refer to the *Manitoba Community Health Assessment Guide* Weblink on the Evolve Web site, pp. 32–34.

Evaluation begins in the planning phase, when goals and measurable objectives are established and goal-attaining activities are identified. After implementing the intervention, the extent of the accomplishment of objectives and the effects of intervention activities have to be assessed. Community health nursing progress notes direct the CHN to perform such appraisals concurrently with implementation. In assessing the data recorded there, the CHN is requested to evaluate whether the objectives were met and the extent that these were met or unmet and whether the intervention activities used were effective. Such an evaluation process is oriented toward community health because the intervention goals and objectives come from the CHN's and the community's ideas about health.

Measurement of outcomes is a particularly important part of the evaluation process. Evaluation needs to be ongoing—that is, process (formative) as well as outcome (summative). This is one reason for placing emphasis on goals and measurable objectives since questions need to be raised about the extent to which they have been met and about the effectiveness or ineffectiveness of community interventions. Questions raised with the community to determine if the health concern has been resolved or the risk reduced are, To what extent have the goals and measurable objectives been met? and What changes, if any, are needed in the goals and objectives? Outcome measures also answer questions about the results of the intervention, such as Which interventions have been effective and why? Which interventions have been ineffective and why? Has the health concern been resolved or the risk reduced? What lessons have been learned? and What changes are needed? Process and outcome evaluation are discussed in greater detail in Chapter 10.

Often data collected over time can provide important outcomes information about health trends within the community. Epidemiological data and trends do not provide the only measure of success, but they do provide important information about the intervention. CHNs need to consider the collection of this type of outcomes data for use as part of the evaluation phase. Outcomes can be measured by looking at changes from before and after the intervention to resolve the health concerns.

In the example of infant malnutrition in Stanfield Township, one would consider the number of cases of infant malnutrition in the community before providing education to other health providers about the assessment of infant development. A time period for evaluation would be chosen, perhaps 1 year later. The number of cases of infant malnutrition would be measured to see if there were fewer cases.

PERSONAL SAFETY IN COMMUNITY HEALTH NURSING PRACTICE

Personal safety is a prerequisite for effective community health nursing practice, and it should be a consideration throughout the process. An awareness of the community and common sense are the two best guidelines for judgement. For example, CHNs need to keep their agency supervisor informed of their planned client contacts with location and timelines. Common sense suggests not leaving anything valuable on public transportation or a car seat or leaving the car unlocked. Calling ahead to schedule meetings helps prevent delays or confusion, and it gives the CHN an opportunity to lay the groundwork for the meeting. During the client contact, the CHN needs to be in a position that allows for easy exiting should an unsafe situation arise. If the client has no telephone or no access to a neighbour's telephone, a time for any future meetings should be established during the initial visit. Regardless of whether telephone contact had been made, rare situations occur that require that the meeting be postponed—for example, if the CHN arrives at a location and is concerned about personal safety because of people unexpectedly loitering by the entrance. Some visits may need to be cancelled at the time of the visit for reasons of personal safety—for example, a threat due to vicious dogs or some exotic animals, allergies to animals or environmental allergens, or illegal drug activities.

For CHNs who are either just beginning their careers as CHNs or who are just starting a new position, the following three groups of information sources will help answer any questions about personal safety:

1. *CHNs, social workers, and health care providers who are familiar with the dynamics of a given community.* They can provide valuable insights into when to visit, how to get there, and what to expect because they also practise in the community.
2. *Community members.* The best sources of information about the community are the community members themselves, and one benefit of developing an active partnership with community members is their willingness to share their insight about day-to-day community life.

3. *The CHN's own observations.* Knowledge gained during the data collection phase of the community health nursing process should provide a solid basis for an awareness of day-to-day community activity. CHNs with experience in practising in the community generally agree that if they feel uncomfortable in a situation, they should trust their feelings and leave.

In summary, CHNs working with the community as the unit of care and as a partner require familiarity with the community where they practise. This familiarity is achieved by conducting a thorough community health assessment using theoretical frameworks and community health assessment guides. Information obtained following this community health assessment will be foundational for health program planning. Program planning, implementation, and evaluation are discussed in the next chapter.

STUDENT EXPERIENCE

1. Examine your community or a community that provides community health assessment data.
2. Compare your findings with those of the *Key Data Findings at a Glance for Central Manitoba* found at http://www.rha-central.mb.ca/data/cha/2/CHASummary.pdf.
3. Prepare key data findings at a glance for your selected community.
4. Identify the sources of data and methods of data collection that will be used for the community health assessment of your selected community. Were similar sources used in your community compared to what was used for Central Manitoba?
5. Purchase an address book, and in it identify and record contact information for the major community health agencies as well as other community resources and assets in your selected community.

REMEMBER THIS!

- A *community* is defined as a locality-based entity composed of systems of formal organizations reflecting societal institutions, informal groups, and aggregates that are interdependent and whose function or expressed intent is to meet a wide variety of collective needs.
- *Community health* as used in this chapter is defined as the meeting of collective needs through identifying community health concerns and managing interactions within the community itself and between the community and the larger society.
- Most changes aimed at improving community health involve, of necessity, partnerships or coalitions among community residents and community health workers from a variety of disciplines.
- Assessing community health requires gathering existing data, generating missing data, interpreting the database, and identifying strengths and health concerns.
- Six methods of collecting data useful to the CHN are informant interviews, focus groups, participant observation, secondary analysis of existing data, surveys, and windshield surveys.
- Gaining entry or acceptance into the community is perhaps the biggest challenge in assessment.
- The CHN is sometimes considered an outsider and may represent to the client an established health care system that is neither known nor trusted by community members, who may react with indifference or even active hostility.
- The planning phase includes analyzing and establishing priorities among community health concerns already identified, establishing goals and objectives, and identifying intervention activities that will accomplish the objectives.
- Once high-priority health concerns are identified, broad, relevant goals and objectives are developed.
- The goal, generally a broad statement of desired outcome, and objectives, the precise statements of the desired outcome, are carefully selected.
- Intervention activities, the means by which objectives are met, are the strategies that clarify what must be done to achieve the objectives, the ways change will be effected, and the way the health concern will be interpreted.
- Implementation, the third phase of the community health nursing process, is transforming a plan for improved community health into the achievement of goals and objectives.
- Evaluation is the appraisal of the effects of some organized activity or program and the extent to which the community health concern has been resolved.

REFLECTIVE PRAXIS

Case Study 1

Alan is a CHN and a member of a committee assigned to assess the health care needs of the aging baby boomers in Woodsbury, a small northern community. The community is located in a scenic area near a large freshwater lake. The winter temperatures can vary from −15° to −40° Celsius. The average snowfall has been declining but is usually around 80 cm. The summers are dry and warm. The major industries in the community are mining and forestry. The unemployment rate has been low, but due to declining demand for some resources, the unemployment rate has been steadily increasing.

Alan and the committee are aware that as the baby-boomer population ages, health care professionals need to prepare for a rapid increase in the number of people older than 65 years. The committee's purpose is to make suggestions to the district health unit or health authority and municipal officials about how to prepare for the increase in health services that will be needed for these older adults.

The ethnic composition of this community is 80% Caucasian (consisting of French Canadians and those of British, Finnish, German, and Dutch descent) and 20% Aboriginal. Currently, 25% of the population in Woodsbury is older than 65 years. However, in 25 years, this percentage is expected to increase to more than 50%. Many of these older adults have practised a lifestyle that included high-fat diets, smoking, and frequent alcohol use. Consequently, many have heart disease or chronic obstructive pulmonary disease. Currently, five primary health care providers are in the community. Waiting times to see these health providers range from 1 to 3 weeks. Only one of these providers specializes in geriatric care. One 54-bed long-term care facility is in the most northern location of the district, located 50 km from Woodsbury. Because of the rural location, there is no public transit system. The long-term-care residents are dependent on family or friends for transportation to appointments in Woodsbury.

1. Define the community.
2. Outline the data collection methods that Alan might decide to use to assess the community.
3. Using the walking or driving windshield survey, present the available data on this community.
4. Identify potential community partners that Alan and the committee might consider working with.

Answers are on the Evolve Web site at http://evolve.elsevier.com/Canada/Stanhope/community/.

Case Study 2

Lily, a CHN in a small city, became aware of the increased incidence of respiratory diseases through contact with families in the community and the local chapter of the Canadian Lung Association. During family visits, Lily noted that many of the parents were smokers. Because most of the families Lily visited had small children, she became concerned about the effects of second-hand smoke on the health of the infants and children among her family caseload.

Further assessment of this community showed that the community recognized several health concerns, including school safety and the risk of water pollution, in addition to the smoking health concern that Lily had identified during her family visits. Talks with different community members revealed that they wanted each of these identified health concerns "fixed," although these same community members also remained uncertain about how to start.

1. In deciding which of the three identified health concerns to address first, which criterion would be most important for Lily to consider?
   a. The amount of money available
   b. The level of community motivation to fix one of the three identified health concerns
   c. The number of people in the community who expressed a concern about one of the three identified health concerns
   d. How much control she would have in the process

Answers are on the Evolve Web site at http://evolve.elsevier.com/Canada/Stanhope/community/.

What Would You Do?

1. Using your own community as a frame of reference, develop examples illustrating the concepts of community, community client, community health, and partnership for health.
2. Read your local newspaper and identify articles illustrating the concepts of community, community client, community health, and partnership for health.

TOOL BOX

evolve

The Tool Box contains useful instruments that can be applied in community health nursing practice. These related resources are found either in the appendices at the back of this book or on the Evolve Web site at http://evolve.elsevier.com/Canada/Stanhope/community/.

Appendices

- Appendix 1: Canadian Community Health Nursing Standards of Practice
- Appendix 8: Community-as-Partner Model

Tools

The Community Development Facilitator's Guide.
This resource is used to facilitate use of *The Community Development Handbook* so that CHNs are able to facilitate workshops in the community.

The Community Development Handbook.
This introductory guide to community development provides information to deepen the CHN's interest in and understanding of community development.

The Community Tool Box.
This Web site is designed to support CHNs by providing more than 6,000 pages of practical information in order to facilitate skill development.

Public Health Agency of Canada. The Community Capacity Building Tool.
This planning tool document assists communities to build community capacity in health promotion projects.

WEBLINKS

evolve

Direct links to these resources can be found on the text's accompanying Evolve Web site at http://evolve.elsevier.com/Canada/Stanhope/community.

Canadian Community Economic Development Network. Information and Communication Tools for Community Economic Development and Social Inclusion: Socio-economic Indicators and Mapping. This site provides a detailed document on socioeconomic indicators, mapping, tools for indicators and mapping, examples of mapping, and other Weblinks to social indicators and mapping resources.

Canadian Community Health Nursing Standards of Practice. This site outlines the standards that the CHN uses in working with the community as client.

Canadian HIV/AIDS Legal Network. Stories of Community Mobilization. Several stories about community mobilization around HIV/AIDS-related stigma and discrimination can be found here. Following a description of community mobilization for each story is a discussion of the factors that contributed to their success in relation to community mobilization.

Canadian Nurses Association. Position statements and backgrounders relevant to this chapter are found at the CNA site.

- CNA Backgrounder: Healthy Communities and Nursing: A Summary of the Issues
- CNA Position Statement: International Health Partnerships

City of Calgary. Rothman's Three Models of Community Organizing. This site provides information on Rothman's three models of community organizing and the purpose for considering the various models.

Community Building Resources. This Alberta Web site contains resources, references to resources, and links pertaining to capacity building and asset mapping.

Community Participation in Local Health and Sustainable Development: Approaches and Techniques. A WHO publication, this Web source provides detailed information on community participation, health, and sustainable development.

Creating S.M.A.R.T. Goals. This site explains the S.M.A.R.T. acronym with some questions that need to be asked in preparing objectives.

Directory of the Networks of Healthy Communities and Cities in Canada. This directory provides a history of the Healthy Cities movement and direct connections to the many cities and communities across Canada that have joined this Canadian network.

First Nations Summit, Indian and Northern Affairs Canada and Ministry of Aboriginal Relations and Reconciliation. *Guide to Community Forums in British Columbia.* For information on planning and conducting community-to-community forums, go to this site. It also has quick tips listed.

Health Canada. *Healthy Canadians: A Federal Report on Comparable Health Indicators.* This Website provides the executive summary of highlights of the report, which includes statistics on findings with identification of areas requiring improvement such as the increased prevalence of diabetes in Canada.

Healthy Cities/Healthy Communities. This site provides information on areas such as the development of healthy cities/communities, how to create a healthy city/community, and international examples of healthy communities and discusses community assessment strategies.

Heart Health Resource Centre. Sustainability. This site defines sustainability and provides insights of its application in Heart Health projects in Ontario.

Human Resources and Social Development Canada. *The Partnership Handbook.* This is an excellent guide for the development and process of partnerships.

Human Resources Development Canada. *Community Learning Asset Mapping: A Guidebook for Community Learning Networks.* This guidebook provides an extensive guideline on using mapping as a tool and provides examples of community mapping.

Kretzmann, J. P., & McKnight, J. L. *Building Communities from the Inside Out: A Path Toward Finding and Mobilizing a Community's Assets.* This Web site provides information on community development using an asset-mapping approach rather than a needs approach.

Manitoba Health and Healthy Living Accountability Support Branch. *Community Health Assessment Guidelines, 2009.* This document provides key considerations on the assessment to evaluation components of a community health assessment.

Ontario Healthy Communities Coalition. This site is an excellent source of information about healthy communities. Many educational publications can be accessed through the e-Resources page, on topics such as healthy food, healthy communities, pathways to a healthy community, inclusive community organizations, and strategies for effective proposal writing.

Province of British Columbia. S.M.A.R.T. Goal Setting. This site provides a brief introduction to writing S.M.A.R.T goals as well as some examples.

Senate Subcommittee on Population Health. *A Healthy, Productive Canada: A Determinant of Health Approach.* This Web site document, specifically pp. 32–38, provides information on the engagement of communities, with particular discussion of some communities in various provinces.

Statistics Canada. At this Government of Canada site, an accurate source of data, you will find profiles of individual communities, a profile of Canada, and detailed data for small groups (such as one-parent families, ethnic groups, occupational groups, and immigrants). The Canadian census is collected every 5 years, and the questions are similar so that comparisons can be made of changes that have occurred in Canada's population over time. The site contains the latest census data (2006) as well as data from previous censuses.

Strong Neighborhoods Task Force. *Putting Theory into Practice: Asset Mapping in Three Toronto Neighbourhoods.* This Web site provides three examples of the application of asset mapping with analysis, reflections, and learnings.

REFERENCES

British Columbia Healthy Communities. (2009). *Funding*. Retrieved from http://www.bchealthycommunities.ca/Content/Funding/Index.asp.

Campaign 2000. (2009). *2009 report card on child and family poverty in Canada: 1989–2009*. Retrieved from http://www.campaign2000.ca/reportCards/national/2009EnglishC2000NationalReportCard.pdf.

Canadian Institute for Health Information. (2006). *How healthy are rural Canadians? An assessment of their health status and health determinants*. Retrieved from http://www.phac-aspc.gc.ca/publicat/rural06/pdf/rural_canadians_2006_report_e.pdf.

Canadian Nurses Association. (2005). *Position statement: International health partnerships*. Retrieved from http://www.cna-aiic.ca/CNA/documents/pdf/publications/PS82_Intl_Health_Partnerships_e.pdf.

Capital Regional District. (2008). *Food and agriculture promoting healthy communities*. Retrieved from http://www.crd.bc.ca/rte/healthycommunities.htm.

Cassells, H. (2007). Community assessment. In M. A. Nies, & M. McEwen (Eds.), *Community/public health nursing: Promoting the health of populations* (4th ed., pp. 74–88). St. Louis, MO: Saunders.

Clark, M. J. (2008). *Community health nursing: Advocacy for population health* (5th ed.). Upper Saddle River, NJ: Pearson Education Inc.

Collier, C. (2010). Long form census change worries researchers. *CMAJ: Canadian Medical Association Journal, 182*(12), E563–E564.

Community Health Nurses Association of Canada. (2008). *Canadian community health nursing standards of practice*. Retrieved from http://www.chnac.ca/images/downloads/standards/chn_standards_of_practice_mar08_english.pdf.

Diem, E. (2005). Collaborative assessment. In E. Diem, & A. Moyer (Eds.), *Community health nursing projects: Making a difference* (pp. 83–121). Philadelphia, PA: Lippincott, Williams & Wilkins.

Dunn, J. R. (2002). *Are widening inequalities making Canada less healthy?*. Retrieved from http://www.opha.on.ca/resources/docs/incomeinequalities/summary.pdf.

Ervin, N. E. (2002). Exploring frameworks and models for guiding community assessment. In N. E. Ervin (Ed.), *Advanced community health nursing practice* (pp. 83–108). Upper Saddle River, NJ: Prentice Hall.

Escoffery, C., Miner, K. R., & Trowbidge, J. (2004). Conducting small-scale community assessments. *American Journal of Health Education, 35*(4), 237–241.

Government of Canada. (2009). *Canadian rural partnership asset mapping: A handbook*. Retrieved from http://www.rural.gc.ca/RURAL/display-afficher.do?id=1230057084263&lang=eng.

Health Canada. (2004). *The Canadian heart health initiative: A policy in action*. Retrieved from www.nhlbi.nih.gov/health/prof/heart/other/paho/prevention_canada.ppt.

Health Canada. (2006). *Healthy Canadians: A federal report on comparable health indicators, 2002*. Retrieved from http://www.hc-sc.gc.ca/hcs-sss/pubs/system-regime/2002-fed-comp-indicat/index-eng.php.

Health Canada. (2010). *Rural places: Variations in health*. Retrieved from http://www.hc-sc.gc.ca/sr-sr/pubs/hpr-rpms/bull/2007-people-place-gens-lieux/rural-ruraux-eng.php.

Horton, J., & MacLeod, M. (2008). The experience of capacity building among health education workers in the Yukon. *Canadian Journal of Public Health, 99*(1), 69–72.

Human Resources and Skills Development Canada. (2006). *Workplace skills strategy: Workplace partners panel*. Retrieved from http://www.hrsdc.gc.ca/eng/ws/wpp_backgrounder.shtml.

Human Resources and Skills Development Canada. (2009a). *Community Partnerships Helping Canadians through community development and partnerships*. Retrieved from http://www.hrsdc.gc.ca/eng/community_partnerships/index.shtml.

Human Resources and Skills Development Canada. (2009b). *Summative Evaluation of the National Homelessness Initiative—May 2008*. Retrieved from http://www.hrsdc.gc.ca/eng/publications_resources/evaluation/2009/nhi/page04.shtml.

Jessup-Falcioni, H., & Viverais-Dresler, G. (2005). *Community health nursing (NURS 2296 EL). On-line course. Envision.* Sudbury, ON: Laurentian University.

Khosla, P. (2005). *Women's poverty in cities.* National Network on Environments and Women's Health. Retrieved from http://www.nnewh.org/images/upload/attach/4832Women%20in%20Poverty%20EN.pdf.

Kretzmann, J. P., & McKnight, J. L. (1993). *Building communities from the inside out: A path toward finding and mobilizing assets.* Evanston, IL: Institute for Policy Research. Retrieved from http://www.oac.state.oh.us/grantsprogs/BuildingCommunitiesEnglish/BuildingCommunities.doc.

Kushner, K. E. (2006). Community-based nursing practice. In J. C. Ross-Kerr, & M. J. Wood (Eds.), *Canadian fundamentals of nursing.* (3rd ed., pp. 51–65). Toronto, ON: Elsevier Mosby.

Maurer, F. A., & Smith, C. M. (2009). *Community/public health nursing practice: Health for families and populations* (4th ed.). St. Louis, MO: Saunders Elsevier.

McKnight, J. L., & Kretzmann, J. P. (2005). Mapping community capacity. In M. Minkler (Ed.), *Community organizing and community building for health.* (2nd ed., pp. 158–172). New Brunswick, NJ: Rutgers University Press.

Mikkonen, J., & Raphael, D. (2010). *Social determinants of health: The Canadian facts.* Retrieved from www.thecanadianfacts.org/.

Minkler, M., & Wallerstein, N. (2005). Improving health through community organization and community building. In M. Minkler (Ed.), *Community organizing and community building for health* (2nd ed., pp. 26–50). New Brunswick, NJ: Rutgers University Press.

Moyer, A. (2005). Building coalitions. In A. Diem, & A. Moyer (Eds.), *Community health nursing projects: Making a difference* (pp. 297–323). Philadelphia, PA: Lippincott, Williams & Wilkins.

Nies, M., & McEwen, M. (2007). *Community/public health nursing: Promoting the health of populations* (4th ed.). St. Louis, MO: Saunders Elsevier.

Ontario Ministry of Health Promotion. (2009). *Healthy communities fund.* Retrieved from http://www.mhp.gov.on.ca/english/healthy_communities/faqs.asp.

Pong, R. W. (2007). *Rural poverty and health: What do we know?.* Retrieved from http://www.cranhr.ca/pdf/Presentation_Senate_Committee_on_rural_poverty_-_May_2007.pdf.

Public Health Agency of Canada. (2008). *The community capacity building tool.* Retrieved from http://www.phac-aspc.gc.ca/canada/regions/ab-nwt-tno/downloads-eng.php.

Raphael, D. (2009). *Social determinants of health: Canadian perspective* (2nd ed.). Toronto, ON: Canadian Scholars' Press.

Rural Communities Impacting Policy (2006). *Healthy and sustainable rural communities.* Retrieved from http://www.ruralnovascotia.ca/backgrounder.asp.

Shah, C. P. (2003). *Public health and preventive medicine in Canada* (5th ed.). Toronto, ON: Elsevier Canada.

Shields, L. E., & Lindsey, A. E. (2002). The community. In N. E. Ervin (Ed.), *Advanced community health nursing practice* (pp. 47–68). Upper Saddle River, NJ: Prentice Hall.

Society and Culture. (2009). *Poverty in Canada.* Retrieved from http://intraspec.ca/povertyCanada_news-and-reports.php.

Statistics Canada. (2009a). *Canadian Community Health Survey (CCHS) Cycle 1-1.* Retrieved from http://www.statcan.gc.ca/concepts/health-sante/index-eng.htm.

Statistics Canada. (2009b). *Census: Spotlight.* Retrieved from http://www12.statcan.gc.ca/census-recensement/index-eng.cfm.

Statistics Canada. (2009c). *Health surveys and statistical programs.* Retrieved from http://www4.statcan.gc.ca/health-sante/fbs-rpe/fbs-rpe-eng.aspx.

Toronto Star. (2009, February 8). *Poor neighbourhoods growing across Toronto.* Retrieved from http://www.thestar.com/News/GTA/article/58420.

Vancouver Coastal Health. (2009). *Healthy communities.* Retrieved from http://www.vch.ca/your_health/population_health/healthy_communities/.

Vollman, A. R., Anderson, E. T., & McFarlane, J. (2008). *Canadian community as partner: Theory and multidisciplinary practice in nursing* (2nd ed.). Philadelphia, PA: Lippincott, Williams & Wilkins.

Winnipeg Regional Health Authority. (2007). *Community development framework.* Retrieved from http://www.wrha.mb.ca/community/commdev/files/CommDev_Framework_07.pdf.

Zotti, M. E., Brown, P., & Stotts, R. C. (1996). Community based nursing versus community health nursing: What does it all mean? *Nursing Outlook, 44*(5), 211–217.

CHAPTER

10 Health Program Planning and Evaluation

KEY TERMS

assessment 291
goals 297
health program 287
health program evaluation process 287
health program implementation process 287
health program management 287
health program planning process 287
objectives 297
operational health planning 288
outcome evaluation 301
outcomes 296
process evaluation 301
strategic health planning 288

See Glossary on page 593 for definitions.

OBJECTIVES

After reading this chapter, you should be able to:

1. Compare the health program management process with the community health nursing process.
2. Explain the health program planning process and its application to nursing in the community.
3. Identify the benefits of health program planning.
4. Explain the components of health program evaluation and application to community health nursing practice.
5. Identify an evaluation method.
6. Identify health program evaluation sources.
7. Describe types of health program evaluation measures.
8. Discuss the social, political, economic, and environmental contexts within which community health assessment, health program planning, and health program evaluation take place.
9. Identify the limitations and advantages of various approaches and practical techniques to carry out effective health program planning and evaluation.

CHAPTER OUTLINE

Health program management is an area in which community health nurses (CHNs) are often involved as essential members of an interdisciplinary team to improve the health of communities. Therefore, it is critical that CHNs become familiar with the processes of health program assessment, planning, implementation, and evaluation. **Health program management** addresses health issues of populations and consists of the four steps: assessing, planning, implementing, and evaluating a health program, in partnership with the client.

The health program management process is similar to the community health nursing process. Like the community health nursing process, it consists of a rational decision-making system designed to help CHNs know the following:

- When to make a decision to develop a health program
- Where they want to be at the end of the health program
- What to do to have a successful health program
- How to develop a plan to go from where they are to where they want to be
- How to know that they are getting to their destination
- How to implement the health program plan
- What to measure to know whether what they are doing is appropriate

This chapter focuses primarily on health program planning, implementation, and evaluation. Although presented in separate discussions, these factors are related and dependent processes that work together to bring about a successful program. Other sections in this book provide examples of implementation. This chapter examines how CHNs, as team members, can be involved in health program planning, implementation, and evaluation. Based on evaluation findings, decisions are made regarding program changes that are needed and whether to modify or terminate programs. Health programs implemented with clients may be health promotion programs, such as weight loss for adults with type 2 diabetes mellitus or an ongoing program to provide community wellness workshops for older adults. Community health programs need to be planned based on the findings of a community health assessment. The community health assessment process, step one, was discussed in Chapter 9 and will be discussed briefly later in this chapter under "Health Program Planning Process."

DEFINITIONS AND GOALS

A **health program** consists of a variety of planned activities to address the assessed health concerns of clients over time and builds on client strengths in order to meet specific goals and objectives. The following are examples of specific health programs in the community that CHNs are involved with:

- Immunization programs for school-aged children
- Hearing screening programs for locomotive engineers
- Family-planning programs for teenagers
- Smoking-cessation programs for women
- Heart Health programs for post–myocardial infarction clients

The following are more broadly based aggregate and population health programs:

- Community school health programs
- Home health care programs
- Disaster management programs
- Occupational health and safety programs
- Environmental health programs
- Community health programs directed at specific health concerns through special interest groups (e.g., Canadian Heart and Stroke Association, Canadian Cancer Society, Canadian Diabetic Association)
- Community wellness programs
- Stress-management programs

A community health assessment is often used to identify the need for specific health programs. The **health program planning process,** the second step in health program management, is the organized approach to identifying and choosing interventions to meet specified goals and objectives that address client health concerns. The goal of planning is to ensure that health care services are acceptable, equitable, efficient, and effective. The **health program implementation process,** the third step in health program management, refers to putting the health program planned activities into action. The **health program evaluation process,** the last step in health program management, is defined as the systematic process of appraising all aspects of a program to determine its impact. The evaluation process of a health program needs to start early and therefore should be designed at the same time as the health program planning process.

HEALTH PROGRAM PLANNING FOR COMMUNITY HEALTH NURSING

Health program planning is a sequence of decisions ranging from broad strategies such as goals to specific objectives that depend on the gathering and analysis of various types of information collected in a variety of ways. Health program planning facilitates how resources (time, money, and people) are used so that they will have the utmost impact, particularly in times of fiscal restraint and limited resources when efficiency is critical. In planning a health promotion program, the CHN needs to ensure that there are opportunities for the continuing participation of key stakeholders in the program decision making and that the process has flexibility to accommodate contextual changes as the program evolves. The intent of health promotion programs is to have a positive impact on knowledge, attitudes, and behaviours of clients.

When CHNs work with clients to address health concerns, health program planning can do the following:

- Benefit clients, CHNs, and the community
- Focus attention on what the CHN and other community partners are attempting to do with the client to address the health concern
- Assist in identifying the community resources and activities that are required to meet the health program objectives
- Reduce role ambiguity (uncertainty) by giving responsibility to the client, the CHN, and other partners to meet health program objectives
- Reduce uncertainty within the health care program environment
- Increase the abilities of the CHN and others involved in the health program to cope with the external environment
- Help the CHN and health program participants (clients) anticipate activities
- Allow for quality decision making and better control over the actual health program results

Strategic health planning involves matching client health needs, client and provider strengths and competencies, and resources. For example, the strategic health planning process would focus on a question such as "How can we attract health professionals to and retain them in rural practice settings?" **Operational health planning** is a process that is used on a smaller scale and starts with a specific objective in relation to health program planning. For example, the operational health planning objective would be "to increase the number of family physicians and CHNs by 20% in the rural primary health care practice setting." Everyone involved with the program health planning can anticipate the following areas for discussion:

- What will be required to implement the health program
- What will occur during implementation
- What will be the health program outcomes

Health planning should involve an assessment of the situation (issue), which should include any literature pertaining to the issue and evaluations of similar proposed program interventions and should also consider socioenvironmental and other determinants of health.

The Web site of the Health Communication Unit (THCU), University of Toronto Centre for Health Promotion, provides information called "Introduction to Health Promotion Program Planning." THCU presents a six-step process that can be used for planning a health promotion program in addition to an online health program planner (see the Tool Box on the Evolve Web site) Three Ontario case study examples of programs implementing THCU's six-step planning process are (1) Child Nutrition Network of Haldimand and Norfolk, (2) Middlesex–London Early Childhood Injury Prevention Project, and (3) Thunder Bay Healthy Weights Strategy; they are also included on THCU's Web site. Within the THCU's health program planning model, a PEEST (*p*olitical, *e*conomic, *e*nvironmental, *s*ocial, and *t*echnological factors) analysis is sometimes used in the community assessment phase to identify any factors that may affect the program. These PEEST factors are often beyond the program planners' control and need to be considered when planning a health program. The THCU site provides further information on program planning, such as webinars on how to develop Program Logic Models and situational assessment guidelines.

Health Program Planning Models for Community Health

Population-based program health planning began with the need for mass immunizations, such as the program to administer the first polio vaccine (Barreto, Van Exan, & Rutty, 2006). Planning models include steps for planning a program that, if used, will likely increase its success. Models provide structure and organization to the planning process. There are many different planning models to choose from that have some common elements but may have different labels. Some models are more applicable to health planning than others.

Some models found in the literature that have been used by CHNs for health program planning are PATCH (Planning Approach to Community Health Model, developed using Green and Kreuter's PRECEDE-PROCEED model); 4-Step Planning Process (Finnegan & Ervin, 1989); Mobilizing for Action through Planning and Partnerships (MAPP); and Targeting Outcomes of Programs (Bennet & Rockwell, 2005). These models, infrequently used in Canada, are described briefly in Table 10-1.

Other planning models are used in community health, and CHNs need to evaluate these models for relevance in relation to health program and community health planning. Questions to determine a models' usefulness would include:

TABLE 10-1 Health Program Planning Models Infrequently Used in Canada

Model & Description	Steps
The **PATCH (Planning Approach To Community Health)** model increases the capacity of members of the community and empowers them to participate, and thus provides the community with a sense of program ownership with the program belonging to the community. The PATCH model is applicable in addressing specific health issues of populations.	I. *Mobilizing the community.* The identified community is organized with community representatives, and working and steering groups providing program information. II. *Collecting and organizing data.* Working and steering groups analyze quantitative and qualitative data to identify community health concerns. III. *Choosing health priorities.* Further data are collected, such as the determinants of health, to assist in stating and selecting health priorities. IV. *Developing a comprehensive intervention plan.* A plan is developed based on the available resources that includes strategies, timelines, and a task list for various activities such as publicizing, recruitment, and program evaluation. V. *Evaluation.* This should be ongoing to assess the progress of the program at each stage as well as the program activities, with feedback of the results directed to the community (Issel, 2008; McKenzie, Neiger, & Thackeray, 2009).
4-Step Planning Process is an organized response to opportunities and challenges for the client as individual, organization, and community.	Steps are the following: 1. *Defining*—Outcome goals are developed based on community desires 2. *Analyzing*—Critical evaluation of multiple data sources to identify need/challenge 3. *Choosing*—Selection of activities to most likely yield desired outcomes 4. *Mapping*—Each implementation step is mapped out with identification of resources and evaluation (Finnegan, & Ervin, 1989)
Mobilizing for Action through Planning and Partnerships (MAPP) is a community-driven strategic planning tool for improving community health and quality of life.	The six MAPP phases are the following: 1. *Organize for Success:* Organizing the planning process and developing the planning partnership 2. *Visioning:* Guiding the community through a collaborative, creative process that leads to a shared community vision and common values 3. *Assessments:* Identifying important information for improving community health 4. *Strategic Issues:* Participants develop an ordered list of the most important issues facing the community 5. *Goals/Strategies:* Formulated as statements related to identified issues with broad strategies for addressing issues and achieving goals identified 6. *Action Cycle:* Links planning, implementation, and evaluation (McKenzie et al., 2009).
Targeting Outcomes of Planning (TOP) focuses on outcomes in planning, implementing, and evaluating programs. TOP assesses needs, targets outcomes, assesses program opportunities, designs programs to achieve stated outcomes, tracks program outcomes, and evaluates outcome achieved.	There are seven levels working downward for the proposal. The downward levels starting with level 7 are resources, activities, participants, reactions, KASA (knowledge, attitudes, skills, aspirations), practices, and SEE (social, economic, and environmental conditions and outcomes) (Bennett & Rockwell, 2005). The seven levels working upward for the results start with level 1, which is SEE. TOPS assists with answering the following four questions: 1. Why have a program? 2. How should it be conducted? 3. Has the program design been implemented? 4. What are the benefits delivered?

are the steps or elements sequential; does the model adapt to stakeholder needs; and will the model support improving health conditions? Two commonly used health program planning models that have demonstrated usefulness in community health are the Program Logic Model and the Green and Kreuter PRECEDE-PROCEED model, which will be discussed and presented diagrammatically.

Program Logic Model (PLM)

The Program Logic Model (PLM) is used in health care as a health program planning, implementation, and evaluation model that describes the effectiveness of programs. It is a communication tool that depicts the process and components in diagrammatic form. This model is useful because it clarifies the logical linkages of program inputs (resources and activities), outputs (products, program deliverables, and audiences or targets), and program outcomes related to a specific health concern or situation. It involves stakeholders such as CHNs who are familiar with the health program and program clients (Vollman, Anderson, & McFarlane, 2008). Program Logic Models depict a cause-and-effect sequence or path toward a stated outcome. In the first stage or "situation element" of the PLM, the relevance of the program is conveyed by a statement of the health concern, such as causes; a description of who is affected by the health concern, such as place of work or connection to the community; and who is interested in the health concern, such as the stakeholders and other projects that might focus on the stated health concern. In the second stage or "input element," resources or investments such as human and fiscal are identified that are required to support the program (facilities, equipment, etc.), and other resources are identified, such as partners who might be involved in the program planning, delivery, and evaluation. The "output element" is the third PLM element; outputs are identified as the product or demonstration of what was done to create an impact from the program and are often captured in publications and workshop-type activities. Program outputs also should provide information about the people who were affected: such as their numbers, their characteristics, and how they participated in the program. The "outcomes element" is the last PLM element. The program outcomes can be short term, intermediate, or long term. Outcomes need to communicate the impacts of the program; they usually include changes in knowledge, behaviours, and situation.

To illustrate the use of the Program Logic Model, a sample schematic diagram using the elements of the model is displayed in Figure 10-1. This figure has been developed based on Statistics Canada data that showed the number of falls by older adults (residing in the psuedo-community of Pine Ridge) was higher than the provincial average. Pine Ridge is a small rural retirement community with a population consisting mainly of older adults. The CHN conducted a community health assessment and determined that there were no educational health programs on the prevention of falls for persons 65 years of age or older who were residing in their own homes. Based on these findings, the CHN conducted focus groups with older adults residing in Pine Ridge and determined that they also identified concerns about the occurrence of falls and the lack of information on prevention of falls. In collaboration with other community health team members, including older adult representatives, it was decided that a health program for this population should be delivered by the CHN and the community occupational health therapist. A Program Logic Model was the chosen planning model for the educational intervention health program. Figure 10-1 identifies the overall program outcome goal for the educational intervention program to prevent falls and provides an example of the basic elements of this educational program using the Program Logic Model. For other examples and more detailed information on logic models, see the University of Wisconsin Program Development and Evaluation Weblink on the Evolve Web site and the *Program Logic Model Workbook* listed in the Tool Box on the Evolve Web site.

PRECEDE-PROCEED Model

The Green and Kreuter PRECEDE-PROCEED model is widely used for planning due to its comprehensiveness; however, for some it can be a complex planning model. It is founded on the disciplines of epidemiology; the social, behavioural, and educational sciences; and health administration. Refer to Figure 10-2 for a pictorial illustration of the PRECEDE-PROCEED model. Originally, PRECEDE was the acronym for Predisposing, Reinforcing, Enabling Constructs in Educational (Environmental) Diagnosis and Evaluation (factors that occur before program implementation). PRECEDE is the process of systematic planning and evaluation of health education programs (Green & Kreuter, 2005). Originally, PROCEED was the acronym for Policy, Regulatory and Organizational Constructs in Educational and Environmental Development (factors that support program implementation). Originally, there were eight phases in the PRECEDE-PROCEED model. Currently, there are nine phases, with the PRECEDE phases being phases 1 to 5 and the PROCEED being phases 6 to 9. The PRECEDE phases set the direction and objectives for the ensuing phases of PROCEED to address the need for health promotion interventions and additionally the traditional educational approaches used to change unhealthy behaviours. These interventions include, for example, political and economic interventions that affect the social environment and its support for healthy lifestyles. Alternatively stated, this model's continuum of phases centre on planning, implementation, and evaluation of a health promotion program plan.

Throughout the PRECEDE-PROCEED model, two basic assumptions are emphasized: (1) health and health risks are caused by multiple factors (determinants of health), and (2) efforts to effect behavioural, environmental, and social change must be multidimensional or multisectoral, and participatory in that the target audience is actively involved in the model (Green & Kreuter, 2005). Using the model starts with a vision of the desired goal or outcome and then works back to identify what is influencing the achievement of that goal (causes) and what precedes it through a series of interdependent parts. Using the data from the Pine Ridge Older Adult Fall Prevention Program, the nine phases of the PRECEDE-PROCEED model are identified and explained in Table 10-2.

FIGURE 10-1 Program Logic Model for Fall Prevention for Older Adults of Pine Ridge

Inputs Resources	Activities	Outputs	Outcomes—Impact Short-term	Outcomes—Impact Intermediate	Outcomes—Impact Long-term
• Have CHN and OT as program lead (in-kind service). • Gain financial support from Provincial Ministry ($10,000.00). • Make fall prevention a priority of the Provincial /Territorial Health Program mandate. • Have as guest speakers community health professionals with expertise in older adult health. • Ensure access to health professionals such as geriatrician, family physician; CHNs (e.g., nurse practitioners, public health nurses, home health nurses) with assessment skills. • Utilize home workers such as Red Cross homemakers. • Utilize community resources such as the older adult centre; clergy; older adults. • Print out resources such as handouts ($2000.00). • Engage in social marketing (community flyers, radio and paper ads) ($2000.00 allocated). • Allocate space for educational sessions. • Provide transportation services ($1000.00 for volunteers' gas allowance). • Provide refreshments for educational session breaks ($300.00). • Pay part-time student salary ($4000.00).	• Recruit older adults as target audience participants. • Recruit older adults as peer educators. • Hire students (part-time) to assist with fall educational program. • Develop age-appropriate fall prevention promotion material for handouts. • Launch marketing program: dissemination of flyers, bulletin board postings, public service announcements, print media. • Inform older adults about fall prevention through dissemination of print materials by health care professionals and clergy. • Educate older adults about fall prevention through six education classes/sessions, including group discussions. • Offer six classes/sessions on fall prevention led by CHN and OT at donated space located at older adult centre. • Prepare for some older adults who may request one 6-week session to be held in the evening.	• 200 community flyers distributed • 10 daily radio public service announcements ×1 week • 1 newspaper announcement • # of older adults enrolled (50) • # of older adults who completed the program (40) • 6 educational classes held per session with one session held in the evenings • 5 sessions held • 5 program participants became peer educators in the community	• By the end of the third class, 80% of Pine Ridge older adults in the fall prevention education program can identify at least two environmental hazards in their home. • By the last class, 90% of Pine Ridge older adults in the fall prevention education program will verbalize appreciation of the safety issues pertaining to their homes.	• By the end of the fall prevention educational program, 90% of Pine Ridge older adults who completed the fall prevention educational program will report having made environmental changes to reduce the risk of the number of falls. • By the end of the fall prevention educational program, 95% of the Pine Ridge older adults who completed the fall prevention program will report more confidence in their mobility in their homes.	• The number of reported falls by Pine Ridge older adults who participated in the fall prevention educational program will be decreased by 80% after 1 year of completion of the fall prevention educational program.

Health Program Planning Process

Planning health programs and planning for the evaluation of health programs are two important activities, whether the health program being planned is a national health program such as seat belt use, a provincial health care program such as immunizations, a local health program such as heart health initiatives for elementary schoolchildren, or a health education program on diet and exercise for a group of obese clients. Regardless of the type of health program, the planning process is the same.

Assessment of Client Health Concern

The initial and most critical step in health program planning is assessing and defining the client health concern. The target population or client to be served by any health program, often referred to as key stakeholders, must be identified and involved in designing the health program to be developed. The interdisciplinary planning team needs to verify that a current health concern exists and is being ignored or unsuccessfully treated in a client group. **Assessment** is defined as a systematic appraisal of the type, depth, and scope of health concerns and strengths as perceived by clients, health providers, or both (see Box 10-1).

Assessment includes the steps in section A1 of the "How To ... Develop a Health Program Plan" box on page 295. The term *client,* used throughout this text, is referred to here. The client should also be defined by biological and psychosocial characteristics, by geographical location, and by the concerns to be addressed. For example, in a community with a large number of preschool children who require immunizations to enter school, the client population may be described as all children between 4 and 6 years of age residing in the Wakefield District who have not had up-to-date immunizations. This example identifies for the CHN who the client is, what the health concern is, how large the population is, and where the client is located.

FIGURE 10-2 PRECEDE-PROCEED Model

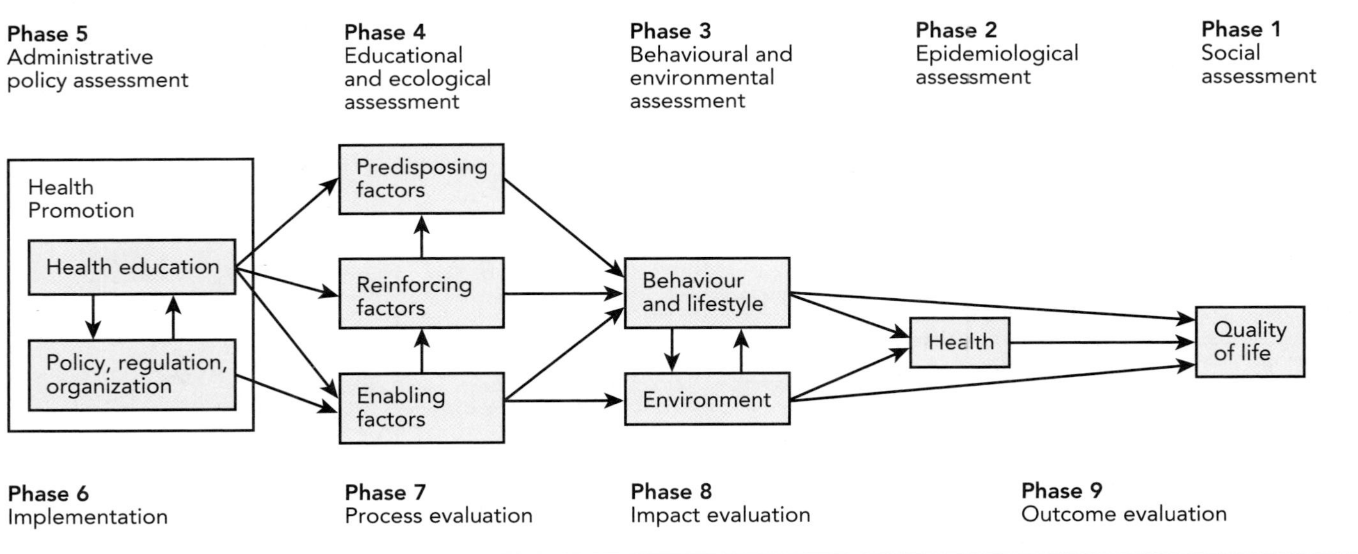

Green, L., & Kreuter, M. (1999). *Health promotion planning: An educational and environmental approach* (3rd ed.). Mountain View, CA: Mayfield Publishing Co. Retrieved from http://www.courseweb.uottawa.ca/pop8910/Outline/Models/Model-Green.PDF.

TABLE 10-2 PRECEDE-PROCEED Model and Its Application to the Pine Ridge Older Adult Fall Prevention Program

Phase	Description	Pine Ridge Fall Prevention Program Data
Phase 1. Social Assessment/ Situational Analysis	Identification of the social challenges affecting target populations using a variety of methods, such as focus groups, surveys, and community forums. The aim is to engage the target population in the identification of their specific needs and aspirations to facilitate their achievement of the best quality of life.	Conduction of a community health assessment that determined there were no educational programs on the prevention of falls for persons 65 years of age or older who were residing in their own home. Focus groups were conducted with older adults residing in Pine Ridge, and they identified concerns about the occurrence of falls and the lack of information on prevention of falls. In collaboration with other community health team members, including older adult representatives, it was decided that a program for this population should be delivered by the CHN and the community occupational health therapist.
Phase 2. Epidemiological Assessment	Determination of health concerns, ranking, and development of objectives using data such as vital statistics, morbidity, and mortality.	Statistics Canada data showed an above-average number of falls by older adults (residing in the pseudo-community of Pine Ridge) when compared to the provincial average.

TABLE 10-2 PRECEDE-PROCEED Model and Its Application to the Pine Ridge Older Adult Fall Prevention Program—Cont'd

Phase	Description	Pine Ridge Fall Prevention Program Data
Phase 3. Behavioural and Environmental Assessment	Personal and environmental factors contributing to health challenge (s) for target population.	Behavioural and lifestyle risk factors such as wearing inappropriate footwear, not appropriately using mobility aids, fear of falling. Environmental risk factors such as inadequate lighting, obstacles such as scatter rugs, too much clutter, and pets.
Phase 4. Educational and Ecological Assessment	Examines the causes of health behaviour according to three kinds of factors: predisposing (knowledge, attitudes, values, beliefs, perceptions); enabling (barriers that help or hinder behavioural and environmental changes); and reinforcing (rewards and feedback that support changes).	Predisposing: value safety in the home by preventing falls in order to prevent injury such as fractures. Enabling: availability of health professionals, community willingness to provide an educational program. Reinforcing: professional, peer support to modify the environment.
Phase 5. Administrative Policy Assessment	Administrative and policy concerns that need to be addressed prior to program implementation include assessment of capabilities and resources that can be used to develop and implement the program, budget allocation, implementation schedule, compatibility of program with organizational objectives, etc.	• $10,000 government funding • A variety of health professionals collaborating to deliver the program • Community resources organized to support the program • Older adult centre donates space for educational program delivery
Phase 6. Implementation	Implementation of the planned activities.	• Development and dissemination of 200 fall-prevention program flyers. • 50 participants enrolled. • Fall-prevention program conducted with 10 older adults per educational session. Each session was made up of 6 weekly classes. Five fall-prevention educational sessions were held. • Five program participants became peer educators in the community. • Some older adults requested a 6-week session of evening classes.
Phase 7. Process Evaluation	Evaluates implementation process.	• Ten older adults dropped out (five due to changes in their health and living arrangements; five due to inability to attend the scheduled evening classes they had originally requested). • Location used provided comfort and accessibility. • Guest speakers were well received.

(Continued)

TABLE 10-2 PRECEDE-PROCEED Model and Its Application to the Pine Ridge Older Adult Fall Prevention Program—Cont'd

Phase	Description	Pine Ridge Fall Prevention Program Data
Phase 8. Impact Evaluation	Evaluates changes in predisposing, enabling, and reinforcing factors, and program effectiveness.	Short-Term Impact Outcomes • By the end of the third class, 80% of the Pine Ridge older adults in the fall-prevention program will identify two or more environmental hazards in their home. • By the last class, 90% of the Pine Ridge older adults in the fall-prevention program will verbalize appreciation of the safety issues pertaining to their homes. Intermediate Impact Outcomes • At the end of the fall-prevention program, 90% of Pine Ridge older adults will report having made environmental changes to reduce the risk of the number of falls. • At the end of the fall-prevention program, 95% of Pine Ridge older adults who completed the fall-prevention program will report more confidence in their mobility in their homes.
Phase 9. Outcome Evaluation	Measures overall changes in achieving program objectives.	Long-term Outcome Evaluation • The number of reported falls by Pine Ridge older adults who participated in the fall-prevention program will be decreased by 80% after 1 year of completion of program.

BOX 10-1 Stages Used in Assessing Client Health Concern

- *Preactive:* projecting future health concerns
- *Reactive:* defining the health concern based on past health concerns identified by the client or the agency
- *Inactive:* defining the health concern based on the existing health status of the population to be served
- *Interactive:* describing the health concern using past and present data to project future population needs

A health education program may be necessary to alert the population to the existing health concern. In the example of the immunization of preschool children, public service announcements on television and radio and in newspapers may be used to alert parents to laws requiring immunizations, to the health concerns of communicable diseases, and to which communicable diseases (e.g., smallpox) have been successfully eradicated by immunization programs. Health concerns to be met for the client population must be identified collaboratively by the client, the CHN, or the interdisciplinary team. If the client does not recognize the health concern or is not involved in the planning, the program usually fails.

The *size and location of a client population* for a health program involves more than counting the number of persons in the community who may be eligible for the health program. More specifically, they involve defining the number of persons with the health concern who are underserved by existing health programs and the number of eligible persons who have and have not taken advantage of existing services. For example, consider again the community need for a preschool immunization program. In planning the health program, the estimates of numbers of preschool children in the district may be

How To... Develop a Health Program Plan

A. Describe the Health Concern

1. Assess the client concern:
   a. Who is the client?
   b. What is the health concern to be met?
   c. What are the client's strengths?
   d. How large is the client population to be served?
   e. Where is the client located?
   f. Are there other health programs addressing the same health concern? (Describe.)
   g. Why is the health concern not being met?
2. Establish health program boundaries:
   a. Who will be included in the health program?
   b. Who will be excluded? Why?
   c. What is the health program goal?
3. Consider health program feasibility:
   a. Who agrees that the health program is required (agency administrator, providers, clients, funders)?
   b. Who does not agree?
4. Determine the resources (general) required:
   a. What personnel are required? What personnel are available?
   b. What facilities are required? What facilities are available?
   c. What equipment is required? What equipment is available?
   d. Is money required? Is money available?
   e. Are resources (printing, paper, medical supplies) being donated? What type and amount?
5. Consider tools used to assess health concern:
   a. Census data
   b. Key informants
   c. Community forums
   d. Existing program surveys
   e. Surveys of client population
   f. Statistical indicators (e.g., morbidity or mortality data)

B. Name the Health Concern

1. List the potential solutions to the health concern.
2. Consider how to use the client strengths.
3. What are the risks of each solution?
4. What are the consequences?
5. What are the outcomes to be gained from the solutions?
6. Draw a decision tree to show the problem-solving process used.

C. Identify Objectives and Activities for Alternatives

1. What are the objectives for each solution to meet the health program goal?
2. What activities will be done to conduct each of the alternative solutions listed under B1 and based on objectives?
3. What are the differences in the resources required for each of the alternative solutions?
4. Which of the alternative solutions would be chosen if the resources described under A4 were the only resources available?

D. Evaluate Solutions for Health Concern

1. Which of the alternative solutions is most acceptable to
   a. The client?
   b. The agency administrator?
   c. The CHN?
   d. The community?
2. Which of the alternative solutions appears to have the most benefits to
   a. The client?
   b. The agency administrator?
   c. The CHN?
   d. The community?
3. Based on costs, which alternative solution would be chosen by
   a. The client?
   b. The agency administrator?
   c. The CHN?
   d. The community?

E. Choose the Health Program Solution

1. Based on the data collected, which of the solutions has been chosen?
2. Why should the agency administrator approve your request? Give your rationale.
3. When can the health program begin? Give a specific date.

obtained from census data or birth certificates. The CHN then needs to determine the number of children underserved and the number of children who have not used services for which they are eligible.

Boundaries for the client population are established by defining the size and location of the client population. The boundaries stipulate who is included in or excluded from the health program. If the fictional immunization program were designed to serve only preschool children of low-income families, all other preschool children would be excluded.

What people think about the need for a health program, or *program feasibility,* might differ among health providers, agency administrators, policy makers, and potential clients. Collecting data on the opinions and attitudes of all persons directly and indirectly involved with the health program's success is necessary to determine the program's feasibility and the need to redefine the health concern, and to decide to develop a new health program or expand an existing one. Before implementing a health program, CHNs need to *identify available resources.* Health program resources include personnel, facilities, equipment, and financing. If any one of the four categories of health program resources is unavailable, the health program is likely to be inadequate to meet the health concerns of the client population.

A number of *assessment* data sources exist to assist the CHN in the assessment process, as discussed in Chapter 9. Some of the major data sources used for assessment, summarized in Table 10-3, are key informants, community forums, surveys of existing community agencies with similar health programs, surveys of residents of the community to be served (client population), and statistical indicators (Rossi, Lipsey, & Freeman, 2004).

The demand for a health program is determined by working with the client. This stage of planning creates options for solving the health concern and considers several solutions. Each option for a health program solution is examined for its uncertainties (risks) and consequences, leading to a set of **outcomes** (the results or impact of health program interventions).

Some alternative solutions to the health concern will present more risks or uncertainties than others, prompting the following considerations:

TABLE 10-3 Summary of Community Health Assessment Data Sources

Name	Definition	Advantages	Disadvantages
Community forum	Community, group, organization, open meeting	Low cost Learn perspectives of large number of persons	Limited data Limited expression of views Discourages less powerful Becomes arena to discuss political issues
Focus groups	Open discussion with small representative groups	Low cost Clients participate in identification of health concern Initiates community support for the program	Time consuming Allows focus on irrelevant or political issues
Key informants	Identify, select, and question knowledgeable leaders	Provides picture of services required	Bias of leaders Community characteristics may be incorrectly perceived by informants
Indicators approach (e.g., census data)	Existing data used to determine health concern	Excellent data on health concerns and characteristics of client groups	Growth and change in population may make data outdated
Survey of existing agencies	Estimates of client populations via services used at similar community agencies	Easy method to estimate size of client group Know extent of services offered in existing programs	All cases of health concern may not be reported Exaggeration of services may occur
Surveys	Measurement of total or sample client population by interview or questionnaire	Direct and accurate data on client population and their health concerns	Expensive Technically demanding Need many interviews or observations Interviews may be biased

- The CHN needs to decide between the solution that involves more risk and the solution that is free of risk.
- A "do nothing" decision is always one with the least risk to the provider.
- When choosing a solution, the CHN looks at whether the desired outcome can be achieved.
- After careful consideration, the CHN rethinks the solutions.
- Information collected with the data source is used to develop these alternative solutions.
- Decision trees are useful graphic aids that give a picture of the solutions and the consequences and risks of each solution.

Health Program Goals and Objectives

Frequently, the terms *goals* and *objectives* are used interchangeably, but, for the purpose of this discussion, goals and objectives are differentiated. **Goals** are defined as broad statements that identify the main purpose(s) for the health program. For example, the goal of an exercise program for middle-aged adults is to help participants to be healthy and participate in regular exercise. **Objectives** are defined as specific measurable statements that identify the steps planned to reach the overall health program goal. For example, in the exercise program for middle-aged adults, a learning objective is that each program participant will increase his or her daily walking by 15 minutes during the first week of the exercise program. Therefore, several objectives (short term, intermediate, and long term) are stated to meet each program goal. Action-oriented verbs are used to specify the change expected. Some examples of action verbs are *identify, define, compare, contrast, apply, decrease, increase, demonstrate,* and *state.*

If the objectives are too general, health program evaluation becomes impossible. The objectives must be specific and stated so that anyone reading them could conduct the health program without further instruction. To be truly effective, the health program plan should begin with a general health program goal and move on to specific objectives. For example, in Wakefield District, a health program goal might be to reduce communicable diseases in the District of Wakefield. Table 10-4 provides one example of an objective to meet this goal. The stated objective is this: The Wakefield District immunization program will decrease the incidence rates of vaccine-preventable illnesses by 10 to 25% by providing immunization clinics in all schools in the district by December 2012. Other objectives would also need to be developed to meet this goal. The objective below is developed using the SMART acronym as a tool to assist in meeting the criteria necessary to write a "good" objective. Some useful Web sites available to help CHNs develop skill in writing objectives using the SMART tool are listed in the Weblinks on the Evolve Web site: *A Guide to Writing Learning Objectives;* and *Bloom's Taxonomy Action Verbs,* which provides a listing of action verbs to be used.

The purpose for a goal is to focus on the major reason for the health program. A general health program goal may be to reduce the incidence of low-birth-weight babies in Wakefield District in 2012 by improving access to prenatal care. Each specific health program objective includes the following:

TABLE 10-4 Using the SMART Acronym to Develop an Objective to Meet the Program Goal "To reduce communicable diseases in the District of Wakefield"

Objectives Using SMART	Criteria	Example Program Objective Using the Wakefield District Data
S = specific	Specific and stated using action-oriented verb to determine behaviour expected	The Wakefield District Immunization program...
M = measurable	Measurable change is identified to know when the objective has been met	will decrease the incidence rates of vaccine-preventable illnesses by 10 to 25% ...
A = achievable/attainable	Can be accomplished by the client or organization	by providing immunization clinics ...
R = realistic	For the situation, the objective can be achieved given the resources	in all schools in the district ...
T = time frame	States the target time or date for accomplishment	by December 2012.

- A measurable behaviour
- The circumstances under which the behaviour is observed
- The minimal acceptable standard for the performance of the behaviour

A specific objective for this Wakefield District health program may be to open a prenatal clinic in each health unit or health authority within the district by January 2012 to serve the population within each census tract of the district. This specific objective is an action-oriented approach to meeting the goal.

Specific health program activities are then planned to meet each specific objective, and resources, such as the number of CHNs, equipment, supplies, and location, are planned for each of the objectives. It is assumed that as each specific objective is met, the general program goal will also be partly achieved. Remember that several specific objectives are required to meet a general health program goal.

It is important for the CHN and other members of the health program planning team to track activities planned and the team member who will work on the various activities. A Gantt chart is a useful tool to visually track the activities pertaining to the achievement of the health program objectives and therefore toward meeting the identified health program goal. The chart indicates the health program activities with the time frame for accomplishment. A Gantt chart is useful to depict the order of tasks, health program progress, and possible dependencies between tasks. A Gantt chart considers the concepts of events and time with events listed on the left side of the chart and time indicated horizontally at the top of the chart showing the planned start and completion dates for health program activities. Time is represented on the chart lines (duration of activity) by using arrows to show start and completion of activity. Because changes in the health program necessitate redrawing the chart, the CHN needs to consider using a computer-generated chart programs such as Microsoft Project or Excel. Figure 10-3 is a Gantt chart for the first objective of the fall-prevention program for older adults of Pine Ridge.

Planning for Implementation

In this planning phase, the CHN, working with the client, considers the possibilities of solving a health concern using one of the solutions identified. The CHN considers the costs, resources, and program activities required for each of the solutions. To illustrate, consider again the immunization scenario. If the proposed solution is to encourage the parents to obtain the immunizations

FIGURE 10-3 Gantt Chart for the First Objective of the Fall-Prevention Program for Older Adults of Pine Ridge

Fall Prevention Program for Pine Ridge Older Adults				
Objective 1: To increase awareness of the fall prevention program by at least 75% of the older adults of Pine Ridge within 3 months				
	January	**February**	**March**	**April**
Develop print resources to be distributed to the local papers	CHN and OT			
Contact local clergy by telephone	CHN			
Develop posters to be displayed at older adults centres and other organizations		CHN		
Prepare newsletter to distribute to the community home care agencies			CHN and volunteers	CHN and volunteers

CHN, Community health nurse; *OT*, occupational therapist.

(the best consequence), examples of activities include developing a script for a health education program and implementing a television program to encourage parents to take children to their health care provider. If one of the other alternatives, such as providing community health nursing clinics at daycare centres (the worst possible consequence) or providing community health nursing clinics at the health unit or health authority for all ages of children were chosen, offering a clinic 8 hours per day at the health unit or health authority and providing a mobile clinic to each daycare centre for 4 hours each day to provide the immunizations would be possible activities.

For each alternative, the CHN lists the resources required to implement each activity. In the example, personnel could include CHNs, volunteers, and clerks; supplies might include handouts, adhesive bandages, medications, records, and consent forms; equipment might include syringes, needles, stethoscopes, and blood pressure cuffs; and facilities might include a television studio for a media blitz on the education program, a room with chairs, and emergency carts. The costs of personnel, supplies, equipment, and facilities for each solution should be listed and considered. As indicated, clients need to review each solution for acceptance.

Deciding on Health Concern Solutions

Each alternative is weighed to judge the costs, benefits, and acceptability of the idea to the client, community, and CHN. The information outlined in section C of the "How to ... Develop a Health Program Plan" box on page 295 would be used to rank the solutions for choice by the client and CHN based on cost, benefit, and acceptability. The solution that would provide the desired outcomes needs to be considered. Looking at available information through literature reviews or interviews might show whether any of the options have been tried in another place or by someone else. The results from other sources would be helpful in deciding whether a chosen solution would be useful.

Choose the Solution

Clients, CHNs, and the interdisciplinary health planning team and agency select the best solution. Working with clients throughout the health planning process helps to promote acceptance of the plan; solutions that are derived from key stakeholders meeting to explore, decide, and commit to possible options that address particular health program needs are more likely to be successful. One type of meeting that could be used is a *charette.* A charette brings people of similar interest together to explore creative ways of addressing a program issue or question. Traditionally, charettes have been used in the arts, where a visual portrayal of ideas can be captured. Charettes are becoming more popular in other fields such as business, urban planning to promote health, and government. (Refer to the Health Canada Web site in the Tool Box on the Evolve Web site for more information on charettes.) Providing a rationale for recommending particular solutions helps the CHN to get support for the plan to be implemented, such as agency and community support.

HEALTH PROGRAM EVALUATION PROCESS

Health Program Evaluation

Health program evaluation is a systematic step-by-step process that examines a program to determine the intended and unintended impacts of a health program (see the "Ethical Considerations" box). Evaluation produces data to inform decision making about ways to support health programs and best use the resources.

The five steps identified by the Public Health Agency of Canada (PHAC) for evaluating public health programs are the following:

- Focus on determining exactly what needs to be known about the health program
- Choose suitable strategies to answer the evaluation questions
- Design or revise data collection tools
- Collect and analyze the data
- Make decisions about the health program based on responses to the evaluation questions (PHAC, 2008)

See the PHAC Guide to Project Evaluation Weblink on the Evolve Web site for further information on PHAC's five steps of evaluation.

The major benefit of health program evaluation is that it shows whether a program is meeting its purpose. It should answer the following questions:

- Are the health needs for which the program was designed being met?
- Are the health concerns it was designed to solve being solved?

Health program justification and continued funding for programs are a result of demonstration through evaluation that the program is meeting its goals. Evaluation is important for health program continuance and improvement. CHNs at all levels of education and preparation can participate in the planning and evaluation of a health program.

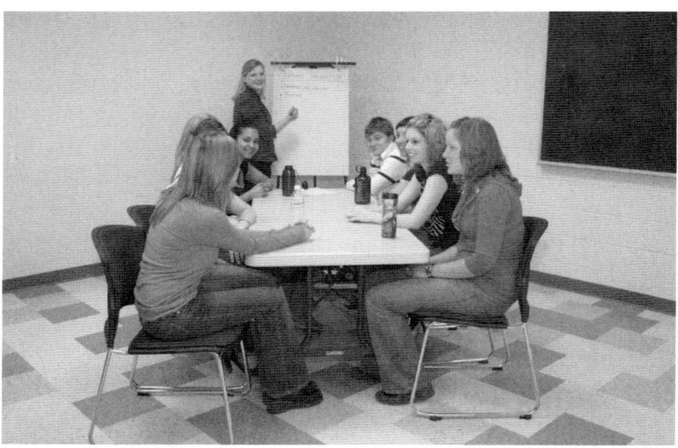

A charette is a meeting of people with a similar interest to explore creative ways of addressing a program issue or a question.

ETHICAL CONSIDERATIONS

A CHN working as a member of an interdisciplinary team is involved in the evaluation of the human papillomavirus (HPV) immunization program implemented by the Public Health Agency of Canada. The team is evaluating the program and has to make sure that the vaccine does no harm.

Ethical principles that apply to the above scenario are the following:

- *Respect for autonomy:* When a community health intervention interferes with the individual rights of persons receiving care, CHNs use and advocate for the use of the least restrictive measures possible for those in their care. CHNs recognize and support a capable person's right to refuse or withdraw consent for care or treatment at any time.
- *Distributive justice:* CHNs ensure that health care is provided with the person's informed consent.

Questions to Consider

1. What ethical considerations does a CHN need to consider when planning health programs?
2. a) In planning for the HPV immunization program, what are the steps taken to ensure that the vaccine is beneficial and not harmful to the target population?
   b) What are the elements to consider in the evaluation stage of the program?

Quality assurance audits are prime examples of formative health program evaluation in health care delivery. Evaluation data are used to justify continuing programs in community health. Health program records—including client evaluations and community indexes—serve as the major source of information for health program evaluation. Surveys, interviews, observations, and diagnostic tests are ways to assess consumer and client responses to health programs. When the planning process begins, health program evaluation starts with assessment—that is, process evaluation. The types of evaluation are process or formative and outcome or summative and these are described in Table 10-5. Process evaluation and outcome evaluation are the terms used in this text.

Health Program Evaluation Sources

Major sources of information for health program evaluation are health program clients, program records, and community indicators. The program participants, or clients, of the service have a unique and valuable role in program evaluation. Whether the clients for whom the program was designed accept the services determines to a large extent whether the program achieves its purpose. Thus, their reactions, feelings, and judgements about the program are important to the evaluation.

To assess the response of participants in a health program, the CHN as evaluator may use a written survey in the form of a questionnaire, an attitude scale, interviews, and observations. *Attitude scales* are probably used most often, and they are usually phrased in terms that will ascertain whether the health program has met its objectives. The client satisfaction survey is an example of an attitude scale often used in the health care delivery system to evaluate the health program objectives.

The second major source of information for health program evaluation is *program records,* especially clinical records. Clinical records provide the CHN evaluator with information about the care given to the client and the results of that care. To determine whether a health program goal has been met, one might summarize the data from a group of records. For example, if one overall goal is to reduce the incidence of low-birth-weight babies through prenatal care, records would be reviewed to obtain the number of mothers who received prenatal care and the number of low-birth-weight babies born to them.

A third major source of health program evaluation is a *community health index.* Health and illness indicators, such as mortality and morbidity data, are probably cited

TABLE 10-5 Types of Health Program Evaluation

Direction of Evaluation	Type of Evaluation	Definition and Purpose	Examples of Some Questions Connected to This Type of Evaluation	Practice Example
	Process/Formative	**Process evaluation** is making a judgement about a program delivery while in development. It begins with an assessment of the need for the program. It focuses on what the program does and for whom. The purpose is to improve the program.	Was the target group reached? Was the target group satisfied with the program? What is working in the program? Why? What is not working in the program and why not? Were the resources used suitable? Which program objectives have not been met and why? What in the program needs to be changed if it is to be implemented elsewhere?	In a weight-loss program for older adults, 20 persons signed up for the program, which was more than the targeted number of 15. Verbal feedback from the group members indicated that 95% were very satisfied with the program and the other 5% were satisfied. Responses showed satisfaction with the time of day, location, program content such as menu preparation, physical activity, and group support. Areas requiring change were the need for more individualized exercises based on individual participant ability, especially for participants over 75 years of age. One consideration for future program delivery would be to conduct a pre-assessment of the older adults physical activity level and abilities.
	Outcome/ Summative	**Outcome evaluation** examines the results of a program—that is, the effects of the program. It also provides information to use in order to decide whether to continue, adjust, or terminate the program (Clark, 2008). Its purpose is to examine the changes that occurred as a result of the program and to determine whether the program is having the intended effect.	To what extent have the short-term objectives been met? To what extent have the intermediate objectives been met? To what extent have the long-term objectives been met? What changes have occurred due to program delivery?	Short-term objectives were fully met—e.g., all participants were able to gradually increase their weekly activity and to follow the recommended total caloric intake and all participants lost at least 3 pounds within the first 3 weeks of the program. The immediate objectives were that all participants indicated that they followed the recommended food preparation and meal plans; however, those over 75 years of age were not able to increase their physical activity. Within 2 months, the participants had each lost a minimum of 10 pounds. The long-term objectives were partially met as 80% of the participants continued with the healthy eating and exercise program, except for those over 75 years of age who continued to be challenged with the physical activity component.

SOURCE: Adapted from Clark, M. J. (2008). *Community health nursing: Advocacy for population health* (5th ed.). Upper Saddle River, NJ: Pearson Prentice Hall.

Evidence-Informed Practice

This study describes a participatory evaluation project, in the field of forensic nursing involving researcher evaluators and sexual assault nurse examiners (SANEs). The evaluation project was developed to determine whether the nursing care provided by SANEs was consistent with a Logic Model of "empowering care." In this program, "empowering care" is referred to as providing health care, support, and resources; treating patients with dignity and respect; believing patients' stories; helping to regain control and choice; and respecting their decisions. An evaluation survey was developed and tested with 52 sexual assault victims in one SANE program to assess their psychological well-being.

Findings concluded that SANE nursing actions included all aspects of empowering care as listed above, such as treating victims with dignity and respect, and believing their stories. As well, sexual assault victims described having positive psychological well-being outcomes. The established partnership in this project led to further collaborative endeavours. This program evaluation process contributed to SANEs' capacity building and therefore sustainability.

Application for CHNs: The Logic Model and other program planning models are tools that the CHN needs to be familiar with. Models are necessary for CHNs so that an organized approach is used in program planning and program evaluation. Program evaluation offers further opportunities for CHNs to communicate and work with clients and to further develop partnerships. The value of partnering has relevance to community health nursing practice.

Questions for Reflection & Discussion

1. What aspects of the Logic Model of "empowering care" do you feel would be appropriate in your own nursing care?
2. As the CHN working on this collaborative team, what process evaluation questions could you ask?
3. Related to evidence-based practice, locate the most recent evidence on SANEs and their use of the Logic Model of care.

Reference: Campbell, R., Patterson, D., Adams, A. E., Diegel, R., & Coats, S. (2008). A participatory evaluation project to measure SANE nursing practice and adult sexual assault patients' psychological well-being. *Journal of Forensic Nursing* 4(1), 19–28.

more frequently than any other single index for health program evaluation. Incidence and prevalence are valuable indexes used to measure program effectiveness and impact (see Chapter 8 for further discussion about rates and ratios).

Health Program Evaluation Criteria

The criteria of health program evaluation are the following: relevance, adequacy, progress, efficiency, effectiveness, impact and sustainability (Veney & Kaluzny, 2005). These criteria are related to the type of evaluation that is conducted in regard to health program evaluations. To conduct a health program evaluation, the first step is to choose the type of evaluation required. Next, identify the goal and objectives for evaluation. Third, decide who will be involved in the evaluation. Last, answer the questions found in Table 10-6. Depending on the answers to the questions, the health program will be found to be successful or not.

In summary, health program planning is evolving as new program planning models are introduced. Furthermore, CHNs need to monitor the quality and necessity of health programs in order to justify existing and proposed program delivery within the current fiscal environment.

TABLE 10-6 Health Program Evaluation Considerations

Criterion	Explanation	Type of Evaluation	Questions to Consider	CHN Implications
Relevance	Is an important component of the initial planning phase. The program is suitable to meet the needs of the target group.	Process evaluation	1. Refer to questions in the "How To … Develop a Health Program Plan" box. 2. Did the community health needs assessment determine that the program is necessary?	As money, providers, facilities, and supplies for delivering health care services are monitored more and more closely, the assessment conducted by the CHN will be used to determine whether the program is required.
Adequacy	Looks at the extent to which the program addresses the entire health concern defined in the assessment. The magnitude of the health concern is determined by vital statistics, incidence, prevalence, and expert opinion.	Process evaluation	1. Does the program have the capacity to positively influence the health concern? 2. Are there clearly identified parameters of the services required to address the target group health concerns?	The CHN will need access to a variety of data sources.
Progress	The monitoring of program activities—such as hours of services, number of providers used, number of referrals made, and amount of money spent to meet program objectives—provides an evaluation of the progress of the program. Progress *evaluation* occurs primarily while implementing the program.	Process evaluation	1. How frequently would activities be monitored? 2. What aspects of the activities would be monitored (e.g., hours of service, clients served, types of providers available)? 3. What is the fit between the program plan and implementation regarding budgeting?	The CHN who completes a daily or weekly log of clinical activities (e.g., the number of clients seen in a clinic or visited at home, number of phone contacts, number of referrals made, number of community health promotion activities such as mass media campaigns) is contributing to the progress evaluation of the community health nursing intervention.
Efficiency	It is the relationship between the program outcomes and the resources spent.	Process evaluation (ongoing) and outcome (end result of the program)	1. Are the costs of this program similar to other programs with the same goal? 2. If the program costs are greater or less than what is planned, is the program needed? 3. Is the program needed if the productivity level is high or low compared to similar programs?	The CHN as evaluator may be able to determine whether the program provides better benefits at a lower cost than a similar program or whether the benefits to the clients or number of clients served justify the costs of the program.

(Continued)

TABLE 10-6 Health Program Evaluation Considerations—Cont'd

Criterion	Explanation	Type of Evaluation	Questions to Consider	CHN Implications
			4. What are benefits of the program to the target group and to the community?	
Effectiveness	An evaluation of program effectiveness may help the CHN determine both client and provider satisfaction with the program activities as well as whether the program met its stated objectives.	Outcome evaluation	1. How satisfied are the providers, target group, and the community with the program outcomes? 2. Are the health concerns of the target group being met?	The CHN determines both client and provider satisfaction with the program activities, as well as whether the program met its stated objectives.
Impact	If an evaluation of impact is the goal, long-term effects such as changes in morbidity and mortality must be investigated.	Outcome evaluation	1. To what extent has (have) the overall goal(s) been met? 2. What changed as a result of the program for the target population?	
Sustainability	The program can be continued if the resources and the program effects can be sustained over time.		1. Did the program receive external funding? 2. What new resources are available to support the program once the initial funding is no longer available?	When program evaluation is completed, dissemination of results is required to be communicated to any funding bodies, appropriate community agencies, stakeholders, and the public. The CHN may be involved with this process.

Source: Based on Veney, A., & Kaluzny, J. (2005). *Evaluation and decision making for health services* (4th ed.). Chicago, IL: Health Administration Press.

CRITICAL VIEW

CHNs, as health program planners, always need to work with the community to achieve the desired results.

1. How would a CHN establish a working group in the community to address an identified health concern?
2. How would you apply the Program Logic Model with a group of grade 5 students to develop a physical activity program in their school?

LEVELS OF PREVENTION

Related to Health Program Planning and Evaluation

PRIMARY PREVENTION

CHNs plan a community-wide program with the local government, health department, and business sector to make all public businesses smoke-free in order to prevent exposure to second-hand smoke.

SECONDARY PREVENTION

Occupational health nurses develop screening programs for all workers in businesses to determine the incidence and prevalence of respiratory illness, cardiovascular diseases, and lung cancer before implementing the smoke-free program.

TERTIARY PREVENTION

Occupational health nurses evaluate the incidence and prevalence of respiratory illness, cardiovascular disease, and lung cancer among nonsmoking workers after the implementation of the smoke-free program and provide programs to reduce complications from identified diseases.

STUDENT EXPERIENCE

You are living in community X. Explore the "Program Logic Model Workbook" and the "How to Make a Gantt Chart Using Microsoft Excel" Web sites listed in the Tool Box on the Evolve Web site.

Program development using the Program Logic Model usually involves the team approach. Your team consists of CHN, health promotion consultant, staff, public health nutritionist, and community key informants (parents, teachers). Analysis by the team of the community health assessment data has identified that childhood obesity is a health concern. The team is in the initial stages of planning a health program to address this health concern.

As the team CHN, you have been designated the role of program coordinator. In this role, you have been asked to coordinate preparation of a two-page draft health program plan using the Program Logic Model and to prepare a one-page Gantt chart. The program goal is to reduce the incidence of childhood obesity in community X. Each team member is to prepare two SMART objectives for this goal that will be discussed and prioritized at the next meeting. Share these objectives with your classmates or team members of community X. As a team, prepare a Program Logic Model and a Gantt chart for your community.

REMEMBER THIS!

- Planning, implementation, and evaluation are essential elements of health program management.
- A health program consists of a variety of planned activities to address the assessed health concerns of clients over time and builds on client strengths in order to meet specific goals and objectives.
- Health program planning is the organized approach to identifying and choosing interventions to meet specified goals and objectives that address client health concerns.
- Health program implementation refers to putting the health program activities into action.
- Health program evaluation is defined as the methods used to determine if a service is required and will be used, whether a program to meet that health concern is carried out as planned, and whether the service actually helps the people it intends to help.
- The two types of program evaluation are process evaluation and outcome evaluation.
- To develop quality health programs, planning should include these essential elements: identification of health concern, assessment of health concern, identification of health concern solutions, analysis and comparison of alternative intervention methods, and selection of the best plan and planning methods.
- The initial and most critical step in planning and evaluating a health program is the assessment of the health concern.
- Some of the major tools used in community health assessment are community forums, surveys of existing community agencies, surveys of community residents, and statistical indicators.
- The major benefit of program evaluation is to determine whether a health program is fulfilling its stated goals.

- Quality assurance programs are prime examples of health program evaluation.
- Plans for implementing and evaluating health programs should be developed at the same time.
- Program records and community indices serve as major sources of information for health program evaluation.
- Planning health programs and planning for their evaluation are two of the most important ways in which CHNs can ensure successful health program implementation.
- The health program management process, like the community health nursing process, is a rational decision-making process.
- Health program planning helps CHNs and agencies focus attention on required community services.
- Health program planning helps all those involved understand their role in working with clients to provide client-directed interventions.
- The criteria for health program evaluation are relevance, adequacy, progress, efficiency, effectiveness, impact, and sustainability.
- Setting goals and writing SMART objectives to meet the goals are necessary to evaluate health program outcomes.

REFLECTIVE PRAXIS

Case Study 1

Jean, a CHN, is the occupational health nurse at the lumber mill in Pine Ridge. She noticed that many of the workers exhibit poor health habits, such as smoking and eating high-fat foods. Through talking with workers who visited the occupational health office, Jean learned that many of them wanted to take better care of themselves but believed they could not because of the long hours they worked and the high stress of their jobs. She decided to investigate whether poor health habits were a problem for everyone working in the mill or if they were common only to those who visited the occupational health office.

Jean sent surveys to all 800 employees at the mill and received responses from 40%. From the surveys, Jean learned that 30% of the workers worked 10 to 12 hours each work day, 40% smoked one-half to two packs of cigarettes a day, and the most recent meal consumed by 85% of the workers did not include any fruits or vegetables.

Jean went to the president of the mill, shared this information with him, and discussed how poor health could decrease productivity. The president supported her suggestion to implement a health promotion program for the mill employees and offered to provide the required space and office materials for the program. Jean is now planning to develop a health education program that will focus on helping the employees to adopt healthy lifestyle behaviours. One of the health program objectives is to have the employees engage in healthy eating behaviours.

1. Using the five elements of the Program Logic Model, write up a health program plan for the healthy eating program objective for the mill employees.
2. Develop a Gantt chart to monitor the accomplishment of the activities.

Answers are on the Evolve Web site at http://evolve.elsevier.com/Canada/Stanhope/community/.

Case Study 2

The following is a real-life example of the application of the program management process by an undergraduate nursing student. This activity resulted in the development and implementation of a CHN-managed clinic for the homeless. This example shows how students as well as providers can make a difference in health care delivery. It also shows that no mystery surrounds the health program management process.

Eva was listening to the radio one Sunday afternoon and heard an announcement about the opening of a soup kitchen within the community for the growing homeless population. She was beginning her nursing course in community health and wanted to find a creative clinical experience that would benefit her as well as others. The announcement gave her an idea. Although it mentioned food, clothing, shelter, and social services, nothing was said about health care.

1. Eva is interested in finding a way to provide community health nursing care and health care services at the soup kitchen. Which of the following should she do?
    a. Talk with key leaders to determine their interest in her idea.
    b. Review the literature to find out the magnitude of the health concern.
    c. Survey the community to find out if others are providing services.
    d. Discuss the idea with members of the homeless population.
    e. Consider potential solutions to the health concerns.

f. Consider where she would get the resources to open a clinic.

g. Talk with church leaders and nurse faculty members to seek acceptance for her idea.

Answers are on the Evolve Web site at http://evolve.elsevier.com/Canada/Stanhope/community/.

What Would You Do?

1. Reflect on the community that you live in and identify one community health concern for a specific client population. For example, a group of high-school students has been observed smoking in the schoolyard. Review the evidence to determine the magnitude of the identified health concern (e.g., the smoking patterns of youth in Canada). Apply the health program planning process for your identified community health concern. Some areas to consider are the key planning team members in working together to address this health concern, what data you would collect to identify client and community health concerns, and the available resources in the community to address the health concern.

TOOL BOX

evolve

The Tool Box contains useful instruments that can be applied in community health nursing practice. See also the Tool Box for this chapter on the book's Evolve Web site: http://evolve.elsevier.com/Canada/Stanhope/community/.

Tools

Canadian Outcomes Research Institute. *How to Prepare a Program Logic Model.*
This site provides links to Program Logic Model information and examples.

The Health Canada Policy Toolkit for Public Involvement in Decision Making.
This site provides information on a charette, how it works, and its logistics.

The Health Communication Unit (THCU). Online Health Program Planner.
Links are provided on this site to tools such as webinars, workbooks, and worksheets on a variety of topics pertaining to health program planning such as situational assessment, Program Logic Models, and objective writing.

How to Make a Gantt Chart Using Microsoft Excel.
This site provides the "how to" for preparing a Gantt chart using a computer-based Microsoft excel program.

The Planning Process. *The Health Planner's Toolkit.*
This excellent resource includes everything required to carry out a program planning process as well as a health impact assessment.

Program Evaluation Tool Kit.
This PHAC site provides a quick-glance tool for program evaluation with links to more detailed information.

Program Logic Model Workbook.
This site provides the step-by-step process for creating and using the Program Logic Model.

WEBLINKS

evolve

Direct links to these resources can be found on the text's accompanying Evolve Web site at http://evolve.elsevier.com/stanhope/community.

Bloom's Taxonomy Action Verbs. This site provides action verbs listed alphabetically to be used when writing SMART objectives.

A Guide to Writing Learning Objectives. This site provides information on objective writing utilizing Bloom's Taxonomy.

The Health Communication Unit (THCU). Evaluation Resources. This excellent Web site provides many links to resources such as a workbook and slideshow on evaluating health promotion programs, a workbook on conducting survey research, and a workbook on conducting focus groups.

Public Health Agency of Canada. *Guide to Project Evaluation: A Participatory Approach.* This Web site provides information on evaluation using five key evaluation questions and five evaluation process steps.

University of Wisconsin Program Development and Evaluation. Logic Models–Examples. This site provides links to logic model examples for various programs such as community nutrition education and treating tobacco addiction.

REFERENCES

Barreto, L., Van Exan, R., & Rutty, C. (2006). Polio vaccine development in Canada: Contributions to global polio eradication. *Biological*, *34*, 91–101.

Bennett, C., & Rockwell, K. (2005). *Targeting outcomes of programs (TOP)*. Retrieved from http://citnews.unl.edu/TOP/english/overviewf.html.

Campbell, R., Patterson, D., Adams, A. E., Diegel, R., & Coats, S. (2008). A participatory evaluation project to measure SANE nursing practice and adult sexual assault patients' psychological well-being. *Journal of Forensic Nursing*, *4*(1), 19–28.

Clark, M. J. (2008). *Community health nursing: Advocacy for population health* (5th ed.). Upper Saddle River, NJ: Pearson Prentice Hall.

Finnegan, L., & Ervin, N. E. (1989). An epidemiological approach to community assessment. *Public Health Nursing*, *6*(3), 147–151.

Green, L., & Kreuter, M. (1999). *Health promotion planning: An educational and environmental approach* (3rd ed.). Mountain View, CA: Mayfield Publishing Co. Retrieved from http://www.courseweb.uottawa.ca/pop8910/Outline/Models/Model-Green.PDF.

Green, L. W., & Kreuter, M. W. (2005). *Health promotion planning: An educational and ecological approach* (3rd ed.). New York: The McGraw-Hill Companies, Inc.

Issel, L. M. (2008). *Health program planning and evaluation: A practical systematic approach for community health* (2nd ed.). Sudbury, MA: Jones & Bartlett.

McKenzie, J. F., Neiger, B. L., & Thackeray, R. (2009). *Planning, implementing, and evaluating health promotion programs: A primer* (5th ed.). San Francisco, CA: Pearson & Benjamin Cummings.

Public Health Agency of Canada. (2008). *Program evaluation tool kit*. Retrieved from http://www.phac-aspc.gc.ca/php-psp/toolkit-eng.php.

Rossi, P., Lipsey, M., & Freeman, H. (2004). *Evaluation: A systematic approach*. (7th ed.). Beverly Hills, CA: Sage.

Veney, A., & Kaluzny, J. (2005). *Evaluation and decision making for health services*. (4th ed.). Chicago, IL: Health Administration Press.

Vollman, A. R., Anderson, E. T., & McFarlane, J. (2008). *Canadian community as partner: Theory and practice in nursing*. Philadelphia, PA: Lippincott Williams & Wilkins.

CHAPTER 11

Working with Vulnerable Populations

OBJECTIVES

After reading this chapter, you should be able to:

1. Define the term *vulnerable populations* and describe selected groups in this category.
2. Describe factors that led to the development of vulnerability in certain populations.
3. Examine ways in which public policies affect vulnerable populations and can reduce health inequities in these groups.
4. Examine the individual and social factors that contribute to vulnerability.
5. Describe strategies that community health nurses can use to improve the health status and eliminate health inequities of vulnerable populations.
6. Describe the social, political, cultural, and environmental factors that influence poverty.
7. Discuss the effects of poverty on the health and well-being of individuals, families, and communities.
8. Discuss how being homeless affects the health and well-being of individuals, families, and communities.
9. Describe the health challenges of importance to Aboriginal peoples in Canada.
10. Describe the ways in which teen pregnancies affect the baby, the parents, and their families.
11. Develop nursing interventions for the prevention of pregnancy concerns that at-risk adolescents might experience.
12. Explain the extent of the concern of clients who have mental illness or who are at risk for mental illness.
13. Explain community health nursing interventions for poor and homeless people, pregnant teens and their significant others, and individuals who are mentally ill or at risk for mental illness.
14. Explain the effect of substance abuse on the community and on people within the community.
15. Discuss the scope of the problem of violence in Canadian communities.

CHAPTER OUTLINE

The Canadian authors wish to acknowledge the contributions of Bonnie Myslik for additions to the mental health content and Catherine Aquino-Russell and Lisa Perley-Dutcher for additions to the content on Aboriginal Peoples.

KEY TERMS

See Glossary on page 593 for definitions

VULNERABILITY: DEFINITION AND INFLUENCING FACTORS

Specific populations who are more vulnerable—that is, at-risk populations who are more susceptible to poor health because of socioenvironmental factors—are often referred to as **vulnerable populations.** Beiser and Stewart (2005) refer to these populations as those who tolerate a larger "burden" of illness and distress than others. Usually included in this group are the poor, homeless, immigrants, refugees, Aboriginal peoples, disabled persons, persons with stigmatizing conditions (physical and mental disabilities, mental illness, substance abuse), the elderly (older adults), children and youth in disadvantaged conditions, persons with low literacy skills, women (particularly those in unsafe situations), gays, lesbians, bisexuals, and transgendered people (Beiser & Stewart, 2005; Canadian Institute for Health Information [CIHI], 2006; Canadian Institutes of Health Research, 2007). The terms *disadvantaged, marginalized, hard to reach,* and *vulnerable populations* are sometimes used to discuss health disparities. Vulnerable populations often are more likely than the general population to experience health disparities. These groups are more inclined to become ill and usually do not receive appropriate care. The vulnerable groups discussed in this chapter are the poor, homeless, youth in disadvantaged conditions, Aboriginal peoples, the mentally ill, substance abusers, and those who experience violence (unsafe situations). **Health disparities** refers to the wide variations in health services and in health status among certain population groups defined by specific characteristics (Canadian Public Health Association, 2005). **Health inequities** refers to differences in health that could be avoided if reasonable action was taken, and therefore these differences were considered to be unfair and socially unjust (World Health Organization [WHO], 2008a). In Canada these inequities are addressed through the five key Ottawa Charter strategies of strengthening community action, creating supportive environments, developing healthy public policy, developing personal skills, and reorienting health systems. A socioenvironmental approach would address social, economic, and environmental factors that contribute to unfair and unjust equity in health.

> *This [health equity] refers to everyone and not just a particular disadvantaged segment of the population. Efforts to promote social equity and health are therefore aimed at creating opportunities and removing barriers to achieving the health potential of all people. It involves the fair distribution of resources needed for health, fair access to the opportunities available, and fairness in the support offered to people when ill.* (WHO, 2007a, p. 5)

Health disparities exist throughout Canada and are related to key factors such as socioeconomic status, education and literacy, employment and working conditions, food security, and genetics. Butler-Jones, in his 2008 Annual Report (Public Health Agency of Canada [PHAC], 2008) discussed these key factors and additional ones that contribute to health inequalities. This PHAC report can be found in the Weblinks on the Evolve Web site. For further information on health inequities, see the Health Officers Council of British Columbia Web site titled *Health Inequities in British Columbia: A Discussion Paper,* listed in the Weblinks on the Evolve Web site. This Web site provides information on the determinants of health and inequities, health inequity policy considerations and options for reducing health inequities, and some stories that depict individual health inequities.

In a society that values self-reliance, individual responsibility, and personal accountability, members of vulnerable groups may not get the respect they deserve. It is important for community health nurses (CHNs) to understand their own beliefs about these groups and to understand the issues surrounding a vulnerable client's illness and/or personal situation. In order to be able to interact effectively with vulnerable groups, CHNs need to identify health care needs, barriers to care, and essential health care services for these groups and for their families as well.

Violence is identified as a health concern and is discussed in reference to how CHNs can help clients cope with and reduce violence and abuse. CHNs work with clients in many settings, including the home. Because CHNs are in key positions to detect and intervene in community and family violence, they need to understand how community-level influences can affect all types of violence.

People living in poverty are frequently exposed to multiple factors that accumulate and lead to poor health. For example, low income leads to difficulty finding affordable housing so these families are forced to live in poorer neighbourhoods often with increased crime rates (social risk); inadequate housing may contribute to lead poisoning from exposure to peeling lead-based paint (environmental risk); and food insecurity leads to poor nutritional status (behavioural risk) and stress leading to family violence (behavioural risk) (Sebastian, 2010). This example also demonstrates that vulnerability results from many interacting factors that individuals do not have control over due to the socioenvironmental variables, including the social determinants of health. Community health nurses often work with clients who are at a greater risk for poorer health than the general population. Some members of vulnerable populations may not be influenced by these health risks; however, it is necessary to identify the factors that contribute to resilience in these populations to gain understanding

CRITICAL VIEW

1. Does resilience result from personal attributes? Explain.
2. What is the connection of resiliency to the sociocultural and economic environments?
3. How do the determinants of health affect resiliency?

of resiliency and to plan appropriate community health nursing interventions. **Resilience** refers to the ability of the client to successfully cope when faced with a threat or hardship. Individuals with low resilience are more inclined to have feelings of hopelessness and may choose suicide as a method to resolve these feelings (Health Canada, 2005a). Support needs to be provided to those with decreased resilience to enhance coping skills and provide a greater sense of personal autonomy. When the CHN places emphasis on client strengths and assets rather than client deficit and susceptibility, resilience is more likely to increase. Resilience applies to any vulnerable population, not only those living in poverty. CHNs have traditionally focused on the identification of health concerns in the populations they work with. Focusing on client strengths or assets or capabilities and working with the client to find solutions to address health concerns is the current focus of community health nursing practice. This assets-based approach has been discussed in Chapters 4 and 9.

Factors Predisposing to Vulnerability (Health Inequities)

Many factors affect the health of populations. Various social determinants of health have greater influence on health than biomedical and behavioural risk factors (Raphael, 2009). The determinants of health have been discussed throughout this text. Social and economic factors predispose people to vulnerability. Refer to the "Determinants of Health" box on page 312 for highlights of some key determinants to consider in relation to this chapter.

Canadians sometimes do not have the financial resources to pay for some costs related to medical care, such as medical supplies, transportation to regional health centres, and associated costs such as meals and accommodation. Some are self-employed or work in small businesses that may not provide health care benefits; they are therefore unable to afford health care because of a lack of or inadequate health insurance coverage. In these situations, the lack of financial resources may cause some people to not seek preventive health services. This leaves them vulnerable and with increased risk of experiencing the effects of preventable illnesses. Certain preventive health tests are not covered by many government health insurances, such as the prostate-specific antigen test for prostate cancer detection; dental health may also be compromised as it is not covered by universal health coverage. Only 25% of Canadians who are poor have dental insurance (Gender & Health Collaborative Curriculum, 2008b).

Age is a factor that contributes to increased vulnerability. For example, the very young and the very old have fewer coping resources (physiological, sociological, psychological), resulting in enhanced health risks such as opportunistic infections and chronic diseases.

DETERMINANTS OF HEALTH: INCOME, GENDER, AND BIOLOGY

Income, gender, and biology are determinants that contribute to being classified as a vulnerable population group. Vulnerable populations are more likely to experience low income and poverty.

Income is a "key to education, community cohesion and inclusion" (Canadian Index of Wellbeing Network, 2009, p. i), so vulnerable populations are disadvantaged and health disparities exist for these populations. The severity of these determinants on the vulnerable varies depending on factors such as geography, support systems, and policies.

DEFINING AND UNDERSTANDING POVERTY

In general, **poverty** refers to having insufficient financial resources to meet basic living expenses: food, shelter, clothing, transportation, and medical expenses. Other items such as personal-care items, school supplies, and telephones are not usually factored in. The Ottawa

CRITICAL VIEW

1. What community health nurse interventions could have a positive impact on the determinants of health that currently affect vulnerable populations?
2. How can the community health nurse "empower" vulnerable populations?

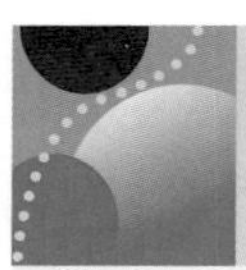

Determinants of Health
Income, Gender, and Biology

- Between 2000 and 2008, the percentage of Canadians earning a minimum wage increased from 4.7% to 5.2% (Institute of Wellbeing, 2009).
- Many Canadians express feelings of belonging and of being "connected to their community," which conveys community vitality (Canadian Index of Wellbeing Network, 2009).
- Food insecurity is experienced by approximately 9% or approximately 2.7 million Canadians (Mikkonen & Raphael, 2010), and Food Banks Canada reported that the monthly use of food banks by Canadians increased by 20% in 2009 (Institute of Wellbeing, 2009). It is a positive that food banks are available for populations that need this service, but more needs to be done to reduce poverty and therefore the need to use food banks. Early childhood development and learning, especially in the first 3 years of life, are negatively affected by food insecurity (Chilton, Chyatte, & Breaux, 2007).
- Approximately 15% of the 2009 Canadian food bank users, although they had a work income, were unable to meet the food security needs of their families (Institute of Wellbeing, 2009). Being employed does not ensure a means to overcome poverty (Campaign 2000, 2009) and therefore an ability to meet one's family's basic human needs. Government policies—such as raising minimum wages and ensuring that healthy foods are affordable to all residents of Canada—are needed to prevent food insecurity challenges for those employed (Mikkonen & Raphael, 2010).
- Canadians earning less than $20,000 annually are three times more likely to experience a decline in self-rated health when compared with Canadians in the highest income bracket (Institute of Wellbeing, 2009). Low-income Canadians have the highest mortality rates and rates for hospitalizations and emergency visits and the lowest life expectancy rates (Institute of Wellbeing, 2009). "Income is a fundamental determining factor regarding health status, mortality rates, birth weights and chronic disease" (Canadian Index of Wellbeing Network, 2009, p. i).
- When compared on incomes, 58% of males on low income have an increased likelihood of being stressed compared with males with higher incomes (Institute of Wellbeing, 2009). When compared on incomes, 25% of females on low income have an increased likelihood of being stressed compared with females with higher incomes (Institute of Wellbeing, 2009). Inequalities in wealth affect the emotional health of both genders but is greater for males. Income affects the abilities of families to meet their food security, housing, and other social determinants of health (Mikkonen & Raphael, 2010).
- Canada ranked 13th out of 17 countries in child poverty in 2009 (Institute of Wellbeing, 2009). Canadians with low incomes usually belong to one of four groups who have significantly reduced well-being. The other three groups are the Aboriginal peoples, visible minorities (racialized groups), and youth (Canadian Index of Wellbeing Network, 2009; Institute of Wellbeing, 2009). Canada needs a comprehensive plan to alleviate poverty and "to prevent families from falling into poverty" (Campaign 2000, 2009).

Charter for Health Promotion indicates that one of the basic prerequisites for health is income. People who are poor (have little or no income) are more likely to live in unsafe environments, to work at high-risk jobs, to eat less nutritious foods, and to have multiple stressors. Canada, in contrast to the United States, does not have an official poverty line, so many researchers use Statistics Canada's before-tax Low-Income Cut-Offs or LICOs, despite some controversy as to this use (Sarlo, 2008). LICOs are usually intended to indicate the income level that a family would have in difficult circumstances after spending the biggest portion of its earnings on food, clothing, and shelter. The controversy over the use of LICOs pertains to areas such as the following: the amount identified for a family of four per year in a large urban area is too high to be considered on the verge of poverty; LICOs measure inequality, not poverty; LICOs do not relate to the actual costs individuals face in purchasing the necessities; and LICOs do not measure regional differentials in costs that matter (Sarlo, 2008). Nevertheless, a comparison of provinces for specific age groups does provide some information using the LICOs. One example for

LICOs in the 18-and-under age group across Canada for 2007 is found in Table 11-1. This table provides information in percentages and numbers for LICOs before tax and after tax.

For years, income level has been used as the criterion that determines whether someone is poor. Three different approaches to defining poverty are *absolute poverty, relative poverty,* and *subjective poverty.* **Absolute poverty** refers to "a deprivation of resources that is life-threatening" (Beckmann Murray, Proctor Zentner, Pangman, & Pangman, 2009, p. 15). **Relative poverty** "refers to a deprivation of some individuals in relation to those who have more" (Beckmann Murray et. al., 2009). **Subjective poverty** refers to individuals and families who perceive that they have insufficient income to meet their expenses (Phipps, 2003).

Most poor Canadian persons or families endure the effects of constant deprivation: a persistent feeling of being trapped and that life is about surviving each day. In this way of life, there is no choice, there is no flexibility, and, if something unexpected happens—a sickness, accident, family death, fire or theft, or rent increase—there is no buffer to deal with the emergency. Life is just today because tomorrow offers no hope. For CHNs, the most significant factor is being able to accept and respect clients and attempt to understand how their life situations, such as the determinants of health, influence their health and well-being. Being poor is one health determinant that must be measured against the presence of other determinants that may increase or decrease the negative effects of poverty. The causes of poverty are complex and interrelated. In recent decades, the numbers of adults and older adults living in poverty have decreased, and Canada's child poverty and overall poverty rate has declined since 1996, with the proportion of Canadians living in poverty falling in 2004 to 4.9% compared with 7.8% in 1996 based on reported incomes (Sarlo, 2006). More than 13% of Canadian families lived at or below the poverty line in 2000, with nearly 70% of these poor people—close to 3.3 million—living in the 25 largest urban areas in Canada (Canadian Council on Social Development, 2007). In 2004, 4.9% of Canadians (close to 1.6 million) were identified as poor (Sarlo, 2006). According to the 2001 census data, 16% of families in Newfoundland were poor, resulting in that province having the highest percentage of poor families in Canada; the provinces of Prince Edward Island and Alberta had the lowest proportion of poor families (Canadian Council on Social Development, 2007). The Fraser Institute publishes *Fraser Alert* online about current issues in public policy and economics. The *Fraser Alert* provides up-to-date information on income and poverty in Canada.

Poverty and Health

There are inequalities in the health status of Canadians who have a lower socioeconomic levels when compared to Canadians from higher socioeconomic levels. According to Phipps (2003), one of the health inequalities is that chronic conditions are more prevalent in poorer areas of the country. For example, 10.1% of adults in Maritime provinces aged 15 to 64 years reported high blood pressure, whereas the national average is 6.8%. Seventeen percent of Maritime children up to the age of

TABLE 11-1 LICOs in Percentages and Numbers for Canada and Across Canada in Ages 18 and Under

LICO Before Tax (18 and under)											
	Canada	NL	PEI	NS	NB	QC	ON	MB	SK	AB	BC
Percentage	15	13	8.3	14.9	16.7	14.9	14.5	18.8	16.7	11.2	18.8
Number	1,009	12	2	26	24	224	395	47	35	87	156
LICO After Tax (18 and under)											
	Canada	NL	PEI	NS	NB	QC	ON	MB	SK	AB	BC
Percentage	9.5	6.5	4.7	8.4	9.4	9.5	9.4	11.1	8.9	6.3	13
Number	637	6	(too unreliable)	15	13	142	257	28	19	49	108

SOURCE: Statistics Canada. (2009). *Income and Canada 2007* (Catalogue No. 75-202-X). Ottawa: Minister of Industry.

CRITICAL VIEW

Refer to the Campaign 2000 Web site titled "End Child and Family Poverty in Canada," found in the Weblinks at the end of this chapter, to assist in answering the following questions:

1. a) Within this Web site, find the link to the province that you reside in. What are the main issues with regard to poverty in your province?
   b) What government strategies have been proposed to deal with poverty in your province?
2. Log on to the Senate Standing Committee Report (Web site listed on the Evolve Web site) to view *In From the Margins: A Call to Action on Poverty, Housing and Homelessness* (2009). Read section 2, titled "Poverty."
   a) What poverty reduction and eradication strategies are recommended by this committee?
   b) What do you believe CHNs can do to deal with poverty and the vulnerable populations affected?

13 years have asthma, compared with 12.7% of Canadian children on the whole. Aboriginal peoples, who have a lower socioeconomic status than non-Aboriginals, more commonly have chronic diseases such as diabetes, heart problems, arthritis, cancer, and hypertension. The poor also have higher rates of infant morbidity and mortality, shorter life expectancies, and more complex health problems (Hwang, 2001; Shah, 2003; Turnbull, Muckle, & Masters, 2007).

Poor health outcomes are often secondary to barriers that impede access to health care, such as geographical location, language barriers, inability to find a health care provider, stigmatization, transportation difficulties, inconvenient clinic hours, lack of information, and negative attitudes of health care providers toward poor clients (Turnbull et al., 2007). Access to health care is especially difficult for the working poor, and many employers, especially those paying low or minimum wage, do not provide health care insurance for their employees. Certain population groups are more likely to be poor—for example, Aboriginal people, unemployed persons, lone parents, recent immigrants, visible minorities, persons with disabilities, children, and elderly women (Curry-Stevens, 2009; Vancouver Island Health Authority, 2006). For information on various aggregates who often experience poverty, see Section 5 ("Over-represented groups") of the Senate Subcommittee on Cities, *In From the Margins* Weblink on the Evolve Web site.

Evidence-Informed Practice

Fuzzy cognitive maps are graphical representations of relationships between concepts that are determined by the "experts" who live the experience. The authors reported on a case study that was a group process demonstrating how fuzzy cognitive maps could be used to pull out, present, and compare the perspectives that a group of Aboriginal peoples had about the determinants or causes of diabetes.

Participants from Mohawk and Miawpukek First Nations communities created fuzzy cognitive maps to describe their perceptions of the various causes of diabetes in their home community. A facilitator worked with the group in mapping their perspectives. Comparison of the fuzzy cognitive maps revealed some significant differences in the perspectives of each group. The Mohawk participants identified social, traditional, and spiritual factors, while the First Nations participants identified personal and lifestyle factors. The determinants that were similar between the groups were healthy diet and physical activity.

Application for CHNs: The study findings demonstrate how fuzzy cognitive maps may be used to uncover and represent different perspectives of complex issues. The opportunity to allow for comparisons among stakeholders or knowledge groups is prevalent in this process. Policy makers must include Aboriginal peoples' perspectives in policies that involve their communities. This type of group strategy is one method of involving communities.

Questions for Reflection & Discussion

1. What other strategy would you use to include Aboriginal peoples in policy decision making?
2. How is this perspective congruent with communities of other peoples?
3. Using the evidence-informed practice approach, how would you apply the client's perspectives from this study when working in your community?

REFERENCE: Giles, B., Haas, G., Sajna, M., & Findlay, C. (2008). Exploring Aboriginal views of health using fuzzy cognitive maps and transitive closure: A case study of the determinants of diabetes. *Canadian Journal of Public Health, 99*(5), 411–417.

CRITICAL VIEW

1. What increases women's vulnerability to poverty?
2. a) How can women's poverty be eliminated?
   b) How can CHNs assist with this plan?

Poverty, while presenting a significant obstacle to health across the lifespan, has an especially negative effect on women. Women, due to their gender, are highly vulnerable to poverty as they are more likely to be paid less because of working in jobs that may pay only minimum wage. In addition, they often have lone-parenting responsibilities. All these factors may result in women being more dependent on social services than men (Canadian Research Institute for the Advancement of Women, n.d.; Raphael, 2009). Income, social status, and gender are important determinants of health nationally (Shah, 2003).

Child poverty rates are dramatically higher amid vulnerable groups. For example, the groups of children 0–14 years at greater risk for poverty are: newly arrived immigrant children, children in ethnic or racially visible families, Aboriginal children, and children with disabilities (Campaign 2000, 2010). Young children under the age of 6 years are at the highest risk for the most harmful effects of poverty, especially in regard to adequate nutrition and brain development. Other risk factors include maternal substance abuse or depression, exposure to environmental toxins, trauma and abuse, and poor-quality daily care (Chilton et al., 2007; Kiernan & Huerta, 2008). See the Evolve Weblink for the PHAC report *Growing up Well—Priorities for a Healthy Future.* Chapter 4 of this report, "Social and Physical Influences on Health," provides information on some of the factors that affect the health of children in Canada, such as income; food security; housing and water; and home, school, and family influences. Refer to the resource Campaign 2000 Web site *Report Card on Child and Family Poverty in Canada: 1989–2009* found in the Weblinks on the Evolve Web site.

Poverty can affect both *urban and rural communities.* Urban inhabitants generally show more signs of healthy behaviours than rural inhabitants (CIHI, 2006). Generally, rural inhabitants demonstrate the following: increased mortality rates, shorter lifespans, increased risk for death from injuries such as suicides and motor vehicle accidents, and increased cardiovascular disease and diabetes (CIHI, 2006). Urban inhabitants, on the other hand, have a higher incidence of cancer, identified less of a sense of "belonging" to the community, and were more inclined to report higher levels of stress (CIHI, 2006). Rural inhabitants had lower educational levels and lower income. Income and education are the socioeconomic determinants of health. In some rural areas, the rural inhabitants demonstrated dietary practices that were not as healthy as those of their urban counterparts, spent less time on physical activity in their leisure time, and had increased smoking rates (personal health practices being a health determinant) (CIHI, 2006).

CRITICAL VIEW

1. What are effective strategies that CHNs can implement to address the health concerns of rural inhabitants?
2. How are the strategies identified in question 1 different for rural inhabitants than for urban inhabitants?

Poor neighbourhoods are often described as having the following characteristics: access to fewer resources, lower levels of education, higher rates of unemployment, lower wage rates, higher incidence of crime and violence, and the presence of more one-parent families (Gender & Health Collaborative Curriculum, 2008b).

DETERMINANTS OF HEALTH: SOCIAL ENVIRONMENT AND VULNERABLE GROUPS

Population health disparities continue in Canada despite some improvements in health (Raphael, 2009). Social determinants of health such as food, income, social status and social support networks, and unemployment are important to the health of Canadians. The "Determinants of Health: Social Environment and Vulnerable Groups" box on the next page identifies some of the factors determining the health of vulnerable groups.

Assumptions are often made by many health care practitioners that clients are heterosexual; therefore, the right health-related questions are not usually asked. Sexual-orientation variations need to be considered by the CHN when working with all clients in reference to health concerns that may be affected by sexual orientation variations, such as the increased risk for depression and sexually transmitted infections (STIs). Some individuals may hesitate, because of sexual orientation, to seek health care services as they may feel reluctant to confide in others who may judge them or minimize their health concerns.

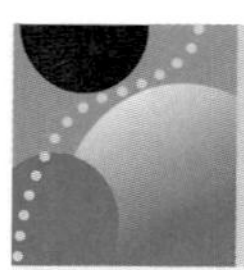

Determinants of Health
Social Environment and Vulnerable Groups

- Canadians view homelessness, street crime, motor vehicle accidents, and unemployment as serious health hazards related to the social environment (Krewski et al., 2006; Lemyre, Lee, Mercier, Bouchard, & Krewski, 2006).
- Homelessness is linked with mental illness and drug dependence (Rosenthal, Mallett, Gurrin, Milburn, & Rotheram-Borus, 2007). The rate of these conditions in the homeless is much greater than in the Canadian general population (Mikkonen & Raphael, 2010), and homelessness threatens the health of this segment of the population. Government policies need to be implemented that will provide affordable, quality housing for the homeless (Mikkonen & Raphael, 2010). Currently, "Canada is the only industrialized country without a national affordable housing strategy" (Campaign 2000, 2009, p. 8).
- Lack of social support groups among women is linked to myocardial infarction (MI) and cerebrovascular accident (stroke) (André-Petersson, Engström, Hedblad, Janzon, & Rosvall, 2007) and, when referred, post-MI women frequently do not attend groups (Gender & Health Collaborative Curriculum, 2008b). Cardiovascular disease morbidity and mortality are almost the same for males and females (Gender & Health Collaborative Curriculum, 2008a). However, many women have work and family responsibilities to balance, which may hinder their attendance, with accessibility and availability being additional hindrances (Gender & Health Collaborative Curriculum, 2008a).
- Black immigrants are at an increased risk for mental health disorders (Williams et al., 2007). Educational programs for this aggregate on early detection, treatments, and community resources could be established by CHNs in their communities.
- Substance use is linked to low academic achievement and poor health in adulthood (Cox, Zhang, Johnson, & Bender, 2007). CHNs need to be aware of this link and, when indicated, conduct an appropriate client assessment.
- Mothers with unresolved sexual abuse issues are likely to abuse their children (Mapp, 2006). Therefore, community health nursing assessment of history of sexual abuse and referral to appropriate community resources are important.
- Older adults, whites, males, depressed individuals, and alcoholics are at increased risk for suicide (Gold, 2005), as well as those living in rural areas (Judd, Cooper, Fraser, & Davis, 2006). Therefore, CHNs need to identify these clients in their daily nursing practice and conduct a depression and suicide assessment.
- Most health care professionals do not assess for and address sexual identity (van Dam, Koh, & Dibble, 2001). CHNs can take the Riddle Homophobia Scale to determine their attitude toward sexual identity persons (refer to http://www.genderandhealth.ca/en/modules/sexandsexuality/gss-homophobia-02.jsp?r=) (Gender & Health Collaborative Curriculum, 2008c). It is important for CHNs to be aware of their biases to provide culturally competent and culturally safe nursing care.
- Gay, lesbian, bisexual, and transgendered persons have higher levels of depression and suicide; have increased use of alcohol, tobacco, and other drugs; and are at greater risk for sexually transmitted infections (Rainbow Health Network, 2007).
- Unemployment negatively affects mental health and physical working capacity (Maier et al., 2006). Becoming unemployed can lead to unhealthy coping behaviours such as smoking and alcohol abuse; mental health conditions such as increased anxiety, increased suicide rates and depression; and poverty and its related consequences (Mikkonen & Raphael, 2010).
- Aboriginal people between the ages of 25 and 54 years experienced increased employment between 1996 (55%) and 2001 (61%) (Treasury Board of Canada, 2004). Employment is one of the social determinants of health.
- When employment was compared, 61% of First Nations adults aged 25 to 54 in 2006 were employed compared to 82% of non-Aboriginal adults (Institute of Wellbeing, 2009).
- For Aboriginal people, life expectancy increased from 1990 to 2001, with males increasing from 66.9 to 70.4 years and females from 74 to 75.5 years (Treasury Board of Canada, 2004).
- In 2009, the percentage of Canadians who became new clients at the nonprofit counselling agency Credit Canada increased by 42% (Institute of Wellbeing, 2009).

CRITICAL VIEW

1. What do your local health unit or regional authority and community have in place to address the health concerns of clients of various sexual orientations?
2. What CHN interventions would be considered to address social inequities? Explain.

THE HOMELESS POPULATION

Homelessness is increasing globally, and not surprisingly, homelessness in Canada is following the same trend. The number of homeless in Canada is difficult to determine for many reasons, with one of the main difficulties being that census data are collected through enumeration of those with addresses. However, it is estimated that in Canada between 150,000 and 300,000 individuals are homeless (Human Resources and Skills Development Canada, 2009; Laird, 2007). Because of the challenge of identifying specific homeless numbers, some cities in Canada (e.g., Vancouver, Toronto, and Calgary) have attempted to determine the numbers of homeless and at-risk persons (Frankish, Hwang, & Quantz, 2005). In 2008, the Government of Canada provided $110 million to the Mental Health Commission of Canada's At Home Research Projects. These projects were launched in 2009 in five Canadian cities to gather information on homelessness and mental illness and to identify ways to provide relevant services to homeless persons (Mental Health Commission of Canada, 2009a). The projects are to be completed by 2013. For further information on the Mental Health Commission of Canada and on the five projects, refer to the Mental Health Commission of Canada Weblink *Out of the Shadows Forever: At Home,* listed on the Evolve Web site.

UNDERSTANDING THE CONCEPT OF HOMELESSNESS

There are many risk factors that can lead to homelessness. Refer to Box 11-1 for some of these factors. For example, if there is limited housing, accommodation prices usually increase and therefore housing becomes unaffordable for the population living on a limited income. Homelessness and poverty are interrelated, and both are affected by the employment rate. When companies close or relocate, workers may go long periods without a steady income. Often these displaced workers seek out full-time work but may be offered only part-time work; these individuals are considered to be underemployed. Increases in part-time jobs mean that there would be a higher number underemployed. Sometimes workers take any job they can find as they may be facing economic hardship; however, some workers might be overqualified for a job they are being offered. This usually occurs with new immigrants who, for a variety of reasons such as language barriers and certification, are unable to work in their field of expertise. Another pattern of interest is that there is an increase in the number of workers who are "overemployed," usually working more than 40 hours per week. Factors such as unemployment, underemployment, and stress at work are associated with poor health (Butler-Jones, 2008). In Alberta, it was determined that the number of underemployed females was greater than the number of underemployed males, with underemployment occurring in younger age groups, persons with lower levels of education, and part-time workers in sales, service, or clerical positions (Pembina Institute, 2005).

BOX 11-1 Contributing Factors to Homelessness

- Lack of affordable housing
- Low income or poverty
- Mental health issues
- Substance abuse or addictions
- Unemployment or underemployment
- Immigration
- Violence
- Ex-offenders
- Family conflict

Many segments of the population experience homelessness. Refer to Box 11-2 for a listing of the most likely aggregates. Homelessness can be considered as absolute homelessness, sheltered homelessness, and hidden homelessness (Laird, 2007). **Absolute homelessness** refers to those people who are perpetually homeless and are sometimes referred to as the *chronic homeless.* These are the people often observed sleeping on park benches,

CRITICAL VIEW

1. What factors need to be considered when developing policy and legislative interventions to reduce homelessness?
2. What educational, behavioural, and environmental strategies could be identified to reduce homelessness and improve the health status of the homeless?

BOX 11-2 Examples of the Homeless Population

- Single males
- Single females
- Female lone-parent families
- Youths
- Children
- Newcomers to Canada
- Mentally ill
- Employed poor
- Aboriginal peoples

sleeping on the sidewalks, and begging on the streets. These homeless persons are experiencing persistent poverty (poverty that is chronic):

- Men and women who experience persistent poverty are chronically homeless and many have mental or physical disabilities.
- This group is most frequently identified with homelessness.
- Physical and mental disabilities often coexist with alcohol and other drug abuses, severe mental illness, other chronic health problems, and chronic family difficulties.
- This group lacks money and family support.
- This group often ends up living on the streets, and they need economic assistance, rehabilitation, and ongoing support.

Sheltered homelessness refers to those persons who need to use emergency shelters either occasionally or regularly for sleeping purposes. **Hidden homelessness** refers to those persons who may be sleeping in their vehicles and/or use the couch or other temporary sleeping cot at a friend's home. These homeless persons are experiencing crisis poverty (temporary transient poverty):

- Lives are generally marked by hardship and struggle.
- Homelessness is often transient or episodic.
- The homeless person may resort to brief stays in shelters or other temporary accommodations.
- Homelessness may result from lack of employment opportunities, lack of education, obsolete job skills, or domestic violence. These issues lead to persistent poverty and need to be addressed, along with efforts to find stable housing.

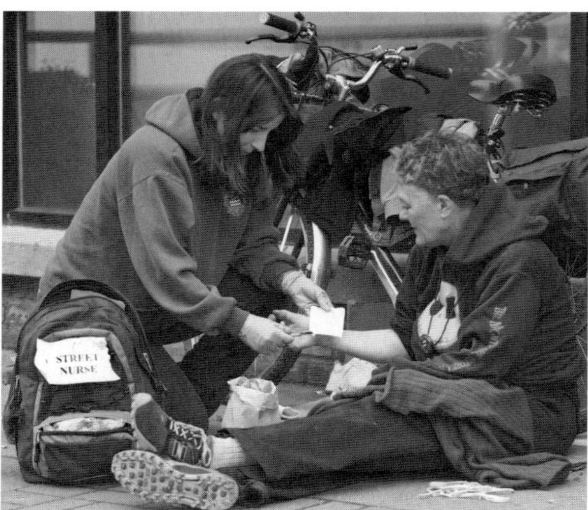

It is important for CHNs to respect the individuality of all clients, including those who are homeless.

Community health nurses may have the opportunity to work with homeless clients in emergency shelters, while home visiting a family who has a homeless person temporarily living with them, or when other community agencies refer homeless clients to the CHN. Although people who have never been homeless usually cannot truly understand what it means to be homeless, CHNs can increase their sensitivity toward the homeless population by examining their own personal beliefs, values, and knowledge of homelessness. Refer to the box below "How To … Evaluate the Concept of Homelessness" for some questions the CHN can reflect on.

How To... Evaluate the Concept of Homelessness

- What is it like to live on the streets?
- What issues might confront a young mother and her children inside a homeless shelter?
- How is it that people are so poor that they have no place to go?
- What really causes homelessness?
- How do you respond to a person on the street asking for money to buy a sandwich or catch a bus?
- How is your response different (or not) when a young mother with children asks you for money?
- How do you react to the smell of urine in a stairwell or elevator?

In 1999, the federal government established the National Homelessness Initiative (NHI) to address the problem of homelessness in Canada. Close to $753 million was assigned over a 3-year period to sustain local, community-based efforts for the identification of priorities and to plan and develop solutions that would be appropriate for the community; this was referred to as Phase I (Human Resources and Skills Development Canada, 2009). The NHI funding was renewed in 2003, with an additional $405 million allocation and was known as Phase 2; a 1-year extension was provided for 2006–2007 with an allocation of $134.8 million in funding (Human Resources and Skills Development Canada, 2009). Evaluation of this project indicated successes in several areas, such as increased community capacity to manage homelessness, the establishment of increased supports and services, and increased understanding of the concept of homelessness.

Another federally funded government of Canada initiative titled "Homelessness Partnering Strategy (HPS)" provided funding to various Canadian communities

CRITICAL VIEW

1. What are the rates and causes of homelessness in your community, and how are these measured?
2. What community health nursing strategies or interventions have been implemented to address the issue of homelessness in your community?

Evidence-Informed Practice

Homelessness and poor health, issues faced by street youth in Canada, are of growing concern for public health. The risks to health of youth living on the street may arise from environmental risks: street experiences, sexual activity, substance abuse, and isolation or lack of social support. The study objective was to describe health risks, outcomes, and use of health services by street youth in Calgary in order to enhance services to this population.

A community-based research approach was used, including community members as part of the research team (street youth [3] and agency representatives [14]). The team participated in the development of the survey instrument and data collection, interview guide, and data analysis. In order to enhance the variability of the sample, nonprobability purposeful sampling was used for the 355 street-involved youth (61% male, 26% Aboriginal) who completed the survey. There were 46% of the respondents currently living on the street, 33% had lived on the street in the past, and 20% were street involved but had not lived on the street. Level of street involvement was related with significant health and health-risk outcome differences. The participants' use of hospitals and walk-in clinics did not differ significantly by level of street involvement; however, youths living on the street were less likely than those who had not lived on the street to visit a physician during office hours. Those youths who had lived on the street were more likely to use mobile clinics, which are services that are specifically targeted to street-involved people.

The researchers concluded that street-involved youths who had not lived on the street showed better health and health-risk outcomes than those who currently or had lived on the street, and health services use showed some differences by level of street involvement.

Application for CHNs: The results of this research highlight the importance of the role of CHNs, specifically public health nurses (PHNs) and other service providers, in providing health care, prevention, safety, or stabilization services for youths at various stages of street life. The availability and accessibility of community health care services need to be based on an assessment of the community with identification of population needs.

Questions for Reflection & Discussion

1. What interventions might be implemented to reduce homelessness in Canada?
2. How can health care services be provided to address the health care needs of the homeless, including street-involved youth?
3. What approaches would you suggest to address the health care needs of the homeless?

   Refer to the Senate Subcommittee report *In From the Margins: A Call to Action on Poverty, Housing and Homelessness* (2009), on the Evolve Web site. Read Section 4, "Homelessness," to assist in answering the above questions.

REFERENCE: Worthington, C., & MacLaurin, B. (2009). Level of street involvement and health and health services use of Calgary street youth. *Canadian Journal of Public Health, 100*(5), 384–388.

in an effort to prevent and reduce homelessness. Sixty-one designated communities, some outreach communities, and some Aboriginal communities were involved in developing community-driven projects based on their specific needs to prevent and reduce homelessness across Canada. Another aspect of this initiative is partnering with provinces, territories, communities, and private and nonprofit organizations with the aim of strengthening community capacity and building sustainability. As well, research is continuing to prevent and reduce homelessness. For further information on designated communities, outreach communities, Aboriginal communities, and knowledge development about homelessness, refer to the Human Resources and Skill Development Canada Weblink "Homelessness Partnering Strategy" on the Evolve Web site. For further information on homelessness and poverty, see the Laird Weblink, *Shelter—Homelessness in a Growth Economy: Canada's 21st Century Paradox*, on the Evolve Web site.

Effects of Homelessness on Health

There are important health implications for homeless Canadians. Homeless people are at increased risk for a wide range of health concerns, such as substance abuse, mental illness, HIV and acquired immunodeficiency syndrome (AIDS), tuberculosis (TB), STIs, unplanned pregnancies, seizures, chronic obstructive pulmonary disease, musculoskeletal disorders, and skin and foot problems (Frankish et al., 2005; Stergiopoulos & Herrmann, 2003). Access to health care services is a problem for many of the homeless. For example, an insulin-dependent diabetic man who lives on the street may sleep in a shelter. Getting adequate rest and exercise, taking insulin on a schedule, eating regular meals, and following a prescribed diet are virtually impossible. How does one purchase an antibiotic without money? How is a child treated for scabies and pediculosis when there are no bathing facilities? How does an older adult with peripheral vascular disease elevate his legs when he must be out of the shelter at 7 A.M. and on the streets all day? These health concerns are often directly related to poor access to preventive health care services. Homeless people devote a large portion of their time to just trying to survive. Health promotion activities are more of a luxury for them than a part of their daily lives.

Homeless persons spend many hours on their feet and often sleep in positions that compromise their peripheral circulation. Hypertension is exacerbated by high rates of alcohol abuse and high sodium content of foods served in fast-food restaurants, shelters, and other meal sites. Crowded living conditions put homeless persons at risk for exposure to viruses and bacteria that cause pneumonia and TB. AIDS is also a growing concern among the homeless population. In addition to its effects on physical health, homelessness also affects psychological, social, and spiritual well-being. Becoming homeless means more than losing a home or a regular place to sleep and eat; it also means losing friends, personal possessions, and familiar surroundings. Homeless people live in chaos, confusion, and fear. Many describe experiencing a loss of dignity, low self-esteem, a lack of social support, and generalized despair. The risk of death is increased for the homeless in Canada. Compared with the general population, mortality rates in Montreal street youth are 9 times higher for males and 31 times higher for females. Homeless men using shelters in Toronto are two to eight times more likely to die prematurely (Frankish et al., 2005).

Homelessness and At-Risk Populations

Being homeless affects health across the lifespan, affecting pregnancy, childhood, adolescence, and older adulthood. Each group has different needs, and CHNs need to be aware of the unique needs of homeless clients at every age.

CHNs need to identify the precursors to homelessness; anticipate the effects of homelessness on physical, emotional, and spiritual well-being; become knowledgeable about resources to assist the homeless; assist the homeless to gain access to needed health care services; work with communities to build capacity to work with this population and to address health inequalities; participate in activities that will facilitate the building of healthy public policies to address homelessness; and work toward reorienting the health system so that it focuses on a socioenvironmental street approach for the homeless population. The work of street nurse Cathy Crowe, discussed in Chapter 3, provides CHNs with a strong example of the importance of the advocacy role of CHNs as a voice for the vulnerable and of working with them to empower, support, and encourage change in the sociopolitical community environment (see the Cathy Crowe Weblink on the Evolve Web site; see also Section 3, "Housing," of the Senate Subcommittee on Cities report Weblink *In From the Margins,* on the Evolve Web site.)

ABORIGINAL PEOPLES IN CANADA

The forced loss of natural resources, including land and therefore a lost relationship to the land, caused a total disconnect with the gathering of traditional foods and resulted in significant dietary changes and practices for Aboriginal peoples. Currently, there has been a marked increase of chronic and degenerative diseases, especially diabetes and cardiovascular disease, among all Aboriginal peoples in Canada (Reading, 2009). Continued oppression, marginalization, and racism over the years have helped to create a looming identity crisis that has also diminished the self-worth of the people (Lavallee & Clearsky, 2006). The mental, spiritual, emotional, and physical well-being of Aboriginal peoples has been jeopardized and continues to manifest itself in multiple health issues. Aboriginal peoples believe that health involves maintaining a balance of the psychological, spiritual, emotional, and physical aspects of the person in relation to others and the environment. Healing practices are diverse among Aboriginal peoples; some healing practices include the sweat lodge, pipe ceremony, smudging, drumming, and using natural medicines from the earth. For further information on the indigenous concepts of health, illness, and healing, see the King Weblink, *An Overall Approach to Health Care for Indigenous Peoples*, on the Evolve Web site.

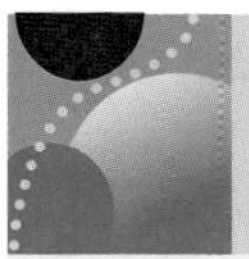

Determinants of Health

Determinants of Health and Aboriginal Peoples

- Aboriginal peoples' not completing high school was 34% compared with 15% for the non-Aboriginal population (Institute of Wellbeing, 2009).
- Aboriginal peoples' completion of university was 8% compared with 23% for the non-Aboriginal population (Institute of Wellbeing, 2009).
- Education is a social determinant of health that affects income, another social determinant of health. The high dropout rate at high-school level for Aboriginal students raises the questions of why these students are not reaching their educational potentials and what community and societal interventions are needed to counter this trend.
- In 2005, the median annual income for Canadian First Nations peoples 15 years of age and older was $14,517, which was approximately $11,000 below the non-Aboriginal population median income of $25,955 (Institute of Wellbeing, 2009). Higher income and higher education lead to longer life expectancy; decreased chronic conditions, including occurrence of diabetes mellitus; and increased reporting of "excellent" and "very good" health (Institute of Wellbeing, 2009).
- Life expectancy for Inuit men is 15 years less than the Canadian average life expectancy (Wilkins, Uppal, Fines, Guimond, & Dion, 2008).
- In 2001, the number of Inuit adults over 15 years of age who rated their health as "excellent" or "very good" was 56% compared with 50% in 2006 (Statistics Canada, 2008b).
- When compared to non-Aboriginals, Aboriginal people are approximately four times more likely to live in overcrowded homes and are three times as likely to require major repairs for these homes (Institute of Wellbeing, 2009). In order to promote population health, the provision of "available, affordable and healthy housing" is essential (Senate Subcommittee on Population Health, 2009).
- When a sense of community belonging and connectedness is measured, 65% of Caucasians have a positive response, whereas 54% of Aboriginal people do (Institute of Wellbeing, 2009).
- Caucasian youth reported levels of well-being two times higher than Aboriginal youth (Institute of Wellbeing, 2009).
- When measuring contact with a physician, 79% of the Canadian general population reported they had had contact, compared with 56% Inuit adults (Statistics Canada, 2008b).
- Seventy percent of Inuit adults who resided in Inuit communities had contact with a nurse (Statistics Canada, 2008b).
- Curriculum development in the Inuit language has been facilitated in Nunavut by providing teacher education programs in their communities (Inuit Tapiriit Kanatami, 2007 cited in Statistics Canada, 2008b).
- The social determinants of health such as poverty, low income, and inadequate and lack of housing for indigenous peoples have disadvantaged them and placed them at increased risk for diseases (Adelson, 2005). Poverty increases the risk of developing chronic diseases and increases the responses to the consequences of these diseases (WHO, 2008b) "because material deprivation, unhealthy living conditions (e.g., poor housing, inadequate food supply) and poor access to health care services predispose people with low socioeconomic status to the development of chronic diseases" (Reading, 2009, p. A-58).

Health Status of Aboriginal Peoples

In 1939, the First Nations and the Inuit became the responsibility and jurisdiction of the federal government of Canada (Auer & Andersson, 2001). This has generally meant that in the areas of health, education, and social services, the Aboriginal population has been organized or "controlled" by others (Auer & Andersson, 2001). The Senate Subcommittee on Population Health in 2008 recommended recognition of Aboriginal peoples' self-determination through the development of regional health authorities funded by federal and provincial funds but led by Aboriginal peoples (Reading, 2009). There is no formal arrangement between the Métis Nation and Health Canada. Further, the Métis Nation is primarily shut out of programming for the Aboriginal people offered by Health Canada, even though the Métis are recognized as one of the three Aboriginal peoples in Canada (Métis National Council, 2004, p. 1).

Health Canada's role in First Nations and Inuit health started in 1945, when services were transferred from the Department of Indian Affairs to Health Canada. Health Canada was providing direct health services to First Nations peoples on reserves and to Inuit communities in northern Canada by 1962. The transfer of health services began for First Nations and Inuit communities in the mid-1980s. Capacity for governance has been increasing over the past decade in all areas of life for these two Aboriginal populations. Many of the communities that have transferred now have health centres that are mainly staffed by Aboriginal people. It is of concern that the Métis peoples have been excluded from access to the same types of health services that the First Nations and Inuit peoples have (Métis National Council, 2004). Attempts are being made to change this (Métis National Council, 2004).

The services offered to First Nations and Inuit peoples range from primary health care services and public health services in varying degrees in each community. Primary health care services are mainly offered in isolated and remote communities and usually include emergency care (Health Canada, 2007). A service referred to as the Non-Insured Health Benefits (NIHB) covers the following benefits: vision, dental, prescription medication, medical supplies, equipment, and short-term mental health crisis intervention. Nursing services such as immunization, communicable disease management, maternal child health services, and home and community care services are provided for those living within the community. Other community-based programs offered in most communities might include personal and support services, environmental health, nonurgent care, children and youth, fetal alcohol syndrome disorder (FASD), prenatal nutrition program, Head Start program, mental health and addictions, National Native Alcohol and Drug Abuse Program (NNADAP), chronic disease and injury prevention, National Aboriginal Youth Suicide Prevention Strategy (NAYSPS), and the Aboriginal Diabetes Initiative. The Inuit face many challenges, one of them a result of geography, which can lead to poor access to health services. Health experts maintain that inadequate housing can be associated with a host of health problems. For instance, hospitalization rates for Inuit children with severe lower respiratory tract infections are the highest in the world, and recent research has shown that crowding, along with poor ventilation, in Inuit homes contributes to these rates (Kovesi et al., 2007). These living conditions can also lead to the transmission of infectious diseases such as TB. TB is still evident in the First Nations and Inuit populations; it is 6 times higher and 17 times higher, respectively, than in the rest of Canada (Health Council of Canada, 2005). Hepatitis A, as well as increased risk for injuries, mental health problems, and family tensions, is also a concern for First Nations and Inuit peoples (Reading, 2009). For specific information on the housing crisis in Nunavut, see the Qulliit Nunavut Status of Women Council 2007 report, *The Little Voices of Nunavut* (pp. 34–38), listed in the Weblinks on the Evolve Web site.

Income plays a role in the health of Aboriginal peoples. The lower incomes for Inuit, compared with the non-Aboriginal population, are significant, especially considering the higher costs of basic needs such as food, housing, clothing, and harvesting supplies when living in the North. Expenses are much higher than in the southern parts of Canada (Inuit Tapiriit Kanatami and Indian and Northern Affairs Canada, 2007). For example, it may cost between $350 and $450 per week to provide a family of four with a nutritious diet, compared to about $200 in the South (Indian and Northern Affairs Canada, 2008).

Determinants of health affect the health of First Nations and Inuit, placing them at high risk for poor health status (see Table 11-2). The National Collaborating Centre for Aboriginal Health (see the Weblinks on the Evolve Web site), located in Prince George at the University of Northern British Columbia, is one of the six national collaborating centres responsible for collecting information that is required by health care practitioners to affect health outcomes for Canadians. The Web site of the centre in Prince George specifically provides information to address Aboriginal health and has uncovered some of the best evidence available for informed practice. The four main topic tabs are setting the context; determinants of health; child and youth health; and emerging priorities. Information is found within each of these tabs specific to Aboriginals in Canada. Although the Inuit population is growing at twice the rate of the general Canadian population and is expected by 2016 to reach more than 60,000 (Kanatami, 2004), the overall health data for this group are limited. However, some of the available data on the Inuit are provided in the "Determinants of Health" box on page 323.

TABLE 11-2 Comparison of Non-Aboriginal, First Nations, Inuit, and Métis Populations in Canada

Criteria	Non-Aboriginal	First Nations	Inuit	Métis
Age	Median age: 40 18% <15 years	Median age: 25 years 33% <15 years 5% seniors >65	Median age: 22 years 35% <15 years	Median age: 30 years
Fertility rates	Low	High	High	High
Employment rate	81.6%	51.9% on reserve 66.3% off reserve	61.2%	74.6%
Median income (2005)	$25,955	$14,517	$16,955	Not available
Report crowded homes and needing major repairs	3%	More likely for those living on reserves	33% more likely	69% live off reserves; 3% and more likely to live in homes needing repairs
Suicide rate	29%	33%	40%	Not available
Percentage deaths per 100,000 population				

Source: Statistics Canada. (2008). *Aboriginal Peoples in Canada in 2006: Inuit, Métis and First Nations, 2006 census* (Catalogue no. 97-558-XIE). Ottawa: Minister of Industry.

Aboriginal people in Canada have varied access to health services depending on their geographic location. Only a few First Nations communities are located within city limits; most communities are in rural and remote locations. Several communities north of 60 degrees latitude are in semi-isolated and isolated (fly-in only) areas of Canada. These geographical challenges are the leading contributing factors hindering access to services for the Aboriginal population. In addition to barriers because of location and travel requirements, there is a lack of access to physicians and other health care providers on northern and rural area reserves and a need for culturally appropriate services (First Nations Centre, 2005). Economic concerns such as transportation, child care, and direct costs of some health services are also barriers (First Nations Centre, 2005).

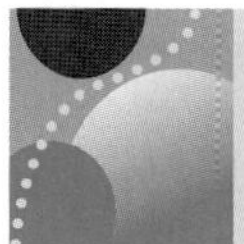

Determinants of Health
Social and Community Factors for the Inuit

- Suicide rates for the Inuit are six times greater than the Canadian average (Kanatami, 2004).
- In the 2006 Aboriginal Peoples survey, approximately 10% of Inuit adults in Inuit Nunaat reported experiencing problems accessing health care (Statistics Canada, 2008b).
- The lung cancer rate in some Inuit regions is 60% higher than the Canadian average (Kanatami, 2004).
- Climate change is negatively affecting Inuit community health (Kanatami, 2004).
- Low income is common, with few opportunities for employment in many Inuit communities (Kanatami, 2004).
- Educational opportunities are limited in Inuit communities (no Inuit region has a university) and high-school dropout rates are higher than for other Canadians (Kanatami, 2004).
- Inuit pay 50% more for groceries than do residents of southern Canada (Kanatami, 2004).
- Environmental contaminants such as persistent organic pollutants and climate change are damaging elements—such as seals and other marine mammals—of the Inuit region's food chain (Kanatami, 2004).
- Changing social conditions and the loss of the dominant culture's language have changed family relationships so that grandparents and grandchildren find it difficult to communicate (Kanatami, 2004).
- Initiatives at the various government levels are required to improve the income, education, employment, housing, health, and social needs of Aboriginal people (Mikkonen & Raphael, 2010).

The Canadian government has identified the health care concerns of First Nations people living on reserves as one of its top priorities, but many First Nations people living off reserves experience poverty, homelessness, and a lack of culturally appropriate health care and access to health care (Health Canada, 2009a). Health Canada (2009a) put forward some suggested interventions for improving the health of First Nations people:

- Strengthening families
- Improving early childhood development
- Improving economic safety measures for families
- Providing early and permanent learning experiences
- Enhancing and encouraging strong development in preteen years
- Establishing supportive, safe, violence-free communities

Visit the various Health Canada and National Aboriginal Health Organization Weblinks on the Evolve Web site for further information on First Nations, Inuit, and Métis health. Health Canada's role in First Nations and Inuit health has been to provide direct health services to the Inuit and First Nations people. Within the past two decades, First Nations and the Inuit have been working with Health Canada to assume more local control for health services. Because health care for First Nations and Inuit is a treaty right, the federal government, through its Health Ministry and the First Nations and Inuit Health (FNIH), provides health services and support for First Nations and Inuit people (King Blood, 2005).

Health and Social Challenges for Aboriginal Peoples

CHNs need to understand the statistical profiles of Aboriginal people. Recently, the health of Aboriginal people has improved; for example, they have been living longer and infant deaths have decreased. However, compared with other Canadians, Aboriginal people have higher rates of injury, suicide, and diabetes (Health Canada, 2007). Health Canada's (2005b) report *Statistical Profile on the Health of First Nations in Canada* provides information that is useful for CHNs and other health professionals, community leaders, and policy makers. Some highlights from this report for 2000 are as follows: the birth rate for First Nations was twice that of non–First Nations persons; the life expectancy for First Nation males was 68.9 years as opposed to 76.3 years for non–First Nation males; the life expectancy for First Nations females was 76.6 years but 81.8 years for non–First Nation females; the infant mortality rate for First Nations was 16% higher than for the rest of Canadian infants; circulatory diseases and injury accounted for nearly half of all mortality among First Nations; unintentional injury and suicide deaths accounted for about 6% of all First Nations deaths (22% of all deaths in youths); potential years of life lost from injury was about 3.5 times higher than for the rest of Canadians; the incidence of TB for First Nations peoples was six times higher than in the Canadian population; and smoking rates (based on 1997 statistics) were 62% compared with 24% for the rest of the Canadian population (Health Canada, 2005b). Refer to Table 11-2 for a comparison of non-Aboriginal and Aboriginal peoples in Canada on health and social variables.

CRITICAL VIEW

1. What are the issues concerning social justice and health disparities related to First Nations, Inuit, and Métis peoples?
2. What health care interventions does the community health nurse need to consider in working with First Nations, Métis, and Inuit peoples at the individual, community, and population levels?

MENTAL HEALTH AND MENTAL ILLNESS IN CANADA

One in five Canadians will experience mental illness in their lifetime (Health Canada, 2006b). The other four will be affected by the mental health of a friend or family member. Mental illness can affect individuals of all ages and does not discriminate between race, culture, sex, socioeconomic status, or educational level. Every year in Canada, 20 to 25% of Canada's workforce is affected by mental illness (Bradley, 2009). In Canada, patients with a primary diagnosis of mental illness accounted for 6% of the 2.8 million hospital stays in 2002–2003 (CIHI, 2005). It has been estimated by the World Health Organization that by the year 2020, depression will be the second leading cause of disability in the developed world. One in four patients will attend health care services having a mental illness that is not diagnosed or treated (WHO, 2009). Mental health is defined as "a state of well-being in which the individual realizes his or her own potential, can cope with the normal stresses of life, can work productively and fruitfully, and is able to make a contribution to his or her own community" (WHO, 2007b). According to the Mental Health Commission of Canada (2009b), "Mental health is more than the absence of mental illness" (p. 1), and furthermore it states, "Mental health contributes to our enjoyment of life, to physical health, as well as to our ability to achieve our goals, in school and in our relationships" (p. 1). Good mental health is an asset because it helps individuals manage stresses in daily living and therefore helps to protect them from mental health issues.

CRITICAL VIEW

It is important to note that early childhood as a determinant of health is a consideration in the development of mental health problems and mental illnesses. It is estimated that approximately 70% of all mental health problems and illnesses have their onset during childhood and adolescence (PHAC, 2006a). Refer to the Government of Canada Weblink *The Human Face of Mental Health and Mental Illness in Canada* on the Evolve Web site, and answer the questions below.

1. a) What is the influence of each of the determinants of health on mental health?
   b) Name and discuss individual, family, and community protective factors that can positively influence a person's mental health.
2. What are examples of health promotion strategies that you could use as a CHN working in community X?

In 2002, Statistics Canada conducted the Mental Health and Well-Being survey (Canadian Community Health Survey [CCHS], Cycle 1.2) (PHAC, 2006a), the first of its kind, to elicit both national and provincial data about mental illness and Canadians. These were some results:

- 10.2% of men and 11.7% of women met the criteria for a mood or anxiety disorder or dependence on substances in the 12 months preceding.
- Women were 1.5 times more likely to have a mood or anxiety disorder.
- Men were 2.6 times more likely to engage in substance abuse.
- Mood disorders were most prevalent in the age group of 15 to 24 years, occurring in 19.8% of women and 17.5% of men.
- Adults aged 25 to 44 years averaged 12.2% mood disorders, with those 45 to 64 years of age averaging only 8.8%.
- Anxiety disorders, including panic disorder, obsessive-compulsive disorder, post-traumatic stress disorder, and phobias, are more common than other mental disorders.
- Schizophrenia is estimated to have a prevalence of 0.2% to 2% of the general population, with the onset occurring between the late teen years and the mid-30s.
- Personality disorders occur, with prevalence estimated at 6 to 9% of Canadians.
- 50% of individuals incarcerated in prison demonstrate antisocial personality disorder (PHAC, 2006a).

Historically, individuals with mental illness were institutionalized and subjected to treatments that are no longer considered effective. In the 1960s, mental health policy changes initiated the deinstitutionalization of hospitalized mentally ill individuals (Davis, 2006). The catalysts for this change included social reform, the goal of reducing the cost of institutional care, and the positive effects of new psychotropic medications on symptom control and advocacy for patient autonomy (Boschma, Groening, & Boyd, 2008). Although these changes were intended to be positive, community support resources were often not in place for individuals displaced from institutional care; the result was many gaps in service, a poverty level income that caused these individuals to have poor living conditions, and a marginalized social status. This has also correlated with a higher risk for negative health outcomes as displayed in Box 11-3.

BOX 11-3 Potential Consequences of Mental Illness

Persons with mental illness are at risk for the following:

- Greater disability rates over a lifetime than those with physical illnesses (Bland, 1998)
- Underemployment and unemployment rates that are high, which contribute to many living in poverty
- More risk for poverty; this may lead to inappropriate dress and unkempt appearance, which can contribute to stigmatization (Wilton, 2003)
- Higher suicide rates, substance abuse and accidental overdoses, and early death from treatable medical conditions, contributing to a higher mortality rate (Arsenault-Lapierre, Kim, & Turecki, 2004)
- Greater risk for homelessness
- Greater risk for personal injury, medical co-morbidities, including HIV/AIDS, hepatitis B and C, hypothyroidism, heart or chronic lung disease, diabetes, and skin conditions (Weber, Cowan, Millikan, & Neibuhr, 2009).
- Increased altercations with law enforcement, often resulting in jail time
- Increased hospital and associated costs
- Increased caregiver burden

SOURCE: Adapted from Davis, S. (2006). *Community mental health in Canada: Policy, theory, and practice*. Vancouver: UBC Press.

In 2006, three major reports related to mental health in Canada were published. The Canadian Alliance on Mental Illness and Mental Health published its report, *Framework for Action on Mental Health and Mental Illness.* The major recommendation to health and social policy leaders of Canada was to develop a national action plan on mental illness and mental health. To date, Canada is the only G8 country without a national mental health strategy. The Kirby report, *Out of the Shadows at Last* (2006) (see the Standing Senate Subcommittee link listed in the Weblinks on the Evolve Web site), is considered one of the premier documents to have been published with regard to mental health and mental illness. The implications of the report are substantial in relation to necessary action and funding mechanisms. Finally, *The Human Face of Mental Health and Mental Illness in Canada* (2006) had as its purpose to raise awareness and increase knowledge and understanding about mental health and mental illness in Canada (PHAC, 2006a). In September 2007, the federal government formed the Mental Health Commission. This commission, which is a nonprofit agency, is poised to act as a catalyst to focus the nation's attention on mental health.

The Mental Health Commission has four key initiatives. The first is to create the first national mental health strategy for Canada. The second is to launch a 10-year anti-stigma and antidiscrimination initiative called "Opening Minds"; it will deal with the dual notions of hope and recovery. The goal is to eliminate stigma and fear of mental illness directed first to youth and health care workers, then expanding to the Canadian workforce and, finally, to seniors, First Nations, Métis, Inuit, and other groups. Third, extensive research on mental health and homelessness will also provide support and housing for homeless individuals. Finally, a knowledge exchange centre will be established providing the general public as well as researchers, educators, and scientists with a Web-based resource for education and exchange of information (Kirby, 2009). These initiatives are the largest in Canada's history and have the goal of truly transforming the promotion of mental health and well-being of all Canadians (see the Mental Health Commission of Canada Weblink *Toward Recovery and Well Being* on the Evolve Web site.) The Canadian Population Health Initiative (CPHI) has chosen the determinants of mental health and resilience as a priority focus for 2007 to 2010 (CIHI, 2006). Its purpose will be to explore positive aspects of mental health, self-perceptions of mental health, coping, self-esteem, and the determinant of mental health. This initiative arises from findings of the major Canadian mental health reports published in 2006 (CIHI, 2006).

Consumer-survivor initiatives have also been important in challenging the status of the current mental health system. A group of agencies collaboratively made a joint recommendation in 2005 that governments need to provide funding for consumer and family initiatives (Canadian Mental Health Association, Ontario; Centre for Addictions and Mental Health, Ontario; Peer Development Initiative; and Ontario Federation of Community Mental Health and Addiction Programs, 2009).

Rockman, Salach, Gotlib, Cord, and Turner (2004) reported that 30 to 40% of clients who access primary care have diagnosable mental health conditions and that approximately one-third of visits to primary care physicians are for mental health problems. In the last 10 years, the model of shared mental health care between primary health care practitioners and psychiatrists has been a strategy to address the need to assist primary care providers in conducting assessment and treatment of individuals who experience mental illness (Craven & Bland, 2002). The model facilitates the education of primary health care providers and provides expert consultation to support the practitioner in the day-to-day care of the mentally ill client. This initiative has been successful in incorporating members of the health team, including community health nurses, into the integrated delivery of mental health care.

CRITICAL VIEW

1. How are the mental health services organized and supported in your province or territory?
2. What are the titles, roles, and functions of community health nurses and mental health nurses who work with the promotion of mental health in your province or territory?
3. How would you envision a role in community health nursing specific to mental health care in your community?

At-Risk Populations for Mental Illness

The 12 determinants of health (PHAC, 2004) are important factors to consider as applied to persons with severe and persistent mental health disorders (see the "Determinants of Health" box on page 327). Davis (2006) indicates that poverty and social isolation are viewed as both cause and effects of psychiatric symptoms.

One-fifth of Canadians will have a mental illness during their lifetime, with the onset usually occurring during adolescence and young adulthood (PHAC, 2002). It is estimated that 14% of children will experience a mental disorder that will have a significant negative impact on their functioning (CIHI, 2009). Types of mental health problems typically diagnosed during childhood

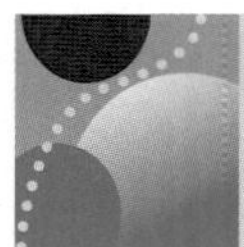

Determinants of Health
Applied to Persons with Mental Disorders

The following excerpt from Davis (2006) relates Health Canada's determinants of health to persons with mental disorders. The author points out that although "biology and genetic endowment" is one of the determinants, many of the other determinants also affect people with mental disorders and therefore represent areas where health care practitioners can help.

(1) Income and social status,

(2) education, and

(3) employment. As socio-economic and educational status [are] strongly associated with better health, it should be noted that persons with serious mental disorders face high rates of unemployment and poverty-level incomes. With the onset of a disorder such as schizophrenia occurring in early adulthood, university education and early career trajectories are cut short in many instances.

(4) Social support networks and

(5) social environments. Social support is associated with better health outcomes, with [the Public Health Agency of Canada, 2004] noting that "the caring and respect that [occur] in social relationships, and the resulting sense of satisfaction and well-being, seem to act as a buffer against health problems." Unfortunately, a large number of those diagnosed with mental disorders face isolation and exclusion, stigma being a major contributing factor. Others face unsafe social environments: frequently residing in poor, inner-city neighbourhoods, psychiatric clients are more likely to be physically and sexually assaulted.

(6) Physical environments. Decent, affordable housing is an urgent need for psychiatric clients, who disproportionately face chronic homelessness, which itself is associated with a host of negative health outcomes.

(7) Coping skills. This term is identified by [the Public Health Agency of Canada, 2004] as "actions by which individuals can ... promote self-care, cope with challenges, develop self-reliance, solve problems and make choices that enhance health." Psychiatric clients may have poorer coping skills because of constitutional factors, because the onset of the disorder interrupted the learning process, and unfortunately because of psychiatric practices that have reinforced dependency.

(8) Healthy child development. A range of adult mental health problems are the result of childhood trauma.

(9) Biology and genetic endowment.*

(10) Health services. Providing comprehensive, effective, and accessible mental health services continues to be a challenge for governments and health authorities in Canada.

(11) Gender. The etiology and expression of mental disorders may differ between the sexes, which has implications for service delivery, one example being the need for programs sensitive to the experiences of sexual assault victims. As the socio-economic status of women remains, on average, lower than that of men, women may be differentially affected by social determinants of health.

(12) Culture. The First Nations have poorer health outcomes in many areas, with substance misuse and higher suicide rates being a particular concern for mental health practitioners.

*It is known that certain mental illnesses may be accounted for by genetics and/or biologic endowment, for example, clinical depression.

SOURCE: Reprinted with permission of the Publisher from *Community mental health in Canada: Policy, theory, and practice*, by Simon Davis © University of British Columbia Press 2006.

are depression, anxiety, and attention deficit disorders. Children may develop depression after a loss, or they may develop behaviour problems from abuse or neglect. Examples of environmental factors include crowded living conditions, violence, separation from parents, and a lack of consistent caregivers. Cohen, Groves, and Kracke (2009) found exposure to community violence to be related to significant stress and depression in children. Currently, there is a shortage of programs designed to prevent mental health problems in children (CIHI, 2009).

The concern for the mental health of adolescents and college students has come to light in the work of Kadison and DiGeronimo (2004). In their unique study of college students in the United States, their findings indicated that 62% of students reported feeling hopeless, 44% said they felt so depressed they could barely function, 79% were very sad, and 9% felt suicidal. To complicate matters, recent research (Jagdeo, Cox, Stein, & Sareen, 2009) has found that young men with a mental illness who are single and socioeconomically challenged had the poorest attitudes toward seeking out mental health services. For this reason, they recommend the need for screening and intervention programs targeted to young adults. The WHO and World Organization of Family Doctors (WONCA) (2008) identify a number of groups that may experience difficulty in accessing mental health care. They include the elderly, children, the homeless, people with chronic physical conditions, and ethnic and cultural groups.

Community mental health nurses (CMHNs) are often found working in Assertive Community Treatment teams. These teams were developed as a mental health strategy to care for individuals with serious and persistent mental illness when deinstitutionalized from long-term psychiatric facilities. This interdisciplinary team-based approach engages the client on a daily basis for ongoing assessment, treatment, and support to reduce hospital readmissions and improve social functioning and quality of life. Research has found that this type of community support has resulted in a decrease of psychiatric symptoms and hospital stays and that social adjustment and housing stability improved (National Alliance on Mental Illness, 2009). Mental health nurses are also employed at nationwide branches of the Canadian Mental Health Association. They provide intensive case management and coordination of care for clients experiencing mental illness.

The Canadian Nurses Association (CNA) position on mental health is found in their paper the *Backgrounder* (2005) titled "Mental Health and Nursing: A Summary of the Issues" and in its position statement titled "Mental Health Services." In these documents the CNA

- distinguishes between mental illness and mental health,
- describes the changes in mental health over the past 40 years in Canada (e.g., changes in treatment regimens and care moving from institution to the community where programs have been developed to address mental illness and promote mental health, consumers and families advocating for appropriate therapeutic regimens, and discussion of addressing the stigma and discrimination of mental illness), and
- describes the coordination of mental health services through projects such as the Canadian Collaborative Mental Health Initiative.

Nurses are advised to direct efforts at prevention (e.g., educate the public about mental health and promote positive attitudes); treatment and management (e.g., include the social determinants of health in planning care and be informed about the latest interventions); and advocacy (e.g., fight for continuity of care and more community resources) (see the "Ethical Considerations" box, above). Further information about these CNA articles can be accessed at the CNA Weblinks listed on the Evolve Web site. The Psychiatric/Mental Health Nursing group is a specialty within the Canadian Federation of Mental Health Nurses, and there are nursing competencies for this group within the CNA certification program. Mental health nurses work in the community across Canada, and their focus and scope of practice are evolving.

CHNs and CMHNs can assist in targeted assessment and interventions of at-risk populations. It is important that CHNs and CMHNs be involved in the establishment of educational programs for the recognition of symptoms, with follow-up assessment for depression and/or psychosis. CHNs and CMHNs also require

ETHICAL CONSIDERATIONS

A CHN has received funding to work with a group of mature second-time mothers experiencing postpartum depression. However, many of the mothers do not want to work in a group format because they are embarrassed and ashamed of their depression, especially since they have beautiful, healthy babies. They are asking the CHN for one-on-one visits, but the CHN has not been funded for individual visits.

Ethical principles that apply to the above case:

- *Distributive justice.* This principle requires fairness in the distribution of resources (Storch, Rodney, & Starzomski, 2004).
- *Beneficence.* This principle requires that we do good, but also acknowledges that we are limited by time, place, and talents in the amount of good we can do.
- *Maintaining privacy and confidentiality.* Maintaining privacy and confidentiality is one of the primary values in the nursing code of ethics. CHNs must be sensitive to clients' need for privacy.

Questions to Consider

1. What is the CHN's ethical responsibility to these women?
2. How can the CHN provide the best care possible under the circumstances?

knowledge of available services such as teen health clinics, crisis help lines, and emergency room mental health services so that referrals can be made to the appropriate service.

Opportunities exist for collaboration with the police (Canadian Mental Healthy Agency [CMHA], 2005). Law-enforcement agencies have taken steps to educate their staff in dealing sensitively with individuals who are mentally ill. The traditional route has been to arrest individuals and put them in jail so they can have access to mental health assessment and treatment. Community mental health nurses have the ability to collaborate with the police in determining the best plan for community follow-up and thus potentially avoid incarceration.

CHNs play an important role in identifying stressful events, assessing stress responses, educating communities, and intervening to prevent or alleviate disability and disease resulting from stress. Although everyone is vulnerable to stressful life events and may develop mental illness, persons with chronic and persistent mental illness have numerous problems. They may not have access to adequate health services or suitable housing. Many accessible and coordinated services are needed to enable people with chronic mental illness to stay in the community, yet these are not always available. Interventions for community survival for those with serious mental illness require a broad range of well-coordinated services, including for mental and physical health, housing assistance, substance abuse treatment for some, and social and vocational rehabilitation. The CHN, by partnering with other community health care professionals and service providers, can facilitate the coordination of these services in the community. The CHN can be an advocate for this vulnerable population. Many mental health service systems exist. They can be found by going to the Health Canada *Healthy Living* Web site, Mental Health section, listed in the Weblinks on the Evolve Web site. This site also provides an overview of mental health and offers online materials on mental health promotion and mental health illness.

CHNs working in community settings, well-child clinics, and home health are well positioned to conduct early mental health assessments that can positively affect clients' mental health. Because many children and adolescents lack services or access to them, community mental health assessment activities are essential. Assessment activities include identifying types of programs available or lacking in places where children and adolescents spend time. Assessments should be performed in schools and in homes of clients served, as well as in daycare centres, churches, and organizations that plan and guide age-specific play and entertainment programs. Assessment data are essential for planning and developing programs that address mental health concerns prevalent from the prenatal period through adolescence. Addressing concerns during these developmental periods can reduce mental health problems in adulthood.

How can CHNs intervene? The general medical sector, including primary care clinics, hospitals, and nursing homes, has long been identified as the initial point of contact for many adults with mental illness; for some, these providers may be the only source of mental health services. Early detection of and intervention for mental health problems can be increased if persons presenting in primary care are assessed for mental health problems. CHNs who work in the general medical sector and in other community settings are in an ideal position to assess and detect mental health problems. CHNs conduct comprehensive biopsychosocial assessments and are often the professionals most trusted with sensitive information by clients in these settings. Screening tools for depression, anxiety, substance abuse, and cognitive impairment can assist the CHN in early detection of and intervention for mental illness. Health Canada provides information on some tools that are used for substance-abuse screening and mental health screening. This information is found on the Health Canada Web sites listed in the Weblinks on the Evolve Web site.

Tertiary prevention targeted at persons with serious mental illness has aimed to reduce the proportion of homeless adults who have serious mental illness, to increase their employment, and to decrease the number of adults with mental disorders who are incarcerated. Brief hospital stays and inadequate community resources have resulted in an increased number of persons with serious mental illness living on the streets or in jail. Some people arrested for nonviolent crimes could be better served if diverted from the jail system to a community mental health treatment program with linkage to mental health services. According to a CIHI (2007) report, 35% of visits to the emergency department by homeless people were related to mental and behavioural disorders, higher than for other patients.

Currently, many people with severe mental disorders live in poverty because they lack the ability to earn or maintain a suitable standard of living. Even people who live with family caregivers or in supervised housing are at risk for inadequate services because the long-term care they require frequently depletes human and fiscal resources. In Canada, the population older than 65 years has been steadily increasing. As the life expectancy of individuals continues to grow, the number experiencing mental illness in later life will increase. This trend will be expensive and will challenge us to deliver the needed mental health services for older adults. Although many older adults maintain highly functional lives, others have mental health deficits associated with normal sensory losses related to aging, failing physical health, difficulty performing activities of daily living, and social deprivation or isolation. Life changes related to work roles and retirement often result in reduced social contacts and support. Other losses are associated with the death of a spouse, other family members, or friends (Beckmann Murray et al., 2009). Reduced social networks and contacts brought about by these life events can influence mood and contribute to serious states of depression. However, depression is not a normal part of aging (Ebersole, Hess, Touhy, & Jett, 2005). It is important for CHNs to recognize that older adults who are depressed usually have a clinically different presentation from clients in other age groups. Older adults who are depressed tend to present with many bodily complaints such as chronic pain, nausea and vomiting, and insomnia and usually do not express feelings of sadness, guilt, or worthlessness (Ebersole et al., 2005).

Activities to improve the mental health status of older adults include public education programs, prevention approaches, and the provision of mental health services in primary care. Specific approaches to reduce stress include use of community support groups, education about lifestyle management, and worksite programs. Nevertheless, most programs currently available for older adults, families, and caregivers with health problems primarily monitor or restore health rather than prevent illness. Two national voluntary organizations that have regional chapters with a mental health focus are included here as examples of resources a CHN might access and refer clients to. The Canadian Mental Health Association (CMHA) has chapters in all provinces and territories. Some of the activities of this voluntary association influence policy on mental health concerns, provide public education, direct services to clients and their families, and support mental health research (CMHA, 2010). The Schizophrenia Society of Canada provides public education for clients with schizophrenia and their families, conducts research on schizophrenia, and assumes an advocacy role to influence public policy (Schizophrenia Society of Canada, 2010). CHNs can refer family caregivers and others to appropriate community mental health resources available in their community. For a comprehensive discussion of information on specific mental illnesses in Canada, refer to a Canadian psychiatric nursing textbook.

SUBSTANCE ABUSE

Identifying high-risk groups helps CHNs design programs to meet specific needs and to mobilize community resources. High-risk groups for abuse of alcohol, tobacco, and other drugs (ATOD) are adolescents, older adults, injection drug users, and drug users during pregnancy (especially alcohol abuse). Children of ATOD abusers or addicts are themselves at a greater risk for childhood physical and sexual abuse (Raising Children Network, 2009).

The **harm reduction model** is a health care approach to address substance-abuse problems by reducing the harm associated with drugs without requiring that all drug use ceases (Davis, 2006). This approach was first used in Great Britain, the Netherlands, Germany, Switzerland, and Australia. Increased interest and momentum are spreading throughout Europe and Canada. This public health model recognizes the following:

- Addiction is a health problem.
- Any psychoactive drug can be abused.
- Accurate information can help people make responsible decisions about drug use.
- People who have substance-abuse problems can be helped.

This approach accepts that psychoactive drug use is endemic, and it focuses on pragmatic interventions, including education, to reduce the adverse consequences of drug use and get treatment for addicts.

It is important for CHNs to identify the underlying roots of various health concerns and plan actions that are realistic, nonjudgemental, holistic, and positive. A harm reduction model for substance-abuse concerns facilitates such an approach. To develop a therapeutic attitude, the CHN needs to realize that any drug can be abused, that anyone may develop drug dependence, and that drug addiction can be successfully treated.

The Registered Nurses Association of Ontario (RNAO) developed a best-practice guideline titled *Supporting Clients on Methadone Maintenance Treatment* (see the Weblinks on the Evolve Web site). In this document, the harm reduction model developed by Cheung is discussed. The harm reduction strategies and programs are also discussed in this document. Specifically, note that pp. 17 to 19 present the harm reduction model and the harm reduction strategies and programs. An example of a harm reduction program is the City of Vancouver's Four Pillars Drug Strategy (see the Weblinks on the Evolve Web site), which is a comprehensive approach to harm reduction with an emphasis on the damage done by substance abuse rather than an emphasis on the substance use itself. It includes programs such as needle exchange and a supervised injection site (SIS). 

CRITICAL VIEW

1. What are some harm reduction approaches that community health nurses can use in the community for substance-abuse concerns?
2. What community health nursing intervention would reflect the Ottawa Charter strategies for health promotion?

Table 11-3 presents commonly used terms regarding substance abuse. The terms *drugs* and *substances* are often used interchangeably when referring to alcohol, tobacco, and so on.

Although any drug can be abused, ATOD abuse and addiction generally involve the **psychoactive drugs.** These drugs, which can alter emotions, are used for enjoyment in social and recreational settings and for personal use to self-medicate for physical or emotional discomfort. Psychoactive drugs are divided into categories according to their effect on the central nervous system and the general feelings or experiences the drugs may induce. The categories are depressants (alcohol, heroin), stimulants (nicotine, cocaine, caffeine, amphetamines), marijuana, hallucinogens (lysergic acid diethylamide [LSD], 3,4-methylenedioxymethamphetamine [MDMA or "ecstasy"], and phencyclidine [PCP]), and inhalants. A pharmacology text or reliable Web-based resource can provide detailed information on these drug categories. Often, if individuals cannot obtain their drug of choice, another drug from the same category is substituted. For example, a person who cannot drink alcohol may begin using a benzodiazepine as an alternative because both are central nervous system depressants.

Caffeine, a stimulant, is one of the most widely used drugs in the world. Caffeine is found in food and beverages such as chocolate, coffee, tea, soft drinks, and some drugs. Table 11-4 lists commonly used substances that are high in caffeine content. Moderate doses of caffeine from 100 to 300 mg per day increase mental alertness and probably have little negative effect on health. Many people take in this amount of caffeine to prevent and manage fatigue and to increase their work productivity. However, higher doses can lead to insomnia, irritability, tremulousness, anxiety, cardiac dysrhythmias, gastrointestinal disturbances, and headaches. Regular use of high doses can lead to physical dependence, and the withdrawal symptoms may include headaches, lethargy, and occasional depression (Lehne, 2007).

Promotion of Healthy Lifestyles and Resiliency Factors

Assisting clients to achieve optimal health includes identifying interventions other than or in addition to the use of drugs whenever possible. Teaching assertiveness and decision-making skills helps clients increase

TABLE 11-3 Commonly Used Terms Related to Drug or Substance Abuse Problems

Term	Definition
Drug or substance abuse	The use of any substance that threatens a person's health or impairs social or economic functioning
Drug or substance dependency	Can be psychological or physical where there is an intense need for continuous use of a substance and if stopped, withdrawal symptoms result
Drug or substance addiction	A pattern of abuse characterized by an overwhelming preoccupation with the use (compulsive use) of a drug or substance and securing its supply, and a high tendency to relapse if the drug is removed
Alcoholism	Addiction to the drug called *alcohol;* alcoholism and drug or substance addiction are recognized as illnesses under a biopsychosocial model
Psychoactive drugs	Drugs or substances that affect mood, perception, and thought
Tolerance	The need for increasing doses of a drug or substance over time to maintain the desired effect; for example, if a person consumes alcohol on a daily basis over time, this person will need to consume more alcohol in order to reach a high blood-alcohol concentration to experience the effects of the alcohol
Mainstream smoke	Smoke inhaled directly by the smoker
Sidestream smoke	Smoke that enters the atmosphere from the lighted end of a cigarette and can be inhaled by others in the vicinity (second-hand smoke)
Denial	A primary symptom of addiction, it involves a refusal to acknowledge that a drug or substance problem exists
Codependency	A stress-induced preoccupation by a partner or friend with the addicted person's life, leading to extreme dependence and excessive concern with the addict
Enabling	The act of shielding or preventing an addict from experiencing the consequences of an addiction

TABLE 11-4 Caffeine Content in Commonly Consumed Substances

Substance	Caffeine Content (mg)
Coffee (148 mL)	
Brewed	60–180
Instant	30–120
Decaffeinated	1–5
Chocolate	
Cocoa (142 g)	2–20
Semisweet (28 g)	5–35
Tea (148 mL)	
Brewed	20–90
Iced	67–76
Soft drinks (355 mL)	
Colas	40–45
Mountain Dew	53
Orange soda, ginger ale, Sprite, 7 Up, and several fruit-flavoured drinks	0
Prescription drugs	
Fiorinal (butalbital, aspirin, and caffeine)	40
Cafergot (ergotamine and caffeine)	100
Over-the-counter drugs	
Anacin (aspirin and caffeine)	32
Excedrin (acetaminophen and caffeine)	65

self-responsibility for health and increase their awareness of the various options. Nagging health concerns such as difficulty sleeping, muscle tension, lack of energy, chronic stress, and mood swings are common reasons people turn to medications, especially the psychoactive drugs. CHNs need to help clients understand that medications may mask concerns rather than solve them. Stress reduction and relaxation techniques along with a balanced lifestyle can address these concerns more directly than medications can. Lack of sleep, improper diet, and lack of exercise contribute to many health complaints. Assisting clients to balance their rest, nutrition, and exercise on a daily basis can reduce these complaints. CHNs provide useful information to groups, assisting the development of community recreational resources or facilitating stress reduction, relaxation, or exercise groups. CHNs need to help persons increase their awareness of drug-free community activities.

Lack of educational opportunities, job training, or both can contribute to socioeconomic stress and poor self-esteem, which can lead to drug use to escape the situation. CHNs help clients identify community resources and solve problems to meet basic needs rather than avoid them. In addition to decreasing risk factors associated with ATOD problems, it is important to increase protective or resiliency factors. CHNs teach parents and teachers how to increase resiliency in youth, using some of the following strategies as prevention guidelines:

- Help them develop an increased sense of responsibility for their own success.
- Help them identify their talents.
- Motivate them to dedicate their lives to helping society rather than believing that their only purpose in life is to be consumers.
- Provide realistic appraisals and feedback, stress multicultural competence, encourage and value education and skills training.
- Increase cooperative solutions to problems rather than competitive or aggressive solutions.

Substance Abuse Education

Nurses are knowledgeable in medication administration and understand the potential dangers of indiscriminate drug use and the inherent inability of drugs to cure all problems. CHNs need to influence the health of clients by destroying the myth of good drugs versus bad drugs. Role playing is useful in teaching many of these skills. This means (1) teaching clients that no drug is completely safe and that any drug can be abused and (2) helping individuals learn how to make informed decisions about their drug use to minimize potential harm. CHNs are educators or advisors to the school systems or community groups to ensure that all relevant areas are addressed.

Several drug education programs such as Drug Abuse Resistance Education (D.A.R.E.), REAL (Refuse, Explain, Avoid, and Leave) and the Harm Reduction Drug Education program approach teach youth decision-making skills about whether, how, and when to use drugs. This youth-targeted approach advises that if drugs are used, they are to be used in a safer and smarter way. A participatory research study was conducted to explore the effectiveness of the harm reduction approach with junior and senior youth in Nova Scotia schools (Poulin & Nicholson, 2005). Of note, the study found that for the younger youth (junior high school), abstinence needs to be the focus for drug education. For older youth (senior high school), abstinence can be one of the decision options in the harm reduction approach. Another

CRITICAL VIEW

1. What drug education programs are included in the school curriculum in your community?
2. What is the effectiveness of these programs, and what can CHNs do to support these programs?

study finding was that senior youth in the study group decreased harmful drug-related behaviours compared with nonstudy youth participants.

Role of the CHN in Substance Abuse Situations

The harm reduction approach to substance abuse focuses on health promotion and disease prevention. Health promotion for ATOD problems includes (1) the promotion of healthy lifestyles and resiliency factors and (2) education about drugs and guidelines for use. CHNs are in an ideal position to use health promotion strategies such as promoting and facilitating healthy alternatives to indiscriminate, careless, and often dangerous drug-use practices and providing education about drugs to decrease harm from irresponsible or unsafe drug-use practices.

To identify substance abuse and plan appropriate interventions, CHNs can assess each client individually. Think of the "4 *H*s" to remember what to ask when assessing drug-use patterns: *h*ow taken (route), *h*ow much, *h*ow often, and *h*ow long. When drug abuse, dependence, or addiction is identified, the CHN needs to assist clients to understand the connection between their drug-use patterns and the negative consequences on their health, family, and the community. The CHN may consider client participation in a self-help group. Referrals may be necessary for some clients. Community programs and services that CHNs might refer clients to are Alcoholics Anonymous (AA), detoxification centres, smoking cessation programs, and drug-awareness programs offered by the Addiction Research Foundation or local mental health centres.

When assessing self-medication and recreational or social drug-use patterns, CHNs need to determine the reason for use. Some underlying health problems (e.g., pain, stress, weight, insomnia) may be relieved by nonpharmaceutical interventions. Ask about the amount, frequency, and duration of use and the route of administration of each drug. To establish the presence of a substance abuse problem, determine if the drug use is causing any negative health consequences or problems with relationships, employment, finances, or the legal system. The box "How To ... Assess Socioeconomic Concerns Resulting from Substance Abuse" lists examples of questions to ask to determine any socioeconomic concerns that are often secondary to substance abuse. If a pattern of chronic, regular, and frequent use of a drug exists, CHNs need to assess the client for a history of withdrawal symptoms to determine if there is physical dependence on the drug. A progression in drug-use patterns and related problems warns about the possibility of addiction. **Denial** is a primary symptom of addiction. Signs of denial include the following:

- Lying about use
- Minimizing use patterns
- Blaming or rationalizing
- Intellectualizing
- Changing the subject
- Using anger or humour
- "Going with the flow" (agreeing that a problem exists and stating that the behaviour will change but not demonstrating any behaviour changes)

Suspect a problem if the client becomes defensive or exhibits other behaviours indicating denial when asked about alcohol or other drug use. Refer to the screening tools found at the Health Canada *Best Practices: Concurrent Mental Health and Substance Use Disorders* Weblink on the Evolve Web site.

The CHN is in a key position to help the addict and the addict's family. The CHN's knowledge of community resources such as detoxification centres, addiction treatment facilities, smoking-cessation programs, and support groups such as AA and the CHN's knowledge of how to mobilize them can significantly influence the quality of care clients receive. The CHN's knowledge can be used to refer the client to the appropriate community resource(s).

Strategies used with clients can vary depending on their readiness for change. Understanding the stages of change, previously discussed in Chapter 4, and assessing the stage of change that a client is at facilitate successful outcomes. After the client has received treatment, the CHN needs to coordinate aftercare referrals and follow up on the client's progress. The CHN needs to provide additional support in the home as the client and family adjust to changing roles and manage the stress involved with such changes. The CHN supports addicted persons who have relapsed by reminding them that relapses may well occur but that they and their families can continue to work toward recovery and an improved quality of life. The CHN assesses and encourages clients, based on readiness, to return for treatment.

How To... Assess Socioeconomic Concerns Resulting from Substance Abuse

If a client admits to use of alcohol, tobacco, or other drugs, ask the following questions:

- Do your family or friends worry or complain about your drinking or using drugs?
- Has a family member gone for help about your drinking or using drugs?
- Have you neglected family obligations as a result of drinking or using drugs?
- Have you missed work because of your drinking or using drugs?
- Does your boss complain about your drinking or using drugs?
- Do you drink or use drugs before or during work?
- Have you ever been fired or quit because of drinking or using drugs?
- Have you ever been charged with driving under the influence or being drunk in public?
- Have you ever had any other legal problems related to drinking and using drugs, such as assault and battery, breaking and entering, or theft?
- Have you had any accidents while intoxicated, such as falls, burns, or motor vehicle accidents?
- Have you spent your money on alcohol or other drugs instead of paying your bills (e.g., telephone, electricity, rent)?

Drug addiction is often a family disease. People in a close relationship with the addict often develop unhealthy coping mechanisms to continue the relationship. The CHN helps families recognize the problem of addiction and helps them confront the addicted member in a caring manner. Whether or not the addicted family member is agreeable to treatment, the family members need to be given some guidance about the literature and services that are available to help them cope more effectively. The CHN helps identify treatment options, counselling assistance, financial assistance, support services, and (if necessary) legal services for the family members. Harm reduction strategies may be needed, such as needle exchange, safe injection sites programs, and shelter-based controlled drinking-reduction programs.

CHILDREN AND YOUTH IN DISADVANTAGED CONDITIONS

Children and youth will be discussed further in Chapter 13. Children who are maltreated (by physical, sexual, or emotional abuse or neglect) are considered a vulnerable group. Regardless of socioeconomic status, gender, age, race, ethnicity, cultural identity, spirituality, personality, sexual orientation, or physical or mental abilities, children are vulnerable to maltreatment (Department of Justice Canada, 2006). Sexually active teenagers who become pregnant are considered a vulnerable group. *Disadvantaged* is a term that is often used in reference to factors such as socioeconomic inequalities, health inequalities, and educational inequalities (Alberta Coalition for Healthy School Communities, 2006). Depending on their circumstances, children and youth may or may not be disadvantaged; however, they are vulnerable.

The four categories of maltreatment or abuse are briefly described as follows:

1. *Physical abuse.* This involves applying force to any part of the body. It includes grabbing, pushing, hitting, shaking, choking, biting, kicking, burning, poisoning, or other dangerous use of force.
2. *Sexual abuse.* This involves using a child or other person for sexual purposes and exploitation. It might include fondling, intercourse, incest, sodomy, exhibitionism, prostitution, or pornographic exposure.
3. *Emotional and psychological abuse.* This involves using emotional behaviours to decrease a person's or child's self-esteem and self-image. It might include verbal threats, social isolation, intimidation, exploitation, terrorizing, manipulation, or consistently making unreasonable demands.
4. *Neglect.* This involves, intentionally or not, failing to provide care for those who are dependent. It might include not attending to their physical, emotional, educational, and medical needs, and abandonment (Northwest Territories Health and Social Services, 2009).

A 1998 study, *Canadian Incidence Study of Reported Child Abuse and Neglect* (CIS), was the first Canadian study to examine the incidence of child abuse and neglect, based on 7,672 cases investigated by Child Welfare Services at 51 sites in all provinces and territories (Trocmé et al., 2005). This first nationwide study provided a snapshot of the extent and types of child maltreatment. The second cycle of this study (CIS-2) was conducted in 2003 to examine the incidence of child abuse and neglect based on 14,200 cases investigated by Child Welfare Services at 63 sites in provinces and territories (excluding Quebec). This study also examined qualities of children and their families. The Canadian domestic and family violence statistics for children reported in this 2003 study were as follows (Trocmé et al., 2005):

- Physical abuse occurred in 5.31 confirmed cases in 1,000 Canadian children compared with 2.56 cases in 1,000 children in 1998.
- Sexual abuse occurred in 0.62 confirmed cases in 1,000 Canadian children compared with 0.89 cases in 1000 children in 1998.
- Neglect occurred in 6.38 confirmed cases in 1,000 Canadian children compared with 3.58 cases in 1,000 children in 1998.
- Emotional maltreatment occurred in 3.32 confirmed cases in 1,000 Canadian children compared with 0.86 cases in 1,000 children in 1998.

In summary, the results of the substantiated cases indicated that the incidence of substantiated maltreatment rose by 125%; physical abuse cases increased from the 1998 findings; sexual abuse cases decreased; neglect cases increased; and emotional maltreatment increased. Final data collection for the third cycle of the study was completed in December 2008. A final report was released in the fall of 2010 (PHAC, 2010). Further information on the CIS 2008 study regarding the child and family features and various types of child abuse and neglect are found at the PHAC Weblink titled 2008 Canadian Incidence Study of Reported Child Abuse and Neglect: Major Findings on the Evolve Web site. Almost a third of Canadian street youth aged 15 to 24 reported having experienced neglect (PHAC, 2006b). All individuals in Canada who suspect child abuse are required to report it to the proper child protection agencies as mandated by law (Department of Justice Canada, 2006). First Nations peoples have their own child protection agencies (Department of Justice Canada, 2006). The Department of Justice Canada (2006) has a fact sheet titled *Child Abuse: A Fact Sheet from the Department of Justice Canada* that defines and discusses the various types of child abuse, provides statistics on the prevalence of child abuse, and discusses the Criminal Code, factors and consequences, and prevention

How To... Identify Potentially Abusive Parents

The following characteristics in couples expecting a child constitute warning signs of actual or potential abuse:

- Denial of the reality of the pregnancy—that is, refusal to talk about the impending birth or to think of a name for the child
- An obvious concern or fear that the baby will not meet some predetermined standard: sex, hair colour, temperament, or resemblance to family members
- Failure to follow through on the desire for an abortion
- An initial decision to place the child for adoption and a change of mind
- Rejection of the mother by the father of the baby
- Family experiencing stress and numerous crises, and the birth of a child may be the "last straw"
- Initial and unresolved negative feelings about having a child
- Lack of support for the new parents
- Isolation from friends, neighbours, or family
- Parental evidence of poor impulse control or fear of losing control
- Contradictory history
- Appearance of detachment
- Appearance of misusing drugs or alcohol
- Shopping for hospitals or health care providers
- Unrealistic expectations of the child
- Verbal, physical, or sexual abuse of mother by father, especially during pregnancy
- Child not biological offspring of stepfather or mother's current partner
- Excessive talk of needing to "discipline" children and plans to use harsh physical punishment to enforce discipline

and management of child abuse. This site, listed in the Weblinks on the Evolve Web site, also provides additional resources on child abuse. Additionally, page 45 of the 2009 PHAC report, *The State of Public Health in Canada: Growing up Well—Priorities for a Healthy Future* (found in the PHAC Weblinks on the Evolve Web site), provides information on abuse and neglect.

Adolescent Sexual Behaviour and Pregnancy

One of the most vulnerable youth groups is sexually active females. One of the risks to sexual activity for teenage girls is pregnancy. Another risk of sexual activity is STIs. Incorrect interpretation by adolescent females about their protection from STIs upon receiving the human papillomavirus (HPV) vaccine may increase teenage pregnancy if this aggregate becomes more sexually active as a result of their perceived STI protection. CHNs need to assess adolescent understanding of HPV immunization and STIs and teach accordingly. Additionally, CHNs when working with teenagers, need to have a discussion of teenage sexual activity, contraceptive use, history of STIs, and any other health concerns pertaining to sexual health (Langille, 2007). Community health nurses explore these areas when working with teenagers in settings such as sexual health clinics and schools.

Teenage pregnancy is an area of public health concern because of its significant effect on communities. See the PHAC *Canadian Guidelines on Sexually Transmitted Infections* Weblink on the Evolve Web site. The 2006 guidelines, revised in 2008, are a reference for professionals for the prevention and management of STIs and now contain information on at-risk populations (vulnerable) populations. Included in this guide are scripts that may be helpful in discussing sexual health. Many factors can lead to teenage pregnancy. Teens can be influenced by peers and by partners. They are more likely to be sexually active if their friends are sexually active (Beckmann Murray, 2009). Other factors influencing teenage pregnancy are a history of sexual victimization, family structure, and parental influences. Some of the factors that can lead to teenage pregnancy are listed in Box 11-4.

For further facts and background information regarding teenage pregnancy, see the Health Canada Weblink *Pro-action, Postponement, and Preparation/Support: A Framework for Action to Reduce the Rate of Teen Pregnancy in Canada* on the Evolve Web site.

CRITICAL VIEW

1. What are the determinants of health associated with teenage pregnancy in your community, your province or territory, and Canada?
2. What programs are available in your community to address these determinants of health?

How To... Recognize Actual or Potential Child Abuse

Be alert to the following:

- An unexplained injury
- Injuries to the skin: burns, old or recent scars, ecchymosis, soft tissue swelling, human bites
- Fractures: recent or older ones that have healed
- Subdural hematomas
- Trauma to genitalia
- Whiplash (caused by shaking small children)
- Dehydration or malnourishment without obvious cause
- Provision of inappropriate food or drugs (alcohol, tobacco, medication prescribed for someone else, foods not appropriate for the child's age)
- Evidence of general poor care: poor hygiene, dirty clothes, unkempt hair, dirty nails
- Unusual fear of CHN and others
- Evidence that child is considered to be a "bad" child
- Inappropriate dress for the season or weather conditions
- Reports or evidence shown by child of sexual abuse
- Injuries not mentioned in history
- Apparent need to take care of the parent and speak for the parent
- Maternal depression
- Maladjustment of older siblings

BOX 11-4 Some Factors That Can Lead to Teenage Pregnancy

- Many teenagers who become pregnant have not used birth control.
- Many teenagers believe erroneously that first-time sex cannot result in pregnancy.
- The earlier the age of sexual activity the less likely the teenager is to have knowledge of and use of birth control.
- Timing (if too late) of school-based sexual health education may contribute to teenage pregnancy.
- Lack of access to services and reproductive health care may be contribute to teenage pregnancy.
- Pressure from peers to be sexually active may contribute to teenage pregnancy.
- Teenagers with a history of sexual abuse are at risk for earlier initiation of voluntary sexual intercourse, are less likely to use birth control, are more likely to use drugs and alcohol at first intercourse, and are more likely to have older sexual partners.
- Teenage pregnancy may be a result of forced sexual intercourse.
- Adolescents raised in lone-parent families are more likely to have intercourse and to give birth than those raised in two-parent families.
- Parenting styles can influence a young woman's risk for early sexual experiences and pregnancy.
- Teenage pregnancy may occur because of poor self-esteem, need for love and belonging, early hormonal changes, and need for independence from the family.
- Media influence may lead to teenage pregnancy, such as high-profile teenagers who are pregnant.
- Conflict in the family, few female friends, and substance abuse by friends and family may contribute to teenage pregnancy.

SOURCE: Adapted from Beckmann Murray, R. (2009). Assessment and health promotion for the adolescent and youth. In R. Beckmann Murray, J. Proctor Zentner, V. Pangman, & C. Pangman (Eds.), *Health promotion strategies through the lifespan* (2nd Canadian ed., pp. 397–453). Toronto: Pearson Prentice Hall.

Early Identification of the Pregnant Teenager

Some teenagers delay seeking pregnancy services because they do not recognize signs such as breast tenderness and a late period. Most young women, however, suspect pregnancy as soon as a period is late. These young women may still delay seeking care since they falsely hope that the pregnancy will just go away. A teenager also may delay seeking care to keep the pregnancy a secret from family members, who may pressure her to terminate the pregnancy, or because she does not want to have a gynecological examination.

Attention needs to be paid to subtle cues that a teenager may offer about sexuality and pregnancy concerns, such as questions about one's fertile period or requests for confirmation that one need not miss a period to be pregnant. Once the CHN identifies the specific concern, information can be provided about how and when to obtain pregnancy testing. The CHN needs to determine how a teenager would react to the possible pregnancy before completing the test. If the test is negative, the CHN needs to take the opportunity to assess whether the young woman would consider birth control counselling to prevent pregnancy. A follow-up visit is important after a negative test to determine if retesting is necessary or if another concern exists.

If the pregnancy test is positive, the CHN needs to refer the pregnant teenager to the family physician or nurse practitioner for a health assessment and pregnancy counselling. Pregnancy counselling usually includes the following:

- Information on adoption, abortion, and child rearing
- Assessment of support systems for the young woman
- Identification of the immediate concerns she might have

Often it is difficult to focus on counselling in any depth at the time of the initial pregnancy testing results. A follow-up visit is usually more productive and should be arranged as soon as possible. A pregnant teenager may be referred to a CHN for follow-up counselling, which could be provided at a public health clinic or school setting. This pregnancy counselling requires that the CHN and young woman explore strengths and weaknesses for personal care and pregnancy options such as abortion, adoption, or parenting the child. If parenting is the choice, the responsibility during a pregnancy and parenting is discussed. Young women vary in their interest in including the partner or their parents in this discussion. Issues to discuss include education and career plans, family finances and qualifications for outside assistance, and personal values about pregnancy and parenting at this time in her life. The CHN needs to ask about violence at each visit because pregnant teenagers are more vulnerable to violence. Violence that begins in pregnancy may continue for several years after, with increasing severity. The CHN needs to observe for physical signs of abuse, as well as for controlling or intrusive partner behaviour. As decisions are made about the course of the pregnancy, the CHN is instrumental in referral to appropriate programs.

CRITICAL VIEW

Explore the Statistics Canada Weblink "Teenage Pregnancy Trends in Canada" on the Evolve Web site. Review this resource and complete the student worksheet within this resource.

1. What did you find useful about this activity?
2. How would you adapt this material for use by CHNs in your community?

CRITICAL VIEW

Visit the *Eating Well with Canada's Food Guide* Web site on Evolve, and answer the following questions:

1. How do the nutritional needs of an adolescent change when she becomes pregnant?
2. a) What are the benefits of taking folic acid during preconception and pregnancy?
   b) How do the folic acid requirements during preconception and pregnancy differ?

The CHN can also begin prenatal education and counselling on nutrition, substance abuse and use, exercise, and special medical concerns.

Special Issues in Caring for the Pregnant Teenager

Community health nursing interventions through education and early identification of concerns may dramatically alter the course of the pregnancy and the birth outcome for pregnant teenagers.

The nutritional needs of a pregnant teenager are especially important. The CHN needs to assess the pregnant teenager's current eating pattern and provide creative guidance to address the issue of the demands of pregnancy on a normally changing teenager's body and a teenager's usual nutritional habits of fast foods and snacking practices. For example, protein can be increased at fast-food establishments by ordering milkshakes instead of soft drinks and broiled chicken sandwiches instead of hamburgers. Healthy snack foods such as granola bars and dried fruits and nuts are suggested. The CHN needs to be familiar with Canada's Food Guide (see the Health Canada *Food and Nutrition* Weblink on the Evolve Web site) and the links to various resources, and needs to discuss nutritional food choices with the pregnant teenager.

Government-funded programs have been developed across Canada to address the nutritional needs of vulnerable women. Some of the programs developed across Canada are Healthy Moms: Healthy Babies, in Whitehorse, Yukon; the *Cap enfants* Family Resource Centre in Wellington, Prince Edward Island; Healthy Baby and Me, in New Brunswick; and BOND—Babies Open New Doors, in Powell River, British Columbia. These programs are similar and include education on a variety of topics related to pregnancy and postpartum issues and child care offered in individual and group sessions. The programs are usually offered to pregnant women under 25 years of age who are considered to be vulnerable based on the determinants of health. These programs are presented under the PHAC project titled "Canada Prenatal Nutrition Program (CPNP)" (see the Weblinks on the Evolve Web site).

The CHN can help prepare the teenager for the transition to motherhood while she is still pregnant—for example, at childbirth education classes. The trend toward early discharge from the hospital has made prenatal preparation even more important. The CHN can enlist the support of the teenager's parents in education about infant care and stimulation. Young fathers-to-be would benefit from this education as well. Adolescents may not know how to communicate with an infant and need help from the CHN to promote mother–neonate attachment. Teenage parents may lack information on neonate and infant growth and development or may have preconceived ideas and unrealistic expectations about their child's development (Beckmann Murray et al., 2009). For example, they may expect that children feed themselves at an early age

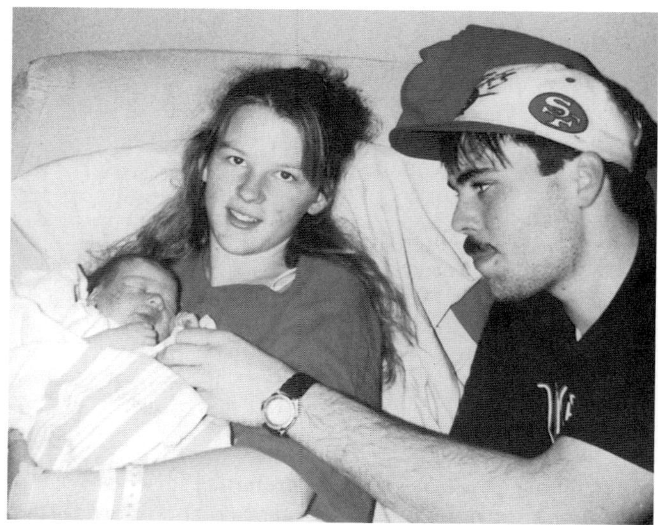

It is important to include both the teenage mother and the father in teaching about child development.

or may think that their child's behaviour is more difficult than what an adult mother might think. These skills can be taught and may prevent the child from later developing academic or behavioural problems.

After the birth of the baby, the CHN needs to observe how the mother responds to infant cues for basic needs and distress. See the PHAC Weblink "First Connections ... Make All the Difference" (on the Evolve Web site) for specific techniques that the new mother can be instructed to use in early child care. This Web site provides information such as behaviours of the infant or child and caregiver that can be observed by the CHN to assess infant attachment and normal infant or child milestones. Within this site, the CHN can access further information for professional use. The CHN could also direct caregivers to this site for information that is directed toward the caregiver on what infant attachment is and how to promote infant attachment. A toll-free help line for caregivers is also included on this site.

The stresses associated with a new role and additional responsibilities of child care can interfere with teenage parents and their ability to concentrate on their school work. There are many community and educational resources that a CHN needs to be familiar with when working in partnership with the school so that teenage mothers are provided with the appropriate supports to achieve school success.

VIOLENCE

Violence is a concern for the CHN. Significant mortality and morbidity result from violence. CHNs often care for the victims, the perpetrators, and those who witness physical and psychological violence. CHNs also can take an active role in the development of community responses to violence by contributing to the development of public policy and needed resources.

Violence is generally defined as those nonaccidental acts, interpersonal or intrapersonal, that result in physical or psychological injury to one or more persons. Violence can be physical, psychological, sexual, financial, or spiritual abuse. In this section, homicides, stalking, bullying, and domestic violence in Canada are discussed.

CRITICAL VIEW

1. What are the resources and supports available in your community for pregnant teenagers?
2. What can CHNs do to promote the use of and compliance with birth control practices?

Homicides and Stalking

The number of homicides in Canada reached a peak in 2005 with 2.04 deaths per 100,000 people (Dauvergne & Li, 2006). Dauvergne and Li (2006) provide the following 2005 Canadian homicide statistics:

- Among provinces, Saskatchewan and Manitoba reported the highest homicide rates, and Prince Edward Island reported no homicides.
- Among cities, Edmonton reported the highest homicide rates, and St. John, Sherbrooke, and Trois-Rivières reported no homicides.
- There was an increase in homicides using firearms.
- Fewer homicides of young children were committed by their parents.
- Slightly fewer spousal homicides occurred.
- There were five times the number of homicides against women than against men.
- There was an increased number of homicides by youth (12 to 17 years of age).

Most frequently, the homicide victim is known to the perpetrator, with approximately one-fifth of homicides committed by a stranger. Statistics Canada (2005) provides the following 2005 Canadian stalking statistics for persons 15 years of age and older:

- About 1.4 million women (11%) reported being stalked to the extent that they feared for their safety or that of someone close to them.
- Approximately 1 million men (7%) reported being stalked to the extent that they feared for their safety or that of someone close to them.
- Nine percent of the women who reported being stalked were stalked by a spouse (current or former) or common-law partner.
- Four percent of the men who reported being stalked were stalked by a spouse (current or former) or common-law partner.

Violent behaviour is predictable and thus preventable, especially with community action. The social determinants of poverty (socioeconomic status), urban crowding (housing), unemployment, and racial inequality (culture) are identified as factors that influence violence. Violence is a major cause of premature mortality and lifelong disability, and violence-related morbidity is a significant factor in health care costs. Further information on violence in children can be found at the United Nations General Assembly Weblink *Report of the Independent Expert for the United Nations Study on Violence Against Children* (on the Evolve Web site). This international report provides the results of an extensive study pertaining to violence against children globally.

Social and Community Factors Influencing Violence

Many factors in a community can support or minimize violence. Changing social conditions, multiple demands on people, economic conditions, and social institutions influence the level of violence and human abuse. The population, community resources, and community facilities can influence the potential for violence.

Population

A community's structure can influence the potential for violence. For example, when people live in crowded conditions and are poor, the potential is greater for community tensions and violence. Communities with a high population density can positively or negatively influence violence. Those with a sense of cohesiveness may have a lower crime rate than areas of similar size that lack social and cultural groups to support unity among members. For example, residents of public housing often form neighbourhood associations to deal with situations common to many or all residents. Tension can often be released in a productive way through projects carried out by the neighbourhood association.

Fear and apathy may cause community residents to withdraw from social contact. Withdrawal can foster crime because many residents assume someone else will report suspicious behaviour, or they fear reprisals for such reports. This tends to happen in larger communities in which the neighbourhood does not lend itself to social interaction and sharing because of highly mobile population patterns and there is an environment that does not promote opportunities for neighbours to interact.

High-population areas may be characterized by a sense of confusion, resulting in disintegration and disorganization. These areas often have transient populations that have limited physical or emotional investment in the community. Lack of community concern allows crime and violence to go unchecked and may become a norm for the area. Also, as crime increases, residents who are able to move leave the area. This increases community disintegration because the residents who leave are often the most capable members of the population.

Community Resources and Facilities

Communities differ in the resources and facilities they provide to residents. Some are more desirable places to live, work, and raise families and have facilities that can reduce the potential for crime and violence. Recreational resources such as playgrounds, parks, swimming pools, movie theatres, tennis courts, basketball courts, walking trails, and bicycle paths provide socially acceptable outlets for a variety of feelings. These resources are adjuncts and residents can use them for pleasure, personal enrichment, and group development. Spectator sports, such as football or hockey, also allow community members to express feelings of anger and frustration. However, viewing physically aggressive sports can encourage a sense of violence as participants hit or shove one another. Familiarity with factors contributing to a community's violence or potential for violence enables CHNs to recognize them and intervene accordingly. It is the CHN's responsibility to work with the citizens and agencies of the community to correct or improve deficits. Factors to be included when assessing a community for violence are shown in Box 11-5.

CRITICAL VIEW

1. What policies and programs are available in your community school to address violence?
2. What are some CHN interventions that could be used in your community to address school violence?

Violence as a Form of Abuse

The potential for violence against individuals or groups (e.g., homicide, robbery, bullying, assault, and sexual assault) or oneself (e.g., suicide) is directly related to the level of violence in the community. Persons living in areas with high rates of crime and violence are more likely to become victims than those in more peaceful areas. The major categories of violence that are most commonly found are homicide and suicide. Homicide was discussed earlier in this chapter; suicide is discussed later. Included next is a discussion of bullying, domestic violence, assault, and sexual assault. Another category, discussed later in this chapter, perceived by some as a violent act, is female genital mutilation.

Bullying

Schools provide many programs to help students learn to deal with violence—for example, classes on bullying and its management, and having a school policy of zero tolerance for violence. Informed parents can assist and support their children to apply what they have learned about handling violence. The incidence of school violence, such as bullying and violent fighting, by school-age children and adolescents has increased (Carter & Stewin, 1999; Joong & Ridler, 2005). There are many forms of bullying such as physical, verbal, social, and electronic bullying, or cyber-bullying. The University of Alberta Weblink on the Evolve Web site provides a PowerPoint presentation on bullying across Canada. See also the Public Safety

BOX 11-5 Indicators of Violence in Individual, Family, and Community Contexts

Individual Factors
- Signs of physical abuse (abrasions, contusions, burns)
- Physical symptoms related to emotional distress
- Developmental and behavioural difficulties
- Presence of physical disability
- Social isolation
- Decreased role performance within the family and in job- or school-related activities
- Mental health concerns such as depression, low self-esteem, and anxiety
- Fear of intimacy with others
- Substance abuse

Familial Factors
- Economic stressors
- Presence of some form of family violence
- Poor communication
- Problems with child-rearing
- Lack of family cohesion
- Recurrent familial conflict
- Lack of social support networks
- Poor social integration into the community
- Multiple changes of residence
- Access to guns
- Homelessness
- Family needs require members to work even though the work may be hated

Community Characteristics
- High crime rate
- High levels of unemployment
- Lack of neighbourhood resources and support systems
- Lack of community cohesiveness
- Media may glamorize or sensationalize violence

Canada Weblink *Bullying Prevention: Nature and Extent of Bullying in Canada* on the Evolve Web site.

The Canadian Teachers' Federation in 2008 adopted a national policy that addresses cyber-conduct and cyber-bullying. Online bullying affects both teachers and students. This unfamiliar milieu for bullying challenges Canadian educators on how to most effectively manage this harmful use of technology. Policy development is a beginning step in curbing cyber-bullying. The policy deals with new and emerging technologies such as cell phones, text messaging, e-mails, blogs, and the use of social network sites such as Facebook (Canadian Teachers' Federation, 2008a).

The Canadian Teachers' Federation conducted a national poll on cyber-bullying and found that 34% of those surveyed in Canada were aware of students in their home community who had been cyber-bullied in the past year, and 20% were aware of teachers who were cyber-bullied (Canadian Teachers' Federation, 2008b). The poll also found that 10% of Canadians surveyed said that they knew someone who was close to them who had experienced cyber-bullying (Canadian Teachers' Federation, 2008b).

Domestic Violence

Domestic violence occurs in children, women, men, same-sex partners, and older adults. It involves any form of real or threatened physical, emotional, or sexual maltreatment and harassment in any relationship that involves intimacy. Approximately 83% of spousal violence victims are females (Statistics Canada, 2009a). The following are some findings according to a 2007 study:

- More serious forms of partner violence are experienced by women.
- Children and youth under the age of 18 years of age were more likely to be assaulted physically or sexually by someone known to them.
- Common assault against older adults accounted for approximately 50% of police-reported family violence.
- Older adult males who experienced family violence most often experienced family violence by their adult children.
- Older adult females who experienced family violence most often experienced family violence by their spouses and their adult children (Statistics Canada, 2009a).

CRITICAL VIEW

1. a) What do you think are the different forms of domestic abuse?
   b) What are the questions that a client might ask a CHN to determine if he or she is in an abusive relationship?
2. What questions would you as a CHN ask a possible victim of abuse to assess if he or she has been or is at risk for abuse?

Explore the Help Guide Weblink on the Evolve Web site, titled "Domestic Violence and Abuse: Signs of Abuse and Abusive Relationships." Review the information presented at this site and compare the information found with your answers.

CHNs need to be alert for signs and symptoms of potential abuse. The Social Services Network manual on elder abuse, *Elder Abuse. See It. Stop It. Prevent It,* is listed in the Weblinks on the Evolve Web site. This resource provides information such as an overview of the different types of elder abuse, and signs, symptoms, and prevention of elder abuse. The information in this document is useful to CHNs as they practise in the community.

There are a variety of risk assessment tools for partner violence. The reason for the assessment should determine which tool to select (Public Safety Canada, 2008). For example, is it to determine a risk assessment of a spousal assault offender, to determine lethality, or to determine spousal assault recidivism? The situation will determine the tool that will be required for the assessment. Recidivism refers to repeat occurrences. The Ontario Domestic Assault Risk Assessment (ODARA) is the first validated domestic-violence risk-assessment tool available to assess the likelihood of wife assault (Government of Ontario, 2007). This 13-question (yes-or-no answer) tool calculates the likelihood of assault based on assaults that are known to police; it can then be used to predict the risk of repeated domestic assault of females by males. The tool compares the male under study with other males who have assaulted their wives. A Likert scale of 0 to 7 ranks the likelihood for repeat domestic assault by the male, with a higher number indicating a greater likelihood of assault. There are two ODARA tools: the ODARA-LE (Ontario Domestic Assault Risk Assessment—Law Enforcement) for police use and the ODARA-C (Ontario Domestic Assault Risk Assessment—Clinical) for use by health professionals.

Family violence that can cause significant injury and death takes the following three forms: sexual abuse, emotional abuse, and physical abuse. These three forms tend to occur together as part of a system of coercive control. Generally, violence within families is perpetrated by the most powerful against the least powerful. Intimate partner violence is directed primarily toward the partner who may be perceived to not be the dominant partner in the relationship (although this partner may fight back physically). Partners can be heterosexual or homosexual.

Assault

In large urban centres, CHNs usually see assaulted persons in home health care with long-term health problems such as head injuries, spinal cord injuries, or stomas from trauma such as motor vehicle accidents or abdominal gunshot wounds. In addition to physical care, CHNs need to address the emotional trauma resulting from the violent attack. This can be done by helping victims talk through their traumatic experience to try to make some sense of the trauma and by referring them for further counselling if anxiety, sleeping problems, or depression persists after the trauma or assault.

Sexual Assault

Often, physically abused women are also being forced into sex. This has implications for the prevention of unintended and adolescent pregnancies, HIV, AIDS, and STIs as well as for women's healthy sexuality and self-esteem. The term *rape* is no longer used in Canada. Instead, according to the Criminal Code of Canada, the term **sexual assault** is used, of which there are the following three levels: sexual assault, sexual assault with a weapon, and aggravated sexual assault. In this text, *sexual assault* is used to refer broadly to all three levels. Sexual assault is one of the most underreported forms of human abuse. The majority of violence against women is intimate partner violence. Sexual assault also happens to men, especially boys and young men, but the statistics on the incidence of male sexual assault vary. It seems reasonable that the emotional trauma for a male sexual assault victim would be at least as serious as that for a woman, but there has been a lack of research in this area.

In the majority of cases, the sexual offenders are known to the victims. Prevention of sexual assault, like that of other forms of human abuse, requires a broad-based community focus for educating both the community as a whole and key groups such as police, health providers, educators, and social workers.

A first step in intervening in the incidence and treatment of sexual assault survivors is to change and clarify misconceptions about sexual assault and the survivors. Sexual assault is a crime of violence, not a crime of passion. The underlying issues are hostility, power, and control rather than sexual desire. The defining issue is lack of consent of the victim. When a woman or man refuses any sexual activity, that refusal means "no." People have the right to change their mind, even when they seemed initially agreeable. Pressure from physical contact, threats, or deliberate inducement of drug or alcohol intoxication is a violation of the law. The myths that women say no to sex when they really mean yes and that the victims of sexual assault are culpable because of the way they dress or act must end. On university and college campuses, negative attitudes toward acquaintance or date rape are slow to change.

During the act of sexual assault, survivors are often hit, kicked, stabbed, and severely beaten. It is this violence, as well as the violation of the sense of self, that most traumatizes people because of the fear for their life and their feelings of helplessness, lack of control, and vulnerability.

People react to sexual assault differently, depending on their personality, past experiences, background, and the support received after the trauma. Some cry, shout, or discuss the experience. Others withdraw and are afraid to discuss the attack. During the immediate as well as follow-up stages, victims tend to blame themselves for what has happened. It is important while working with sexual assault victims to help them identify the issues behind self-blame. Although fault should not be placed on survivors, they should be taught to take control, learn assertiveness, and therefore believe that they can take certain actions to prevent future sexual assaults. Survivors need to talk about what happened and to express their feelings and fears in a nonjudgemental atmosphere. Nonjudgemental listening is important. In any psychological trauma, the right to privacy and confidentiality is crucial. Sexual assault victims should be given privacy, respect, and assurance of confidentiality; told about health care procedures conducted immediately after the sexual assault; and offered a complete physical examination, usually by a sexual assault nurse examiner (SANE). SANEs were discussed in Chapter 3.

CHNs often provide continuous care once a victim enters the health care system. Because many victims deny the sexual assault once the initial crisis is past, a single-session debriefing should be completed during the initial examination. The health assessment and debriefing should be carried out by specially trained providers who have obtained the consent of the victim prior to using the sexual assault evidence kit. In some provinces and territories, nurses trained in sexual assault examination (SANEs) perform the health assessment in the emergency department to gather evidence, usually using a sexual assault kit for criminal prosecution of sexual assault (refer to Chapter 3 for information about this kit). This is an important community health nursing intervention, and it often takes time, which allows the SANE the opportunity to begin communication with the victim. The evidence collected by the SANE is credible and effective in resultant court proceedings. Certain tests should be offered to all sexual assault victims, such as a pregnancy test and tests for STIs. Sexual assault is a situational crisis for which advance preparation is rarely possible. Therefore, CHNs need to help victims cope with the stress and disruption of their lives caused by the attack. Counselling focuses on the crisis and the fears, feelings, and issues involved. CHNs help survivors learn how to regroup personal forces. If post-traumatic stress disorder has developed, professional psychological or psychiatric treatment is indicated.

Many sexual assault victims need follow-up mental health services to help them cope with the short-term and long-term effects of the crisis. The time after a sexual assault is one of disequilibrium, psychological breakdown, and reorganization of attitudes about the safety of the world. Common, everyday tasks often tax a person's resources. Many individuals forget or fail to keep appointments. CHNs need to make appropriate referrals and obtain permission from the sexual assault victim to remain in contact through telephone conversations, which allows for ongoing assessment of the victim's needs and opportunities to intervene when needed. For further information on domestic violence (all forms of abuse), refer to the Government of Canada Weblink *Domestic Violence* on the Evolve Web site. This Web site provides extensive links for sites organized alphabetically according to topic that cover topics related to domestic violence, such as action plans on abuse, the Criminal Code of Canada, abuse and neglect of older adults, battered men, child abuse, emotional abuse, family violence, how to stay safe, neglect, possible indicators of abuse, transition housing, and violence against Aboriginal people.

Suicide

Like mental illness, suicide in present-day society is stigmatizing (Austin & Boyd, 2008). Annually, approximately 3,700 Canadians commit suicide (Health Canada, 2009b). Refer to Table 11-5 for the suicide rates in Canada from 2001 to 2005, which demonstrates the suicide trend in Canada for all age groups. Suicide rates in Canada vary between genders and ages (see Table 11-6); however, suicide occurs in all age groups, cultures, and social classes. Suicide occurs nearly four times more frequently in men than in women; women are more likely to attempt suicide; men more frequently use more lethal methods such as hanging or using firearms while women are more likely to use overdoses or poisoning (Health Canada, 2009b). Suicide is a leading cause of all deaths in Canada; it is the leading cause of death in 25- to 29-year-old men, 40- to 49-year-old men, and 30- to 40-year-old women; and it is the second leading cause of death in 10- to 24-year-old females (Austin & Boyd, 2008). In the 15- to 24-years age group, at least one in five deaths is due to suicide, and approximately 3% of persons 15 years of age and older reported attempted suicide (Health Canada, 2009b). Some Aboriginal communities have reported higher suicide rates than the non-Aboriginal communities (Health Canada, 2009b). Refer to Table 11-7, which shows the number of suicides in Canada from 2002 to 2005 by province and territory.

It is documented that Aboriginal people living in their communities have higher suicide rates than do

TABLE 11-5 Suicides in Canada by Sex and by Age Group from 2001 to 2005

	2001	2002	2003	2004	2005
	Both Sexes Number of Suicides				
All ages[1]	3,692	3,650	3,765	3,613	3,743
10 to 14	27	35	27	28	43
15 to 19	207	215	216	210	213
20 to 24	296	277	306	270	296
25 to 29	288	265	245	275	228
30 to 34	326	325	295	316	283
35 to 39	441	415	434	390	381
40 to 44	452	432	463	409	495
45 to 49	457	437	454	446	476
50 to 54	389	378	404	393	407
55 to 59	258	267	292	275	294
60 to 64	154	174	187	174	166
65 to 69	104	121	142	121	138
70 to 74	125	115	105	108	99
75 to 79	91	83	85	88	113
80 to 84	36	58	53	63	66
85 to 89	30	37	34	36	31
90 and older	11	16	23	11	13

[1]*"All ages" includes suicides of children under age 10 and suicides of persons of unknown age.*

SOURCE: Statistics Canada. (2010). *Suicides and suicide rate, by sex and by age group*. CANSIM, table 102-0551 and Catalogue no. 84F0209X. Retrieved from http://www40.statcan.ca/l01/cst01/hlth66a-eng.htm.

TABLE 11-6 Suicides in Canada by Age Group and Gender

Age	Number of Suicides by Age Group and Gender, Canada, 2005	
	Males	Females
10–14	18	25
15–19	147	66
20–24	231	65
25–29	195	33
30–34	220	63
35–39	296	85
40–44	375	120
45–49	377	99
50–54	293	114
55–59	221	73
60–64	130	36
65–69	105	33
70–74	83	16
75–79	86	27
80–84	47	19
85–89	23	8
90 and older	9	4
All Ages	2,857	886

SOURCES: Statistics Canada. (2010). *Suicides and suicide rate, by sex and by age group—Males* (Catalogue no. 84F0209X). Ottawa, ON. Retrieved from http://www40.statcan.ca/l01/cst01/hlth66b-eng.htm; Statistics Canada. (2010). *Suicides and suicide rate, by sex and by age group—Females* (Catalogue no. 84F0209X). Ottawa, ON. Retrieved from http://www40.statcan.ca/l01/cst01/hlth66c-eng.htm.

people in the rest of Canada (Health Canada, 2009b). Although there is variation among Aboriginal communities, youth suicide rates for First Nations and Inuit Canadians are higher overall than the rest of Canada (Health Canada, 2006a). For example, First Nations youth suicide rates are between five and seven times higher than non-Aboriginal Canadian youth, and Inuit youth suicide rates are eleven times higher than the rest of Canada, with this latter group having the highest suicide rate in the world (Health Canada, 2006a). (For further information on youth suicide and how it should be addressed in First Nations, see the Health Canada—First Nations and Inuit Health Weblink *Acting on What We Know: Preventing Youth Suicide in First Nations*, on the Evolve Web site.) However, it is noted that a few studies of Canadian Aboriginal communities have different findings (Bagley, Wood, & Khumar, 1990; Chandler & Lalonde, 1998). These latter studies of Aboriginal communities have found large regional variations in the rates of suicide, with some Aboriginal communities having minimal to no suicides and others having numbers greatly exceeding the national average. Chandler and Lalonde (1998) identified the following factors as contributing to lower suicide rates in Aboriginal communities in British Columbia: some self-government responsibilities, land claims, and resources such as educational services, police and fire services, health services, and cultural facilities. They propose that having three or more of these factors contributes to reduced suicides in the community. Having some aspects of self-government and land claims implies a feeling of empowerment, which is known to contribute to health promotion. Many

TABLE 11-7 Suicides in Canada, by Province and Territory, from 2002 to 2005

Province	2002	2003	2004	2005
BC	495	450	465	412
AB	443	441	450	412
SK	106	112	111	115
MB	129	165	132	166
ON	947	1038	1021	1115
PQ	1247	1260	1153	1237
NB	97	91	89	101
NS	98	99	90	86
NL	34	48	53	55
PE	14	14	8	13
YK	6	6	6	5
NT	8	10	11	4
NU	25	31	24	20

SOURCE: Statistics Canada. (2009). *Mortality, Summary List of Causes: 2005* (Catalogue no. 84F0209X). Retrieved from http://www.statcan.gc.ca/bsolc/olc-cel/olc-cel?catno=84F0209X&CHROPG=1&lang=eng.

TABLE 11-8 Suicide Risk Factors

Factors	Conditions
Gender	Male
Age	Adolescents Older adults
Marital status	Unmarried men have a greater risk than married men
Employment	Unemployment
History	Previous suicide attempts Family history of suicide
Social	Violence Social seclusion (loneliness) Poverty School troubles Homelessness Loss of a spouse or significant other
Biological and lifestyle	Mental illness, such as mood disorder (major depression); schizophrenia; organic brain syndrome Substance abuse (alcohol use, marijuana use) Homosexuality Physical illness

Canadians take these community supports and resources for granted.

Suicide is tragic because it can often be prevented, and such a loss causes grief for family members and friends. Mental illness and unemployment are two factors that precipitate risk for suicide in men and women (Austin & Boyd, 2008). Table 11-8 shows selected suicide risk factors. See the Health Canada Weblink *Healthy Living: Suicide Prevention* on the Evolve Web site for background information on suicide, factors in suicidal behaviour, and how to minimize the risk.

Many suicides can be prevented by early recognition and interventions. Often there are warning signs prior to suicides and the CHN needs to be aware of these warning signs. The CHN can establish risk, provide early client intervention, and advocate for suicide-prevention programs (Myslik, 2005). Some common warning signs for people at risk for suicide are found in the Registered Nurses' Association of Ontario best-practices guideline for suicide prevention (see the Weblinks on the Evolve Web site). This guideline is an excellent resource for CHNs on the recognition of suicide potential based on risk factors and warning signs, suicide assessment considerations, and interventions to consider. For example, some of the warning signs for suicide are making statements about death, describing methods of harming self, developing a suicide plan, giving possessions away, mood changes, and withdrawal and social isolation (RNAO, 2009). These signs may apply to any person who is at risk for suicide, who has problems with daily interactions such as family relationships, or who is experiencing personal problems. Many available tools are also included and discussed in the RNAO Web site. Warning signs for adolescent suicide ideation could include a loss of interest in usual activities, acting-out behaviours, and unnecessary risk taking.

Despite the widespread use of telephone crisis lines, school-based intervention programs, and antidepressants, high rates of suicide continue. All suicide attempts should be taken seriously. The CHN's goals and some examples are as follows:

- Detect risk factors
- Promote safety (establish suicide contract, supportive environments; decrease access to lethal means)
- Prevent self-harm (identify and discuss risk factors and risk-reduction strategies)
- Make appropriate referrals (support groups, mental health services)
- Help people return to health (empower clients to promote hopefulness)

CRITICAL VIEW

Visit the Statistics Canada Weblink "Suicides and Suicide Rates" on the Evolve Web site. Review this resource and complete the student worksheet located within this resource.

1. Using your findings from completing this activity, what did you find were the differences in this information compared to the most recent Statistics Canada data?
2. How would you update and adapt this material for use by CHNs in your community?

At a community level, CHNs need to be involved in a coordinated response to the prevention of suicide and the care of those who have attempted suicide. In their roles in community health nursing, CHNs need to be involved in the development of policies and protocols for suicide prevention across the lifespan. Community health nursing care may focus on family members and friends of suicide victims. Survivors often feel anger toward the dead person, yet frequently turn the anger inward. Likewise, survivors often question their own liability for the death. The impact of suicide can affect family, friends, co-workers, and the community. Beyond the anger some survivors feel, they and others may have difficulty dealing with their feelings toward the dead person. They may have difficulty concentrating and may limit their social activities because it is difficult for both survivors and their friends to talk about the suicide. CHNs help survivors cope with the trauma of the loss and make referrals to a counsellor or support group. Suicide affects the community. For information on community assessment, planning, and implementation considerations in First Nations communities, see the Health Canada tool kit listed in the Toolbox on the Evolve Web site. This tool kit was prepared to assist First Nations Peoples address suicide in their communities.

Female Genital Mutilation

Female genital mutilation (FGM) is common in many African countries and certain Asian and Middle Eastern countries. Global prevalence rates vary; for example, it is estimated to be as widespread as 97% usage in Egypt, 90% in North Sudan, 71% in Mauritius, 23% in Yemen, and 5% in Ghana (UNICEF, 2005). FGM is a practice that is centuries old. Banned in the early 1990s in Somalia, FGM is now at an all-time high in that country because of its preoccupation with civil war. Justification for FGM is related to tradition, power inequities, and the compliance of women to community norms or law (WHO, 2010). In countries where this act of violence is practised against women, it is considered to be an important part of a woman's access to marriage and child-bearing.

FGM can take several forms, ranging from the excision of the clitoris with partial or total removal of the labia minora to the severe form, in which the labia majora are fused following the removal of the clitoris and labia minora (WHO, 2010). These procedures are associated with morbidity related to substantial complications such as severe pain, hemorrhage, infection, tetanus, and septicemia. Long-term effects of FGM include impaired urinary and menstrual functioning, chronic genital pain, cysts, risk of childbirth complication and newborn deaths, urinary incontinence, and infertility (WHO, 2010). Increasingly, women who have been mutilated are immigrating to Canada, mostly residing in urban centres. This procedure is illegal in Canada and other developed countries such as France and the United States (UNICEF, 2005). CHNs need to be familiar with the practices of immigrants in their communities. For further information, see the WHO and UNICEF Weblinks on female genital mutilation, found on the Evolve Web site.

COMMUNITY HEALTH NURSING PROCESS USED WITH VULNERABLE CLIENTS

CHNs who work with specific populations requiring socioeconomic considerations need well-developed assessment skills, current knowledge of available resources, and the ability to plan care based on client concerns and receptivity to help. They also need to be able to show respect for the client. The CHN needs to assess the *living environment* and *neighbourhood surroundings* of vulnerable families and groups for environmental hazards such as lead-based paint, asbestos, water and air quality, industrial wastes, and the incidence of crime. Working with community leaders, CHNs are able to assess community strengths and assets, identify any limitations with a health plan, and identify what will be required to address client concerns.

Because members of vulnerable populations often experience multiple stressors, assessment must balance the need to be comprehensive with a focus on only the information that a CHN needs and that the client is willing to provide. The CHN needs to include questions about the client's perceptions of his or her *socioeconomic resources,* including identifying people who can provide support and financial resources. Support from other people may include caregiving, emotional support, and

LEVELS OF PREVENTION

Related to Vulnerable Populations

PRIMARY PREVENTION

Community health nurses (CHNs) provide influenza and pneumococcal vaccinations to vulnerable populations such as clients with human immunodeficiency virus or acquired immunodeficiency syndrome, who are immunocompromised (unless contraindicated), or vulnerable populations prone to communicable diseases.

SECONDARY PREVENTION

CHNs conduct screening clinics for vulnerable populations. For example, CHNs who work in homeless shelters, prisons, and substance-abuse treatment facilities need to know that these groups are at high risk for acquiring communicable diseases. For example, both clients and staff need routine screening for TB.

TERTIARY PREVENTION

- CHNs refer severely mentally ill adults to a therapy group.
- CHNs work with abused women to help them enhance their levels of self-esteem.
- CHNs advocate for rehabilitation and recovery services for vulnerable populations.

help with instrumental activities of daily living, such as transportation, shopping, and babysitting. Financial resources may include the extent to which the client can pay for any additional health services and medications, as well as questions about eligibility for third-party payment. The CHN needs to ask the client about the perceived adequacy of both formal and informal support networks.

Vulnerable populations need to be assessed for *congenital* and *genetic predisposition* to illness and either receive education and counselling as appropriate or be referred to other health professionals as necessary. For example, pregnant adolescents who are substance abusers need to be referred to programs to help them quit using addictive substances during their pregnancy and, ideally, after delivery of their infant as well. Pregnant women older than 35 years need to be encouraged to consider amniocentesis testing to determine if genetic abnormalities exist in their fetus.

When necessary, assessment may include evaluation of a client's *preventive health needs,* including age-appropriate screening tests, such as immunization status,

CRITICAL VIEW

1. What screening tests are conducted by the CHN in your province or territory?
2. What referrals will be necessary for the screening tests not conducted by the CHN, and how are these arranged?

blood pressure, weight, serum cholesterol, Papanicolaou smears, breast examinations, mammograms, prostate examinations, glaucoma screening, and dental evaluations. It may be necessary to make referrals to have some of these tests done for clients.

The CHN needs to assess also for the amount of *stress* the person or family is having. Does the family have healthy coping skills and family interaction? Are some family members able and willing to care for others? What is the level of mental health in each member? Also, are diet, exercise, and rest and sleep patterns conducive to good health?

In some situations, the CHN works with individual clients. The CHN also develops programs and policies for vulnerable populations. In both examples, planning and implementing care for members of vulnerable populations involve partnerships between the CHN and the client. CHNs who direct and control the client's care cannot establish a trusting relationship and may inadvertently foster a cycle of dependency and lack of personal health control. In fact, the most important initial step is for CHNs to establish that they are trustworthy and dependable. For example, CHNs working in a community clinic for substance abusers must overcome any suspicion that clients may have of them and eliminate any fears clients may have of being manipulated.

The relationship with the client depends on the nature of the contact. Some are seen in clinics, others in homes, in schools, and at work. Regardless of the setting, the following key community health nursing actions need to be used:

- *Create a trusting environment.* Trust is essential since many of these individuals have previously been disappointed in their interactions with health care and social systems. It is important to follow through and do what you say you are going to do. If you do not know the answer to a question, the best reply is "I do not know, but I will try to find out."
- *Show respect, compassion, and concern.* Vulnerable persons have been defeated again and again by life's circumstances. They may have reached a point where they question if they even deserve to get care.

Listen carefully, since listening is a form of respect as well as a way to gather information to plan care.

- *Do not make assumptions.* Assess each person and family. No two people or groups are alike.
- *Coordinate services and providers.* Getting health and social services is not always easy. Often clients feel like they are travelling through a maze. In most communities, a large number of useful services exist. Clients who need them may simply not know how to find them. For example, clients may need help finding a food bank or a free clinic or obtaining low-cost or free clothing through churches or in second-hand stores. Clients often need help determining if they meet the eligibility requirements. If gaps in service are found, CHNs can work with others to try to get the needed services established.
- *Advocate for accessible health care services.* Vulnerable clients have trouble getting access to services. Neighbourhood clinics, mobile vans, and home visits can be valuable for them. Also, coordinating services at a central location is helpful. These multiservice centres can provide health care, social services, daycare, drug and alcohol recovery programs, and case management. When working with vulnerable populations, it is a good idea to arrange to have as many services as possible available in a single location and at convenient times. This "one-stop shopping" approach to care delivery is helpful for populations experiencing multiple social, economic, and health-related stresses.
- *Focus on prevention.* Use every opportunity to teach about preventive health care. Primary prevention may include child and adult immunization and education about nutrition, foot care, safer sex, contraception, and the prevention of injuries or chronic illness. It may also include providing prophylactic anti-TB drug therapy for HIV-positive clients who live in homeless shelters or giving the influenza vaccine to people who are immunocompromised or adults older than 65 years. Secondary prevention would include screening for health problems such as TB, diabetes, hypertension, foot problems, anemia, drug use, or abuse.
- *Know when to "walk beside" the client and when to encourage the client to "walk ahead."* At times it is hard to know when to do something for clients and when to teach or encourage them to do it for themselves. Community health nursing actions range from providing encouragement and support to providing information and active intervention. It is important to assess for the presence of strength and the ability to problem-solve, cope, and access services. For example, CHNs may provide information and encouragement to clients about immunization and influenza clinics and schedule the clinics at varying times and places in the community that are easy to access. It is then up to the client to access these clinics to acquire the intervention.
- *Know what resources are available.* It is important to be familiar with community agencies that offer health and social services to vulnerable populations. Also, follow up after you make a referral to ensure the client was able to obtain the needed help. Examples of agencies found in most communities are health units or authorities, community mental health centres, voluntary organizations such as the Canadian Red Cross, missions, shelters, soup kitchens, food banks, nurse-managed or free clinics, social service agencies such as the Salvation Army, and church-sponsored health and social services.
- *Develop your own support network.* Working with vulnerable populations can be challenging, rewarding, and at times exhausting. CHNs need to find their sources of support and strength. This can come from friends, colleagues, hobbies, exercise, poetry, music, and other sources.

In addition to the community health nursing actions described, the "How To ... Intervene with Vulnerable Clients" box summarizes goals, interventions, and evaluating outcomes with vulnerable populations. In general, more agencies are needed that provide comprehensive services with nonrestrictive eligibility requirements. Communities often have many agencies that restrict eligibility to make it difficult for more people to receive services. For example, shelters may prohibit people who have been drinking alcohol from staying overnight and sometimes limit the number of sequential nights a person can stay. Food banks usually limit the number of times a person can receive free food. Agencies are often specialized as well. This means that vulnerable individuals and families must go to several agencies to obtain services for which they qualify and that meet their health concerns. This is tiring and discouraging, and people may forgo help because of these difficulties, which also include the added expense of travel.

ROLES OF THE COMMUNITY HEALTH NURSE WORKING WITH VULNERABLE CLIENTS

As discussed in Chapter 3, CHNs fulfill a variety of roles. CHNs need to know about community agencies that offer various health and social services. It is important

How To... Intervene with Vulnerable Clients

Goals

- Set reasonable goals that are based on the baseline data you collected. Focus on reducing disparities in health status among vulnerable populations.
- Work toward setting manageable goals with the client. Goals that seem unattainable may be discouraging.
- Set goals collaboratively with the client as a first step toward client empowerment.
- Set family-centred, culturally sensitive goals.

Interventions

- Set up outreach and case-finding programs to help increase access to health services by vulnerable populations.
- Do everything you can to minimize the "hassle factor" connected with the interventions planned. Vulnerable groups do not have the extra energy, money, or time to cope with unnecessary waits, complicated treatment plans, or confusion. CHNs, as an advocate for clients, need to identify what hassles may occur and develop ways to avoid them. For example, this may include providing comprehensive services during a single encounter, rather than asking the client to return for multiple visits. Multiple visits for more specialized aspects of the health concerns of a client, whether individual or family group, reinforce a perception that health care is fragmented and organized for the professional's convenience rather than the client's.
- Work with clients to ensure that interventions are culturally sensitive and competent.
- Focus on teaching clients skills in health promotion and disease prevention. Also, teach them how to be effective health care consumers. For example, role-play with a client on how to ask questions when in a physician's office or with other health care professionals.
- Help clients learn what to do if they cannot keep an appointment with a health care or social service professional.

Outcomes

- It is often difficult for vulnerable clients to return for follow-up care. Help clients develop self-care strategies for evaluating outcomes. For example, teach homeless clients the signs and symptoms of infection and intervention strategies they can use or when to seek additional assistance.
- Remember to evaluate outcomes in terms of the goals you have mutually agreed on with the client. For example, one outcome for a homeless person receiving isoniazid therapy for TB might be that the person return to the clinic daily for direct observation of compliance with the drug therapy.

also that they follow up with the client after a referral to ensure that the desired outcomes were achieved. Sometimes, excellent community resources may be available but impractical because of transportation or other access issues. CHNs need to identify these potential concerns by following through with referrals, and they can also work with other team members to make referrals as convenient and realistic as possible. Although clients with social problems such as financial needs should be referred to social workers, it is useful for CHNs to understand the close connections between health and social problems and to know how to work effectively with other professionals. A list of community resources can often by found in the telephone directory, and many communities publish these lists and have the resources online. The following are examples of agency resources found in most communities:

- Health units or health authorities
- Community mental health centres
- Canadian Red Cross and other voluntary organizations
- Food and clothing banks
- Missions and shelters
- Nurse-managed neighbourhood clinics
- Social service agencies such as the Salvation Army
- Church-sponsored assistance

Specific populations are often resourceful and creative in managing multiple stressors. CHNs work with clients to help them identify and draw on their own strengths when managing their health concerns. Also, clients may be able to depend on informal support networks. Even though social isolation is a health concern for many vulnerable clients, CHNs should not assume that they have no one who can or will help them.

Case management involves linking clients with services and providing direct community health nursing services, including teaching, counselling, screening, and immunizing. Linking health services is accomplished by making appropriate referrals and by following up with clients to ensure that the desired outcomes from the referral were achieved. See the box "How To ...Coordinate Health and Social Services for Members of Vulnerable Populations." CHNs are effective case managers in community nursing clinics, health departments, hospitals, and various other health care agencies. They emphasize health promotion and illness prevention with vulnerable clients and focus on helping them avoid unnecessary hospitalization.

As can be seen, many of these community health nursing actions are in the realm of case management, in which the CHN makes referrals and links clients with other community services. In the case manager role, the CHN often is an advocate for the client or family. The CHN serves as an advocate when referring clients to other agencies, when working with others to develop health programs, and when trying to influence legislation and health policies that affect vulnerable population groups. Referring clients to community agencies involves much more than simply making a phone call or completing a form. CHNs need to ensure that the agency to which they refer clients is the right one to meet the clients' concerns. CHNs can do more harm than good by referring stressed, discouraged clients to an agency from which they are not really eligible to receive services. See the box "How To... Use Case Management in Working with Vulnerable Populations." The CHN helps clients learn how to get the most from the referral by working with the clients to ensure that the necessary information about their health concern is written out in chronological order, including any health assessments and other relevant client information.

It is helpful to provide comprehensive services in locations where people live and work, including schools, churches, neighbourhoods, and workplaces. **Comprehensive services** are health services that focus on more than one health concern. For example, some CHNs use mobile outreach clinics to provide a wide

How To... Coordinate Health and Social Services for Members of Vulnerable Populations

Community health nurses who work with vulnerable populations often need to coordinate services across several agencies for members of these groups. It is helpful to have a strong professional network of people who work in other agencies. Effective professional networks make it easier to coordinate care smoothly and in ways that do not add to clients' stress. Community health nurses can develop strong networks by participating in community coalitions and attending professional meetings. When one is making referrals to other agencies, a phone call can be a helpful way to obtain information that clients will need for the visit. When possible, having an interdisciplinary, interagency team plan of care for clients at high risk for health problems can be quite effective. It is crucial to obtain clients' written and informed consent before engaging in this kind of planning because of confidentiality issues. The following list of tips can be helpful:

- Be sure to involve clients in making decisions about the kinds of services they will find beneficial and can use.
- Work with community coalitions to develop plans for service coordination for targeted vulnerable populations.
- Collaborate with legal counsel from the agencies involved in the coalitions to ensure that legal and ethical issues related to care coordination have been properly addressed. Examples of issues to address include privacy and security of clinical data.
- Develop policies and protocols for making referrals, following up on referrals, and ensuring that clients receiving care from several agencies experience the process as smooth and seamless.

How To... Use Case Management in Working with Vulnerable Populations

- Know available services and resources.
- Find out what is missing; look for creative solutions.
- Use your clinical skills.
- Develop long-term relationships with the families you serve.
- Strengthen the family's coping and survival skills and resourcefulness.
- Be the road map that guides the family to services and help them get the services.
- Communicate with the family and the agencies that can help them.
- Work to change the environment and the policies that affect your clients.

array of health promotion, illness prevention, and illness management services to geographically remote areas. A single client visit may focus on an acute health concern such as influenza, but it may also include health education about diet and exercise, counselling for smoking cessation, and a follow-up appointment for immunizations once the influenza is over. The shift away from hospital-based care includes a renewed commitment to the health services that vulnerable populations need to prevent illness and promote health, such as the reduction of environmental hazards and violence and assurance of safe food and water.

Some examples of care to clients, families, and groups follow: (1) a CHN in a mobile clinic might administer a tetanus booster to a client who has been injured by a piece of farm machinery and may also check the client's blood pressure during the same visit; (2) a home health nurse seeing a family referred by the courts for child abuse might weigh the child, conduct a nutritional assessment, and help the family learn how to manage anger and disciplinary problems; (3) a public health nurse working in a school might lead a support group for pregnant adolescents and conduct a birthing class; and (4) public health nurses working with clients in the community being treated for TB might monitor drug treatment compliance to ensure that clients complete their full course of therapy.

CHNs focus also on advocacy and social justice concerns. CHNs may function as advocates for vulnerable populations by working for the passage and implementation of policies that lead to improved public health services for these populations. For example, one CHN may serve on a local coalition for homeless uninsured people, and another may work to develop a plan for sharing the provision of free or low-cost dental health care by local health care organizations and providers. CHNs who function in advocacy roles and facilitate change in public policy are intervening to promote social justice. CHNs need to be advocates for policy changes to improve social, economic, and environmental factors that predispose populations to poor health.

CHNs have a critical role in the delivery of health care to poor, homeless, mentally ill, and other high-risk populations. To be effective, CHNs need strong physical and psychosocial assessment skills, current knowledge of available resources, and an ability to convey respect, dignity, and value to each person. CHNs need to be able to work with their clients to prevent illness and promote, maintain, and restore health. CHNs need to be prepared to look at the whole picture (upstream thinking): the person, the family, and the community interacting with the environment. The assessment may take place in the home or in a community site. Visiting in the home provides a great deal of useful information about the family, its resources, support systems, and knowledge of common housekeeping and health issues. For example, the CHN needs to assess for the adequacy of heating and cooling, water supply, cleanliness, cooking facilities, food storage, sleeping arrangements, and safety issues such as loose rugs, fire extinguishers, and fire alarms.

CHNs working with vulnerable populations may fill numerous roles (including those listed in Box 11-6):

- Identify vulnerable individuals and families through outreach and case finding
- Encourage vulnerable groups to obtain health services
- Develop community programs that respond to client health concerns
- Teach vulnerable individuals, families, and groups strategies to prevent illness and promote health
- Counsel clients about ways to increase their sense of personal power and help them identify strengths and resources
- Direct care to clients and families in a variety of settings, including storefront clinics, mobile clinics, shelters, homes, neighbourhoods, worksites, churches, and schools
- Serve as population health advocates

BOX 11-6 Community Health Nurse Roles When Working with Vulnerable Clients

- Case finder
- Health educator
- Counsellor
- Direct-care provider
- Population health advocate
- Community assessor and developer
- Monitor and evaluator of care
- Case manager
- Advocate
- Health program planner
- Participant in developing health policies

- Work with local, provincial or territorial, or federal groups to develop and implement healthy public policy
- Collaborate with other community members and serve as community assessors and developers; monitor and evaluate care and health programs
- Function as case managers for vulnerable clients, making referrals and linking them with community services
- Serve as advocates when they refer clients to other agencies
- Work with others to develop health programs
- Influence legislation and health policies that affect vulnerable populations

The nature of a CHN's roles varies depending on whether a client is a single person, family, group, community, or population. For example, a CHN might teach an HIV-positive client about the need for prevention of opportunistic infections, may help a family with an HIV-positive member understand myths about the transmission of HIV, may work with a community group concerned about HIV transmission among students in the schools, and may work with the community to identify priorities for action to prevent and reduce transmission of HIV. In each case, the CHN teaches how to prevent infectious and communicable disease and considers that the size of the group and the teaching methods will differ for each group.

Health education is often used in working with vulnerable populations. The CHN needs to teach members of populations with low educational levels what they need to do to promote health and prevent illness rather than directing health education to groups that the CHN *thinks* might be at high risk, despite the fact that there is no evidence to support the perception. A new concern for CHNs is whether the populations with whom they work have adequate health literacy to benefit from health education. It may be necessary to collaborate with a health educator, an interpreter or translator, or an expert in health communications to design messages that vulnerable populations can understand and use.

It is important for CHNs to understand the three levels of prevention and health promotion related to vulnerable populations (see the "Levels of Prevention" box related to vulnerable populations, on p. 347). Most importantly, CHNs need to consider the determinants of health in all program planning and health care interventions organized using knowledge of the health disparities of the vulnerable. CHNs need to influence political and social policies and programs such as affordable housing, community outreach services, preventive health services, and other assistance programs for their clients.

CRITICAL VIEW

1. Which Canadian Community Health Nursing Standards of Practice apply when working with vulnerable populations?
2. What can CHNs do to affect the determinants of health for vulnerable clients within the identified Standards of Practice?

Levels of Prevention and the CHN

Primary preventive services include affordable housing, housing subsidies, effective job-training programs, employer incentives, preventive health care services, multisystem case management, birth control services, safer-sex education, needle-exchange programs, parent education, and counselling programs. As a primary prevention for mental health problems, CHNs provide education about stress-reduction techniques to older adults attending a health fair. They also form networks with other health professionals to educate policy makers and the public about the value of these preventive services. These programs could provide health education and other forms of care to strengthen community residents and consequently prevent many devastating sequelae.

Secondary preventive activities are aimed at reducing the prevalence or pathological nature of a condition. They involve early diagnosis, prompt treatment, and the limitation of disability. For example, these services might target those on the verge of becoming high risk because of the threat of homelessness, as well as those who are newly homeless. Examples include supportive and emergency housing, targeted case management, housing subsidies, soup kitchens and meal sites, and comprehensive physical and mental health services. CHNs can work with homeless and near-homeless aggregates to provide education about existing services and strategies for influencing public policy that will provide more comprehensive services for homeless and near-homeless persons.

Tertiary prevention efforts attempt to restore and enhance functioning and reduce disabilities. On a community level, these might include the support of affordable housing, promotion of psychosocial rehabilitation programs, and involvement in advocacy groups for the mentally ill or homeless population. Tertiary prevention of homelessness includes comprehensive case management, physical and mental health services, emergency-shelter housing, needle-exchange programs, and drug and alcohol treatment. It is important to know about the social and political environments in which problems occur. CHNs need to influence politicians and other policy makers at the federal, provincial and territorial, and local levels about the plight of vulnerable populations in their community.

The old saying "All men [and women] are created equal" is really not true. People have different genetic compositions, social and environmental resources, skills, and access to health services. People with lower incomes and less education tend to be at higher risk for health problems. Health initiatives need to focus on the elimination of health disparities by expanding access to health care for vulnerable or at-risk populations. The determinants of health need to be addressed before the health of vulnerable populations in Canada can be improved.

STUDENT EXPERIENCE

STELLA'S STORY

Why is Stella in the psychiatric unit?

Because she slashed her wrists.

Why did she slash her wrists?

Because she does not want to live.

Why doesn't she want to live?

Because she feels hopeless.

Why does she feel hopeless?

Because social services took her children away.

Why did they take her children away?

Because she cannot feed and clothe her children.

Why can't she feed and clothe her children?

Because what little she gets from welfare she spends on alcohol and drugs.

Why does she spend her money on alcohol and drugs?

Because she needs to escape the reality of her own childhood memories.

Why does she need to escape her childhood memories?

Because she was taken away from her family and was put into a residential school.

Why was she put in a residential school and taken from her family?

Because the government made it a policy to assimilate and destroy Aboriginal culture.

But why?

Although Stella is a fictionalized character, she represents the experience of thousands of Aboriginal people in Canada who suffered trauma as a direct result of forced education through the residential schools.

1. So what does our health care system do with people like Stella?
2. Why is knowing the history of Aboriginal people in Canada helpful in understanding Stella and her situation?
3. What should be a CHN approach in helping Stella?

SOURCE: Dutcher, L. (2006). *Nursing leadership: Providing cultural competent care to Aboriginal people.* Unpublished paper for the University of New Brunswick.

REMEMBER THIS!

- All countries have population subgroups that are more vulnerable to health threats than the general population.
- Vulnerable populations are more sensitive to risk factors than those who are more resilient since they are often exposed to cumulative risk factors. These populations include the poor, the homeless, immigrants, refugees, Aboriginal peoples, the disabled, persons with stigmatizing conditions (physical and mental disabilities, mental illness, substance abuse), the elderly (older adults), children and youth in disadvantaged conditions, persons with low literacy skills, women (particularly those in unsafe situations), gays, lesbians, bisexuals, and transgendered people.
- Poverty has a direct effect on health and well-being across the lifespan. Poor people have higher rates of chronic illness and infant morbidity and mortality, a shorter life expectancy, and more complex health problems.
- Mental health care is increasingly moving into the community. This began with deinstitutionalization of the severely mentally ill population and is continuing today as hospitals reduce in-patient stays. Vulnerable populations need a wide variety of services, and because these are often provided by several community agencies, CHNs coordinate and manage the service needs of vulnerable groups.
- Socioeconomic problems, including poverty and social isolation, physiological and developmental aspects of age, poor health status, and highly stressful life experiences, predispose people to vulnerability. Vulnerability can become a cycle, where the predisposing factors lead to poor health outcomes, chronic stress, and hopelessness. These outcomes increase vulnerability.
- CHNs assess vulnerable individuals, group aggregates, families, populations, and communities to determine which socioeconomic, physical, biological, psychological, and environmental factors are problematic for clients. They work as partners with vulnerable clients to identify client strengths, assets, and health concerns and to develop intervention strategies designed to break the cycle of vulnerability.
- At present, the following populations often constitute the homeless in both rural and urban areas: families, single mothers and their children, single women, recently unemployed persons, substance abusers, adolescent runaways, mentally ill individuals, and single men.
- Factors contributing to homelessness include an increase in the number of persons living in poverty, diminishing availability of low-cost housing, increased unemployment, substance abuse, a lack of treatment facilities for mentally ill individuals, domestic violence, and family situations causing children, youth, and women to run away.
- The complex health concerns of homeless persons include the inability to get adequate rest, exercise, and nutrition; environmental exposure; infectious diseases; acute and chronic illnesses; infestations; trauma; and mental health concerns.
- Factors such as a history of sexual victimization, family dysfunction, substance use, and failure to use birth control can influence whether a young woman becomes pregnant.
- Adolescents, especially those who become pregnant, have special nutritional needs.
- The pregnant teenager will need support during and after the pregnancy from family and friends, from the father of the baby, and from health professionals such as CHNs.
- Incidence rates and prevalence rates for mental health problems are very high, and people are at risk for threats to mental health at all ages across the lifespan.
- Low-income and minority groups are often at an increased risk for mental illness because they frequently lack access to services.
- CHNs have a critical role in the delivery of care to persons who are high risk. CHNs bring to each client encounter the ability to assess the client in context and to intervene in ways to prevent, restore, maintain, or promote health.
- Substance abuse is a major community health concern, linked to numerous forms of morbidity and mortality.
- Harm reduction is an approach to ATOD problems; it deals with substance abuse primarily as a health concern rather than as a criminal problem.
- Social conditions such as a fast-paced life, excessive stress, and the availability of drugs influence the incidence of substance abuse.
- Important terms to understand when working with individuals, groups, or communities for whom substance abuse is prevalent are *drug dependence, drug addiction, alcoholism, psychoactive drugs, depressants, stimulants, marijuana, hallucinogens,* and *inhalants.*

- Health promotion for substance abuse includes education about drugs and guidelines for use as well as the promotion of healthy alternatives to drug use, whether for recreation or to relieve stress.
- CHNs need to play a key role in developing drug-abuse community-prevention programs for the community.
- Secondary prevention depends heavily on a careful assessment of a client's use of drugs. This should be part of all basic health assessments.
- Substance abuse is often a family and community concern, not merely an individual concern.
- *Codependency* describes a companion illness to the addiction of one person in which the codependent member is addicted to the addicted person.
- CHNs are in ideal roles to assist with tertiary prevention for both addicted individuals and their family and work with the community to establish and support programs.

REFLECTIVE PRAXIS

Case Study 1*

Nina lives with her children—a daughter, 12; a son, 5; and infant twin girls—and her common-law husband, Gerry, in subsidized housing. The public health nurse (PHN), Anna-Rosa, has been impressed with Nina's friendliness and confidence despite the many challenges she faces, including uncontrolled diabetes, chronic fatigue syndrome, and, now, a prolapsed uterus. Nina's 12-year-old daughter has recently been diagnosed with attention deficit hyperactivity disorder, depression, and a hearing deficit. At age 5, the son has not learned his letters or numbers. Neither adult has a job right now; finances are very tight. They cannot afford a phone, and often they run out of diapers. Nina's family lives close by and provides some help when they can.

Anna-Rosa began working with this family because one twin was diagnosed with failure to thrive at her 6-month checkup. A priority was to determine if there was enough food in the home and why one twin was so much smaller than the other. The PHN needed to communicate her compassion for the family by listening carefully when taking histories on each family member. She needed to show concern and care by monitoring the smaller twin's growth and development each week. In addition, it was a priority to improve Nina's health so that she could take care of her children and herself in the future.

Anna-Rosa's interventions included assessing Nina's blood sugar level and the family's diet at each visit. Referral to a local food bank was necessary on occasion. Anna-Rosa helped Nina with careful diet planning for the whole family. Also, Anna-Rosa found local tutoring programs to help the older children with their learning needs and arranged for hearing aids for the older girl, as well as visits to a psychiatrist to treat her depression. Anna-Rosa found an infant development program to bring support workers into the home and to show Nina how to stimulate the twins' normal development. When summer approached, Anna-Rosa found community children's programs that would provide the older two children with some learning opportunities and supervision while Nina recuperated from the scheduled hysterectomy to repair her prolapsed uterus. Anna-Rosa showed Nina and Gerry materials to assist them to be more qualified for jobs.

1. Identify strengths in this family.
2. Based on this client situation, which actions by the PHN relate to the Canadian Community Health Nursing Standards of Practice (see Appendix 1)?

Answers are on the Evolve Web site at http://evolve.elsevier.com/Canada/Stanhope/community/.

Case Study 2

Sally, a 46-year-old farm worker pregnant with her fifth child, has come to the clinic requesting treatment for swollen ankles. During your assessment, you learned that she had seen the primary health care nurse practitioner (PHC-NP) at the local health unit 2 months ago. The PHC-NP gave her some sample vitamins, but Sally lost them. She has not received regular prenatal care and has no plans to do so. Her previous pregnancies were essentially normal, although she said she was "toxic" with her last child. She also said that her middle child was "not quite right." He is in grade 7 at age 15. Sally is 157 cm (5 ft. 2 in.) tall, weighs 81.6 kg (180 lb.), and has a blood pressure of 160/90. She has pitting edema of the ankles and a mild headache.

Sally says that she usually takes chlorpromazine hydrochloride (Thorazine) but has run out of it and cannot afford to have her prescription refilled. She says that she has been a client in several mental hospitals in the past and that she has become more agitated and now has problems managing her daily activities. As her agitation grows, she says that she usually hears voices and this really makes her aggressive.

*This case study was originally created by Deborah C. Conway and adapted by the Canadian authors.

None of Sally's children live with her, and she has no plans for taking care of the infant. She thinks she will ask the child's father, a truck driver, to help her since she usually travels around the country with him.

1. What additional information do you need to help you adequately assess Sally's health status and current needs?
2. What community health nursing activities would you suggest, given her history, physical examination, and psychological descriptions?

Answers are on the Evolve Web site at http://evolve.elsevier.com/Canada/Stanhope/community/.

Case Study 3

A local agency for youth requested the assistance of Kristen, a CHN, in the implementation of a new high school–based program for pregnant and teenage girls who are parents. The primary goal of the program is to keep these teenagers in school through graduation. The secondary goal is to provide knowledge and skills about healthy pregnancy, labour and delivery, and parenting. After delivery, students enrolled in this program were paid for school attendance; this money could be used to defray the costs of child care.

A CHN was the ideal choice to conduct the educational sessions. The group met weekly during the lunch hour. The curriculum that was developed had topics from early pregnancy through the toddler years. Occasionally, Kristen brought in outside speakers such as a labour and delivery nurse or an early intervention specialist.

Kristen also met individually with each enrolled student to provide case management services. Ideally, she would ensure that each student had a health care provider for prenatal care, that each was visited at home by a CHN, and that both the pregnant teenager and her partner knew about other parenting and support groups.

One educational session that was particularly interesting was the discussion about the postpartum course—provided 6 weeks after delivery. There were many lively discussions about labour experiences, as well as some emotional discussions about the reality of coming home with a baby and changes in the relationship with their male partner. Many girls benefited from understanding the normalcy of postpartum blues, but one young woman recognized that she had a more serious and persistent depression and privately approached Kristen for assistance.

At the end of the first school year, the dropout rate for pregnant and parenting teenagers had been reduced by half and preterm labour rates had also declined. The local school board and a local agency serving youth joined together to provide financial support to continue this program for an additional 2 years. Kristen was asked to expand the educational programs and interventions she had developed.

1. What are some directions in which Kristen might expand the program? List four.

Answers are on the Evolve Web site at http://evolve.elsevier.com/Canada/Stanhope/community/.

Case Study 4

Janiz, a CHN, is a home health case manager in a large, low-income housing area in her local community. She designs care plans and coordinates health care services for clients who need health care at home. She makes the initial visits to determine the level and frequency of care needed and then acts as supervisor of the volunteers and health care workers who perform most of the day-to-day care. One-parent families are the norm, and drug dealing is commonplace in this housing area.

Janiz made a home visit to Anne, a 26-year-old mother of three. Anne takes care of her 62-year-old maternal grandfather, Gino, who is recovering from cardiac bypass surgery. Gino has a smoking history of two packs per day for almost 40 years. Since his surgery, he has decreased to one pack per day, but he refuses to quit. He had a history of alcohol dependence, reportedly consuming up to "40 oz." (1.1 L) of liquor a day, and a history of withdrawal seizures. Four years ago, Gino went through alcohol detoxification, but he refused to stay at the facility for continued treatment, stating he could stay sober on his own. Since that time, he has had several binge episodes, but Anne says he has not been drinking since the surgery. A widower for 5 years, Gino now lives with his granddaughter and her children.

Anne is a widow and has two sons, ages 3 and 9 years, and a daughter, age 5 years. The oldest son's father is an alcoholic who is currently incarcerated for manslaughter (while driving under the influence of alcohol), and the father of her two youngest children was killed by a stray bullet in a cocaine bust 3 years ago. She and her husband had smoked crack cocaine for several months, but both stopped when she became pregnant with their youngest child and remained cocaine-free. Anne has been angry at the community and frightened of police officers ever since the drug raid in which her husband was killed. Other residents were also hurt, and less than $500 worth of cocaine was found three apartments away from hers.

Anne does not consume alcohol, but she smokes one to two packs of cigarettes per day. She quit smoking during her pregnancies but restarted soon after each birth.

1. What type of interventions can Janiz provide for Gino regarding his smoking?
2. How can Janiz help Anne cope with the potential risk of Gino's continuing to drink when he progresses to more independence?
3. How can Janiz help Anne with her cigarette smoking?

4. Knowing that there is a genetic link to alcoholism and being aware of the high rate of substance abuse in the housing area, how can Janiz help prevent Anne and her children from developing substance abuse problems?
5. What can Janiz do to help make the environment safer and more nurturing?

Answers are on the Evolve Web site at http://evolve.elsevier.com/Canada/Stanhope/community/.

What Would You Do?

1. Using Web-based resources, examine health statistics and demographic data for your geographical area to determine which vulnerable groups predominate in your area. Look through your telephone book for examples of agencies that you think provide services to these vulnerable groups. Prepare a table with your findings. Do a literature search to identify recommended state-of-the-art interventions for poor and homeless persons. Compare the recommended programs and interventions with those available in your target area. How does your area measure up? Give some specific recommendations about how you would fill the gaps.
2. For 1 week, keep a list of incidents related to mental health problems that you learn about in the local media. Categorize the incidents according to age, sex, and socioeconomic, ethnic, or minority status.
3. Explore the resources in your community that are available for clients and families requiring mental health services. Prepare a chart of these services with the contact information and eligibility criteria to share with your classmates.
4. Select one of the vulnerable populations discussed in this chapter. Search the literature for two evidence-based articles that identify one aspect of community health nursing care for that population. Prepare a summary of your articles, outlining the health care components for CHN use.
5. Search the literature for information pertaining to vulnerabilities of Aboriginal women and children. Identify and list your findings and bring them to class.
6. Review the CNA Position Statement "Violence" found in the Weblinks on the Evolve Web site. Prepare in chart form the roles of nurses, employers, unions, and government to manage or eliminate violence. Focus on the roles of the nurse as outlined in the CNA document and relate these to the roles of a CHN as outlined in the *Canadian Community Health Nursing Standards of Practice* (see Appendix 1).

TOOL BOX

evolve

The Tool Box contains useful instruments that can be applied in community health nursing practice. These related resources are found either in the appendices at the back of this book or on the Evolve Web site at http://evolve.elsevier.com/stanhope/community/.

Appendices

- Appendix 1: Canadian Community Health Nursing Standards of Practice

Tools

Gender & Health Collaborative Curriculum. *Gender and Health Modules.*
This site provides interactive learning modules about gender and health in reference to poverty and diseases such as cardiovascular disease and depression. It also includes the topics of sex and sexuality and trauma, with other modules being developed.

Health Canada. *Assessment and Planning Tool Kit for Suicide Prevention in First Nations Communities.*
This tool kit has been prepared to assist First Nations Peoples address suicide in their communities. The tool kit provides information and research on suicide prevention such as community assessment, community risk factors, and how to develop a healing plan.

Sexuality and U: Teaching Tools for the Classroom.
This site contains links to tools useful for health care professionals and educators when teaching about sexual health.

Social Planning Council of Winnipeg. *Campaign 2000 Poverty Primer.*
This tool kit provides resources on how to advocate to end poverty.

WEBLINKS

evolve

Direct links to these resources can be found on the text's accompanying Evolve Web site at http://evolve.elsevier.com/stanhope/community.

Campaign 2000. End Child and Family Poverty in Canada. This site provides information on child and family poverty for all provinces. Scroll down under the current issues section to locate the links.

Campaign 2000. *Report Card on Child and Family Poverty in Canada: 1989–2009.* A review of the history of poverty development in Canada can be found here.

Canada Without Poverty. The organization providing this site was formerly called National Anti-Poverty Organization (NAPO). It is a nonprofit organization working to eradicate poverty in Canada. The site has several tab choices. Selecting the "Poverty in Canada" tab takes the reader to short stories of individuals who have experienced poverty in their lives.

Canadian Child Welfare Research Portal. Canadian Incidence Study. This site provides information on the CIS studies, particularly the 2008 study, regarding the child and family and various types of child abuse and neglect.

Canadian Journal of Public Health. Reducing Health Disparities in Canada. This special supplement issue of the journal contains articles pertaining to vulnerable populations and issues such as health disparities, homelessness, and literacy and health research.

Canadian Nurses Association: Position Statements and Backgrounders can be accessed from the CNA site.

- CNA Backgrounder: *Children's Health and Nursing: A Summary of the Issues*
- CNA Position Statement: *Mental Health and Nursing: A Summary of the Issues*
- CNA Position Statement: *Mental Health Services*
- CNA Position Statement: *Violence*. The CNA's position on violence and the roles and responsibilities of nurses, employers, unions, and government are presented.

Cathy Crowe. This site takes the name of the activist and street nurse Cathy Crowe. Crowe has assumed an activist role in working toward a national housing program that is affordable for the homeless. The Web site provides information on Crowe's work and provides connections to some additional resources on homelessness, including Crowe's book, titled *Dying for a Home: Homeless Activists Speak Out.*

Centre for Suicide Prevention. Are You in Crisis? This site provides information on the problem of suicide among young Aboriginal people and strategies for suicide prevention.

Centre of Excellence for Child Welfare. *2003 Canadian Incidence Study of Reported Child Abuse and Neglect* (CIS-2003). This site provides information on the CIS-2003 study regarding the child and family and features various types of child abuse and neglect. The complete report and several short information sheets, including a PowerPoint presentation, are provided.

City of Vancouver's Four Pillars Drug Strategy. This site provides information on a coalition-driven comprehensive approach to harm reduction with an emphasis on the damage done by substance abuse rather than an emphasis on the substance use itself. It includes programs such as needle exchange and supervised injection site (SIS).

Department of Justice Canada. *Child Abuse: A Fact Sheet from the Department of Justice Canada.* This site defines and discusses the various types of child abuse, provides statistics on the prevalence of child abuse, and discusses the Criminal Code, factors and consequences, and prevention and management of child abuse. It also provides additional resources on child abuse.

Directory of Canada Alcohol and Drug Education and Prevention Programs. This site provides extensive links to a variety of services across Canada to address alcohol and drug abuse.

Feminist Research Education Development and Action Centre for Research on Violence against Women and Children. This site provides research that focuses specifically on violence against women and children. Collaborative partnerships between communities and academics who are working to end this type of violence resulted in the research.

First Nations Centre, National Aboriginal Health Care Organization. This site provides an assessment and planning framework for suicide prevention in First Nations communities. Also provided is information and research on suicide prevention.

The Fraser Institute. This site provides access to the *Fraser Alert* that contains the most up to date information on poverty in Canada.

Gender & Health Collaborative Curriculum. Gender and Health Modules. This site provides interactive learning modules pertaining to gender and health in reference to poverty and includes diseases such as cardiovascular disease and depression. It also includes topics such as sexuality and trauma.

Government of Canada. Domestic Violence. Extensive Weblinks for sites are organized alphabetically. The topics are related to domestic violence and include action plans on abuse, the Criminal Code of Canada, abuse and neglect of older adults, battered men, child abuse, emotional abuse, family violence, how to stay safe, neglect, possible indicators of abuse, transition housing, and violence against Aboriginal people.

Government of Canada. *The Human Face of Mental Health and Mental Illness in Canada.* This report provides information for Canadians to increase their awareness of mental illness and mental health and provides specific information on topic areas such as eating disorders, suicidal behaviour, substance dependency, and Aboriginal health and well-being.

Health Canada. *Best Practices. Concurrent Mental Health and Substance Use Disorders.* This site provides best-practice guidelines for health professionals screening for substance use and mental health disorders, assessment and treatment of people with concurrent disorders, and implications of best-practice guidelines. Assessment measures are discussed with reference to assessment tools.

Health Canada—First Nations and Inuit Health. *Acting on What We Know: Preventing Youth Suicide in First Nations.* This report on the examination of the issues of youth suicide in First Nations communities identifies recommendations on how to address these issues, and suggests strategies for how to implement these recommendations in First Nations communities.

Health Canada. First Nations, Inuit & Aboriginal Health. This site includes a wealth of information targeted at First Nations and Inuit peoples about how to stay healthy; disease threats and health conditions; substance use and help with addictions; drug, dental, and medical benefits; and programs and funding available for First Nations and Inuit peoples in Canada.

Health Canada. *Food and Nutrition.* The Canada Food Guide is found on this site, with links to the guide in 10 different languages and to the Canada Food Guide specific for First Nations, Inuit, and Métis; as well, it provides information for educators and health care professionals who use the Canada Food Guide with students and clients.

Health Canada. *Healthy Living: Mental Health.* This site provides an overview of mental health and provides online materials on mental health promotion, mental health problems, and mental disorders and includes service systems available to address mental health issues such as health, housing, and income support.

Health Canada. *Healthy Living: Suicide Prevention.* This site provides background information on suicide, factors in suicidal behaviour, and how to minimize the risk.

Health Canada. *Pro-action, Postponement, and Preparation/Support: A Framework for Action to Reduce the Rate of Teen Pregnancy in Canada.* This document provides facts on teenage pregnancy, presents a profile of teenagers who become pregnant, discusses the factors contributing to teenage pregnancy with a discussion of the consequences of teenage pregnancy, and provides a framework to reduce the rate of teenage pregnancy.

Health Officers Council of British Columbia. *Health Inequities in British Columbia: A Discussion Paper.* This document provides information on the determinants of health and inequities, health inequity policy considerations, and options for reducing health inequities, plus some stories that depict individual health inequities.

Help Guide. *Domestic Violence and Abuse: Signs of Abuse and Abusive Relationships.* This site provides information on domestic violence and abuse such as the types of abuse, recognizing an abusive relationship, abuser tactics to manipulate the victim, common warning signs of abuse, and how to intervene when an abusive situation is suspected.

Human Resources and Skill Development Canada. Homelessness Partnering Strategy. This site provides information on the designated communities, the outreach communities, Aboriginal communities, and knowledge development about homelessness in Canada.

King, M. An Overall Approach to Health Care for Indigenous Peoples. The author provides a socioenvironmental overview of the indigenous concepts of health, illness, and healing, such as living in harmony with the community and the spiritual world, the balance of the person and others and the environment, and the impact of the social determinants of health on indigenous health and well-being.

Laird, G. *Shelter—Homelessness in a Growth Economy: Canada's 21st Century Paradox.* This document provides information on the Canadian government's actions or lack of actions on housing and homelessness in the past 10 years. The report contains statistical information and specifics on homelessness and poverty in Vancouver, Calgary, Toronto, Ottawa, and Iqaluit.

Lee, K. Canadian Council on Social Development. *Urban Poverty in Canada: A Statistical Profile.* CHNs can use this resource to gain an understanding of poverty in Canada. Statistical information related to poverty is provided for visible minorities, immigrants, and Aboriginal peoples, among others.

Mental Health Commission of Canada. *Out of the Shadows Forever: At Home.* This site provides information on the Mental Health Commission of Canada's At Home Research Demonstration Projects, which were launched in 2009 in five Canadian cities to gather information on homelessness and mental illness to identify ways to provide relevant services and housing to homeless persons. This site also provides links for the projects in each of the five cities (Moncton, Montreal, Toronto, Vancouver, and Winnipeg) with their specific foci.

Mental Health Commission of Canada. *Toward Recovery and Well-Being: A Framework for a Mental Health Strategy for Canada.* In this 2009 document, seven interconnected goals are presented with the intent to foster mental health in Canada. This document is the first phase in developing a mental health strategy for Canada.

National Aboriginal Health Organization (NAHO). *Social Determinants of Métis Health.* This resource provides information on the determinants of health for Canada's Aboriginal people and specifically speaks to Métis social determinants of well-being.

National Collaborating Centre for Aboriginal Health. This site, run from the University of Northern British Columbia at Prince George, is one of the six national collaborating centres responsible for providing some of the best evidence available for informed practice that is required by health care practitioners to impact health outcomes for Canadians. The site specifically provides information to address Aboriginal health. The four main topic tabs are setting the context, determinants of health, child and youth health, and emerging priorities. Information is found within each of these tabs specific to Aboriginals in Canada.

Public Health Agency of Canada. Canada Prenatal Nutrition Program (CPNP). This site provides information about programs that have been developed for vulnerable pregnant women in Canada to reduce the incidence of unhealthy birth weights, improve the health of mother and infant, and encourage breastfeeding.

Public Health Agency of Canada. *Canadian Guidelines on Sexually Transmitted Infections.* This site provides a reference for professionals for the prevention and management of STIs with additional information on at-risk populations—that is, vulnerable populations.

Public Health Agency of Canada. *The Chief Public Health Officer's Report on the State of Public Health in Canada: 2008 Addressing Health Inequalities.* At this site, key socioeconomic determinants of health (SEDOH) are discussed in Chapter 4. It provides a definition of health inequalities; a summary of the statistics on SEDOH for Canadians; a summary of each of the determinants and their effect on the health of the Canadian population and specific aggregates; and examples of Canadian programs and policies that have been implemented as interventions to reduce these key determinants.

Public Health Agency of Canada. *The Chief Public Health Officer's Report on the State of Public Health in Canada: 2009 Growing up Well—Priorities for a Healthy Future.* This site provides the second annual report by Dr. David Butler-Jones, Chief Public Health Officer of Canada. The focus of this report is on the health of the children of Canada.

Public Health Agency of Canada. First Connections … Make All the Difference. Access "What Professionals Need to Know" for information, such as behaviours of the infant or child and caregiver to observe in order to assess infant attachment and normal infant and child milestones. The CHN can access further information that is for professional use and also direct caregivers to this site for information on what infant attachment is and how to promote infant attachment. A toll-free help line for caregivers is included.

Public Health Agency of Canada. *Reducing Health Disparities—Roles of the Health Sector, Discussion Paper, 2004.* This site provides information on the health disparities in Canada, including the history of disparities and opportunities for reducing them.

Public Health Agency of Canada. *2008 Canadian Incidence Study of Reported Child Abuse and Neglect: Major Findings.* This site contains a report, published in the fall of 2010, which examined child abuse and neglect across Canada.

Public Safety Canada. *Bullying Prevention: Nature and Extent of Bullying in Canada.* This site defines bullying and provides a summary of a variety of research studies conducted on bullying, delinquency, and risk factors of bullying. Some strategies to prevent bullying are included. It also discusses the fourth *R* in a school curriculum, which is skills for youth *r*elationships.

Qulliit Nunavut Status of Women Council. *The Little Voices of Nunavut: A Study of Women's Homelessness North of 60 Territorial Report.* This research report provides qualitative study findings on Nunavut women's homelessness north of 60 degrees latitude as well as the determinants of homelessness for this study population. Recommendations for change are also provided in this extensive report.

Registered Nurses' Association of Ontario. *Assessment and Care of Adults at Risk for Suicide Ideation and Behaviour.* This guideline is an excellent resource for CHNs on the recognition of suicide potential based on risk factors and warning signs, suicide assessment considerations, and interventions to consider. Many available tools are also presented and discussed.

Registered Nurses' Association of Ontario. *Nursing Best Practice Guideline: Crisis Intervention Supplement.* This resource is useful for CHNs who must intervene in mental health or other crises. This guideline can be used to standardize community practice.

Registered Nurses' Association of Ontario. *Supporting Clients on Methadone Maintenance Treatment.* This document provides information on the harm reduction model developed by Cheung with further discussion of the harm reduction strategies and programs.

Senate Subcommittee on Cities. *In From the Margins: A Call to Action on Poverty, Housing and Homelessness.* This site provides information on poverty, housing, and homelessness and makes recommendations on ways to eradicate poverty and deal with the housing and homelessness issues.

Social Services Network. *Elder Abuse. See It. Stop It. Prevent It.* This resource provides information such as an overview of the different types of elder abuse, signs and symptoms, and prevention of elder abuse. The information in this document is useful to CHNs as they practise in the community.

Standing Senate Committee on Social Affairs, Science and Technology. *Out of the Shadows at Last: Transforming Mental Health, Mental Illness and Addiction Services in Canada.* This is the report, chaired by the Honourable Michael J. L. Kirby, and is often referred to as the Kirby report on mental health. It is a voice for those living with mental illness and covers topics ranging from living with the stigma and discrimination to dealing with legal issues and includes brief stories of what it is like to live with mental illness.

Statistics Canada. Suicides and Suicide Rates. This site provides a learning resource for health care professionals and educators whose work pertains to suicide.

Statistics Canada. Teenage Pregnancy Trends in Canada. This site provides a learning resource for health care professionals and educators working with teenagers to assist in the prevention of teenage pregnancy.

UNICEF. *Female Genital Mutilation/Cutting: A Statistical Exploration.* This site provides extensive information on the issue of female genital mutilation and cutting. It increases understanding of this issue and its connection to gender equality and social justice. Global prevalence rates are provided with the socioeconomic and demographic factors affecting this issue.

United Nations General Assembly. *Report of the Independent Expert for the United Nations Study on Violence against Children.* This international report provides the results of an extensive study pertaining to violence against children globally. Refer to pages 38–80 (settings in which violence against children occurs).

University of Alberta. *A Look at Bullying in Canada.* This site provides a PowerPoint presentation on bullying in Canada that covers topics such as statistics, definitions, family characteristics of bullies and victims, myths, and interventions.

World Health Organization. *Media Centre Fact Sheet: Female Genital Mutilation.* This site provides a fact sheet of information on female genital mutilation and includes information such as key facts, procedures, health consequences, who is at risk, causes, international response, and the WHO response to this issue.

World Health Organization. Sexual and Reproductive Health: Female Genital Mutilation and Other Harmful Practices. This site provides many links to publications related to advocacy, clinical guides, evidence, policy, and programs, including problems with programs.

REFERENCES

Adelson, N. (2005). The embodiment of inequity-health disparities in Aboriginal Canada. *Canadian Journal of Public Health, 96*(S-2), 45–61.

Alberta Coalition for Healthy School Communities. (2006). *Socioeconomic disadvantage: Health and education outcomes for school-aged children and youth*. Retrieved from http://www.achsc.org/download/ACHSC%20Background%20Paper_SES_Health_Educ_SCY(June%2015,06).pdf.

André-Petersson, L., Engström, G., Hedblad, B., Janzon, L., & Rosvall, M. (2007). Social support at work and the risk of myocardial infarction and stroke in women and men. *Social Science and Medicine, 64*(4), 830–841.

Arsenault-Lapierre, G., Kim, C., & Turecki, G. (2004). Psychiatric diagnoses in 3,275 suicides: A meta-analysis. *BMC Psychiatry, 4*(37), 1186/1471. Retrieved from http://www.biomedcentral.com/content/pdf/1471-244X-4-37.pdf.

Auer, A. M., & Andersson, R. (2001). Canadian Aboriginal communities: A framework for injury surveillance. *Health Promotion International, 16*(2), 169–177.

Austin, W., & Boyd, M. A. (2008). *Psychiatric nursing: Contemporary practice* (3rd ed.). Philadelphia, PA: Lippincott, Williams & Wilkins.

Bagley, C., Wood, M., & Khumar, H. (1990). Suicide and careless death in young males: Ecological study of an aboriginal population in Canada. *Canadian Journal of Community Mental Health*, *9*(1), 127–142.

Beckmann Murray, R. (2009). Assessment and health promotion for the adolescent and youth. In R. Beckmann Murray, J. Proctor Zentner, V. Pangman, & C. Pangman (Eds.), *Health promotion strategies through the lifespan* (2nd Canadian ed., pp. 397–453). Toronto: Pearson Prentice Hall.

Beckmann Murray, R., Proctor Zentner, J., Pangman, V., & Pangman, C. (2009). *Health promotion strategies through the lifespan* (2nd ed). Toronto: Pearson Prentice Hall.

Beiser, M., & Stewart, M. (2005). Reducing health disparities: A priority for Canada. *Canadian Journal of Public Health*, *96*(Suppl. 2), S4–S5.

Bland, R. (1998). Psychiatry and the burden of mental illness. *Canadian Journal of Psychiatry*, *43*, 801–810.

Boschma, G., Groening, M., & Boyd, M. A. (2008). Psychiatric and mental health nursing from past to present. In W. Austin, & M. A. Boyd (Eds.), *Psychiatric nursing for Canadian practice* (pp. 3–17). Philadelphia, PA: Lippincott, Williams & Wilkins.

Bradley, L. (2009). *The recession's impact on the mental health of workers and their families: A global perspective*. Retrieved from http://www.mentalhealthcommission.ca/SiteCollectionDocuments/Key_Documents/en/2009/LB_QIISP_Kingston_18Aug09_FINAL_for%20web%20_2_.pdf.

Butler-Jones, D. (2008). *The Chief Public Health Officer's report on the state of public health in Canada: Addressing health inequalities*. Retrieved from http://www.phac-aspc.gc.ca/publicat/2008/cphorsphc-respcacsp/cphorsphc-respcacsp07c-eng.php.

Butler-Jones, D. (2009). *The Chief Public Health Officer's report on the state of public health in Canada: Growing up well—priorities for a healthy future*. Retrieved from http://www.phac-aspc.gc.ca/publicat/2009/cphorsphc-respcacsp/pdf/cphorsphc-respcacsp-eng.pdf.

Campaign 2000. (2009). *Report card on child and family poverty in Canada: 1989–2009*. Retrieved from http://www.campaign2000.ca/reportCards/national/2009EnglishC2000NationalReportCard.pdf.

Campaign 2000. (2010). *Report card on child and family poverty in Canada: 1989–2010*. Retrieved from http://www.campaign2000.ca/reportCards/national/2010EnglishC2000NationalReportCard.pdf.

Canadian Child Welfare Research Portal. (2009). *Canadian incidence study, 2008*. Retrieved from http://www.cecw-cepb.ca/cis-2008.

Canadian Council on Social Development. (2007). *Almost 3 million households paying more than they can afford for housing*. Retrieved from http://www.ccsd.ca/media/2007/pr_com_profiles.htm.

Canadian Index of Wellbeing Network. (2009). *How are Canadians really doing? A closer look at select groups: Special report*. Retrieved from http://www.ciw.ca/en/media/09-12-16/df39996f-52af-4c21-a004-823133c15744.aspx.

Canadian Institute for Health Information. (2005). *One in seven hospitalizations in Canada involve patients diagnosed with mental illness*. Retrieved from http://secure.cihi.ca/cihiweb/dispPage.jsp?cw_page=media_12oct2005_e.

Canadian Institute for Health Information. (2006). *The Canadian population health initiative: Action plan 2007–2010*. Retrieved from http://secure.cihi.ca/cihiweb/products/action_plan_2007_2010_e.pdf.

Canadian Institute for Health Information. (2007). *Mental disorders account for more than half of hospital stays among the homeless in Canada*. Retrieved from http://www.cihi.ca/cihiweb/dispPage.jsp?cw_page = media_30aug2007_e.

Canadian Institute for Health Information. (2009). *Children's mental health in Canada: Preventing disorders and promoting population health*. Retrieved from http://secure.cihi.ca/cihiweb/en/downloads/waddell_summary2009_e.pdf.

Canadian Institutes of Health Research. (2007). *Reducing health disparities and promoting equity for vulnerable populations*. (Archived). Retrieved from http://www.cihr-irsc.gc.ca/e/4277.html.

Canadian Mental Health Association. (2005). *Police and mental illness: Models that work*. Retrieved from http://www.cmha.bc.ca/files/4-models.pdf.

Canadian Mental Health Association. (2010). *About CMHA*. Retrieved from http://www.cmha.ca/bins/content_page.asp?cid=7&lang=1.

Canadian Mental Health Association, Ontario; Centre for Addiction and Mental Health, Ontario; Peer Development Initiative; & Ontario Federation of Community Mental Health and Addiction Programs. (2009). *Consumer/survivor initiative: Impact, outcomes and effectiveness*. Retrieved from http://info.wlu.ca/~ wwwpsych/gnelson/csi%20advocacy%20paper%20july%202005.pdf.

Canadian Nurses Association. (2005). Mental health and nursing: A summary of the issues. In *CNA Backgrounder*. Ottawa, ON: Canadian Nurses Association.

Canadian Public Health Association. (2005). *Reducing health disparities—Roles of the health sector: Recommended policy directions and activities*. Retrieved from http://www.phac-aspc.gc.ca/ph-sp/disparities/pdf06/disparities_recommended_policy.pdf.

Canadian Research Institute for the Advancement of Women. (n.d). *Women and poverty* (3rd ed.). Retrieved from http://www.criaw-icref.ca/WomenAndPoverty.

Canadian Teachers' Federation. (2008a). *Addressing cyberconduct: A brief to the Department of Justice Canada*. Retrieved from http://www.ctf-fce.ca/publications/Briefs/BRIEF-Justice-reCyberconduct-eng.pdf.

Canadian Teachers' Federation. (2008b). *Cyberbullying in schools: National poll shows Canadians' growing awareness*. Retrieved from http://www.canadiansafeschools.com/content/documents/Link/Safe%20Schools%20in%20the%20News/cyberbullyinginschools-july1108.pdf.

Carter, S. P., & Stewin, L. L. (1999). School violence in the Canadian context: An overview and model for intervention. *International Journal for the Advancement of Counselling*, *21*(4), 267–277.

Chandler, J. J., & Lalonde, C. (1998). Cultural continuity as a hedge against suicide in Canada's First Nations. *Transcultural Psychiatry*, *35*(2), 191–219.

Chilton, M., Chyatte, M., & Breaux, J. (2007). The negative effects of poverty and food insecurity on child development. *Indian Journal of Medical Research*, *126*, 262–272.

Cohen, E., Groves, B. M., & Kracke, K. (2009). *Understanding children's exposure to violence. The Safe Start Centre Series on Children Exposed to Violence. Issue Brief #1*. Retrieved from http://www.safestartcenter.org/pdf/IssueBrief1_UNDERSTANDING.pdf.

Cox, R. G., Zhang, L., Johnson, W. D., & Bender, D. R. (2007). Academic performance and substance use: Findings from a state survey of public high school students. *Journal of School Health*, *77*(3), 109–115.

Craven, M. A., & Bland, R. (2002). Shared mental health care: A bibliography and overview. *Canadian Journal of Psychiatry*, *47*(2 Suppl. 1). Retrieved from http://ww1.cpa-apc.org:8080/Publications/CJP/supplements/april2002_sharedCare/toc.asp.

Curry-Stevens, A. (2009). When economic growth doesn't trickle down: The wage dimensions of income polarization. In D. Raphael (Ed.), *Social determinants of health* (pp. 41–60). Toronto, ON: Canadian Scholars' Press.

Davis, S. (2006). *Community mental health in Canada: Theory, policy and practice*. Vancouver, BC: UBC Press.

Dauvergne, M., & Li, G. (2006). Homicides in Canada, 2005. *Canadian Centre for Justice Statistics*, *26*(6), 1–26.

Department of Justice Canada. (2006). *Child abuse: A fact sheet from the Department of Justice Canada*. Retrieved from http://www.justice.gc.ca/eng/pi/fv-vf/facts-info/child-enf.pdf.

Dutcher, L. (2006). *Nursing leadership: Providing cultural competent care to Aboriginal people*. Unpublished paper for the University of New Brunswick.

Ebersole, P., Hess, P., Touhy, T., & Jett, K. (2005). *Gerontological nursing and healthy aging* (2nd ed). St. Louis, MO: Mosby.

First Nations Centre. (2005). *First Nations regional longitudinal health survey (RHS) 2002/2003: Results for adults, youth and children living in First Nations communities*. Ottawa, ON: First Nations Centre at the National Aboriginal Health Organization.

Frankish, C. J., Hwang, S. W., & Quantz, D. (2005). Homelessness and health in Canada: Research lessons and priorities. *Canadian Journal of Public Health*, *96*(Suppl. 2), S23–S29.

Gender & Health Collaborative Curriculum. (2008a). *Gender and cardiovascular disease*. Retrieved from www.genderandhealth.ca/en/modules/cardiovascular/.

Gender & Health Collaborative Curriculum. (2008b). *Gender and poverty*. Retrieved from www.genderandhealth.ca/en/modules/poverty/.

Gender & Health Collaborative Curriculum. (2008c). *Gender and sexual diversity*. Retrieved from www.genderandhealth.ca/en/modules/sexandsexuality/.

Giles, B., Haas, G., Sajna, M., & Findlay, C. (2008). Exploring Aboriginal views of health using fuzzy cognitive maps and transitive closure: A case study of the determinants of diabetes. *Canadian Journal of Public Health*, *99*(5), 411–417.

Gold, L. H. (2005). Gender issues in suicide. *Psychiatric Times*, *22*(11), 64–72.

Government of Ontario. (2007). *The Ontario Domestic Assault Risk Assessment (ODARA)*. Retrieved from http://www.mhcp-research.com/odarasum.htm.

Health Canada. (2005a). *Acting on what we know: Preventing youth suicide in First Nations*. Retrieved from http://www.hc-sc.gc.ca/fniah-spnia/pubs/promotion/_suicide/prev_youth-jeunes/.

Health Canada. (2005b). *Statistical profile on the health of First Nations in Canada*. Retrieved from http://www.hc-sc.gc.ca/fniah-spnia/intro-eng.php.

Health Canada. (2006a). *First Nations, Inuit and Aboriginal health: Suicide prevention*. Retrieved from http://www.hc-sc.gc.ca/fniah-spnia/promotion/suicide/index-eng.php.

Health Canada. (2006b). *Mental health—Mental illness: It's your health*. Retrieved from http://www.hc-sc.gc.ca/hl-vs/iyh-vsv/diseases-maladies/mental-eng.php.

Health Canada. (2007). *First Nations and Inuit health: Program compendium*. Retrieved from http://www.hc-sc.gc.ca/.

Health Canada. (2009a). *A statistical profile on the health of First Nations in Canada: Determinants of health, 1999 to 2003*. Retrieved from http://www.hc-sc.gc.ca/fniah-spnia/pubs/aborig-autoch/index-eng.php.

Health Canada. (2009b). *Suicide prevention: It's your health*. Retrieved from http://www.hc-sc.gc.ca/hl-vs/iyh-vsv/diseases-maladies/suicide-eng.php.

Health Council of Canada. (2005). *The health status of Canada's First Nations, Métis and Inuit Peoples: A background paper to accompany health care renewal in Canada: Accelerating change*. Toronto, ON: Health Council of Canada.

Human Resources and Skills Development Canada. (2009). *Summative evaluation of the national homelessness initiative—May 2008*. Retrieved from http://www.rhdcc-hrsdc.gc.ca/eng/publications_resources/evaluation/2009/nhi/page03.shtml.

Hwang, S. W. (2001). Homelessness and health. *Canadian Medical Association Journal*, *164*(2), 229–233.

Indian and Northern Affairs Canada. (2008). *Revised northern food basket—Highlights of price survey results for 2006–2007*. Retrieved from http://www.ainc-inac.gc.ca/nth/fon/fm/ar/hpsr0607-eng.asp.

Institute of Wellbeing. (2009). *How are Canadians really doing: A closer look at select groups*. Retrieved from http://www.ciw.ca/Libraries/Documents/ACloserLookAtSelectGroups_FullReport.sflb.ashx.

Inuit Tapiriit Kanatami and Indian and Northern Affairs Canada. (2007). *Inuit social trends series: Levels and sources of individual and household level income for Inuit in Canada, 1980–2000*. Indian and Northern Affairs Canada, Catalogue R2-461/2007E-PDF. Ottawa, ON: Minister of Public Works and Government Services Canada.

Jagdeo, A., Cox, B. J., Stein, M. B., & Sareen, J. (2009). Negative attitudes toward help seeking for mental illness in 2 population-based surveys from the United States and Canada. *Canadian Journal of Psychiatry*, *54*(11), 757–765. Retrieved from http://publications.cpa-apc.org/media.php?mid = 874&xwm = true.

Joong, P., & Ridler, O. (2005). School violence: Perception and reality. *Education Canada*, *45*(4), 61–63.

Judd, F., Cooper, A., Fraser, C., & Davis, J. (2006). Rural suicide—people or place effects? *Australian and New Zealand Journal of Psychiatry*, *40*(3), 208–216.

Kadison, R., & DiGeronomo, T. (2004). *College of the overwhelmed, the campus mental health crisis and what to do about it*. San Francisco, CA: Jossey-Bass.

Kanatami, T. (2004). *Backgrounder on Inuit health*. Retrieved from http://www.itk.ca/roundtable/pdf/20041105-sectoral-health-backgrounder-en.pdf.

Kiernan, K. E., & Huerta, M. C. (2008). Economic deprivation, maternal depression, parenting and children's cognitive and emotional development in early childhood. *British Journal of Sociology*, *59*(4), 783–806.

King Blood, R. J. (2005). Aboriginal Canadians. In L. Stamler, & L. Yiu (Eds.), *Community health nursing: A Canadian perspective* (pp. 239–246). Toronto, ON: Pearson Education Canada.

Kirby, M. (2009, November 4). *Speaking notes for the Honourable Michael Kirby, Chair, Mental Health Commission of Canada*. Retrieved from www.senate-senat.ca/SOCIAL.asp.

Kirby, M. J. L. (2006). *Out of the shadows at last: Highlights and recommendations. Final report of the Standing Senate Committee on Social Affairs and Technology*. Retrieved from http://www.parl.gc.ca/39/1/parlbus/commbus/senate/com-e/soci-e/rep-e/pdf/rep02may06part1-e.pdf.

Kovesi, T., Gilbert, N., Stocco, C., Fugler, D., Dales, R., Guay, M., & Miller, J. (2007). Indoor air quality and the risk of lower respiratory tract infections in young Canadian Inuit children. *Canadian Medical Association Journal*, *177*(2), 155–160.

Krewski, D., Lemyre, L., Turner, M. C., Lee, J. E. C., Dallaire, C., Bouchard, L., & Mercier, P. (2006). Public perception of population health risks in Canada: Health hazards and sources of information. *Human and Ecological Risk Assessment*, *12*(4), 626–644.

Laird, G. (2007). *Shelter—Homelessness in a growth economy: Canada's 21st century paradox*. Calgary, AB: Sheldon Chumir Foundation for Ethics in Leadership. Retrieved from www.chumirethicsfoundation.ca.

Langille, D. B. (2007). Teenage pregnancy: Trends, contributing factors, and the physician role. *Canadian Medical Association Journal*, *176*(11), 1601–1602. Retrieved from http://www.cmaj.ca/cgi/reprint/176/11/1601.pdf.

Lavalee, D., & Clearsky, L. (2006). Commentary. 'From Woundedness to Resilience': A critical review from an Aboriginal perspective. *Journal of Aboriginal Health*, 4–6. Retrieved from http://www.naho.ca/jah/english/jah03_01/commentary.pdf.

Lehne, R. A. (2007). *Pharmacology for nursing care* (6th ed.). St. Louis, MO: Saunders Elsevier.

Lemyre, L., Lee, J. E. C., Mercier, P., Bouchard, L., & Krewski, D. (2006). The structure of Canadians' health risk perceptions: Environmental, therapeutic and social health risks. *Health, Risk and Society*, *8*(2), 185–195.

Maier, R., Egger, A., Barth, A., Winker, R., Osterode, W., Kundi, M., et al. (2006). Effects of short- and long-term unemployment on physical work capacity and on serum cortisol. *International Archives of Occupational and Environmental Health*, *79*(3), 193–198.

Mapp, S. C. (2006). The effects of sexual abuse as a child on the risk of mothers physically abusing their children: A path analysis using systems theory. *Child Abuse and Neglect*, *30*(11), 1293–1310.

Mental Health Commission of Canada. (2009a). *Out of the shadows forever: At home*. Retrieved from http://www.mentalhealthcommission.ca/English/Pages/homelessness.aspx.

Mental Health Commission of Canada. (2009b). *Summary: Toward recovery & well-being: A framework for a mental health strategy for Canada*. Retrieved from http://www.mentalhealthcommission.ca/SiteCollectionDocuments/strategy/MHCC_Summary_EN.pdf.

Métis National Council. (2004). In *Prime Minister's Aboriginal roundtable briefing note on Métis health issues*. (p. 1). Retrieved from www.metisnation.ca.

Mikkonen, J., & Raphael, D. (2010). *Social determinants of health: The Canadian facts*. Retrieved from http://www.thecanadianfacts.org/.

Myslik, B. (2005). Suicide. In L. Stamler, & L. Yiu (Eds.), *Community health nursing: A Canadian perspective* (pp. 317–324). Toronto, ON: Pearson Education Canada.

National Alliance on Mental Illness. (2009). *About treatments and supports: Assertive community treatment (ACT)*. Retrieved from http://www.nami.org/Template.cfm?Section=About_Treatments_and_Supports&template=/ContentManagement/ContentDisplay.cfm&ContentID=8075.

Northwest Territories Health and Social Services. (2009). *Types of abuse*. Retrieved from http://www.hlthss.gov.nt.ca/english/services/family_violence/types_of_abuse/default.htm.

Pembina Institute. (2005). *Underemployment*. Retrieved from http://pubs.pembina.org/reports/16.Underemployment.pdf.

Phipps, S. (2003). *The impact of poverty on health: A scan of research literature*. Retrieved from http://secure.cihi.ca/cihiweb/products/CPHIImpactonPoverty_e.pdf.

Poulin, C., & Nicholson, J. (2005). Should harm minimization as an approach to adolescent substance use be embraced by junior and senior high schools? Empirical evidence from an integrated school- and community-based demonstration intervention addressing drug use among adolescents. *International Journal of Drug Policy*, *16*, 403–414.

Public Health Agency of Canada. (2002). *A report on mental illness in Canada*. Retrieved from http://www.phac-aspc.gc.ca/publicat/miic-mmac/chap_2_e.html.

Public Health Agency of Canada. (2004). *What determines health?*. Retrieved from http://www.phac-aspc.gc.ca/ph-sp/determinants/index-eng.php.

Public Health Agency of Canada. (2006a). *The human face of mental health and mental illness in Canada, 2006*. Retrieved from http://www.phac-aspc.gc.ca/publicat/human-humain06/pdf/human_face_e.pdf.

Public Health Agency of Canada. (2006b). *Street youth in Canada: Findings from enhanced surveillance of Canadian street youth, 1999–2003*. Retrieved from http://www.phac-aspc.gc.ca/std-mts/reports_06/pdf/street_youth_e.pdf.

Public Health Agency of Canada. (2010). *2008 Canadian incidence study of reported child abuse and neglect: Major findings*. Retrieved from http://www.phac-aspc.gc.ca/ncfv-cnivf/pdfs/nfnts-cis-2008-rprt-eng.pdf.

Public Safety Canada. (2008). *The validity of risk assessments for intimate partner violence: A meta-analysis*. Retrieved from http://www.publicsafety.gc.ca/res/cor/rep/vra_ipv_200707-eng.aspx.

Rainbow Health Network. (2007). *Social determinants of health*. Retrieved from www.rainbowhealthnetwork.ca.

Raising Children Network. (2009). *Parenting as a drug user*. Retrieved from http://raisingchildren.net.au/articles/parenting_as_a_drug_user.html.

Raphael, D. (2009). *Social determinants of health* (2nd ed). Toronto, ON: Canadian Scholars' Press.

Reading, J. (2009). *A life course approach to the social determinants of health for Aboriginal Peoples for the Senate Sub-Committee on Population Health*. Retrieved from http://www.parl.gc.ca/40/2/parlbus/commbus/senate/com-e/popu-e/rep e/appendixAjun09-e.pdf.

Registered Nurses' Association of Ontario. (2009). *Assessment and care of adults at risk for suicide ideation and behaviour*. Retrieved from http://www.rnao.org/Storage/58/5263_Suicide_-Final-web.pdf.

Rockman, P., Salach, L., Gotlib, D., Cord, M., & Turner, T. (2004). Shared mental health care model for supporting and mentoring family physicians. *Canadian Family Physician*, *50*, 397–402.

Rosenthal, D., Mallett, S., Gurrin, L., Milburn, N., & Rotheram-Borus, M. J. (2007). Changes over time among homeless young people in drug dependency, mental illness and their co-morbidity. *Psychology, Health and Medicine*, *12*(1), 70–80.

Sarlo, C. (2006). *Fraser alert: Poverty in Canada: 2006 update*. Retrieved from http://www.fraserinstitute.org/commerce.web/product_files/PovertyinCanada2006.pdf.

Sarlo, C. (2008). *Measuring poverty in Canada*. Retrieved from http://www.fraserinstitute.org/Commerce.Web/product_files/Measuring_Poverty_in_Canada.pdf.

Schizophrenia Society of Canada. (2010). *A reason to hope: The means to cope*. Retrieved from http://www.schizophrenia.ca/heimEnglish1.htm.

Sebastian, J. G. (2010). Vulnerability and vulnerable populations: An overview. In M. Stanhope, & J. Lancaster (Eds.), *Foundations of nursing in the community: Community-oriented practice* (pp. 385–399). St. Louis, MO: Mosby Elsevier.

Senate Subcommittee on Population Health. (2009). *A healthy, productive Canada: A determinant of health approach*. Ottawa, ON: The Senate. Retrieved from http://senate-senat.ca/health-e.asp.

Shah, C. (2003). *Public health and preventive medicine in Canada* (5th ed.). Toronto, ON: Elsevier Saunders.

Statistics Canada. (2005). *Family violence in Canada: A statistical profile*. Retrieved from http://www.statcan.ca/Daily/English/050714/d050714a.htm.

Statistics Canada. (2008a). *Aboriginal Peoples in Canada in 2006: Inuit, Métis and First Nations, 2006 census* (Catalogue no. 97-558-XIE). Ottawa: Minister of Industry.

Statistics Canada. (2008b). *Aboriginal peoples survey 2006: Inuit health and social conditions*. Retrieved from http://www.statcan.gc.ca/pub/89-637-x/89-637-x2008001-eng.htm.

Statistics Canada. (2009a). *Family violence in Canada: A statistical profile*. Retrieved from http://dsp-psd.pwgsc.gc.ca/collection_2009/statcan/85-224-X/85-224-x2009000-eng.pdf.

Statistics Canada. (2009b). *Income in Canada, 2007* (Catalogue no. 75-202-X). Ottawa, ON: Minister of Industry.

Statistics Canada. (2010a). *Suicides and suicide rate, by sex and by age group*. CANSIM, table 102-0551 and Catalogue no. 84F0209X. Retrieved from http://www40.statcan.ca/l01/cst01/hlth66a-eng.htm.

Statistics Canada. (2010b). *Suicides and suicide rate, by sex and by age group—Females* (Catalogue no. 84F0209X). Ottawa, ON. Retrieved from http://www40.statcan.ca/l01/cst01/hlth66c-eng.htm.

Statistics Canada. (2010c). *Suicides and suicide rate, by sex and by age group—Males* (Catalogue no. 84F0209X). Ottawa, ON. Retrieved from http://www40.statcan.ca/l01/cst01/hlth66b-eng.htm.

Stergiopoulos, V., & Herrmann, N. (2003). Old and homeless: A review and survey of older adults who use shelters in an urban setting. *Canadian Journal of Psychiatry*, *48*(6), 374–380.

Storch, J. L., Rodney, P., & Starzomski, R. (2004). *Toward a moral horizon: Nursing ethics for leadership and practice*. Toronto, ON: Pearson Prentice-Hall.

Treasury Board of Canada. (2004). *About Canada's performance 2004*. Retrieved from http://www.tbs-sct.gc.ca/report/govrev/04/cp-rc1_e.asp.

Trocmé, N., Fallon, B., MacLaurin, B., Daciuk, J., Felstiner, C., Black, T., & Cloutier, R. (2005). *Canadian incidence study of reported child abuse and neglect*. Ottawa, ON: Minister of Public Works and Government Services. Retrieved from http://www.canadiancrc.com/PDFs/Canadian_Incidence:Study_Child_Abuse_2003e.pdf.

Trocmé, N., MacLaurin, B., Fallon, B., Daciuk, J., Billingsley, D., Tourigny, M., & McKenzie, B. (2001). *Canadian incidence study of reported child abuse and neglect: Final report*. Retrieved from http://www.phac-aspc.gc.ca/publicat/cisfr-ecirf/pdf/cis_e.pdf.

Turnbull, J., Muckle, W., & Masters, C. (2007). Poverty and human development: Homelessness and health. *Canadian Medical Association Journal*, *177*(9), 1065–1066.

UNICEF. (2005). *Female genital mutilation/cutting: A statistical exploration*. Retrieved from http://www.childinfo.org/files/fgmc_U83FGM_9_web_Finalversionprinted.pdf.

van Dam, M. A. A., Koh, A. S., & Dibble, S. L. (2001). Original research: Lesbian disclosure to health care providers and delay of care. *Journal of the Gay and Lesbian Medical Association*, *5*(1), 11–19.

Vancouver Island Health Authority. (2006). *Understanding the social determinants of health*. Retrieved from http://www.crd.bc.ca/reports/regionalplanning_/generalreports_/housingaffordability_/buildingthehousingaf_/miscellaneous_/understandingsociald/understanding_social_determinants_of_health_05082006.pdf.

Weber, N. S., Cowan, D. N., Millikan, A. M., & Neibuhr, D. W. (2009). Psychiatric and general medical conditions comorbid with schizophrenia in the national hospital discharge survey. *Psychiatric Services*, *60*, 1059–1067. Retrieved from http://psychservices.psychiatryonline.org/cgi/content/abstract/60/8/1059.

Wilkins, R. S., Uppal, P., Fines, S., Guimond, S. E., & Dion, R. (2008). Life expectancy in the Inuit-inhabited areas of Canada:1989–2003. *Health Reports*, *19*(1), 7–19.

Williams, D. R., Haile, R., Neighbors, H., González, H. M., Baser, R., & Jackson, J. S. (2007). The mental health of black Caribbean immigrants: Results from the national survey of American life. *American Journal of Public Health*, *97*(1), 52–59.

Wilton, R. (2003). Poverty and mental health: A qualitative study of residential care facility clients. *Canadian Journal of Community Mental Health*, *39*(2), 139–156.

World Health Organization. (2007a). *Concepts and principles for tackling social inequities in health: Levelling up Part 1*. Retrieved from http://www.euro.who.int/document/e89383.pdf.

World Health Organization. (2007b). *What is mental health?*. Retrieved from http://www.who.int/features/qa/62/en/index.html.

World Health Organization. (2008a). *Closing the gap in a generation: Health equity through action on the social determinants of health*. Retrieved from http://whqlibdoc.who.int/hq/2008/WHO_IER_CSDH_08.1_eng.pdf.

World Health Organization. (2008b). *Part two: The urgent need for action*. Retrieved from http://www.who.int/chp/chronic_disease_report/part2_ch2/en/index5.html.

World Health Organization. (2009). *Mental health: Depression*. Retrieved from http://www.who.int/mental_health/management/depression/definition/en/.

World Health Organization. (2010). *Media centre fact sheet: Female genital mutilation*. Retrieved from http://www.who.int/mediacentre/factsheets/fs241/en/.

World Health Organization (WHO) & World Organization of Family Doctors (WONCA). (2008). *Integrating mental health into primary care: A global perspective*. Retrieved from http://www.who.int/mental_health/policy/Mental%20health%20+%20primary%20care-%20final%20low-res%20120109.pdf.

Worthington, C., & MacLaurin, B. (2009). Level of street involvement and health and health services use of Calgary street youth. *Canadian Journal of Public Health*, *100*(5), 384–388.

CHAPTER 12

Working with Family

OBJECTIVES

After reading this chapter, you should be able to:

1. Explain the importance of family nursing in the community setting.
2. Describe family demographics.
3. Define family, family nursing, family health, and healthy, unhealthy, and resilient families.
4. Analyze changes in family function and structure.
5. Explain how the determinants of health affect family.
6. Compare and contrast the four family social science theoretical frameworks.
7. Compare and contrast the four ways to view family nursing.
8. Explain the Calgary Family Assessment Model (CFAM).
9. Explain the Calgary Family Intervention Model (CFIM).
10. Outline how to promote capacity building with the family.
11. Describe the various barriers to family nursing.
12. Outline the important considerations for planning, conducting, and evaluating family home visits.
13. Analyze the various approaches to defining and conceptualizing family health.
14. Analyze the major risks to family health.
15. Analyze the interrelationships among individual health, family health, and community health.
16. Explain the application of the community health nursing process (assessment, planning, implementation, evaluation) to reducing family health risks and promoting family health.

CHAPTER OUTLINE

KEY TERMS

See Glossary on page 593 for definitions.

The family as a client unit is fundamental to the practice of community health nursing, and community health nurses (CHNs) are responsible for promoting healthy families in society. Family nursing is practised in all settings. The trend in the delivery of health care has been to move health care to community settings; thus, family nursing is incorporated in community health nursing practice. Families in the twenty-first century continue to be more diverse. **Family nursing** is a specialty area that has a strong theory base and is more than just "common sense" or viewing the family as the context for individual health care. Family nursing consists of community health nurses and families working together to ensure the success of the family and its members in adapting to health and illness.

Working as partners with families, CHNs focus on capacity building, that is, recognize family strengths and use these strengths to deal with health concerns. The family as a client unit is fundamental to the practice of community health nursing, and CHNs are responsible for promoting healthy families in society. Societal support contributes to healthier families. CHNs need to be involved in community assessment, planning, development, and evaluation activities that emphasize family issues and the family's ability to sustain itself.

The family is both an important environment affecting the health of individuals and a social unit whose health is basic to that of the community and the larger population. It is within the family that health values, health habits, and health risk perceptions are developed, organized, or performed. Individuals' health behaviours are affected by and acted out within the family environment, the larger community, and society. For example, if a child is raised in a home where the parents demonstrate healthy eating with daily physical activity and are nonsmokers, the child is more likely to adopt these healthy behaviours and to maintain them into adulthood. The risks to individual and family health are affected by the family social norms—in this example, the norm is practising healthy living. In the same manner, it is in the context of community norms and values that family health habits are developed. For example, healthy communities with walking trails, bicycle paths, smoke-free spaces, and community gardens are supportive environments for families.

To intervene effectively and appropriately with families to reduce their health risk and promote their health, it is necessary to view the family as the unit of care, to understand family structure and functioning, family theory, nursing theory, and models of health risk. It is usually necessary to go beyond the individual and the family and understand the complex environment in which the family exists. Increasing evidence of the effects of social, biological, economic, and life events on health suggests a broader approach be taken in addressing health risks for families.

The purpose of this chapter is to present a current overview of families and family nursing, theoretical frameworks, and strategies for assessing and intervening with families in the community; to note the influences, both individual and in society, that place families at risk for poor health outcomes; and to discuss how positive outcomes for families can be accomplished based on the family strengths. Options are explored for structuring community health nursing interventions with families to decrease health risks and to promote health and well-being. The Wright and Leahey (2009) Calgary Family Assessment Model (CFAM) is introduced as an assessment and an organizing framework for working with families. The Wright and Leahey (2009) Calgary Family Intervention Model (CFIM) is discussed in regard to promoting healthy family functioning.

FAMILY NURSING IN THE COMMUNITY

Health care decisions are made within the family, the basic social unit of society. Families are responsible for providing or managing the care of family members. In the current health care system, families are significant members of health care teams since they are the ever-present factor. Currently, families are expected to take more responsibility for assisting in the health care of ill family members.

CHNs partnering with families are responsible for the following:

- Helping families promote their health and healing
- Assisting with their identification of family strengths and health concerns
- Assisting and supporting families to cope with health concerns within the context of the existing family structure, family strengths, and community resources
- Identifying, enhancing, and promoting family resiliency (Black & Lobo, 2008)
- Collaborating with families to develop useful interventions
- Referring to community resources as agreed upon by the family
- Facilitating family evaluation of strengths and progress made in reference to health concerns

CHNs need to be knowledgeable about family structures, family developmental stages, functions, processes, and roles. As a partner, it is important that the CHN acknowledge that the family is the expert in relation to their health concern and in the selection of interventions most likely to work for them. Although the family is expert as to what is most important to them and their health, the CHN uses evidence-informed practice when working with the family in decision making about health intervention choices. In addition, CHNs need to be aware of and understand their own personal values and attitudes pertaining to their own families, as well as being open to different family structures and cultures.

FAMILY DEMOGRAPHICS

Family demographics is the study of the structure of families and households and the family-related events, such as marriage and divorce, that alter the structure through their number, timing, and sequencing. An important use of family demography by CHNs is to forecast stresses and developmental changes experienced by families and to identify possible solutions to family health concerns. It is important to note that the structure of families has changed over time from traditionally defined families (e.g., nuclear and extended families) to include blended families and partners (heterosexual couples who are not married), homosexual or same-sex partners, and, more recently, commuter families, and an increased number of "skipped-generation" families (grandmothers caring for grandchildren). Fuller-Thompson (2005) has prepared a research document on skipped-generation families for the Program for Research on Social and Economic Dimensions of an Aging Population (SEDAP). This document is the result of interdisciplinary research located at McMaster University in Hamilton, Ontario, but it is a collaboration project between 17 universities in Canada and internationally. In this document, titled *Grandparents Raising Grandchildren in Canada: A Profile of Skipped Generation Families,* statistics, research findings, and trends in Canada and elsewhere are presented. Implications such as the economic and health factors and cultural variations are raised and discussed. (See the Fuller-Thompson Weblink on the Evolve Web site. The CANGRANDS Weblink on the Evolve Web site provides links to available support groups across Canada to support, educate, and empower grandparents raising their grandchildren. Choose the link on the map of Canada to learn whether your community has such a group.)

Table 12-1 provides examples of the various family forms most common in Canada. In Canada, same-sex marriages were legalized nationally in July 2005 (Statistics Canada, 2007). Most persons view families and their experiences through the lens of their own family of origin. It is important to be aware of and attempt to understand other family variations. The rapid changes that occurred at the close of the twentieth century have implications for family relationships and the ability of families to meet the changing needs of their members. There is limited available published literature on same-sex unions; however, some of the available literature indicates that lesbian and gay relationships are frequently stable despite the couples usually experiencing less social support from families and communities; furthermore, children raised by same-sex partners are undifferentiated from children of heterosexual-parent partnerships (Keita, 2009; Pawelski et al., 2006; Sauvé, 2003). The Vanier Institute of the Family (2010) report identifies major changes in the Canadian family in the following aspects: structural, functional, and affective. Some of the changes, primarily based on the 2006 Canadian census data reported by the Vanier Institute, are as follows:

- There was a decreased percentage of females legally married by age 30 years (55% of those born in 1970 compared with 88% born in 1948).
- There was an increase in the ages for both females and males at time of first marriage.

TABLE 12-1 Examples of Different Family Forms in Canada

Type of Family	Description
Nuclear	• Mother, father, and children living together
Lone parent (single parent or one parent)	• Unmarried, separated, or divorced mother or father living alone with his/her children
Extended	• Nuclear family and relatives of the nuclear family
Blended (stepfamily)	• A widowed or divorced spouse with some or all of his/her children lives with a new spouse from another union with some or all of his/her children (spouses are of the opposite sex)
Commuter	• Couple with or without children live in separate residences in two different geographic locations most of the time because of work commitments. They are in a committed relationship as a couple.
Living apart together (LAT)	• A couple who are in a caring relationship, and for a variety of reasons, keep their own residences
Same sex	• Partners of the same sex living together who may or may not have children
Grandparent-led (skip generation)	• Grandparent is caring for grandchild/children within a three-generation family
Cohabiting (common-law)	• Unmarried couples living together

SOURCE: The Vanier Institute of the Family. (2010). *Families count: Profiling Canada's families IV.* Retrieved from http://www.vifamily.ca/media/node/371/attachments/Families_Count.pdf.

- There was an increase in ages in both genders for same-sex marriages compared with heterosexual marriages.
- Family size decreased.
- The percentage of lone parents increased.
- In Newfoundland and Labrador and Ontario, approximately 50% of young adults between 20 and 29 years of age resided with their parents compared with 33% in Alberta and Saskatchewan
- More immigrant population numbers in larger urban centres is a contributing factor to increased numbers of young adults residing with their parents.
- An increased percentage of young adults between the ages of 20 to 24 years of age reside with their parents (approximately 60% compared with 40%).
- Canadian families showed an increased adaptability and resiliency.

For more detailed description and discussion of the changing patterns in the Canadian family, refer to the report titled "Families Count: Profiling Canada's Families IV," available at the Vanier Institute of the Family Weblink on the Evolve Web site. The Statistics Canada "2006 Census—Families" Weblink on the Evolve Web site provides demographics of families based on 2006 census data.

Evidence-Informed Practice

Recently, child development researchers have been exploring a broader range of issues raised by different kinds of lesbian and gay families because these types of families are becoming more prevalent in our society. A convenient sample of 80 families (55 lesbian parents and 25 heterosexual parents) completed a mailed questionnaire. The study found that adolescents living with same-sex parents were similar in adjustment and on self-reported assessments of their psychological well-being when compared with opposite-sex parents; engagement in romantic relationships and in sexual intercourse was found to be equal in both groups; self-reported substance abuse, delinquency, and peer bullying findings were found to be similar in both groups; those with same-sex parents were found to have a better connection with school contacts than those with heterosexual parents (only statistically significant difference); and the qualities of the family relationships were more important than the sexual orientation of the parents for adolescent development. More research is needed about economic, religious, racial, ethnic, and cultural diversity in gay and lesbian families, as well as research findings about the ways in which gay and lesbian parents and children manage their multiple identities. There is a paucity of research on gay men and lesbians who have adopted children after "coming out." There is also a need for a study about the effects of heterosexism and homophobia on parents and children in lesbian and gay families and how they cope with ignorance and prejudice that they undoubtedly encounter. Results of future research on such issues will have the potential to increase our knowledge about nontraditional family forms and about the impact on children. These studies will stimulate innovations in theoretical understanding of human development. Research done in this area will also inform legal rulings and public policies that are relevant for gay and lesbian parents and their children.

Application for CHNs: The information gained from this type and focus of research is important for CHNs as our society is changing to include a greater number of "nontraditional" families. CHNs in their practice need to respect the differences in nontraditional families in order to work effectively with these groups. It is through enhanced tolerance and understanding that CHNs can integrate and appreciate each family unit for "who they are" rather than labelling and judging them. The quality of family relationships is an important part of the CHN's family assessment, and CHNs work with families to identify their strengths and use these to further improve their health.

Questions for Reflection & Discussion

1. What challenges do you think families headed by gays and lesbians might experience in your community?
2. What strategies does a CHN need to use when caring for a family that is nontraditional?
3. Conduct a literature search using the words *transgendered families, gay families,* and *lesbian families.* What new strategies did you find for working with nontraditional families?

REFERENCE: Patterson, C. J. (2005). Children of lesbian and gay parents. *Child Development, 63,* 1025–1042.

DEFINITION OF FAMILY

The definition of family is critical to the practice of community health nursing. Family has traditionally been defined using the legal concepts of relationships such as genetic ties, adoption, guardianship, or marriage. Since the 1980s, a broader definition of family has been used that moves beyond the traditional blood, marriage, and legal constrictions. "**Family** refers to two or more individuals who depend on one another for emotional, physical, and/or financial support. The members of the family are self-defined" (Harmon Hanson, 2005, p. 7). Wright and Leahey (2009) state, "The family is who they say they are" (p. 50), which moves beyond the traditional definitions. Based on these definitions, it is important to recognize that a family is a group and is therefore two or more people, with *people* being defined by the family. Therefore, it is critical that CHNs working with families ask the family members who they consider to be their family and then include those members in health care planning. The family may range from traditional nuclear and extended families to such "postmodern" family structures as one-parent families, stepfamilies, same-sex families, neighbours, and friends.

FAMILY STRUCTURE

Family structure refers to the characteristics and demographics (gender, age, number) of individual members who make up family units. More specifically, the structure of a family defines the family members (who is in this family), what the relationships are between these members, and family context. Wright and Leahey (2009) further divide family structure into internal, external, and contextual categories, with specific subcategories within each. Figure 12-1 is a branching diagram from the Calgary Family Assessment Model that outlines the structural, developmental, and functional categories of family assessment.

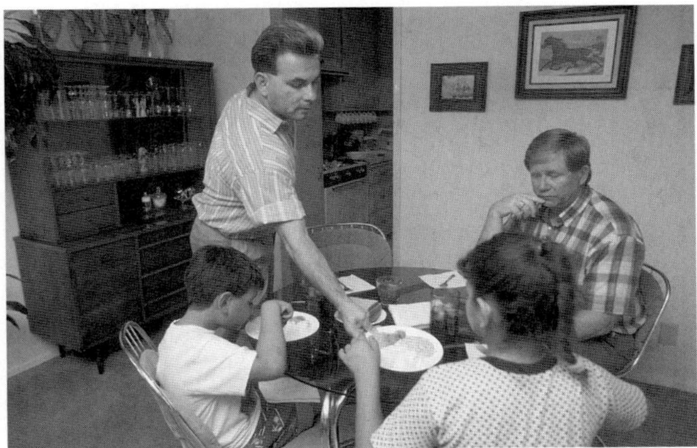

People view families and their experiences based on their own family of origin. However, it is important to be aware of and understand other family variations.

CRITICAL VIEW

1. What do you think is the difference between the terms *gender* and *sex*?
2. What legislation is in place, if any, in your province or territory to prevent discrimination based on gender?
3. What is the difference between gender discrimination, gender sensitivity, and gender mainstreaming?

After you have answered these questions, go to the Gender and Health Collaborative Curriculum Weblink: http://www.genderandhealth.ca/difference.jsp. Click to start the video.

DETERMINANTS OF HEALTH

Health and illness are influenced by family. The determinants of health need to be considered when working with families in the community. Housing is part of the physical environment (man-made), which is one of the determinants of health. Income is another determinant of health. Adequate income is related to the ability to purchase affordable housing and to meet food security and other needs. The determinants of health "personal health practices and coping skills" also incorporate lifestyle choices that affect the family. Gender and social environments are determinants of health that also have an impact on the family. The "Determinants of Health" box on page 373 provides some examples of available information on the determinants of health for CHNs to consider when working with families. See also the "Ethical Considerations" box on page 373.

FAMILY HEALTH

Despite the focus on family health within nursing, the meaning of family health lacks consensus and is not precise. The term *family health* is often used interchangeably with the concepts of family functioning, healthy families, or familial health. **Family health** refers to

FIGURE 12-1 Branching Diagram of the Calgary Family Assessment Model

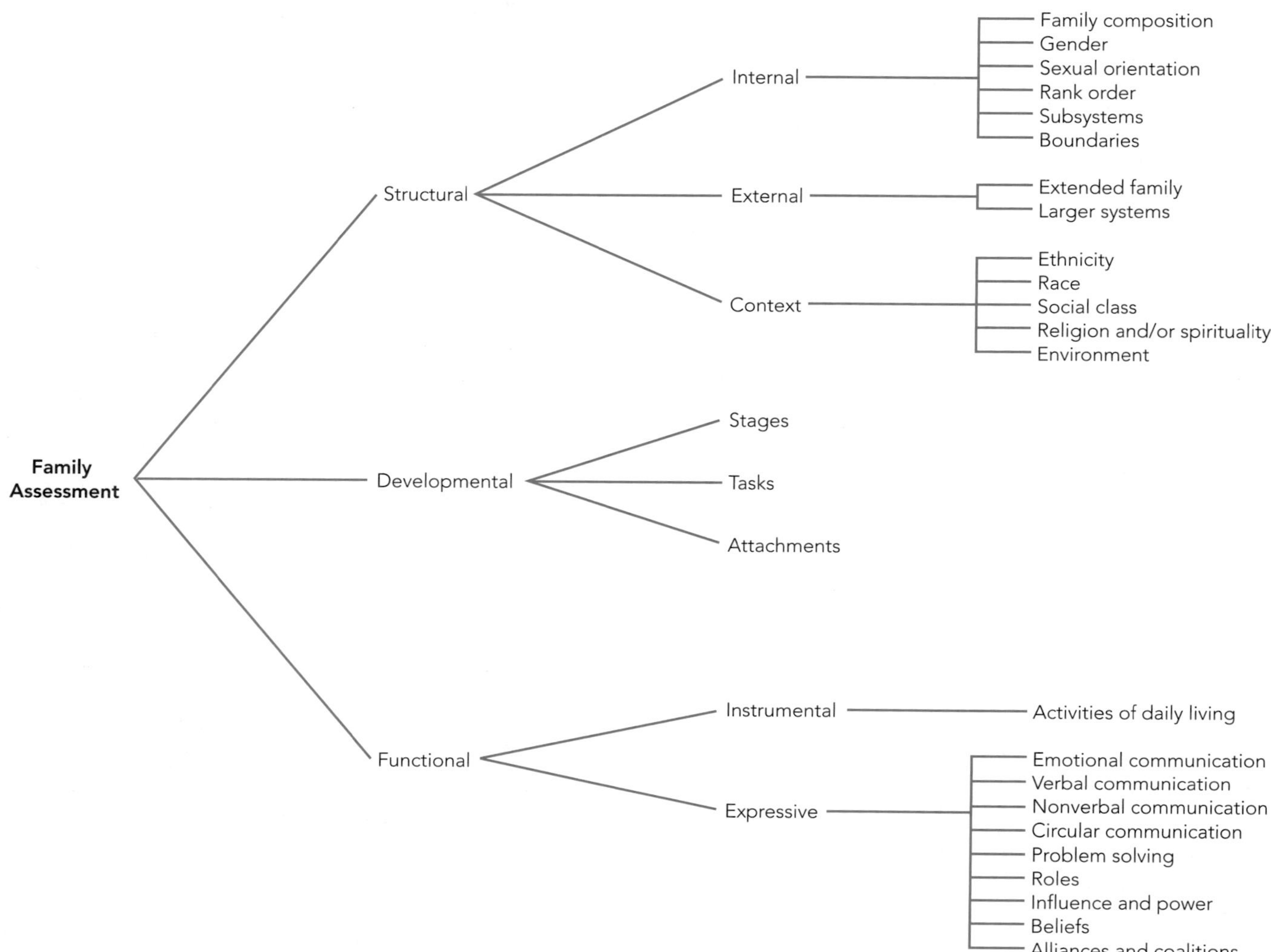

Wright, L. M., & Leahy, M. (2009). *Nurses and families: A guide to family assessment and intervention* (5th ed., p. 48). Philadelphia, PA: F. A. Davis.

the health of a family system that is ever changing and encompasses a holistic focus that includes biological, psychological, sociological, cultural, and spiritual factors (Harmon Hanson, 2005).

This holistic approach refers to individual members as well as the family unit as a whole. An individual's health (wellness–illness continuum) affects the entire family's functioning, and, in turn, the family's functioning affects the health of the individuals. Thus, assessment of family health involves simultaneous assessment of individual family members and the family system as a whole. For CHNs, it is important in clinical practice to distinguish between caring for "the individual as client," with the family as the context for care, and the "family as client" and, therefore, the unit of care. For example, in the former instance, the individual family member is the unit of care, with the family members in the background in their context as resource; in the latter instance, the family is the unit of care and the individual is in the background (Harmon Hanson, Gedaly-Duff, & Rowe Kaakinen, 2005; Wright & Leahey, 2009).

Family Health and Functionality

Terms related to "healthy" versus "unhealthy" families have varied in the literature. Table 12-2 contrasts characteristics of healthy and unhealthy families. Health professionals have tended to classify families dependent on their coping skills as a unit into two groups: "good families," or functional families, and "bad families," or

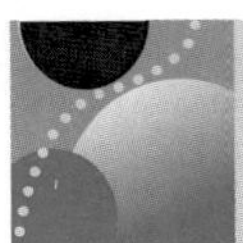

Determinants of Health
Families

- The 2006 census enumerated 45,345 same-sex couples; 16.5% were married couples. Approximately 54% of these same-sex married spouses were male, compared with approximately 46% who were female (Statistics Canada, 2007). These findings support the changing face of families to include "nontraditional" family structure forms.
- The 2006 census data for married-couple families reported an increase of only 3.5% from 2001. Common-law-couple families increased 18.9%, and the number of lone-parent families increased 7.8% (Statistics Canada, 2007). These findings also support the changing face of families to include nontraditional family structure forms.
- Approximately half (52%) of low-income children in Canada live in female lone-parent families (Campaign 2000, 2006). Poverty is more likely to be experienced by female lone-parent families in Canada. In fact, most female lone-parent families in Canada have an income that is at least "$9,400 below the poverty line" and "the gap between the incomes of low income families and well-off families has continued to widen" (Campaign 2000, 2006, p. 4).
- Children who live with family violence have an increased risk of developing psychological and behavioural problems (Bedi & Goddard, 2007); therefore, more community strategies are needed to prevent, reduce, and possibly eliminate family violence.
- Inadequate housing and income are linked with domestic violence (Christy-McMullin & Shobe, 2007). Women with lower incomes experience physical abuse more frequently than women with higher incomes (Christy-McMullin & Shobe, 2007). Canada does not yet have a strategy on affordable housing, and vulnerable populations are most affected by this lack of policy.
- It is anticipated that the number of families will decrease, with a growth of approximately 15% between 2005 and 2026 (Vanier Institute of the Family, 2006).
- Lifestyle choices are linked to patterns learned from parents (Baxter, Bylund, Imes, & Scheive, 2005). Strategies such as creating supportive environments are essential to encourage healthy lifestyles.

ETHICAL CONSIDERATIONS

The CHN works with low-income young mothers in her community. The CHN organized a 6-week educational program about breastfeeding and healthy nutrition. During the time of the program delivery, she noticed that the majority of the single-parent mothers did not attend these sessions.

Ethical principles that apply to this scenario:

- *Beneficence*. Do good. It relates to health improvement in populations, not just individuals. In assessing the health improvement benefits of a given action, consideration is given to the importance, the causation, and the potential preventability of the issue or issues concerned (Tannahill, 2008).
- *Nonmaleficence*. Do no harm. It is not always possible to avoid harm entirely, but CHNs act according to the standards of due care in making sure to produce the least amount of harm possible.

Questions to Consider

1. a) How would you apply the principles of beneficence and nonmaleficence to this client situation?

   b) Are there other ethical considerations in relation to this client situation? Explain.
2. Are there moral issues to consider in this client situation? Explain.

TABLE 12-2 Features of Healthy and Unhealthy Families

Healthy	Unhealthy
Family is stable and copes with its physical, psychosocial, and spiritual needs, and growth and development needs.	Family is unstable with ineffective family coping to meet family needs.
Family works together, members are sensitive, encourage and support each other, especially during problem solving and decision making, thereby strengthening family relationships and unity.	Family members do not support each other and may act as if other family members do not matter. Member individuality is often lost because of extremely close or distant relationships among some members in the family. There is lack of problem solving and decision making by the family.
Families with children practise healthy child-rearing and discipline.	Families with children are too permissive or restrictive with child-rearing practices. One example of unhealthy practices would include child abuse.
Parents are positive role models for children in the family.	Lack of positive role modelling. Children assume parental roles because parents are unable to do so.
Boundary is flexible so family and its external systems are able to exchange information.	Boundary is too rigid so that there is very limited family and individual member contacts with external systems, or boundary is too flexible and family system is overwhelmed with information from outside sources.
Power structure, roles, and rules are clear and relevant.	Unclear lines of authority with roles and rules that are unclear and/or not relevant, often resulting in derogatory comments among family members.
Power is appropriately shared with family members.	Family members are domineering with each other and do not respect rights and abilities of its members.
Communication among family members is open and direct; actively listen to its members and are respectful of member individuality.	Lack of communication among family members, or family arguments occur that negate family members.
Family is sufficiently open, flexible, adaptable, and resilient so it can manage a variety of demands on its unit.	Family home is insecure with high anxiety levels; scapegoating and blaming of others for individual and/or family problems is common.
Family demonstration of growth producing community relationships.	Family has limited or no involvement with the community.
Family is open to accepting outside help when appropriate and recognizes limitations.	Family often denies problems or tries to solve all its own problems and is unwilling to accept outside help.

SOURCE: Adapted from McEwen, M., & Pullis, B. (2009). *Community-based nursing: An introduction* (3rd ed.). St. Louis, MO: Saunders Elsevier.

dysfunctional families. **Functional families** are effective coping family units that provide autonomy and are responsive to the particular interests and needs of individual family members. Dysfunctional families are ineffective coping family units that inhibit clear communication within family relationships and do not provide psychological support for individual members. A term that has been used for unhealthy families is *dysfunctional families;* they are also referred to as *noncompliant, resistant,* or *unmotivated.* These terms denote families that are not functioning well within the family unit or in society. The use of the term *dysfunctional family* has been challenged by some family writers (Bell, 1995; Cooley, 2009). CHNs would be well advised to avoid thinking in these terms because it suggests pathology with deficits, versus family capacity building based on strengths, and therefore tends to encourage helplessness in the family. The term encourages CHNs to assign blame and to use "why" questions, which are linear and suggest causation, instead of "how" questions to explore possible interventions. CHNs might consider referring to these families as families with health challenges. Although the two terms, *functional* and *dysfunctional*, are far from ideal when referring to family functioning, they are often used in the family and nursing literature.

CRITICAL VIEW

1. What are some examples of healthy families in today's sociopolitical environmental context?
2. To be a healthy family, do you need to have all the characteristics identified in Table 12-2? Explain.
3. Using an "equity lens," identify what factors might contribute to health disparities in lone-parent families.

FOUR APPROACHES TO FAMILY NURSING

Central to the practice of family nursing is conceptualizing and approaching the family from four perspectives (Harmon Hanson et al., 2005). All have legitimate implications for nursing assessment and intervention (see Figures 12-2 and 12-3). Which approach CHNs use is determined by many factors, including the health care setting, family circumstances, and CHN values, beliefs, and resources:

1. *Family as the context, or structure.* This has a traditional focus that places the individual first and the family second. The family as context serves as either a resource or a stressor to individual health and illness. A CHN using this focus might ask an individual client, "How has your diagnosis of insulin-dependent diabetes affected your family?" or "Will your need for medication at night be a problem for your family?"
2. *Family as the client.* The family is first, and individuals are second. The family is seen as the sum of individual family members. The focus is concentrated on each individual as he or she affects the family as a whole. From this perspective, a CHN might say to a family member who has just become ill, "Tell me about what has been going on with your own health and how you perceive each family member responding to your mother's recent diagnosis of liver cancer."
3. *Family as a system.* The focus is on the family as client, and the family is viewed as an interacting system in which the whole is more than the sum of its parts. This approach simultaneously focuses on individual members and the family as a whole at the same time. The interactions between family members become the target for nursing interventions (e.g., the direct interactions between the parents, or the indirect interaction between the parents and the child). The systems approach to family always implies that when something happens to one family member, the other members of the family system are affected. Questions CHNs ask when approaching a family as system are "What has changed between you and your spouse since your child's head injury?" or "How do you feel about the fact that your son's long-term rehabilitation will affect the ways in which the members of your family are functioning and getting along with one another?"
4. *Family as a component of society.* The family is seen as one of many institutions in society, along with health, education, religious, and financial institutions. The family is a basic or primary unit of society, as are all the other units, and they are all a part of the larger system of society. The family as a whole interacts with other institutions to receive, exchange, or give services and communicate. CHNs have drawn many of their tenets from this perspective as they focus on the interface between families and community agencies.

THEORETICAL FRAMEWORKS FOR FAMILY NURSING

An important consideration for community health nursing practice is an awareness that approaches to family nursing stem from family theory. Within the family social science tradition, four conceptual approaches have dominated the field of marriage and family: structure–function theory, systems theory, developmental theory, and interactional theory (Maurer & Smith, 2009). These theories are constantly evolving and being tested, which helps make this knowledge base stronger and more user-friendly for working with families. Table 12-3 summarizes the four major family social theories and what they have contributed to **family nursing theory,** whose function is to characterize, explain, or predict phenomena (events) evident within family nursing. Table 12-4 provides information on the assessment and interventions, strengths, and weaknesses of each of these theories.

Each of the four major theories is briefly summarized. The structure–function theory perspective is a useful framework for assessing families and health. Illness of a family member results in the alteration of the family structure and function. If a single mother is ill, she cannot carry out her various roles, so grandparents or siblings may have to assume child care responsibilities. Family power structures and communication patterns are affected when a parent is ill. However, the family system theory perspective encourages CHNs to view clients as participating members of a family. CHNs using this perspective determine the effects of illness or injury on the entire family system—that is, the family as the unit of care. Emphasis is on the whole rather than on individuals. In comparison, the developmental

FIGURE 12-2 Approaches to Family Nursing

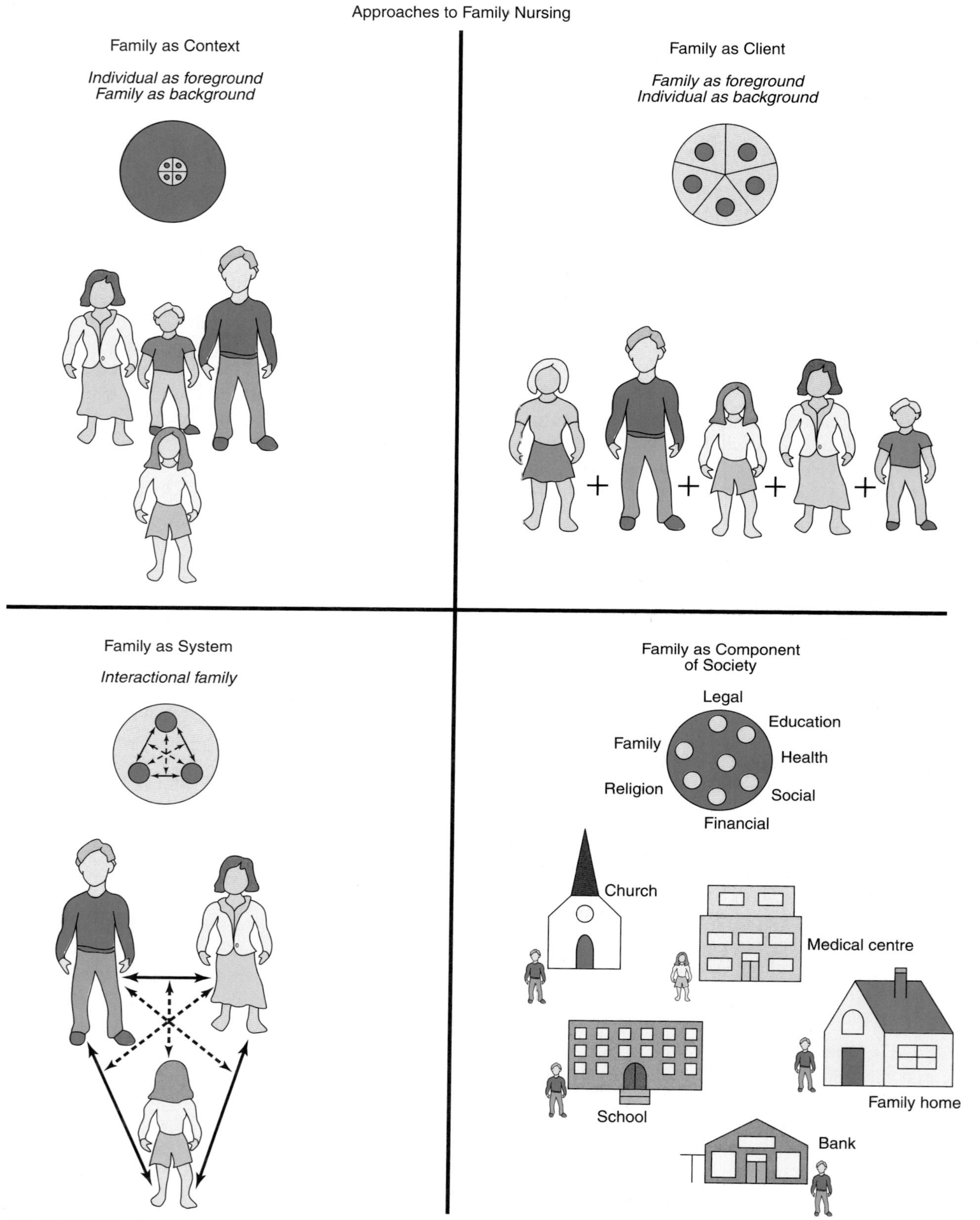

Harmon Hanson, S. M. (2005). Family health care nursing: An introduction. In S. M. Harmon Hanson, V. Gedaly Duff, & J. Rowe Kaakinen (Eds.), *Family health care nursing: Theory, practice and research* (3rd ed., p. 12). Philadelphia, PA: F. A. Davis.

FIGURE 12-3 Four Views of the Family

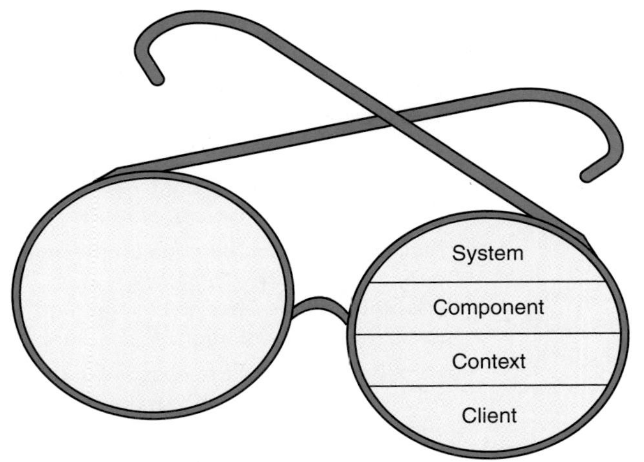

Harmon Hanson, S. M. (2005). Family health care nursing: An introduction. In S. M. Harmon Hanson, V. Gedaly Duff, & J. Rowe Kaakinen (Eds.), *Family health care nursing: Theory, practice and research* (3rd ed., p. 13). Philadelphia, PA: F. A. Davis.

framework assists CHNs in anticipating clinical health concerns in families, identifies family strengths, serves as a guide in assessing the family's developmental stage, assesses the extent to which the family is fulfilling the tasks associated with its respective stage, assesses the family's developmental history, and assesses the availability of resources essential for performing developmental tasks. Finally, CHNs using the interactional theory would explore individual family members' perceptions, their interactions and communication processes with other members. The CHN would analyze family roles, expectations, conflicts, problem solving, and decision making (Beckmann Murray, Zentner, Pangman, & Pangman, 2009).

The International Council of Nurses has prepared a document titled *Tools for Action,* listed in the Tool Box on the Evolve Web site. This document provides information on three family assessment models and a short tool that agencies can use to assess family satisfaction with their services.

FAMILY ASSESSMENT MODELS AND APPROACHES

Many family assessment models and approaches are available, and three of these are discussed below. One of these family assessment models and approaches—the Friedman Family Assessment Model (Short Form)—integrates the structure–function framework and developmental and systems theories. The Friedman Family Assessment Model (Short Form) is presented in Appendix E-4 on the Evolve Web site accompanying this text. The model takes a broad approach to family assessment, which views families as a subsystem of society. The family is viewed as an open social system. The family's structure (organization) and functions (activities and purposes) and the family's relationship to other social systems are the focus of this approach. The assumptions underlying this model are presented in Table 12-3.

This assessment approach is important for CHNs because it enables them to assess the family system as a whole, as part of the whole of society, and as an interaction system. The guidelines for the Friedman Family Assessment Model (Friedman, Bowden, & Jones, 2003) consist of the following six broad categories of interview categories:

TABLE 12-3 Key Points and Assumptions of Selected Theoretical Frameworks for Family Nursing

Name of Theory Type	Key Points	Assumptions
Structure-Function Theory	• Defines family as a social system • Family is viewed as open to the outside system but boundaries are maintained • Family is viewed as passive in adapting to outside system and therefore is not viewed as a change agent • Examines families in terms of: a) relationships with, for example, government, health care, and religious institutions b) family patterns in relation to society c) how well the family structure performs its functions	• A family is a social system with functional requirements. • A family is a small group that has basic features common to all small groups. • Social systems, such as families, accomplish functions that serve the individuals in addition to those that serve society. • Individuals act within a set of internal norms and values that are learned primarily in the family through socialization.

(Continued)

TABLE 12-3 Key Points and Assumptions of Selected Theoretical Frameworks for Family Nursing—Cont'd

Name of Theory Type	Key Points	Assumptions
Systems Theory	• Influenced by theory from physics and biology • A system is composed of a set of interacting elements. • Each system can be identified and is distinct from the environment in which it exists. • An open system exchanges energy and matter with the environment (negentropy). • A closed system is isolated from its environment (entropy). • Systems depend on both positive and negative feedback to maintain a steady state (homeostasis). • Seeking therapy when the marital relationship is strained is an example of using negative feedback to maintain a steady state.	• Family systems are greater than and different from the sum of their parts. • There are many hierarchies within family systems and logical relationships between subsystems (e.g., mother–child, family–community). • There are boundaries in the family system that can be open, closed, or random. • Family systems increase in complexity over time, evolving to allow greater adaptability, tolerance to change, and growth by differentiation. • Family systems change constantly in response to stresses and strains from within and from outside environments. There are structural similarities in different family systems (isomorphism). • Change in one part of family systems affects the total system. • Causality is modified by feedback; therefore, causality never exists in the real world. • Family systems patterns are circular rather than linear; change must be directed toward the cycle. • Family systems are an organized whole; therefore, individuals within the family are interdependent. • Family systems have homeostasis features to maintain stable patterns that can be adaptive or maladaptive.
Developmental Theory	• Principles of individual development are applied to the family unit. • Stage of family unit is determined by age of the oldest child. • Identified family tasks need to be accomplished during each stage of family development. • Developmental concepts include moving to a different level of functioning, implying progress in a single direction. • Family disequilibrium and conflicts are described as occurring during transition periods from one stage to another. The family has a predictable natural history designated by stages, beginning with the simple husband–wife pair. • The group becomes more complex with the addition of each new child. • The group again becomes simple and less complex as the younger generation leaves home. • The group comes full circle to the original husband–wife pair. • At each family life-cycle stage, there are developmental needs of the family and tasks that must be performed. • Achievement of family developmental tasks helps individual members accomplish their tasks.	• In every family, there are both individual and family developmental tasks that need to be accomplished for every stage of the individual and family life cycle that are unique to that particular group. • Families change and develop in different ways because of internal and environmental stimulations. • Developmental tasks are goals to work toward rather than specific jobs to be completed at once. • Each family is unique in its composition and complexity of age–role expectations and positions. • Individuals and families are a function of their history, as well as the current social structure. • Families have commonalities despite the way they develop over the family lifespan. • Families may arrive at similar developmental levels through different processes.

TABLE 12-3 Key Points and Assumptions of Selected Theoretical Frameworks for Family Nursing—Cont'd

Name of Theory Type	Key Points	Assumptions
Interactional Theory	• Family is viewed as interacting personalities. • Family is examined by the symbolic communications by which family members relate to one another. • Within the family, each member occupies a position to which a number of roles are assigned. • Members define their role expectations in each situation through their perceptions of the role demands. • Members judge their own behaviour by assessing and interpreting the actions of others toward them. • Central to the interaction approach is the process of role taking. • The ability to predict other family members' expectations for one's role enables each member to have some knowledge of how to react in the role and indicates how other members will react to performing the role.	• Complex sets of symbols having common meanings are acquired through living in a symbolic environment. • Individuals distinguish, evaluate, and assign meaning to symbols. • Behaviour is influenced by meanings of symbols or ideas rather than by instincts, needs, or drives; therefore, the meaning an individual assigns to symbols is important to understanding behaviour. • The self continues to change and evolve over time through introspection caused by experience and activity. • The evolving self has several dimensions: the physical body and characteristics and a complex social self. The "me" is a conventional, habitual self that consists of learned, repetitious responses. The "I" is spontaneous to the individual. • Individuals are actors as well as reactors; they select and interpret the environment to which they respond. • Individuals are born into a dynamic society. • Individuals learn from the culture and become the society. • Individuals' behaviour is a product of their history, which is continually being modified by new information.

TABLE 12-4 Information on Assessment and Interventions, Strengths and Weaknesses of Selected Theoretical Frameworks for Family Nursing

Theory Name	Assessment and Interventions	Strengths	Weaknesses
Structure–Function	• Determine if changes resulting from the illness influence the family's ability to carry out its functions. • Sample assessment questions are "How did the death alter the family structure?" and "What family roles were changed with the onset of the chronic illness?" • Interventions become necessary when a change in the family structure alters the family's ability to function. • Examples of interventions using this model include helping families use existing support structures and helping families modify the way they are organized so that role responsibilities can be distributed.	• Comprehensive approach that views families in the broader community in which they live	• Static picture of the family, which does not allow for dynamic change over time

(Continued)

TABLE 12-4 Information on Assessment and Interventions, Strengths and Weaknesses of Selected Theoretical Frameworks for Family Nursing—Cont'd

Theory Name	Assessment and Interventions	Strengths	Weaknesses

Systems	• Assessment is made of the following:
	  • Individual members
	  • Subsystems
	  • Boundaries
	  • Openness
	  • Inputs and outputs
	  • Family interactions
	  • Family processing
	  • Adaptation or change abilities
	• Assessment questions include "Who is in the family system?" and "How has one member's critical illness affected the entire family system?"
	• Interventions need to assist individual, subsystem, and whole family functioning.
	• Examples include establishing a mechanism for providing families with information about their family members on a regular basis and discussing ways to provide for a "normal" family life for family members after someone has become ill.
		• Views families from both a subsystem and a suprasystem approach
		• Views the interactions within and among family subsystems as well as the interactions among families and the larger supersystems, such as community, world, and universe
			• Focus is on the interaction of the family with other systems rather than on the individual, which is sometimes more important

Developmental	• Several questions can be asked, for example, "Where does this family place on the continuum of the family life cycle?" and "What are the developmental tasks that are not being accomplished?" • Typical kinds of community health nursing intervention strategies using this perspective help the family understand individual and family growth and development stages and deal with the normal transitions between developmental periods (e.g., tasks of the school-age family member versus tasks of the adolescent family member).	• Provides a basis for forecasting what a family will be experiencing at any period in the family life cycle (e.g., role transitions and family structure changes)	• Model was developed at a time when the traditional nuclear family was emphasized

Interactional	• Emphasis is on interaction between and among family members and family communication patterns about health and illness behaviours appropriate for different roles.
	• Nursing strategies focus on the following (Bomar, 2004):
	  • Effectiveness of communication among members
	  • Ability to establish communication between community health nurses and families
	  • Clear and concise messages between members
	  • Similarities between verbal and nonverbal communication patterns
	  • Directions of the interaction
	• Observe how family members interact with one another to help explain family communication, roles, decision making, and problem solving (Friedman, Bowden, & Jones, 2003).
		• Focus on internal processes within families, such as roles, conflict, status, communication, responses to stress, decision making, and socialization
		• Processes, rather than end products, of social interactions are major focus; thus, this framework used by many nurse scholars
			• Broadness and lack of agreement about concepts and assumptions of the theory, which has made it difficult to refine
			• Families considered as closed units with little relation to the outside society

1. Identifying data
2. Developmental family stage and history
3. Environmental data
4. Family structure, including communication, power structures, role structures, and family values
5. Family functions, including affective functions, socialization, and health care
6. Family coping

Each category has several subcategories. The Friedman Model was developed to provide guidelines for family nurses who are interviewing a family to gain an overall view of what is going on in the family. The questions are extensive, and it may not be possible to collect all the data at one visit. All the categories may not be pertinent for every family.

The second family assessment model and approach discussed is Wright and Leahey's (2009) CFAM model. CFAM is a **family systems nursing model** that takes a holistic approach to assessment of family health (see Appendix 9). As a family systems nursing model, the focus is on the family unit as client. This family systems nursing approach consists of a structural, developmental, and functional assessment of the family. The structural assessment includes the categories of the internal and external structures and context of the family. Refer to Figure 12-1 (see page 372) for the branching diagram of CFAM, which outlines the subcategories in the structural assessment. The genogram and ecomap are two commonly used structural assessment tools used in this model; they are presented later in this chapter.

The developmental assessment contains the family life-cycle stages, tasks usually achieved in relation to life-cycle stages, and attachments for the family. The family life stages are as follows: leaving home as a single young adult, family joining as a new couple, families with children, families with adolescents, children leaving home and moving forward, and families in later life. The hypothesis is that the family is always at a new stage and facing new transitions as they deal with new issues of development (Wright & Leahey, 2009). **Transition** is the movement from one developmental or health stage or condition to another that may be a time of potential risk for families.

For example, a family with an adolescent and also a young child is developmentally at the stage of "families with adolescents." *Attachments* refers to particular emotional bonds formed between specific members and does not refer to right or wrong attachments (Wright & Leahey, 2009). Hypotheses are formed about these attachments in relation to family development.

Functional assessment includes the categories of instrumental and expressive functioning. *Instrumental family functioning* refers to the activities of everyday living. *Expressive family functioning* refers to the emotional functioning, communication types, and other areas as outlined in the CFAM branching diagram. Wright and Leahey (2009) have developed the Calgary Family Intervention Model (CFIM), the first nursing family intervention model, for CHNs to use to facilitate functioning in the cognitive, affective, and behavioural domains of family functioning. In this nursing model, family strengths are identified through the use of **commendations,** which means the health professional praises the family for patterns in behaviour that are family strengths within the family unit. Using commendations as an intervention helps to change family functioning in the cognitive domain. Commendations frequently help families to begin viewing the family unit in a different, more positive light. In fact, Sittner, Hudson, and Defrain (2007) indicate that when nurses use a family strengths approach, the family focuses on its visions and hopes for the future instead of focusing on factors related to family health concerns.

Circular communication happens between people as each person influences the behaviour of the other. Difference, behavioural effect, hypothetical and future-oriented, and triadic questions are the four types of circular questions used to change family behaviour (Wright & Leahey, 2009). Examples for each domain are presented in Table 12-5. Wright and Leahey (2009) provide a detailed discussion of CFAM and CFIM.

The third family assessment model and approach presented is the McGill Model of Nursing, which was initially developed by Dr. Moyra Allen and others and then was further developed by Ford-Gilboe and colleagues (Ford-Gilboe, 2002). This developmental model of health in nursing explores contextual factors of health work, health potential, style of nursing, competence in health behaviour, and health status. It is described by Bomar (2004) as having the potential to become a health promotion model as it focuses on increasing the unity of the

CRITICAL VIEW

1. What are some culturally competent considerations that you, as a CHN, would consider when working with culturally diverse families?
2. a) What are some family stressors that could challenge this unit of care?

   b) How would you as the CHN assist the family to deal with these family stressors?

Evidence-Informed Practice

The purpose of this evaluation project was to uncover nurses' and families' experiences about the family–nurse relationship when practice was guided by a family systems nursing (FSN) approach. In the FSN approach, the family–nurse relationship is an equal partnership whereby each partner brings expertise to the relationship, with reciprocity being an important component of this relational partnership. The aim of FSN is to create partnerships for mutual trust, communication, and cooperation between the nurse and family.

Nurses in the current study were introduced to the FSN approach in an educational workshop. Following the workshop, the evaluation, involving 17 nurses and 13 parents, was completed over an 8-week period of the hospitalization of the parent-participants' children in a pediatric rehabilitation centre. Questionnaires and semi-structured interviews were the data-collection methods. Nurses also completed journals reflecting their experiences with families. Content analysis was used in the analysis of the qualitative data. The results of the study indicated that FSN had a positive impact on nurses' views about their practice with families, and families were more positive about the family–nurse interaction. The differences for nurses, as they describe their nursing practice, were being more focused on the whole family as a unit of care, having increased communication and interactions with family, and creating enhanced professional practice and self-esteem. Families reported nurses to be more open and caring in their communication. Families also perceived nurses to be more receptive about their expertise regarding their family function.

Application for CHNs: The study findings support the importance of family as client, an approach that has relevance for community health nursing. Family system nursing is an important approach for CHNs to use when working with families in the community.

Questions for Reflection & Discussion

1. How might you apply the study findings in your community health nursing practice?
2. What has been your experience in working with family as the unit of care?
3. Based on your further review of the family systems nursing literature, what are the findings that would be applicable to your community health nursing practice in relation to the family as expert and partner?

REFERENCE: LeGrow, K., & Rossen, B. (2005). Development of professional practice based on a family systems nursing framework: Nurses' and families' experiences. *Journal of Family Nursing, 11*(1), 38–58.

family unit and also its quality of life. Harmon Hanson et al. (2005) describe this interactional model as a family health promotion model that empowers clients toward improvements in their health. Rather than focusing on the deficits or dysfunctional family, the CHN using this assessment model identifies family strengths considering individual family members, family as the unit of care, and external resources to plan interventions.

The CHN works in partnership with the client to promote health. Each family nursing assessment model and approach is unique and creates a database upon which to plan interventions. Select family assessment models have been presented and are not all-inclusive. Many other models exist, but the focus in this text is on the Canadian CFAM, one of the most frequently used nursing family models. Loveland-Cherry (2006), in her editorial, reviewed the family intervention literature to determine where nursing is at with regard to the evaluation of family interventions. This researcher found that the quantitative studies included randomized clinical trials, longitudinal studies, and comparative studies and also some qualitative studies. Based on the review of the research, Loveland-Cherry concluded that family at the time of review was considered to influence health and that funding agencies were supporting this area of research.

FAMILY HOME VISITS

CHNs work with families in a variety of settings, including clinics, schools, support groups, and offices. However, an important aspect of the CHN's role in reducing health risks and promoting the health of populations has been the tradition of providing services to families in their homes. The Canadian Community Health Nursing Standards of Practice provide further guidance on the CHN's responsibilities under the various standards when dealing with family

TABLE 12-5 Types of Circular Questions

Type of Question	Cognitive	Affective	Behavioural
	Examples to Elicit Change in Domains		
Difference Question			
Explores differences between people, relationships, time, ideas, or beliefs	What is the best advice given to you about supporting your son with AIDS? What is the worst advice that you received?	Who in the family is most worried about how AIDS is transmitted?	Which family member is best at getting your son to take his medication on time?
Behavioural Effect Question			
Explores communications between how one family member's behaviour affects other members	What do you know about the effect of life-threatening illness on children?	How does your son show that he is afraid of dying?	What could you do to show your son that you understand his fears?
Hypothetical/Future-Oriented Question			
Explores family options and alternative actions or meanings in the future	What do you think will happen if these skin grafts continue to be painful for your son?	If your son's skin grafts are not successful, what do you think his mood will be? Angry? Resigned?	When will your son engage in treatment for his contractures?
Triadic Question			
Question posed to a third person about the relationship between two other people	If your father were not drinking daily, what would your mother think about his receiving treatment for alcoholism?	What does your father do that makes your mother less anxious about his condition?	If your father were willing to talk with your mother about solutions to his addiction, what could he say?

AIDS = Acquired immunodeficiency syndrome.

Source: Adapted from Wright, L. M., & Leahy, M. (2009). *Nurses and families: A guide to family assessment and intervention* (5th ed., p. 148). Philadelphia, PA: F. A. Davis. Reproduced with permission.

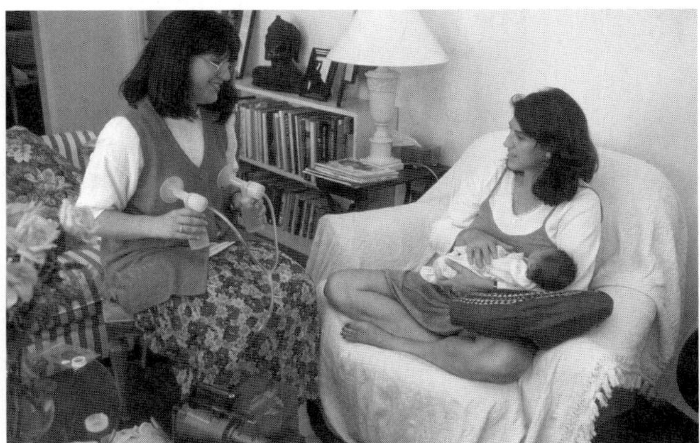

An advantage of the community health nurse meeting the family in the home is that it allows family members to feel comfortable and be themselves.

as client. The CHN works with families within the context of care to an individual and in many instances within the context of family as the unit of care. The standards also give direction as to the strategies to use when working with families, such as forming partnerships, promoting capacity building, empowering families, and advocating for families. Using a family assessment model needs to be the first step CHNs take in identifying family strengths, health risks, and health concerns when working with the family to implement health promotion interventions.

Planning for Home Visits

Before contacting the family to arrange for the initial appointment, the CHN decides the best place to meet with the family, which might be in the home, clinic, or office. Often this decision is dictated by the type of agency with which the CHN works (e.g., home health is conducted in the home, or a mental health agency may

CRITICAL VIEW

Refer to the five Canadian Community Health Nursing Standards of Practice: promoting health; building individual and community capacity; building relationships; facilitating access and equity; and demonstrating professional responsibility and accountability. Then answer the questions below:

1. How do these standards guide the community health nurses' practice with families? Provide specific examples.
2. From your experience as a member of a family and based on readings about family, what, if any, gaps exist in care of the family in relation to the Canadian Community Health Nursing Standards of Practice?

choose to have the family meet in the neighbourhood clinic office). The CHN needs to review the agency policy about home visiting before the decision is made to contact the family to make arrangements regarding where and when to meet.

Advantages to meeting in the family home include the following:

- Meeting in the home allows for viewing the everyday family environment.
- Family members are likely to feel more relaxed and therefore demonstrate typical family interactions.
- Meeting with a family in their home emphasizes that the health concern is the responsibility of the whole family and not one family member.
- Conducting the interview in the home may increase the probability of having more family members present.

The following are two possible disadvantages of meeting in the family's home:

1. Perception of invasion of privacy. Their home may be the only sanctuary or safe place for the family or its members to be away from the scrutiny of others.
2. Meeting with a family on their ground requires the CHN to be highly skilled in communication, setting limits, and guiding the interaction.

Conducting the family appointment in the office or clinic allows easier access to other health care providers for consultation. An advantage of using the clinic may be that the family situation is so intense that a more formal, less personal setting may be necessary for the family to begin discussion of emotionally charged issues. A disadvantage of not seeing the everyday family environment is that it may reinforce a possible culture gap between the family and the CHN.

After the decision is made regarding where to meet the family, the CHN contacts the family. It is important to remember that the family gathers information about the CHN from this initial phone call to arrange a meeting, so the CHN should be confident and organized. After the introduction, the CHN concisely states the reason for requesting the family visit and encourages all family members to attend the meeting. Several possible times for the appointment can be offered, including late afternoon or evening, allowing the family to select the most convenient time for all members to be present (see the "How To... Set an Appointment with the Family" box).

Usually, a home visit is initiated as the result of a referral from a health or social agency. A **home visit** is the provision of community health nursing care where

How To... Set an Appointment with the Family

The assessment process starts immediately upon referral. The following are suggestions that will make the process of arranging a meeting with the family easier:

1. Remember that the assessment is reciprocal and the family will be making judgements about you when you call to make the appointment.
2. Introduce yourself and state the purpose for the contact.
3. Do not apologize for contacting the family. Be clear, direct, and specific about the need for an appointment.
4. Arrange a time that is convenient for the greatest possible number of family members.
5. Confirm the place, time, date, and directions to the selected meeting place.

the individual resides. However, a family may request services, or the CHN may initiate the home visit as a result of case-finding activities. The CHN would need to clarify with the referral agency and family the reason for the visit request. The first contact between the CHN and the family provides the foundation for an effective therapeutic relationship. The CHN needs to be aware that families may feel that they are being "checked up on," that they are seen as being inadequate or dysfunctional, or that their privacy is being impinged on. These potential areas of concern underlie the need for sensitivity on the part of the CHN, the need to clarify information regarding the reason for visits, and the need to establish collaborative, trusting relationships with the family members. Subsequent home visits should be based on need and mutual agreement between the CHN and the family. Frequently, CHNs are not sure of the reason for the visit. This carries with it the potential for the visit to be compromised and to come aimlessly or abruptly to a premature halt. Regardless of the reason for the home visit, it is necessary that the CHN be clear about the purpose for the visit and that this purpose or understanding be shared with the family.

Preparing for the visit has several components. For the most part, these are best accomplished in order, as presented in the "How To... Prepare for the Home Visit" box (below).

The possibility exists that the family may refuse a home visit. Less experienced CHNs or students may mistakenly interpret this as a personal rejection. Families make decisions about when and which outsiders are allowed entry into their homes. The CHN needs to explore the reasons for the refusal, considering the following:

- There may be a misunderstanding about the reason for a visit.
- There may be a lack of information about services.

As the CHN plans for the first family visit, he or she begins hypothesizing about what the possible family

How To... Prepare for the Home Visit

- First, if at all possible, the CHN needs to contact the family by telephone before the home visit to introduce himself or herself, to identify the reason for the contact, and to schedule the home visit. A first telephone contact should be a maximum of 15 minutes. The CHN needs to give name and professional identity—for example, "This is Karen Smith. I'm a community health nurse from the health unit or health authority."
- The family needs to be informed of how they came to the attention of the CHN—for example, as the result of a referral or a contact from observations or records in the school setting. If a referral has been received, it is important and useful to ascertain whether the family is aware of the referral.
- A brief summary of the CHN's knowledge about the family's situation will allow the family members to clarify their health concerns. For example, the CHN might say, "I understand that your baby was discharged from the hospital yesterday and that you requested some assistance with learning more about how to care for your baby at home."
- A visit needs to be scheduled as soon as possible. Letting the family know agency hours available for visits, the approximate length of the visit, and the purpose of the visit is helpful to the family in determining when to set the visit. Although the lengths of home visits may vary, depending on circumstances, approximately 30 minutes to 1 hour is usual.
- If possible, the visit needs to be arranged for a time when as many family members as possible will be available for the entire visit.
- The telephone call can terminate with a review by the CHN of the time, place, and purpose for the visit, directions to the meeting place, and a means for the family to contact the CHN in case they need to verify or change the time for the visit, or to ask questions. If the family does not have a telephone, another method for setting up the visit can be used. A note can be dropped off at the family home or sent by mail informing the family of when and why the home visit will occur and providing a way for the family to contact the CHN if necessary.

health concerns might be. **Hypothesizing** is the development of a hunch based on information collected about the family that the CHN decides to explore further. Hypothesis generation starts in the planning stage and continues throughout the home visits. Refer to Box 12-1 for questions the CHN could ask the family when hypothesizing about the family and its health concern(s). Based on the information gathered, the CHN will be able to validate or invalidate hunch "hypotheses."

The stages of a home visit utilizing CFAM and CFIM are summarized in Table 12-6. Building a trusting relationship with the family client is the cornerstone of successful home visits. The following five skills are fundamental to effective home visits:

1. Observing
2. Listening
3. Questioning
4. Probing
5. Prompting

The need for these skills is evident in all stages of the home visit process.

Engagement

Engagement is the beginning of the interview process with a family, where the focus is on the establishment of the nurse–client relationship. The first visit to the home affords the CHN the opportunity to assess the family's neighbourhood and community resources, as well as the home and family interactions. The actual home visit includes several components, as follows:

- The CHN provides professional identification and tells the client the location of the agency.
- A brief social conversation helps establish rapport.
- The CHN describes his or her role, responsibilities, and limitations.
- The CHN determines the client's expectations (an important step).

BOX 12-1 Questions That Invite Hypothesizing about the Family (System) and Their Health Concern (Problem)

Who

Who is in the system? Who are the key players?

Who first noticed the health concern?

Who is concerned about the health concern?

Who is affected by the health concern? (most, least)

Who referred the family?

What

What is the health concern at this time?

What is the meaning that the health concern has for the family and for different members of the family?

What solutions have been attempted?

What question(s) do I feel obliged to ask?

What beliefs perpetuate the health concern?

What beliefs might be identified as core beliefs?

What beliefs are perpetuated by the health concern?

What concerns and solutions perpetuate the beliefs?

Why

Why is the family presenting at this time?

Where

Where has the information about this health concern come from?

Where does the family see the health concern originating?

Where does the family see the health concern and the family going if there is no change or if there is change?

When

When did the health concern begin?

When does the health concern begin in relation to another phenomenon of the family?

When does the health concern not occur?

How

How might a change in the health concern affect other parts of the family (key members, relationships, beliefs)?

How does a change in one part of the family affect another part of the family or the health concern?

How will I know when my work with this family is over?

How might my work with this family constrain the system from finding its solution?

Adapted from: Wright, L. M., & Leahey, M. (2009). *Nurses and families: A guide to family assessment and intervention* (5th ed., p. 189). Philadelphia, PA: F. A. Davis.

TABLE 12-6 Stages and Activities of a Home Visit

Stage	Activity
1. Engagement	Introduce self and professional identity
	Clarify source of referral for visit
	Clarify purpose for home visit
	Share information on reason and purpose of home visit with family
	Establish shared perception of purpose with family
	Establish nurse–client relationship
2. Family assessment	Apply CFAM to identify family health concerns
	Work with family to identify mutually agreeable goals
	Work with the family to identify solutions
3. Family intervention	Implement nursing interventions using CFIM
	Continue to work on nurse–client relationship
4. Termination and evaluation	Review visit with the family
	Evaluate the extent to which the goals have been met
	Provide referral to other community resources as needed
	Plan for future visits (if need is identified during evaluation)
5. Postvisit documentation	Record visit

CFAM = Calgary Family Assessment Model; *CFIM* = Calgary Family Intervention Model.

The major portion of the home visit involves establishing the relationship and implementing the community health nursing process. Too much disclosure of personal family information during the early contacts between the family and CHN may threaten the family. The CHN needs to slow the process down and take time to build trust. Assessment, planning, intervention, and evaluation are ongoing. Assessment is interactive. As the CHN evaluates families, the families evaluate the CHN. The reason for the visit determines what then occurs in the home visit.

It is important that the CHN be realistic about what can be accomplished in a home visit. In some situations, one visit may be all that is possible or appropriate. In this instance, health concerns and the resources available to meet them are explored with the family and it is determined whether further services are desired or indicated. If further services are indicated and the CHN's agency is not appropriate, the CHN can assist the family in identifying other services available in the community and can help in initiating referrals. Although it is not unusual to have only one home visit with a family, often multiple visits are made. The frequency and intensity of home visits vary, not only with the health concerns of the family but also with the eligibility of the family for services as defined by agency policies and priorities. It is realistic to expect an initial assessment and at least the beginning of building a relationship on a first visit.

Families may or may not be able to control interruptions during the visit. Telephones ring, pets join in the visit, people come and go, and televisions are left on. The CHN can ask that, for a limited time, televisions be turned off or that other disruptive activities be limited. Families may be so accustomed to the background noises and routine activities that they do not recognize them as being potentially disruptive.

Personal safety is an issue that may arise either in approaching the family home or once the family has opened the door to the CHN:

- CHNs need to examine personal fears and objective threats to determine if safety is indeed an issue.
- Certain precautions can be taken in known high-risk situations (e.g., carry a cellular phone).
- Agencies may provide escorts for CHNs or have them visit in pairs.
- In rare instances, it may be necessary to make home visits accompanied by a police or security officer.

How To... Plan for the Assessment Process

Assessment of families requires an organized plan before meeting the family. This planning includes the following:

1. What is the reason for the visit?
2. Who will be present during the interview?
3. Where will the visit take place, and how will the space be arranged?
4. What is going to be assessed?
5. How are the data going to be collected?
6. What will be done with the information found by the community health nurse?

- Readily identifiable uniforms may be required.
- A sign-out process indicating the timing and location of home visits may be used routinely.
- CHNs' driving routes can be registered with the agency.

CHNs are most often perceived as helpful, caring health professionals with specialized skills working with clients in the community in a supportive capacity, and as guests in client homes CHNs are usually perceived as nonthreatening (Smith, 2009). Home visits are generally safe; however, as with all worksites, the possibility of violence exists. Therefore, CHNs need to use caution. If a reasonable question exists about the safety of making a visit, a CHN should not make the visit alone. Box 12-2 outlines some safety considerations and behaviours for use by CHNs to avoid dangerous situations.

Family Assessment

Family nursing assessment is the cornerstone for family nursing interventions. By using a systematic process, family health concerns are identified and family strengths are emphasized as the building blocks for interventions. Building the interventions with family-identified health concerns and strengths allows for equal family and provider commitment to the solutions and ensures more successful interventions.

CHNs need to use a systematic format for family assessment. At times, the CHN may need to make modifications to a framework so that a complete individualized family assessment can be conducted. Keep in mind, cultural assessments are conducted with the client as individual, family, and community. Therefore, when conducting a family assessment, CHNs need to consider culture and should include relevant areas from a cultural assessment tool. For example, a more in-depth cultural or spiritual assessment might be indicated, and, therefore, parts of these tools might be integrated into the family assessment model. During the family visit, it is critical that the CHN be sufficiently familiar with the chosen family assessment model so that complete data are collected along with the development of the nurse–client relationship. There are many assessment frameworks, but the focus of this chapter is on the CFAM by Wright and Leahey. In certain situations, it is appropriate to conduct a family assessment interview of 15 minutes or less (Wright & Leahey, 2009). Wright and Leahey (2009) present two clinical examples that demonstrate the use and effectiveness of the brief family interviews. Following the collection of data, a CHN analyzes the data collected and develops a prioritized list of family health concerns and strengths; nursing interventions are planned and implemented in partnership with the family (whenever possible).

Contracting With Families

Increasingly, health professionals look at working with clients in an interactive, collaborative style. This approach is consistent with a more knowledgeable public and the recent self-care movement. However, it may not be consistent with other cultures that look to health care providers for more direct guidance; therefore, it is important to determine the family's value system before assuming that contracting will work.

Contracting, which is making an agreement between two or more parties, involves a shift in responsibility and control toward a shared effort by the client and professional as opposed to an effort by the professional alone. The premise of contracting is family control. It is assumed that when the family has legitimate control, their ability to make healthful choices is increased. Contracting is a strategy aimed at formally involving the family in the community health nursing process and jointly defining the roles of both the family members and the health professional.

The contract is a working agreement that is continuously renegotiable and may or may not be written. It may be either a contingency or a noncontingency contract, as follows:

- A *contingency contract* states a specific reward for the client after completion of the client's portion of the contract.
- A *noncontingency contract* does not specify rewards.

BOX 12-2 Safety Concerns for the CHN to Consider for Family Home Visits

1. Possible unsafe situations
   - Clients or family members have a pattern of violent behaviour such as domestic violence (physical, verbal, emotional).
   - Clients or family members are known substance abusers.
   - Persons with communicable diseases are in the home.
   - There are environmental risks, such as an unsafe built environment, threatening animals, and second-hand smoke.
2. Actions taken to promote safety
   - Arrange the visit by telephone with the family so family members have given permission to visit.
   - Have another CHN accompany you on the visit, if necessary.
   - If the neighbourhood is unsafe, arrange to meet the family in a neutral, safe area such as a clinic.
   - Leave a schedule of your home visits with the supervisor at your agency.
   - Certain areas may be safer during certain times of the day, so consider this when planning home visits.
   - Know the directions to the family home.
   - Dress in a professional manner.
   - Have a cell phone that is readily accessible and functional.
   - Drive on main highways or roads and drive or walk in heavily travelled areas.
   - When walking, avoid areas where people are loitering.
   - Keep supplies, equipment, and other necessary items easily accessible and not in the trunk, to avoid taking time to locate them.
   - Keep purse or other valuables in a locked trunk.
   - Do not wear expensive jewelry.
   - Check the front and back seats before getting into your vehicle.
   - Keep a nearly full tank of gasoline.
   - Keep your vehicle in a well-maintained order.
   - Look for suspicious behaviour such as individuals following you, and contact the police.
   - Avoid offering rides to home visit family members or strangers.
   - At all times keep the vehicle locked with the windows up.
   - If vehicle problems occur, remain in your vehicle and phone for help.
3. Precautions to use in the home
   - When ascending stairs, follow the client.
   - If you have concerns about client behaviour, always visit when other family members are present.
   - Listen to your intuition and if you are feeling unsafe, leave the family situation.
   - If the family or visitors behave in a threatening or inappropriate manner terminate the home visit immediately.
   - Ask that pets be moved to another room if they are threatening or bothersome.

Source: Adapted from McEwen, M., & Pullis, B. (2009). *Community-based nursing: An introduction* (3rd ed.). St. Louis, MO: Saunders Elsevier; Smith, C. M. (2009). Home visiting: Opening the doors for family health. In F. A. Maurer & C. M. Smith, *Community/Public health nursing practice: Health for families and populations* (4th ed., pp. 302–325). St. Louis, MO: Saunders Elsevier.

The implied rewards are the positive consequences of reaching the goals specified in the contract.

For family health risk reduction, it is essential that the contract be made with all responsible and appropriate members of the family. Involving only one individual is not sufficient if the goal is family health risk reduction, which requires a total family system effort and change. Scheduling a visit with all family members present may require extra effort; if meeting with the entire family is not possible, each family member can review a contract, give input, and sign it. This allows active participation by all family members without having to find a time when everyone involved can be present.

Contracting is a learned skill on the part of both the CHN and the family. All persons involved need to know the purpose and process of contracting. The three general phases are *beginning, working,* and *termination.* The three phases can be further divided into a total of eight sets of activities, as summarized in Table 12-7.

TABLE 12-7 Phases and Activities in Contracting

Phase	Activity
1. Beginning phase	Mutual data collection and exploration of needs and problems
	Mutual establishment of goals
	Mutual development of a plan
2. Working phase	Mutual division of responsibilities
	Mutual setting of time limits
	Mutual implementation of plan
	Mutual evaluation and renegotiation
3. Termination	Mutual termination of contract

The first activity is collection and analysis of data, and it involves both the family and the CHN. An important aspect of this step is obtaining the family's view of the situation and its health concerns. The CHN can do the following:

- Present his or her observations
- Validate the observations with the family
- Obtain the family's view

It is important that goals be mutually set and realistic. A pitfall for CHNs and clients who are new to contracting is to set overly ambitious goals. The CHN needs to recognize that there may be discrepancies between professional priorities and those of the client and determine whether negotiating is required. Because contracting is a process characterized by renegotiating, the goals are not static.

Throughout the process, the CHN and family continually learn and recognize what each can contribute to meeting health concerns. The exploring of resources allows both parties to become aware of their own and one another's strengths and requires a review of the CHN's skills and knowledge, the family support systems, and community resources.

Developing a plan to meet the goals involves the following:

- Specifying activities
- Prioritizing goals
- Selecting a starting point
- Deciding who will be responsible for which activities (decision is made by the CHN and the family)
- Setting time limits that involve deciding on a deadline for accomplishing (or evaluating progress toward accomplishing) a goal and the frequency of contacts

At the agreed-on time, the CHN and family together evaluate the progress in both process and outcome. The contract can be modified, renegotiated, or terminated on the basis of the evaluation.

Advantages and Disadvantages of Contracting

Contracting takes time and effort and may require the family and CHN to reorient their roles. Increased control on the part of the family also means increased responsibility. Some CHNs may have difficulty relinquishing the role of the controlling expert professional. Contracts are not always successful, and contracting is neither appropriate nor possible in some cases. Some clients do not want to have this kind of involvement; they prefer to defer to the "authority" of the professional. The following are included in this group:

- Individuals with minimal cognitive skills
- Those who are involved in an emergency situation
- Those who are unwilling to be more active in their care
- Those who do not see control or authority for health concerns as being within their domain

Some of these clients may learn to contract; others never will. Contracting is one approach that depends on the following:

- The value of input from both the CHN and the family
- The competency of the family
- The family's ability to be responsible
- The dynamic nature of the process

Contracting not only allows for but also requires continual renegotiating. Although it may not be appropriate in all situations or with all families, contracting can give direction and structure to health risk reduction and health promotion in families.

Family Interventions

When the family assessment is completed and interventions are warranted to facilitate positive family change, the CHN would use the CFIM with the family. Solutions need to be identified by partnering with the family to change the most pressing health concern within a particular domain. Further information on nursing interventions to promote change in the cognitive, affective, and behavioural

BOX 12-3 Helpful Hints about Interventions

- Interventions are the core of clinical work with families.
- They should be devised with sensitivity to the family's ethnic and religious background.
- They can only be *offered* to families. The CHN cannot direct change but can create a context for change to occur.
- They are offered in the context of collaborative conversations as the CHN and family together devise solutions to find the most useful fit.
- When the CHN's ideas are not a good fit for the family, the CHN should be open to offering other ideas rather than becoming blameful of self or the family because the intervention was not chosen.

SOURCE: Adapted from Wright, L., & Leahey, M. (2009). *Nurses and families: A guide to family assessment and intervention* (5th ed., p. 238). Philadelphia, PA: F. A. Davis.

BOX 12-4 Factors to Consider When Devising Interventions

- What is the agreed-on problem* to change?
- At what domain of family functioning is the intervention aimed?
- How does the intervention match the family's style of relating?
- How is the intervention linked to the family's strengths and previous useful solution strategies?
- How is the intervention consistent with the family's ethnic and religious beliefs?
- How is the intervention new or different for the family?

*"Problem" refers to health concern.

SOURCE: Wright, L., & Leahey, M. (2009). *Nurses and families: A guide to family assessment and intervention* (5th ed., p. 238). Philadelphia, PA: F. A. Davis.

domains of family functioning is presented in the book by Wright and Leahey (2009). Boxes 12-3 and 12-4 provide the CHN with considerations in relation to family interventions. Interventions by CHNs when dealing with families include roles such as direct care, health promoter, health educator, counsellor, and advocate. An elaboration of these and additional roles for CHNs' consideration when partnering with families is presented by the International Council of Nurses at the Web site listed in the Tool Box on the Evolve Web site.

CRITICAL VIEW

1. How would you introduce to a family their need for a referral to an agency for additional help?
2. a) How would you introduce to a family the idea of referral as a unit for family therapy?
   b) How would you introduce to a family the idea of referral for speech therapy for the benefit of an individual family member?

Termination and Evaluation

When the purpose of the visit has been accomplished, the CHN reviews with the family what has occurred and what has been accomplished. This is the major focus of the **termination phase,** and it provides a basis for evaluating whether further home visits are needed or referrals to community resources are required:

- Ideally, termination of the visit and, ultimately, termination of service begin at the first contact with the establishment of a goal or purpose.
- If communication has been clear to this point, the family and CHN can now plan for future visits, specifically the next visit.

CHNs need to engage in evaluation that involves critical, creative, and concurrent reflection about the client situation. Evaluation has two components, that is, process (formative) and outcome (summative). The termination home visit phase involves outcome evaluation (summative).

CHNs may send a letter, sometimes referred to as a *closing* or *therapeutic letter,* to families that summarizes their strengths and health concerns and encourages them to continue working on their health goals (see Box 12-5). These letters also provide health care clinicians with the opportunity of reflective thinking (Erlingsson, 2009). The use of therapeutic letters is one strategy used by students working with families to assist them in connecting theory to practice (Erlingsson, 2009). In these letters, commendations are offered to the family, changes made are emphasized, summary of efforts and accomplishments during therapeutic interactions are provided, and the ideas and interventions that were discussed are addressed (Wright & Leahey, 2009).

BOX 12-5 Example of a Therapeutic Letter

Dear W, H, and T,

First I want to thank all of you for allowing me the opportunity to get acquainted with your family. I appreciated your openness and willingness to talk with me.

During our time together, we discussed several issues that were important to your family. One of these issues was the ongoing possibility of H losing his job due to the seasonal nature of his work. We explored the effects of potential job loss on a personal and family level.

H, you expressed some concern about your ability to adequately provide for your family. You indicated a personal constraining belief that a lack of steady employment meant that you were letting your family down and not providing for them. We discussed the idea that a paying job is only one part of the entire family support system that you provide. We explored some examples of noneconomic means of support, such as specific tasks related to the farm chores, household management, and child care. If your job situation changes again, I hope you will find some of these suggestions helpful.

W, I was so impressed with your ability to juggle your nursing job with home, farm, kids, and spouse. I can't think of many women who could handle all of that with such strength and grace. With all that you do, it's not surprising that there isn't much time left over for your own personal endeavours. We discussed your constraining belief that you had to be responsible for everything. You envisioned the possibility of letting go of certain tasks and suggesting ways to share other tasks more equitably among family members. If you and your family choose to implement some task-sharing ideas, I sincerely hope this will work for all of you.

T, you have mapped out a path to higher education and a future career. You have every reason to expect success. We briefly touched upon what "success" might mean for you and whether success depends on the university attended. I hope you will consider my thoughts in this regard. Whatever the outcome, you have the love and support of your parents.

Finally, I would like to commend all of you for your deep devotion to each other and for putting family first. You value family time and you strive to communicate in a way that sustains a close relationship with each other.

I would like to invite W and H to consider a suggestion regarding making time for just the two of you. "Couple time" is easy to overlook when you're focused on creating a loving, stable home for T and helping to launch T into higher education. Please remember that you two are the solid foundation of your family; the stronger your relationship, the stronger your whole family can be.

As a result of our time spent together, I came away with a feeling that your family is exceptionally strong, deeply committed to one another, and fully capable of adapting to any of life's challenges. Thank you again for your time.

Best wishes to you and your family,

Suzanne Ahn, R.N., Family Nurse Practitioner (FNP) Student

SOURCE: Harmon Hanson, S. M. (2005). Family health care nursing: An introduction. In S. M. Harmon Hanson, V. Gedaly-Duff, & J. Rowe Kaakinen (Eds.), *Family health care nursing: Theory practice and research* (3rd ed., p. 231). Philadelphia, PA: F. A. Davis.

Post-visit Documentation

Even though the CHN has now concluded the home visit and left the client's home, the responsibility for the visit is not complete until the interaction has been recorded. Visit recording is a basic element needed for legal and clinical purposes. It is important that the recording be current, dated, and signed. The format may consist of the following:

- Narratives
- Flow sheets
- Problem-oriented medical records
- Subjective, objective, assessment plans
- A combination of formats

The CHN needs to use theoretical frameworks that are appropriate to the family-centred community health nursing process with the family as the unit of care. Therefore, the health concern needs to be a family health concern and not an individual health concern. Examples are the following: a family that needs to accomplish the stage-appropriate task of providing a safe environment for a preschooler; a couple with communication difficulties has a desire for improved communication with an adolescent daughter; and a couple interested in improving their parenting skills with their toddler. At times, it may be necessary to address individual health concerns, too. However, as mentioned, the emphasis needs to be on the individual as a member of and within the structure of the family as a unit.

Clinical Judgement

Critical thinking and clinical judgements are required throughout the application of the community health nursing process when working with families. In making clinical judgements or evaluating the outcome, CHNs engage in critical thinking. When an outcome is not achieved, the CHN and the family work together to determine the barriers. Family apathy and indecision are known to be barriers in family nursing (Friedman, Bowden, & Jones, 2003; Harmon Hanson et al., 2005), and other family barriers identified by Harmon Hanson et al. (2005) are hopelessness as perceived by the family; fear of failure; fears and mistrust of the health care system; minimal access to monetary resources; and minimal access to other resources and support. Friedman, Bowden, and Jones (2003) also identified the following nurse-related barriers to achieving the outcome:

- CHN imposes ideas
- CHN uses negative labels
- CHN does not identify family strengths
- CHN neglects cultural or gender implications

Family apathy may occur because of value differences between the CHN and the family, because the family is overcome with a sense of hopelessness, because the family views the health concerns as too overwhelming, or because family members have a fear of failure (Harmon Hanson et al., 2005). The giving of commendations (by the CHN), which identify strengths seen in the family, often helps the family to feel empowered and hopeful. Additional factors to be considered are that the family may be indecisive because of the following:

- Members cannot determine which course of action is better.
- They have an unexpressed fear or concern.
- They have a pattern of making decisions only when faced with a crisis.

An important part of the judgement step in working with families is the decision to terminate the relationship between the CHN and the family. Termination is phasing out the CHN from family involvement. When termination is built into the interventions, the family benefits from a smooth transition process. The family is given credit for the outcomes of the interventions that they helped design. Strategies often used in the termination component are as follows:

- Decreasing contact with the CHN
- Extending invitations to the family for follow-up
- Making referrals when appropriate

The termination should include a summative evaluation meeting in which the CHN and family put a formal closure to their relationship. When termination with a family occurs suddenly, it is important for the CHN to determine the forces bringing about the closure. The family may be initiating the termination prematurely, which requires a renegotiating process. Regardless of how termination comes about, it is an important aspect in working with families.

FAMILY HEALTH RISK REDUCTION

Several factors contribute to the development of healthy or unhealthy outcomes. Clearly, not everyone exposed to the same event will have the same outcome. The factors that determine or influence whether disease or other unhealthy results occur are called **health risks. Risk** is the probability of some event or outcome within a specified period of time. Controlling health risks is done through disease prevention and health promotion efforts.

Although single risk factors can influence outcomes, the combined effect of several risks has greater influence. For example, a family history of cardiovascular disease is a single biological risk factor that is affected by smoking (a behavioural risk that is more likely to occur if other family members also smoke) and by diet and exercise. Diet and exercise are influenced by family and society's norms. The determinants of health such as culture, biology, and income can also influence diet and exercise. The combined effect of a family history, determinants of health, family behavioural risks, and society's influences is greater than each of the three individual risk factors (smoking, diet, exercise). **Social risks** refer to risky social situations that can contribute to the stressors experienced by families. If adequate resources and coping processes are not available, breakdowns in health can occur.

Health risk appraisal refers to the process of assessing and analyzing for the presence of specific factors in each of the categories that have been identified as being associated with an increased likelihood of an illness developing such as cancer, or *an unhealthy event,* such as an automobile accident. **Health risk reduction** is based on the assumption that decreasing the number of risks or the magnitude of risk will result in a lower probability of an undesired event. For example, to decrease the likelihood of adolescent substance abuse, family behaviours such as parents not drinking, alcohol not being available in the home, and family contracts related to alcohol and drug use may be useful. Health risks can be reduced through a variety of approaches. It is important to note the specific risk and the family's tolerance of it. Risk reduction is a complex process that requires knowledge of the specific risk and the family's perceptions of the nature of the risk.

A **family crisis** occurs when the family is not able to cope with an event and becomes disorganized; the demands of the situation exceed the resources of the family. When families experience a crisis or a crisis-producing event, they attempt to gather their resources to deal with the demands created by the situation. Examples of family resources are money and extended family who are available to them. Families cope by using known processes and behaviours to help them manage or adapt to the problem. Thus, if a family's main wage earner were to experience an unexpected illness, family resources might include financial assistance or emotional support from relatives. Family coping strategies, in contrast, would include whether the family were able to ask a relative to loan them emergency funds or were able to talk with relatives about the worries they were experiencing. (Refer to the Registered Nurses' Association of Ontario [RNAO] Best Practice Guidelines *Crisis Intervention* and *Supporting and Strengthening Families Through Expected and Unexpected Life Events* Weblinks on the Evolve Web site.)

Family Resilience

Family resilience helps families to adapt to crisis. **Family resiliency** is defined as "the ability to cope with expected and unexpected stressors" (Potter, Perry, Ross-Kerr, & Wood, 2006, p. 300). In 1993, McCubbin and McCubbin developed the Family Resiliency Model to assess family stress and family adjustment and adaptation. This model was a further development of the previously available family stress theories such as the Family Adjustment and Adaptation Response (FAAR) Model. The McCubbin and McCubbin model explores family adaptation as it adjusts to stressors on the family system in an attempt to regain equilibrium. This model considers family strengths as the family copes with their changed situation and attempts to maintain family functioning (Danielson, McEwen, & Pullis, 2009).

Black and Lobo (2008) describe family resilience as "the successful coping of family members under adversity that enables them to flourish with warmth, support, and cohesion" (p. 33). These authors reviewed the family literature and identified the following factors found in resilient families:

- Positive outlook—Overcoming challenges with an optimistic lens; sense of humour present
- Spirituality—Using a sense of purpose to deal with stressors
- Family member accord—Family working together in a supportive manner
- Flexibility—Ability to adapt to interchangeable roles and functions when needed, such as during times of change
- Family communication—Family collaborates to problem-solve; uses direct, open channels of communication and open expression of emotion
- Financial management—Able to manage family finances; when confronted with financial challenges family caring is maintained
- Family time—Working together to complete daily family tasks and functions
- Shared recreation—Enjoying leisure activities as a family
- Routines and rituals—Routines and rituals are maintained even during times of stress
- Support networks—Use of, and contribution to maintenance of, support networks (Black & Lobo, 2008)

FAMILY HEALTH RISK APPRAISAL

Risks to a family's health arise in three major areas:

1. Biological and age-related risks
2. Environmental risks
3. Behavioural risks

In most instances, a risk in one of these areas may not be enough to threaten family health but a combination of risks from two or more categories could lead to a family crisis. For example, if a family presents with a family history of cardiovascular disease, this health risk is often increased by an unhealthy lifestyle and the presence of determinants of health such as coping skills and social environment. An understanding of each of these categories provides the basis for a comprehensive approach to family health risk assessment and intervention.

CRITICAL VIEW

1. a) Would you add the determinants of health to the risk categories identified above? If yes, explain the relationship between the determinants and family health risks.
   b) What programs exist in your community that would address the determinants of health for families?
2. a) Compare the family health risk approach with the family assets approach.
   b) How would your approach with the family as a CHN differ when you use a family assets approach?

Assessment of family health risk requires many approaches. As in any assessment, the first and most important task is to get to know the family, their strengths, and their health concerns.

Biological and Age-Related Risk

The family plays an important role in both the development and management of a disease or condition. Some illnesses can be related to either genetics or lifestyle patterns. These factors contribute to the **biological risk** for certain conditions. Patterns of cardiovascular disease, for example, can often be traced through several generations of a family; such families are said to be at risk for cardiovascular disease. How or whether cardiovascular disease is found in a family is often influenced by the lifestyle of the family. CHNs, as family nurses, need to recognize that family history data can provide the genetic information required by families to make relevant decisions. Van Riper (2006) believes that family nurses need to "become involved in some aspects of genomic health care ... [p. 111] and assume leadership roles in the family history initiatives" (p. 116).

Biological Health Risk Assessment

One of the most widely used techniques for assessing the patterns of health and illness in families is the genogram (Friedman et al., 2003). Briefly, a **genogram** is a drawing that shows the family unit of immediate interest to the CHN and includes at least three generations of family members with gender and age, their relationships, health status, and mortality, using a series of circles, squares, and connecting lines. Basic information about the family, relationships in the family, and patterns of health and illness can be obtained by completing the genogram with the family. The following is shown in Figure 12-4:

- A square indicates a male.
- A circle indicates a female.
- An X through either a square or a circle indicates a death.
- Marriage is indicated by a solid horizontal line.
- Offspring or children are noted by a solid vertical line.
- A broken horizontal line indicates a divorce or separation.
- Dates of birth, marriage, death, and other important events can be indicated where appropriate.
- Major illness or conditions can be listed for each individual family member.

It is important to include a legend on the genogram that conveys the meaning of the various symbols used—this is because there are variations in acceptable symbols and by providing a legend, communication is enhanced. Patterns can be quickly assessed by reviewing the genogram information and providing a guide for the health interviewer about health areas that need further exploring.

The genogram in Figure 12-4 was completed for a fictional family, the Grahams. Some of the interesting health patterns that can be seen from the genogram are the repetition of the following:

- Hypertension
- Adult-onset diabetes
- Cancer
- Hypercholesterolemia

Completing a genogram requires interviews with as many family members as possible. If possible, it is important to collect family history data dating back three generations in order to develop a complete picture of the family and their health patterns. Frequently, as families complete the genogram with the CHN, they experience an awareness of strengths in their family health status. This can have an empowering effect.

A more intensive and quantitative assessment of a family's biological risk can be achieved through the use of a standard family risk assessment. Because such assessments involve other areas in addition to biological risk, one will be described later, after the description of other types of risk assessment.

Both normative and non-normative life events pose potential risks to the health of families. Even events that are generally viewed as being positive require changes and can place stress on a family. The normative event of the birth of a child, for example, requires considerable changes in family structures and roles. Furthermore, family functions are expanded from previous levels, requiring families to add new skills and establish additional resources. **Family functions** are behaviours or activities performed to maintain the integrity of the family unit and to meet the family's needs, individual members' needs, and society's expectations. These changes can in turn result in strain and—if adequate resources are not available—stress. Therefore, to adequately assess life risks, both normative and non-normative events occurring in the family need to be considered. Community-level support groups have been successful in assisting families in dealing with a variety of stressful situations and crises (e.g., Families Anonymous, Bereaved Parents, Parents and Friends of Lesbian and Gay Persons, and Single Parents) that arise from both life events and age-related events. CHNs have been instrumental in developing and moderating such groups.

FIGURE 12-4 Genogram of the Graham Family

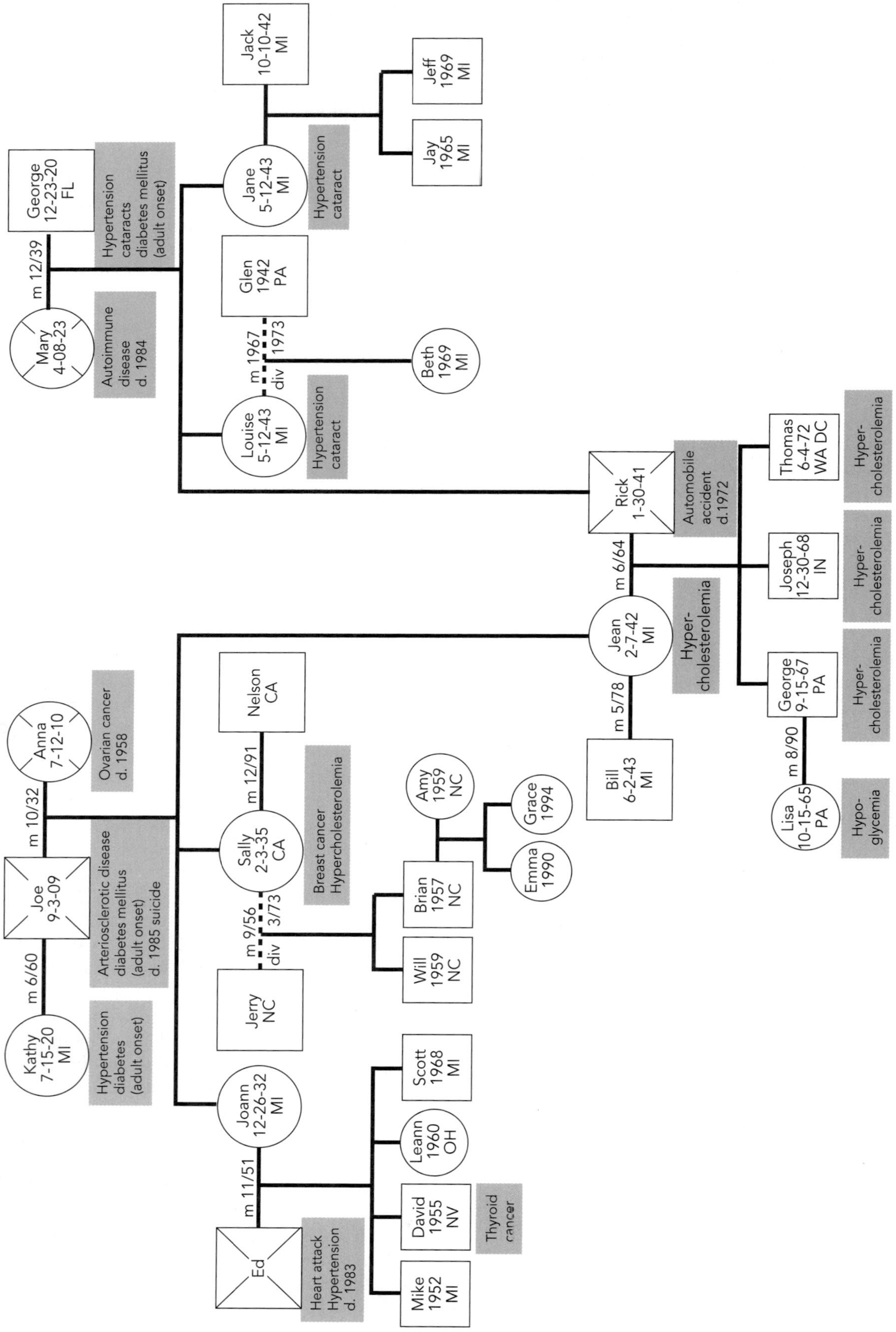

Kathy 7-15-20 MI
Hypertension diabetes (adult onset)
m 6/60
Joe 9-3-09
Arteriosclerotic disease diabetes mellitus (adult onset) d. 1985 suicide
m 10/32
Anna 7-12-10
Ovarian cancer d. 1958

Mary 4-08-23
Autoimmune disease d. 1984
m 12/39
George 12-23-20 FL
Hypertension cataracts diabetes mellitus (adult onset)

Ed
Heart attack Hypertension d. 1983
m 11/51
Joann 12-26-32 MI
Mike 1952 MI
David 1955 NV
Thyroid cancer
Leann 1960 OH
Scott 1968 MI

Jerry NC
m 9/56
div 3/73
Sally 2-3-35 CA
Breast cancer Hypercholesterolemia
m 12/91
Nelson CA
Will 1959 NC
Brian 1957 NC
Amy 1959 NC
Emma 1990
Grace 1994

Louise 5-12-43 MI
Hypertension cataract
m 1967
div 1973
Glen 1942 PA
Beth 1969 MI

Jane 5-12-43 MI
Hypertension cataract
Jack 10-10-42 MI
Jay 1965 MI
Jeff 1969 MI

Bill 6-2-43 MI
m 5/78
Jean 2-7-42 MI
Hyper-cholesterolemia
m 6/64
Rick 1-30-41
Automobile accident d.1972

Lisa 10-15-65 PA
Hypo-glycemia
m 8/90
George 9-15-67 PA
Hyper-cholesterolemia
Joseph 12-30-68 IN
Hyper-cholesterolemia
Thomas 6-4-72 WA DC
Hyper-cholesterolemia

Developed by Carol Loveland-Cherry. In Stanhope, M., & Lancaster, J. (2008). *Community and public health nursing* (7th ed.). St. Louis, MO: Mosby.

Environmental Risk

The importance of social risks to family health is gaining increased recognition. A family's health risk increases if they are living in the following:

- High-crime neighbourhoods
- Communities without adequate recreation or health resources
- Communities that have major noise pollution or chemical pollution
- Other high-stress environments

Information on environmental considerations is discussed in Chapter 15. Family preparedness in disaster management will be discussed in Chapter 16.

One social stress is discrimination, whether racial, cultural, or other. The psychological burden resulting from discrimination is itself a stressor, and it adds to the effects of other stressors. The implication of these examples of risky social situations is that they contribute to the stressors experienced by the families. If adequate resources and coping processes are not available, breakdowns in health can occur.

Persons with low income are at greater risk for health problems. **Economic risk,** which is related to social risk, is determined by the relationship between family financial resources and the demands on those resources. Having adequate financial resources means that a family is able to purchase the necessary services and goods related to health, such as the following:

- Adequate housing
- Clothing
- Food
- Education
- Health or illness care

The amount of money that a family has available is related to situational, cultural, and social factors. A family may have an income well above the poverty level, but because of the devastating illness of a family member, they may not be able to meet financial demands. Likewise, families from ethnic populations or families with same-sex parents frequently experience discrimination in finding housing. Even if they find housing, they may not be welcome and may be harassed, resulting in increased stress. A Campaign 2000 report titled *Oh Canada: Too Many Children in Poverty for Too Long* was released in March 2007 and reports on 2006 data (see the Weblinks on the Evolve Web site). This report card provides statistics, including information on Aboriginal child poverty and government programs to address poverty in children.

CRITICAL VIEW

1. What initiatives are available in your community to provide a supportive environment for families?
2. What healthy public policies are currently in place, and which policies are still needed to provide supportive environments for families?

Environmental Risk Assessment

Assessment of environmental health risk is less defined and developed. Information on relationships that the family has with others such as relatives and neighbours; their connections with other social units such as church, school, work, clubs, and organizations; and the flow of energy, positive or negative, can be assessed through the use of an ecomap. It is also important to assess the environmental social risks such as high-crime neighbourhoods, communities without adequate recreation and health resources, communities that have major noise pollution or chemical pollution, and other high-stress environments.

An **ecomap** represents the family's interactions with other groups and organizations, accomplished by using a series of circles and lines. In Figure 12-5, a legend box is included in the bottom left corner. Consider the family of interest (the Graham family [see Figure 12-5]):

- It is represented by a circle in the middle of the page.
- Other groups and organizations are then indicated by other circles.
- Lines, representing the flow of energy, are drawn between the family circle and the circles representing other groups and organizations.
- An arrowhead at the end of each line indicates the direction of the flow of energy (into or out of the family).
- The weight of the line indicates the intensity of the energy.

The Graham family ecomap indicates that much of the family energy goes into work (also a source of stress for the parents). Major sources of energy for the Grahams are their immediate and extended families and friends.

In addition to the support network shown by the ecomap, other aspects of social risk include characteristics of the neighbourhood and community where the family lives. A CHN who has worked in the general geographical area may already have conducted a community health assessment and have a working knowledge of the neighbourhood and community. It is important, however, for the CHN to obtain information from the

FIGURE 12-5 Ecomap of the Graham Family

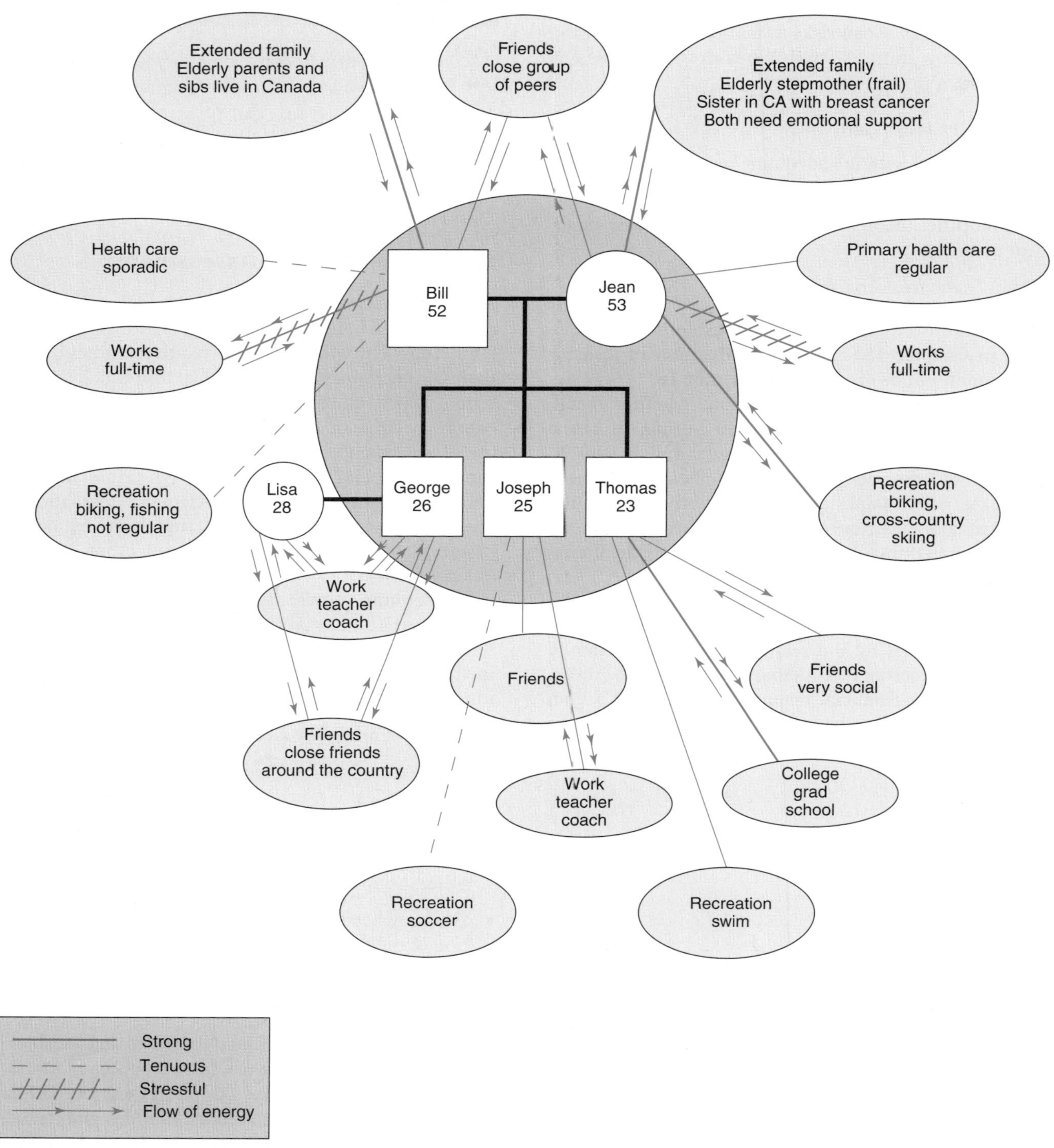

Developed by Loveland-Cherry, C. In M. Stanhope, J. Lancaster. (2008). *Community and public health nursing* (7th ed.). St. Louis, MO: Mosby.

family to understand their perceptions of the community; information about the origins of the family, which is useful to understand other social resources and stressors; information about how long the family has lived in their current location; and the immigration patterns of the family and their ancestors, which provide insight into pressures they may experience.

Economic risk is one of the foremost predictors of health. Families often consider financial information private, and both the CHN and the family may be uncomfortable when discussing finances. It is not necessary to know actual family income except in instances when it is needed to determine whether families are eligible for programs or benefits. It is useful to know whether the family's resources are adequate to meet their needs. And it is important to understand that the family may be quite comfortable with their finances and standard of living, which may be different from those of the health care provider. CHNs should not impose their financial values onto the family.

With regard to health risk, it is important to understand the resources that families have to obtain health and illness care; adequate shelter, clothing, and food; and access to recreation. Families with limited resources may qualify for social programs. Families with wage earners with medical benefits and those with enough income are usually able to afford adequate health care. Unfortunately, in a growing number of families, the main wage earner is employed but receives no additional health care insurance benefits, and the salary is not sufficient for health promotion or illness-related care. This is a policy issue, and CHNs can contribute to the drafting of legislation and provide testimony related to the stories of families in their caseloads.

Behavioural (Lifestyle) Risk

Personal health habits continue to contribute to the major causes of morbidity and mortality in Canada. The pattern of personal health habits, known as **behavioural risk,** defines individual and family health status. The family is the basic unit within which health behaviour—including health values, habits, and risk perceptions—is developed, organized, and performed. Families maintain major responsibility for the following:

- Determining what food is purchased and prepared
- Setting sleep patterns
- Planning family activities
- Setting and monitoring norms about health and health risk behaviours
- Determining when a family member is ill
- Determining when health care should be obtained
- Carrying out treatment regimens

Families can structure time and activities for family members. It is helpful when the community in which they live promotes exercise by having accessible parks and walking or biking paths; these help families select activities that provide moderate, regular physical exercise rather than sedentary activities in the home setting.

CRITICAL VIEW

Adolescents who have close, supportive interactions with their family, have clearly set and enforced rules, and have parents who are involved with their children are at a decreased risk for alcohol use or misuse. These family patterns can be enhanced through family-focused intervention sessions in the home.

1. Using the Calgary Family Assessment Model (CFAM), what family assessment data would you collect with a family in this developmental stage?
2. What family-focused interventions could contribute to decreased alcohol use or misuse?

Behavioural (Lifestyle) Health Risk Assessment

Families are the major source of factors that can promote or inhibit positive lifestyles. They regulate time and energy and the boundaries of the system. A number of tools exist for assessing individuals' lifestyle risks, but few are available for assessing family lifestyle patterns. Although assessment of individual lifestyle contributes to determining the lifestyle risk of a family, it is important to look at risks for the family as a unit. One approach is to identify family patterns for lifestyle components. In the areas of health promotion, health protection, and preventive services, lifestyle can be assessed in several dimensions. From the literature on health behaviour research, the critical dimensions include the following:

- The value placed on the behaviour
- Their knowledge of the behaviour and its consequences
- The effect of the behaviour on the family
- The effect of the behaviour on the individual
- Barriers to performing the behaviour
- Benefits of the behaviour

It is important to assess the frequency, intensity, and regularity of specific behaviours, as well as to evaluate the resources available to the family for implementing behaviours. Thus, items for assessment of physical activity include the following:

- The value that a family places on physical activity
- The hours that a family spends exercising
- The kinds of exercise the family does
- Resources available for exercise

HEALTH PROMOTION WITH FAMILIES

A risk assessment takes a behavioural approach; more recently an asset approach with families is promoted. An asset approach focuses on family competencies and family strengths rather than risks and deficits. The CFAM framework encompasses a family strength-based orientation. Table 12-2 identifies family strengths listed as features of a healthy family that CHNs need to consider when working with families. These strengths may be present or may have been present in the past in the family and may be helpful as interventions to promote, protect, or maintain family health. Family strengths are "positive behaviours or qualities that help maintain family health" (Smith, 2009, p. 355). **Family strengths** and resources can be used to help families deal with health concerns and to promote their health. Health promotion is most likely to occur when a family is able to define health holistically and with a wellness or well-being focus rather than health as the absence of disease. For example, a family with a father who has been newly diagnosed with diabetes mellitus agrees to follow the diabetic diet as a family, to promote family nutritional wellness. Another example is a family with a health promotion focus who purchases a family membership at the local sports complex. The family commits to participating in the public swimming for families.

Empowering Families

Empowerment is a process that CHNs use to promote and protect the health of families, encourage autonomy, and provide families with information to actively involve them so that they can make informed choices about their health (Pender, Murdaugh, & Parsons, 2006). Help-giving interventions do not always have positive outcomes for clients. If families do not perceive a situation as a health concern, offers of help may cause resentment. Help-giving also may have negative consequences if there is no match between what is expected and what is offered. A CHN's failure to recognize a family's competencies (strengths) and to not define an active role for them can contribute to the family's dependency and lack of growth. This can be frustrating for both the CHN and the family. For families to become active participants, they need to feel a sense of personal competence and a desire for and willingness to take action. Definitions of *empowerment* reflect the following three characteristics of the empowered family seeking help:

- Access and control over needed resources
- Decision-making and problem-solving abilities
- Abilities to communicate and obtain needed resources

Empowerment requires a viewpoint that may conflict with the views of many helping professions, including nursing. Empowerment's underlying assumption is one of a partnership between the professional and the client as opposed to one in which the professional is dominant. Families are assumed to be either competent or capable of becoming competent. This implies that the professional is not an unchallenged authority who is in control. Empowerment promotes an environment that creates opportunities for competencies to be used. Finally, families need to identify that their actions result in behaviour change. A community health nursing intervention that incorporates the principles of empowerment meets the following requirements:

- It is directed toward the building of nurse–family partnerships.
- It emphasizes health risk reduction and health promotion.

The CHN's approach to the family needs to be capacity building, positive, and focused on competencies and strengths rather than on health concerns, deficits, or pathology. The interventions need to be consistent with family cultural norms and the family's perception of the health concern. Rather than making decisions for the family, the CHN supports the family in primary decision making and bolsters their self-esteem by recognizing and using family strengths and support networks. Interventions that promote desired family behaviours increase family competency, decrease the need for outside help, and result in families seeing themselves as being actively responsible for bringing about desired changes. The goal of such an empowering approach is to create a partnership between the CHN and the family characterized by cooperation and shared responsibility. Bell (2009) states, "Family Systems Nursing occurs in a relationship between an individual/family and a nonjudgmental nurse who prefers collaborative, nonhierarchical relationships and who believes in the legitimacy of multiple realities" (p. 127).

Community Resources

Families have varied and complex health concerns. The CHN is often involved in mobilizing several resources to effectively and appropriately meet family health promotion issues. Identifying resources in a community requires time and effort. One valuable source is the telephone book. Often community service organizations, such as the local Chamber of Commerce and health unit or health authority, publish community resource listings. Regardless of how a resource is identified, the CHN needs to be familiar with the types of services offered and any requirements or costs involved. If this information is not available, the CHN can contact the resource.

Locating and using these systems often requires skills and patience that many families lack. CHNs work with families to identify community resources, and as client advocates they help families learn to use the resources. This may involve the following:

- Sharing information with families
- Rehearsing with families what questions to ask
- Preparing required materials
- Making the initial contact
- Arranging transportation

The appropriateness and effectiveness of resources need to be evaluated with families afterward. It is important to remember that navigating the maze of resources is often difficult for the CHN. If a family is in crisis or does not have a phone or a home base from which to call or receive return calls, this process is even more difficult and the family's sense of helplessness may be increased. Therefore, the CHN's assistance, while promoting the family's sense of empowerment, is both necessary and complex.

Each family is an unexplored mystery, unique in the ways in which it meets the needs of its members and of society. Healthy and vital families are essential to the world's future because family members are affected by what their families have invested in them or failed to provide for their growth and well-being. Families will continue to survive and serve as the basic social unit of society.

LEVELS OF PREVENTION

Related to Families and Child Abuse

PRIMARY PREVENTION

Community health nurses use a family genogram to identify family strengths and health risks and plan with the family strategies to prevent disease.

Community health nurses provide programs in child development for families at risk for child abuse, such as one-parent households.

SECONDARY PREVENTION

During a home visit, community health nurses screen for warning signs of abuse in the family.

Community health nurses provide programs in child development and behaviour management for families who have not abused their children but whose children are brought to the attention of social authorities for aggressive behaviour problems.

TERTIARY PREVENTION

Community health nurses develop programs with the family to change nutritional patterns to reduce complications from obesity.

Community health nurses refer abusive families to family therapy.

STUDENT EXPERIENCE

1. Define your family or a family you visited in the community.
2. a) Develop a genogram for your family. The following Web site may prove useful: http://www.childsafety.qld.gov.au/adoption/education/intercountry/module7/family-tree.html#familytree. Be sure to include a legend in the genogram.

   b) What have you found out about your family's health and illness patterns?
3. a) Develop an ecomap for your family. The previous site also includes an ecomap. Be sure to include a legend in the ecomap.

   b) What have you found out about your family's connections outside their family boundary with the community?
4. Write a therapeutic letter to your family.

REMEMBER THIS!

- Families are the context within which health care decisions are made. CHNs are responsible for assisting families in meeting health care needs.
- Family nursing is practised in all settings.
- Family nursing is a specialty area that has a strong theoretical base and is more than just common sense.
- Family demographics is the study of the structures of families and households as well as events that alter the family, such as marriage, divorce, births, cohabitation, and dual careers.
- A variety of family forms exist such as nuclear, lone parent, extended, blended, commuter, living apart together, same sex, grandparent led, and cohabitating.
- Traditionally, families have been defined as a nuclear family: mother, father, and young children. A variety of family definitions now exist, such as a group of two or more, a unique social group, and two or more persons joined together by emotional bonds.
- Family structure refers to the characteristics, gender, age, and number of the individual members who make up the family unit.
- Family health is difficult to define, but it includes the biological, psychological, sociological, cultural, and spiritual factors of the family system.
- The four approaches to viewing families are family as context, family as client, family as a system, and family as a component of society.
- Structure–function theory views the family as a social system with members who have specific roles and functions.
- Systems theory describes families as a unit of the whole, composed of members whose interactional patterns are the focus of attention.
- Family developmental theory is one theoretical framework used to study families. This approach emphasizes how families change over time and focuses on interactions and relationships among family members.
- Interactional theory focuses on the family as a unit of interacting personalities and examines the communication processes by which family members relate to one another.
- CHNs need to ask clients whom they consider to be family and then include those members in the family interviews.
- It is important for the CHN to recognize that the family has the right to make its own health decisions.
- The CHN, in working with families, must evaluate the family outcomes and responses to the plan, not just the success of the interventions.
- The importance of the family as a major client system for CHNs in reducing health risks and promoting the health of individuals and populations is well documented.
- The family system is a basic unit within which health behaviour, including health values, health habits, and health risk perceptions, is developed, organized, and performed.
- Knowledge of family structure and functioning is fundamental to implementing the community health nursing process with families in the community.
- CHNs need to go beyond the individual and family and to understand the complex environment in which the family functions to be effective in reducing family health risks. Categories of risk factors that are important to family health are biological risk, environmental risk, and determinants of health and behavioural risk.
- Several factors contribute to the experience of healthy or unhealthy outcomes. Not everyone exposed to the same event will have the same outcome. The factors that influence whether disease or other unhealthy results occur are called health risks. The accumulated risks are synergistic; their combined effect is more important than individual effects.
- An asset approach focuses on family competencies and family strengths rather than risks and deficits.
- Family strengths and resources can be used to help families deal with their health concerns and to promote their health.
- An important aspect of the role of the community health nursing in reducing health risk and promoting the health of populations has been the tradition of providing services to families in their homes.
- Home visits afford the opportunity to gain a more accurate assessment of the family structure and behaviour in the natural environment. Home visits also provide opportunities to observe the home environment and to identify both barriers and supports to reducing health risks and reaching family health goals.
- Increasingly, health professionals are working with clients in a more interactive, collaborative style.
- Contracting, which is making an agreement between two or more parties, involves a shift in responsibility and control, from the professional alone to a shared effort by client and professional.
- Families have varied and complex health concerns. The CHN often mobilizes several resources to effectively and appropriately meet family health concerns.

REFLECTIVE PRAXIS

Case Study 1

The initial contact between a community health nursing service and a family provides limited information, and the situation that develops may be much more complex than anticipated. The following example, based on an actual case, illustrates the issues and approaches outlined in this chapter.

The Valley View Health Unit was notified that Amy, age 16, had been referred by the school counsellor at the local high school for prenatal supervision. Amy is 4 months pregnant, in apparently good health, in grade 10, and living at home with her mother, stepfather, and younger sister. The family lives in a rural area outside of a small farming community. The father of the baby also lives in the community and continues to see Amy on a regular basis. The referral information provides the community health nurse (CHN) with a beginning, but limited, assessment of the family situation.

1. What would you do first as the CHN assigned to this family?
2. How would you help this family empower themselves to take responsibility for this situation?
3. After the initial contact, how would you extend the assessment to the entire family system?
4. Would you contract with this family? How? On what terms?
5. What developmental stage is this family in? Use the Calgary Family Assessment Model (CFAM) to guide your decision.

Answers are provided on the Evolve Web site at http://www.evolve.elsevier.com/Canada/Stanhope/community/.

Case Study 2

The Mitchell family consists of Harry (father), 46, Shirley (mother), 42, 18-year-old Annie, 15-year-old Michelle, 13-year-old Sean, and 7-year-old Bobby. Harry is the pastor of Faith Baptist Church, where he has served the past 15 years. Shirley is the homemaker and primary caretaker for the children.

For the past year, Shirley has felt tired and "run down." At her annual physical, she describes her symptoms to her physician. After several tests, Shirley is diagnosed with stomach cancer. She starts to cry and says, "How will I tell my family?"

Shirley's primary physician refers the family to Trisha, a CHN. Trisha calls the household and speaks with Shirley to arrange a home visit. Shirley confides to Trisha that it has been 2 weeks since she received the cancer diagnosis, but she has yet to tell her husband and children. Shirley asks Trisha if she can help her tell her family and explain what it all means. Trisha makes an appointment for a home visit with the family.

1. If you were the CHN, how would you plan for this home visit?
2. What developmental stage is this family in? Use CFAM to guide your decision.
3. Using CFAM, what data would you plan to collect in your family assessment under structural, developmental, and functional areas?
4. What specific community health nursing interventions would you use? Provide a rationale.

Answers are provided on the Evolve Web site at http://www.evolve.elsevier.com/Canada/Stanhope/community/.

What Would You Do?

1. Describe how a family assessment is different from an individual client assessment.
2. What kind of difficulties could you experience when arranging for a family assessment interview?
3. Discuss factors to be considered when determining the place to conduct a family assessment interview. Include pros and cons.
4. Complete a family genogram and ecomap on your family and identify major health risks. Summarize your findings.
5. Search the literature and select one refereed journal article to share in class pertaining to CFAM or the Calgary Family Intervention Model. Come to class prepared to present a summary of the article. Include your reflections on the new learning gained from reading this article.
6. Using Web-based resources, find statistics on the following: types of Canadian families, such as married couples, common-law families, one-parent families, step-families, blended families, same-sex marriages; family size; birth rates; marriage and divorce rates; low-income families; and working mothers. Statistics Canada would be a good starting point. Prepare a chart to include the identified statistics with the sources referenced and bring this information to class for discussion.

TOOL BOX

evolve

The Tool Box contains useful instruments that can be applied in community health nursing practice. These related resources are found either in the appendices at the back of this book or on the book's Evolve Web site at http://evolve.elsevier.com/Canada/Stanhope/community/.

Appendices

- Appendix E-4: Friedman Family Assessment Model (Short Form)
- Appendix 9: The Calgary Family Assessment Model

Tools

Ecomap Construction.
This link contains an example of an ecomap, which is used to delineate the external structure of the family.

International Council of Nurses.
A document titled *Tools for Action* is available on this site. It provides information on three family assessment models and a short tool that agencies can use to assess family satisfaction with their services.

Introduction to the Genogram.
This link contains information on the background for use of genograms.

Understanding Families: Simple Guide to Genograms.
This link contains instructions for constructing genograms.

WEBLINKS

evolve

Direct links to these resources can be found on the text's accompanying Evolve Web site at http://evolve.elsevier.com/Canada/Stanhope/community/.

Campaign 2000. This Web site report, titled *Oh Canada: Too Many Children in Poverty for Too Long* (2006) and released in March 2007, provides statistics about child poverty, including a discussion of children in Aboriginal communities and government programs.

CANGRANDS. This site provides links to available groups across Canada that support, educate, and empower grandparents raising their grandchildren. Choose the site on the map of Canada to learn whether your community has such a group.

Fuller-Thompson, E. *Grandparents Raising Grandchildren in Canada: A Profile of Skipped Generation Families.* This site provides statistics, research findings, and trends in Canada and elsewhere. Implications such as the economic and health factors and cultural variations are raised and discussed.

Registered Nurses' Association of Ontario. Best Practice Guidelines titled *Crisis Intervention* and *Supporting and Strengthening Families Through Expected and Unexpected Life Events* are found at this RNAO Web site. Select the "Nursing Best Practice Guidelines" link and use the search option to find these documents.

Statistics Canada. Using census data, this site provides statistics on various family forms in Canada.

Statistics Canada. *2006 Census—Families, Marital Status, Households and Dwelling Characteristics.* Based on 2006 census data, a variety of demographic information on families in Canada is provided.

Understanding Families. This site provides information for professionals and parents about the development of families and how to work with families.

The Vanier Institute of the Family. This site provides information on contemporary family trends such as characteristics of one-parent families and same-sex marriages and on family and transitions. To navigate the site, use the search engine and the key words "family," "health," and "statistics."

The Vanier Institute of the Family. *Families Count: Profiling Canada's Families IV.* This site provides information based primarily on the 2006 census data on the changes in the structure and function of the Canadian family.

REFERENCES

Baxter, L. A., Bylund, C. L., Imes, R. S., & Scheive, D. M. (2005). Family communication environments and rulebased social control of adolescents' healthy lifestyle choices. *Journal of Family Communication*, *5*(3), 209–227.

Beckmann Murray, R., Zentner, J. P., Pangman, V., & Pangman, C. (2009). *Health promotion strategies throughout the lifespan* (2nd Canadian edition.). Toronto, ON: Pearson Education Canada.

Bedi, G., & Goddard, C. (2007). Intimate partner violence: What are the impacts on children? *Australian Psychologist*, *42*(1), 66–77.

Bell, J. M. (1995). The dysfunction of "dysfunctional". *Journal of Family Nursing*, *1*(3), 235–237.

Bell, J. M. (2009). Family systems nursing: Re-examined. *Journal of Family Nursing*, *15*(2), 123–129.

Black, K., & Lobo, M. (2008). A conceptual review of family resilience factors. *Journal of Family Nursing*, *14*(1), 33–55.

Bomar, P. J. (2004). *Promoting health in families: Applying family research and theory to nursing practice* (3rd ed.). Philadelphia, PA: Saunders.

Campaign 2000. (2006). *Oh Canada! Too many children in poverty for too long…2006 report card on child and family poverty in Canada*. Retrieved from http://www.canadiancrc.com/PDFs/Campaign2000_06NationalReportCard_EN.pdf.

Christy-McMullin, K., & Shobe, M. A. (2007). The role of economic resources and human capital with woman abuse. *Journal of Policy Practice*, *6*(1), 3–26.

Cooley, M. L. (2009). A family perspective in community/public health nursing. In F. A. Maurer, & C. M. Smith (Eds.), *Community/Public health nursing practice: Health for families and populations* (4th ed., pp. 327–344). St. Louis, MO: Saunders Elsevier.

Danielson, C. B., McEwen, M., & Pullis, B. (2009). *Community-based nursing: An introduction* (3rd ed.). St. Louis, MO: Saunders Elsevier.

Erlingsson, C. (2009). Undergraduate nursing students writing therapeutic letters to families: An educational strategy. *Journal of Family Nursing*, *15*(1), 83–101.

Ford-Gilboe, M. (2002). Developing knowledge about family health promotion by testing the developmental model of health and nursing. *Journal of Family Nursing*, *8*(2), 140–156.

Friedman, M. M., Bowden, V. R., & Jones, E. G. (2003). *Family nursing: Research, theory and practice* (5th ed.). Upper Saddle River, NJ: Prentice Hall.

Fuller-Thompson, E. (2005). *Social and economic dimension of an aging population*. Retrieved from http://socserv.mcmaster.ca/sedap/p/sedap132.pdf.

Harmon Hanson, S. M. (2005). Family health care nursing: An introduction. In S. M. Harmon Hanson, V. Gedaly-Duff, & J. Rowe Kaakinen (Eds.), *Family health care nursing: Theory practice and research* (3rd ed., pp. 3–37). Philadelphia: F. A. Davis.

Harmon Hanson, S. M., Gedaly-Duff, V., & Rowe Kaakinen, J. (2005). *Family health care nursing: Theory practice and research* (3rd ed.). Philadelphia, PA: F. A. Davis.

Keita, G. P. (2009). Contributing to the debate over same-sex marriage. *Monitor on Psychology*, *40*(4). Retrieved from http://www.apa.org/monitor/2009/04/itpi.html.

LeGrow, K., & Rossen, B. (2005). Development of professional practice based on a family systems nursing framework: Nurses' and families' experiences. *Journal of Family Nursing*, *11*(1), 38–58.

Loveland-Cherry, C. J. (2006). Guest editorial: Where is the family in family interventions? *Journal of Family Nursing*, *12*(1), 4–6.

Maurer, F. A., & Smith, C. M. (2009). *Community/Public health nursing practice: Health for families and populations* (4th ed.). St. Louis, MO: Saunders Elsevier.

Patterson, C. J. (2005). Children of lesbian and gay parents. *Child Development*, *63*, 1025–1042.

Pawelski, J. G., Perrin, E. C., Foy, J. M., Allen, C. E., Crawford, J. E., Del Monte, M., & Vickers, D. L. (2006). The effects of marriage, civil union, and domestic partnership laws on the health and well-being of children. *Pediatrics*, *118*(1), 349–364.

Pender, N. J., Murdaugh, C. L., & Parsons, M. A. (2006). *Health promotion in nursing practice* (5th ed.). Upper Saddle River, NJ: Prentice Hall.

Potter, P. A., Perry, A. G., Ross-Kerr, J. C., & Wood, M. J. (2006). Family nursing. In J. C. Ross-Kerr, & M. J. Wood (Eds.), *Canadian fundamentals of nursing* (3rd ed., pp. 296–314). Toronto, ON: Elsevier.

Sauvé, R. (2003). *Marriage and legal recognition of same-sex unions: A discussion paper*. Vanier Institute of the Family. Retrieved from http://www.vifamily.ca/commentary/samesexpr.html.

Sittner, B. J., Hudson, D. B., & Defrain, J. (2007). Using the concept of family strengths to enhance nursing care. *American Journal of Maternal/Child Nursing*, *32*(6), 353–357.

Smith, C. M. (2009). Home visiting: Opening the doors for family health. In F. A. Maurer, & C. M. Smith (Eds.), *Community/Public health nursing practice: Health for families and populations* (4th ed., pp. 302–325). St. Louis, MO: Saunders Elsevier.

Stanhope, M., & Lancaster, J. (2008). *Community and public health nursing* (7th ed.). St. Louis, MO: Mosby.

Statistics Canada. (2007). *2006 Census: Families, marital status, households and dwelling characteristics*. Retrieved from http://www.statcan.gc.ca/daily-quotidien/070912/dq070912a-eng.htm.

Tannahill, A. (2008). Beyond evidence-to ethics: A decision-making framework for health promotion, public health and health improvement. *Health Promotion International*, *23*(4), 380–390.

Van Riper, M. (2006). Guest editorial: Family nursing in the era of genomic health care: We should be doing so much more! *Journal of Family Nursing*, *12*(2), 111–118.

Vanier Institute of the Family (2006). *Contemporary family trends: The effects of the changing age structure on households and families to 2026*. Retrieved from http://30645.vws.magma.ca/media/node/392/attachments/Effects_changing_age_structure.pdf.

Vanier Institute of the Family (2010). *Families count: Profiling Canada's Families IV*. Retrieved from http://www.vifamily.ca/media/node/371/attachments/Families_Count.pdf.

Wright, L. M., & Leahey, M. (2009). *Nurses and families: A guide to family assessment and intervention* (5th ed.). Philadelphia, PA: F. A. Davis.

Working with Client as Individual: Health and Wellness Across the Lifespan

CHAPTER 13

OBJECTIVES

After reading this chapter, you should be able to:

1. Integrate the determinants of health throughout the life stages.
2. Discuss major health issues of children and adolescents.
3. Evaluate the role of the community health nurse with specific at-risk populations in the community.
4. Describe ways to promote child and adolescent health within the community.
5. Describe men's health and women's health issues.
6. Discuss health issues in men's health and women's health.
7. Explain how women's and men's lifestyles affect their health.
8. Define terms commonly used to refer to older adults.
9. Explain the chronic health problems that are often experienced by older adults.
10. Describe the assessment and interventions for depression, delirium, and dementia.
11. Explain caregiver burden.

CHAPTER OUTLINE

KEY TERMS

See Glossary on page 593 for definitions.

The Canadian authors wish to acknowledge Mary-Louise Batty and Margaret Milburn for their contribution to the Comprehensive School Health Project section.

LIFESTYLE APPROACH

This chapter examines the health status of populations and of individuals across the lifespan. The emphasis is on population health and health promotion, but consideration is also given to health status, health risks, and lifestyle considerations. A behavioural approach is usually taken when lifestyle is the focus of change. Healthy lifestyle is important because it can reduce the occurrence and outcomes of certain chronic diseases and therefore contributes to the quality of life for Canadians. However, it is important to keep in mind that lifestyle is affected by factors such as the determinants of health and societal foci, and that public policies can also influence the development and impact of chronic diseases in the population. Lyons and Langille (2000) proposed a new definition of *lifestyle*—that is, lifestyle as a "resource for quality of life and coping" (p. 43)—which does consider many of the aforementioned factors. They maintained that it is an all-inclusive concept—more than changing areas such as diet, alcohol, and exercise. These authors proposed that lifestyle needs to include consideration of the social conditions in communities and determinants of health such as socioeconomic status and social networks (Lyons & Langille, 2000). They maintained that for healthy lifestyles to occur, a balance is needed between the assuming of personal responsibility ("What can I do?"), social responsibility ("What can we do?" and "What can I do for those around us?"), and government responsibility (what is done to promote "healthy environments," "healthy public policy" development, and "reductions in social inequities"). There is general agreement in Canada that lifestyle changes and health promotion need to go beyond the focus on the individual. However, we need to keep the individual as part of the whole in health promotion. Strategies that community health nurses (CHNs) can use to meet health concerns with an emphasis on health promotion and disease prevention are introduced in this chapter. Specifics about growth and development and particular diseases are not the focus of this chapter. These areas will have been covered elsewhere in the literature and in nursing programs; however, several Weblinks have been provided on the Evolve Web site that give access to this information.

Major chronic diseases in adults such as cancer, diabetes, and respiratory and cardiovascular diseases are a concern globally, accounting for approximately 60% of all deaths (World Health Organization [WHO], 2010). Globally, in 2005, half of these deaths from chronic diseases occurred in persons under 70 years of age (WHO, 2010). In Canada, more than 75% of adult deaths resulted from these chronic diseases (Public Health Agency of Canada [PHAC], 2005a). The economic burden of chronic disease in Canada is enormous (Patra et al., 2007). For example, annually for the years 1995 to 2003 in Canada, premature deaths from cardiovascular diseases cost approximately $9.2 billion (Patra et al., 2007).

In North America, actions are being taken to improve health outcomes by reducing preventable risk factors for diseases that require lifestyle changes such as ceasing of physical inactivity, unhealthy eating, and smoking. In Canada, a greater focus on the socioenvironmental approach with a population focus, discussion of health disparities, and discussion of the need for policy changes has shifted the Canadian thinking more in the direction of the "big picture." However, much of the focus has been at the discussion level with the beginnings of application at a health policy level. In 2005, a collaborative healthy living strategy was approved by federal, provincial, and territorial ministers of health. This plan, called *The Integrated Pan-Canadian Healthy Living Strategy,* has a goal of increasing by 20% the number of Canadians who have healthy diets, are physically active, and have healthy body weights (PHAC, 2007). Currently, it is believed that lifestyle patterns are learned in childhood; therefore, prevention is key during the formative years in order to work toward reducing the number of chronic illnesses that occur in adulthood. Some researchers, however, have challenged the belief of lifestyle behaviours as the major contributors to certain chronic diseases, such as cardiovascular diseases, cancers, and respiratory illness (Hertzman & Power, 2003; Hertzman, Power, Matthews, & Manor, 2001; Raphael & Farrell, 2002a, 2002b). They suggest a life-course perspective, which considers latent effects (risk that begins prenatally and continues throughout the lifespan); cumulative effects (repeated exposures over time that affect health); and pathway effects (exposure to certain factors at one stage in the life course increases the chances for other exposures later in life) (Hertzman & Power; 2003; Hertzman et al., 2001). Canada's Chief Public Health Officer, in the report titled *The Chief Public Health Officer's Report on the State of Public Health in Canada, 2009: Growing up Well—Priorities for a Healthy Future* (Butler-Jones, 2009), provides further examples for latent, cumulative, and pathway effects. Furthermore, Butler-Jones maintains that the impact of the life-course perspective in Canada has contributed to a greater focus on improving the living conditions and opportunities for children so the future health outcomes of the Canadian population will be significantly improved (Butler-Jones, 2009). In the life-course perspective, these effects contribute to chronic diseases in adulthood. Refer to Chapter 2 of the Butler-Jones 2009 report (available at the PHAC Weblink on the Evolve Web site) for a definition and description of the life-course trajectory and a discussion on how public health influenced this trajectory.

As mentioned earlier, Canada has developed a strategy for promoting healthy living. The current priorities of the Healthy Living Strategy are in areas such as physical activity and healthy eating and their relation to weight; tobacco reduction; and prevention of diabetes and other chronic diseases (PHAC, 2007). The vision is to create a healthy Canadian population based on healthy living. The two primary goals are to reduce health disparities and improve overall health outcomes in each of the areas of emphasis by using a population health approach. The objectives of the Healthy Living Strategy (priority 1) are to increase by 20% the number of Canadians who eat healthily, participate in regular physical activity, and have healthy body weights. Since the emphasis in this Healthy Living Strategy is a population health approach, consideration has been given to the interrelationship between a person's behaviour and socioeconomic factors such as environment, poverty, education, and employment. Actions on these social determinants of health will contribute to improved population health and not just focus on changing individual behaviours. The strategies to reach the objectives include intersectoral collaboration for policy and community development, research development and transfer, and providing public information. Healthy living priorities for mental health and injury prevention are part of the long-term planning and priorities for the PHAC. Further information on the Pan-Canadian Healthy Living Strategy is available at the PHAC Weblink *The 2007 Report on the Integrated Pan-Canadian Healthy Living Strategy* listed on the Evolve Web site. This is the first annual report of healthy living initiatives across Canada pertaining to the following four strategic directions: leadership and policy development, knowledge development and transfer, community development and infrastructure, and public information (PHAC, 2007). This site provides information on the progress made for each province and territory for the Healthy Living strategic directions. Refer to Figure 13-1 for the diagram depicting the Integrated Pan-Canadian Healthy Living Strategy Framework.

FIGURE 13-1 Integrated Pan-Canadian Healthy Living Strategy Framework Diagram

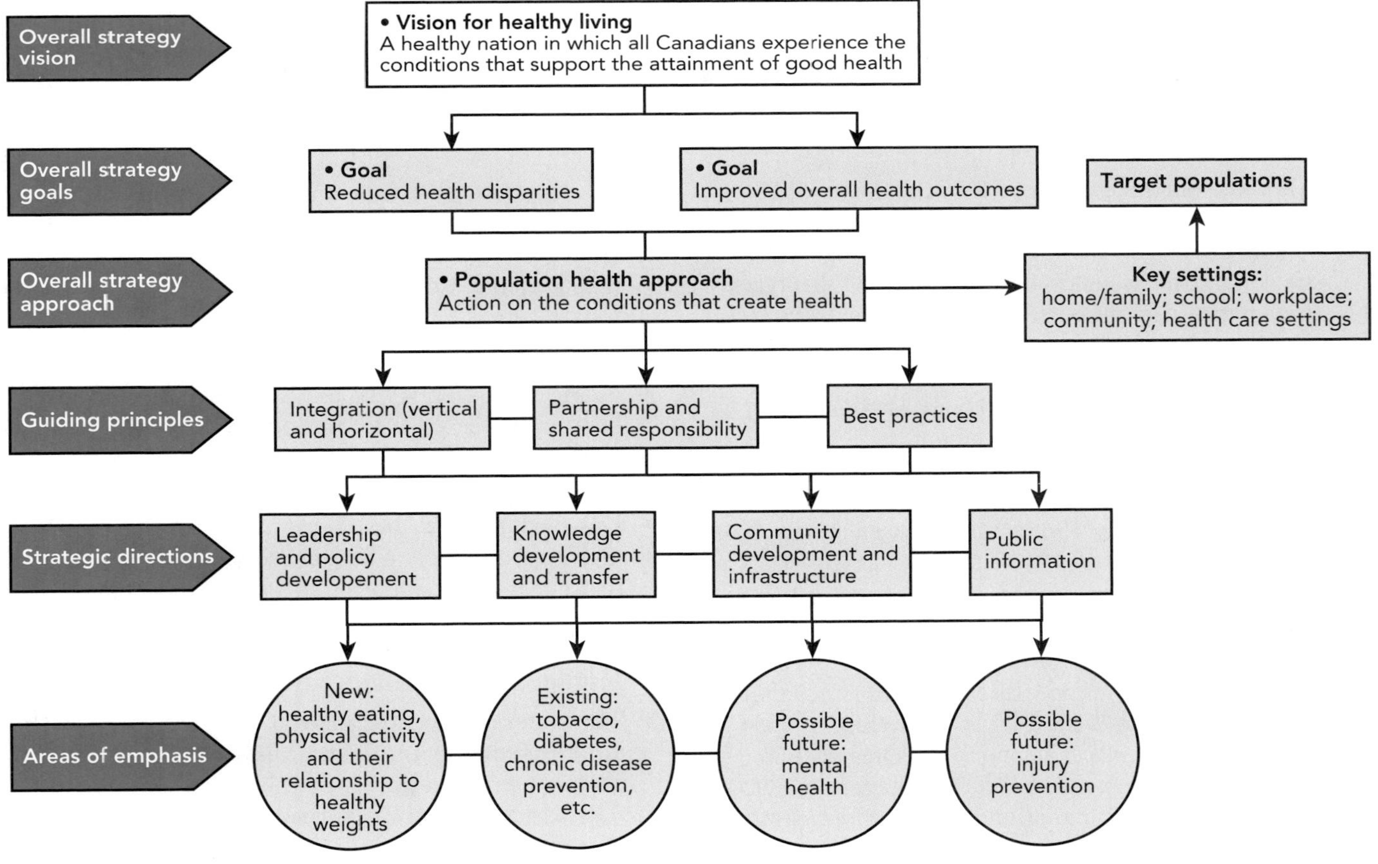

Public Health Agency of Canada. (2005). *Integrated Pan-Canadian Healthy Living Strategy Framework.* Ottawa, ON: Minister of Health (p. 9, Framework diagram). Retrieved from www.http://origin.phac-aspc.gc.ca/hl-vs-strat/hl-vs/diagram_bg-eng.php. Reprinted with permission of the Minister of Public Works and Government Services Canada, 2010.

Throughout this chapter, the areas of emphasis identified in the Integrated Pan-Canadian Healthy Living Strategy framework are addressed within the following lifespan groups: children and youth, adults, women, men, and older adults. Consideration is given to populations and individuals within a socioecological context with consideration of the strategic directions as outlined in the framework. Within each age group, certain health issues, conditions, and concerns are discussed in more detail because of their higher risk at certain time frames in the lifespan. For further information on integration of the healthy living strategies in Canada, refer to the PHAC "Healthy Living Fund" (see Weblinks on the Evolve Web site).

EARLY CHILD DEVELOPMENT AS A DETERMINANT OF HEALTH

Child poverty is increasing, lower-income families experience more illnesses than higher-income Canadians, and early child development affects health (Campaign 2000, 2009). According to the National Collaborating Centre for Determinants of Health (2009), early child development is the most important determinant of health. For further support on this position, refer to the WHO's *Total Environment Assessment Model for Early Child Development* listed in the Weblinks on the Evolve Web site. This model, for consideration by health care professionals, researchers, and policy makers, describes how the socioenvironmental determinant is fundamental to early child development, which is the most important determinant of health.

Some influences on healthy child development are found in Box 13-1 (see also the Canadian Nurses Association [CNA] *Healthy Child Development* Weblink on the Evolve Web site). Key factors that contribute to health inequalities are discussed in more depth in the document titled *Report on the State of Public Health in Canada 2009: Growing up Well—Priorities for a Healthy Future* (Butler-Jones, 2009). This report (at the PHAC Weblink on the Evolve Web site) highlights six areas of concern that have the greatest impact on the health of Canadian children: socioeconomic status and developmental opportunities; abuse and neglect; prenatal risks; mental health and disorders; obesity; and unintentional injuries (Butler-Jones, 2009).

BOX 13-1 Influences on Healthy Child Development

- Although playtime is essential for healthy child development, many children do not get enough time to play due to increased academic demands, fewer and/or shorter recesses at school, hurried lifestyles, and changes in family structure (Ginsburg, 2007). Play positively influences children's physical (e.g., provides exercise), cognitive (e.g., learning problem-solving skills), social (e.g., establishing interpersonal relationships), mental (e.g., helps to build self-esteem), and psychometric (e.g., develops and improves muscle strength) development (Beckmann Murray, Proctor Zentner, Pangman, & Pangman, 2009).
- Children with challenges such as autism have difficulty with social development (Ozonoff, Williams, & Landa, 2005). There is limited government support for social integration of persons with disabilities into Canadian society (Mikkonen & Raphael, 2010). In fact, in this area Canada ranks 27th among the 29 Organization for Economic Co-operation and Development (OECD) nations on public spending, and these authors identify the need for federal government policies to "meet the costs" (Mikkonen & Raphael, 2010, p. 51).
- Regulated child care is accessible to only 17% of Canadians (Mikkonen & Raphael, 2010). Since regulated child care is important for early child development, government policies need to ensure Canadian families access to affordable and quality child care regardless of socioeconomic status (Mikkonen & Raphael, 2010).
- Abused children are more likely to experience poor health in adulthood (Cromer & Sachs-Ericsson, 2006).
- Young children residing in poor neighbourhoods have an increased risk for illnesses as a result of exposure to environmental toxins and second-hand smoke (PHAC, 2005c).
- Low birth weights, disability and death, behavioural problems, and mental health disorders are more likely to occur in children born into low socioeconomic environments and these conditions can contribute to poor health for the rest of their lives (Canadian Institute for Health Information [CIHI], 2008).
- The material, social, structural, or community environments that influence the socioeconomic status of children lead to poor health as adults (Conroy, Sandel, & Zuckerman, 2010).
- "All Canadians would benefit from improved early childhood development in terms of improved community quality of life, reduced social problems and improved Canadian economic performance" (Mikkonen & Raphael, 2010, p. 24).

CHILD AND ADOLESCENT HEALTH

Children's health includes the health of children from infancy to adolescence. The future of Canada depends on how our children are cared for. Focusing on the health needs of children increases the chances of future adults who value and practise healthy lifestyles and who are healthier (Butler-Jones, 2009). Refer to the PHAC Weblink *Report on the State of Public Health in Canada 2009: Growing up Well—Priorities for a Healthy Future* on the Evolve Web site (specifically Chapter 3, which describes some key considerations about Canadian children's health; Chapter 4, which discusses, family and environmental factors influencing health; and Chapter 5, which provides information on various community and government programs available in Canada and internationally that have been implemented to facilitate a healthy life for children and their families).

CHNs have the following two major roles to fulfill in the area of child and adolescent health:

1. Provision of direct services to children and their families: assessment, management of care, education, and counselling
2. Assessment of the community and the establishment of programs to ensure a healthy environment for its children

Many opportunities arise for CHNs to teach healthy lifestyles to children and caregivers and to provide family-centred care in the community. Specific issues that may arise during adolescence such as teenage pregnancy and sexually transmitted infections were discussed earlier in Chapter 11 and will be discussed again in Chapter 17 of this text.

Ongoing growth and development make this age group unique. Table 13-1 provides a brief review of some common health concerns from infancy to adolescence. Physical, cognitive, and emotional changes occur more rapidly during childhood and adolescence than at any other time in the lifespan. Health visits should be scheduled at key ages to monitor these changes. Many available resources provide this information in detail, such as the PHAC Weblink "Maternal and Infant Health" on the Evolve Web site. Community health nursing assessments for child health (see Box 13-2) include assessing growth and health status, development, quality of the parent–child relationship, and family support systems.

CHNs such as a nurse practitioner in a community clinic or a public health nurse visiting with families (newborns and other age groups) may need to conduct an assessment of any of the following age groups: infant, toddler, schoolchild, and adolescent (some individual assessment tools are provided in Appendix E-6, found on the Evolve site, such as Infant, Child, and Youth Screening Tools). During these contacts, the CHN needs to actively involve the parent(s) throughout the assessment process, and the developmental stages need to be part of the assessment. This parental involvement will facilitate data collection, empower the parent(s), and encourage parental identification of health concerns. The community health nurse and parent(s) partner to identify appropriate interventions to address all health concerns, and strategies for follow-up and evaluation are planned. The CHN, in collaboration with the parent(s), may determine the need for a referral to a specific community agency. The CHN would follow the referral process as outlined earlier in Chapter 3.

The CHN considers the developmental stages, as previously mentioned, as part of the child and family assessment (see Table 13-2). Also, the developmental stages are considered by CHNs in order to provide anticipatory guidance to parents so that the developmental stage progression is maximized. For example, during a home visit to a family with a newborn, a CHN would most likely assess for indicators of the development of trust between the parent(s) and the newborn. The CHN could counsel the parent(s) on ways to promote the development of trust during parent–newborn interactions. The CHN would also discuss issues surrounding development of trust during infancy. Provision of resources to the parent(s) may be indicated to assist in acquiring parental skills to promote the development of trust. One resource that

BOX 13-2 Community Health Nursing Assessment for Child Health

- Physical assessment
- Psychosocial assessment
- Nutritional needs
- Elimination patterns
- Sleep behaviours
- Development and behaviour
- Safety issues
- Parenting concerns

CRITICAL VIEW

Currently, more children are being diagnosed with type 2 diabetes mellitus, which is most commonly found in older adults.

1. Why do you think this new pattern is developing?
2. Are the incidence and prevalence of type 2 diabetes mellitus on the increase in Caucasian children? Explain.

TABLE 13-1 Common Health Concerns—Infancy Through Adolescence

Age Group	Common Health Concerns	Age Group	Common Health Concerns
Infant (1 to 12 months)	• Atopic dermatitis • Diaper dermatitis	Schoolchild (6 to 12 years)	• Accommodative esophoria • Otitis externa
Newborn (1 to 4 weeks) not included in this table	• Seborrheic dermatitis ("cradle cap") • Oral candidiasis ("thrush") • Constipation • Iron-deficiency anemia • Roseola infantum • Colic		• Serous otitis media • Allergic rhinitis • Asthma • Herpes type 1 • Contact dermatitis • Tinea corporis (ringworm of the nonhairy skin) • Tinea capitis (ringworm of the head) • Warts • Pediculus humanus capitis (head lice) • Mumps • Diabetes type 1 • Fifth disease (erythema infectiosum) • Hand-foot-and-mouth disease • Pityriasis rosea
Toddler (12 months to 3 years)	• Umbilical cord granuloma • Myopia • Astigmatism • Strabismus • Hearing impairment • Otitis media • Dental caries • Malabsorption syndrome • Impetigo • Pharyngitis • Acute nonspecific gastroenteritis (simple diarrhea) • Varicella (chickenpox) • Rubella (3-day measles) • Pinworms *(Enterobius vermicularis)* • Miliaria rubra ("heat rash" or "prickly heat") • Viral croup (laryngotracheobronchitis)	Acolescents (13 to 21 years)	• Hordeolum (stye) • Epistaxis (nosebleed) • Acne vulgaris • Dental caries and gingivitis • Aphthous stomatitis • Tinea cruris • Tinea pedis (athlete's foot) • Infectious mononucleosis • Hepatitis A, B, and C virus • Rocky Mountain spotted fever • Lyme disease • Sexually transmitted infections
Preschooler (3 to 5 years)	• Measles • Diarrhea • Postural problems • Juvenile hypertension • Hypochromic anemia		

Source: Adapted from Beckmann Murray, R. B., Zentner, J. P., Pangman, V., & Pangman, C. (2006). *Health promotion strategies through the lifespan* (Canadian ed.), pp. 330, 359–361, 435–438, 492–494. Toronto, ON: Pearson.

could be provided is the PHAC *First Connections... Make All the Difference* resource kit listed in the Tool Box on the Evolve Web site. This kit includes resources for professionals and also information for parents and primary caregivers regarding promoting infant attachment.

Transitions are life events that occur from infancy and continue as a person ages. These transitions, often referred to as turning points in life (with the potential to create crisis), can present as challenges that sometimes require support to move forward. The Health Canada resource *Growing Healthy Canadians: A Guide for Positive Child Development* (also listed in the Tool Box on the Evolve Web site) is an excellent source of information on transition from infancy to adulthood. Information is provided on the role of communities, research on the determinants of health, and factors that influence development.

Overweight and Obesity

"Overweight and obesity are conditions that occur at different points of weight gain, can have very different outcomes, and possibly different determinants and risk factors" (Clinton, 2009, p. 7). Approximately 36% of Canadian adults are overweight and 24% are obese, and approximately 26% of Canadian children and adolescents are overweight and 8% are obese (PHAC, 2005a). These numbers have increased over the years, with obesity now being referred to as a major public health issue (PHAC, 2009b). "Obesity is sometimes defined as the condition of an individual who is 20% or more above ideal weight" (Beckmann Murray et al., 2009, p. 362). However, obesity is more than an individual health issue. Many factors contribute to obesity. Societal changes led

TABLE 13-2 Developmental Stages—Infancy Through Adolescence

Age Group	Freud (Psychosexual)	Erickson (Psychosocial)	Piaget (Logical, Cognitive, and Moral)	Kohlberg (Moral)
Infant (1 to 12 months)	Oral stage	Trust versus mistrust	Period I (sensorimotor)	
Newborn (1 to 4 weeks) not included in this table			Beginning development of motor and cognitive skills	
Toddler (12 months to 3 years)	Anal stage	Autonomy versus shame and doubt	Period I (sensorimotor) (beginning of preoperational): child is egocentric; beginning of parallel play	Level 1 (preconventional) Stage 1: punishment and obedience orientation
Preschooler (3 to 5 years)	Phallic stage (Oedipus complex; Electra complex)	Initiative versus guilt	Period II (preoperational): rapid language development	
Schoolchild (6 to 12 years)	Latent stage	Industry versus inferiority	Period III (concrete operations) Ability to perform mental operations	Level 1 (preconventional) Stage 2: instrumental relativist orientation
Adolescents (13 to 21)	Genital stage	Identity versus identity diffusion	Period IV (formal operations): stages -abstract thinking develops -increased ability to reason about consequences	Level 2 (conventional) Stage 3: good boy, nice girl orientation Stage 4: society maintaining orientation Level 3 (postconventional) Stage 5: social contact orientation Stage 6: universal ethical principle orientation

SOURCE: Modified from Potter, P. A., Perry, A. G., Ross-Kerr, J. C., and Wood, M. J. (2009). *Canadian fundamentals of nursing* (4th ed.), pp. 317–322. Toronto, ON: Elsevier/Mosby.

to the proliferation of fast-food availability to meet the demands of working families, easier access to vending machines containing fast foods, and increased plate sizes, which has led to increased portions or "supersizing" with extra calories. Vending machines with fast-food choices are common in schools. Colas and sugary fruit punch add empty calories. Snacking on high-sugar and high-fat foods is a problem. Advertising directed at children also glorifies poor food choices.

Additionally, because of increased awareness for child safety pertaining to walking to school and out-of-school activities, parents have increasingly taken to driving their children to school and to after-school activities. Also, transportation for taking children to school through busing rather than walking has resulted in decreased physical activity levels of children and adolescents. In Canada, over 50% of school children and adolescents (5 to 17 years of age) are driven to school either by car or by bus (Heart & Stroke Foundation, 2009). As all this was happening, some schools decreased or discontinued physical education programs in the schools. Furthermore, there has been an increase in sedentary lifestyle of children and youth due to technological changes that have precipitated increased time spent in nonphysical activities such as watching television and playing computer games (PHAC, 2009b). Because the rates of child obesity (2 to 17 years) tripled from 1978 to 2004 (Shields, 2006), actions have been taken at various levels. Most schools have maintained or reintroduced physical activity education programs as well as increased healthy food choices in schools. Governments have introduced new health promotion policies such as bans on trans fats and the introduction of the Children's Fitness Tax Credit. Communities are planning for and providing physical activity opportunities, such as connecting neighbourhoods with walking trails. There is also more control over children's good eating advertising. For further information on the influence of the built environment on promoting healthier outcomes for Canadians, refer to the Evolve Web site for the PHAC Weblink, "Bringing Health to the Planning Table—A Profile of Promising Practices in Canada and Abroad." For information on alternatives for physical activity modes of travel to school, visit the School Travel Planning News Weblink on the Evolve Web site.

The medical consequences of obesity vary, with obese children and teens having an increased prevalence of the following:

- Hypertension
- Respiratory problems
- Hyperlipidemia
- Bone and joint difficulties
- Hyperinsulinemia
- Menstrual problems

The psychosocial disadvantages of being overweight in the young may include the following:

- Teasing
- Scholastic discrimination
- Low self-esteem
- Negative body image

There is a downward spiral of overweight, poor self-image, increasing isolation, and decreasing activity, which together lead to obesity. Long-term risks include cardiovascular disease, diabetes, and cancer. For further information on the issue of overweight and obesity in Canada and the ecological approach to addressing obesity and its determinants, refer to the Canadian Population Health Initiative report Weblink on the Evolve Web site. The Government of Canada Weblink (on the Evolve Web site), *Healthy Weights for Healthy Kids: Report of the Standing Committee on Health,* contains information on what determines healthy weights, what works for healthy weight control, and issues pertaining to Aboriginal and Inuit populations.

Physical Activity

As previously indicated, television and computer time contribute to a sedentary lifestyle and increase the tendency of children and youth to be overweight and obese (PHAC, 2005b; PHAC, 2009a). As these passive activities such as playing with a computer rather than with others increase, obesity in Canadian children and youth also increase (PHAC, 2005a). Interventions need to be based on goals of lifestyle changes for the entire family. The goal is to modify the way the family eats, exercises, and plans daily activities. Guidelines for managing childhood obesity are discussed in Box 13-3. The goal of managing weight in children and adolescents is to normalize weight. This may involve the following:

- Slowing the rate of weight gain
- Allowing children to "grow into" their weight
- Improving dietary habits
- Increasing physical activity
- Improving self-esteem
- Improving parent relationships

For information on the recommended physical activity levels for Canadian children and youth, refer to the PHAC Weblink *Canada's Physical Activity Guides for Children and Youth* on the Evolve Web site. Along with

BOX 13-3 Guidelines for Managing Childhood Obesity

- Set goals related to healthier lifestyle, not dieting.
- Keep objectives realistic and obtainable.
- Modify family eating habits to include low-fat food choices. Serve calorie-dense foods that incorporate the Canada Food Guide: whole grains, fruits, vegetables, lean-protein foods, and low-fat dairy products.
- Encourage family members to stop eating when they are satisfied. Encourage recognizing hunger and satiation cues.
- Schedule regular times for meals and snacks. Include breakfast and do not skip meals.
- Have low-calorie, nutritious snacks ready and available. Avoid having empty-calorie junk foods in the home.
- Encourage the keeping of food intake and activity diaries.
- Promote physical activity. Make daily exercise a priority. Encourage family participation. Find ways to make the activity fun. Include peers.
- Limit television viewing. Do not allow snacking while watching television.
- Scale back computer time. Replace sedentary time with hobbies, activities, and chores.
- Recognize healthier food choices when eating out. Order broiled, roasted, grilled, or baked items. Split orders or take home "doggy bags."
- Praise and reward children for the progress they make in reaching nutrition and activity goals. Emphasize the unique positive qualities of each child.
- Understand the genetic features of the child's or adolescent's body type. Acceptance of the child who has a higher range of abdominal girth measurement may be a part of reaching health goals.

CRITICAL VIEW

1. How does the Children's Fitness Tax Credit address childhood obesity?
2. Does the Children's Fitness Tax Credit potentially widen the differential that exists between low-income and higher-income families? Explain.

the guides are support resources such as family and teacher guides for physical activity promotion for children and youth. Additionally, there is a link to the Department of Finance Canada for information on the Children's Fitness Tax Credit, which became effective on January 1, 2007, to support children's participation in all programs that will contribute to their physical fitness.

Nutrition

Promoting good nutrition and dietary habits is one of the most important aspects of maintaining child health. The first 6 years in a child's life are the most important for developing sound lifetime eating habits. The quality of nutrition has been widely accepted as an important influence on growth and development. It is now becoming recognized as an important role in disease prevention.

Atherosclerosis begins during childhood. Other diseases such as obesity, diabetes, osteoporosis, and cancer may have early beginnings also. Low-income and minority families are at increased risk for poor nutrition, but all groups show poor dietary habits.

The child and family both provide a range of variables that influence nutritional habits. Ethnic, racial, cultural, and socioeconomic factors influence what the parents eat and how they feed their children. The child brings individual issues to the nutritional arena, such as the following:

- Slow eating
- Picky patterns
- Food preferences
- Allergies
- Acute or chronic health problems
- Changes with acceleration and deceleration of growth

Parents often have unrealistic expectations of what children should eat. Health Canada's *Eating Well with Canada's Food Guide* (see the Weblinks on the Evolve Web site) offers guidelines for daily food requirements for all ages. The latest version addresses, for the first time, gender difference in nutritional requirements and suggests portion sizes and food choices based on quality. Physical growth serves as an excellent measure of adequacy of the diet. Height, weight, and head circumference of children younger than 3 years are plotted on appropriate growth curves at regular intervals to allow assessment of growth patterns. Good nutritional intake supports physical growth at a steady rate.

A 24-hour diet recall by the parent is a helpful screening tool to assess the amount and variety of food intake of children. If the recall is fairly typical for the child, the CHN can compare the intake with basic recommendations for the child's age. CHNs will want to ask about the family's and the child's concerns regarding diet and look at the family's meal patterns. In some situations, the CHN could direct the family to the interactive Web component of the Canada Food Guide titled "My Food Guide," where the family can plan food intake based on age, sex, food preferences, and culture. A key area of nutrition assessment includes the child's and family's exercise patterns. Behaviour problems that occur during meals may also be an issue.

Growth charts are one tool available to assess whether a child is growing within the "normal" range for age. They also provide the opportunity to monitor a child's growth over time. These charts are used during well-child assessments. The results can be used to reassure parents regarding their child's growth and also to provide an opportunity to teach about the normal range that contributes to individual child differences. Further information about the health of children, including calculating growth using growth charts and height calculators, can be found at the Keep Kids Healthy Web site listed in the Tool Box on the Evolve Web site.

The increased occurrence of type 2 diabetes mellitus in childhood, especially in children who are obese, supports the need for school and other community programs to promote healthy lifestyles and therefore diabetes prevention in this population. One study in Nova Scotia explored the risk factors for childhood weight problems based on school and family factors (Veugelers & Fitzgerald, 2005). One finding of note was that students who skipped breakfast were more likely to have weight issues and to eat unhealthy foods at lunch at school. One recommendation by these authors that relates to one of the determinants of health and families was that "preventive public health actions should be targeted first toward low-income neighbourhoods" (p. 612). It is known that poverty puts populations at increased risk for poorer health.

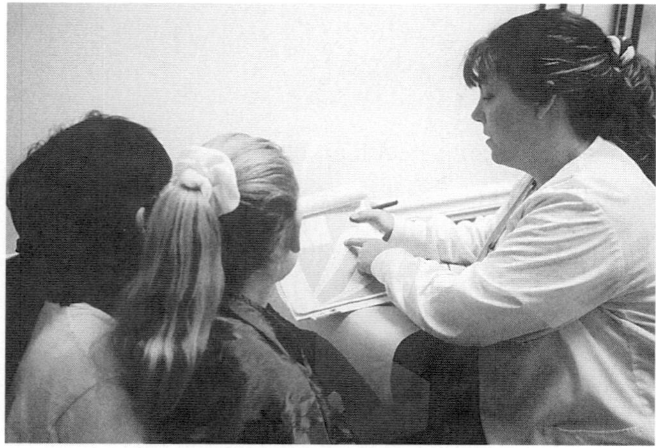

A community health nurse explains the growth patterns on a growth chart to a child and her mother.

CRITICAL VIEW

Reflect on and record your food intake and physical activity for the previous 48 hours. Be sure to include all meals, liquids, and snacks consumed.

1. a) How would you describe your nutritional intake and physical activity level over the past 48 hours?
   b) Compare your nutritional intake and activity level to the recommendations provided in the revised Canada Food Guide (Health Canada, 2007b).
2. Based on your findings, what nutritional and physical activity level changes would you need to implement to meet the Canada Food Guide (Health Canada, 2007b) recommendations?

Community and government interventions are needed to address the health disparities in which poor Canadians live and work if their health is to be improved. Food is one of the prerequisites for health identified in the Ottawa Charter on health promotion. CHNs can advocate for healthy public policies to reduce inequities in income. This might be accomplished by partnering with other community groups to influence the various government levels and through involvement with nursing professional organizations to lobby for change. Of note for CHNs is the discussion on the need for relevant research to identify policy priorities to address obesity in Canada (PHAC, 2009b). This discussion should include recognition of the determinants of health, such as food insecurity; inequitable access to physical activity; and environmental determinants of health. For example, rural and Aboriginal children tend to be overweight and obese because of living on lower incomes and residing in areas where nutritious foods are either unavailable or very expensive and unaffordable (Butler-Jones, 2009). The PHAC's "Obesity in Canada: Snapshot" Weblink (on the Evolve Web site) provides information such as the obesity trends in Canada, factors influencing prevalence of obesity, and the economic costs of obesity. Additionally, the PHAC document *Obesity: An Overview of Current Landscape and Prevention-Related Activities in Ontario* (see Evolve Weblinks) presents statistics on overweight and obesity in Canadian children, youth, and adults, as well as the contributing factors to obesity and related health concerns and presents an obesity-prevention approach. Also, CHNs could initiate the development of community programs such as school breakfast and healthy snack programs and food bank programs at higher-education institutions. Health educational programs on nutritious foods and physical activity requirements in the community could also be offered by CHNs.

One of the national research initiatives of significance for Canadian communities is the Early Learning and Child Care (ELCC) experiences in selected cities across the nation. The study was funded by Social Development Canada and the cities of Toronto and Vancouver (Mahon, Jenson, & Mortimer, 2006). Participating cities were St. John's, Newfoundland; Halifax, Nova Scotia; Montreal, Quebec; Sherbrooke, Quebec; Toronto, Ontario; Sudbury, Ontario; Winnipeg, Manitoba; Saskatoon, Saskatchewan; Calgary, Alberta; Vancouver, British Columbia; and Whitehorse, Yukon. It was found that (1) most successful programs target all children under 12 years and not just the high-risk groups; (2) even with community partnerships, ELCC requires more support than is offered by cities to be able to expand services to all children and families; (3) inconsistency exists across the cities in relation to the sufficiency of the provision of child programs; (4) cities with more resources are better able to access funding; (5) high-quality programs are needed for out-of-school children, such as those before and after the school day; and (6) cities are responsible for recreational facilities for this latter group. The study findings show that these city programs require government funding at all levels so that parents are supported and early learning and child care needs are met. As well, the study findings indicate the need for cities to form partnerships that focus on health promotion and population health if communities are to address lifestyle changes through supportive environments.

CRITICAL VIEW

1. How can CHNs contribute to the reduction of societal inequalities?
2. What community-based programs are available in your community to address social disparities?

The Comprehensive School Health Approach

Healthy child development can be promoted through the Comprehensive School Health Framework (CSHF). This approach to child health moves beyond the behavioural and lifestyle approach, to, as its name implies, a comprehensive framework for health promotion. Central to the philosophy of comprehensive school health (CSH) is the belief that "healthy learners are better learners" (Murray, Low, Hollis, Cross, & Davis, 2007). This link between comprehensive school health and academic success is evidenced by research (Dukowski, 2009; Murray et al., 2007). Comprehensive school health focuses on school children as a population; the use of the CSHF is relevant as children spend approximately one-third of each weekday in school. Thus, opportunities to access the population and build capacity are plentiful (Canadian Association for School Health, 2006). The concept of CSH has been endorsed by the WHO and is recognized internationally. The term *comprehensive school health* is most commonly used in Canada. Similar frameworks exist in other countries and are known as "health promoting schools" or "coordinated school health" (Canadian Association for School Health, 2006).

Comprehensive school health has its roots in population health, particularly the 1986 World Health Organization's seminal Ottawa Charter for Health Promotion. The Ottawa Charter helped change the focus of health promotion from focusing on individual responsibility and lifestyle change to emphasizing the importance of understanding the broader influences on health. In line with the Ottawa Charter, the CSH approach promotes health in and out of the classroom. Comprehensive school health drew particularly on the Ottawa Charter's focus on development of personal skills (Stewart-Brown, 2006). This and the other four tenets of the Ottawa Charter remain one side of the Population Health Promotion Model (Hamilton & Bhatti, 1996) previously discussed in Chapter 4. Community health nurses practising within CSHF recognize that programs that focus on helping individual children in the classroom, without acknowledging the importance of the environments within which the children live, as well as the sociopolitical context of those environments, will not be as effective in long-term promotion of health (Health Nexus, 2008; Labonte, 2003). For example, a community health nurse working within the CSHF might want to provide students with some health information about nutrition. Therefore, a classroom presentation about nutrition might be supplemented by a school breakfast program and a district-wide nutrition policy that supports provision of healthy foods to the children in the schools. In addition, the CSH community health nurse might work with parent or guardian support groups at the school to encourage fundraisers that do not involve foods with a low nutritional rating (e.g., selling gift baskets instead of chocolate bars). The CSH community health nurse might educate teachers and staff about alternatives to food rewards (e.g., stickers or other low-cost items). The CSH community health nurse might also participate as a member of a multidisciplinary group that advocates for legislation of a nationwide breakfast program for children.

Children's health is recognized as being influenced by the relationships of children with family, school, and community. Community health nurses who work within the comprehensive school health framework must be supportive of these relationships, as well as be cognizant of the following four CSH cornerstones:

- Social and physical environment (e.g., programs support physical activity, environments are inclusive and welcoming, schools are built in environmentally safe areas)
- Teaching and learning (programs are typically universal and upstream in their approach; programs build developmental assets, nurture development of protective factors and resilience, and also target students' knowledge, attitudes, skills, and behaviours)
- Healthy school policy (e.g., nutrition policies, tobacco-free policies)
- Partnerships and services (includes intersectoral and interdisciplinary partnerships between the school and community and considers accessibility of health services within the school, particularly primary and secondary prevention) (Avison, 2009; Joint Consortium for School Health, 2010; PHAC, 2008a)

Stewart-Brown (2006), commissioned by the WHO, conducted an extensive literature review that focused on the evidence-informed practice of CSH. The report concluded that, in order to be most effective, CHNs who work within the CSHF should promote injury prevention, nutrition, physical activity, and mental health. Programs should involve families, the community, and the school when possible. In addition, CHNs should support programs that are delivered by students to students (peer-delivered) as they can be as effective as those facilitated by an adult.

Comprehensive school health CHNs spend significant amounts of time engaging in both primordial and primary prevention. Although the concept of primary prevention is commonly found in health promotion literature, the concept of *primordial prevention,* or preventing risk factors for health issues from ever occurring, is seen less frequently. A similar pattern exists in discussions about the CSHF. Ironically, the concept is not new and was first suggested by Strasser (1978). **Primordial prevention** focuses on the prevention of health issues in a population at a stage early enough to avoid risk factors arising and thus preventing the health issue from developing within a population. It includes creating supportive environments and helping populations develop personal skills (Centers for Disease Control [CDC], 2008). This level of prevention was used in a significant study that continues to be relevant, titled "The Children and Adolescent Trial of Health (CATCH)." Randomized control trials were conducted on elementary school children between 1987 and 2000. Researchers engaged schoolchildren in activities designed to promote cardiovascular health. Programs focused on physical activity, nutrition, and smoking (Child Trends, 2007). Research about the importance of primordial prevention continues to demonstrate its importance for policy development and population health promotion. Findings from the Labarthe, Dai, Day, Fulton, and Grunbaum (2009) longitudinal study on children aged 8 to 18 years supported the effectiveness of obesity-prevention programs beginning in the elementary school population.

Comprehensive School Health Project in New Brunswick

Since September 2008, nursing students and their instructor at the University of New Brunswick have partnered with local CSH/Public Health Nurse Marg Milburn to create and implement health promotion programs grounded in primordial and primary prevention at Park Street Elementary School. Content for each presentation is based on epidemiology and surveillance literature (Canadian Council on Social Development, 2007; Leitch, 2007; PHAC, 2008a) and supported by evidence from New Brunswick Wellness Surveys (New Brunswick Wellness, Culture and Sport, n.d.). Wellness programs in New Brunswick focus on four pillars: healthy eating, tobacco-free living, mental fitness and resilience, and physical activity. Outcomes for each presentation are matched to the provincial education curriculum outcomes for each grade. Some topics include handwashing, healthy active learning, nutrition, injury prevention, healthy friendships, smoking prevention, and hygiene. Nursing students visit the same classrooms each week and build relationships with schoolchildren and school staff. Presentations follow a predictable pattern, beginning with deep breathing and stretching activities. Nursing students also build capacity by becoming involved with the home and school, drawing on experts within the community (e.g., a mother whose daughter has severe allergies discusses her experiences and demonstrates the use of an anaphylaxis kit), and contributing to the school newsletter. Nursing students include both teachers and the children in the evaluation of the presentations. Preparation for the clinical experience encourages nursing students to transfer knowledge from previous and current coursework and to build on their own strengths and interests. For example, they draw on theory from the previous years about healthy child development, common pediatric chronic and acute health challenges, and mental health challenges. Knowledge transfer from concurrent theory courses includes epidemiology, immunizations, communicable diseases, leadership, effective communication and presentation skills, community development, and more.

As the nursing students learn in the classroom about community assessment through asset mapping (Ryan & Bourke, 2008), they learn in the clinical site about the Developmental Asset Framework that is supported by school districts across the province (Ryan & Bourke, 2008). The focus for presentations is strength based and positive in approach. Students learn in the theory courses about population health and the importance of evidence-informed practice, and they use epidemiology and research when creating or modifying their clinical classroom presentations. As well, they learn about the importance of building capacity, relationship building, and working with the community. In the clinical settings, they have the opportunity to build relationships by visiting the same classrooms each week, including the voices of the children and teachers in evaluating the presentations, and extending the relationship outside the classroom to the broader school community. As students learn in the theory courses about primary health care, social justice, and citizenship, they learn in clinical settings about healthy public policy within the school district and across Canada. They also discuss poverty, inclusion, citizenship initiatives, and capacity-building initiatives at the school (e.g., "Leader in Me Program"). Nursing students are also encouraged to bring their strengths and interests to the program. One example is of a student who loved to sing and had a degree in music, and who was able to record herself singing safety and handwashing songs for future presentations. Another student who enjoyed sewing was able to make beanbags for a game that was developed by the group.

Nursing students have commented positively about the experience, and other schools have requested partnerships. The direction for the ongoing planning of the partnership is based on recent, local research (Morrison, Kirby, Losier, & Allain, 2009). For example, in 2006 and 2007, wellness behaviours of students from grades 5 to 12 were surveyed provincially by the New Brunswick Department of Wellness, Culture and Sport in collaboration with the New Brunswick Department of Education, the University of New Brunswick, and the Université de Moncton. Students' mental fitness needs were assessed. The researchers concluded that there is substantial evidence that students who meet their needs for relatedness, competence, and autonomy are more likely to participate in healthy lifestyle choices. More work in the field of mental fitness is developing in schools and through the Department of Wellness, Culture and Sport. Comprehensive school health community health nurses continue to be inspired by the belief that "children are critically important. We must keep them healthy and help them when they are not" (Leitch, 2007, p. 17).

Injuries and Accidents

Injuries and accidents are the most common causes of preventable disease, disability, and death among children. Most accidents occur in the home; therefore, measures to promote home safety are important. In Canada, injuries and accidents in children 1 to 14 years of age are the leading causes of death (Safe Kids Canada, 2007). Most injuries and accidents are preventable. A 2006 Safe Kids Canada survey found that most parents were unaware of the serious risks of injury to children under 14 years of age (Safe Kids Canada, 2007).The key to changing behaviours is teaching age-appropriate safety. Often, CHNs take the lead role in providing education on the prevention of accidents and injuries and work with partners such as teachers, police safety officers, and social workers. The CHN identifies risk factors by assessing the characteristics of the child, family, and environment. Interventions include anticipatory guidance, environmental modification, and safety education. Education should focus on age-appropriate interventions based on knowledge of leading causes of death and risk factors. Injury prevention topics are listed in Box 13-4. For further information on unintentional injuries, refer to the Safe Kids Canada Weblink, "Child & Youth Unintentional Injury: Ten Years in Review." This Web site provides statistical information and fact sheets on unintentional injuries that would be useful to CHNs, other professionals working in the area of childhood safety, and parents. The CNA position statement *Determinants of Health* (see the Evolve Weblinks) presents the CNA position on the determinants of health such as the need for increased funding for chronic disease prevention and increasing research on the determinants of health. The effects of the determinants of health, including individual behaviour and physical environment and genetics, are identified in this document as important considerations for nurses to influence the health outcomes of Canadians.

The CNA provides a summary of the built environment in relation to the issue of injury prevention. This issue is recognized as significant in Canadian public health because of the morbidity and mortality implications, including premature mortality. The various age groups are discussed in reference to economic implications based on the types of injuries that most commonly occur in Canada. Refer to the CNA Backgrounder *The Built Environment, Injury Prevention, and Nursing: A Summary of the Issues* (listed in the Weblinks on the

BOX 13-4 Injury Prevention Topics

- Car restraints, seat belts, airbag safety
- Preventing fires, burns, frostbite
- Preventing poisoning
- Preventing falls
- Preventing drowning; water safety
- Bicycle safety
- Safe driving practices
- All-terrain vehicle and snowmobile safety
- Sports safety
- Pedestrian safety
- Gun control
- Decreasing gang activities
- Crime prevention
- Substance-abuse prevention
- Playground safety
- School bus safety
- Rail safety

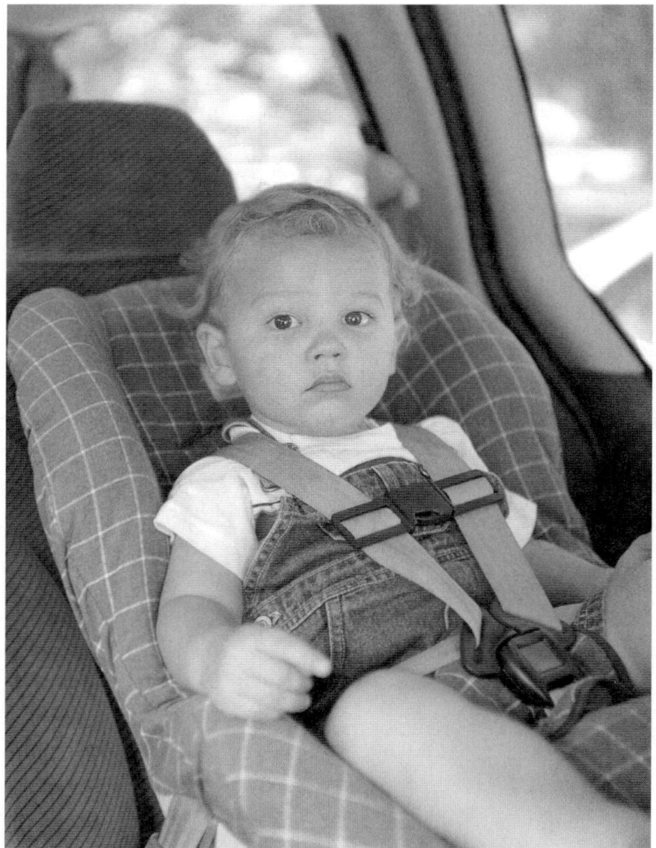

Children should always be restrained while riding in a vehicle.

Evolve Web site), which provides information on the role of the nurse in primary, secondary, and tertiary unintentional injury prevention.

From a community perspective, the National Strategy on Community Safety and Crime Prevention has been established by the Government of Canada to develop approaches to prevent crimes and increase community safety (Public Safety Canada, 2010). This national strategy is based on a social development approach that addresses the underlying causes of crime. It provides funding and support to communities to develop projects and partnerships through the Safer Community Initiative. Funding occurs at several levels and involves a multisectoral approach. Within the initiative, communities are mobilized, what works is tracked, organizations are involved in resource preparation, and businesses and professional associations are partners in the process (see the Public Safety Canada Weblink on the Evolve Web site).

Injury in children and youth is an important community issue and requires continued injury prevention strategies to reduce and prevent its occurrence. More government programs are required, as well as policies instituted to reduce income disparities. At a community level, strategies need to be directed toward environmental improvements such as safe playgrounds; mass educational programs on home, vehicle, and community safety measures; and provision of safer highways. One issue raised is whether these government programs should be directed to aggregate groups such as "high-risk" groups or provided to the total population in this age group. Refer to the PHAC "Child Health" Weblink on the Evolve Web site, which provides several links to areas on child and adolescent health and programs available to address these issues. For further information on resources available for families and practitioners, refer to the Canadian Child Care Federation Weblink on the Evolve Web site. This federation is a bilingual provincial and territorial association that promotes the use of the best health care practices.

Tobacco Use

Smoking is a risk factor for cardiovascular disease (CVD), cancer, and lung disease. Smoking has been identified as one of the major preventable causes of morbidity and mortality in Canada. From 2007 to 2008, based on the previous 3 years of smoking rates, only a 1% decrease in smokers 15 years of age and older occurred compared to the usual 1% decline on average per year (Canadian Cancer Society, 2010b). In 2008, 18% of Canadians 15 years of age and older were smokers and youth smoking rates (age 15 to 19 years) were steady at 15%

(Canadian Cancer Society, 2010b). The decline has been slow because of easy access to cheaper contraband cigarettes (Canadian Cancer Society, 2010). The rates were highest in adults between 20 to 44 years of age with a higher percentage of men smoking than women, and similar rates were found for males and females under 20 years of age (Statistics Canada, 2008). Some factors likely to account for the decline are sociopolitical policies—for example, the implementation of policies for smoke-free spaces; social marketing strategies to affect public attitudes about smoking; and education about the dangers of smoking. Smoking patterns varied from province to province, with British Columbia and Ontario reporting the lowest rates (Statistics Canada, 2008).

Second-hand smoke—smoke exhaled or given off by a burning cigarette—is toxic (Health Canada, 2007a). Second-hand smoke is also referred to as "environmental tobacco smoke" or "sidestream smoke." In 2005, 8.7% of nonsmoking Canadians reported being exposed to second-hand smoke in their home, and 8.1% in vehicles and/or public places (Human Resources and Skills Development Canada, 2010). Parents often do not understand or believe the effects of smoking on children. Children exposed to second-hand smoke experience increased episodes of ear and upper respiratory tract infections. Children of smokers are more likely to take up smoking. Tobacco use is the single most preventable cause of lung cancer (Lung Association of Saskatchewan, 2009). Primary prevention is of utmost importance. Smoking-cessation strategies such as national ad campaigns aimed at altering the perception of smoking as "cool," education, and self-help groups have led to decreased tobacco use. Therefore, these efforts need to be continued. Lung cancer is the leading cause of cancer death for both men and women, and the total cases of lung cancer in men and women combined are greater than those for breast cancer and prostate cancer (Canadian Cancer Society, 2009a).

Advertisements in the media and on billboards of tobacco products have been eliminated, and public display of tobacco products has been banned or restricted. Efforts to manage the media exposure of youth and adults to tobacco advertising is one strategy in the campaign to prevent individuals from starting to smoke and to encourage them and support them in their efforts to quit. CHNs spend a great deal of time working with clients to assist them to deal with the effects of smoking or of second-hand smoke. The CHN is in a strategic position to support and act as a positive role model when working to reduce smoking behaviours.

Interventions to discourage smoking focus on the parent, the child or adolescent, and public policy. CHNs need to offer the following:

- Educational programs dealing with the negative effects of smoking on children
- Interventions to stop smoking
- Ways to create a smoke-free environment
- Behaviour-modification techniques

Anti-smoking programs directed at children and teenagers are more successful if the focus is on short-term rather than long-term effects. Developmentally, children and teenagers cannot visualize the future to imagine the consequences of smoking. Also, teenagers often perceive themselves to be invincible and believe "it will not happen to me." The immediate health risks and the cosmetic effects need to be emphasized. Teaching should include how advertising puts pressure on people to smoke. Music, sports, and other activities, including stress-reducing techniques, need to be encouraged. Teaching social skills to resist peer pressure is critical. For information on peer-led support groups of trained senior youth who lead group sessions on smoking prevention, see the Health Canada "Youth and Tobacco" Weblink on the Evolve Web site, which provides information on and links to several smoking-prevention and -cessation programs targeted at youth across Canada.

CHNs can become politically active in the following areas by lobbying for

- Banning tobacco advertising
- Enforcing restrictions of sale of tobacco to minors
- Increasing funds for antismoking education
- Restricting public smoking to reduce the incidence of smoking and exposure to second-hand smoke

For further information on tobacco and health, refer to the Physicians for a Smoke Free Canada Weblink on the Evolve Web site, which contains information on who smokes in Canada and provides statistics on the leading causes of preventable deaths and the health impacts of smoking.

Immunization

Immunization is an important preventive measure that needs to be initiated in infancy and continued throughout the lifespan as recommended for specific ages. Routine immunization of children has been very successful in preventing selected diseases. The routine immunization schedules for Canadians are presented in Appendix E-5. These schedules provide Canadian immunization guidelines; however, variances occur within provinces and territories. For further information on the administration of vaccines and the latest immunization schedules, refer to the PHAC "National Advisory Committee on Immunization" Weblink, which provides information on timely medical, scientific, and public health advice pertaining to the use of vaccines and their use in Canada, as well as a link to the latest *Canadian Immunization Guide.*

CRITICAL VIEW

1. a) What is the immunization schedule in your province/territory?
   b) How does it vary from the Canadian immunization schedule?
   c) What are the implications, given the variances or differences?
2. a) What are the roles of the CHN in relation to immunization?
   b) What specifically might the CHN educate parents about immunizations?

There are several resources found in Appendix E-6 on the Evolve site accompanying this text that the CHN can use to assess and screen children and youth: "Infant, Child, and Youth Screening Tools," "Accident Prevention in Children," "Screening for Common Orthopedic Problems," "Vision and Hearing Screening Procedures," "Development Characteristics: Summary for Children,"] "Development Behaviours: Summary for School-Age Children," and "Tanner Stages of Puberty."

Information on the priority areas for action pertaining to children and youth is available on the Evolve Web site. View the PHAC Weblink *The Chief Public Health Officer's Report on the State of Public Health in Canada, 2009,* Chapter 6, for discussion of the following four priority areas: "better data and information; improved and ongoing education and awareness; healthy and supportive environments; and coordinated, multi-pronged and sustained strategies" (Butler-Jones, 2009, p. 70).

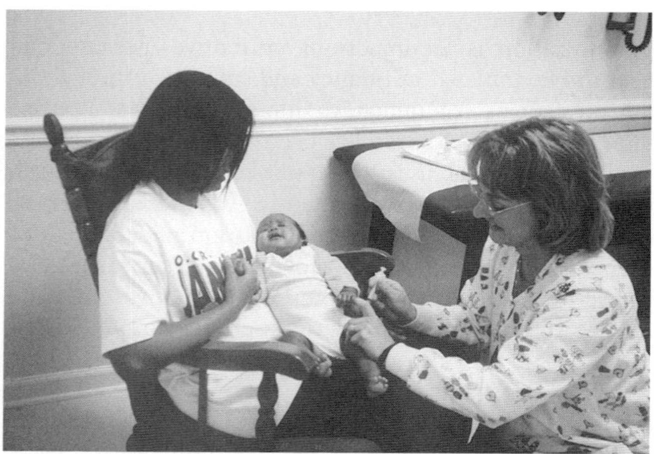

An infant receives a regularly scheduled immunization.

ADULT HEALTH

Increases in adult overweight and obesity are major public health concerns in Canada and other developed countries. Lifestyle practices such as sedentary lifestyle, smoking, and alcohol use place these adults at increased risk for type 2 diabetes mellitus and cardiovascular diseases due to dyslipidemia, hypertension, and certain cancers. Preventive community health nursing strategies directed at aggregates, populations, communities, and individuals are needed to address the increasing unhealthy lifestyle practices.

Women's Health

To understand women's health issues, one must first understand the term *women's health.* **Women's health** addresses health promotion, health protection and disease prevention, and health maintenance in adult women. This term recognizes that the health of women is holistic and is related to the biological, psychosocial, spiritual, and cultural dimensions of women's lives. Moreover, women's normal life events or rites of passage, such as menstruation, childbirth, and menopause, are considered part of normal female development rather than syndromes or diseases requiring medical treatment only. This broad emphasis on women's health is in contrast to the view of women solely in relation to their reproductive health or their role in parenting children. For information on women's health issues, refer to the Society of Obstetricians and Gynaecologists of Canada (SOGC) Weblink on the Evolve Web site.

Unfortunately, millions of people, particularly women, do not have access to basic health-related resources. In most countries, women live longer than men, but women are generally less healthy. This gender difference in health is often related to poverty. For example, approximately 24% of Canadian women who are raising children on their own are poor; 14% of single older women are poor; and there is a 9% poverty rate among children (Townson, 2009). Although women have made some strides toward financial equality during the past decade, progress has been slow. Worldwide, the education of women is the single most important factor in the improvement of the health of women and their families. As women are educated, their socioeconomic status improves and mortality rates decline. Because women's financial stability is closely linked to health outcomes, it is essential to promote policies that support the advancement of women. Because CHNs are visible and involved in the community with individuals and groups of women, there are many opportunities to provide women with the knowledge and skills to take charge of their own health. For example, CHNs can influence women through their assessments, educate women about primary prevention strategies, and advocate for policy change through their professional associations and other avenues.

Breast Self-Examination

In 2001, the Canadian Task Force on Preventive Health Care, based on a review of evidence about breast self-examination (BSE), recommended that the routine teaching of BSE be excluded from the periodic examination for women between the ages of 40 and 69 years. This decision was based on insufficient evidence to support doing BSE because various international research studies were showing that mortality rates were not decreased and that there were higher rates of benign breast biopsies performed. Controversy arose internationally and across Canada. Internationally, women's groups and cancer societies were gravely concerned about this change and its impact on women's health and loss of empowerment. In 2003 and 2005, systematic reviews and meta-analysis by the Cochrane Collaboration supported the task-force decision that no benefit was found to performing BSE and good evidence existed to show that harm could occur (SOGC, 2006b). The harm referred to was for some women the result of having a diagnostic test, the breast biopsy; for others, it was the emotional responses when a lump is found and there is a need for additional testing (SOGC, 2006b). These authors do not recommend routine teaching of BSE. However, they stress the need to (1) consider the wishes of women who request BSE teaching; (2) counsel women on the risks of performing BSE; (3) teach BSE with a focus on how, when, and why to do it; expected normal findings; early signs of cancer; and the importance of reporting any changes or concerns immediately; (4) have women demonstrate the technique and convey their understanding of BSE; and (5) refer to a trained health professional for teaching of BSE, if indicated. Refer to the Canadian Cancer Society Web site listed in the Tool Box on the Evolve Web site for information on the technique for BSE. It is important that women learn the correct technique before doing BSE. Often, the CHN has the skills to do this teaching; however, referrals can be made to family physicians or breast screening programs in communities.

Reproductive Issues

Women often use health care services for reproductive issues or problems, and CHNs are frequently the health professionals they encounter. CHNs are in a unique position to advocate for policies that increase women's access to services for reproductive health. In addition, many CHNs discuss contraception with women of child-bearing age. Contraceptive counselling requires accurate knowledge of current contraceptive choices and a nonjudgemental approach. The goal of contraceptive counselling is to ensure that women have appropriate instruction to make informed choices about reproduction. The choice of method depends on many factors, including the woman's health, frequency of sexual activity, number of partners, and plans to have children.

The problem of unintended pregnancy exists among adolescents as well as adult women. CHNs need to use caution and not assume that any woman is fully informed about contraception and that a method is used correctly and consistently. The CHN needs to consider many factors when planning for contraceptive assessment and education. Some of these factors are culture, health status, socioeconomic status, and client literacy. Preconception counselling addresses risks before conception and includes education, assessment, diagnosis, and interventions. The purpose is to reduce or eliminate health risks for women and infants. Another concern critical to preconception awareness is exposure to health-endangering substances, including alcohol. A major preventable cause of birth defects, mental retardation, and neurodevelopmental disorders is fetal exposure to alcohol during pregnancy. To adequately address substance use during pregnancy, community health nursing interventions need to address substance use, nutrition, physical activity, environmental exposures, and intimate-partner violence.

Related to women's reproductive health is access to prenatal care. For many women, barriers to prenatal care include the following:

- Lack of transportation
- Difficulty accessing the health care system
- Lack of child care

CHNs can serve as advocates not only to encourage their clients to use prenatal care services but also to work toward the establishment of services that are accessible, affordable, and available to all pregnant women. CHNs also need to be able to respond to clients who may be experiencing infertility issues. Smaller communities often do not have fertility experts, and women may need to travel for specialized care. The CHN needs to consider how to support infertile women through individual counselling sessions or the establishment of community self-help support groups.

Menopause

Another developmental phase for women is **menopause,** also referred to as *the change* or *change of life,* the time when the levels of the hormones *estrogen* and *progesterone* change in a woman's body. Women's attitudes toward menopause vary greatly and are influenced by culture, age, support, and the recounted experiences of other women. Menopause has been viewed on a continuum from a normal progression of aging, to a disease state, a time of imbalance, or ill health.

Hormone replacement therapy (HRT) was approved by Health Canada for the relief of some of the menopausal symptoms experienced by women (Health Canada, 2006a). Many women started taking these medications, and the benefits were remarkable for the majority. Most women continued HRT for several years, some up to 20 years. Some early research studies suggested that HRT had the added value of heart protection and the prevention of osteoporosis. However, a longitudinal study (1991 to 2004) by the American Women's Health Initiatives concluded that there is no benefit of heart protection (Health Canada, 2006a). The study results led to changes in the use of HRT; for example, in Canada, HRT with combined estrogen and progestin is now recommended only in specific individual client situations. The decision to use HRT in postmenopausal women is based on consideration of benefits versus harm, and HRT is aimed at improving quality of life using the lowest possible effective dosage in the short term (Health Canada, 2006a; SOGC, 2006a). Some of the study findings have suggested a possible increase in mild cognitive impairment and dementia in some women over 65 years of age taking the combined HRT of estrogen and progestin (Health Canada, 2006a). This possible outcome continues to be monitored.

With the change in hormones during menopause, women are at risk for bone mass and tissue deterioration, which can lead to osteoporosis. Nearly one out of four women over 50 years in Canada have osteoporosis (Health Canada, 2009). Preventive measures that can significantly reduce osteoporosis in the future are for children, youth, and young adults to eat foods high in calcium, to take vitamin D, and to be physically active with weight-bearing exercises and involvement in sports, plus avoid smoking and excessive intake of caffeine and alcohol (Osteoporosis Canada, 2010).

Primary osteoporosis-prevention activities aimed at women need to include the following:

- Diets rich in calcium and vitamin D
- Exposure to sunlight for 20 minutes a day, recommended as an alternative source of vitamin D
- Daily intake of vitamin D based on age
- Exercise, especially weight-bearing activities such as walking, running, stair climbing, and weight lifting, to improve bone density. Refer to the Osteoporosis Canada site "60-Second Osteoporosis Risk Quiz" found in the Tool Box on the Evolve Web site. This quiz can help determine the risk for developing osteoporosis; a calcium calculator tool is also included.

Cardiovascular Disease

Once considered a disease of men, cardiovascular disease is now the number-one killer of women in Canada (Women's Health Matters, 2008) and is the major cause of disability (Health Canada, 2006b). "Compared to men, the onset of cardiovascular disease (CVD) in women is somewhat later, by approximately 10 years, and women are less likely to seek care, be investigated and treated with as wide a range of interventions as are men" (British Columbia Centre of Excellence for Women's Health, 2008, p. 6). CVD refers to heart disease and stroke. According to Health Canada (2006b), some notable statistics about CVD in Canadian women are these:

- Two out of three women have at least one major risk factor for heart disease.
- Twenty-six percent of females 15 years of age and older smoked in 1996, and 71% of women 18 to 34 years of age were on oral contraceptives, which increases their risk for CVD.
- The mortality of 40% of Canadian women is due to CVD.
- The risk of mortality from heart disease increases four times after menopause.
- Inactive women are twice as likely to die from CVD.

Women not only wait longer than men to go to an emergency department but may also have a different clinical presentation for myocardial infarction. Both genders may present with chest pain (Health Canada, 2006b; Heart & Stroke Foundation, 2007); however, women may be more vague in describing their pain (Heart & Stroke Foundation, 2007), and women more often present with nonspecific chest pain and atypical symptoms than men (British Columbia Centre of Excellence for Women's Health, 2008). Also, compared with men, women may experience symptoms such as nausea, back pain, and indigestion (Health Canada, 2006b). Other symptoms specific to women are fatigue, sleep disturbance, and weakness (McSweeney et al., 2003; University of Michigan, 2008).

Many factors predispose women to CVD. Factors that are thought to contribute to the development of CVD include the following (British Columbia Centre of Excellence for Women's Health, 2008; Shah, 2003):

- Smoking
- High blood cholesterol levels
- Diabetes mellitus
- Obesity
- Hypertension
- Diets high in fat and low in fibre
- Physical inactivity
- Family history

Sociocultural factors have a significant influence on women and CVD. It is known that a lower socioeconomic status correlates with low levels of knowledge and understanding about health, limited health maintenance and preventive care, and decreased access to care (British Columbia Centre of Excellence for Women's Health, 2008). The following factors for women have a significant impact on increasing their risk for CVD: increasing age; Aboriginal women, South Asian women, lower income women, and women with an addiction or mental illness (British Columbia Centre of Excellence for Women's Health, 2008).

The key to addressing this alarming epidemic of heart disease is education aimed at certain populations and focusing on risk-factor modification such as diet, smoking, physical activity, and stress management. CHNs can partner with communities to promote heart health initiatives. Community heart health initiatives need to address all income levels with a focus on the determinants of health such as unemployment and education. As well, communities need to provide supportive environments such as walking paths. Public policies dealing with health should be initiated. CHNs need to be aware that heart disease is a health concern not just for men. Dissemination of information about the various factors that influence the development of CVD can be accomplished through prevention and outreach activities. Intervention efforts should reflect the diversity of age, environment, and ethnicity in the community. CHNs can also do a careful family history assessment, which can highlight situations that might place an individual at a higher level of risk. CHNs can initiate the development of heart health programs for groups. Group education programs for high-risk individuals save money, reach greater numbers with time savings, and have the benefit of sharing experiences among group members that might allay fears and provide support. For further information on CVD information specific to women's health, see the British Columbia Centre of Excellence for Women's Health report titled *Women's Heart Health: An Evidence Review* (listed in the Evolve Weblinks), which provides an overview of CVD in women.

Diabetes Mellitus

The diagnosis of diabetes mellitus in the Canadian population in 2005 occurred in 1.8 million adults, or 5.5% of the Canadian population (PHAC, 2008b). Those populations who have a greater risk of developing diabetes are Aboriginal peoples and other special populations such as Asians, Hispanics, Africans, and older adults (PHAC, 2008b). Obesity and physical inactivity increase the risk of onset of type 2 diabetes mellitus and also affect the progression of this disease. Preventing or managing obesity and increasing physical activity can prevent or delay the onset of type 2 diabetes. Type 1 diabetes is not preventable, but it can be controlled.

Over the past 50 years, lifestyles in Aboriginal communities have changed mainly due to adapting to a non-Aboriginal way of life. Prior to European contact, Aboriginal people led physically active lifestyles that included hunting, fishing, and surviving off the land. Aboriginal people currently lead much more sedentary lives and eat foods high in fat and sugar. These changes have contributed profoundly to the health of many Aboriginal people today and in particular to the increased incidence of type 2 diabetes (Ontario Ministry of Health and Long-Term Care, 2006). Type 2 diabetes and obesity are considered rampant in most Aboriginal communities. Diabetes is three to five times more common among First Nations people than in the general population (Assembly of First Nations [AFN], 2007). Rates for Inuit peoples are increasing. Statistics concerning those with diabetes who are Métis is at 7% of the population compared with the total population, which is at 4% (Janz, Seto, & Turner, 2009).

Diabetes is the most reported and documented disease in Aboriginal health and is relatively "new," with an increased frequency and distribution (Reading, 2009). In general, the prevalence of diabetes differs between southern Canada, where it is higher than in northern Canada. Women are diagnosed with diabetes more often than men. As well, those who are less educated are being diagnosed at a higher rate than those who are educated and acculturated. With these higher rates, the impact of diabetes on the health of future generations of Aboriginal people is of concern. The trend in the earlier onset of diabetes and higher rates in the Aboriginal population is of concern to the health of future generations (Reading, 2009). In fact, some believe that if these trends do not change, the number of Canadian Aboriginal people with diabetes will increase threefold by the year 2016 (Jin, Martin, & Sarin, 2002) (see the Health Canada "First Nations, Inuit and Aboriginal Health" Weblink on the Evolve Web site).

Risk factors for diabetes mellitus are more prevalent in women than in men (PHAC, 2008b). Risk factors include low socioeconomic status, less formal education, smoking, decreased physical activity, and being overweight (Canadian Diabetes Association, 2008). Diabetes is a potentially debilitating disease. Some examples of group projects that are community based and pertain to diabetes are found at the Health Canada Web site titled *Making Change Happen: Stories from British Columbia* found on the Evolve Web site. These stories demonstrate creative approaches for how to involve aggregates with diabetes to promote health and prevent disease.

Gestational diabetes mellitus (GDM) is a condition characterized by a carbohydrate intolerance that is first identified or first develops during pregnancy. In Canada, the prevalence varies from 3.7% in the non-Aboriginal population to 8 to 18% in the Aboriginal populations (Canadian Diabetes Association, 2008). Women with GDM have a 25 to 45% greater risk for recurrence of diabetes in subsequent pregnancies (Reading, 2009). They also have a higher risk of developing diabetes in later life. Many First Nations women who are diagnosed with diabetes are also diagnosed with GDM. When a mother has diabetes, the birth weight of her newborn is very likely to be high (Reading, 2009). For those children, obesity can lead to diabetes in later life. As well, maternal obesity may be a factor in determining children's obesity (Boney, Verma, Tucker, & Vohr, 2005). The income gap between Aboriginal peoples and non-Aboriginal peoples continues to grow, and so does the poor health status in Aboriginal children and adults (Adelson, 2005). Community and government interventions are needed to address the health disparities in which poor Canadians live and work if their health is to be improved. Food is one of the prerequisites for health identified in the Ottawa Charter on health promotion. CHNs can advocate for healthy public policies to reduce inequities in income. This might be accomplished by partnering with other community groups to influence the various government levels and through involvement with professional nursing organizations to lobby for change. Of note for CHNs is the discussion on the need for relevant research to identify policy priorities to address obesity in Canada (PHAC, 2009b). This discussion includes recognition of the determinants of obesity such as food insecurity, inequitable access to physical activity, and environmental determinants of health. Also, CHNs could initiate the development of community programs, such as school breakfast and healthy snack programs, and food bank programs at higher-education institutions. Health educational programs on nutritious foods and outlining physical activity requirements in the community could also be offered by CHNs. CHNs are in a position to have a positive effect on the lives of women and children at risk by focusing on family history as well as on the personal health history.

CHNs are in a position to have a positive effect on the lives of women with diabetes. Assessing for a history of GDM in women, especially women of colour, is important. Focusing on family history as well as on the personal health history provides an opportunity for the CHN to identify those at high risk. Primary prevention activities include interventions aimed at educating women about diabetes, nutrition, and the risks of obesity, smoking, and physical inactivity. Community interventions that address healthy eating, exercise, and weight reduction benefit women who are at risk for diabetes. Screening for diabetes is an example of secondary prevention. Screening activities include a finger-stick blood glucose test or a full glucose-tolerance test. Screening is also accomplished through a thorough history-taking and physical examination. CHNs need to be well versed in understanding the health disparities among women to target those at greater risk. Tertiary prevention includes activities that are aimed to reduce the complications of the disease process. Examples of tertiary prevention for women with diabetes include intense monitoring of blood glucose levels, modification of diet and medications as indicated, and efforts to prevent long-term complications such as those mentioned previously.

For further information on diabetes, refer to the Canadian Diabetes Association's *2008 Clinical Practice Guidelines for the Prevention and Management of Diabetes in Canada* (see Weblinks on the Evolve Web site), which provides professional guidelines for all aspects of management of diabetes. A second site worth exploring is PHAC's *Diabetes in Canada: Highlights from the National Diabetes Surveillance System 2004–2005* (see the Weblinks on the Evolve Web site), which provides extensive data on age-standardized statistical findings from Canada's national diabetes surveillance system; these data include prevalence and incidence rates, hospitalizations, and mortality related to diabetes.

Mental Illness

Mental health issues have also been discussed in previous chapters. CHNs who view health holistically recognize that mental health is as important as physical health in the daily functioning of all individual clients. Individual clients who have physical illnesses frequently develop mental health problems as they endeavour to cope with their physical health challenges and those who have mental health problems may also experience physical health challenges. Mental illness occurs when a person has changes in thinking, mood, or behaviour that results in impaired functioning or difficulty coping over a period of time. Although both men and women suffer from mental illness, women experience certain conditions more often than men. Depression is a particularly serious health concern for women. A number of factors contribute to depression in women; possible contributors being researched are biological factors, including genetics and gonadal (sex) hormones, and psychosocial factors such as life stress, trauma, and interpersonal relationships. Risk factors for depression include being female, having a family history of depression, being unemployed, and having a chronic disease. CHNs can encourage health professionals in their communities to screen and treat depression among women and to work for the development of other services that decrease stress and generally improve the mental well-being of women. The PHAC's *A Report on*

Evidence-Informed Practice

Type 2 diabetes is a relatively new disease for people living in Inuit communities. This qualitative research study focused on the experiences and perceptions of Inuit participants who live with diabetes. A case-study approach was undertaken with four in-depth interviews, field observations, and informal interviews. Data were transcribed and analyzed using a holistic thematic analysis and open coding. Participants described accessibility issues related to the inability to obtain healthy foods and health services. Language interpretation was also an issue. The importance of cross-cultural communication was predominant in the findings, as were issues related to trust and rapport when diabetes care was discussed. Findings suggested a paucity of health education and services in Inuit communities. The importance of including the voices of Inuit peoples when providing and directing diabetes education and health services delivery is stressed.

Application for CHNs: Partnering with clients is extremely important as a CHN, and this article reinforces how essential this undertaking is when working with clients with diabetes. For clients residing in rural and remote areas, lack of available and perhaps affordable foods is a barrier to healthy eating as a diabetic. Other barriers can be language, cultural differences, and lack of health services. These barriers can present challenges for CHNs in their nursing practice.

Questions for Reflection & Discussion

1. What questions might you ask a person who lives in a rural and remote community about their experiences living with diabetes?
2. How does this research study relate to what you have read about rural and remote community health nursing practice?
3. What key terms would you use to find the latest evidence on cross-cultural competence in Inuit communities?

Reference: Bird, S., Wiles, J., Okalik, L., Kilabuk, J., & Egeland, G. (2008). Living with diabetes on Baffin Island: Inuit storytellers share their experiences. *Canadian Journal of Public Health, 99*(1), 17–21.

Mental Illness in Canada (see Evolve Weblinks) provides statistics and information on the various forms of mental illness and additional links for information, including hospitalization patterns. The WHO Weblink *Mental Health: New Understandings, New Hope* discusses socio-economic factors, demographic factors, family environment, the presence of major physical diseases, and serious threats as factors affecting mental health.

Cancer

Cancers are noted to be the second leading cause of death among all women. Lung cancer death rates continue to climb among women while decreasing among men (Canadian Cancer Society, 2009b). In Canadian women, breast cancer is the most common cancer (Canadian Cancer Society, 2009a). Although it is known that women suffer from other cancers, especially ones that are unique to women such as cervical and ovarian cancers, what will be addressed here are only the top three cancers that lead to illness and death in women.

A diagnosis of cancer is a life-changing event and is considered a life transition. Upon diagnosis, a woman is confronted with many decisions that often leave her feeling overwhelmed and out of control (in crisis). Breast cancer is one of the leading causes of cancer deaths among all Canadian women, and this type of cancer has had screening programs devoted to its detection. Screening activities (the secondary level of prevention) include mammography and breast examination by a health care professional. Early detection may mean cure, whereas late detection often means a limited prognosis. Colorectal cancer is another leading cause of cancer deaths in Canadian women. Primary prevention and early detection are the keys to surviving colorectal cancer. CHNs can inform women of their risks, the signs and symptoms to be aware of, and screening opportunities in their communities.

Cervical cancer is another common cancer diagnosis for Canadian women. Cervical cancer prevention rates can be improved through regular screening. Common risk factors for cervical cancer are inadequate screening, multiple sexual partners, smoking, the sexual behaviour of a male partner(s), a young age at first intercourse, and infection with human papillomavirus (HPV), a weakened immune system, multiple births, and long-term use of birth control pills (Canadian Cancer Society, 2010a). For further information on the prevention of cervical cancer, refer to the PHAC "Cervical Cancer" Weblink on the Evolve Web site, which provides information on the incidence, risk factors, and management of cervical cancer in Canada.

Obesity

The number of overweight women in Canada is on the rise. Obesity is a major health concern among women because it is linked to the development of diabetes mellitus, hypertension, CVD, and other medical problems. The CHN can provide education about the risks to health from overweight and obesity. The educational offerings can be fashioned after a community health model using the levels of prevention to establish effective interventions for women at risk for weight control issues.

Because obesity in women is such a stigma in Western culture, women are at high risk for suffering adverse social and psychological consequences of obesity. Even as children, women begin to fear obesity. These consequences can include social as well as financial discrimination. More women enter weight-loss programs for their perceived loss of attractiveness than for health concerns. In today's North American culture, being thin is often identified with competence, success, control, power, and sexual attractiveness. The culture's focus and preoccupation with the thinness and shape of women can be seen in the media and the entertainment industry, where beautiful is equated with very thin women. These idealistic and often unrealistic images perpetuate women's dissatisfaction and preoccupation with their bodies.

Many women are dissatisfied with their body weight, but despite their unhappiness with their current shape and weight only a few of them go on to develop a serious eating disorder. CHNs are in a key position to include assessment for eating disorders and referral for treatment into their routine clinical practices. Included in this assessment would be an abdominal girth measurement (waist circumference) and waist-to-hip ratio measurement. It is important to note that calculation of a body mass index (BMI) is frequently replaced with measuring waist circumference. For information on how to calculate body fat, refer to Health Canada's *Canadian Guidelines for Bodyweight Classification in Adults—Quick Reference Tool for Professionals* (found in the Tool Box section on the Evolve Web site). This resource provides information on how to calculate and interpret body mass assessments. The goal of the CHN is to identify not only women who have eating disorders but also those women at risk for developing eating disorders. Through a comprehensive physical and psychosocial assessment, as well as a history of dietary practices, the CHN may be able to identify women with eating disorders and provide appropriate referrals. CHNs can promote healthy eating habits and regular physical activity as a weight-control strategy. At a population level, CHNs can discourage advertising that promotes exceptionally thin bodies for women. They can also promote exercise and healthy eating programs in their communities.

CRITICAL VIEW

Refer to the article titled "The Expanded Chronic Care Model: An Integration of Concepts and Strategies from Population Health Promotion and the Chronic Care Model" found in your library or at the following Web site: http://www.primaryhealthcarebc.ca/phc/pdf/eccm_article.pdf.

1. a) What are the key components of this expanded chronic care model?
   b) What are the advantages of using this expanded model?
2. How would you apply this model when working with a group of women who want to maintain their employment despite experiencing a chronic condition such as osteoarthritis?

Men's Health

Men have a lower life expectancy than women and a higher mortality rate (Mikkonen & Raphael, 2010). When men are compared to women, the following differences are noted:

- Fewer episodes of chronic diseases
- More accidents
- More extreme forms of social exclusion such as homelessness and substance abuse
- Four times greater suicide rates
- More frequently experience robbery and physical assault
- More frequently are perpetrators of crime
- Are more likely to engage in antisocial behaviour and criminal offences, particularly disadvantaged young males
- View masculinity in terms of aggressiveness, dominance, and excessive self-reliance, which negatively affect men's health (Mikkonen & Raphael, 2010)

Although men and women have similar ideas about health, there are some distinct differences. Most people view health as being closely associated with well-being. Both men and women define *health* comprehensively and refer to it as a state or condition of well-being, and they often relate this condition to capacity, performance, and function. Refer to the Canadian Institutes of Health Research (CIHI) document *Gender and Sex-Based Analysis in Health Research: A Guide for CIHR Researchers and Reviewers* (see Evolve Weblinks) for some of the research based on sex and gender, specifically men's health.

Men frequently engage in compensatory, aggressive, and risk-taking behaviour predisposing them to illness, injury, and even death. Men tend to avoid medical help as long as possible, leading to serious health problems. A preventive focus is a wise one because men have been identified as a high-risk group.

Men need to openly express their health care concerns. Health care professionals can help men explore their concerns by encouraging them to discuss non-health problems as well as health care problems and by promoting preventive health care. Although some men are apprehensive about discussing health concerns with professionals, strategies can be used to reduce men's anxiety. CHNs can remove physical barriers separating themselves from the client, use handouts and other written information to support verbal instructions, and show a genuine interest in men's needs.

In Canada, men's life expectancy for all ages is the third-highest in developed countries, although lower than Canadian women's. Table 13-3 lists life expectancies for men and women in selected countries. Accidents, homicides and other violence, cancers, circulatory system diseases, and infectious and parasitic diseases account for most deaths in developed countries. Refer to Table 13-4 for facts on cancer in Canada.

Testicular cancer is a commonly found solid tumour malignancy most often found in men 15 to 35 years of age. The etiology of this cancer, the testicular germ cell, is unknown. Many possible explanations exist:

- Age
- Family history
- Endocrine problems
- Genetic disorders
- Human immunodeficiency virus
- Cryptorchidism
- Occupational factors

TABLE 13-3 Life Expectancies for Men and Women in Selected Countries

Country	Men (Years)	Women (Years)
Canada	78	83
Japan	78	85
Netherlands	79	86
Norway	78	83
Sweden	79	83
United States	77	81

Source: From United Nations, Department of Economic and Social Affairs, Population Division. (2009). *World population prospects: The 2008 revision.* Retrieved from http://unstats.un.org/unsd/demographic/products/socind/health.htm.

TABLE 13-4 Facts on Cancer in Canada

Type of Cancer and Gender Affected	(Estimated New Cases for the Year 2009	Mortality Rate (Estimates for the Year 2009)	Other
Breast Cancer			
Females	22,700	5,400	Most common cancer among Canadian women
Males	180	50	
Prostate Cancer	25,500	4,400	Most common cancer among Canadian men
Lung Cancer			
Females	10,700	9,400	
Males	12,800	11,200	
Colorectal Cancer			
Females	9,900	4,200	
Males	12,100	4,900	

Source: From Canadian Cancer Society's Steering Committee. (2009). *Canadian cancer statistics, 2009.* Toronto: Canadian Cancer Society, 2009. Retrieved from http://www.cancer.ca/canada-wide/about%20cancer/cancer%20statistics/~/media/CCS/Canada%20wide/Files%20List/English%20files%20heading/pdf%20not%20in%20publications%20section/Stats%202009E%20Cdn%20Cancer.ashx.

The most common presenting symptom is a painless, firm scrotal mass or swelling that is accidentally discovered. Low back pain may result with retroperitoneal lymph node involvement. The CHN needs to teach men who are at risk for testicular cancer a preventive strategy as part of a comprehensive testicular educational program. Instructions on how to perform a monthly **testicular self-examination** (TSE) (a self-examination of the testicles to assess for any unusual lumps or bumps) are provided in Figure 13-2 and in Box 13-5. A program may consist of audiovisual aids and pamphlets followed by step-by-step procedures and return demonstrations. These approaches lead to increased frequency of TSE and enhanced comfort levels of the men performing the procedure. If tumours are found, the most common form of management is retroperitoneal lymph node dissection and chemotherapy for metastases larger than 3 cm.

FIGURE 13-2 Performing a Testicular Self-Examination

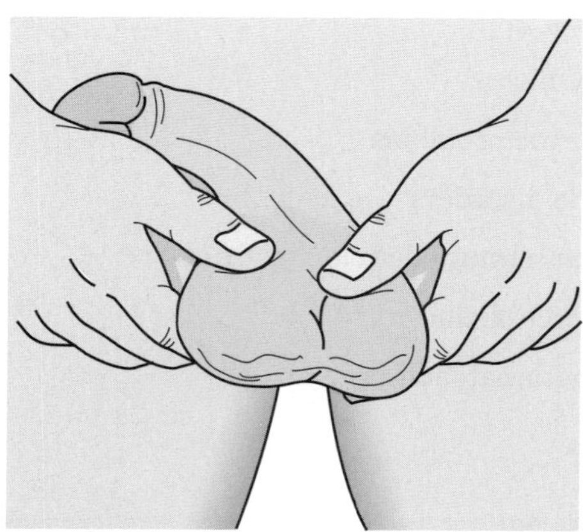

BOX 13-5 Performing a Step-by-Step Monthly Testicular Self-Examination

1. Perform the testicular self-examination during a warm bath or shower. Be sure your hands are warm.
2. Roll each testicle between your thumb and fingers. Testicles should be egg-shaped, 4 cm, oblong, and similar in size and have a rubbery texture; the left dangles lower than the right.
3. Check the epididymis for softness and slight tenderness.
4. Check the spermatic cord for firm, smooth, tubular structure.

Refer to the PHAC's "Prostate Cancer" Weblink (in the Tool Box on the Evolve Web site) for statistics, signs, and symptoms, and management of prostate cancer. The Health Canada "Just for You—Men" Weblink has information pertaining to several health issues for men, such as heart health, mental health, work-life balance, and diseases and conditions. 

OLDER ADULTS' HEALTH

The growth of the population aged 65 years and older in Canada has steadily increased since the turn of the century. As Canada's population continues to increase, the proportion of older adults in the older age range will also increase (Shah, 2003). This increase is the result of aging of baby boomers. It is predicted that in Canada, by 2016, older adults will outnumber children under age 14; by 2026, 50% of Canada's population will be "over the age of 43.6" years; and by 2051, the "median age will be 46.2" (Shah, 2003, p. 105). Currently, many older adults live into their 80s and 90s (Ebersole, Hess, Touhy, & Jett, 2005; Shah, 2003), and an increased number of older adults reach 100 years of age (Ebersole et al., 2005). This latter group is referred to as *centenarians* (Ebersole et al., 2005). Since most health care for older adults is now delivered outside of an acute-care setting, CHNs in particular provide nursing care to an increased proportion of this aging population, that involves specialized knowledge, skills, and abilities in gerontology. Furthermore, the increasing proportion of those over 65 years of age will continue, a change that has implications for health promotion strategies such as creating healthy environments, reorienting health services, and increasing prevention. Also, increasing health care resources, such as skilled home care personnel (Boal & Loengard, 2007) to meet the needs of this aggregate group, may prove challenging with the current limited fiscal resources.

CRITICAL VIEW

1. What community services for older adults exist in your community? What are the gaps in services for this population?
2. Currently, are older adult Canadians as a population considered poor? Explain your thinking.

Aging, if defined purely from a physiological perspective, has been described as a process of deterioration of body systems. This definition is obviously inadequate to describe the multidimensional aging process in older adults. **Aging** can be more appropriately defined as the total of all changes that occur in a person with the passing of time. It is known that aging starts from the time of birth, not just when a person reaches age 65 years. Influences on how one ages come from several domains that include the physiological as well as psychological, sociological, and spiritual processes. The physiological declines associated with aging have been easier to understand than aging as a process of growth and development.

Myths associated with aging have evolved over time. Some of the common myths involve the perception that all older adults are infirm and senile and cannot adapt to change and learn new behaviours or skills. These myths are easily debunked by older adults who run marathons, learn to use the Internet, and are vibrant members of society. **Ageism,** a term coined by Robert Butler in the 1960s, denotes discrimination toward older people because of their age (Ebersole et al., 2005; Millar, 2004). Ageism may be obvious or subtle, and it fosters a stereotype that does not allow older adults to be viewed realistically and denies the diversity of aging. It classifies all older adults as being the same (a homogeneous group) and therefore denies the individuality of older adults (a heterogeneous group).

Gerontology is the specialized study of the processes of growing old (Meiner & Leueckenotte, 2006; Beckmann Murray et al., 2006) with a focus on what is "normal" and "successful" aging (Millar, 2004). *Geriatrics* is the study of disease in old age. **Gerontological nursing** is the specialty of nursing concerned with assessment of the health and functional statuses of older adults, planning and implementing health care and services to meet the identified needs, and evaluating the effectiveness of such care (Meiner & Lueckenotte, 2006).

The client experiences aging in many ways: physiologically, psychologically, sociologically, and spiritually. Physiological changes occur in all body systems with the passing of time. How and when these processes occur between individuals varies widely, as well as the degree of aging within the various body systems in the same individual. Table 13-5 highlights common physiological changes with the aging of body systems and the nursing implications of these changes. The effect of these physiological changes overall may result in a diminished physiological reserve, a decrease in homeostatic mechanisms, and a decline in immunological response. These changes require adaptation by older adults, but it is also important to recognize that aging is not a disease (Ebersole et al., 2005; Meiner & Lueckenotte, 2006). Intellectual capacity does not usually decline with age.

No known intrinsic psychological change occurs with aging. The influences of the environment and culture on personal development and maturation are substantial and further limit the ability of the CHN to predict how an individual ages psychologically. Some known and some disputed changes in brain function over time may influence cognition and behaviour. Reaction speed and psychomotor response are somewhat slower, both of which can be related to the neurological changes with aging. This is demonstrated particularly during timed tests of performance in which speed is an influencing variable. It has also been demonstrated in simulated tests of driving skills, where speed of response, perception, and attention slow with age. Typically, older individuals can learn and perform as well as younger individuals, although they may be slower and it may take them longer to accomplish a specific task. It is therefore important for CHNs to consider these changes when providing education programs to older adults.

Intellectual capacity does not normally decline with age as was previously thought. An age-associated memory impairment, benign senescent forgetfulness, involves very minor memory loss. This is not progressive and does not cause dysfunction in daily living. Reassurance by formal caregivers such as CHNs is important for the older adult and families since anxiety often exacerbates the problem of mild memory impairment. Memory aids (e.g., mnemonics, signs, and notes) may help the older adult compensate for this type of impairment.

The later years for many older adults mark a period of changing social dynamics. Social networks provide the structure for social support. Most older people continue to respond to life situations as they did earlier in their lives. Aging does not bring about radical changes in beliefs and values. How individuals stay involved in activities and with people who bring their lives meaning and support is a major factor that can contribute to ongoing health and vitality.

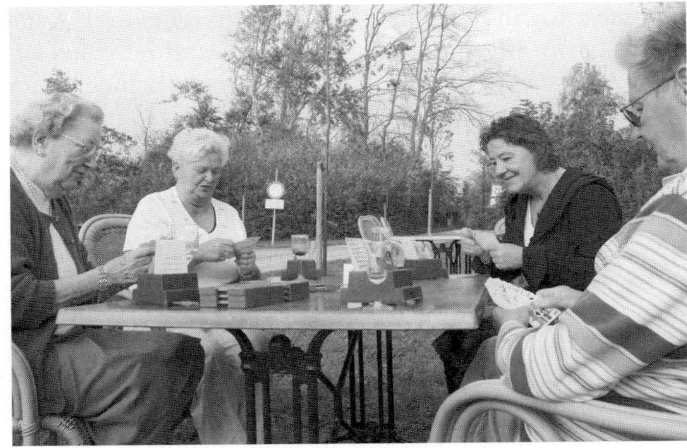

Older adults may be at an increased risk for depression and should be encouraged to participate in social experiences.

TABLE 13-5 Physiological Age-Related Changes in Body Systems

System	Age-Related Change	Implication for Nursing
Skin	Thinning of the skin Atrophy of sweat glands Decrease in vascularity	Skin breakdown and injury Increased risk of heat stroke Frequent pruritus, dry skin
Respiratory	Decreased elasticity of lung tissue Decreased respiratory muscle strength	Reduced efficiency of ventilation Atelectasis and infection
Cardiovascular	Decrease in baroreceptor sensitivity Decrease in number of pacemaker cells	Orthostatic hypotension and falls Increased prevalence of dysrhythmias
Gastrointestinal	Dental enamel thins; loss of teeth and presence of caries Gums recede Delay in esophageal emptying Decreased muscle tone Altered peristalsis	Periodontal disease Swallowing dysfunction Constipation
Genitourinary	Decreased number of functioning nephrons Reduced bladder tone and capacity Prostate enlargement	Modifications in drug dosing may be required Incontinence more common May compromise urinary function
Neuromuscular	Decrease in muscle mass Decrease in bone mass	Decrease in muscle strength Osteoporosis, increased risk of fracture
Sensory	Loss of neurons and nerve fibres Decreased visual acuity, depth perception, adaptation to light changes Loss of auditory neurons Altered taste sensation	Altered sensitivity to pain May pose safety issues Hearing loss may cause limitation in activities May change food preferences and intake
Immune	Decrease in T-cell function Appearance of autoantibodies	Increased incidence of infection Increased prevalence of autoimmune disorders

As older adults adapt and cope with the challenge of aging, especially the successive losses and changes that occur for many, an increased spiritual awareness and consciousness can occur (Ebersole et al., 2005). *Spirituality* refers to the need to transcend physical, psychological, and social identities to experience love, hope, and meaning in life, and it is more than religion. Having a purpose in life, religious affiliations, and religious rituals are aspects of spirituality that can include other activities and relationships. Caring for pets and plants or experiencing nature through a walk outdoors can also foster spiritual growth. Physical and functional impairments and fear of death may challenge one's spiritual integrity. Having a strong sense of spirituality enables individuals who are physically and functionally dependent on others to avoid despair by appreciating that they are still capable of giving and deserving of receiving love, respect, and dignity.

CHNs are pivotal to older adults having access to health care. It is important to build relationships in a caring manner. Once that relationship is developed, the CHN can work with the individual and family to promote the health of the older adult, to initiate actions to prevent disease, to facilitate access to community resources, and in many cases to provide palliation (see the "Ethical Considerations" box, page 433). The Community Health Nurses Association of Canada Standard of Practice 3, "Building Relationships," further discusses the principles of "connecting and caring" and provides the CHN with strategies for implementation (see Appendix 1).

Health care in general is oriented toward acute illness. Chronic illness requires a shift in perspective compared with the rapid onset and focus on curing an acute problem. In chronic illness, cure is not expected, so community health nursing activities need to be more holistic, addressing function, wellness, and psychosocial issues. With chronic illness, the focus is on *healing* (a unique process resulting in a shift in the body, mind, and spirit system) rather than *curing* (elimination of the signs and symptoms of disease).

Chronic illnesses occur over a long period with occasional acute exacerbations and remissions. They can

ETHICAL CONSIDERATIONS

An older adult who has been diagnosed with final-stage lung cancer asks the CHN if she should go to the palliative-care unit "when my time is near" or "should I die at home?" She appears to wish to die at home, even if it might require her to spend her own money to do it. Her family members have said that they would prefer that she go to the palliative-care unit.

Ethical principles that apply to this scenario:

- *Promoting and respecting informed decision making (CNA Code of Ethics).* According to this primary value, CHNs recognize and promote a person's right to be informed and involved in decision making about his or her health. Therefore, CHNs value the giving of health information to clients in their care in an open, accurate, and transparent manner.
- *Preserving dignity (CNA Code of Ethics).* This value requires that CHNs relate to all persons with respect and, during decision making, take into account their unique values, beliefs, and social and economic circumstances.
- *Distributive justice.* If the decision is for the client to die at home, are the necessary resources accessible in her community to support her and her family?

Questions to Consider

1. What information can the CHN provide to the client and her family that might help them reach a decision together?
2. The client asks the CHN to explain the differences between the three acronyms CPR, DNAR, AND, so she can make an informed decision. What are the ethical principles to consider in these three end-of-life examples?

CRITICAL VIEW

1. What strategies found within the Community Health Nurses Association of Canada standards would be most applicable to older adults? Explain.
2. What issues might a community health nurse advocate for when working with an older adult population?

affect several systems and be discouraging because of symptoms such as chronic pain and also because of the losses in functioning and often social interactions too. The prevalence of chronic disease rises with lengthening of lifespan and highly technical medical care. Not only do chronic illnesses cause disability and activity restriction, they also often require frequent hospitalizations for exacerbations.

Many older adults adjust to the changes associated with aging and actually experience health and wellness with aging. Often, their definitions of health change with aging (Ebersole et al., 2005). These authors maintain that even though many older adults experience chronic illnesses, they can experience wellness (Ebersole et al., 2005). It is also noteworthy that not all older adults have a chronic illness. It has become evident that to be effective in the prevention of chronic illnesses and the promotion of health, the focus on education at individual and population levels also requires supportive environments (Shah, 2003). Supportive physical environments, for example, are needed to allow older adults to stay physically active and to eat nutritious meals. Supportive social environments—for example, family members, the availability of older adult centres, and government pensions based on financial need—are needed to assist older adults in communities.

CRITICAL VIEW

1. a) Do you agree with the premise that even though older adults experience chronic illness, they can still be healthy and even experience wellness? Explain your position.

   b) What factors do you think would contribute to older adults "being healthy"?
2. a) What are the dimensions of wellness?

   b) What factors do you think would contribute to older adults experiencing wellness?

Ebersole et al. (2005) indicate the importance of mobility for older adults as it "provides opportunity for exercise, exploration, and pleasure and is the crux of maintaining independence" (p. 455). At the present time, the majority of older adults live outside of institutions, are considered "healthy" and require "minimal assistance" (Shah, 2003). Communities with a commitment to health promotion for older adults will provide such things as safe sidewalks for walking, shopping malls for winter walking, and parks with walking trails. Also, communities need to ensure that home services such as Meals on Wheels and outdoor home-maintenance services are available. The CHN might partner with the community for planning these services if they are lacking in the community. CHNs provide education programs to individual and aggregate older adults about the benefits of nutritious eating and physical activity. The PHAC publication, *Physical Activity Guide to Healthy Active Living for Older Adults* (see Evolve Weblinks) provides information about choices concerning physical activity to promote health and to prevent disease for older adults. Immobility can be caused by a variety of chronic illnesses such as degenerative joint disease, osteoporosis, cerebrovascular accidents, Parkinson's disease, and neuromotor disorders (Ebersole et al., 2005). Chronic illnesses can result in pain, stiffness, loss of balance, psychological problems, a fear of falling, and falls, all of which may contribute to immobility. Many factors contribute to older adults falling, and several of them can be prevented. For information on falls, refer to the Registered Nurses' Association of Ontario (RNAO) guideline *Prevention of Falls and Fall Injuries in the Older Adult* (see Weblinks on the Evolve Web site). The Home Safety Assessment Tool (listed in the Tool Box on the Evolve Web site) can be used by CHNs in the home setting to assess the home environment for safety, including risk of falls. CHNs are in a prime position to educate the public, older adults and their caregivers, and aggregates of older adults in the community about fall prevention.

Management of some of the chronic illnesses can be aided by the provision of opportunities for physical activity through community recreational programs such as swimming, water aquatics for older adults, and mall walking. For many older adults, these activities can prevent or at least slow down disabilities from chronic illness. In addition, physical activity can contribute to improved a sense of well-being (Ebersole et al., 2005). Also, involvement in these activities encourages independence.

In the management of chronic illness, the focus is on the development of self-management skills. The CHN is in partnership with the client, paying attention to the client's self-concept and self-esteem as well as to the resources that are needed to manage the disease outside the medical system. Goals for care are structured to help clients adjust their day-to-day choices to maintain the highest level of functional ability possible within the limits of their conditions (Ebersole et al., 2005; Millar, 2004). The motivation to make the lifestyle changes that are necessary to cope with chronic illness may stem from a fear of death, disability, pain, negative effects on activities of daily living, and family.

Urinary incontinence often contributes to institutional care and social isolation. For that reason, it is difficult to estimate the numbers of individuals and cost of incontinence. It is important to address continence routinely in the assessment process, identify the type of incontinence, and intervene appropriately. Minor memory loss, or "forgetfulness," can be due to "normal" aging changes. However, more than a minor loss is possible due to disease processes. New cognitive theories of aging are developing, and the current debate is whether intellectual skills—for example, memory games and other forms of memory training—can enhance cognitive functioning and perhaps even prevent cognitive deterioration (Millar, 2004). A significant memory loss in older adults is likely because of one or more of the **three Ds** of intellectual impairment (Ebersole et al., 2005):

1. ***D**ementia* (progressive intellectual impairment)
2. ***D**epression* (mood disorder)
3. ***D**elirium* (acute confusion)

Delirium and dementia are often referred to as cognitive impairment. See the RNAO Web site (see Evolve Weblinks) for the best practice guidelines titled *Screening for Delirium, Dementia and Depression in Older Adults* and *Caregiving Strategies for Older Adults with Delirium, Dementia and Depression.* These guidelines were developed for nurses who work with older adults experiencing cognitive impairment and their caregivers. These two guidelines differentiate between the three Ds, provide screening tools for use with older adults, and discuss nursing considerations in caring for these older adults and in working with their caregivers.

For older adults experiencing any of the three Ds, CHNs need to be aware of the existing community services such as outpatient clinics, daycare services, and self-help groups. If services are lacking and needed in the community, CHNs can initiate partnerships in the communities so that these become available based on input from clients. As well, CHNs can initiate education programs at the aggregate and community levels.

Medication use in the older adult is an important consideration for CHNs. The changes that come with aging can alter the pharmacokinetics and pharmacodynamics of medications in older adults (Ebersole et al., 2005; Millar, 2004) and can result in health and safety issues. In addition, many older adults take several prescription and over-the-counter medications for the treatment of their chronic illnesses and are thus at an increased risk for iatrogenic drug reactions (Ebersole et al., 2005; Millar, 2004). Nonadherence to prescribed medications is often identified in the literature as a concern with older adults.

CHNs need to assess medication use with older adults and educate this aggregate group as indicated. One strategy is to ask to see the medications that older adults are taking and to discuss with the older adults their understanding of these medications and their pattern of use. If not visiting the older adult in their homes, many CHNs use the "brown bag approach"—older adults are asked to bring all their medications (prescription and nonprescription) to the CHN. Together, the CHN and the older adult review the medications to determine client knowledge and skill in taking medications, and safety issues can be addressed.

CRITICAL VIEW

Polypharmacy can be a concern when working with some older adults in the community. *Polypharmacy* refers to the taking by an individual of multiple prescription drugs and/or over-the counter medications (Ramage-Morin, 2009).

Hazards of polypharmacy include possible drug interactions, side effects, and overmedication, which can contribute to chemically induced impairment.

1. Why do you think many older adult Canadians are taking multiple medications?
2. What can the CHN do to assess, manage, and intervene in situations of polypharmacy?

Refer to the article by Planton, J., & Edlund, B. (2010). Strategies for reducing polypharmacy in older adults. *Journal of Gerontological Nursing, 36*(1), 8–12; and the article by Ramage-Morin (2009) at the Web site http://www.statcan.gc.ca/pub/82-003-x/2009001/article/10801-eng.pdf to further develop your reflections on this topic.

One often-overlooked concern of older adults is that of abuse. *Elder abuse* encompasses physical, psychological, financial or material, spiritual, and sexual abuse and neglect (Department of Justice, 2005; Health Canada, 2008). *Abuse* consists of the willful infliction of physical pain or injury, debilitating mental anguish and fear, theft or mismanagement of money or resources, or unreasonable confinement or the deprivation of services. **Neglect** refers to intentionally or unintentionally not providing care or a lack of services that are necessary for the physical, spiritual, social, and mental health of an older adult who is dependent on a caregiver. Older adults can make independent choices with which others may disagree. Their right to self-determination can be taken from them if they are declared incompetent. *Exploitation* is the illegal or improper use of a person or their resources for another's profit or advantage. During the assessment process, CHNs need to be aware of incongruence between injuries and the explanation of their causes, dependency issues between the client and caregiver, and substance abuse by the caregiver. Refer to the Department of Justice Canada "Family Violence Initiative: Abuse of Older Adults" Weblink (on the Evolve Web site).

The majority of older adults live in homes alone, with spouses, or with other family or friends. Female spouses represent the largest group of family caregivers of the older adult family caregivers. *Stress, strain,* and *burnout* are words that are used to reflect the negative effects of the family caregiver burden. Issues involve the work itself, past and present relationships, the effect on others, and the caregivers' lifestyle and well-being. For many families, the caregiving experience is a positive, rewarding, and fulfilling one. Community health nursing intervention can facilitate good health for older adults and their caregivers and contribute to meaningful family relationships during this period. Caregiving situations can vary from grandparents caring for grandchildren or other relatives to older adult spouses taking care of their partners or their own elderly parents (Ebersole et al., 2005). Older adults are living longer, with many older adults delaying institutionalization, and some family members and friends are assuming the caregiver role at home.

Caregiving roles can be formal (professional or personal care providers) or informal (family and friends). Women are often the caregiver, with women who are employed outside the home acting as informal caregivers as often as women who work in the home (Beckmann Murray et al., 2006). Caring for someone in the home, such as someone with Alzheimer's disease, on a continual basis can be very stressful and challenging. Family and friend caregivers are often not health care professionals, and the stress they experience may not be recognized. CHNs need to be alert for signs of caregiver stress and assist caregivers to reduce their stress or refer caregivers to community resources for support and assistance in dealing with their stress and their caregiving responsibilities, such as adult daycare services, Meals on Wheels, and respite care in the home and in many institutions. Some signs of caregiver stress are denial, anger, withdrawing socially, anxiety, depression, exhaustion, sleeplessness, emotional reactions, lack of concentration, and health concerns (Alzheimer Society, 2008). Further information on these signs and ways to reduce caregiver stress is found on the Alzheimer Society site listed in the Evolve Weblinks. The information is directed to those who care for people with Alzheimer's disease; however, the signs of stress and the ways to reduce stress are applicable to all caregiver situations. The CHN needs to be familiar with the respite care available in the community and refer caregivers as needed.

CRITICAL VIEW

Caring for a dependent older adult can be very stressful and can lead to caregiver burden. Answer the following:

1. What do you think are some of the stresses on the client, the caregivers, and the family?
2. a) What determinants of health are most relevant to the health of caregivers and why?
   b) How do the determinants of health affect caregiver burden?

Go to the Alzheimer Society of Canada Web site listed in the Evolve Weblinks to compare your answers to the above questions.

There is an abundance of health information and related resources for older adults and health care providers, such as information on health promotion and injury prevention and numerous publications on a vast array of topics. Refer to the Government of Canada "Seniors Canada: Working for Seniors" and the PHAC "Seniors' Health" Weblinks on the Evolve Web site.

LIVING HEALTHY IN ALL LIFE STAGES

CHNs have many resources available to assist them in their many roles and to facilitate and support clients in striving to achieve healthy living throughout the life stages. The RNAO Web site (see the Evolve Weblinks) provides best practice guidelines that direct nurses in their practice with clients. These guidelines include breastfeeding best practice guidelines for nurses, enhancing adolescent development, nursing management of hypertension, prevention of falls and fall injuries in the older adult, and supporting and strengthening families through expected and unexpected life events. Many other Web-based resources provide information that is useful to the CHN pertaining to various age groups. Working with individuals and families experiencing life's developmental stages is challenging for any CHN; however, it is also a very rewarding experience as the CHN has the opportunity to influence and facilitate healthy life choices at the micro and macro levels.

When working with all clients, CHNs need to continue to put an emphasis on illness prevention and on promotion of healthy living. This requires maintaining an "upstream" comprehensive approach that considers the influence of the determinants of health and provision of socioenvironmental multilevel strategies that are evidence-informed. Healthy living patterns are learned, acquired behaviours; therefore, if this trend of decreasing health is to be reversed, efforts must be directed toward the Canadian population, especially families and children.

STUDENT EXPERIENCE

Visit the World Health Organization's "Total Environment Assessment Model for Early Child Development" (see Evolve Weblinks). This site provides information on a model being proposed for consideration for health care practitioners, researchers, and policy makers to emphasize the importance of recognizing early child development as the most important determinant of health. The model is called "The Total Environment Assessment Model for Early Child Development (TEAM-ECD)" and identifies some of the inequities that exist that affect early childhood development.

Read through the document and familiarize yourself with the guiding principles of the model, model components, model application, and the story about Antoinette.

Answer the questions found on page 12 of the Web site.

REMEMBER THIS!

- Good nutrition is essential for healthy growth and development and influences disease prevention in later life. The adolescent population is at greatest risk for poor nutritional health.
- The family is critical to the growth and development of the child. Social support is one of the most powerful influences on successful parenting.
- Accidents and injuries are the major cause of health concerns in the child and adolescent population. Most are preventable. CHNs have a major role in anticipatory guidance and prevention.
- Smoking is a risk factor for a number of major health problems, including lung cancer, heart disease, osteoporosis, and poor reproductive outcomes.
- Men engage in more risk-taking behaviours, such as physical challenges and illegal behaviours, than do women.
- The most significant death-rate differences between men and women are for acquired immunodeficiency syndrome, suicides, homicides, and accidents.
- Men tend to avoid the diagnosis and treatment of illnesses, which may result in serious health concerns.
- Most older adults live in the community. The last few years of life often represent a functional decline. CHNs strive to help older adults maximize functional status and minimize costs through direct care and appropriate referral to community resources.
- CHNs address the chronic health concerns of older adults with a focus on maintaining or improving self-care and preventing complications to maintain the highest possible quality of life.
- Assessing the older adult incorporates physical, psychological, social, cultural, and spiritual domains.
- Individual and community-focused interventions involve all three levels of prevention through collaborative practice.

REFLECTIVE PRAXIS

Case 1

Sonya, a 79-year-old widow, lives alone in a seniors' high-rise apartment building. Sonya's neighbours and the administrator of the apartment building reported to the community health nurse who visits residents in the apartment building that no one had been observed coming or going from Sonya's apartment recently. The neighbours reported that when they did see Sonya, she appeared unkempt and did not appear to recognize them.

When the CHN made a visit to the apartment, Sonya answered the door and was very pleasant. The CHN validated the unkempt appearance of both Sonya and the apartment and detected an odour of urine. Sonya was mobile without the use of aids. Sonya was hesitant and unsure in her answers. Her history revealed medical problems. Sonya said that she has a son and daughter-in-law living in the next town who usually phone her at least once a week. Their phone number was taped on a table beside the phone.

Information found in the family assessment was that Sonya's son is an alcoholic, her daughter-in-law has the beginning symptoms of CVD, and her great-grandchild has asthma and is cared for by Sonya's son and daughter-in-law. Several pill bottles were observed on the kitchen counter, with the names of a local physician and pharmacist.

The CHN noted that both Sonya and her clothes were dirty and that she moved without aids and appeared steady on her feet. The kitchen was littered with unwashed dishes and empty fast-food boxes. Sonya could not recall buying or having the dinners delivered. A billfold with several bills was lying open on the kitchen counter, as well as an uncashed Canada pension cheque.

1. What should the CHN do about the situation she found?
   a. Call adult protective services and get an emergency order to put Sonya in a nursing home.
   b. Call Sonya's son and see if his mother can move in with him since she cannot take care of herself.
   c. Complete physical and mental examinations to first determine the cause of Sonya's situation.
   d. Call Sonya's pharmacist to see what medications she is taking.
   e. Call Sonya's son to discuss the situation with him and to make plans with him and his mother for her future.
2. What factors make this a difficult situation?

Answers are on the Evolve Web site at http://evolve.elsevier.com/Canada/Stanhope/community/.

What Would You Do?

1. Log on to the following Web site about osteoporosis: http://www.osteoporosis.ca/english/For %20Health%20Professionals/Related%20Links/default.asp?s=1. Prepare a chart that includes information on the following: statistics on this disease for males and females, the major and minor risk factors, and the health promotion or disease prevention interventions. Bring your chart to class for discussion.
2. Log on to the following Web site about diabetes mellitus: http://www.diabetes.ca/cpg2003/chapters.aspx. Prepare a chart that includes information on the following: screening and risk factors for type 2 diabetes and gestational diabetes, and nutritional and lifestyle counselling. Bring your chart to class for discussion.
3. Log on to the following Web site about suicide: http://www.hc-sc.gc.ca/hl-vs/iyh-vsv/diseases-maladies/suicide-eng.php. Prepare a chart that includes information on the following: statistics; the warning signs; the predisposing, precipitating, contributing, and protective factors to suicide behaviour; and suicide prevention programs.
4. Log on to the following Web site about men's health: http://www.hc-sc.gc.ca/hl-vs/jfy-spv/men-hommes-eng.php. Prepare a chart that includes information on the following: statistics on common diseases and conditions, "risky" behaviours, strategies to achieve healthier living, risk factors for heart disease, and teaching required to address these risk factors. Bring your chart to class for discussion.
5. Log on to the following Web site about seniors' health: http://www.hc-sc.gc.ca/hl-vs/jfy-spv/seniors-aines-eng.php. Prepare a chart that includes information on the following: why physical activity is important, ways to increase physical activity in seniors, how much and what types of exercise are healthy, and supports in your community for seniors to maintain a healthy lifestyle. Bring your chart to class for discussion.
6. Search for clinical practice guidelines for your province or territory. Prepare a list and bring it to class for discussion.

TOOL BOX

evolve

The Tool Box contains useful instruments that can be applied in community health nursing practice. These related resources are found either in the appendices at the back of this book or on the Evolve Web site at http://evolve.elsevier.com/Canada/Stanhope/community/.

Appendices

- Appendix 1: Canadian Community Health Nursing Standards of Practice
- Appendix E-5: Canadian Required Immunization Schedule
- Appendix E-6: Infant, Child, and Youth Screening Tools
- Appendix 9: The Calgary Family Assessment Model and the Calgary Family Intervention Model

Tools

Canadian Cancer Society.
This site contains information that can be used to teach women about BSE, including how to perform a BSE. Conduct a search for and choose the link to "Breast Self-Examination: What You Can Do."

Health Canada. *Canadian Guidelines for Bodyweight Classification in Adults—Quick Reference Tool for Professionals.*
This site provides a tool that gives the calculations for the body mass index and the waist circumference measure.

Health Canada. Growing Healthy Canadians: A Guide for Positive Child Development.
This guide is a collection of information to promote the well-being of children.

Health Canada. *Healthy Living. Reaching for the Top: A Report by the Advisor on Healthy Children and Youth.*
This Health Canada report presents five key recommendations and 95 sub-recommendations that will have an impact on health care programs to improve the health of children and youth.

Health Canada. Making It Work: A Program Checklist.
This site provides information on how to set up health promotion programs and presents an example of a program on healthy weights for women.

Keep Kids Healthy: *Children's Growth Charts.*
This link contains growth charts for boys and girls. These tools are useful for CHNs to monitor the development of children under their care.

Osteoporosis Canada.
Choose the links to a calcium calculator and calcium recipes. This is an excellent tool to share with clients because they can enter their daily food and fluid intake and then calculate the amount of calcium taken. Also, clients will likely find some of the recipes helpful.

Osteoporosis Canada. Osteoporosis 60-Second Risk Quiz.
This quiz can be useful for clients in determining their risk for developing osteoporosis. CHNs can use this screening tool to determine clients at risk and refer them for appropriate medical care.

Public Health Agency of Canada. *First Connections... Make All the Difference.*
This resource provides a checklist of information for health care professionals to assess infant attachment.

Public Health Agency of Canada. *The Physical Activity Readiness Questionnaire.*
This tool is used to determine if it is safe to become more physically active. It can be used by CHNs to screen for clients at risk before recommending that they increase their level of physical activity.

Public Health Agency of Canada. *Promising Pathways—A Handbook of Best Practices.*
This tool can be used by CHNs to assess a home environment for safety, including falls.

Public Health Agency of Canada. Prostate Cancer.
This site provides information specifically on prostate cancer, with statistics, advice for managing with prostate cancer, and the risk factors.

WEBLINKS

evolve

Direct links to these resources can be found on the text's accompanying Evolve Web site at http://evolve.elsevier.com/Canada/Stanhope/community.

Alzheimer Society of Canada. 10 Signs of Caregiver Stress. This site provides indicators of caregiver stress and ways to reduce it.

British Columbia Centre of Excellence for Women's Health. ***Women's Heart Health: An Evidence Review.*** This site provides an overview of CVD for women, with topics such as health promotion and prevention, diagnosis and treatment, as well as women's heart health and policy issues for the province of British Columbia. The information is useful for consideration in other provinces and territories.

Canadian Child Care Federation. This bilingual provincial and territorial association promotes the use of the best health care practices, and builds on capacity-building collaborations, networks, and partnerships to address issues in child care. The site provides links to resources for families and child care practitioners that will support children's social well-being with regard to issues such as self-esteem, language and literacy, and supporting children's positive behaviour.

Canadian Diabetes Association. ***Canadian Diabetes Association 2008 Clinical Practice Guidelines for the Prevention and Management of Diabetes in Canada.*** Professional guidelines for all aspects of the assessment, diagnosis, and management of diabetes with all age groups and for special populations such as pregnant women, Aboriginal peoples, the elderly, and high-risk ethnic populations.

Canadian Institutes of Health Research. ***Gender and Sex-Based Analysis in Health Research: A Guide for CIHR Researchers and Reviewers.*** This site explores the definition of gender and sex-based analysis and research and ethical considerations and discusses some of the research based on sex and gender.

Canadian Nurses Association. ***Backgrounder: The Built Environment, Injury Prevention, and Nursing: A Summary of the Issues.*** This backgrounder provides a summary of the built environment in relation to the issue of injury prevention. From the CNA home page, click on "Position Statements," then choose "CNA Backgrounders," on the left.

Canadian Nurses Association. Healthy Child Development. This site provides some information on the CNA position on healthy child development and links to other sites providing data and research findings on initiatives on child and youth development in Canada and issues affecting them such as smoking, immunization, and bullying prevention in schools.

Canadian Nurses Association. Position Statement: Determinants of Health. This site presents the CNA position on the determinants of health such as the need for increased funding for chronic disease prevention and increasing research on the determinants of health. The effects of the determinants of health, including individual behaviour and physical environment and genetics, are identified in this document as important considerations for nurses to influence the health outcomes of Canadians.

Canadian Population Health Initiative. *Overweight and Obesity in Canada: A Population Health Perspective.* This report covers information related to (1) the health issue of obesity, (2) the impact of obesity, (3) a population health perspective on the determinants of obesity, (4) how effective approaches have been for addressing obesity and its determinants, and (5) identification of priorities for future policy research pertaining to obesity for reducing population obesity levels.

Department of Justice Canada. *Family Violence Initiative: Abuse of Older Adults.* This site provides fact sheets about the abuse of older adults on specific topics such as epidemiology, potential warning signs, and prevention and suggests resources about the abuse of older adults.

Government of Canada. *Healthy Weights for Healthy Kids: Report of the Standing Committee on Health.* This report contains information on what determines healthy weights, what works for healthy weight control, and issues pertaining to Aboriginal and Inuit populations. The report also contains the committee's 12 recommendations the federal government needs to take to reduce the prevalence of childhood obesity by 2020. Some of these recommendations are establishing healthy weight targets, initiating a comprehensive public awareness campaign, simplifying food labelling, limiting use of trans fats, and increasing knowledge exchange on healthy weights for children.

Government of Canada. Seniors Canada: Working for Seniors. This site provides information on issues such as health matters, legal matters, retirement, transportation, and leisure time.

Health Canada. *First Nations, Inuit and Aboriginal Health: Diabetes.* This site provides clearly organized specific information on diabetes for First Nations, Inuit, and Aboriginal peoples.

Health Canada. *Food and Nutrition—Eating Well with Canada's Food Guide.* This site presents the Canada Food Guide, information on food choices, tips on using the Food Guide, and developing healthy habits. It also provides the opportunity for creating individualized eating plans.

Health Canada. Healthy Living. This is the home page for extensive resources pertaining to healthy living for Canadians across the lifespan with links for healthy babies, safety and injuries, mental health, physical activity, and healthy eating. The information provided is to assist Canadians make healthy living choices.

Health Canada. Just for You—Men. This site provides extensive links on information specifically for men.

Health Canada. *Making Change Happen: Stories from British Columbia (Diabetes Project).* These stories from British Columbia demonstrate creative partnership approaches on how to involve aggregates with diabetes to promote health and prevent disease. From the link, choose "Communities Act!" in the feature box and then click on the pdf file "Making Change Happen: Stories from British Columbia."

Health Canada. Youth and Tobacco. This site provides information on and links to several smoking prevention and cessation programs targeted at youth across Canada.

Heart and Stroke Foundation. *2010 Heart and Stroke Foundation Annual Report on Canadians' Health.* The annual Heart and Stroke report titled *A Perfect Storm of Heart Disease Looming on Our Horizon* gives information on the risk factors and changes that are placing a burden on the cardiovascular health of Canadians. The report identifies disparities between the health of Canadians and the lack of a comprehensive approach required to address these disparities.

Physicians for a Smoke Free Canada. *Smoking in Canada: A Statistical Snapshot of Canadian Smokers.* This site contains information on who smokes in Canada and provides statistics on one of the leading causes of preventable deaths and the health impacts of smoking.

Public Health Agency of Canada. Bringing Health to the Planning Table—A Profile of Promising Practices in Canada and Abroad. This site provides information in the form of profile case studies of lessons learned for 13 Canadian communities where collaborative approaches related to the built environment were used to improve health outcomes.

Public Health Agency of Canada. *Canada's Physical Activity Guide for Older Adults.* Information about physical activity choices to promote health and to prevent disease for older adults can be found here.

Public Health Agency of Canada. *Canada's Physical Activity Guides for Children and Youth.* This site provides links to guides and support resources such as family and teacher guides for physical activity promotion for children and youth and a link to the Department of Finance Canada for information on the Children's Fitness Tax Credit.

Public Health Agency of Canada. Cervical Cancer. This site provides information on the incidence, risk factors, and management of cervical cancer in Canada.

Public Health Agency of Canada. ***The Chief Public Health Officer's Report on the State of Public Health in Canada, 2009: Growing up Well—Priorities for a Healthy Future.*** This second annual report by Dr. Butler-Jones highlights six areas of concern that have the greatest impact on the health of Canadian children.

Public Health Agency of Canada. Child Health. A wide variety of links to online resources on many issues that affect child and youth health are found on this Web site.

Public Health Agency of Canada. ***Diabetes in Canada: Highlights from the National Diabetes Surveillance System 2004–2005.*** This site provides extensive data on age-standardized statistical findings from Canada's national diabetes surveillance system pertaining to diabetes, such as prevalence and incidence rates, hospitalizations, and mortality.

Public Health Agency of Canada. Healthy Living Fund. This site provides information on healthy activities as part of the chronic diseases initiative and provides links to projects that address activities of healthy living for Alberta and the NWT regions.

Public Health Agency of Canada. Maternal and Infant Health. This site provides information such as nutrition during pregnancy, including folic acid; congenital anomalies; and physical abuse during pregnancy.

Public Health Agency of Canada. National Advisory Committee on Immunization. Information on the use of vaccines and their use in Canada for humans is presented, as well as the identification of groups at risk for vaccine-preventable disease for whom vaccine programs should be targeted. This site also provides a link to the latest *Canadian Immunization Guide.*

Public Health Agency of Canada. ***Obesity: An Overview of Current Landscape and Prevention-Related Activities in Ontario.*** This site presents statistics on overweight and obesity in Canadian children, youth, and adults. The site also discusses the contributing factors to obesity and related health concerns and presents an obesity-prevention approach.

Public Health Agency of Canada. Obesity in Canada: Snapshot. This site provides information such as the obesity trends in Canada, factors influencing prevalence of obesity, and the economic costs of obesity.

Public Health Agency of Canada. ***A Report on Mental Illnesses in Canada.*** An overview of mental illnesses in Canada, this in-depth discussion includes information on specific forms of mental illness such as mood disorders, schizophrenia, anxiety, and personality and eating disorders. Information on suicide is also presented.

Public Health Agency of Canada. Seniors' Health. This site provides extensive information for older adults such as health promotion strategies and injury prevention, as well as numerous publications to support older adults.

Public Health Agency of Canada. ***The 2007 Report on the Integrated Pan-Canadian Healthy Living Strategy.*** This first annual report of healthy living initiatives across Canada pertains to the following four strategic directions: leadership and policy development; knowledge development and transfer; community development and infrastructure; and public information. This site provides information on the progress made for each province and territory for these strategic directions.

Public Safety Canada. ***Summative Evaluation of the National Strategy on Community Safety and Crime Prevention, Phase ll—Summary Report.*** This site provides information on the federal government initiatives and strategies to prevent crime.

Registered Nurses' Association of Ontario. ***Caregiving Strategies for Older Adults with Delirium, Dementia and Depression.*** This RNAO best practice guideline addresses how to care for older adults with delirium, dementia, and depression.

Registered Nurses' Association of Ontario (RNAO). Clinical Practice Guidelines. This site provides nursing best practice guidelines developed for the RNAO, including the following: primary prevention of childhood obesity; enhancing healthy adolescent development; asthma care guidelines for nurses regarding promoting control of asthma and promoting asthma control in children; breastfeeding best practice guidelines for nurses; nursing management of hypertension; integration of smoking cessation into daily nursing practice; screening for delirium, dementia, and depression; caregiving strategies for older adults with delirium, dementia, and depression; and prevention of falls and fall injuries in the older adult. From the main menu on the RNAO home page, select "Nursing Best Practice Guidelines" and click on "Clinical Practice Guidelines Program" and then "Guidelines and Fact Sheets."

Registered Nurses' Association of Ontario. ***Prevention of Falls and Fall Injuries in the Older Adult.*** This best practice guideline provides information for the health care provider to assist in the prevention of falls in the older adult.

Registered Nurses' Association of Ontario. ***Screening for Delirium, Dementia and Depression in Older Adults.*** This document is an RNAO best practice guideline.

Safe Kids Canada. Child & Youth Unintentional Injury: Ten Years in Review. Statistical information and fact sheets on unintentional injuries that would be useful to CHNs, other professionals working in the area of childhood safety, and parents can be accessed here.

School Travel Planning News. This site provides information on implementation strategies for the Canadian School Travel Planning pilot project that was initiated in four Canadian provinces (Alberta, British Columbia, Ontario, and Nova Scotia) to promote safe methods of physical activity related to modes of travel to schools.

Society of Obstetricians and Gynaecologists of Canada. Women's Health Information. This site provides evidence-informed information for the public to help women make informed choices about their health.

Statistics Canada. Canadian Community Health Survey, 2003. A report of the findings of the Canadian Community Health Survey of 2003 on smoking, obesity, health perception, sexual orientation, and access to medical care in rural areas is at this site.

World Health Organization. *Mental Health: New Understandings, New Hope.* This site discusses mental health as a public health issue, a burden for those experiencing these disorders, and policies and services needed to solve mental health problems.

World Health Organization. *Total Environment Assessment Model for Early Child Development.* This site provides information on a model being proposed for health care practitioners, researchers, and policy makers to use to emphasize the importance of recognizing early child development as the most important determinant of health.

REFERENCES

Adelson, A. N. (2005). The embodiment of inequity: Health disparities in Aboriginal Canada. *Canadian Journal of Public Health*, *96*(Suppl. 2), S45–S61.

Alzheimer Society of Canada. (2008). *10 signs of caregiver stress media kit*. Retrieved from http://www.alzheimer.ca/english/media/cgstress99-brochure-signs.htm.

Assembly of First Nations (AFN). (2007). *Backgrounder on diabetes in First Nations communities: State of diabetes among First Nations peoples*. Retrieved from http://www.afn.ca/article.asp?id=3604.

Avison, C. (2009). Comprehensive school health in Canada. *The Canadian Association of Principals Journal*, *17*(2), 6–7.

Beckmann Murray, R., Proctor Zentner, J., Pangman, V., & Pangman, C. (2009). *Health promotion strategies through the lifespan* (2nd Canadian ed.). Toronto, ON: Pearson Prentice Hall.

Beckmann Murray, R. B., Zentner, J. P., Pangman, V., & Pangman, C. (2006). *Health promotion strategies through the lifespan* (Canadian ed.). Toronto, ON: Pearson.

Bird, S., Wiles, J., Okalik, L., Kilabuk, J., & Egeland, G. (2008). Living with diabetes on Baffin Island: Inuit storytellers share their experiences. *Canadian Journal of Public Health*, *99*(1), 17–21.

Boal, J., & Loengard, A. (2007). Home care. In R. J. Ham, P. D. Sloane, G. A. Warshaw, M. A. Bernard, & E. Flaherty (Eds.), *Primary care geriatrics: A case-based approach* (5th ed., pp. 172–178). Philadelphia, PA: Mosby.

Boney, C. M., Verma, A., Tucker, R., & Vohr, B. R. (2005). Metabolic syndrome in childhood: Association with birth weight, maternal obesity, and gestational diabetes mellitus. *Pediatrics*, *115*(3), e290–e296.

British Columbia Centre of Excellence for Women's Health. (2008). *Women's heart health: An evidence review*. Retrieved from http://synthesis.womenshealthdata.ca/uploads/topic204_0.pdf.

Butler-Jones, D. (2009). *The chief public health officer's report on the state of public health in Canada 2009: Growing up well—priorities for a healthy future*. Public Health Association of Canada. Retrieved from http://www.phac-aspc.gc.ca/publicat/2009/cphorsphc-respcacsp/index-eng.php.

Campaign 2000. (2009). *2009 Report card on child and family poverty in Canada: 1989–2009*. Retrieved from www.campaign2000.ca.

Canadian Association for School Health. (2006). *CSH consensus statement*. Retrieved from http://www.cash-aces.ca/index.asp?Page=Consensus.

Canadian Cancer Society. (2009a). *Breast cancer statistics 2009*. Retrieved from http://www.cancer.ca/Canada-wide/About%20cancer/Cancer%20statistics/Stats%20at%20a%20glance/Breast%20cancer.aspx?sc_lang=en.

Canadian Cancer Society. (2009b). *Lung cancer statistics*. Retrieved from http://www.cancer.ca/Canada-wide/About%20cancer/Cancer%20statistics/Stats%20at%20a%20glance/Lung%20cancer.aspx.

Canadian Cancer Society. (2010a). *Causes of cervical cancer*. Retrieved from http://www.cancer.ca/canada-wide/about%20cancer/types%20of%20cancer/causes%20of%20cervical%20cancer.aspx?sc_lang=en.

Canadian Cancer Society. (2010b). *Tobacco statistics in Canada*. Retrieved from http://www.cancer.ca/canada-wide/prevention/quit%20smoking/canadian%20tobacco%20stats.aspx.

Canadian Council on Social Development. (2007). *Growing up in North America: Child health and safety in Canada, the United States and Mexico*. Retrieved from http://www.ccsd.ca/pubs/2006/cina/trihealth.pdf.

Canadian Diabetes Association. (2008). *Canadian Diabetes Association 2008 clinical practice guidelines for the prevention and management of diabetes in Canada*. Retrieved from http://www.diabetes.ca/files/cpg2008/cpg-2008.pdf.

Canadian Institute for Health Information. (2008). *Reducing gaps in health: A focus on socio-economic status in urban Canada*. Retrieved from http://secure.cihi.ca/cihiweb/products/Reducing_Gaps_in_Health_Report_EN_081009.pdf.

Centers for Disease Control and Prevention. (2008). *A public health plan to prevent heart disease and stroke*. Retrieved from http://www.cdc.gov/DHDSP/library/action_plan/full_appendix_a.htm.

Child Trends. (2007). *Child and adolescent trial for cardiovascular health (CATCH)*. Retrieved from http://www.childtrends.org/Lifecourse/programs/ChildandAdolescentTrialforCardiovascularHealth.htm.

Clinton, K. (2009). Preventing youth overweight and obesity: A population health perspective. *Transdisciplinary Studies in Population Health Series, 1*(1), 7–21. Retrieved from http://www.iph.uottawa.ca/eng/transdis/files/001-PREVENTING%20YOUTH %20OVERWEIGHT %20 AND%20OBESITY- %20A%20POPULATION%20 HEALTH%20PERSPECTIVE.pdf.

Conroy, K., Sandel, M., & Zuckerman, B. (2010). Poverty grown up: How childhood socioeconomic status impacts adult health. *Journal of Developmental & Behavioral Pediatrics, 31*(2), 154–160.

Cromer, K. R., & Sachs-Ericsson, N. (2006). The association between childhood abuse, PTSD, and the occurrence of adult health problems: Moderation via current life stress. *Journal of Traumatic Stress, 19*(6), 967–971.

Department of Justice Canada. (2005). *The national strategy on community safety and crime prevention*. Retrieved from http://www.justice.gc.ca/en/news/nr/1998/newsbckg.html.

Dukowski, L. (2009). Comprehensive school health—Why should we care? *Canadian Association of Principals Journal, 17*(2), 4–5.

Ebersole, P., Hess, P., Touhy, T., & Jett, K. (2005). *Gerontological nursing and healthy aging* (2nd ed.). St. Louis, MO: Elsevier Mosby.

Ginsburg, K. R. (2007). The importance of play in promoting healthy child development and maintaining strong parent-child bonds. *Pediatrics, 119*(1), 182–191.

Hamilton, N., & Bhatti, T. (1996). *Population health promotion: An integrated model of population health and health promotion*. Health Promotion Development Division, Health Canada.

Health Canada. (2006a). *Benefits and risks of hormone replacement therapy (estrogen with or without progestin)*. Retrieved from http://www.hc-sc.gc.ca/iyh-vsv/med/estrogen_e.html.

Health Canada. (2006b). *Women and heart health*. Retrieved from http://www.hc-sc.gc.ca/hl-vs/pubs/women-femmes/heart-cardiovasculaire-eng.php.

Health Canada. (2007a). *Cigarette smoke: It's toxic*. Retrieved from http://hc-sc.gc.ca/hc-ps/tobac-tabac/second/fact-fait/tox-eng.php.

Health Canada. (2007b). *Food and nutrition*. Retrieved from http://www.hc-sc.gc.ca/fn-an/food-guide-aliment/index_e.html.

Health Canada. (2008). *Just for you—Seniors*. Retrieved from http://www.hc-sc.gc.ca/hl-vs/jfy-spv/seniors-aines-eng.php.

Health Canada. (2009). *Osteoporosis awareness month*. Retrieved from http://www.hc-sc.gc.ca/ahc-asc/minist/messages/_2009/2009_11_02b-eng.php.

Health Nexus and Ontario Chronic Disease Prevention Alliance. (2008). *Primer to action: Social determinants of health*. Retrieved from http://www.healthnexus.ca/projects/primer.pdf.

Heart & Stroke Foundation. (2007). *Heart attack warning signals*. Retrieved from http://www.heartandstroke.com/site/c.ikIQLcMWJtE/b.2796497/k.BF8B/Home.htm?src=home.

Heart & Stroke Foundation. (2009). *On the pulse news: Why aren't more children walking or biking to school?*. Retrieved from http://www.heartandstroke.com/site/apps/nlnet/content2.aspx?c=ikIQLcMWJtE&b=3485821&ct=7506431.

Heart & Stroke Foundation. (2010). *2010 Heart & Stroke Foundation annual report on Canadians' health*. Retrieved from http://www.heartandstroke.com/atf/cf/%7B99452D8B-E7F1-4BD6-A57D-B136CE6C95BF %7D/Jan23_EN_ReportCard.pdf.

Hertzman, C., & Power, C. (2003). Health and human development: Understandings from life-course research. *Developmental Neuropsychology, 24*(2&3), 719–744.

Hertzman, C., Power, C., Matthews, S., & Manor, O. (2001). Using an interactive framework of society and lifecourse to explain self-related health in early childhood. *Social Science & Medicine, 53*(12), 1575–1585.

Human Resources and Skills Development Canada. (2010). *Indicators of well-being in Canada*. Retrieved from http://www4.hrsdc.gc.ca/.3ndic.1t.4r@-eng.jsp?iid=12.

Janz, T., Seto, J., & Turner, A. (2009). *Aboriginal peoples survey, 2006: An overview of the health of the Métis population*. Retrieved from http://www.metisnation.ca/PDF-May2009/press/APS%20M%C3%A9tis%20article%202006%20English.pdf.

Jin, A., Martin, D., & Sarin, C. (2002). Diabetes mellitus in the First Nations population of British Columbia, Canada: Part 1. Mortality. *International Journal of Circumpolar Health, 61*, 251–264.

Joint Consortium for School Health. (2010). *What is comprehensive school health?* Retrieved from http://eng.jcsh-cces.ca/index.php?option=com_content&view=article&id=40&Itemid=62.

Labarthe, D. R., Dai, S., Day, S., Fulton, J. E., & Grunbaum, J. A. (2009). Findings from project heartbeat! Their importance for CVD prevention. *American Journal of Preventive Medicine, 37*(1S), S105–S115.

Labonte, R. (2003). *How our programs affect population health determinants: A workbook for better planning and accountability*. Saskatchewan, SK: Population Health and Evaluation Research Unit for Health Canada.

Leitch, K. (2007). *Reaching for the top: A report by the Advisor on Healthy Children and Youth. Health Canada*. Retrieved from http://www.hc-sc.gc.ca/hl-vs/pubs/child-enfant/advisor-conseillere/index-eng.php.

Lung Association of Saskatchewan. (2009). *Lung cancer*. Retrieved from http://www.sk.lung.ca/content.cfm?edit_realword=lungcancer.

Lyons, R. D., & Langille, L. (2000). *Healthy lifestyle: Strengthening the effectiveness of lifestyle approaches to improve heath*. Retrieved from http://www.ahprc.dal.ca/lifestylefinal.pdf.

Mahon, R., Jenson, J., & Mortimer, K. (2006). *Learning from each other: Early learning and child care experiences in Canadian cities*. Retrieved from http://www.toronto.ca/children/pdf/elreseachreport.pdf.

McSweeney, J. C., Cody, M., O'Sullivan, P., Elberson, K., Moser, D. K., & Garvin, B. J. (2003). Women's early warning symptoms of acute myocardial infarction. *Circulation*, *108*(21), 2619–2623. Retrieved from http://circ.ahajournals.org/cgi/content/full/108/21/2619.

Meiner, S. E., & Lueckenotte, A. G. (2006). *Gerontological nursing* (3rd ed.). St. Louis, MO: Mosby.

Mikkonen, J., & Raphael, D. (2010). *Social determinants of health: The Canadian facts*. Toronto, ON: York University School of Health Policy and Management. Retrieved from www.thecanadianfacts.org/.

Millar, C. A. (2004). *Nursing for wellness in older adults: Theory and practice* (4th ed.). Philadelphia, PA: Lippincott Williams & Wilkins.

Morrison, W., Kirby, P., Losier, G., & Allain, M. (2009). Conceptualizing psychological wellness: Addressing mental fitness needs. *Canadian Association of Principals Journal*, *17*(2), 19–21.

Murray, N., Low, B., Hollis, C., Cross, A., & Davis, S. (2007). Coordinated school health programs and academic achievement: A systematic review of the literature. *Journal of School Health*, *77*(9), 589–599.

National Collaborating Centre for Determinants of Health. (2009). *Early child development as a determinant of health*. Retrieved from http://nccdh.ca/work/earlychildhood.html.

New Brunswick Wellness, Culture and Sport (n.d.). *Wellness*. Retrieved from http://www.gnb.ca/0131/wellness-e.asp.

Ontario Ministry of Health and Long-Term Care. (2006). *Aboriginal diabetes strategy*. Retrieved from http://www.health.gov.on.ca/english/public/pub/ministry_reports/oads_06/oads_06.pdf.

Osteoporosis Canada. (2010). *Facts and statistics about osteoporosis*. Retrieved from http://www.osteoporosis.ca/index.php/ci_id/8867/la_id/1.htm.

Ozonoff, S., Williams, B. J., & Landa, R. (2005). Parental report of the early development of children with regressive autism: The "delays-plus-regression" phenotype. *Autism: The International Journal of Research and Practice*, *9*(5), 461–486.

Patra, J., Popova, S., Rehm, J., Bondy, S., Flint, R., & Giesbrecht, N. (2007). *Economic cost of chronic disease in Canada: 1995–2003*. Retrieved from http://www.ocdpa.on.ca/docs/OCDPA_EconomicCosts.pdf.

Planton, J., & Edlund, B. (2010). Strategies for reducing polypharmacy in older adults. *Journal of Gerontological Nursing, 36*(1), 8–12.

Potter, P. A., Perry, A. G., Ross-Kerr, J. C., & Wood, M. J. (2009). *Canadian fundamentals of nursing* (4th ed.). Toronto, ON: Elsevier Mosby.

Public Health Agency of Canada. (2005a). *Integrated pan-Canadian healthy living strategy*. Retrieved from http://www.phac-aspc.gc.ca/hl-vs-strat/pdf/hls_e.pdf.

Public Health Agency of Canada. (2005b). *Integrated strategy on healthy living and chronic disease*. Retrieved from http://www.phac-aspc.gc.ca/media/nr-rp/2005/2005_37bk3-eng.php.

Public Health Agency of Canada. (2005c). *Backgrounder: How healthy are Canadians?*. Retrieved from http://www.phac-aspc.gc.ca/ph-sp/report-rapport/toward/pdf/3howe.pdf.

Public Health Agency of Canada. (2007). *The 2007 report on the integrated Pan-Canadian Healthy Living Strategy*. Retrieved from http://www.phac-aspc.gc.ca/hl-vs-strat/pancan/index-eng.php.

Public Health Agency of Canada. (2008a). *Comprehensive school health*. Retrieved from http://www.phac-aspc.gc.ca/dca-dea/7-18yrs-ans/comphealth-eng.php.

Public Health Agency of Canada. (2008b). *Diabetes in Canada: Highlights from the National Diabetes Surveillance System, 2004–2005*. Retrieved from http://www.phac-aspc.gc.ca/publicat/2008/dicndss-dacsnsd-04-05/index-eng.php.

Public Health Agency of Canada. (2009a). *Obesity in Canada: Snapshot*. Retrieved from http://www.phac-aspc.gc.ca/publicat/2009/oc/pdf/oc-eng.pdf.

Public Health Agency of Canada. (2009b). *Obesity: An overview of current landscape and prevention-related activities in Ontario*. Retrieved from http://www.ocdpa.on.ca/docs/OCDPA_PHAC-%20Obesity_Prevention_Final.pdf.

Public Safety Canada. (2010). *National crime prevention strategy*. Retrieved from http://www.publicsafety.gc.ca/prg/cp/ncps-eng.aspx.

Ramage-Morin, P. (2009). *Medication use among senior Canadians*. Retrieved from http://www.statcan.gc.ca/pub/82-003-x/2009001/article/10801-eng.pdf.

Raphael, D., & Farrell, S. E. (2002a). Beyond medicine and lifestyle: Addressing the societal determinants of cardiovascular disease in North America. *Leadership in Health Services*, *15*(4), i–v.

Raphael, D., & Farrell, S. E. (2002b). Income inequality and cardiovascular disease in North America: Shifting the paradigm. *Harvard Health Policy Review*, *3*(2).

Reading, J. (2009). *A life course approach to the social determinants of health for Aboriginal Peoples for the Senate Sub-Committee on Population Health*. Retrieved from http://www.parl.gc.ca/40/2/parlbus/commbus/senate/com-e/popu-e/rep-e/appendixAjun09-e.pdf.

Ryan, G. & Bourke, C. (2008). *Community connection asset mapping process*. Wethersfield, CT: The Connecticut Assets Network.

Safe Kids Canada. (2007). *Child & youth unintentional injury, 1994 to 2003: 10 years in review*. Retrieved from http://www.mhp.gov.on.ca/English/injury_prevention/skc_injuries.pdf.

Shah, C. P. (2003). *Public health and preventive medicine in Canada* (5th ed.). Toronto, ON: Elsevier Saunders.

Shields, M. (2006). Overweight and obesity among children and youth. *Health Reports*, *17*(3), 27–42.

Society of Obstetricians and Gynaecologists of Canada. (2006a). *The journalist's menopause handbook: A companion guide to the Society of Obstetricians and Gynaecologists of Canada menopause consensus report*. Retrieved from http://www.sogc.org/media/pdf/advisories/Menopause-journalists-guide_e.pdf.

Society of Obstetricians and Gynaecologists of Canada. (2006b). SOGC Committee opinion: Breast self-examination. *Journal of Obstetrics and Gynaecology*, *181*, 728–730.

Statistics Canada. (2008). Canadian community health survey. *The Daily*, Wednesday June 18, 2008. Retrieved from http://www.statcan.gc.ca/daily-quotidien/080618/dq080618a-eng.htm.

Stewart-Brown, S. (2006). *What is the evidence on school health promotion in improving health or preventing disease and specifically, what is the effectiveness of the health promoting schools approach?*. Copenhagen: WHO Regional Office for Europe (Health Evidence Network report). Retrieved from http://www.euro.who.int/document/e88185.pdf.

Strasser, T. (1978). Reflections on cardiovascular diseases. *Interdisciplinary Science Review, 3*, 225–230.

Townson, M. (2009). *Women's poverty and the recession.* Retrieved from http://www.policyalternatives.ca/publications/reports/women%E2%80%99s-poverty-and-recession.

United Nations, Department of Economic and Social Affairs, Population Division. (2009). *World population prospects: The 2008 revision*. Retrieved from http://unstats.un.org/unsd/demographic/products/socind/health.htm.

University of Michigan. (2008). *Myocardial infarction (heart attack). Adult health advisor, 4*. Retrieved from http://www.med.umich.edu/1libr/aha/aha_myoinf_car.htm.

Veugelers, P. J., & Fitzgerald, A. L. (2005). Prevalence of and risk factors for childhood overweight and obesity. *Canadian Medical Association Journal, 173*(6), 607–613.

Women's Health Matters. (2008). *Cardiovascular health.* Retrieved from http://www.womenshealthmatters.ca/centres/cardio/index.html.

World Health Organization. (2010). *Chronic diseases.* Retrieved from http://www.who.int/topics/chronic_diseases/en/.

CHAPTER 14

Working with Groups, Teams, and Partners

KEY TERMS

collaborative client-centred practice 458

group 448

group process 449

interdisciplinary team 448

intradisciplinary team 448

leadership 452

multidisciplinary team 448

partnership 458

team 448

See Glossary on page 593 for definitions.

OBJECTIVES

After reading this chapter, you should be able to:

1. Examine the concepts of group, teams, and partnerships.
2. List and define the key characteristics of effective groups, teams, and partnerships.
3. Explain the factors affecting the ability of groups, teams, and partnerships to function effectively.
4. Name and describe the stages of group development.
5. Explain the various leadership styles and their influence on group functioning.
6. List and define the various leadership roles used in groups.
7. Evaluate the composition and performance of a group.
8. Define and give examples of group conflict.
9. Identify ways to resolve group conflict.
10. Explain the importance of collaboration in multidisciplinary, interdisciplinary, and intradisciplinary teams and interprofessional partnerships.
11. Discuss key concepts of effective team building.
12. Examine the CHN role in working with groups and as a member of a health team.
13. Discuss evaluation of interprofessional education.
14. Compare intraprofessional collaboration and interprofessional collaboration

CHAPTER OUTLINE

Working with Groups
- Group Process
- Group Development
- Group Roles
- Group Norms
- Group Leadership
- Group Conflict
- Group Evaluation

Working with Health Care Teams and Partners
- Team Building
- Partnerships
- Interprofessional Partnerships
- Interprofessional Education

The ability to work collaboratively with diverse groups, teams, and partners is an important skill required in community health nursing. CHNs work with a variety of groups to address the health needs of client as aggregate, community, population, and society. Groups can be an effective way to address clients' health concerns. It is essential that CHNs develop skill in working with groups, and therefore they need to understand groups, group dynamics, and team building. The CHNAC Standards of Practice identify the practice expectations for CHNs when working with groups, teams, and in partnerships (see Appendix 1). Some of the information required to work with groups is provided in this chapter; however, readers are encouraged to consult other resources that provide detailed information on group structure and function.

WORKING WITH GROUPS

CHNs work in teams, which in this text, is considered to be a type of group. Some examples of different types of small groups that CHNs might work with in practice are family, self-help groups, community groups, health care teams, professional associations, and committees. Regardless of the type of group that the CHN is working with, the structure and functioning of the group is of utmost importance. Groups can be instrumental in bringing about changes to improve the health and well-being of individuals, populations, and communities. Refer to Table 14-1 for some examples of CHNs working with a variety of small groups.

Working effectively with groups requires that CHNs understand and apply group concepts. When working with groups, it is important to consider areas such as purpose of the group, group membership, group dynamics, group process, group leadership, group size, and group task and maintenance functions.

Throughout this text, *client* is defined as society, community, population, aggregate/group, family, and individual. The term *aggregate/group* refers to a large group such as a group of schoolchildren or older adults. The CHN may also work with a subgroup of aggregates, often referred to as a small group. Usually a small group is less

TABLE 14-1 Selected Examples of CHNs Working with Groups

Type of CHN	Target Group	Main Purpose
Nurse practitioner (NP)	Family	1. Promote family and individual behaviour change to manage health challenges 2. TB screening for follow-up and monitoring treatment of family
Public health nurse (PHN)	Family	1. Disease prevention as follow-up with the family regarding an infectious disease 2. Health promotion regarding family adaptation to birth of a high-risk neonate
Home health nurse (HHN)	Family	1. Family support and family empowerment regarding care of family member with a chronic disease 2. Provide health teaching to family regarding care of family member dealing with a health challenge
Occupational health nurse (OHN)	Workplace group	1. Promote healthy lifestyle 2. Policy development that supports healthy workplace environments
PHN	Community group	Provision of health education for expectant parents
NP	Community self-help group	Support and empowerment to members of substance abuser group
HHN	Student group	Health education regarding a specific health issue common to the group that provides information on management of their health issue and prevention of complications
NP	Team, e.g., primary health care	Coordination and delivery of the most effective client interventions by an interdisciplinary team
PHN	Team, e.g., heart health	Participation of professional and nonprofessional team members to address issues pertaining to heart health in their community
HHN	Team, e.g., palliative care	Coordination and delivery of the most effective client interventions
CHN	Professional association, e.g., Canadian Nurses Association (CNA)	Advocate for healthy public policy such as crib safety
CHN	Committee, e.g., Healthy Communities	To promote the health of the community

than 20 members; 12 group members is considered ideal. However, every group is unique, and the level of involvement of all members and the purpose and goals of the group will help determine the membership size in a small group. Thelen (1954) provided guidelines for "least group size" in which he determined that a group should contain the least number of members to accomplish the task, to build and maintain the group, and to reach the group's goals (cited in Dimock & Kass, 2008). A **group** is a collection of two or more individuals in face-to-face interactions with a common purpose(s) and who are in an interdependent relationship (Diem & Moyer, 2005; Maurer & Smith, 2009). Each group member influences and is, in turn, influenced by every other member. Also, since relationships exist and affect a group, the group needs to work at relationship building if it is to be an effective group. Key elements in this definition of group are member interactions, group purpose, and interdependence. Therefore, a random collection of individuals such as a number of persons standing at a bus stop or sharing an elevator are not a group. **Team** is defined as a specialized group working toward a common goal or activity. CHNs participate most often as a member of an interdisciplinary team (often also referred to as an interprofessional team). Saltman, O'Dea, Farmer, Veitch, Rosen, and Kidd (2007) maintain that a group and a team in health care settings are two separate entities. It is noted that their definition of a team reflects this text's *group* definition. An **interdisciplinary team** contains members who have expertise from a variety of disciplines, such as nurses, social workers, dietitians, physiotherapists and physicians, who work together during the assessment, planning, implementation, and evaluation of client care; the client is considered a member of the team (Kelly & Crawford, 2008; Mauk, 2009). A **multidisciplinary team** contains members who have expertise from a variety of disciplines, such as nurses, social workers, dietitians, physiotherapists, and physicians, working independently who come together to make client-based decisions. An **intradisciplinary team** refers to nurses working with other nurses. For example, an intradisciplinary team could be a group of registered nurses and a group of registered practical nurses.

Evidence-Informed Practice

In this journal article, a description of how emotional intelligence affects interdisciplinary team effectiveness is discussed. To be effective a team requires "both emotional intelligence and expertise, including technical, clinical, social and interactional skills" (McCallin & Bamford, 2007, p. 386). *Emotional intelligence* is defined using Goleman, Boyatzis, and McKee (2002) team competencies as including self-awareness, self-management, social awareness, and social skills. In this grounded theory study, the purposes were to identify the main concerns of health professionals from different disciplines working on interdisciplinary teams in two main acute care teaching hospital settings and to explain how these team members handled workplace practice concerns. The sample consisted of 44 health team members from seven disciplines. Data were collected by interview and participant observation. It was found that in interdisciplinary teams, professional competence was especially valued; personalities often contributed to having to deal with problems and dysfunctional team members; team members focused less on social factors affecting team process and outcome; team members focused more on tasks that affected team effectiveness; many team members focused on individuality and individual expertise; avoidance of conflict was used; supporting interdisciplinary colleagues was seldom done; psychosocial safety within the teams was threatened as new discipline alignments were formed; professional boundaries were blurred; and technical expertise, cognitive intelligence, and emotional intelligence were identified as required to work effectively with all other team members

Application for CHNs: CHNs are members of a variety of interdisciplinary teams. It is important for CHNs when working with teams to consider the competencies of emotional intelligence, that is, self-awareness, self-management, social awareness, and social skill. CHNs as members of interdisciplinary teams need to be open to and encourage teams to examine how team members are managing the emotional-intelligence aspects of their team because of its influence on team effectiveness and client care outcomes.

Questions for Reflection & Discussion

1. What emotional-intelligence competencies do you bring to a team? Provide examples.
2. How would you approach group conflict as an interdisciplinary team member?
3. What key search words would you use when searching the evidence-informed practice literature about effectiveness of interdisciplinary teams? Explain your choices.

REFERENCE: McCallin, A., & Bamford, A. (2007). Interdisciplinary teamwork: Is the influence of emotional intelligence fully appreciated? *Journal of Nursing Management, 15*(4), 386–391.

BOX 14-1 Group Dimensions That Significantly Influence Group Process

- Group physical and emotional climate
- Group involvement
- Group interaction
- Group cohesion
- Group productivity

SOURCE: Adapted from Dimock, H. G., & Kass, R. (2007). *How to observe your group* (4th ed.). Concord, ON: Captus Press.

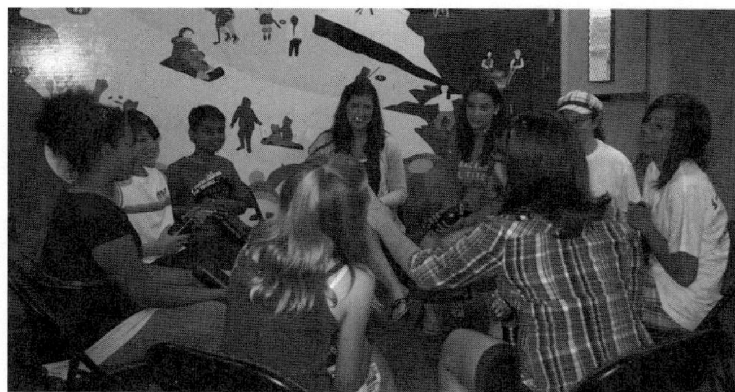

Group members interact and influence each other, whether formally or informally, such as this group of youth meeting at a community centre.

Group Process

Group process refers to how the group as a unit is working and how group members interact with one another (Dimock & Kass, 2007). Group process occurs at every group interaction. There are five dimensions in a group that are interrelated and that significantly influence group process (Dimock & Kass, 2007). Box 14-1 lists these five dimensions.

Group physical and emotional climate refers to the physical and emotional milieu. For group meetings, CHNs need to consider physical milieu factors such as adequate lighting, appropriate temperature and ventilation, comfortable chairs, and limiting distractions. Another consideration is the physical arrangement of the seating for group members; it should encourage and support decision making, verbal and nonverbal communication, and expression of feelings. The CHN, in selecting the type of seating arrangement, needs to consider the group and its purpose. For example, if it is a committee meeting where note taking and decision making are required, a table and chairs are suggested; however, if it is a self-help group meeting, an open circle of chairs is suggested so that all members can see and hear each other. This latter approach is more likely to encourage expression of feelings (Dimock & Kass, 2007). It is important to meet the safety and security needs of group members through the group's emotional milieu. The CHN contributes to this emotional milieu by being welcoming and open to contributions from all members and being respectful and supportive, thereby increasing trust and decreasing member anxiety. This milieu encourages group members to participate, take risks, and share resources.

Group involvement refers to the degree of attraction and commitment by group members to the achievement of group goals. The extent of group member involvement is demonstrated by respecting group meeting times, group participation, and commitment to group work. Effective groups are groups in which members have been highly involved and have therefore developed group cohesiveness and solidarity. The CHN as group facilitator can encourage involvement by acknowledging the unique contributions to the group by members. The leadership style of the CHN can also contribute to group involvement when members are encouraged to take part in setting the group goals and processes.

Group interaction refers to how the group members connect and relate to each other. The physical and emotional climate has an impact on group interaction. Therefore, the CHN needs to influence the physical and emotional climate. The more frequent the interactions, the more likely it is that the groups will be productive. The CHN needs to assess the patterns of communication and the roles of group members to gain a sense of group interaction and intervene as needed.

Group cohesion is the attraction between individual members and the group, a sense of togetherness often described as a sense of "we-ness" (Boyd & Ewashen, 2008). Similarity among members tends to increase group attraction, whereas differences tend to decrease it. Groups that are supportive of their members, set and work toward the same goals, see themselves as a work group, work through challenges, and celebrate successes are often seen as a highly unified group. Often, group work is attractive to members when there are clearly stated group goals and the group is cohesive. Dimock and Kass (2007) identify cohesion as a product of the three previously described dimensions in a group. CHNs support group cohesion by assisting the group to identify its purpose. Also, the CHN can assess the extent that the group perceives itself and its sense of "we-ness."

Group productivity refers to the activities that a group uses to reach its task and process goals and therefore to accomplish maximum effectiveness. Productivity is a motivator for retaining group membership and maintaining positive group interaction. Leadership style and the sharing of group member roles influence productivity. The CHN needs to consider the leadership style in the group and also evaluate the group member roles and their influence on group productivity so that appropriate interventions can be implemented if required.

Group Development

As a group works together to meet its identified purpose, the group goes through a process in its development. Several theories about group development have been proposed. Tuckman (1965) and Tuckman and Jensen's (1977) classic five stages of group development will be discussed and are also briefly presented in Box 14-2. The first stage, *forming,* starts when the group has its first meeting. Usually group members are polite to each other and cautious about expressing their own opinions and feelings, so conflict is avoided. The group tends to take a task focus—for example, setting meeting times, clarifying its purpose, and setting the agenda for the next meeting. Stage 2, *storming,* occurs as the group works on the task and related issues and some comfort is established; feelings and thoughts are expressed by some group members with some of this expression possibly causing conflict over goals and procedures. Sometimes, this is referred to as "testing others." Some group members will be very silent during this expression of conflict. Some members are passive and others respond to the threat by expressing anger (Smith, Meyer, & Wylie, 2006). The perception of power and threat in the group may influence the kind of group member behaviour (Kamans, Otten, & Gordijn, 2010). *Norming,* the third stage, occurs when group members recognize the benefits of group work, and group members begin to accept differing members' viewpoints, skills, and experiences. A sense of "we-ness" exists. In an effective group, conflict is dealt with (Marquis & Huston, 2006). In stage 4, *performing,* the group works together, trust exists among members, the work gets done, and flexibility is evident (Marquis & Huston, 2006). Interdependence within the group is evident as task and maintenance roles are shared by group members. The group is described as effective and well-functioning. Although this stage is the aim of all groups, it is important to note that not all groups reach this stage. The final stage as identified by Tuckman and Jensen (1977) is *adjourning,* which occurs when, based on group evaluation, it is determined that the group purpose has been completed and therefore the group will be terminated. Although group members are satisfied with the group and its accomplishments, many or all group members recognize this potential loss of their group, experience the grieving process, and begin to withdraw from the task and emotional aspects of group interactions.

BOX 14-2 Five Stages of Group Development

- **Stage 1: Forming:** Group members, as strangers, focus on getting to know each other.
- **Stage 2: Storming:** Group members begin to express their feelings as real issues are focused on.
- **Stage 3: Norming:** Group members start to feel part of the group and recognize the benefits of the group reaching its goal.
- **Stage 4: Performing:** Group members focus on the group work with sharing of ideas in a supportive group environment.
- **Stage 5: Adjourning:** Group members recognize the need for termination of the group and therefore work toward completion of the tasks and disengage from other group members.

SOURCE: Based on Tuckman, B. W., & Jensen, M. A. C. (1977). Stages of small group development revisited. *Group and Organizational Studies, 2*(4), 419–427.

Group Roles

Task, maintenance, and nonfunctional roles may be assumed by group members as the group develops and works on its tasks. The use of these roles in the group can be facilitators or barriers to group functioning (Dimock & Kass, 2007) (see Table 14-2). Examining group roles, a part of group process, provides the CHN with an understanding of how well the group is functioning and meeting its work as a group. Part of group process includes task and maintenance functions. Task functions in a group help the group to work toward completion of the task and therefore reaching the identified purpose and goals. For example, in an effective group, a group member needs to assume the role of problem definer in order to ensure that the group gets started by clarifying the purpose of a group; an information seeker helps to clarify what some of the unclear areas are so that the group can keep working on the task. In task functions, the focus is on problem solving and decision making (Dimock & Kass, 2008). Maintenance functions in a group help to create a comfortable climate and facilitate group interaction. For example, in an effective group, an encourager, a maintenance role, provides praise to the group members for their contributions, and the maintenance role of compromiser helps to decrease group conflict. Nonfunctional roles are individual roles used in the group that hinder group cohesiveness and productivity. For example, the aggressor who verbally attacks other group members or makes jokes about the group task is likely to hinder the group process, and the dominator may take over the task and present their point of view as the best and only worthwhile way to proceed.

Group Norms

Group norms are the rules and standards that set the stage for how the group will proceed in reference to how decisions are made, how work is assigned, and what acceptable member behaviour is. For example, in an effective group, the norms could be these:

TABLE 14-2 Selected Examples of Roles Assumed in Groups

Type	Example	Explanation
Task roles	Problem definer	The purpose of the group is clarified and defined.
	Information seeker	Asks for factual information about group work, procedures, or suggestions made.
	Information giver	Offers information about group work, procedures, or suggestions.
	Opinion seeker	Asks for group members' opinions about group work.
	Opinion giver	Offers own opinions related to group work.
	Elaborator	Provides examples related to suggestions on how these might work.
	Recorder	Tracks in writing the activities and accomplishments of the group.
	Evaluator	Raises questions about group activities and accomplishments and compares to a standard.
	Feasibility tester	Checks for reality and how practical suggested solutions are.
Group-building and maintenance roles	Coordinator	Statements are clarified and related to previous comments made.
	Harmonizer	Mediates differences and attempts to reconcile these often by pointing out similarities in views.
	Encourager	Warm and responsive to viewpoints and conveys praise for contributions made.
	Orienter	Monitors so group stays focused and identifies departures from goals, procedures, etc. May make suggestions for improvements in group functioning.
	Follower	Listens and accepts suggestions of group members and expresses agreement.
	Compromiser	In a group conflict situation decides to go along with the group.
	Gatekeeper	Encourages participation and open communication by all group members.
	Commentator	Tracks in writing group process and conveys findings to the group.
Individual roles by group members (nonfunctional roles)	Blocker	Hinders group functioning by arguing, disagreeing, or not accepting ideas beyond reason or focusing on dead issues.
	Aggressor	Conveys disapproval of group members' beliefs or feelings.
	Digressor	Moves the group away for group work by moving away from the topic under discussion.
	Recognition seeker	Focuses attention on self.
	Dominator	Focuses on controlling and manipulating the group.
	Confessor	Expresses personal situation in the group.
	Help seeker	Focuses on self-weaknesses to gain group sympathy.
	Withdrawer	Uses behaviours to withdraw from group such as daydreams, whispering to another group member, or leaving the group temporarily.

SOURCES: Adapted from Dimock, H. G., & Kass, R. (2007). *How to observe your group* (4th ed.). Concord, ON: Captus Press; and Marquis, B. L., & Huston, C. J. (2006). *Leadership roles and management functions in nursing: Theory and application* (5th ed.). Philadelphia, PA: Lippincott, Williams & Wilkins.

- Members show respect and trust by actively listening to others' points of view.
- Members are transparent and avoid hidden agendas.
- Meetings start on time and end on time.
- Members are open, sharing positive and negative feelings about what is happening in the group.
- Members focus on the task so that the group's purpose and goals are reached.

- Members demonstrate accountability and responsibility to the group.

Group norms and rules often follow a standard form of decision making. *Robert's Rules of Order* addresses procedures on how to conduct a group meeting, covering topics about the order of business for the meeting such as approval of minutes and agenda setting.

All groups need to determine the decision-making process, such as consensus decision making, majority decisions, or leader-only or single-member-only decisions. Consensus decision making is the most difficult and most time-consuming method; however, all the resources in the group are used, each member has supported the decision, and therefore each member is committed to the decision, encouraging group solidarity. Decision making by majority vote is less time consuming, and those group members (the majority) who supported the decision will commit to it; however, those who did not support the motion or abstained may or may not be committed to the decision. If the decision making is by leader only or single member only, group support and commitment to follow through will vary depending on how much the group has put in into the decision and their support of the leader or individual member to make the decision. CHNs need to be cognizant of group norms and how to conduct meetings and need to use consensus decision making in groups whenever feasible.

Group Leadership

Leadership in a group refers to influencing and directing others and includes acts that assist the group to meet its goal(s) (Dimock & Kass, 2007) and influence group actions to maintain the group. Group leaders play an active role to help the group fulfill its purpose and goals (Boyd & Ewashen, 2008). Leaders are constantly attentive to the group process and facilitate it; they have to carefully decide when it is appropriate to intervene in the case of an individual or the group as a whole (Boyd & Ewashen, 2008). Strong leadership is essential for groups to function effectively. It may come from one person or may be shared by a number of people depending on the situation.

Some of the advantages of shared leadership are increased productivity, enhanced group cohesion, and satisfaction with group membership. The leader can assume various behaviours. Refer to Box 14-3 for some examples of leadership behaviours.

Leadership styles may vary; some examples of leadership styles are autocratic, laissez-faire, democratic, shared, bureaucratic, charismatic, task-oriented, people-oriented, situational, and transactional. In the early 1930s, Kurt Lewin introduced the first three different styles of leadership; the fourth leadership style was recently introduced by Pearce and Conger.

The first four leadership styles are most often used in health care and are briefly discussed next. First is an *authoritarian* leadership style, also referred to as paternalistic or autocratic leadership. In this style of leadership, the leader maintains control in the group; communication is from the leader to the members; coercion of the group members is the motivator; work demands and not work requests are made; decision making does not involve others; the leader makes the decisions; the leader is the "I" and the group members are the "you"; and punitive criticism is often used (Marquis & Huston, 2006). This leadership style is best used in situations where decisions need to be made quickly or when high productivity is needed. For example, this style of leadership is best used in emergency or crisis situations such as CHNs involved in disaster management circumstances, such as the SARS outbreak, or CHNs working on projects with short project deadlines, such as planning a vaccination program for the

BOX 14-3 Examples of Leadership Behaviours

- *Advising:* Providing direction on the basis of knowledgeable opinion
- *Analyzing:* Reviewing what has occurred as encouragement to examine behaviour and its meaning
- *Clarifying:* Checking the meanings of interaction and communication through questions and restatement
- *Confronting:* Presenting behaviour and its effects to the individual and the group to challenge existing perceptions
- *Evaluating:* Analyzing the effect or outcome of action or the value of an idea based on some standard
- *Initiating:* Introducing topics, beginning work, or changing the focus of a group
- *Questioning:* Encouraging analysis of a view or views through questions that support examination
- *Reflecting behaviour:* Giving feedback on how a certain behaviour appears to others
- *Reflecting feelings:* Naming the feelings that may be behind what is said or done
- *Suggesting:* Proposing or bringing an idea to a group
- *Summarizing*: Restating discussion or group action in brief form, highlighting important points
- *Supporting:* Giving emotionally comforting feedback that helps a person or group continue actions

SOURCE: Lassiter, P. G. (2006). Working with groups in the community. In M. Stanhope and J. Lancaster (Eds.), *Foundations of nursing in the community: Community oriented practice* (p. 306). St. Louis, MO: Mosby Elsevier.

H1N1 immunizations. although with this style of leadership group member frustration levels are reduced, so too are "creativity, self-motivation, and autonomy" (Marquis & Huston, 2006, p. 51), group cohesiveness does not develop, and members do not learn independence or value the benefits of group work.

Second is a *laissez-faire* leadership style, which is a nondirected delegative leadership style. In this style of leadership, the leader assumes little or no group control; permissiveness prevails; minimal or no direction is provided by the leader; two-way communication occurs among group members; decision making is shared by the group; the emphasis is on the "you" for the group; and criticism is usually withheld (marquis & huston, 2006). this leadership style is best used in situations when problem solving requires generating alternative solutions and when group members are self-directed and committed to the goal without strict time constraints—for example, a group of home health nurses brainstorming how best to address the shortage of long-term care beds in their community. This leadership style can encourage creativity and increase productivity when group members are self-directed and committed; however, it can result in group frustration, apathy, and loss of interest (Marquis & Huston, 2006).

The third leadership style is referred to as *democratic* or *participative* style leadership. In this style of leadership, the leader maintains some group control; communication is two-way; suggestions and guidance direct group members; group members are involved in decision making; the emphasis is on the "we" for the group; and constructive criticism is used (Marquis & Huston, 2006). This leadership style is best used in groups who meet for a long period of time, whose members have a variety of experiences, when coordination and cooperation is needed, and when thorough problem solving is required and promotes group member growth (Marquis & Huston, 2006). This style is time consuming, may be frustrating for group members looking for quick solutions, or can be ineffective if all group members are inexperienced, such as a PHN working with a school's student council to develop sexual-health curriculum content delivery strategies.

The fourth leadership style is referred to as *shared*- or *distributed*-style leadership. This is a recent leadership style that has not been well studied in practice (Barr & Dowding, 2008). In this style of leadership, there is a balance of power; there is a shared purpose or goal; leadership roles are shared so that group work is done; there is a working together with a "we"; there is shared communication among members, a collaborative decision-making process, and cooperative interactions; and constructive criticism is used (Pearce, Conger, & Locke, 2007; Woods, 2004). This leadership style is best used in groups that work together for an extended period of time, are knowledgeable, and are highly committed to the goal, and the group and group members are empowered,

CRITICAL VIEW

1. How can group leaders modify their leadership style to meet the needs of different groups?
2. What particular situations would warrant such a modification of leadership style?

which can lead to increased productivity, positive group climate, and group cohesiveness; however, this style takes more time and is frustrating for members looking for quick solutions or when some group members are looking to be the designated leader—for example, NPs involved in interdisciplinary primary health care team meetings organized to assess and plan client care in their community. The examples provided indicate that leadership styles need to vary depending on each situation.

Group Conflict

Conflict is an inevitable part of most group interactions, and most group members do not welcome conflict (Chinn, 2008; Dimock & Kass, 2007). Chinn (2008) maintains that there are ways to transform conflict. The three ways are these:

- Using the power of diversity, which refers to supporting flexibility, creativity, and diverse viewpoints
- Using the power of solidarity, which refers to incorporating variety within the group through sharing of leadership and promoting communication skill development
- Using the power of shared responsibility, which refers to group member accountability for their own actions, encouraging reflection and evaluation of self and group on the basis of concern for the group and individual members (Chinn, 2008)

The three types of conflict in groups are intrapersonal, interpersonal, and intergroup. *Intrapersonal conflict* refers to conflict that occurs within an individual (Barr & Dowding, 2008; Pangman & Pangman, 2010). For example, a CHN working with a group of teenagers regarding sexual health and pregnancy may not personally support abortion and therefore experiences internal conflict about providing information about this option and the available community clinics providing abortion (see the "Ethical Considerations" box on page 454). *Interpersonal conflict* refers to conflict between two or more people who have different values and beliefs (Barr & Dowding, 2008; Pangman & Pangman, 2010). For example, a home health nurse supports a palliative care client's decision to die at home; however, the family physician and the social worker both believe that

ETHICAL CONSIDERATIONS

A CHN working with a group of teenagers regarding sexual health and pregnancy does not personally support abortion.

Ethical principles that apply to this interpersonal conflict are the following:

- *Distributive or social justice.* This principle recognizes that all citizens have an equal opportunity in the benefits and burdens in society. When providing care, CHNs do not discriminate on the basis of a person's race, ethnicity, culture, political and spiritual beliefs, social or marital status, gender, sexual orientation, age, health status, place of origin, lifestyle, mental or physical ability, or socioeconomic status or any other attribute.
- *Veracity.* The principle of veracity identifies the need to be truthful, which promotes trust in the CHN–client relationship. CHNs are honest and practise with integrity in all their professional interactions.
- *Respect for autonomy.* CHNs, to the extent possible, provide persons in their care with the information they need to make informed decisions related to their health and well-being. They also work to ensure that health information is given to individuals, families, groups, populations, and communities in their care in an open, accurate, and transparent manner.
- *Respect for autonomy.* CHNs in their professional capacity relate to all persons with respect. The CHN permits the individuals to choose those actions and goals that fulfill their life plans.

Questions to Consider

1. The CHN finds in the course of working with teenagers that they do not share her beliefs about abortion. In relation to each of the ethical considerations discussed above, how should the CHN respond?
2. When working with this aggregate, what are some strategies CHNs can use to demonstrate integrity in their practice?

the client should be hospitalized. *Intergroup conflict* refers to conflict between two or more groups (Barr & Dowding, 2008; Pangman & Pangman, 2010). For example, a municipal council has decided to close a community swimming pool, and a Healthy-Community citizens group is opposing this decision.

Additionally, conflict in groups can occur because of relationship, task, and process difficulties. In relationships, interpersonal frictions can develop among group members due to their differing personalities. For example, some competitive group members disagree with each other on many different discussions and therefore have an impact on group dynamics. In task groups, friction occurs because of disagreement about the work to be done by the group. For example, conflicts occur when there are goal differences such as when some group members are reflective and want to defer decision making so more time can be spent reviewing the issue and other group member want a quick decision without further discussion. In this process, friction occurs because of disagreement about how to manage and complete the work. For example, all group members refuse to assume the role of recorder due to their time commitments, so it has been suggested that a secretary be used for this process. Some group members support the financing of this while others do not.

When conflict occurs within a group, a group response is needed if conflict is to be transformed (Chinn, 2008). Frequently, members try to deal with conflict in the group. Some common strategies used in a group are to avoid, compete, compromise, accommodate, or collaborate (Barr & Dowding, 2008). See Table 14-3 and Figure 14-1 for examples of group conflict resolution strategies. The order of the strategies flows from what is perceived as a very individual group member

CRITICAL VIEW

1. What have been your experiences in working with groups?
2. How has conflict been managed in the groups you have participated in?

FIGURE 14-1 Examples of Group Conflict Resolution Strategies

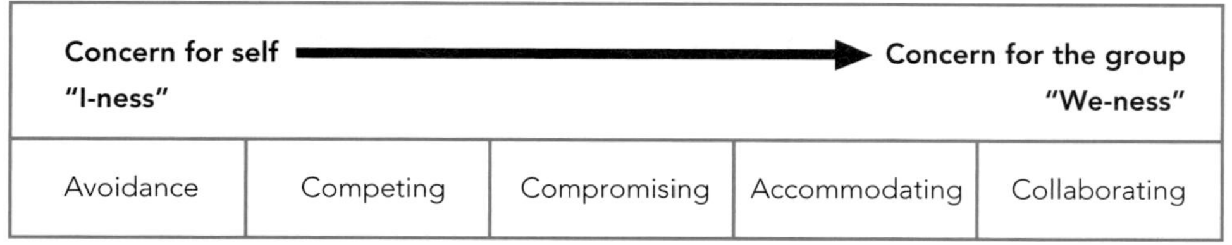

Based on Barr, J., & Dowding, L. (2008). *Leadership in health care.* Los Angeles, CA: Sage.

TABLE 14-3 Examples of Group Conflict Resolution Strategies

Type	Description	Example
Avoidance	Group members are aware of the conflict but do not address it.	Conflict has occurred and further discussion of this topic does not occur, with the group moving in another direction.
Competing	Some group members use power to have their own needs met rather than the needs of the group.	A newly established group trying to determine meeting times and frequency has members in conflict over availability. The leader in the organization uses power and states that they are available only on Tuesday mornings so that is when the meetings must be held.
Accommodating	Group members who are in conflict resolve the difference by one member cooperating and giving in to the other members for the benefit of the group.	Conflict has occurred between group members about group goals. The group members in the conflict situation agree to the suggested goals so that the team can move the task forward.
Compromising	Group members explore solutions to a conflict and negotiate a solution where members have equal gain.	Group A and Group B need to meet. The travel distance between the two groups is 200 km and neither group wants to spend the resources or time to travel. After considerable negotiation, both groups decide to meet halfway.
Collaborating	Group members examine the differences that exist and work together to establish an acceptable solution that is beneficial to all group members.	A group of community members at their first meeting are planning location of meetings, and a member suggests that travelling to the proposed meeting site is not equitable for all group members for time spent and resources spent to travel. Rotation of meeting sites among member agencies is suggested. The group discusses this idea and agrees to rotate the sites so that all members share in the travel expenses and time spent to get to meetings.

SOURCE: Based on Barr, J., & Dowding, L. (2008). *Leadership in health care*. Los Angeles, CA: Sage.

How To... Handle Group Conflict

- Remain calm and positive.
- Use direct and objective communication.
- Use positive body language and tone of voice.
- Focus on the problem not the group member(s).
- Recognize that outcomes of conflict can result in member and group growth.
- Group members need to express their feelings about the conflict without blaming. Start statements with "I feel. . . ."
- Group members need to clarify in a factual manner what happened in the conflict situation without blaming. Start statements with "When (such and such happened). . . ."
- Each group member shares (preferably seated in a circle) how they wish the group to proceed so the conflict situation is resolved. Start statements with "I want. . . ."
- Group members verbalize the mutually shared beliefs and agreements that are evident in the conflict situation and how the conflict situation will influence or positively change the group's principles of solidarity. Start statements with "Because. . . ."

SOURCE: Barr, J., & Dowding, L. (2008). *Leadership in health care*. Los Angeles, CA: Sage; and Chinn, P. L. (2008). *Peace and power: Creative leadership for building community* (7th ed.). Sudbury, MA: Jones and Bartlett.

focus to a focus on the group as a unit. See the "How To . . . Handle Group Conflict" box on how to handle group conflict.

Group Evaluation

The CHN when working with groups needs to observe and examine how the group is functioning to determine group effectiveness. Refer to Figure 14-2. The CHN could also have each group member complete this group evaluation form so that group strengths and weaknesses are identified and interventions initiated to improve group effectiveness. The group evaluation form can be used for the formative and summative evaluation of a group.

WORKING WITH HEALTH CARE TEAMS AND PARTNERS

Team Building

Team building is discussed in this chapter with reference to interdisciplinary teams. An interdisciplinary team consists of health care professionals with a variety of knowledge, skills, and areas of expertise. An interdisciplinary health care team consists of members such as CHN, client, physician, physiotherapist, occupational therapist, dietitian, and pharmacist. Since interdisciplinary teams are a group, team development follows the same stages as group development with the structure and processes of a group, and the team also experiences conflict. Since it is a group, it has a clearly stated team purpose and goals. A team often performs at an advanced level of unity than what is required of a group (Barr & Dowding, 2008). According to Kreitner, Kinicki, and Cole (2007) [cited in Pangman & Pangman, 2010], the goal of team building is to develop highly efficient teams that would demonstrate the following salient characteristics:

- Participative leadership—Empowers team members to promote team interdependence
- Shared responsibility—All team members take responsibility for team work
- Aligned on purpose—Team shares a common goal
- Strong communication—Develops an atmosphere of openness, respect, trust, honest communication among all team members
- Future focused—Change is seen as an opportunity for professional and personal growth
- Focused on task—Team is results-oriented by staying on task
- Creative talents—Each member's creativity and talents are encouraged and applied
- Rapid response—Possibilities are identified and acted upon

Yoder-Wise (2007) proposes that effective teams that are able to work together efficiently contribute to improved health care.

CHNs often fulfill the role of team facilitator. Based on the role of facilitator as described by Kelly and Crawford (2008), the CHN needs to reflect on the following questions:

- How has the atmosphere or environment contributed to successful team building?
- How have the team members demonstrated mutual respect, trust, and honesty with each other?
- How have team members actively participated in the problem-solving and decision-making work of the team?
- Is each team member familiar with the purpose, goal, and objectives of the team?
- How do all team members encourage and support creativity and new ideas?
- How productive is the team?
- How is the team progressing toward goal attainment?
- Do team meetings begin and end on time?
- How does the team leader motivate the team?
- How is the team vision promoted by the leader?

For information on health teams, see the Evolve Weblinks for the Health Council of Canada's "Teams in Action" and the Canadian Health Services Research Foundation's *Teamwork in Healthcare*, as well as the Physician Integrated Network "Primary Care Interdisciplinary Team Toolkit," found in the Tool Box on the Evolve Web site.

Partnerships

Partnerships are formed for a variety of reasons but some of the most common are to build capacity in the system in the most appropriate ways, for cost reduction and containment, to avoid duplication of services, to coordinate services, and to most effectively address client health

CRITICAL VIEW

1. What are some teams that the community health nurse would be a member of in your community?
2. What would be their main role and function?

FIGURE 14-2 Group Evaluation Form

GROUP EVALUATION FORM

Group: ______________________ Date: ______________________

Time: ______________________ Observer: ______________________

For each area, place an "X" in the box that most nearly describes the group.

1. **UNITY** (degree of unity, cohesion, or "we-ness")
   - ❒ Group is just a collection of individuals or subgroups; little group feeling.
   - ❒ Some group feeling. Unity stems more from external factors than from friendship.
   - ❒ Group is very close, and there is little room or felt need for other contacts and experience.
   - ❒ Strong common purpose and spirit based on real friendships. Group usually sticks together.
2. **SELF-DIRECTION** (group's own motive power)
   - ❒ Little drive from anywhere, either from members or designated leader.
   - ❒ Group has some self-propulsion but needs considerable push from designated leader.
   - ❒ Domination from a strong single member, a clique, or the designated leader.
   - ❒ Initiation, planning, executing, and evaluating comes from total group.
3. **GROUP CLIMATE** (extent to which members feel free to be themselves)
   - ❒ Climate inhibits good fun, behaviour, and expression of desire, fears, and opinions.
   - ❒ Members express themselves but without observing interests of total group.
   - ❒ Members freely express needs and desires: joke, tease, and argue to detriment of the group.
   - ❒ Members feel free to express themselves but limit expression to total group welfare.
4. **DISTRIBUTION OF LEADERSHIP** (extent to which leadership roles are distributed among members)
   - ❒ A few members always take leadership roles. The rest are passive.
   - ❒ Some of the members take leadership roles, but many remain passive followers.
   - ❒ Many members take leadership, but one or two are continually followers.
   - ❒ Leadership is shared by all members of the group.
5. **DISTRIBUTION OF RESPONSIBILITY** (extent to which responsibility is shared among members)
   - ❒ Everyone tries to get out of jobs.
   - ❒ Responsibility is carried by a few members.
   - ❒ Many members accept responsibilities but do not carry them out.
   - ❒ Responsibilities are distributed among and carried out by nearly all members.
6. **PROBLEM SOLVING** (group's ability to think straight, make use of everyone's ideas, and decide creatively about its problems)
   - ❒ Not much thinking as a group. Decisions made hastily, or group lets leader or worker do most of the thinking.
   - ❒ Some cooperative thinking, but group gets tangled up in pet ideas of a few. Confused movement toward solutions.
   - ❒ Some thinking as a group but not yet an orderly process.
   - ❒ Good pooling of ideas and orderly thought. Everyone's ideas are used to reach final plan.
7. **METHOD OF RESOLVING DISAGREEMENTS WITH GROUP** (how group works out disagreements)
   - ❒ Group waits for the designated leader to resolve disagreements.
   - ❒ Strongest subgroup dominates through a vote and majority rule.
   - ❒ Compromises are affected by each subgroup giving up something.
   - ❒ Group as a whole arrives at a solution that satisfies all members and that is better than any single suggestion.
8. **MEETS BASIC NEEDS** (extent to which group gives a sense of security, achievement, approval, recognition, and belonging)
   - ❒ Group experience adds little to the meeting of most members' needs.
   - ❒ Group experience contributes to some degree to basic needs of most members.
   - ❒ Group experience contributes substantially to basic needs of most members.
   - ❒ Group contributes substantially to basic needs of all members.
9. **VARIETY OF ACTIVITIES**
   - ❒ Little variety in activities—stick to same things.es.
   - ❒ Some variety in activities.
   - ❒ Considerable variety in activities. Try out new activities.
   - ❒ Great variety in activities. Continually trying out new ones.

(Continued)

10. DEPTH OF ACTIVITIES (extent to which activities are gone into in such a way that members can use full potentials, skills, and creativity)

- ❒ Little depth in activities—just scratching the surface.
- ❒ Some depth but members are not increasing their skills.
- ❒ Considerable depth in activities. Members able to utilize some of their abilities.
- ❒ Great depth in activities. Members find each a challenge to develop their abilities.

11. LEADER–MEMBER RAPPORT (relations between the group and the designated leader)

- ❒ Antagonistic or resentful.
- ❒ Indifferent toward leader. Friendship neither sought nor rejected. Noncommunicative.
- ❒ Friendly and interested. Attentive to leader's suggestions.
- ❒ Intimate relations: openness and sharing. Strong rapport.

12. ROLE OF THE LEADER (extent to which the group is centred around the designated leader)

- ❒ Activities, discussion, and decisions revolve around interests, desires, and needs of leader.
- ❒ Group looks to leader for suggestions and ideas. Leader decides when member gets in a jam.
- ❒ Leader acts as stimulator—suggests ideas or other ways of doing things. Helps group find ways of making own decisions.
- ❒ Leader stays out of discussion and makes few suggestions of things to do. Lets members carry the ball themselves.

13. STABILITY

- ❒ High absenteeism and turnover; influences group a great deal.
- ❒ High absenteeism and turnover; little influence on group growth.
- ❒ Some absenteeism and turnover with minor influence on group.
- ❒ Low absenteeism rate and turnover. Group very stable.

care concerns. A **partnership** is a relationship between individuals, groups, or organizations, in which the partners are actively working together in all stages of planning, implementation, and evaluation.

Interprofessional Partnerships

Some of the attributes found in the literature that contribute to effective interprofessional partnerships are the following:

- Each partner recognizes the purpose and the need for the partnership.
- A collegial relationship is valued, and partner members convey reciprocity, mutual respect, trust, genuineness, open communication, and equality and are committed to conflict management.
- Interdependency exists among partner members and includes sharing, cooperation, "presence of synergy," and flexible boundaries.
- Power and leadership are shared by the partners and are based on the knowledge and expertise of partners, and decision making is by consensus and is egalitarian (Butt, Markle-Reid, & Browne, 2008).

For effective and sustainable partnerships, some general principles need to be followed (refer to Box 14-4). CHNs need to be aware of these principles when working with partners. Partnerships and teamwork are types of collaboration (Butt, Markle-Reid, & Brown, 2008; Vollman, Anderson, & McFarlane, 2008). Collaboration is also involved when working in groups. Collaboration is defined as the commitment of two or more partners, such as agency, client, and professional, who are in a power-sharing partnership. Collaboration is differentiated from coordination and cooperation (Vollman et. al., 2008); however, they are interdependent and are necessary to build relationships in groups, teams, and partnerships. Vollman et al. (2008) include collaboration and partnership as links to strengthening community action, one of the Ottawa Charter strategies to reach Canada's population health goals. **Collaborative client-centred practice** is the active involvement of health care professionals from various disciplines working together collaboratively to improve client health outcomes. This model of health care practice facilitates improvement of population health; client health; access to health care; communication among health care professionals; client and health care professional satisfaction; and better utilization of human health care resources (Health Canada, 2004). For further information on interdisciplinary collaboration in primary health care, refer to the Enhancing Interdisciplinary Collaboration and Primary Health Care (EICP) Evolve Weblink *Interdisciplinary Primary Health Care: Finding the Answers—A Case Study Report.*

BOX 14-4 Some Principles for Effective and Sustainable Partnerships

- Partnership members discuss and agree on the mission, values, goals, outcomes, and activities.
- Partners agree that partnerships take time to develop.
- Communication between partners is clear, frequent, open, and evaluative.
- Social justice and equity will be considered in all communication and activities agreed to.
- Partner relationships are built on mutual respect, trust, caring, acceptance, and commitment.
- Partnerships work with strengths and assets and address weaknesses.
- Recognition of the diverse and vital contributions of partner members is acknowledged.
- Partners share resources and agree on power distribution and use within the partnership (power may not be equally distributed).
- All members agree to be partners, share the recognition for the successes, and accept responsibility for any associated risks.
- All partners review and determine partner roles and responsibilities.
- Flexibility in the partnership structure will allow for changing needs.

SOURCES: Centre for Addiction and Mental Health. (2008). *Recommendations of the Building Equitable Partnerships (BEP) symposium 2008*. Retrieved from http://www.camh.net/News_events/CAMH_Events/BEP%20Symposium%20Recommendations.pdf; Vollman, A. R., Anderson, E. T., & McFarlane, J. (2008). *Canadian community as partner: Theory & multidisciplinary practice* (2nd ed.). Philadelphia, PA: Lippincott, Williams, & Wilkins.

CRITICAL VIEW

Retrieve the following online document and answer the questions below:

Canadian Interprofessional Health Collaborative. (2010). *A National Interprofessional Competency Framework*. Available at http://www.cihc.ca/files/CIHC_IPCompetencies_Feb1210.pdf.

1. a) What is interprofessional collaboration?
   b) What are the essential prerequisites for effective collaboration to occur?
2. a) What are the interprofessional competencies necessary for the interprofessional collaboration?
   b) What is the National Competency Framework and its usefulness in community health nursing?

Retrieve the following online article and answer the questions below:

Takahashi, S., Brissette, S., & Thorstad, K. (2010). Different roles, same goal: Students learn about interprofessional practice in a clinical setting. *Nursing Leadership, 23*(1), 32–39. Available at http://www.longwoods.com/content/21727.

1. What are some of the key requirements for effective interdisciplinary practice?
2. a) What do you think are some of the benefits of interprofessional learning?
   b) What are some barriers to the provision of interprofessional education?

Interprofessional Education

Butt et al. (2008) have identified professional education as one of the systematic moderating factors in interprofessional health and social service partnerships. *Interprofessional education* (IPE) has been defined as "occasions when two or more professions learn with, from and about each other to improve collaboration and the quality of care" (Barr, Freeth, Hammick, Koppel, & Reeves, 2006, p.1).

An interprofessional health care education movement was introduced in Canada in 2003 (Health Canada, 2004). It focuses on IPE, providing the opportunity for learning with and about a variety of disciplines through students sharing their discipline perspectives in learning environments (Buring et al., 2009). There is some evaluation evidence that indicates the interprofessional education can lead to effective interprofessional partnerships, but further evaluative studies are needed (Freeth, Reeves, Koppel, Hammick, & Barr, 2005). For further information on evaluating interprofessional education partnerships, see the Freeth, Reeves, Koppel, Hammick, and Barr document entitled *Evaluating Interprofessional Education: A Self-Help Guide* in the Evolve Weblinks. It is believed that through this collaborative learning, graduates in health care will be better prepared to work in interprofessional partnerships such as the primary health care team.

This chapter has provided knowledge and skills that CHNs need to work effectively in partnership with health care professionals and clients. Health care reform in Canada has placed a greater emphasis on teams and partnerships as a future direction for community health care nursing practice. Therefore, it is vital that CHNs develop group and team building skills and initiate partnership development that is effective and sustainable.

STUDENT EXPERIENCE

Form a group of at least four students. You are part of a newly formed team of interagency health care partners from social and health agencies who have identified the issue of low literacy levels in their community. Community health assessment data that led to identification of this issue were higher population of newcomers, higher incidence of high school dropouts, lower educational levels in the community, higher unemployment rates, and poorer levels of health based on census data.

1. Identify who the key interagency partners are in this team. Each student member will assume a role for one of the identified agencies.
2. The overall team goal is to increase literacy in their community.
3. As a group of students, wearing an interagency hat, work together to assess and plan how your team will work together to meet this goal. Included in this planning should be consideration of the required group processes and team building, other partners that may need to be invited to join the team, and additional required assessment data, etc.
4. Evaluate how your team functioned using the Group Evaluation form (Figure 14-2).
5. Discuss the team task and maintenance roles assumed by group members and the effect on team functioning.

REMEMBER THIS!

- Working with diverse groups, teams, and partners is an important skill required in community health nursing.
- A group is a collection of two or more individuals in face-to-face interactions with a common purpose(s) and who are in an interdependent relationship.
- A team is a specialized group working toward a common goal or activity. CHNs work with interdisciplinary, multidisciplinary, and intradisciplinary teams.
- Interdisciplinary teams are often referred to as interprofessional.
- A partnership is a relationship between individuals, groups, or organizations, in which the partners are actively working together in all stages of assessment, planning, implementation, and evaluation.
- An interdisciplinary team contains members who have expertise from a variety of disciplines, such as nurses, CHNs, social workers, dietitians, physiotherapists, and physicians, and also includes the client in the assessment, planning, implementation, and evaluation of client care.
- An understanding of group process is important for CHNs.
- Group process refers to how the group as a unit is working and how group members interact with one another.
- The five dimensions of group climate, group involvement, group interaction, group cohesion, and group productivity can significantly influence group process.
- CHNs need to be familiar with the task, maintenance, and nonfunctional group roles and consider group norms and group leadership when working with groups, with teams, and in partnerships.
- Group conflict is inevitable and can result in growth of the group if handled effectively.
- Group and team evaluation is important when working in community health nursing practice.
- Team building is an essential skill for a CHN.
- CHNs need to consider the general partnership principles so that effective and sustainable partnerships can be developed and promoted.
- Collaboration is the commitment of two or more partners, such as agency, client, and professional, who are in a power-sharing partnership.
- Collaboration and partnership are linked to strengthening community action, one of the Ottawa Charter strategies to reach Canada's population health goals.
- Interprofessional education is necessary to promote collaborative client-centred practice.

REFLECTIVE PRAXIS

Case Study

Mark, a public health nurse (PHN), and Mary, a social worker, conduct parenting classes for parents of teenagers with discipline problems. The 2-hour class meets every Wednesday for 5 weeks. At the first class, Mark and Mary outline to the parents that the classes will cover areas such as how to enhance teen self-esteem; developing good decision-making skills; developing cooperation and successful attitudes; effective disciplining; and dealing with teens' angry and disruptive behaviours. At the beginning of each class, Mark and Mary ask the group if they have any questions or concerns they would like to discuss in the class. Generally, the first hour includes Mark and Mary lecturing with the aid of a PowerPoint presentation of key points and often includes video vignettes of parent–teen interactions. The second hour of the class is a group discussion of an assigned parenting challenge with some role playing on how to intervene with the challenge. During week 4, Andrea, a 33-year-old single parent of a 15-year-old daughter, starts to cry when the group is assigned the topic of handling angry disruptive teens. Andrea shares with the group that her daughter left home that evening in an angry state and will not be back. It is not the first time this has happened, but Andrea is worried because the first time her daughter left it was warmer weather. This time the weather is cold and she is worried about how her daughter was dressed and where she was going, as most of her friends do not live with their parents. Susan, a fellow group member, leans over and hugs Andrea and says, "I had that experience with my daughter 2 months ago and that is why I am here—to try and figure out how to cope with this type of situation. You're not alone. If you ever want to talk, we can meet at Tim Hortons for coffee anytime."

The discussion focuses on how to find support when it is needed and how to cope with a teen who leaves home when she is angry. Mark and Mary identify agencies in the area providing ongoing services for parents, such as discipline classes and educational support resources, as well as identify some 800-numbers that are 24-hour access providing telecounselling. The class ends on a positive note with the members agreeing to talk more about their worries and feelings about parenting at the start of the next class.

1. Identify the task and maintenance behaviours evident in this group meeting.
2. Identify Mark and Mary's roles in working with (a) parents and (b) group situations, such as the parenting classes. Find an evidence-informed article to direct and support your discussion about the role of the CHN in working with this client group.
3. Do you think that Susan's response to Andrea would be reassuring? Provide a rationale for your answer.
4. If you were the PHN in this situation, how would you handle the situation so that the group continues to move forward? Provide specific examples with rationales.

Answers are on the Evolve Web site at http://evolve.elsevier.com/Canada/Stanhope/community/.

What Would You Do?

1. Consider two groups where you are or have been a member. What is the stated purpose of each one? Are you aware of unstated but clearly understood purposes? How do members interact in each group? What task and maintenance roles are evident in each group?
2. Locate one article from a refereed journal for each of the following community health nursing practice areas:

- Home health nursing (VON and one private agency)
- Parish nursing
- Occupational health nursing
- Outpost nursing
- Primary health care nurse practitioner and acute care nurse practitioner (tertiary care)
- School nursing
- Telehealth nursing
- Public health nursing

In chart form, identify for each of these community health nursing practices the nursing roles and functions that relate to community health nursing. Bring your findings to class for further discussion.

TOOL BOX

The Tool Box contains useful instruments that can be applied in community health nursing practice. These related resources are found either in the appendices at the back of this book or on the Evolve Web site at http://evolve.elsevier.com/Canada/Stanhope/community/.

Appendices

Appendix 1: Canadian Community Health Nursing Standards of Practice

Tools

The Community Toolbox. Building Teams: Broadening the Base for Leadership.
This Tool Box site contains further links to sites with information, such as group facilitation, team building, and what makes a good team.

ELL ToolBox.
This Tool Box provides examples of activities that group members can practice to enhance their group skills, such as listening, providing clear directions, and information analysis.

Interprofessional Team Development for Diabetes Care—Discussion Paper.
The Diabetes Toolkit Task Group created this document to assist Family Health Teams in Ontario with guidelines on how to address chronic care management programs for diabetes from a primary care team perspective.

Physician Integrated Network. *Primary Care Interdisciplinary Team Toolkit.*
This tool kit provides fact sheets on various health care disciplines. These fact sheets provide an overview of some specific discipline information that may facilitate inclusion of that discipline as a partner member in a primary health care interdisciplinary team.

WEBLINKS

Direct links to these resources can be found on the text's accompanying Evolve Web site at http://evolve.elsevier.com/Canada/Stanhope/community.

Canadian Health Services Research Foundation. *Teamwork in Healthcare: Promoting Effective Teamwork in Healthcare in Canada: Policy Synthesis and Recommendations.* This site answers questions about teamwork, such as determining effectiveness, sustainability, and implementation. Challenges of building and maintaining teamwork are identified along with the current policy implications on teams.

Enhancing Interdisciplinary Collaboration and Primary Health Care (EICP). *Interdisciplinary Primary Health Care: Finding the Answers—A Case Study Report.* This comprehensive report provides information on a definition of interdisciplinary collaboration, how it is practised, and challenges; it also provides case studies and discussion.

Freeth, D., Reeves, S., Koppel, I., Hammick, M., & Barr, H. *Evaluating Interprofessional Education: A Self-Help Guide.* This comprehensive guide provides information with examples and questions to consider, to help with decision making about evaluation of interprofessional education. Information is also provided on evaluation tools and on interprofessional educational studies with a listing of additional Web sites.

Health Council of Canada. *Teams in Action: Primary Health Care Teams for Canadians.* This site provides information about primary health care teams in Canada and the positive effects of team-based care and includes five in-depth case studies of effective teams, with four representing Canada and one representing Finland.

REFERENCES

Barr, H., Freeth, D., Hammick, M., Koppel, I., & Reeves, S. (2006). The evidence base and recommendations for interprofessional education in health and social care. *Journal of Interprofessional Care, 20*(1), 75–78.

Barr, J., & Dowding, L. (2008). *Leadership in health care.* Los Angeles, CA: Sage.

Boyd, M. A., & Ewashen, C. (2008). Interventions with groups. In W. Austin, & M. A. Boyd (Eds.), *Psychiatric nursing for Canadian practice* (pp. 255–269). Philadelphia, PA: Lippincott, Williams & Wilkins.

Buring, S. M., Bhushan, A., Broeseker, A., Conway, S., Duncan-Hewitt, W., Hansen, L., & Westberg, S. (2009). Interprofessional education: Definitions, student competencies, and guidelines for implementation. *American Journal Pharmaceutical Education, 73*(4), 59–64.

Butt, G., Markle-Reid, M., & Browne, G. (2008). Interprofessional partnerships in chronic illness care: A conceptual model for measuring partnership effectiveness. *International Journal of Integrated Care, 8*(14). Retrieved from http://www.ijic.org/.

Centre for Addiction and Mental Health. (2008). *Recommendations of the Building Equitable Partnerships (BEP) symposium 2008*. Retrieved from http://www.camh.net/News_events/CAMH_Events/BEP%20Symposium%20Recommendations.pdf.

Chinn, P. L. (2008). *Peace and power: Creative leadership for building community* (7th ed.). Sudbury, MA: Jones and Bartlett.

Diem, E., & Moyer, A. (2005). *Community health nursing projects: Making a difference*. Philadelphia, PA: Lippincott, Williams & Wilkins.

Dimock, H. G., & Kass, R. (2007). *How to observe your group* (4th ed.). Concord, ON: Captus Press.

Dimock, H. G., & Kass, R. (2008). *Leading and managing dynamic groups* (4th ed.). Concord, ON: Captus Press.

Freeth, D., Reeves, D., Koppel, I., Hammick, M., & Barr, H. (2005). *Evaluating interprofessional education: A self-help guide*. London: Higher Education Academy Health Sciences and Practice Network. Retrieved from http://www.health.heacademy.ac.uk/publications/occasionalpaper/occp5.pdf.

Goleman, D., Boyatzis, R., & McKee, A. (2002). The emotional reality of teams. *Journal of Organizational Excellence*, *21*(2), 55.

Health Canada. (2004). *Interprofessional education for collaborative patient-centred practice: Research synthesis paper*. Retrieved from http://www.hc-sc.gc.ca/hcs-sss/hhr-rhs/strateg/interprof/synth-eng.php.

Kamans, E., Otten, S., & Gordijn, E. H. (2010). *Power and threat in intergroup conflict: How emotional and behavourial responses depend on amount and content of threat*. Group Processes and Intergroup Relations. Retrieved from http://gpi.sagepub.com/content/early/2010/09/03/1368430210372525.full.pdf + html1.

Kelly, P., & Crawford, H. (2008). *Nursing leadership and management* (first Canadian ed.). Toronto, ON: Nelson Education Ltd.

Lassiter, P. G. (2006). Working with groups in the community. In M. Stanhope, & J. Lancaster (Eds.), *Foundations of nursing in the community: Community oriented practice* (pp. 301–317). St. Louis, MO: Mosby Elsevier.

Marquis, B. L., & Huston, C. J. (2006). *Leadership roles and management functions in nursing: Theory and application* (5th ed.). Philadelphia: Lippincott Williams & Wilkins.

Mauk, K. (2009). *Gerontological nursing: Competencies for care*. Boston: Jones and Bartlett Publishers.

Maurer, F. A., & Smith, C. M. (2009). *Community/public health practice: Health for families and populations* (4th ed.). St. Louis, MO: Saunders Elsevier.

McCallin, A., & Bamford, A. (2007). Interdisciplinary teamwork: Is the influence of emotional intelligence fully appreciated? *Journal of Nursing Management*, *15*(4), 386–391.

Pangman, V. C., & Pangman, C. (2010). *Nursing leadership from a Canadian perspective*. Philadelphia, PA: Lippincott, Williams & Wilkins.

Pearce, C. L., Conger, J. A., & Locke, E. A. (2007). Theoretical and practitioner letters: Shared leadership theory. *Leadership Quarterly*, *18*, 281–288. Retrieved from www.sciencedirect.com.

Saltman, D. C., O'Dea, N. A., Farmer, J., Veitch, C., Rosen, G., & Kidd, M. R. (2007). Groups or teams in health care: Finding the best fit. *Journal of Evaluation in Clinical Practice*, *13*, 55–60.

Smith, D., Meyer, S., & Wylie, D. (2006). In J. M. Hibberd & D. L. Smith, *Nursing leadership and management in Canada* (3rd ed., pp. 519–547). Toronto, ON: Elsevier Canada.

Tuckman, B. (1965). Developmental sequence in small groups. *Psychological Bulletin*, *63*, 384–399.

Tuckman, B. W., & Jensen, M. A. C. (1977). Stages of small group development revisited. *Group and Organizational Studies*, *2*(4), 419–427.

Vollman, A. R., Anderson, E. T., & McFarlane, J. (2008). *Canadian community as partner: Theory & multidisciplinary practice* (2nd ed.). Philadelphia, PA: Lippincott, Williams & Wilkins.

Woods, P. A. (2004). Democratic leadership: Drawing distinctions with distributed leadership. *International Journal of Leadership in Education*, *7*(1), 3–26.

Yoder-Wise, P. S. (2007). *Leading and managing in nursing* (4th ed.). St. Louis, MO: Mosby Elsevier.

CHAPTER

15 Environmental Health

KEY TERMS

See Glossary on page 593 for definitions

OBJECTIVES

After reading this chapter, you should be able to:

1. Describe the various environmental pollutants that can influence the quality of the environment.
2. Explain how the environment, as a determinant of health, influences human health and disease.
3. Describe how environmental ethics and justice influence the health status of Canadians.
4. Explain the role of the community health nurse in environmental health.
5. Apply the community health nursing process to the practice of environmental health.
6. Identify Canadian legislative and regulatory policies that have influenced the effects of the environment on health and disease patterns.
7. Describe the skills needed by community health nurses practising in environmental health and be prepared to apply them in practice.

CHAPTER OUTLINE

In watching diseases, both in private homes and in public hospitals, the thing which strikes the experienced observer most forcibly is this, that the symptoms or the sufferings generally considered to be inevitable and incidental to the disease are very often not symptoms of the disease at all, but of something quite different—of the want of fresh air, or of light, or of warmth, or of quiet, or of cleanliness, or of punctuality and care in the administration of diet, of each or of all of these. (Nightingale, 1859, p. 8)

The environment is as influential on health in this century as it was in previous centuries. The environment is everything around us, and our lives depend largely on its quality. Much of our time is spent in our home, school, workplace, and community environments. Often we take the environment for granted and fail to see the hazards in front of us. For example, how many of us know for certain that our drinking water is safe or that the air we breathe is free from pollutants that aggravate our individual respiratory functions? If children are in the home, are all the toxic cleaning materials and insecticides out of reach? In recent years, environmental health issues have increased in Canada—for example, the contaminated water supplies in Walkerton, Ontario, and North Battleford, Saskatchewan. Another issue is greenhouse gas (GHG) emissions, which rose 24% from 1990 to 2003, with Alberta and Ontario having the highest emissions of all provinces in 2003, and the provinces with the highest percentage increases in emissions since 1990 being Saskatchewan, New Brunswick, and Alberta (Statistics Canada, 2006). As a result, the Public Health Agency of Canada (PHAC), in 2004, announced the establishment of a National Collaborating Centre for Environmental Health (PHAC, 2005). Also, in 2004, the Government of Canada (Environment Canada, Statistics Canada, and Health Canada) promised to establish federal indicators for GHG emissions as well as air and water quality so that Canadians would have dependable information about their environment and links to human activity (Statistics Canada, 2005). The 1999 National Consensus Conference on Population Health Indicators identified the health indicators connected to environmental factors, such as air quality, water quality, exposure to second-hand smoke, toxic waste, and ecological footprint, and recommended that these factors required future research and monitoring (Pong, Pitblado, & Irvine, 2002). In 2004, the Government of Canada initiated annual reporting on Canadian indicators for air quality, GHG emissions, and fresh water quality (Environment Canada, 2006a). Exposure to environmental hazards in the air, water, and soil can contribute to illnesses, particularly in children and young adults, such as cancers, asthma, and birth defects (Canadian Partnership for Children's Health and Environment, 2008). The psychosocial environment also contributes to the morbidity and mortality of Canadians. Some examples of psychosocial environmental hazards are stress in the workplace, violence in the home, and bullying in the school setting. Therefore, it is critical that collaborative intersectoral environmental partnerships be formed to explore ways of reducing modern and traditional environmental health hazards that would improve the health of Canadians and people globally because of the connected ecosystem that exists.

CRITICAL VIEW

1. a) Community health nurses practise within a sociopolitical environmental context. What are the implications for community health nursing practice in environmental health?
   b) How do the Canadian Community Health Nursing Standards of Practice address environmental health?
2. How would a socioecological model be used by community health nurses to address environmental health issues?

Many of the environmental pollutants are known or suspected *neurotoxins*—that is, toxins that destroy nerves or nervous tissue. It is important that there be an awareness of environmental hazards such as food contaminants. Community health nurses (CHNs) need to consider aspects of food consumption and other environmental pollutants by questioning the following: Are people in the community eating above the Health Canada recommended servings of fish such as shark, swordfish, and fresh or frozen tuna that are known to contain high mercury levels? What toxic exposures can be identified in homes? What pesticides are used in homes and in the community? Are the homes old, possibly containing lead-based paint and lead pipes? Is the paint chipping or peeling, or are home renovations being done? Have homes been tested for radon gas levels? Is medical equipment containing mercury, such as mercury thermometers and sphygmomanometers, still being used? What environmental hazards might be present in workplaces?

In the air we breathe, the water we drink, the food we eat, and the products we use, we are exposed to chemical, biological, and radiological elements that affect our health. CHNs need to know how to assess for environmental health risks and develop educational and other health promotion interventions to help clients understand and, where possible, decrease the risks. CHNs also need to be aware of the effect of the forces of globalization on the environment. This chapter provides information that will assist CHNs with addressing environmental hazards and provides an introduction to the concepts of environmental health, environmental hazards and impacts, environmental assessment and referral, and the role of the CHN in environmental health.

CRITICAL VIEW

1. a) What are some examples that would demonstrate an individual approach to improving environmental health?

   b) What are some examples that would demonstrate a population approach to improving environmental health?
2. What are some possible roles for the community health nurse on environmental issues using health promotion strategies as outlined in the Ottawa Charter for Health Promotion?

ENVIRONMENT AND HEALTH

In order to work with environmental health issues, CHNs need to understand some basic terms and concepts, such as *environment, environmental health, climate change, toxicology, epidemiology,* and *environmental principles.* The **environment** can be defined as all those factors internal and external to the client that constitute the context in which the client lives and works that influence and are influenced by the host and agent–host interactions—the sum of all external conditions affecting the life, development, and survival of an organism. With reference to hazards found in the work or nonwork environment, the CHN needs to consider the different environmental hazards clients are exposed to that affect their health. **Environmental health** is defined as the achievement of health and wellness and the prevention of illness and injury from the exposure to physical or psychosocial environmental hazards. **Climate change** refers to a change in weather patterns over time in a geographic area related to changes in the amount of GHGs and can be the result of natural or human causes.

CRITICAL VIEW

Dr. Margaret Chan, Director-General of the World Health Organization, stated: "Climate change is one of the greatest challenges of our time . . . and will affect, in profoundly adverse ways, some of the most fundamental determinants of health: food, air, water" (Chan, 2007).

1. What have been some of the impacts of climate change in your community?
2. Who are the community partners working together to address these environmental impacts?

The physical environment is an important determinant of children's health and well-being; therefore, when children experience ill health due to a poor physical environment, their quality of life is affected (Commission for Environmental Cooperation, 2006). In 2002, the environment ministers of Canada, Mexico, and the United States agreed to protect children from environmental risks. They set a "cooperative agenda" between the three countries to select and publish a foundational set of indicators for North America of children's health and the environment (Commission for Environmental Cooperation, 2006). The first report (see the "Government of Canada" link in the Evolve Weblinks) was released in 2006 as a result of this cooperative agenda; it outlined the available environmental health indicators and measures for Canada. This Canadian research report contains case studies on subpopulations of children who may be unreasonably affected by environmental contaminants. The report also provides extensive information on the environmental health indicators related to the health of children, such as air pollution; lead and other chemicals, including pesticides; drinking water; and water-borne diseases. The Canadian Nurses Association (CNA) publication *The Environment and Health: An Introduction for Nurses* (see the Evolve Weblinks) provides an excellent background of environmental issues and implications for nurses with one area of focus being exposure to lead among children and its impact on children's health. Minimizing exposure to lead from contaminant sources such as water, home renovations, arts and crafts items, consumer products, and soil usually involves educating children and parents on its harmful effects.

Toxicology is the science that studies the poisonous effects of chemicals. **Poisons** are toxic substances that cause injury, illness, or death to humans and other organisms. For example, **acid rain,** a toxic material found in the environment and originating from the atmosphere, releases toxic substances such as aluminum into the soil; aluminum is toxic to trees and fish (U.S. Environmental Protection Agency, 2007) and therefore if ingested by humans can lead to illness and possibly death. For further information on acid rain, see the Environment Canada and U.S. Environmental Protection Agency Weblinks on the Evolve Web site. The Environment Canada Web site is organized in a question-and-answer format and provides information on what acid rain is, where it is a problem in Canada, and the sources of emissions that contribute to acid rain. For example, Eastern Canada is more affected by acid rain, and certain provinces are more greatly affected because of their topography because hard-rock areas cannot effectively neutralize the acid rain naturally. The U.S. Environmental Protection Agency Web site elaborates on some areas discussed at the Canadian site and provides a pictorial view of the affects of the gases that contribute to acid rain.

Pollution sources are characterized as point or nonpoint sources. A pollutant from a **point source** is released into the environment from a single site, such as a smokestack, a hazardous waste site, or an effluent pipe into a waterway. **Hazardous waste** is any waste material that poses actual or potential harm to the environment and to humans. A **nonpoint source** of pollution is more diffuse—for example, traffic, fertilizer, or pesticide runoff into waterways (whether from large-scale farming operations or from individual lawns and gardens). Another nonpoint source is animal waste, from wildlife or confined animal operations for food production (e.g., swine, poultry), that can get into nearby water bodies, resulting in coliform contamination and nutrient overload.

Climate change such as global warming is an environmental issue. Air pollution and GHGs in our environment markedly influence population health. For example, epidemiological studies have concluded that exposure to air pollution increases a population's risk for cardiovascular and respiratory diseases; air pollution contributes to more than 5,000 premature deaths per year in Canada; and annually in Ontario approximately 60,000 visits to the emergency department and approximately 17,000 hospital admissions are attributable to air pollution (Environment Canada, 2009b). It is important to understand the health effects of climate change on the health of Canadians and possible future implications. For further information, see the Health Canada "Environmental and Workplace Health" Weblink on the Evolve Web site.

GHGs are naturally occurring gases in the atmosphere that assist in regulating the earth's temperatures for habitation. The GHGs are water vapour, ozone, carbon dioxide, methane, and nitrous oxide. GHGs are produced from sources such as the agricultural sector, transportation sector, and industrial sectors. See the Environment Canada "Information on Greenhouse Gas Sources and Sinks" Weblink on the Evolve Web site, which provides information on various GHG sources such as the oil and gas industry, electric power generation sites, transportation emissions, and sinks. A **sink** is "any process, activity or mechanism which removes a greenhouse gas, an aerosol, or a precursor of a greenhouse gas from the atmosphere" (Environment Canada, 2006b, p. 1).

You may be well informed about environmental issues; however, did you know the following:

- One city bus can take 40 vehicles off the road.
- One city bus can save 70,000 litres of fuel.
- One city bus can keep 168 tonnes of pollutants out of the atmosphere each year.
- On-road vehicles contribute up to 35% of the emissions involved in smog formation.
- On-road vehicles contribute up to 19% of Canada's total GHG emissions (Environment Canada, 2009b, p. 1).

Further facts can be found at the Environment Canada Weblink on the Evolve Web site.

At the United Nations Framework Convention held in Kyoto, Japan, in 1997, the Kyoto Protocol on Climate Change was developed with the goal to decrease GHGs emissions globally (Environment Canada, 2006b). In 1998, Canada signed the Kyoto Protocol and ratified it in 2002; and in 2005, it became a legally binding agreement (Environment Canada, 2006b). Under this agreement, Canada committed to reduce GHG emissions between 2008 and 2012 to a level of 6% below 1990 levels.

The Canadian federal government increased its commitment to a 20% reduction target by 2020 of GHG emissions from the 2006 levels (Environment Canada, 2009c). To reach this target, its action plan, called "Eco-Action on Climate Change and Air Pollution" (see the Government of Canada Weblink on the Evolve Web site), outlined reduction targets by the years 2012 to 2015 with specific caps for the various air pollutants and GHGs. Indoor pollutants were also considered. The cost implications, health benefits, and the responsibilities for Canadians are also briefly discussed. For example, incentives are provided to assist Canadians to improve their homes so indoor quality of air is improved. Some proposed health benefits of these new government actions are decreased incidence of respiratory and cardiovascular diseases and decreased hospital admissions.

In the Government of Canada document *Turning the Corner: Regulatory Framework for Industrial Greenhouse Gas Emissions,* additional stringent industrial regulatory targets to reduce GHGs were outlined (Government of Canada, 2008b). These targets were set as a result of in-depth consultations with the various stakeholders.

Globally, 2% of the total GHG emissions annually are produced by Canada (Environment Canada, 2009a). Canada has initiated some partnerships globally to address climate change issues (Government of Canada, 2009). However, many environmentalists agree much more needs to be done to reduce GHG emissions and address climate change.

Despite Canada's efforts to deal with environmental issues, in 2009 Canada ranked near the bottom (15th out of 17 countries) for its overall environmental performance (Conference Board of Canada, 2009). Only Australia and the United States were of lower ranking. Geography and its industrial structures were considered to affect the performance of these lower-ranking three countries, but it was identified that overall "Canada is not taking the necessary steps toward environmental sustainability" (Conference Board of Canada, 2009, p. 2). It also reported that Canada has improved in air quality—that is, less acid rain and smog—and has decreased its energy intensity, but emissions and waste generation per capita are the highest in the world.

Some debate exists as to whether climate change is actually occurring at a faster rate than would normally be expected. One school of thought supports the belief that climate change is real and affects the environment and health of the population globally. For example, proponents such as David Suzuki propose that if we continue to live as we currently do and to pollute the environment, our future generations will be immensely affected negatively with regard to climate changes. Conversely, others adhere to the school of thought that climate change is happening at a usual, expected rate and is minimally affecting the environment and the health of populations globally. Suzuki refers to these proponents as the "skeptics" of climate change (David Suzuki Foundation, 2009). Claims have been made that proponents of this latter group are members of industries or have been funded by industries that are contributing to pollution and the resultant negative environmental changes (David Suzuki Foundation, 2009).

Humans' ecological and environmental footprint measures their consumption of natural resources and the waste absorption of the earth's ecosystem over a specific time frame. Carbon footprints are a subset of ecological footprinting; the term refers to a measurement of carbon dioxide emitted during a specific time frame. Footprinting allows countries to monitor their annual use of resources to determine if their consumption of resources exceeds the earth's ability to regenerate. If consumption of resources continues at the current levels, the earth will be unable to meet the resource demands. If interventions are introduced early enough, ecological assets can be used more effectively to sustain the ecosystem. For further information on ecological and environmental and carbon footprinting, see the Global Footprint Network in the Weblinks on the Evolve Web site.

It is important to consider how environmental exposures affect community members. For example, children are more vulnerable to virtually all pollutants. The most vulnerable to food-borne and water-borne pathogens are immunocompromised persons such as (1) those infected with human immunodeficiency virus (HIV), (2) those who have acquired immunodeficiency syndrome (AIDS), (3) those who are taking chemotherapeutic drugs, and (4) those who are organ recipients. When assessing a community's environmental health status, it is important to review the general health status of the community to identify members who may have higher risk factors and to assess the environmental exposures.

Knowing about chemicals and being able to use that information in practice can seem like a huge task. Fortunately, chemicals can be grouped into families, and it is possible to understand the actions and risks associated within these groups. The following are group examples:

- Metals and metallic compounds such as arsenic, cadmium, chromium, lead, and mercury
- Hydrocarbons such as benzene, toluene, ketones, formaldehyde, and trichloroethylene
- Irritant gases such as ammonia, hydrochloric acid, sulphur dioxide, and chlorine
- Chemical asphyxiants that include carbon monoxide, hydrogen sulphide, and cyanides
- Pesticides such as organophosphates, carbamates, chlorinated hydrocarbons, and bipyridyls

As you may recall, *epidemiology* is the science that helps us understand the strength of an association between exposures and health effects in human populations. For example, the Maternal-Infant Research on Environmental Chemicals (MIREC) national longitudinal study was conducted between 2008 and 2010 with approximately 2,000 pregnant women from across Canada (Canadian Partnership for Children's Health and Environment, 2008). This epidemiological study explored associations between exposure during pregnancy and lactation and specific environmental chemicals.

Environmental epidemiology, a useful tool for CHNs, is the study of the effect on human health of physical, chemical, and biological factors in the external environment. By examining specific populations or communities exposed to different ambient environments, environmental epidemiology seeks to clarify the relationships between physical, chemical, and biological factors and human health. Environmental epidemiology explains risks such as the risk of respiratory illness resulting from exposure to forest fire particulate matter (Moore et. al., 2006); risk of various cancers in humans related to several pollutants (Boffetta, 2006); and the risk of respiratory disease due to exposure to outdoor air pollutants (Curtis, Rea, Smith-Willis, Fenyves, & Pan, 2006). Environmental surveillances, such as childhood lead registries, use epidemiological methods to track and analyze incidence, prevalence, and health outcomes. Exposure to lead can cause premature births, learning disabilities in children, hypertension in adults, and other health problems (Shah, 2003). Factors contributing to the reduction of lead levels in Canada include the reduction of lead in gasoline, a reduction in the number of manufactured food and drink cans and household plumbing components containing lead solder, lead-screening laws, and the elimination of lead in paint and lead paint–abatement programs in communities. It is important to note that lead-based paint is found only in older homes, and lead in gasoline is used only in older vehicles. In addition, often plumbing used for the water supply in older homes was lead based. Therefore, older homes need to be assessed for the use of lead products, such as paint and pipes. **Surveillance** is systematic and ongoing observation and collection of data concerning disease occurrence to describe phenomena and detect changes in frequency or distribution. CHNs need to be aware of their environment and recognize the value of their observations in contributing to an increased awareness of any abnormal or unusual disease phenomena that may need to be studied further.

An **environmental scan** assesses both the internal and external environments and is frequently used by researchers to assess population health issues; by organizations to develop, evaluate, and revise programs; and by policy makers to address social, economic, technological, and political issues (Graham, Evitts, & Thomas-MacLean, 2008). An environmental scan assesses the internal requirements and assets of a community (micro level) along with assessing the environment external to the community (meso and macro levels). The information provided by an environmental scan is used to identify whether adequate internal resources are available to achieve goals or to identify priorities. The internal environmental scan includes looking at community resources such as people, education, employment, housing, leisure, geography, and culture. The external environmental scan looks at what affects a community at the following levels: regional, provincial, territorial, national, and global. Information gathered that affects communities should include policies, economic climate, environmental factors, social (population and lifestyle trends), and technological factors, or what is known as a **PEEST** analysis (Public Health Agency of Canada, 2009). A PEEST analysis can be organized into a **SWOT** format, which identifies Strengths(S), Weaknesses(W), Opportunities (O), and Threats (T) for a community. Further information on the SWOT analysis and environmental scan can be found on the Health Canada Web site "Situational Analysis," listed in the Weblinks. The term *environmental scan* is used in various ways and is sometimes used instead of the term *community assessment.* For an example of development and use of an environmental scan, visit the B.C. Injury Research and Prevention Unit Weblink on the Evolve Web site.

CRITICAL VIEW

1. a) How would a community health nurse work with an epidemiologist to conduct an environmental scan?
   b) What other community partners would be involved as team members in conducting an environmental scan?
2. How would this collaboration be initiated by the community health nurse?

As discussed in Chapter 3, three major epidemiological concepts are agent, host, and environment, which form the classic epidemiological triangle (see Chapters 3 and 8). An *agent* is a causative factor invading a susceptible host through an environment favourable to produce disease, such as a biological or chemical agent. A *host* is a living human or animal organism in which an infectious agent can exist under natural conditions. The epidemiological triangle model belies the often complex relationships among *agent,* which may include chemical mixtures (i.e., more than one agent); *host,* which may refer to a community spanning different ages, genders, ethnicities, cultures, and disease states; and *environment,* which may include dynamic factors such as air, water, soil, and food, as well as temperature, humidity, and wind. This epidemiological triangle when applied to avian influenza (commonly known as "bird flu") would depict the initial host as the bird (most common in fowl such as ducks, geese, and chickens), the agent as the avian influenza virus H5N1, and the environment as the place of interaction (an example of a geographical environment would be Fraser Valley, British Columbia). Avian flu may be passed to humans through contact with infected poultry or contaminated surfaces. In bird-to-human transmission, the host is the person, the agent is the avian influenza virus H5N1, and the environment is the place of interaction (e.g., China, Indonesia, Thailand, Vietnam, or Egypt). Refer to Box 15-1 for other examples of the application of the epidemiological triangle.

Interdisciplinary practice makes it unnecessary for the CHN to be an in-depth expert in environmental science, and it is important that the CHN collaborate with other environmental team members such as environmental health inspectors, epidemiologists, and microbiologists. CHNs, however, need to have knowledge of four environmental principles, and how they explain environmental threats to health is important. A discussion of each of the four environmental principles with some examples follows.

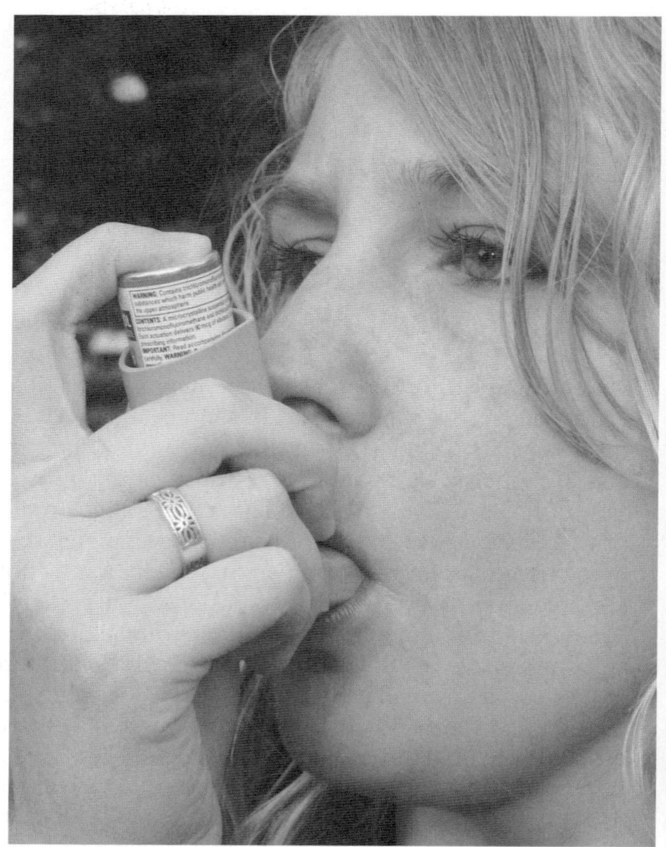

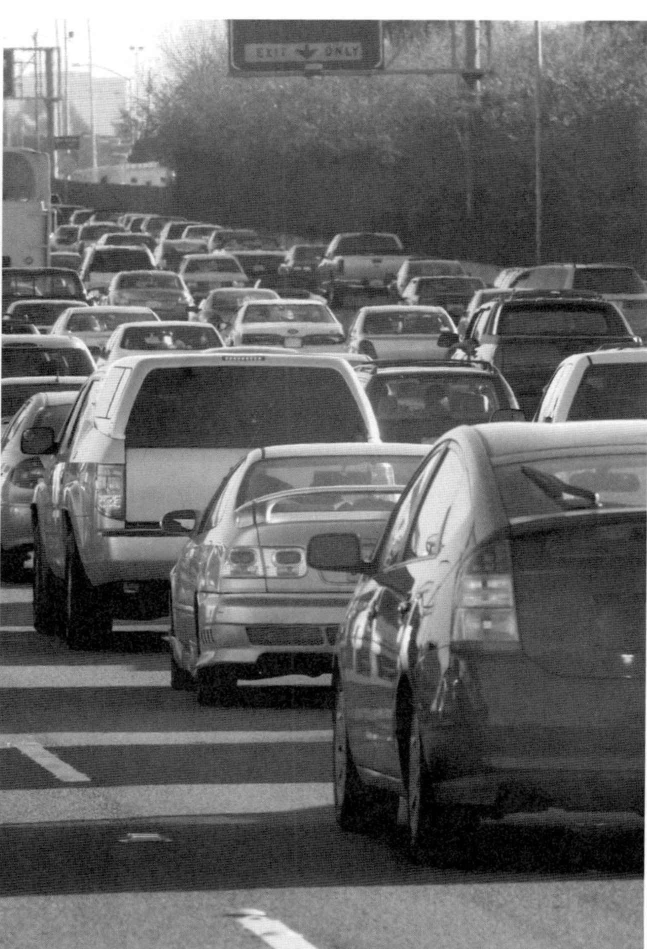

Environmental epidemiology is the study of the effect on human health of physical, chemical, and biological factors in the external environment. Air pollution caused by vehicle emissions and other sources contributes to many health concerns, including the increasing prevalence of respiratory problems such as asthma.

BOX 15-1 Environmental Health Examples Using the Agent–Host–Environment Triad

Agent	Host	Environment
Speeding automobile	Intoxicated drivers	Poor street lighting; unenforced speed limits
Poor-fitting shoes	Older adult with impaired vision and decreased muscular agility	Inadequate lighting; stairs
High-powered snowmobiles	Young adult risk-taking males	Early spring unsafe ice conditions on lakes
High-caloric consumption; sedentary lifestyle	Children	Access to high-caloric foods; lack of nutritional information; peer pressure
Tobacco	Youth	Peer pressure; access to tobacco products; unclear health messaging

Environmental Principle 1: Everything Is Connected to Everything Else

The principle that everything is connected to everything else is introduced in elementary-school science when students are taught about the water cycle of evaporation and condensation. Lead in paint is a good example: although it is banned, it is still present in older homes in poorer neighbourhoods and in restored homes in more affluent communities. When lead-containing paint chips are sanded and scraped, they become airborne in breathing space for a brief time and then end up on the floor or in nearby soil. Children play in these areas, where their hand-to-mouth activity results in exposure to lead, which has developmental and behavioural effects. In Canada, unborn children and children up to the age of 6 years are at a greater risk of the negative health effects of even low levels of lead (Health Canada, 2008a; Shah, 2003). The remedies for lead contamination have a required chain of their own: education for prevention, screening (of both the victim and the source), treatment (in the individual and the environment), and authority for regulatory and remedial action in public policy. The principle of connectedness is the essence of tracking exposures and risks (see Box 15-2). It is significant to know that simply the presence of a contaminant at a site does not automatically constitute a risk. In order for a risk to exist, the following conditions must be met: (1) the presence of contaminants that can cause toxic or adverse biological effects and (2) exposure pathways (a route a contaminant may take to come in contact with a receptor) by which receptors (person, animal, or plant) may be exposed to the contaminants. A single contaminant could follow a few exposure pathways; for example, contaminants in the soil may be inhaled, absorbed through the skin, ingested directly, or ingested indirectly after accumulating in food grown on site. A risk assessment would evaluate this interaction at a specific site and determine the resulting risk.

BOX 15-2 Environmental Harm

For persons to be harmed by something in the environment, several factors must be in place and connected:

- A source of harm that has chemical or physical properties
- An environmental medium for transport—air, water (surface or groundwater), or soil
- A receptor population within the exposure pathway for harm to human health
- A route of exposure—humans can be exposed to environmental contaminants through only three routes: inhalation, ingestion, and skin absorption
- An adequate amount (dose) of the chemical to result in human harm

Environmental Principle 2: Everything Has to Go Somewhere

The principle that everything has to go somewhere means that matter cannot be created or destroyed. Once waste products are generated, they must be disposed of in one of the following three ways:

1. *Incineration.* Burning can change the chemical composition through heat, but the products of burning, such as ash and air emissions, must be controlled and disposed of in one of the following two options.
2. *Water discharge.* To interrupt the exposure pathway, the products to be disposed of in water must be treated to ensure that the dose in the water is not great enough to do harm.
3. *Placement in a landfill or burial in the soil.* Protections must be put in place, such as liners and leachate pumps and monitors, to avoid seepage of harmful doses into groundwater or air.

Each of the options for waste disposal is intended to either provide a way to alter the waste product to a less toxic form through chemical intervention (biodegradation) or store the product in a bio-unavailable form or place. Because both the options for disposal can be a problem, prevention is desirable.

One additional point of emphasis is that human effects are intensified in the most sensitive, vulnerable environments, such as estuaries and the nurseries for much of sea and coastal plant and animal life. Some of the most valued food sources are also the most sensitive to pollution. Shellfish are very efficient filters of contaminants in the water in which they live. For example, oysters filter and retain almost all contaminants from the water in which they grow. It is impossible to rid them of contaminants after harvesting. The only protection for humans is to grow oysters in environments free from harmful contamination. Safe seafood depends on clean water. This example leads to the third principle.

Environmental Principle 3: The Solution to Pollution Is Dilution

Reflecting on the element of dose in human exposure reveals the truth in environmental principle 3: the solution to pollution is dilution. The use of this principle can be seen in historical environmental and sanitation measures. Garbage was moved from streets to the nearest body of water. Early industries went from dumping wastes outside their buildings to piping them to the nearest stream or river. Human wastes followed the same paths and pipelines. The problem with this principle is that it was tied to a world view that saw the environment as an unlimited resource, a limitless repository for whatever was useless. The dilution capacity of large rivers and certainly the ocean seemed boundless. The belief in the capacity of air to dilute resulted in such "solutions" as taller smokestacks to release pollutants higher into the atmosphere. The reality, which becomes more evident every day, is that this planet's capacity to assimilate by-products of human civilization is far from limitless. It is, in fact, fragile and delicately balanced, and the knowledge and practice about how to live peacefully within that balance without doing harm is far from adequate. The fourth principle reflects this insight.

Environmental Principle 4: Today's Solution May Be Tomorrow's Problem

Environmental principle 4 states that today's solution may be tomorrow's problem. As in almost every aspect of life, environmental scientists and regulators are dealing with incomplete information and insufficient science. The brief history of organized environmental protection is filled with examples. Garbage that went from the streets into unlined landfills is now a source of groundwater contamination. Gasoline tanks that were buried underground to avoid an ugly landscape were found to leak over time. New solutions of lined landfills and double-walled storage tanks, with sensors for leaks and monitoring wells, have emerged, as has the increasing work of cleaning up the earlier "mistakes." **Monitoring** is the periodic or continuous surveillance or testing to determine the level of compliance with statutory requirements or pollutant levels in various media or in humans, plants, and animals.

What can now be called "mistakes" were not necessarily the result of malicious carelessness or insensitivity. Decisions were based on the best information available at the time. The "best information" is often likely to be incomplete and imperfect. That is why research continues to be so necessary. An encouraging trend in industry's new product development is engineering analysis of the full life cycle of the product, from raw material to waste disposal. Up-front consideration of the costs and effects throughout the cycle can lead to choices that prevent future problems.

One of the greatest challenges and a major source of concern in today's environmental picture is the solutions themselves. The growing number and complexity of chemicals that are part of everyday life exemplify this. Chemicals are used in industry, household, and medical settings, and there is no doubt that chemicals have been part of the solution to numerous problems. The problem with the enormous growth in chemicals is that the effects of new chemicals on the environment are unknown. People living in neighbourhoods that are in proximity to industrial parks are concerned that, even when only allowable levels of each chemical are released, no one is able to say what the health effects of exposure to even small amounts of chemicals may be over time.

ENVIRONMENTAL HEALTH IN CANADA

Canada is part of the global community, connected through economic interactions, cultural diversity and diffusion, communication exchange through technology, and travel. Environmental impacts currently threaten the health of future generations on all continents. Environmental health indicators have been developed by Environment Canada, Statistics Canada, and Health Canada with input from the provinces and territories to measure the relationship between the environment and health (Environment Canada, 2006a). These annual reports addressed the three main indicators of air quality, greenhouse gas emissions, and air quality and are referred to as the Canadian Environmental Sustainability Indicators (CESI) (Environment Canada, 2006a). According to Statistics Canada (2006), the indicators are described as follows: air quality monitors exposure to ozone, a harmful air pollutant in smog affecting Canadians; GHG emissions indicator monitors the GHGs (carbon dioxide, methane, nitrous oxide, sulphur hexafluoride, hydrofluorocarbons, perfluorocarbons) that contribute to climate change; and freshwater quality indicator monitors the pollution of water from discharge wastes such as chemicals and monitors the quality of water for the protection of aquatic life. The evaluation of environmental program objectives (outcome performance measurements) is usually subjective rather than objective. Monitoring health trends in the context of environmental exposure and risk factors can assist with the decision making on health policy.

Health Canada has input into the development of environmental regulations and guidelines; however, Environment Canada enforces the *Canadian Environmental Protection Act.* The *Canadian Environmental Protection Act* oversees pollution prevention and protection of the environment and human health. It ensures that environmental assessments are completed on all substances not regulated under other Canadian acts. It also ensures that these substances meet Canadian health, safety, and **environmental standards**—governmental guidelines or rules that impose limits on the amount of pollutants or emissions produced. It has the authority to effect change in pollution from emissions caused by a variety of toxic substances. Health Canada has total or partial responsibility for several acts—for example, the *Controlled Drugs and Substances Act, Department of Health Act, Food & Drugs Act,* and *Hazardous Products Act.* For a listing of additional acts falling under Health Canada and for access to the full text of many of the acts, refer to the Health Canada "About Health Canada: Acts" Weblink on the Evolve Web site. Health Canada may also be involved in educating the public about risks and risk reduction.

There is a process of developing legislation, regulations, guidelines, and agreements in Canada. The CHN needs to be familiar with these processes as there are many opportunities to be involved in the development of policies. Table 15-1 provides information on some of the most common stages in policy development. It is essential for CHNs to differentiate between agreements, guidelines, regulations, and legislation and to gain an understanding as to how these processes are implemented in policy change.

Some federal, provincial and territorial, and regional agencies that have responsibilities related to environmental health are presented in Table 15-2. Nonenvironmental information for these agencies has also been included. Web sites for provinces and territories and regions have not been included due to the variance of titles and contact information for these areas.

TABLE 15-1 Health Canada Legislation, Regulations, Guidelines, and Agreements

Type	Description	Web Site
Legislation	Legislation, often referred to as *acts* or *statutes*, are written laws. They are passed by the legislative body of government, that is, parliament. A bill, or draft legislation, when it is brought to parliament for approval, requires the assent of the House of Commons, the Senate, and the Crown (Governor General) to become law.	http://www.hc-sc.gc.ca/ahc-asc/legislation/index-eng.php
	Bills are debated in parliament by all party members during what are officially known as first reading, second reading, and third reading. Also, bills are presented to a parliamentary committee for appraisal. This committee as a rule asks for the views of interested parties, including the public. Lastly, a bill becomes law (an act) in the course of a formal procedure known as proclamation, which is done by the governor in council (cabinet, i.e., the prime minister and his or her federal ministers).	http://www.hc-sc.gc.ca/ahc-asc/legislation/acts-lois/index-eng.php
Regulations	Regulations are like acts and are a way of making laws that must reflect policy objectives. Regulations are made by a delegate of parliament. Regulations cannot go beyond what the act provides and may be viewed as the operational part of a law, such as what is meant by certain terms used in an act, actions and procedures that have to be followed, standards that should be met, etc., in order to conform with an act.	http://www.hc-sc.gc.ca/ahc-asc/legislation/reg/index-eng.php
Guidelines	Guidelines are departmental documents that are used to understand legislation or regulation. Guidelines do not have the force of law, even though they result from legislation.	http://www.hc-sc.gc.ca/ahc-asc/legislation/index-eng.php
Agreements	Agreements may be referred to as *accords, conventions, declarations, final acts, general acts, pacts,* and *protocols.* Other types of agreements consist of letters of agreement, letters of intent, various types of memoranda, and mutual recognition agreements.	http://www.hc-sc.gc.ca/ahc-asc/legislation/agree-accord/index-eng.php
	Health Canada is involved in a number of mutual and multiparty agreements and planning measures with the intent to achieve defined objectives. Such agreements, depending on their nature, may be legally binding.	

Source: Adapted from Health Canada. (2006). *Legislation and guidelines.* Retrieved from http://www.hc-sc.gc.ca/ahc-asc/legislation/index-eng.php.

TABLE 15-2 Canadian Government Agencies Involved with Environmental Health Issues

Federal Government Agencies			
Agency	**Responsible for:**	**Branch of Agency**	**Responsible for:**
Health Canada http://www.hc-sc.gc.ca/index-eng.php	• Providing national leadership in the development of health policy, the enforcement of federal health regulations, the prevention of disease, and the promotion of healthy living • Collaborating with other federal departments to reduce health and safety risks • Participating in international knowledge development, surveillance, and regulatory activities	Healthy Environments and Consumer Safety http://www.hc-sc.gc.ca/ahc-asc/branch-dirgen/hecs-dgsesc/index-eng.php	• Reducing the harm caused by tobacco, alcohol, controlled substances, environmental contaminants, and unsafe consumer and industrial products to assist Canadians to maintain and improve their health by promoting healthy and safe living, working, and recreational environments
		Pest Management Regulatory Agency http://www.hc-sc.gc.ca/ahc-asc/branch-dirgen/pmra-arla/index-eng.php	• Protecting human health and the environment by pesticide regulation
		Health Products and Food Branch http://www.hc-sc.gc.ca/ahc-asc/branch-dirgen/hpfb-dgpsa/index-eng.php	• Minimizing health risk factors associated with health products by monitoring for safety, quality, and effectiveness of vaccines, drugs, medical devices, natural health products, and therapeutic products • Monitoring the safety and quality of foods • Providing information to Canadians so they can make informed decisions about their health
		Environmental & Workplace Health http://www.hc-sc.gc.ca/ewh-semt/index-eng.php	• Providing information on many environmental factors that influence health, such as air quality, climate change, noise, occupational health and safety, and water quality

Public Health Agency of Canada http://www.phac-aspc.gc.ca/index-eng.php	• Promoting health • Preventing and controlling chronic diseases and injuries • Preventing and controlling infectious diseases • Preparing for and responding to public health emergencies • Strengthening public health capacity	Health Promotion & Chronic Disease Prevention Branch	• Providing leadership in Canada and globally in health promotion, chronic disease prevention, and control • Coordinating the monitoring of chronic diseases and their risk factors and early disease detection • Developing and evaluating programs addressing common risk factors and concerns for specific aggregates (i.e., older adults, youth) • Educating the public and professionals • Managing contributions and grants
		Planning & Public Health Integration Branch	• Providing specialized policy advice and coordination • Managing policy partnerships with various stakeholders • Managing the agency's communication plans and strategies • Ensuring compliance with relevant federal legislation and policies • Providing expert advice and services re: human resources, information management and technology expertise, and leadership, as well as safety and security
		Infectious Disease & Emergency Preparedness Branch	• Preventing, eliminating, and controlling infectious diseases, including responsibility for pandemic preparedness and response • Maintaining the safety and health security of people both nationally and internationally
Environment Canada http://www.ec.gc.ca/default.asp?lang=En&n=FD9B0E51-1	• Protecting and conserving the natural environment • Protecting water resources • Forecasting weather • Monitoring climate change • Promoting sustainable development		• Providing leadership in health promotion and undertaking programs designed to help Canadians stay healthy, reduce their risks for developing chronic illnesses, and prevent disease progression for those living with chronic diseases • Designing programs to help Canadians stay healthy by reducing their risks of developing chronic illnesses and preventing disease progression for those with chronic illness

Continued

TABLE 15-2 CANADIAN GOVERNMENT AGENCIES INVOLVED WITH ENVIRONMENTAL HEALTH ISSUES —CONT'D

Provincial and Territorial Government Agencies*			
Agency	**Responsible for:**	**Branch of Agency**	**Responsible for:**
Environment Ministry	• Ensuring provision of clean, safe drinking water • Protecting air by supporting climate change initiatives • Managing waste to reduce risks to humans and the environment		
Health Ministry Responsibility of each provincial and territorial ministry guided by the *Canada Health Act*	• Administering the health care system • Providing services such as health insurance programs, drug benefits, assistive devices, care for the mentally ill, long-term care, home care, community and public health, and health promotion and disease prevention • Regulating hospitals and nursing homes • Providing medical laboratories • Coordinating emergency health services • Protecting and promoting health, including environmental health	Ministry of Labour, Occupational Health & Safety, Workplace Safety & Insurance	• Organizing and enforcing workplace health and safety standards for the prevention of workplace deaths, injuries, and disease by setting, communicating, and enforcing standards
Local and Regional Agencies*			
Local and Regional Boards of Health	• Enforcing local bylaws • Conducting complaint investigations and risk assessments • Inspecting premises to ensure compliance with pertinent legislations such as safe food handling, land use, and traffic		

**Due to variances in titles and contact information across provinces and territories and regions, Web sites have not been included.*

SOURCE: Based on Clarke, C. (2008). Environmental Health in Canada. In M. Stanhope, J. Lancaster, H. Jessup-Falcioni, & G. Viverais-Dresler. *Community health nursing in Canada*. Toronto: Mosby Elsevier (pp. 167–169), and data collected by the Canadian authors.

CRITICAL VIEW

1. What can community health nurses do to strengthen the capacity of clients (community, populations, aggregates, groups and families, individuals) to promote environmental health?
2. What can community health nurses do to enhance collaboration with communities on environmental health issues?

The CHN, when working with the client as partner, can facilitate and support health policy development. Policy development can be done by engaging and supporting the client in capacity building. Capacity building enhances the ability of the client to use knowledge and skills that will effectively address environmental health threats, issues, and concerns. The development of health policy involves using tactics to achieve select goals. Policy development usually involves partnering and collaborating with organizations, conferring with stakeholders (community), working with designated officials, looking at the environment, gathering and analyzing data, and writing reports. Consideration needs to be given to the social, political, and economic costs of a proposed policy. Furthermore, awareness is needed that there may be resistance to the policy by individuals and groups, such as organizations, agencies, and corporations, that may try to prevent the policy from development or delay its action while a "cover-up" of the environmental problem occurs. For example, there has been a lot of resistance to smoke-free workplaces and public places by citizens and tobacco companies, who confronted the health experts' evidence on the negative effects of smoking and second-hand smoke with their own "scientific experts" to state the contrary. Legislation for smoke-free public and workplace policy was delayed for many years; however, through the collaborative efforts of concerned citizens in their communities and health care professionals, these policies were developed. Currently, policies such as smoke-free spaces are in place in many communities to promote and protect the health of their community members.

ENVIRONMENT AS A DETERMINANT OF HEALTH

The physical and psychosocial environment has an impact on the health of the client. Physical environment refers to the natural and human-built environment and the factors that influence health such as the quality of air, water, and soil. The psychosocial environment refers to the psychosocial hazards and the factors that influence health such as stress and support networks.

The "Determinants of Health" box on p. 478 provides examples of various physical and psychosocial environmental factors in the natural and built environments that can influence health. (See the "Making Environmental Health Happen in the Community" Weblink on the Evolve Web site. This program is a guide on how to incorporate environmental health as a determinant into health activities. It also provides an example of the socio-environmental model.)

ENVIRONMENTAL HEALTH ASSESSMENT

Health Canada's role is to ensure identification and evaluation of the environment to minimize safety risks to Canadians involved in proposed development projects such as roadways, mines, and energy (Health Canada, 2008b). This is done using an environmental assessment with responsibilities falling within the mandate of the Environmental Assessment Division (EAD) as directed by the *Canadian Environmental Assessment Act.* Some of these responsibilities are listed in Box 15-3.

BOX 15-3 Health Canada's Responsibilities in the Environmental Assessment Process

- Maintaining environmental assessment process involvement of Health Canada
- Analyzing the health component within federal environmental assessment projects
- Ensuring that scientific health information is prepared for presentation to other departments and public review panels or mediators
- Encouraging public participation in the environmental assessments
- Disseminating assessment and assessment process knowledge with other countries
- Promoting health impact assessments

SOURCE: Health Canada. (2008). *Environmental and workplace health.* Retrieved from http://www.hc-sc.gc.ca/ewh-semt/eval/index-eng.php.

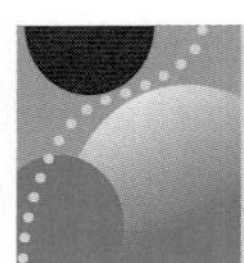

Determinants of Health
Physical and Social Environments

- Street vendors are at risk for respiratory and other adverse health symptoms due to traffic-related air pollution (Kongtip, Thongsuk, Yoosook, & Chantanakul, 2006). Prohibiting vehicle engines from running when the vehicle is stopped for longer than 10 seconds (not at intersections) would help to minimize the risk of exposure to air pollution (Health Canada, 2005). Therefore, a city bylaw that prohibits leaving vehicles running would help to reduce street vendors' exposure to air pollutants.
- Agricultural activities have a negative impact on groundwater quality (Twarakavi & Kaluarachchi, 2006). These activities can result in contaminants such as chemicals, livestock wastes, and fertilizers in surface and groundwater supplies, which has public health and environmental implications, such as unsafe drinking water supplies or unsafe recreational areas (Government of Alberta, 2010).
- Contaminated drinking water can lead to the acquisition of disease, which can lead to death (Hrudey, Hrudey, & Pollard, 2006).
- *Salmonella* poisoning can occur through handling or consuming contaminated foods or contact with pets carrying the organism (Finley, Reid-Smith, & Weese, 2006).
- Mercury, a nerve toxicant, can be found in swordfish, marlin, shark, and tuna sold in Canadian supermarkets (Forsyth, Casey, Dabeka, & McKenzie, 2004). Some benefits of eating fish in moderation include omega-3 fatty acids for heart health and getting minerals such as selenium, iodine, and magnesium. However, the type of fish and its amount of mercury, frequency of ingestion, and meal portion size need to be considered (Health Canada, 2008c).
- Respiratory health problems in humans may be due to diesel engines as they contribute to urban particulate matter, which can carry carcinogens (Environment Canada, 2009b).
- Injuries in the workplace are occurring from exposure to hazardous materials and perceived work overload (Breslin et al., 2007), so it is important that CHNs working in occupational health conduct a workplace environmental assessment and that education be provided for employers and workers to prevent workplace injuries.
- Perceptions of heavy work demands or long hours of work have caused Canadian workers to report excess worry or stress in the workplace (Canadian Policy Research Network, 2009).

The nature of environmental health requires an interdisciplinary approach to assess and decrease environmental health risks. For instance, to assess and address a case of lead-based paint poisoning, the team might include a housing inspector with expertise in lead-based paint to assess the lead-associated health risks in the home; clinical specialists to mandate the clients' health needs; laboratory workers to assess lead levels in the clients' blood as well as in the paint, house dust, and drinking water; and lead-based paint remediation specialists to reduce the lead-based paint risk in the home. This approach could potentially involve the local health department, the provincial department of environmental protection, the housing department, a rehabilitation setting, and laboratories. The CHN would need to understand the roles of each respective agency and organization, know the public health laws (particularly as they pertain to lead-based paint and lead pipe poisoning), and work with the community to coordinate services to address the community's needs. The CHN might also set up a screening program to check levels of lead in people's blood, educate local health providers to encourage them to systematically test children for lead poisoning, work with local landlords to improve the condition of their housing, and educate the community on the most current evidence about lead contamination from all sources.

Assessment and Referral

Assessment activities by CHNs can range from individual health assessments to full participation in community assessment or partnering in a specific environmental site assessment. *Referral* resources may vary in communities. One starting point may be the environmental epidemiology or toxicology unit of the local or provincial health department or environmental agency.

When environmental exposures are assessed, the environment can be divided into functional locations such as home, school, workplace, and community. In each of these locations, there may be unique environmental exposures as well as overlapping exposures. For instance, ethylene oxide, the toxic gas that is used to sterilize equipment in hospitals, would typically be found only in a workplace. However, pesticides might be found in all four areas. When assessing environments, the CHN determines whether an exposure is in the air, water, soil, or food (or a combination) and whether it is a physical, chemical, biological, ergonomic, or psychological exposure. Refer to Table 15-3 for examples of health hazards found in the home, school, workplace, and community.

Exposures may occur in any settings where people spend time; be sure to conduct a complete assessment. Two tools are commonly used to conduct the history-taking of environmental exposure and take the form of a mnemonic. A *mnemonic* is a device such as an acronym, a visual association, or a rhyme to classify or organize information in a systematic manner, and these two were developed to help health professionals remember the questions to ask when taking an environmental history. The first is CH^2OPD^2 (*c*ommunity, *h*ome, *h*obbies, *o*ccupation, *p*ersonal habits, *d*iet, *d*rugs), and the second is I PREPARE (*i*nvestigate potential exposures, *p*resent work, *r*esidence, *e*nvironmental concerns, *p*ast work, *a*ctivities, *r*eferrals and resources, *e*ducate). Both tools can be used when assessing an individual, family, or community. Box 15-4 explains the I PREPARE mnemonic. See the Marshall, Weir, Abelsohn, and Sandborn Weblink on the Evolve Web site for more information on the CH^2OPD^2 mnemonic.

The Ottawa Charter refers to health as the interaction between person and environment and identifies the social elements of peace, shelter, education, food, income, social justice, and equity as essential for health. The Charter also identifies that our physical environment is significant to health and indicates that a supportive environment (psychosocial environment) should be established. Following the Charter, the World Health Organization (WHO) Healthy Cities movement adopted a collaborative approach to include many development sectors and agencies such as housing, industry, transport, and planning to address health issues. In the late 1980s, the Healthy Communities Project was developed in Canada as a joint venture to assist communities to commit to healthy environments. In 1992, in Rio de Janeiro, the United Nations Conference on Environment and Development (Earth Summit) was held, and out of this conference an action plan, called Agenda 21, was proposed and adopted. This plan was to guide future strategies for health and environment activities and was

LEVELS OF PREVENTION

Related to Unhealthy Environments

PRIMARY PREVENTION

Community health nurses work with a community group to prepare a draft proposal for a municipal bylaw change to ban all pesticide use in the community to prevent foods from becoming contaminated with pesticides.

SECONDARY PREVENTION

Community health nurses work with community groups such as the hearing society, concerned parents, and school representatives to organize mass screening programs at local high schools to detect hearing loss in grade 12 students as a result of continual exposure to high-decibel noise related to the use of audio-player earphones.

TERTIARY PREVENTION

Occupational health nurses initiate a support group for injured workers.

How To... Apply the Community Health Nursing Process to Environmental Health

If as a CHN you suspect that a client's health concern is being influenced by environmental factors, follow the community health nursing process and note the environmental aspects of the health concern in every step of the process as follows:

1. *Assessment.* Include inventories and history questions that cover environmental issues as a part of the general assessment.
2. *Goal setting.* Include outcome measures that mitigate and eliminate the environmental factors.
3. *Planning.* Look at community policy and laws as methods to facilitate the care needs for the client; include environmental health personnel in the planning.
4. *Intervention.* Coordinate medical, nursing, and public health actions to meet the client's needs.
5. *Evaluation.* Examine criteria that include the immediate and long-term responses of the client, as well as the recidivism of the problem for the client.

TABLE 15-3 Environmental Health Hazards

	Physical	Chemical	Biological (Biohazard)	Ergonomic	Psychological
Home	Noise Aerosol sprays Unsafe physical structures Electromagnetic radiation (computers, microwaves)	Bleach Lead paint Paint thinners and solvents Carbon monoxide	Mouse droppings Mould and fungi Dust mites Pet dander	Improper work methods Improper workstations Incorrect techniques Repetition Incorrect posture	Stress Threat of violence Fatigue
School	Noise Laser pointers Poor ventilation Variations in temperature	Asbestos Photocopier ink Perfumes Cleaning solutions	Bacteria Mould and fungi Viruses Dust mites	Repetition Improper play and workstations Incorrect posture	Interpersonal problems Bullying School violence
Workplace	Noise Vibrating equipment Variations in temperature Ionizing radiation (X-rays, etc.) Electromagnetic radiation (computers)	Industrial cleaners Perfumes Carbon monoxide	Viruses Biomedical waste products Viruses Latex products	Material handling Improper work methods Improper workstations Incorrect techniques Repetition Incorrect posture	Workplace stress Harassment Job dissatisfaction Shift work Social and physical isolation Inadequate equipment
Community	Noise Variations in temperature Poorly planned structural defects Poorly constructed roads Gas emissions	Pesticides Poorly stored chemical Chemicals in public pools	Birds and animals Plants Ticks Mosquitoes	Poor community planning and design Poor transit design Lack of traffic control	Violence Unemployment Poverty Lack of housing

adopted by over 150 member states of the WHO. The WHO agreed that "good" health could not be attained or maintained in hazardous or deteriorating environments (Health Canada, 2004a). Agenda 21 found that population, consumption, and technology are the principal moving forces of environmental change and identified what needs to occur to reduce wasteful consumption patterns in some countries while encouraging improved but sustainable development in other countries (U.N. Department of Economic and Social Affairs, 2009). For sustainability to occur, factors such as social, economic, and political issues need to be addressed. Assessment needs to be made of the impact these factors have on health, and this is done through an environmental health assessment, sometimes known as an Environmental Impact Assessment, often associated with a Health Impact Assessment. These latter two assessments include factors such as population growth and impact on ecosystems, poverty, unsafe and inadequate amount of drinking water, inadequate shelter, and food insecurity, with risk assessment being a critical assessment piece (Health Canada, 2004a). These assessments have moved beyond the usual assessment of hazards in air, water, food, and soil and include the impacts that development has on the other determinants of health. For further information on environmental assessments, such as what they are and how they affect us, potential sources that affect our health, and federally funded environmental assessment projects across Canada, refer to the Health Canada "Environmental Health Assessment" Weblink on the Evolve Web site.

A "windshield survey," or environmental scan, is a helpful first step that CHNs can use to initiate understanding of the potential environmental health risks in a community. If the community is urban, the age and condition of the housing and potential garbage problems (and the associated pest problems) can be easily determined by driving around the neighbourhood. CHNs can also note proximity to factories, dump sites, major transportation routes, and other sources of pollution. In rural communities, attention should be

BOX 15-4 The "I PREPARE" Mnemonic

An exposure history should identify current and past exposures, have a preliminary goal of reducing or eliminating current exposures, and have a long-term goal of reducing adverse health effects. The "I PREPARE" mnemonic consigns the important questions to categories that can be easily remembered.

I Investigate potential exposures

Investigate potential exposures by asking the following:

- Have you ever felt sick after coming in contact with a chemical, pesticide, or other substance?
- Do you have any symptoms that improve when you are away from your home or work?

P Present work

Ask questions about the client's present work:

- Are you exposed to solvents, dusts, fumes, radiation, loud noise, pesticides, or other chemicals?
- Do you know where to find material safety data sheets on the chemicals you work with?
- Do you wear personal protective equipment?
- Do you wear work clothes home?
- Do co-workers have similar health problems?

R Residence

Inquire about the client's place of residence:

- When was your residence built?
- What type of heating do you have?
- Have you recently remodelled your home?
- What chemicals are stored on your property?
- Where does your drinking water come from?

E Environmental concerns

Ask about the client's living environment:

- Are there environmental concerns in your neighbourhood (i.e., air, water, soil)?
- What types of industries or farms are near your home?
- Do you live near a hazardous waste site or landfill?

P Past work

Inquire about the client's past work:

- What are your past work experiences?
- What is the longest job you held?
- Have you ever been in the military, worked on a farm, or done volunteer or seasonal work?

A Activities

Ask about your client's activities:

- What activities and hobbies do you and your family engage in?
- Do you burn, solder, or melt any products?
- Do you garden, fish, or hunt?
- Do you eat what you catch or grow?
- Do you use pesticides?
- Do you engage in any alternative healing or cultural practices?

R Referrals and resources

Use these key Canadian referrals and resources:

- Environment Canada (www.ec.gc.ca)
- Environmental Search Guide (www.oen.ca/dir/searchguide.html)
- Greenpeace Canada (www.greenpeace.org/canada/en/)
- National Pollutant Release Inventory (www.ec.gc.ca/inrp-npri/)
- Library and Archives Canada (www.collectionscanada.ca)
- PHAC (www.phac-aspc.gc.ca)
- Disease Surveillance Online (www.phac-aspc.gc.ca/dsol-smed/index.php)
- Canadian Centre for Occupational Health and Safety (www.ccohs.ca)
- Health Canada (www.hc-sc.gc.ca)
- Environmental and Workplace Health (www.hc-sc.gc.ca/ewh-semt/index_e.html)
- Local health department, environmental agency, and poison control centres

E Educate

Use this checklist of educational materials:

- Are materials available to educate the client?
- Are alternatives available to minimize the risk of exposure?
- Have prevention strategies been discussed?
- What is the plan for follow-up?

Source: Prepared by Grace Paranzino, RN, MPH, for the Agency for Toxic Substances and Disease Registry (www.atsdr.cdc.gov); with additional resources by Heather Jessup-Falcioni and Gloria Viverais-Dresler.

given to the use of aerial and signage regarding types of pesticide and herbicide sprayings. In addition to the tools used for a general community assessment, the specific tools, I PREPARE and CH²OPD² mnemonics, as previously discussed, are available to detect the environmental health risks within a community. See Appendix E-1 on the Evolve site accompanying this text for a comprehensive occupational and environmental health history tool.

Environmental issues are global issues and are therefore the concern of nongovernmental agencies such as Greenpeace and international, national, provincial, and municipal governments. Environmental hazards have the greatest impact on air, water, and food sources in the environment, which, in turn, have an impact on health. The economic impact of the environment on these sources is extremely costly as a result of lost productivity at work, pain and suffering due to illness, health treatment and rehabilitation costs, and clean-up and prevention costs, to name a few.

Provincial and territorial governments establish the environmental protection acts required in their provinces or territories to ensure the quality of air, water, and soil; the regulation of industrial emissions; toxic waste disposal; and the surveillance of environmental health hazards. Local governments have the responsibility for following the provincial or territorial environmental protection acts and may also set local bylaws to control environmental health hazards in their own communities. Public health departments are funded by the municipal and provincial or territorial governments and therefore follow and enforce the mandated environmental regulations. Environmental hazards may vary from community to community as do some bylaws to control them, such as pesticide control bylaws. Therefore, it is important that CHNs keep abreast of the environmental health issues by using evidence-informed data often available at their local health unit or health authority.

Air

Outdoor and indoor air pollution is a major consideration in environmental health. An international panel on climate change with representatives from around the world has been established to deal with the adverse effects of climate change and its influence on health.

Motor vehicles have been a major cause of outdoor air pollution; however, due to recent technologies such as the use of catalytic converters in vehicles, introduction of unleaded gasoline, and increased numbers of citizens using public transit systems, the effects of motor vehicle pollution have declined. The Healthy Cities movement has been supportive and instrumental in the use of such strategies to reduce air pollution. Polluted air produced and emitted by certain industries has decreased. This is still an area that needs further research, development, and cooperation. Forest fires are one of the major natural sources of air pollution. Health effects associated with air pollution include asthma and other respiratory diseases, cardiovascular diseases (including heart disease and hypertension), cancer, immunological effects, reproductive health problems including birth defects, and neurological problems.

Indoor air quality is a measure of the chemical, physical, or biological contaminants in indoor air; indoor air quality in the workplace, schools, and homes is a growing concern, especially relating to children (see the "Ethical Considerations" box, p. 483). Asthma is the most common chronic respiratory disease in children in Canada (The Lung Association, 2010). Both the Asthma Society of Canada and Health Canada provide excellent resource materials on indoor air quality. The Asthma Society of Canada has centres across the country that provide media clips, responses to frequently asked questions, and a paper-based resource kit for parents and teachers. The objectives and material presented by this society are developed based on the Canadian Asthma Consensus Guidelines. Health Canada has an action kit for schools known as the Indoor Air Quality Tools for Schools Action Kit. This tool kit helps schools to understand and check for problems with indoor air quality by using a variety of checklists (see Tool Box on the Evolve Web site).

The major culprits contributing to poor indoor air are carbon monoxide, dust, moulds, dust mites, cockroaches, pests and pets, cleaning and personal care products (particularly aerosols), lead, and environmental tobacco smoke. It is important to assess both the environmental exposures and the human health status in a community. Because most Canadians spend a great deal of time indoors, the quality of air can have a major effect on their health. One of the most harmful indoor air hazards is tobacco smoke. The effects of second-hand smoke have been widely documented (Kovesi et al., 2006; Ward et al., 2005). CHNs are key players in dealing with this air quality issue. Recently, there has been major progress in the area of policy development to deal with the effects of second-hand smoke in public places and enclosed spaces. Enclosed spaces such as cars and homes remain hazardous places to smoke, especially when children are present, and assessment and education for individuals and families by CHNs are required. An excellent resource that provides CHNs with detailed information about factors affecting indoor air quality is the Health Canada "Indoor Air Quality" Web site, listed in the Evolve Weblinks.

Outdoor air quality is affected by both natural and human sources. Natural sources are contaminants usually resulting from forest fires and volcano eruptions. Human sources result from the burning of fossil fuels

ETHICAL CONSIDERATIONS

A group of CHNs wanted to know more about the indoor air that children with respiratory diseases were exposed to at home. They found that many of these children lived in poor-quality housing. They also found that the levels of environmental tobacco smoke were high.

Ethical principles that apply to the environmental health perspective:

- *Respect for autonomy.* This is fundamental to the equality and diversity dimension of health improvement efforts; it covers the protection and promotion of self-respect and self-esteem among individuals, groups, and communities, as part of both promoting a sense of well-being and protecting against unhealthful influences (Tannahill, 2008).
- *Nonmaleficence.* Do not harm; the CHN needs to support environmental preservation and restoration and advocate for initiatives that reduce environmentally harmful practices (Code of Ethics).

Question to Consider

1. Given the ethical considerations, what actions should be taken by the CHNs in order to provide "respiratory care" to these children?

(e.g., release of oxides, such as sulphur, carbon, and nitrogen) (Health Canada, 2006a) and use of toxic metals, such as manganese and lead (Health Canada, 2006a; Shah, 2003). The most common contributors to outdoor air pollution that have serious adverse health effects have been identified as ozone pollution, smog, and acid rain (Health Canada, 2006a; Shah, 2003). For an in-depth discussion of each of these contributors to deterioration of outdoor air quality, visit the Health Canada Weblink (on the Evolve Web site) entitled "Let's Talk About Health and Air Quality." Air quality must be carefully and regularly monitored, and the authors of the site suggest approaches to reduce the presence of air pollutants—for example, restrictions on idling of vehicles and considering use of alternative fuels.

Water

People's lives are tied to safe and adequate water. Water is necessary for all life forms. It is necessary for the production of food—also essential to life. The quality of the soil is affected by its water supply, the chemicals that are intentionally added by humans, and the deposition of pollutants from the air. Soil that is free from harmful contaminants and pathogens is essential for good health. Health Canada publishes drinking water guidelines that are the benchmarks for maintaining water quality. These guidelines can be accessed at the Health Canada "Drinking Water" Weblink (see the Evolve Web site).

In most parts of Canada, fluoride has been added to the municipal drinking water to prevent tooth decay. Some controversy exists about the negative effects of fluoride on health. It is important for CHNs to assess for other sources of fluoride intake. Some questions to ask the individual or family would be these: Does your drinking water have fluoride (the health unit or health authority would know this answer if the client does not), and what other sources of fluoride are you exposed to (toothpaste, mouthwash, fluoride tablets, or drops)?

Discharges into water bodies from industries, farm animal waste, and wastewater treatment systems can contribute to the degradation of water quality. Water quality is also affected by nonpoint sources of pollution, such as storm water runoff from paved roads and parking lots, erosion from clear-cut tracts of land (after timbering and mining), and runoff from chemicals added to soils, such as fertilizers. The chain of potential damage continues with the additives to farm produce and to animal diets, such as antibiotics and growth hormones (which are then consumed by humans).

Food

Food and food production continue to be a source of concern. In recent years, food-borne illnesses have been associated with *Salmonella* and *Escherichia coli* in chicken, eggs, and hamburger. Good food preparation practices, such as washing and adequate cooking temperature and time, can prevent food-borne illnesses associated with most pathogens. Other food worries include the presence in food of pesticides, bovine growth hormones (given to dairy cows), and low-level antibiotics (given to beef cattle, pigs, and chickens); the irradiation of food; and the emerging use of genetically modified organisms and genetically engineered crops.

In 2008, a Canada-wide food recall was put into place as a result of an outbreak of listeriosis, a food-borne illness. The outbreak, which claimed four lives in Canada, was linked to processed meats from one major Canadian meat processing company. The Canadian Food Inspection Agency (CFIA) and the Public Health Agency of Canada were involved with testing the recalled meat samples to determine the source of the listeriosis. The investigation involved the Canadian Food Inspection Agency, provincial, territorial, and local health authorities.

Governments need to enhance efforts to deal with environmental threats to food safety. In Canada, the CFIA is the regulatory agency for food, plant, and animal

CRITICAL VIEW

Food sources in Canada are safe; however, contamination of food in the environment is a major food issue. "Food contamination accounts for up to 95% of our daily intake of persistent toxic chemicals whereas air contributes approximately 15% and drinking water contributes very little" (Shah, 2003, p. 297).

1. a) What is being done to ensure food security (adequate quality and quantity of food) in your community?
   b) What more could be done to improve food security in your community?
2. Are there risks associated with genetically modified foods? Support your position.

safety. This agency is committed to protecting human health through safe food. The CFIA applies many key strategies to ensure that its goals are met (CFIA, 2008).

Risk Assessment

A process called *risk assessment* is used to develop health-based standards. **Risk assessment** refers to a qualitative and quantitative evaluation of the risk posed to human health or the environment by the actual or potential presence or use of specific pollutants. Information on human health effects from exposure to various materials in the environment is collected in Canada to determine human health risks to Canadians. Based on this information, leading authorities, such as Health Canada, the Government of Canada, and Environment Canada, set policies and regulations to protect the Canadian public. Some of Health Canada's activities include developing and providing tools to be used in risk assessments for chemical, radiological, and biological contamination; providing training to governmental departments on risk assessment; developing Canadian soil quality guidelines; and disseminating toxicological reference values used in human health risk assessments (Health Canada, 2009). For further information on Health Canada's approach to risk assessment and management, drinking and recreational water quality, and links to assessment tools, see the "Human Health Risk Assessment" Weblink listed on the Evolve Web site. The Government of Canada is involved in several aspects of risk assessment and management. Its involvement in risk assessment and management related to chemical substances includes determination of how substances get into the environment, who is using these chemicals and in what capacity, and implementation of relevant tools to address actual and potential risks to humans due to chemicals (Government of Canada, 2008a).

Governmental policy currently incorporates the **precautionary principle,** which suggests that when credible doubt exists action should be on the side of caution (Chaudry, 2008). Bisphenol A (BPA) has been added to the toxic substances list by Environment Canada (Young-Reuters, 2010; Mittelstaedt, 2010). Bisphenol A is now considered a toxin like asbestos and lead. In Canada, in humans, BPA is primarily obtained through dietary intake such as continued use of foods from polycarbonate containers and some food packaging, and also through environmental sources such as toys, drinking water, and indoor air (Young-Reuters, 2010; Environment Canada Health Canada, 2008).

Care and caution should be exercised prior to implementing change that may have ecological harm (there may be insufficient scientific evidence indicating harm). Potential threats should be identified and caution exercised before proceeding with the intended action. New products should be proven safe before being introduced onto the market. Some products may not be identified as being unsafe to the environment but may produce symptoms in humans. For example, populations living close to industrial wind turbines have experienced Wind Turbine Syndrome. Some of the symptoms identified are headache, tinnitus, dizziness, nausea, irritability, sleep disturbance, and problems with memory (Pierpont, 2010).

Risk Communication

Risk is defined as the chance that a specific health problem will develop in a client because of exposure to certain factors. It is a familiar term in community health nursing practice. CHNs, as risk communicators, inform or counsel in areas such as safe drinking water, handwashing techniques,

CRITICAL VIEW

Access the following article:

Chaudry, R. V. (2008). The precautionary principle, public health, and public health nursing. *Public Health Nursing, 25*(3), 261–268.

Answer the following questions:

1. a) How would the precautionary principle guide CHNs in the practice of safe environmental disposal of client medications?
   b) What are possible CHN roles regarding the safe disposal of client medications?
2. What is the relevance of the precautionary principle to public health interventions?

food preparation, risks of pregnancy, communicable diseases (especially sexually transmitted infections), unintentional injury, and personal health-related choices (e.g., smoking, alcohol consumption, diet). Risk assessment in environmental health has focused on characterizing the hazard (i.e., the source), its physical and chemical properties, its toxicity, and the presence of (or potential for) other elements in the exposure pathway—mode of transmission, route of exposure, receptor population, and dose.

Environmental hazards often produce fear because they create risk situations and heighten risk perception, which can lead to public feelings of outrage. **Outrage** is the emotional public response to the perception of risk related to an environmental issue; trust in authorities is weak. Outrage is a concept that has been familiar in the United States since the 1970s. Within the past three decades in Canada, interest in public outrage has become more evident. It has escalated particularly because of unforgettable environmental events such as contaminated water in Walkerton, Ontario, and North Battleford, Saskatchewan, and the outbreak of severe acute respiratory syndrome in Toronto. Unforgettable environmental events create an awareness with the public and increase the need for information and action on the particular risk associated with the event. The media, in the aforementioned cases, were instrumental in magnifying the risks due to their reactionary reporting of such events, often raising questions of culpability, responsibility, and accountability. As a result, fear was heightened and outrage resulted from this chain of events. Table 15-4 outlines some of the factors that can affect perception of risk.

Communication of risk involves consideration of the outrage factors relevant to the risk. These factors and the action to be taken to alleviate them can be incorporated into the message. Action is taken to ensure that safety is increased and unnecessary fear is reduced. **Risk communication** includes all the principles of good communication in general and the exchange of information about health or environmental risks. It is a combination of the following:

- *The right information.* Accurate and relevant information in a language that audiences can understand for shaping the message.
- *To the right people.* The communication is directed at those affected and those who may not be affected but are worried. Information about the community is essential: the geographical boundaries, who lives there (demographics), how they get information (flyers or newspapers, radio, television, word of mouth), where they get together (school, church, community centre), and who within the community can help plan the communication.
- *At the right time.* Communication must allow for timely action or allay fear.

TABLE 15-4 Important Attributes Affecting the Perception of Risk

Involuntary	A risk that is involuntarily imposed (e.g., building an industrial plant without community input) will be judged less acceptable than a risk that is voluntarily assumed (e.g., smoking).
Uncontrollable	The inability to control a risk decreases the judgement of its acceptability.
Industrial versus natural	An industrial risk (e.g., nuclear power) is judged less acceptable than a natural risk (e.g., lightning strike).
Unfamiliar	An exotic or unfamiliar risk (e.g., biotechnology) is judged less acceptable than a familiar risk (e.g., household cleanser).
Memorable	A risk that is embedded in a remarkable event (e.g., airplane crash) is judged to be less acceptable than one that is not.
Dreaded	A risk that is highly feared (e.g., cancer) is judged less acceptable than one that is not (e.g., household accident).
Catastrophic	A catastrophic risk (e.g., airplane crash) is judged less acceptable than diffuse or cumulative risks (e.g., vehicle collision).
Unfair	If a risk is thought to be inequitably or unfairly placed upon a group, it is judged as less acceptable. This is particularly true if that group happens to be children.
Untrustworthy	If the source of the risk is untrustworthy, the risk is judged less acceptable.
Uncertain	A risk that has high uncertainty and that we know little about is judged less acceptable than one that is not.
Immoral	A risk that is deemed to be unethical or immoral is judged less acceptable than one that is not.

SOURCE: Hill, S. (2005). *Appendix A: Some factors affecting the perception of risk. Risk communication literature review: Summary report.* Ottawa: Treasury Board of Canada Secretariat. Retrieved from http://www.tbs-sct.gc.ca/rm-gr/rc-cr/report-rapport_e.asp#two. Reproduced with permission.

(For more on how to perform an effective risk communication, refer to the Hill Weblink on the Evolve Web site.)

In 2004, the government of Newfoundland and Labrador took an ecological approach to the management of drinking water in its province and developed guidelines and strategies to ensure the safety of drinking water based on an assessment study of community health needs and resources conducted between 1997 and 2004 (Pike-MacDonald, Best, Twomey, Bennett, & Blakeley, 2007). The study explored the "health beliefs and practices, satisfaction with health and related community services, and community health concerns" for residents residing in various communities in Newfoundland and Labrador (Pike-MacDonald et al., 2007, p. 15). One of the most serious concerns expressed by these study participants was the quality of drinking water. CHNs need to ensure that drinking water is safe (e.g., monitor reports on water quality in their community), partner with communities to inform the public (e.g., work with mass media campaigns to include risks associated with drinking contaminated water), build healthy public policy (e.g., advocate or lobby decision makers), and strengthen community actions (e.g., visually and verbally explain in detail the technique for effectively boiling water). (The authors of the Newfoundland and Labrador study elaborate further on the role of the CHN in environmental health; refer to their article for a greater discussion.)

ENVIRONMENT AND CHILDREN'S HEALTH

Children are very vulnerable to adverse health effects because of their underdeveloped brains and other organs, undeveloped detoxification systems and more rapid breathing rate, and behaviours such as hand-to-mouth activity. Other factors putting children at risk are their genetic makeup and where they live. Currently, the health of children in Canada is improving; however, some disorders, due in part to environmental exposures, are on the rise. These conditions include asthma, learning and behaviour disorders, some cancers, and obesity (Canadian Partnership for Children's Health & Environment [CPCHE], 2008). Children today are also at risk for environmental hazards because of factors such as poverty, lack of access to health care, and the dangerous environmental situations in the communities where they live. Environmental toxins, such as lead, pesticides, mercury, air pollution, solvents, asbestos, and radon, get into homes, schools, child care centres, and playgrounds (CPCHE, 2008; Shah, 2003).

Children are not just little adults with regard to their responses to environmental exposures. Infants and young children breathe more rapidly than adults and thus have a proportionally greater exposure to air pollutants. While infants' lungs are developing, they are particularly susceptible to environmental toxicants. Because children are short, their breathing zones are lower than those of adults, so they have closer contact with the chemical and biological agents that accumulate on floors and carpeting. Children's bodies also operate differently. Some protective mechanisms that are well developed in adults, such as the blood–brain barrier, are immature in young children, making them more vulnerable to the effects of toxic chemicals. And, finally, the kidneys of young children are less effective at filtering out undesirable, toxic chemicals, which then continue to circulate and accumulate.

Many children are injured by falls, which result in, on average, $630 million in health care expenses per year in Canada (CNA, 2005). Reducing occurrences of these injuries would entail redesigning the **built environment**—anything physical in the environment that is built or produced by humans, such as playgrounds—and increasing prevention by teaching about safety in the home and teaching children ways to fall more safely to minimize injury. The leading cause of death in children and youth in Canada is injury, frequently in the home (CNA, 2005; PHAC, 2008). Young children under 4 years of age experience 40% of all playground injuries, specifically from using slide equipment. Road vehicle injuries involving Canadian cyclists under the age of 20 years account for 25% of hospitalizations (CNA, 2005).

Toxic chemicals can have different effects, depending on the timing of exposure. During fetal development, there are periods of great sensitivity to the effects of toxic chemicals. During such times, even very small exposures can prevent or change a process that may permanently affect normal development. The brain undergoes rapid structural and functional changes during late pregnancy and in the neonatal period. Therefore, it is extremely important to safeguard women's environments when they are pregnant.

The PHAC, in its Division of Childhood and Adolescence (Safe, Healthy Environments), provides resources for health care professionals to help decrease the incidence of death and hospitalizations in Canadian children and youth (PHAC, 2008). Issues such as the influence of built environments, safe transportation, water and air quality, and toxic substances are addressed by this division.

A nutritionally balanced diet is important, and fish is a good source of protein; however, the effects of mercury are of extreme concern for Canadians because fish is the main source of mercury. Therefore, Health Canada recommends Canadians consume limited weekly amounts of certain fish such as shark, tuna, and swordfish. The recommendations for pregnant women, women of child-bearing age, and young children are more stringent (Ontario Ministry of Natural Resources, 2009).

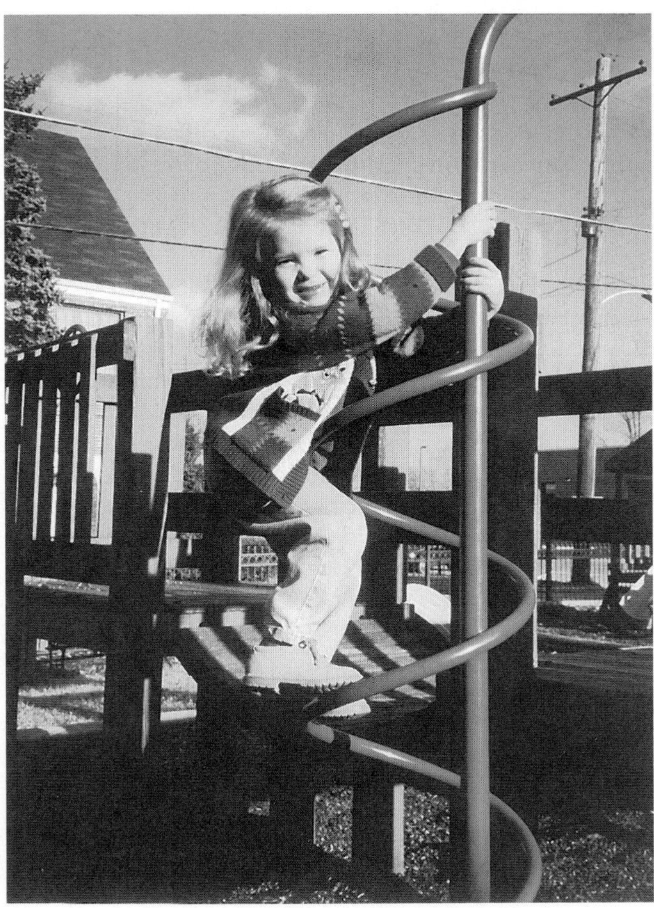

Playground injuries are frequent among young children.

Waterfowl and other wildlife also eat contaminated fish and may be additional sources of mercury to people. Exposure to mercury most often affects the nervous system, the cardiovascular system, the immune system, and the kidneys, with fetal mercury exposure possibly leading to neurodevelopmental problems in children (Health Canada, 2007). Mercury is a metal that occurs naturally with low levels found in air, water, rocks, soil, and plant and animal matter, and was used widely in industry with reductions of its use being initiated in the late 1960s (Ontario Ministry of Natural Resources, 2009). Industrial use of mercury was a source that created residual water contamination; in addition, some quantities of man-made and natural mercury sources currently are entering the aquatic environment from the atmosphere (Ontario Ministry of Natural Resources, 2009).

Of the many tens of thousands of synthetic chemicals that are in air, water, food, workplaces, and consumer products, only a small percentage have undergone sufficient toxicity testing (Shah, 2003). Companies are not required to divulge all the results of their private testing. A full battery of neurotoxicity tests is not required even for pesticides that may be sprayed in nurseries and labour and delivery areas of hospitals, not to mention in our homes. Complicating matters even further, risks from multiple chemical exposures are rarely considered when regulations are drafted. Such an omission ignores the reality that children (as well as adults) are exposed to many toxic chemicals, often concurrently. The only exception to this is in the case of regulations regarding pesticides that are used on food supplies. The Canadian federal government established the Pest Management Regulatory Agency in 1995 to scrutinize the effect of pesticides on our food supply and health. In addition, several Canadian municipalities have set regulations limiting or banning pesticide use. Health Canada and the Canadian Food Inspection Agency (CFIA) are responsible for guaranteeing the safety of Canada's food supply. CFIA, as previously mentioned, monitors the amount of contaminants in our food supply. The National Chemical Residue Monitoring Program, a branch of CFIA, monitors the chemicals in our food supply (Health Canada, 2004b). Health Canada is responsible for the setting and modifying of food standards. The Pest Management Regulatory Agency, a branch of Health Canada, registers and regulates pest control products (Health Canada, 2010).

REDUCING ENVIRONMENTAL HEALTH RISKS

Preventing problems is less costly than "fixing" them, whether the cost is measured in resources consumed or health effects. Education is a primary preventive strategy. When a CHN is examining the sources of environmental health risks in communities and planning intervention strategies, it is important to apply the basic principles of disease prevention. For a home with lead-based paint, the primary prevention strategy would be to remove that specific source of lead. Good surveillance, a secondary prevention strategy, would not prevent lead exposure, but it might help with early identification of rising levels of lead in blood. For a symptomatic child brought to a health care provider, a system should be in place for specialists familiar with lead poisoning to provide immediate care; swift medical interventions to reduce blood levels of lead can reduce the risk of further harm. This might be a tertiary prevention response.

Risk Management

For workplaces, community health professionals work with a list of precautions for avoiding or minimizing employees' exposure to potentially hazardous chemicals. Once it is established that a human health threat exists, a plan of action needs to be developed to eliminate or manage (reduce) the risk. Risk management

Evidence-Informed Practice

A pilot study was conducted to examine indoor air quality–related risk factors for respiratory infections in young Inuit children under the age of 2 years living in Nunavut. The main foci were to assess the indoor air quality in their homes and the children's respiratory health status and to explore risk factors for lower respiratory tract infection (LRTI). This population group is more susceptible to permanent lung injury following a severe LRTI. Young Inuit children are prone to severe LRTIs. Twenty homes in Nunavut were included in this study. A respiratory health questionnaire was used, a structured housing inspection was conducted, and various measures of indoor air quality were taken.

Study findings were as follows: (1) homes were small and single storey, lacked basements, and were above ground level; (2) several people resided in each home, with young children often sharing a bed for sleeping; (3) many household residents were smokers; (4) air exchange rates were reduced; (5) fungi levels in mattresses were elevated; (6) dust mite levels were minimal; and (7) 25% of the study sample had been hospitalized for chest illnesses. The finding of second-hand smoke in the home and increased LRTIs in young children is well supported in the literature. Also, LRTIs in young children due to exposure to fungi and dampness are also supported in the literature. Many public health suggestions were proposed on the basis of the study findings. It was suggested that additional homes be built with better ventilation systems and the opportunity for less sharing of homes and beds by young Inuit children, that there be more frequent turning of mattresses to reduce the fungi, and that public education be provided to address the issue of second-hand smoke in the home.

Application for CHNs: The community health nurse would need to work with this population to develop strategies that are culturally and geographically appropriate to address the findings. Community health nurse interventions that could be offered, in consultation with community partners such as Inuit lay visitors, would include individual and group educational sessions in the community to reduce the smoking patterns in the home; working with families and community partners to facilitate the acquisition of cribs; working with community partners to address the building standards of the current homes in the community; and working with community partners, when necessary, to facilitate the acquisition of new housing.

Questions for Reflection & Discussion

1. Which determinants of health are evident in this Nunavut community?
2. What community health nurse interventions can be implemented to address the identified determinants of health? Elaborate.
3. What type of qualitative research question might you develop to discover what the Inuit family members' perceptions are about the air quality in their homes and respiratory infections their children have?

REFERENCE: Kovesi, T., Creery, D., Gilbert, N. L., Dales, R., Fugler, D., Thompson, B., Randhawa, V., & Miller, J. D. (2006). Indoor air quality risk factors for severe lower respiratory tract infections in Inuit infants in Baffin Region, Nunavut: A pilot study. *Indoor Air*, *16*(4), 266–275.

should be informed by the risk assessment process. **Risk management** involves the selection and implementation of a strategy to reduce risks. This can take many forms—for example, the "Four Rs for Reducing Environmental Pollution," which are as follows, in order of effectiveness:

1. *Reduce.* Reducing consumption lessens waste and unnecessary packaging and nonessentials.
2. *Reuse.* Choosing reusable rather than disposable products creates less waste (e.g., using glass dishes rather than paper ones or choosing used products such as those found at second-hand stores and yard sales).
3. *Recycle.* The simple activity of recycling paper, glass, and cans to be used to produce new items is one good way to decrease pollution.
4. *Recover.* Recover involves retrieving energy from waste materials such as through the incineration of waste to produce a new energy.

In Canada, legislation covers hazardous materials used in the workplace. The Workplace Hazardous Materials Information System (WHMIS) was implemented in Canada effective October 31, 1988, through federal, provincial, and territorial legislations (Canadian Centre for Occupational Health and Safety, 2005). WHMIS provides information in the form of product labels, material

CRITICAL VIEW

Shah (2003) states, "It is estimated that after recycling plastic, glass and metal containers, and paper products, backyard composting could reduce the volume of remaining residential waste in Canada by up to 60%" (p. 308).

1. a) What are you doing to reduce, reuse, and recycle?
   b) What is your community doing to reduce, reuse, and recycle?
2. What more could you be doing?

safety data sheets, and worker education programs on the safe use of hazardous materials used in Canadian workplaces.

There are other forms of risk reduction. One is to reduce the risk from exposure to ultraviolet rays. People should avoid being outside during peak sun hours and need to wear protective clothing or use sunblock. To reduce exposure to dangerous heavy metals, special processes can be employed at water filtration plants that supply the public water. In the home, one can run the cold water tap for 1 or 2 minutes each morning before collecting water for coffee or drinking to reduce the presence of lead that may have leached from old pipes (or the solder used on them) overnight. Individuals, communities, and nations can reduce risks; in recent years, there have been global agreements to reduce persistent pollutants and decrease global warming.

Community Health Nursing Interventions

Community health nursing interventions to reduce environmental health risks can also take many forms. One mode of action is education. By working with an array of community members, CHNs can explain the relationship between harmful environmental exposures and human health and guide the community toward risk reduction based on both individual behaviour changes and community-wide approaches. A second mode of action by CHNs is that of advocacy. In this role, CHNs work with the community, governmental agencies, and other stakeholders to develop environmental health policies that support changes to improve environmental health. CHNs need to work with community partners in the following ways: advocate, inform, consult, and involve the community in reducing environmental risks such as consumer products (e.g., cosmetic products), radiation, and chemicals; identify community assets, constraints, opportunities, and capacities; and identify the economic, political, and social factors as well as the determinants of health that affect or are affected by the environment so that environmental risks to client health can be removed or minimized.

Environmental Ethics and Environmental Justice

As discussed in Chapter 6, understanding ethics is essential for CHNs in making their own choices, in describing issues and options, and in advocating for ethical choices. When the competing commodities (e.g., jobs versus environmental protection; production versus conservation) are of concern, the skillful CHN can change the discussion from "either/or" to "both" by opening new possibilities for ethical and mutually satisfactory outcomes. Some ethical issues likely to arise in environmental health decisions are these:

- Who has access to information and when?
- How complete and accurate is the available information?
- Who is included in decision making and when?
- What and whose values and priorities are given weight in decisions?
- How are short- and long-term consequences considered?
- Is there a conflict of interest?

Recently, discussion of environmental health concerns has included discussion about environmental justice. Environmental justice originated as a social movement in the United States. More recently, in Canada, in venues such as academia and advocacy movements, it is a concept that has gained merit, especially in the discussions about vulnerable populations (Canadian Public Health Association [CPHA], 2008). **Environmental justice,** from a population health perspective, is the effort to reduce the impact of health inequalities and socioeconomic marginalization of persons resulting from environmental conditions affecting adequate nutrition, shelter, sanitation, and safe working conditions (CPHA, 2008).

Colonialism, urbanization, and the increase in the natural resource economy has most greatly affected and disadvantaged the following populations: resource-dependent communities, which are usually small towns and regions; First Nations communities often affected by close proximity to toxic industries or being excluded from the benefits of development; low-income and ethnoracial communities within urban centres who are often found in deteriorated parts of the city, are excluded from easy access to food and green space, and are not part of the planning and decision making; and biologically vulnerable populations such as older adults and children who are not properly protected by policies and standards (CPHA, 2008). Further information on environmental justice in Canada may be found at the Canadian Public Health Association Weblink on the Evolve Web site. Refer also to the Canadian Policy Research Networks Weblink "Environmental Justice in Canada—It Matters Where You Live," for further environmental justice examples, plus information on the development and implementation of environmental justice policy.

Evidence-Informed Practice

Canada has experienced infectious disease outbreaks as a result of water-borne pathogens. A quantitative study was conducted because of the questions raised about water safety after two recent tragedies in Canada. In Walkerton, Ontario, an outbreak of gastroenteritis occurred as a result of *Escherichia coli* in the municipal water supply in May to June 2000. In North Battleford, Saskatchewan, in 2001, *Cryptosporidium,* which causes gastroenteritis, was found in the local drinking water supply, raising questions about the quality and safety of water.

The objectives of this retrospective study were to review available data on water-borne outbreaks in Canada from 1974 to 2001 to determine the contributing factors and the implications for public health and disease occurrences. Data were collected through a review of the reports of outbreak investigations, which resulted in a sample size of 288 outbreaks of disease due to contaminated drinking water.

The findings were as follows: outbreaks occurred in public (municipal) water systems (99), semipublic systems (private systems with public access, such as at campgrounds; 138), and private systems (e.g., wells; 51); outbreaks usually occurred in spring (79) and summer (93); the organisms most commonly found, starting with the most frequent, belonged to *Giardia lamblia, Campylobacter, Cryptosporidium,* Norwalk-like viruses, *Salmonella,* and hepatitis A virus, and contributing factors included extreme weather events (e.g., heavy rainfall), insecure wells, animal populations (e.g., livestock) and farming operations in the vicinity of water sources, the presence of environmental disease-causing bacteria, and inadequate water treatment processes, including treatment failures and human error. It is important to note that in many of the cases, more than one factor was present. For example, in Walkerton, most of the listed factors were present.

One of the study findings of note is that because of inconsistencies in the actual reporting and the detail of reporting among provinces and territories, there was limited data collection. For example, the researchers were unable to determine the disease burden and the details of contributing factors due to water-borne outbreaks. Therefore, the researchers recommend the development of a federal surveillance system for consistent reporting of outbreaks.

Application for CHNs: Community health nurses will encounter clients in their community who may present with gastrointestinal symptoms that have not responded to the usual treatments. Community health nurses play a key role in the surveillance of disease patterns and environmental data in their community in order to appropriately administer the public health interventions and follow up when necessary.

Questions for Reflection & Discussion

1. a) What are some major chemical contaminants found in water?
   b) What is the role of the community health nurse in preventing exposure to these chemical contaminants?
2. What actions could be taken to promote an environmentally responsible community?
3. With the knowledge you have gained from Schuster et al.'s study, how would you frame your question to search for the most recent and available evidence on contributors to infectious disease outbreaks?

Reference: Schuster, C. J., Ellis, A. G., Robertson, W. J., Charron, D. F., Aramini, J. J., Marshall, B. J., & Medeiros, D.T. (2005). Infectious disease outbreaks related to drinking water in Canada, 1974–2001. *Canadian Journal of Public Health*, *96*(4), 254–258.

CRITICAL VIEW

1. What are some of the environmental injustices in your community?
2. a) What can CHNs do to address these environmental injustices?
   b) What roles might CHNs assume in addressing environmental injustices?

COMMUNITY HEALTH NURSES' ROLES IN ENVIRONMENTAL HEALTH

Currently, CHNs have not played a significant role in environmental health. However, CHNs could be involved in a number of roles in environmental health, in full-time work, as an adjunct to existing roles, and as informed citizens. Environmental health activities could include the following:

- *Community involvement and public participation.* Organizing, facilitating, and moderating and making public notices effective, public forums accessible and welcoming of input, information exchange understandable, and problem solving acceptable to culturally diverse communities are valuable assets CHNs contribute. Skills in community organizing and mobilizing can be essential to a community having a meaningful voice in decisions that affect it.
- *Individual and population risk assessment.* Community health nursing assessment skills are used to detect potential and actual exposure pathways and outcomes for clients cared for in acute, chronic, and healthy communities of practice.
- *Risk communication.* Interpreting and applying principles to practice, CHNs may serve as skilled risk communicators within agencies, working for industries or working as independent practitioners. As risk communicators, CHNs fulfill the roles of educators for clients about environmental risks and possible preventive activities pertaining to the risks. In this role, CHNs must be knowledgeable of community resources and make appropriate referrals.
- *Epidemiological investigations.* CHNs have the skills to respond in scientifically sound and sensitive ways to community concerns about cancer, birth defects, and stillbirths that citizens fear may have environmental causes.
- *Policy development.* CHNs propose, inform, and monitor action from agencies, communities, and organization perspectives.

As CHNs learn more about the environment, opportunities for integration of environmental considerations into their practice, educational programs, research, advocacy, and policy work will become evident. Opportunities abound for those pioneering spirits within the nursing profession who are dedicated to creating healthier environments for their clients and communities. The CNA work plan for 2007–2010 identifies six strategic directions to be addressed (CNA, 2007). One direction is to "identify the importance to health status of social determinants including childcare, housing and environmental safety" (CNA, 2007). This work will expand on past efforts in promoting healthy social policies such as national child care strategies and health and environmental safety; proceeding with a strategy to address national housing by initially looking at available resources; and providing healthy child development evidence on its Web site, information on the effects of poverty, and suggestions for reduction of poverty. In addition, it will address environmental issues such as climate change by continuing to work with environmental partners such as Environment Canada to provide Web-based information on climate change and the CNA position statements on the environment (CNA, 2007).

Appendix 10, "The CNA Position Statement: Nurses and Environmental Health" (2009), discusses the environment as a determinant of health and its impact on the health of Canadians as well as the role of the nurse regarding environmental issues. The "CNA/CMA Joint Position Statement on Environmentally Responsible Activity in the Health Sector" presents the CNA and the Canadian Medical Association's (CMA) intent to encourage environmentally responsible activities in the health sector for various reasons, such as economic, health enhancement, and ethical reasons. This statement describes the role of individual practitioners and professional associations and includes resolutions to address the issue of health and the environment. The CNA 2009 position statement titled "Climate Change and Health" discusses nurses' many roles in working with clients to help them adapt to climate change and reduce their ecological footprint. The CNA document "The Role of Nurses in Addressing Climate Change" provides information on climate change and social justice; the impact of and adaptation to climate change; mitigation strategies; and nurses' involvement in policy pertaining to climate change. The CNA document "The Role of Nurses in Greening the Health System" provides information on energy use, GHGs disposal of wastes, and toxic substance use. The CNA backgrounder "The Built Environment, Injury Prevention and Nursing: A Summary of the Issues" identifies injury as one of the leading causes of death in Canada for those aged 1 to 44 years. The backgrounder discusses injury as an important issue for children, workers, and older adults; reports that CHNs are prepared to help reduce the risk of injury in these aggregates; and suggests primary, secondary, and tertiary interventions. For access to these CNA documents, refer to the CNA Web sites listed in the Evolve Weblinks.

CHNs, with continued nursing leadership, use of established partnerships, and the establishment of new multilevel-approach partnerships, will continue to have a positive impact on the environmental hazards and risks that affect health. In addition, CHNs, when working with populations, screen, manage outbreaks, educate, and use surveillance techniques for early detection, the reduction of harm, and the promotion of health (Pike-MacDonald et al., 2007). CHNs need to be environmentally responsible in their practice and encourage and facilitate environmental responsibility in their workplace and community. An international coalition of health care professionals, Health Care without Harm (see the Weblinks on the Evolve Web site), has a platform of environmentally responsible health care with a focus on environmental issues and their health impact.

Advocacy

Canadian nurses have a strong voice for environmental change. As informed citizens, CHNs can take a variety of actions to protect the environmental health of clients. Although every CHN cannot be an expert in all aspects of environmental health, every CHN does have a basic education in human health and can identify those who may be most vulnerable to environmental insult. CHNs' thoughts about the potential effects of new laws on the health of clients are valuable to legislators. As advocates for environmental issues, CHNs can do the following:

- Write letters to local newspapers responding to environmental health issues affecting the community.
- Serve as credible sources of information at community gatherings, formal governmental hearings, and professional nursing forums.
- Actively participate as committee members on community committees that focus on environmental health issues.
- Volunteer to serve on municipal, provincial, territorial, or federal environmental health commissions.
- Use resources such as the CNA Presentation Toolkit about environmental health (see Tool Box on the Evolve Web site).
- Know and support the zoning and permit laws that regulate the effects of industry and land use on the community, plus environmental laws applying to the community.
- Read, listen, and ask questions. Then, they will be leaders, fostering community action to address environmental health threats.

As a professional body, the CNA has advocated significantly to promote environmental health. CNA contributions have included passing resolutions on some of the effects of environmental health hazards; creating policy and position statements on the responsibilities of health professionals regarding environmental health activities; and being a member of environmental committees such as the Environmental Health Coalition, the Canadian Coalition for Green Health Care, and the Expert Advisory Board on Children's Health for the Commission for Environmental Co-operation (CNA, 2005). The CNA identifies nurses' involvement at the three levels of prevention in relation to environmental health as outlined in the "Levels of Prevention" box.

Nurses are taking action on environmental health issues. Through CNA, they have formed a group called Canadian Nurses for Health and the Environment (CNHE) (CNA, 2011). CHNs care about the population's health and ways to convey this is through involvement in environmental health issues, especially policy issues, and by assuming roles in prevention and reduction of environmentally related health concerns. In their opening message at the first CNHE national conference, Swirsky and Hanley stated, "We must assume a leadership role by taking opportunities, through our practice in advocating for policies and practices, that protect human health and the enviornment over the long term. Collaboration is fundamental in planning for our future...." (2010, p. 1).

LEVELS OF PREVENTION

Related to Environmental Health

PRIMARY PREVENTION

Community health nurses:

- Counsel women of child-bearing age about reducing their exposure to environmental hazards
- Support the development of exposure standards for toxins and other contaminants
- Advocate for safe air, water, and soil
- Teach avoidance of ultraviolet exposure and use of sunscreen
- Support programs for waste reduction and recycling, as well as energy conservation in communities and workplaces

SECONDARY PREVENTION

Community health nurses:

- Assess homes, schools, worksites, and communities for environmental hazards
- Review water and soil results
- Monitor air quality reports

TERTIARY PREVENTION

Community health nurses:

- Support the cleanup of toxic waste sites and removal of other hazards
- Refer homeowners to approved programs that eliminate contaminants such as lead and asbestos

SOURCE: Adapted from Canadian Nurses Association. (2005). *Backgrounder—The ecosystem, the natural environment, and health and nursing: A summary of the issues.* Retrieved from http://www.cna-aiic.ca/CNA/documents/pdf/publications/BG4_The_Ecosystem_e.pdf. Reprinted with permission.

STUDENT EXPERIENCE

1. What are your beliefs about climate change and the associated environmental issues?
2. What have your contributions been to reduce the ecological and environmental footprint?
3. Refer to the following Web site: http://www.davidsuzuki.org/what-you-can-do/reduce-your-carbon-footprint/. Click on "Food and climate change; Cut your energy use; Four places to cut carbon; and Get on your bike and off oil." How do you plan to reduce your environmental footprint?
4. Calculate your ecological footprint at http://footprint.wwf.org.uk/.
5. What additional steps could you take to further reduce your environmental footprint?

REMEMBER THIS!

- CHNs have responsibilities to be informed consumers and advocates in their community regarding environmental health issues.
- Models describing the determinants of health acknowledge the role of the environment in health and disease.
- For many chemical compounds, whether new or familiar, scientific evidence of possible health effects is lacking.
- Each community health nursing assessment should include questions and observations about intended and unintended environmental exposures.
- Environmental databases facilitate the easy and immediate access to environmental data useful in environmental assessment.
- Advocacy skills are important for CHNs in environmental health practice.
- Risk assessment is a qualitative and quantitative evaluation of the risk posed to human health or the environment by the actual or potential presence or use of specific pollutants.
- One form of risk management is the 4Rs—that is, reduce, reuse, recycle, recover.
- Risk communication is an important skill and must acknowledge the outrage factor experienced by communities with environmental hazards.
- Municipal, provincial, territorial, and federal laws and regulations exist to protect the health of citizens and workers from environmental hazards.
- A PEEST analysis can be organized into a SWOT format.
- Environmental health practice engages multiple disciplines, and CHNs are important members of the environmental health team.
- Environmental health practice includes principles of health promotion, disease prevention, and health protection.
- At present, vulnerable populations are at risk for environmental hazards because of factors such as poverty, lack of access to health care, and dangerous neighbourhoods and homes in which they live.
- CHNs need to assume a more active role in environmental health.

REFLECTIVE PRAXIS

Case Study 1

Skylark, a 28-year-old First Nations female, lives in a small community in Newfoundland. Her only child, a 10-year-old son named Randy, likes to go fishing for brook trout and for Arctic char with his father. Randy is a healthy young male who enjoys many activities such as biking, fishing, hockey, and spending time with his extended family. Skylark comes to the community health nursing clinic to talk with the community health nurse about her recent reading that eating certain fish can cause health problems. She tells the nurse that she eats brook trout and Arctic char at least twice a week and that she has some concerns and questions.

1. According to Environment Canada, what is a healthy amount of Arctic char and brook trout for Skylark to eat?
2. What would be a healthy amount of these fish for her son to eat?
3. What symptoms should the community health nurse ask Skylark about to determine if mercury poisoning is present in her immediate family?

Answers are on the Evolve Web site at http://evolve.elsevier.com/Canada/Stanhope/community/.

Case Study 2

A citizen calls the local health department to report that his drinking water, from a private well, "smells like gasoline." A water sample is collected, and analysis reveals the presence of petroleum products. A nearby rural store with a service station has removed its old underground gasoline storage tanks and replaced them, as required by law. Contaminated soil from the old leaking tank has been removed, and a well to monitor groundwater contamination is scheduled for installation. However, sandy soil has allowed rapid movement of the contamination through the groundwater, and the plume has reached the neighbour's drinking-water well in levels that exceed the standard.

1. What are some possible short- and long-term actions to deal with the current situation?

Answers are on the Evolve Web site at http://evolve.elsevier.com/Canada/Stanhope/community/.

What Would You Do?

1. If you thought that the drinking water in your community was contaminated from polluted sources, how would you go about verifying your concern? Who would you contact? What would your sources of information be? If you found that you were correct, what steps would you take to remedy this environmental health problem?
2. Think of your community and identify the types of hazardous wastes that are produced. What actions would need to be taken in your community to reduce the amount of identified hazardous wastes?
3. You have been asked to join a municipal environmental health promotion committee newly organized by the mayor's office. You volunteer to determine the health hazards of prominence in your community. What information will you collect from your local public health department? What are the roles of the various public health professionals employed by that agency who work with environmental health issues?

TOOL BOX

evolve

The Tool Box contains useful instruments that can be applied in community health nursing practice. These related resources are found either in the appendices at the back of this book or on the Evolve Web site at http://evolve.elsevier.com/Canada/Stanhope/community/.

Appendices

- Appendix 10: CNA Position Statement: "Nurses and Environmental Health"
- Appendix E-1: Comprehensive Occupational and Environmental Health History

Tools

Canadian Nurses Association. CNA Presentation Toolkit.
This site provides tools that can be used by nurses to educate about environmental health. Resources include PowerPoint slides, videos, handouts, posters, and bookmarks.

Environmental Handbook for Community Development Initiatives.
This handbook by the Canadian International Development Agency is a guide to assist with environmental assessment, mostly for smaller initiatives.

Health Canada. *Indoor Air Quality Tools for Schools Action Kit.*
This is an easy-to-use tool intended for use by school teaching and administrative staff to enable them to address concerns about indoor air quality.

WEBLINKS

evolve

Direct links to these resources can be found on the text's accompanying Evolve Web site at http://evolve.elsevier.com/Canada/Stanhope/community.

Asthma Society of Canada. The society provides media clips, responds to frequently asked questions, and provides games and stories for children with asthma and a paper-based resource kit for parents and teachers.

B.C. Injury Research and Prevention Unit. ***Interior Health Injury Prevention Environmental Scan: A Final Report.*** This site describes the development of an environmental scan in order to identify capacity, service needs, and possible partnerships and coalitions within the scan area. The focus in this document is on youth suicide and abuse.

Canadian Centre for Occupational Health and Safety. The centre's site takes you to the Canadian enviroOSH legislation, which provides a listing of health, safety, and environmental legislations for all Canadian federal, provincial, and territorial jurisdictions. Note that there is limited access.

Canadian Environmental Network. This site is a link to major sources of environmental groups, organizations, Web sites, and resources in Canada, arranged by themes such as environmental action alerts, ecoshop/greenlist directory, and special environmental projects.

Canadian Institute of Child Health. This organization focuses on improving the health of children and youth in Canada. The focus is on monitoring, education, and advocacy for policies and practices affecting children and youth health.

Canadian Institute for Health Information (CIHI). ***Housing and Population Health: The State of Current***

Research Knowledge. This site provides information about housing and its connection to population health.

Canadian Nurses Association: Backgrounders, Position Statements, and Other Related Documents.

- CNA Backgrounder: *The Built Environment, Injury Prevention and Nursing: A Summary of the Issues*
- CNA Backgrounder: *The Ecosystem, the Natural Environment, and Health and Nursing: A Summary of the Issues*
- *CNA/CMA Joint Position Statement on Environmentally Responsible Activity in the Health Sector*
- CNA Position Statement: *Climate Change and Health*
- CNA: *The Environment and Health: An Introduction for Nurses*
- CNA: *The Role of Nurses in Addressing Climate Change*
- CNA: *The Role of Nurses in Greening the Health System*

Canadian Partnership for Children's Health & Environment. *First Steps in Lifelong Health.* This resource provides information on health concerns affecting the health of children in Canada. Also included is information on strategies such as research, policies, and protection to address some of the health concerns.

Canadian Policy Research Networks. *Environmental Justice in Canada—It Matters Where You Live.* This site provides information on environmental justice, with examples, and discusses development and implementation of environmental justice policy.

Canadian Public Health Association. *Environmental Justice in Canada? Identifying a Role for Public Health Research and Practice.* This document provides information on environmental justice in Canada. Case examples of ongoing environmental disputes in Canada such as the Sydney tar ponds in Nova Scotia and the Athabasca oil sands in Alberta are provided.

Canadian Public Health Association. *A Guide to Collaborative Processes in Health Policy Development and Their Implications for Action.* The Canadian Public Health Association's Voice Project site hosts a guide with information involving a wide range of situations and issues in health policy development. The guide can be used as a reflective tool and an action tool. Within the guide are many excellent Weblinks to other similar guides. From the link provided, select "Planning Tools" from the main menu, and then choose "A Guide to Collaborative Processes."

Environment Canada. *Acid Rain and...the Facts.* This site, presented in a question-and-answer format, provides information on what acid rain is, where in Canada it is a problem, and the sources of emission that contribute to it.

Environment Canada. *Air.* This site provides information on the many pollutants affecting indoor and outdoor air quality and health. From the Environment Canada home page, click on "Air."

Environment Canada. *Canadian Environmental Quality Guidelines.* This site identifies what is done at Environment Canada and provides the Environmental Quality Guidelines.

Environment Canada. *Information on Greenhouse Gas Sources and Sinks.* This site provides information on various GHG sources such as the oil and gas industry, electric power generation sites, transportation emissions, and sinks.

Global Footprint Network. *World Footprint.* This site provides snapshots of the global footprint of nations and cities. For information on Canada, check the 2008 data tables under North America.

Government of Canada. *Chemical Substances: What Is Risk Management?* This site provides information on how to minimize the risks associated with chemicals and it provides examples of risk management tools.

Government of Canada. *Children's Health and the Environment in North America: A First Report on Available Indicators and Measures.* This Canadian report contains case studies of research on subpopulations of children who may be unreasonably affected by environmental contaminants. The report also provides extensive information related to children, such as asthma and respiratory diseases, lead, and chemicals, as well as pesticides and water-borne diseases.

Government of Canada. Eco-Action on Climate Change and Air Pollution. This online document outlines the federal government's action plan for significantly reducing GHG emissions by 2020.

Health Canada. *About Health Canada: Acts.* This site explains the process of how a bill becomes law or an act. Also found is a listing of acts falling under Health Canada and an access link to the full text of many of the acts under the responsibility of Health Canada.

Health Canada. *Drinking Water.* This site provides information on published reports, including the safe drinking water guidelines.

Health Canada. *Drinking Water and Wastewater.* This site provides information regarding the quality of water, monitoring of drinking water, and the responsibility of the federal government for the provision of quality drinking water to First Nations, Inuit, and Aboriginal peoples. There are excellent related links at the end of this site.

Health Canada. *Environmental Health Assessment.* Links at the site will allow you to access information on how to conduct an environmental health assessment and information about the *Canadian Environmental Health Act.*

Health Canada. *Environmental and Workplace Health.* Environmental and workplace health is one of the areas listed in the Health Canada directory identified on the left of the screen. When you select this choice, you will find numerous topics such as air quality, climate change and health, contaminated sites, environmental contaminants, environmental health assessment, environmental impact initiative, environmental radiation, noise, occupational health and safety, radiation, and water quality. If you were to choose another area such as First Nations and Inuit health, you would gain valuable information about Health Canada's role in health care for these peoples, plus statistical data on their health.

Health Canada. *Fluorides and Human Health.* This Health Canada site provides the health benefits and health risks of using fluoride and the role government plays in fluoridation.

Health Canada. *The Health and Environment Handbook for Health Professionals.* This document provides information on environmental risk and quality of water, air, food, and soil.

Health Canada. Human Health Risk Assessment. Risk assessment tools and guidance materials.

Health Canada. *Indoor Air Quality.* This site provides information on how to assess the indoor air quality to determine the health impact of the presence of items such as formaldehyde, carbon monoxide, and radon.

Health Canada. Let's Talk about Health and Air Quality. This site focuses on the major outdoor air pollutants and the quality of outdoor air in Canada.

Health Canada. *Situational Analysis.* This site discusses conducting situational analysis that includes an environmental scan and a SWOT analysis.

Health Care Without Harm. This is an international coalition of health care systems and professionals, community groups, labour unions, environmental health organizations, and religious groups with a mission to transform the health care industry worldwide so that it is ecologically sustainable and no longer a source of harm to public health and the environment.

Making Environmental Health Happen in the Community: The Story of South Riverdale Community Health Centre's Environmental Health Program. This site provides a Web manual that documents some characteristics of an environmental health program at the South Riverdale Community Health Centre in Toronto. This program is a guide for how to incorporate environmental health as a determinant into health activities. From the link given, click on the document.

Marshall, L., Weir, E., Abelsohn, A., & Sandborn, M. D. (2002). ***Identifying and Managing Adverse and Environmental Health Effects: 1. Taking an Exposure History.*** This article discusses the reasons for taking an environmental health history and speaks to the use of the CH^2OPD^2 mnemonic (*c*ommunity, *h*ome, *h*obbies, *o*ccupation, *p*ersonal habits, *d*iet, *d*rugs).

Pollution Probe. *Clean Air. Clean Water.* This Canadian environmental organization's site deals with the research, education, and advocacy needs of the public regarding environmental issues. The site lists publications on the various environmental issues. One of the reports available is a discussion of Canadian environmental standards.

U.S. Environmental Protection Agency. *Acid Rain.* This site elaborates on acid rain issues and provides a pictorial view of the effects of the gases that contribute to acid rain.

REFERENCES

Asthma Society of Canada. (2005). *Asthma facts and statistics.* Retrieved from http://www.asthma.ca/corp/newsroom/pdf/asthmastats.pdf.

B.C. Injury Research and Prevention Unit. (2007). *Interior health injury prevention environmental scan: A final report.* Retrieved from http://www.injuryresearch.bc.ca/admin/DocUpload/3_20090616_100720IH%20ENVT%20SCAN%20FINAL_May.9.07.pdf.

Boffetta, P. (2006). Human cancer from environmental pollutants: The epidemiological evidence. *Mutation Research, 608*(2), 157–162.

Breslin, F. C., Day, D., Tompa, E., Irvin, E., Bhattacharyya, S., Clarke, J., & Wang, A. (2007). Non-agricultural work injuries among youth: A systematic review. *American Journal of Preventive Medicine, 32*(2), 151–162.

Canadian Centre for Occupational Health and Safety. (2005). *OSH answers.* Retrieved from http://www.ccohs.ca/oshanswers/.

Canadian Food Inspection Agency. (2008). *Canadian Food Inspection Agency: 2008–2009 corporate business plan.* Retrieved from http://www.inspection.gc.ca/english/corpaffr/busplan/2008-09/plan200809_2e.shtml.

Canadian Nurses Association. (2005). *Backgrounder: The ecosystem, the natural environment, and health and nursing: A summary of the issues.* Retrieved from http://www.cna-nurses.ca/CNA/documents/pdf/publications/BG4_The_Ecosystem_e.pdf.

Canadian Nurses Association. (2007). *Joint letter on 2007 work plan*. Retrieved from http://www.cna-nurses.ca/CNA/documents/pdf/publications/Open-Letter-Joint-Workplan-e.pdf.

Canadian Nurses Association. (2009). *Position statement: Climate change and health*. Retrieved from http://www.cna-nurses.ca/CNA/documents/pdf/publications/PS100_Climate_Change_e.pdf.

Canadian Nurses Association. (2011). *Nursing and environmental health*. Retrieved from http://www.cna-aiic.ca/CNA/issues/environment/action/default_e.aspx.

Canadian Partnership for Children's Health & Environment. (2008). *First steps in lifelong health*. Retrieved from http://www.healthyenvironmentforkids.ca/img_upload/13297cd6a147585a24c1c6233d8d96d8/CPCHE_VandS.pdf.

Canadian Policy Research Network. (2009). *Stress and hours of work*. Retrieved from http://www.jobquality.ca/indicators/environment/phy5.shtml.

Canadian Public Health Association. (2008). *Environmental justice in Canada? Identifying a role for public health research and practice*. Retrieved from http://www.pchr.net/media/CNEHSE%20CPHA%20WORKSHOP%20REPORT.doc.

Chan, M. (2007). *Address to the Regional Committee for the Western Pacific*. Retrieved from http://www.who.int/dg/speeches/2007/20070910_korea/en/index.html.

Chaudry, R. V. (2008). The precautionary principle, public health, and public health nursing. *Public Health Nursing*, *25*(3), 261–268.

Commission for Environmental Cooperation. (2006). *Children's health and the environment in North America: A first report on available indicators and measures*. Retrieved from http://www.cec.org/files/PDF/POLLUTANTS/CEH-Indicators-fin_en.pdf.

Conference Board of Canada. (2009). *How Canada performs: Environment overview*. Retrieved from http://sso.conferenceboard.ca/HCP/overview/environment-overview.aspx.

Curtis, L., Rea, W., Smith-Willis, P., Fenyves, E., & Pan, Y. (2006). Adverse health effects of outdoor air pollutants. *Environment International*, *32*(6), 815–830.

David Suzuki Foundation. (2009). *Science: The skeptics*. Retrieved from http://www.davidsuzuki.org/Climate_Change/Science/Skeptics.asp.

Environment Canada. (2006a). *CESI 2006 Feature report*. Retrieved from http://www.ec.gc.ca/indicateurs-indicators/default.asp?lang=En&n=667DD94F-1&offset=23&toc=show.

Environment Canada. (2006b). *Information on greenhouse gas sources and sinks*. Retrieved from http://www.ec.gc.ca/pdb/ghg/about/FAQ_e.cfm.

Environment Canada. (2009a). *About climate change*. Retrieved from http://www.ec.gc.ca/cc/default.asp?lang=En&n=9C2CF393-1.

Environment Canada. (2009b). *Cleaning the air in Canadian cities*. Retrieved from http://ec.gc.ca/scitech/4B40916E-16D3-4357-97EB-A6DF7005D1B3/EnvTech_Air_Story_8.5x11EN.pdf.

Environment Canada. (2009c). *News release: Government of Canada to reduce greenhouse gas emissions from vehicles*. Retrieved from http://www.ec.gc.ca/default.asp?lang=En&n=714D9AAE-1&news=29FDD9F6-489A-4C5C-9115-193686D1C2B5.

Environment Canada Health Canada. (2008). *Screening assessment for the challenge phenol, 4,4'-(1-methylethylidene) bis-(Bisphenol A)*. Retrieved from http://www.ec.gc.ca/substances/ese/eng/challenge/batch2/batch2_80-05-7_en.pdf.

Finley, R., Reid-Smith, R., & Weese, J. S. (2006). Human health implications of *Salmonella*-contaminated natural pet treats and raw pet food. *Clinical Infectious Diseases*, *42*(5), 686–691.

Forsyth, D. S., Casey, V., Dabeka, R. W., & McKenzie, A. (2004). Methylmercury levels in predatory fish species marketed in Canada. *Food Additives and Contaminants*, *21*(9), 849–856.

Government of Alberta. (2010). *Surface water quality program*. Retrieved from http://www.environment.alberta.ca/01256.html.

Government of Canada. (2008a). *Chemical substances: What is risk management?*. Retrieved from http://www.chemicalsubstanceschimiques.gc.ca/manage-gestion/what-quoi/index_e.html.

Government of Canada. (2008b). *Turning the corner: Regulatory framework for industrial greenhouse gas emissions*. Retrieved from http://www.ec.gc.ca/doc/virage-corner/2008-03/pdf/COM-541_Framework.pdf.

Government of Canada. (2009). *ecoAction*. Retrieved from http://www.ecoaction.gc.ca.

Graham, P., Evitts, T., & Thomas-MacLean, R. (2008). Environmental scans. *Canadian Family Physician*, *54*, 1022–1023.

Health Canada. (2004a). *The Canadian handbook on health impact assessment, Volume 1: The basics*. Retrieved from http://www.hc-sc.gc.ca/ewh-semt/pubs/eval/handbook-guide/index-eng.php.

Health Canada. (2004b). *The national chemical residue monitoring program*. Retrieved from http://www.inspection.gc.ca/english/fssa/microchem/resid/residfse.shtml.

Health Canada. (2005). *Road traffic and air pollution*. Retrieved from http://www.hc-sc.gc.ca/hl-vs/iyh-vsv/environ/traf-eng.php.

Health Canada. (2006a). *Chemical residue annual reports*. Retrieved from http://www.inspection.gc.ca/english/fssa/microchem/chemchime.shtml.

Health Canada. (2006b). *Legislation and guidelines*. Retrieved from http://www.hc-sc.gc.ca/ahc-asc/legislation/index-eng.php.

Health Canada. (2007). *Mercury: Your health and the environment*. Retrieved from http://www.hc-sc.gc.ca/ewh-semt/pubs/contaminants/mercur/q35-q42-eng.php.

Health Canada. (2008a). *Effects of lead on human health*. Retrieved from http://www.hc-sc.gc.ca/hl-vs/iyh-vsv/environ/lead-plomb-eng.php#he.

Health Canada. (2008b). *Environmental and workplace health*. Retrieved from http://www.hc-sc.gc.ca/ewh-semt/eval/index-eng.php.

Health Canada. (2008c). *Human health risk assessment of mercury in fish and health benefits of fish consumption.* Retrieved from http://www.hc-sc.gc.ca/fn-an/pubs/mercur/merc_fish_poisson-eng.php#4.4.

Health Canada. (2009). *Human health risk assessment.* Retrieved from http://www.hc-sc.gc.ca/ewh-semt/contamsite/risk-risque-eng.php#tools.

Health Canada. (2010). *About the pest management regulatory agency (PMRA).* Retrieved from http://www.hc-sc.gc.ca/cps-spc/pest/faq-eng.php#abo.

Hill, S. (2005). *Appendix A: Some factors affecting the perception of risk. Risk communication literature review: Summary report.* Ottawa: Treasury Board of Canada Secretariat. Retrieved from http://www.tbs-sct.gc.ca/rm-gr/rc-cr/report-rapport_e.asp#two.

Hrudey, S. E., Hrudey, E. J., & Pollard, S. J. T. (2006). Risk management for assuring safe drinking water. *Environment International*, *32*(8), 948–957.

Kongtip, P., Thongsuk, W., Yoosook, W., & Chantanakul, S. (2006). Health effects of metropolitan traffic-related air pollutants on street vendors. *Atmospheric Environment*, *40*(37), 7138–7145.

Kovesi, T., Creery, D., Gilbert, N. L., Dales, R., Fugler, D., Thompson, B., & Miller, J. D. (2006). Indoor air quality risk factors for severe lower respiratory tract infections in Inuit infants in Baffin Region, Nunavut: A pilot study. *Indoor Air*, *16*(4), 266–275.

The Lung Association. (2010). *Asthma in children.* Retrieved from http://www.on.lung.ca/Page.aspx?pid = 428.

Marshall, L., Weir, E., Abelsohn, A., & Sandborn, M. D. (2002). Identifying and managing adverse and environmental health effects: 1. Taking an exposure history. *Canadian Medical Association Journal*, *166*(9), 1049–1055.

Mittelstaedt, M. (2010, October 13). Canada first to declare Bisphenol A toxic. *The Globe and Mail.* Retrieved from http://www.theglobeandmail.com/news/national/canada-first-to-declare-bisphenol-a-toxic/article1755272/.

Moore, D., Copes, R., Fisk, R., Joy, R., Chan, K., & Brauer, M. (2006). Population health effects of air quality changes due to forest fires in British Columbia in 2003. *Canadian Journal of Public Health*, *97*(2), 105–108.

Nightingale, F. (1859). *Notes on nursing: What it is and what it is not.* London: Harrison.

Ontario Ministry of Natural Resources. (2009). *Guide to eating Ontario sport fish.* Toronto, ON: Queen's Printer for Ontario.

Pierpont, N. (2010). *Wind Concerns Ontario.* Retrieved from http://windconcernsontario.wordpress.com/2010/04/24/wind-turbine-syndrome-excerpts-from-the-executive-summary/.

Pike-MacDonald, S., Best, D. G., Twomey, C., Bennett, L., & Blakeley, J. (2007). Promoting safe drinking water. *Canadian Nurse*, *103*(1), 15–19.

Pong, R. W., Pitblado, J. R., & Irvine, A. (2002). *A strategy for developing environmental health indicators for rural Canada.* Retrieved from http://www.cranhr.ca/pdf/CJPH_2002.pdf.

Public Health Agency of Canada. (2005). *National collaborating centres for public health?.* Retrieved from http://www.phac-aspc.gc.ca/media/nr-rp/2005/2005_15bk1-eng.php.

Public Health Agency of Canada. (2008). *Safe healthy environments.* Retrieved from http://www.phac-aspc.gc.ca/dca-dea/allchildren_touslesenfants/she_main-eng.php.

Public Health Agency of Canada. (2009). *Key element 1: Focus on the health of populations.* Retrieved from http://cbpp-pcpe.phac-aspc.gc.ca/population_health/key_element_1-eng.html.

Schuster, C. J., Ellis, A. G., Robertson, W. J., Charron, D. F., Aramini, J. J., Marshall, B. J., & Medeiros, D. T. (2005). Infectious disease outbreaks related to drinking water in Canada, 1974–2001. *Canadian Journal of Public Health*, *96*(4), 254–258.

Shah, C. P. (2003). *Public health and preventive medicine in Canada* (5th ed.). Toronto, ON: Elsevier Saunders.

Stanhope, M., & Lancaster, J. (2004). *Community and public health nursing* (6th ed.). St. Louis, MO: Mosby.

Statistics Canada. (2006). *Canadian environmental sustainability indicators.* Retrieved from http://www.statcan.gc.ca/pub/16-251-x/16-251-x2005000-eng.htm.

Swirsky, H., & Hanley, F. (2010). *Canadian nurses for health and the environment: 2010 national conference.* Retrieved from http://www.cnhe-iise.ca/conference.html.

Tannahill, A. (2008). Beyond evidence—to ethics: A decision-making framework for health promotion, public health and health improvement. *Health Promotion International*, *23*(4), 380–390.

Twarakavi, N. K. C., & Kaluarachchi, J. J. (2006). Sustainability of ground water quality considering land use changes and public health risks. *Journal of Environmental Management*, *81*(4), 405–419.

U.N. Department of Economic and Social Affairs. (2009). *Agenda 21.* Retrieved from http://www.un.org/esa/dsd/agenda21/res_agenda21_02.shtml.

U.S. Environmental Protection Agency. (2007). *Acid rain.* Retrieved from http://www.epa.gov/acidrain/what/index.html.

Ward, M. S., Sahai, V. S., Tilleczek, K. C., Fearn, J. L., Barnett, R. C., & Zmijowskyj, T. (2005). Child and adolescent health in Northern Ontario: A quantitative profile for public health planning. *Canadian Journal of Public Health*, *96*(4), 287–290.

Young-Reuters, J. (2010, October 13). BPA declared toxic by Canada. *CBC News.* Retrieved from http://www.cbc.ca/health/story/2010/10/13/bpa-toxic.html.

CHAPTER

16 Disaster Management

KEY TERMS

Centre for Emergency Preparedness and Response (CEPR) 508

disaster 501

disaster preparedness 507

disaster prevention and mitigation 506

disaster recovery 519

disaster response 517

disaster vulnerability 507

Emergency Measures Organization (EMO) 510

human-made disasters 504

influenza pandemic 511

natural disasters 503

triage 518

See Glossary on page 593 for definitions

OBJECTIVES

After reading this chapter, you should be able to:

1. Explain the various types of disasters.
2. Evaluate the effects of disasters on people and their communities.
3. Describe the disaster management phases of prevention and mitigation, preparedness, response, and recovery and explain the community health nurse's role in each phase.
4. Describe the considerations for personal and professional preparedness in disasters.
5. Identify how community groups and other organizations such as the Canadian Red Cross can work together to prepare for, respond to, and recover from disasters.
6. Describe pandemic preparedness.
7. Describe the role and responsibilities of community health nurses in preparing for and responding to disasters.

CHAPTER OUTLINE

The Canadian authors gratefully acknowledge the work of contributor Vicki Morley for additions to the H1N1 content.

DISASTERS

Disasters are events that usually occur suddenly and unexpectedly. They seldom can be fully prevented, nor can they be adequately prepared for by those who will be affected. They are destructive events that disrupt the normal functioning of a community and create vulnerabilities for those experiencing the disaster (Raholm, Arman, & Rehnsfeldt, 2008). Often those who experience being in major disasters are confronted with their own death and the deaths of loved ones and encounter situations they have never been faced with before (Raholm et al., 2008).

Accidents, acts of war or terrorism, and environmental mishaps cause disasters. The most recent disasters in this century are associated with global instability, economic downturns, political upheaval with its often accompanying wars or collapse of governments, famine, mass population displacements, violence, and civil conflicts (Veenema, 2003). The tsunami that devastated areas of Asia in 2004 illustrates the unpredictable nature of disasters. Raholm et al. (2008) studied the lived experiences of this tsunami disaster. Unfortunately, disasters are inevitable; however, there are ways to prevent or manage how people respond (Raholm et al., 2008). Raholm et al. (2008) suggest that reviewing the literature on the experiences of disaster survivors can help health professionals gain an understanding so that strategies for future disasters can be developed. This chapter describes management techniques to be used in the prevention and mitigation, preparedness, response, and recovery phases of disaster. The community health nursing role is discussed for each phase. Some Web-based resources are provided throughout this chapter as supplemental resources. One resource of note is the Royal Roads University Web site (see the Weblinks on the Evolve Web site), "Disaster and Emergency Management."

Types of Disasters

A **disaster** is any human-made or natural event that causes destruction and devastation that cannot be relieved without assistance. The event need not cause injury or death to be considered a disaster. For example, a hurricane may cause millions of dollars in damage without causing a single death or injury. Table 16-1 lists examples of natural and human-made disasters.

Although natural disasters cannot be prevented, much can be done to prevent further increases in accidents, death, and destruction after impact. A concise, realistic, and well-rehearsed disaster plan is essential. There needs to also be open, clear, and ongoing communication among involved workers and organizations. Also, many of the human-made disasters listed in Table 16-1 can be prevented (e.g., major transportation accidents and fires resulting from substance abuse). For further information, refer to the Government of Canada Weblink (on the Evolve Web site) "SafeCanada.ca—Emergencies and Disasters." This is an excellent Web site that CHNs would use and provide to clients who have Internet access.

TABLE 16-1 Types of Disasters

Natural	Human
Biological	**Conflict**
Epidemic/pandemic	Civil unrest
Infestation	School violence
	Terrorism/bioterrorism
	Technological
	Accident—industrial
	Accident—other
	Accident—transport
	Computer viruses
	Fire
	Hazardous chemicals
	Structural collapse
Meteorological and hydrological	
Cold wave	
Drought	
Flood, hail/thunderstorm	
Heat wave/cold wave	
Hurricane/typhoon	
Snow avalanche	
Storm surges	
Storm—freezing rain	
Storm—unspecific or other	
Storm—winter	
Tornado	
Wildfire	
Geological	
Earthquake	
Landslide/mudslide	
Tsunami	

Disasters can affect a single family or a small group, as in a house fire, or they can kill thousands and have economic losses in the millions, as with floods, earthquakes, tornadoes, hurricanes, and bioterrorism. *Bioterrorism* refers to the threat of use, or use, of biological agents to frighten or coerce individuals, groups, or populations as a whole. Recent hurricanes, the tsunami of 2004, the 2009 earthquake in Haiti, and the 2011 extensive flooding in Australia have escalated the loss of lives, homes, businesses, and even towns and villages. In Canada, over the past 25 years, six disasters cost over $22 billion (Etkin, Haque, Bellisario, & Burton, 2004).

People in industrialized countries are becoming less self-sufficient because they rely heavily on technology and social and economic systems within their community. People who live on the brink of disaster every day, physically, emotionally, or economically, are among the first to be affected when disaster strikes. Disasters affect the health of a community in many ways—they may do the following (Veenema, 2003):

- Cause premature deaths, illnesses, and injuries in the affected community
- Destroy the local health care infrastructure and prevent an effective response to the emergency
- Create environmental imbalances, thereby increasing the risk of communicable diseases and environmental hazards
- Affect the psychological, emotional, and social well-being of the people
- Cause shortages of food and water
- Displace populations of people

SARS

The occurrence of severe acute respiratory syndrome (SARS) in 2003 demonstrated the effect that a disaster can have on a community, especially when it leads to premature deaths and illnesses and an awareness of imbalances in the infrastructure. SARS occurred initially in Asia, but it rapidly became a disease of international significance because of its communicability, lack of available diagnostic tests, and increased world travel. The SARS outbreak heightened awareness of the enormous financial and human costs due to the lack of readiness for this type of event. It created international and national economic effects, with a cost of $500 billion worldwide, 8,098 cases worldwide with 774 deaths, and 252 cases in Canada with 44 deaths (Canadian Paediatric Society, 2006; University of British Columbia, 2003). In addition to patient deaths, the SARS outbreak also resulted in the deaths of two nurses and one physician in Ontario and led to families experiencing major stress and fear (Registered Nurses' Association of Ontario [RNAO], 2004). The extent of fear experienced by health care workers has been described as overwhelming. The RNAO (2004) provides an extensive report on nurses' experiences and emotions due to the SARS outbreak, provides a chronological development of the events, talks about lessons learned, and makes recommendations. This report is available in the Weblinks on the Evolve Web site. SARS will also be discussed in Chapter 17.

Mr. Justice Archie Campbell of the Ontario Superior Court of Justice, who was appointed commissioner by the Government of Ontario, released a report in December 2006 titled *The SARS Commission—Spring of Fear: Final Report* (Campbell, 2006). (See the Weblinks on the Evolve Web site.) This report focused primarily on the management of SARS in Ontario and its impact so that preparedness for similar outbreaks could be implemented. Some of the most significant findings and recommendations from this lengthy report are the following:

- This was a system failure (e.g., lack of preparedness against infectious disease, challenges to public health due to lack of resources, health system failures to protect their workers).
- Failures occurred in the occupational safety and infection control systems in the health care sector.
- There was a failure of the system to respond by providing the necessary resources.
- There were financial costs to the government and health care system; however, the emotional losses related to illness, pain and suffering, separation from support systems, and death need to be recognized.
- One aspect of infection control was related to airborne transmission, and Ontario decided to defer use of protective equipment because the scientific evidence was not available. Campbell refers to this system weakness as ignoring the "precautionary principle," that is, to initiate prevention actions to reduce risks even though the scientific evidence is not yet available.
- Vancouver suffered significantly fewer losses from SARS because of system-wide commitment to the precautionary principle.
- Readiness for "the unseen" is one of the most significant lessons learned from SARS.

SARS was a catalyst to implement change in the preparation for future infectious disease outbreaks such as SARS and pandemic flu (Campbell, 2006). Following the outbreak of SARS, Dr. A. Naylor, appointed by Health Canada, assumed the position as Chair of the National Advisory Committee on SARS and Public Health (Krawchuk, 2003). This committee produced the Naylor Report, which included numerous recommendations on improving public health. In the follow-up to the Naylor Commission recommendations, Canada has improved its ability to respond to public health care emergencies. The Public Health Agency of Canada (PHAC, 2008) identified the following significant changes as follow-up to the Naylor Commission recommendations:

- September 2004—Public Health Agency of Canada (PHAC) established. Canada's first Chief Public Health Officer, Dr. David Butler-Jones, appointed
- 2004—Canadian Public Health Network Council established in a partnership and collaboration between all levels of government. Provides a forum to discuss key public health issues

- 2006—Expanded planning and emergency preparedness with revision of the Canadian Pandemic Influenza Plan, coordinated by the PHAC, with input from all levels of government
- 2006—Government of Canada stockpiled antiviral drugs and secured a domestic vaccine supplier as part of a multifaceted approach to protecting Canadians during influenza pandemic
- 2006—Enacted the new *Quarantine Act* that has enhanced the capacity to reduce and prevent the spread of serious infectious diseases by sick individuals entering or leaving Canada through establishment of Quarantine Services at key airports across the country
- 2007—Multidisciplinary National Health Emergency Response Teams established by PHAC within the Centre for Emergency Preparedness and Response to be deployed across Canada to provide medical surge capacity caused by a public health crisis
- Increase infectious disease surveillance and response with development of Global Public Health Intelligence Network established by PHAC as a secure Internet-based early-warning system monitoring global media sources for reports of public health significance in seven languages in real time 24 hours a day. Reports are analyzed by public health officials.
- Development of Canadian Network for Public Health Intelligence by PHAC's Centre for Infectious Disease Prevention and Control and National Microbiology Lab. It is a secure Web-based framework of applications and resources with capabilities of collecting and processing laboratory and epidemiological surveillance data from sources such as pharmacy sales and emergency room visits, analyzing the information, and providing alerts when significant trends emerge.
- Development of a Canadian Integrated Outbreak Surveillance Centre, a Web-based alert system that efficiently provides public health professionals with time-sensitive information
- Development of Web-based information sites such as Fluwatch by PHAC, which uses surveillance systems to assess influenza severity, vaccine effectiveness, and antiviral resistance that may be occurring across Canada
- Augmented capacity of the National Microbiology Laboratory to respond to outbreaks

The SARS outbreak in Ontario (discussed in Chapter 17) led to many significant and necessary changes regarding the management of such disasters in other provinces and territories and at the federal level. Figure 16-1 provides a timeline of the structures and strategies developed in the wake of SARS. The outbreak was the catalyst for the establishment of many committees at the provincial and federal levels, many of which generated a number of noteworthy reports. Examples include the Naylor Report, the Kirby Report, the Campbell Report, and the Walker Report (Mildon, 2004). As a result of these reports, a number of significant changes were made in the way in which disasters are prepared for and managed in Canada, including the appointment of a minister of Public Safety and Emergency Preparedness and a minister of state for Public Health and the creation of a Canadian Public Health Agency, to name just a few (Mildon, 2004).

Natural Disasters

The urbanization and overcrowding of cities have increased the danger of **natural disasters** (destruction or devastation caused by natural events) because communities have been built in areas that are vulnerable to disasters, such as in known tornado zones or near rivers (see Table 16-1). Population increases and the investing of money in areas vulnerable to natural disasters have led to major increases in insurance payouts in Canada and many other countries around the world in the past several decades. The ice storm of 1998 in the provinces of Ontario and Quebec affected more than five million people by creating power outages. The short-term economic costs reported by McCready (2004) were estimated at $1.6 billion. The total costs of the Saguenay flooding in the province of Quebec were estimated at $1.5 billion (Library and Archives Canada, 2006). Projections suggest that by 2050, at least 46% of the world's population will live in areas vulnerable to natural floods, earthquakes, and severe storms.

Many Canadians reside in areas that are prone to natural disasters such as flooding, earthquakes, tornadoes, landslides, or hail (Natural Resources Canada, 2009). Table 16-1 gives examples of natural disasters such as hail storms, wildfires, droughts, avalanches, and floods and human-made disasters such as transportation accidents and various types of warfare that can negatively affect the health of a community. Table 16-2 provides a chronology of some of the best-known or worst Canadian natural and human-made disasters.

Unfortunately, developing countries experience a disproportionate burden from natural disasters. These countries are usually poor and have limited resources for dealing with the effects of disaster. Disasters create the most devastation in developing countries, where the death rate is up to 12 times higher than in developed countries. The poor suffer the most because their houses are less sturdy and they have fewer social security supports. On January 12, 2010, Haiti, a Caribbean

FIGURE 16-1 In the Wake of the Outbreak of Severe Acute Respiratory Syndrome (SARS): Structures and Strategies—A Timeline

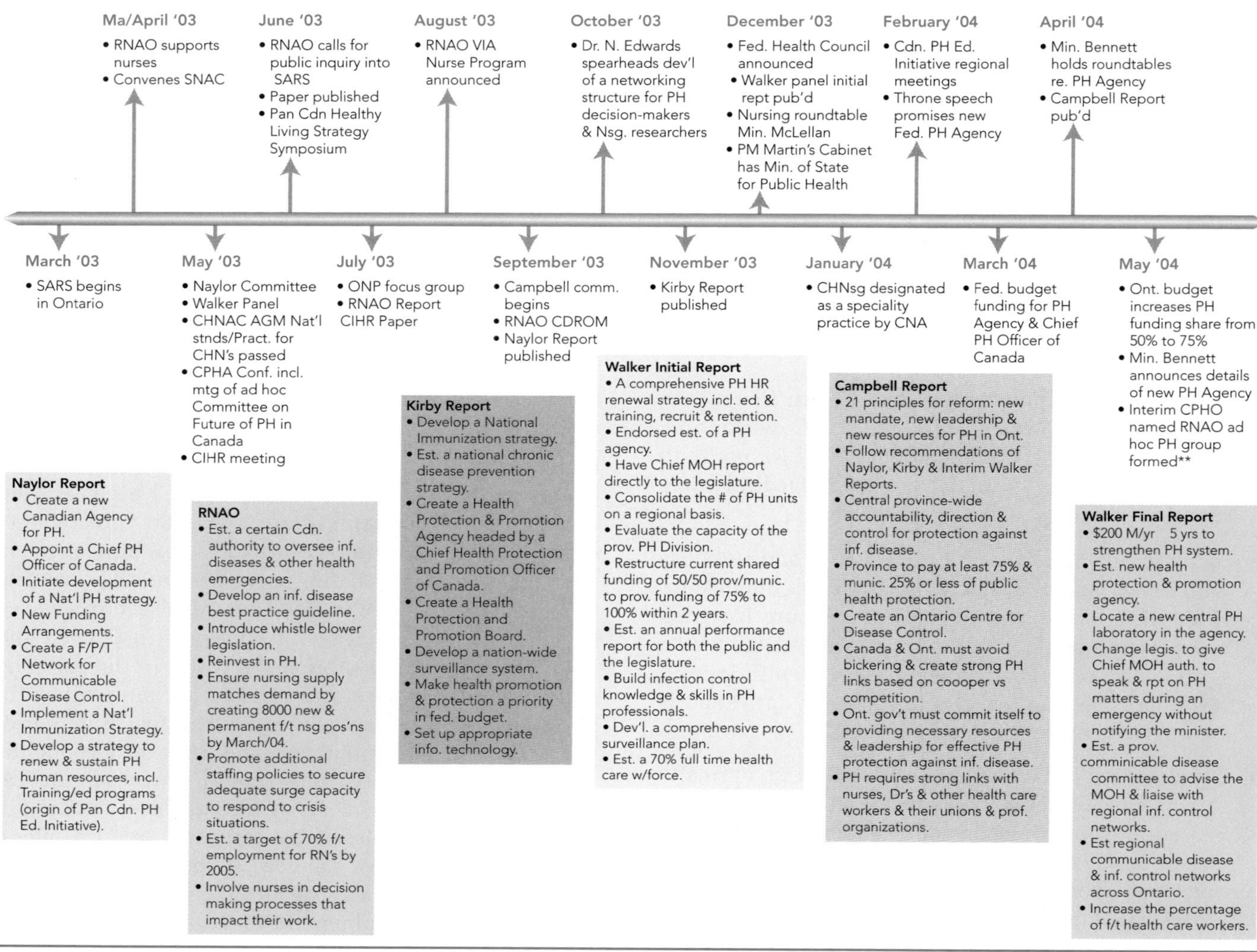

From Mildon, B. (2004). *Community Health Nurses Association of Canada Newsletter, 6*(3), 10–11. Retrieved from www.communityhealthnursescanada.org/Newsletters/CHNAC%20Newsletter-June%203rd%202004.doc. Reprinted with permission.

island and one of the poorest countries in the Western hemisphere (Foreign Affairs and International Trade Canada, 2010), experienced a 7.0 magnitude earthquake. This earthquake resulted in a natural disaster of horrific proportions for an island that has been hit often by natural disasters such as hurricanes. The extent of the damage was mostly due to the poorly constructed homes and public buildings (ABC News, 2010).

Human-made Disasters

Overcrowding and urban development have also increased **human-made disasters** (destruction or devastation caused by humans). The stress caused by overcrowding has led to civil unrest and riots. In some parts of the world, modern wars waged over land rights and space have markedly increased the risk of injury and death from disaster.

In Canada and other countries, school violence, a human-made disaster, has increased in intensity and magnitude. In Canada, there have been several violent incidents of school shootings. The first mass school shooting, known as the Montreal Massacre, occurred in 1989 at l'École Polytechnique in Montreal. Fourteen female engineering students were killed by a 25-year-old Montreal man. In 1999, at W. R. Myers High School in Taber, a small town in Alberta, two high school students were shot by a former classmate. The shootings left one dead and one student seriously wounded. In September 2006, a school shooting occurred at Dawson College in

TABLE 16-2 Best-Known or Worst Canadian Disasters

Year	Disaster and Place*	Approximate Number of Canadian Deaths
1825	Forest fire, Miramichi, NB	160
1851	Sinking ship, PEI	300
1862	Smallpox epidemic	20,000
1885	Smallpox epidemic, Montreal, QC	6,000
1903	Frank rock slide, Turtle Mountain, AB	70
1910	Avalanche, Rogers Pass, Bear Creek, BC	62
1912	Tornado, Regina, SK	30
1917	Harbour explosion, Halifax, NS	2,000
1918	Spanish influenza epidemic ("Spanish flu")	30,000 to 50,000
1922	Wildfire, Timiskaming District, ON	43
1929	Tsunami, Burin Peninsula, NL	30
1942	Building fire, Knights of Columbus hostel, St. John's, NL	100
1947	Train derailment, Dugald, MB	40
1954	Hurricane Hazel, ON	81
1958	Mining accident, Springhill, NS	75
1974	Bus crash, St. Joseph de la Rive, QC	13
1974	Airplane crash, Rea Point, NWT	32
1985	Airplane crash (plane from Toronto, ON, crashed in the North Atlantic off Ireland coast)	280
1987	Tornado, Edmonton, AB	27
1992	Westray mining accident, Plymouth, NS	26
1996	Floods, Saguenay, QC	10
1997	Bus crash, St. Joseph de la Rive, QC	43
1998	Plane crash, Peggy's Cove, NS	230
1998	Ice storm, Eastern Ontario, Quebec, Maritimes	35
1999	Contaminated water, Walkerton, ON	7
2000	Tornado, Pine Lake, AB	16
2003	Severe acute respiratory syndrome, Toronto, ON	44
2003	Hurricane Juan, Atlantic Canada	8
2005	Outbreak of Legionnaires disease, Toronto, ON	21
2006	Overpass collapse, Laval, QC	5
2008	Outbreak of listeriosis, Toronto, ON	20
2008	Motor vehicle accident, Bathhurst, NB	8
2009	Cougar helicopter crash, off St. John's, NL	17
2009	H1N1	83

SOURCE: Jones, R. L. (2009). *Canadian disasters: An historical survey.* Retrieved from http://web.ncf.ca/jonesb/DisasterPaper/Table2.html; Historica Foundation of Canada. (2010). *The Canadian encyclopedia.* Retrieved from http://www.thecanadianencyclopedia.com/index.cfm?PgNm=TCE&Params=A1ARTA0002313; and Public Health Agency of Canada. (2009). *Flu watch.* Retrieved from http://www.phac-aspc.gc.ca/fluwatch/09-10/w41_09/index-eng.php.

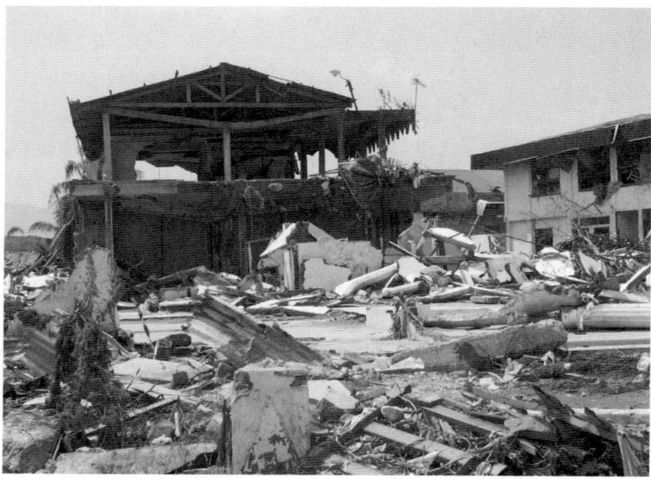

Underdeveloped areas are most at risk after a natural disaster has occurred; their infrastructure and housing quality are often inadequate to begin with, and inhabitants of such areas often have limited resources for coping with a disaster.

Montreal that left one deceased victim and 20 injured. In Toronto, a shooting incident occurred in May 2007 when a 14-year-old grade 9 student at C. W. Jefferys Collegiate Institute in Toronto was killed, and also in September 2008 a shooting left a 16-year-old student of Bendale Business and Technical Institute seriously injured. For further information on school violence in Canada, see the Government of Canada Web site "School Violence," listed in the Weblinks on the Evolve Web site.

THE FOUR STAGES OF DISASTER INVOLVEMENT

Canadian federal, provincial, territorial, and local agencies have partnered during the past decade to work proactively for disaster reduction to save lives and property. Etkin et al. (2004) suggest that Canada has the ability to lessen the probability of disasters occurring and to increase disaster preparedness and the ability to respond and recover from disasters. Canada has established a national emergency management system that includes all federal departments and authorities and partners with provincial and territorial governments (Public Safety Canada, 2008). One outcome of this partnership has been the development of an emergency management framework. It includes the development of an all-hazards approach to deal with natural and human hazards and disasters (Public Safety Canada, 2008). This emergency management framework was jointly developed by the federal, provincial, and territorial governments with the aim of coordinating all systems required to manage emergency and disaster situations. A regular 5-year review process has been put into place.

The framework identifies initiatives that address the four stages of disaster management in Canada. These four stages are prevention and mitigation, preparedness, response, and recovery (Etkin et al., 2004; Public Safety Canada, 2008). Figure 16-2 shows the disaster management cycle. This depiction demonstrates that the four stages in disaster management are central to reduce risk and therefore promote safer communities. Each of these stages will be discussed in further detail later in this chapter.

Disaster Prevention and Mitigation

The United Nations declared the 1990s the decade of natural disaster reduction. It initiated a campaign to educate people on ways to reduce their risk of injury and death caused by national disasters. This campaign led to increased public–private partnering that emphasized disaster mitigation. Stage one of the disaster management cycle is **disaster prevention and mitigation,** which refers to ongoing activities aimed at minimizing or eradicating risks of natural or human-made disasters before the disasters occur (Public Safety Canada, 2009).

FIGURE 16-2 The Disaster Management Cycle

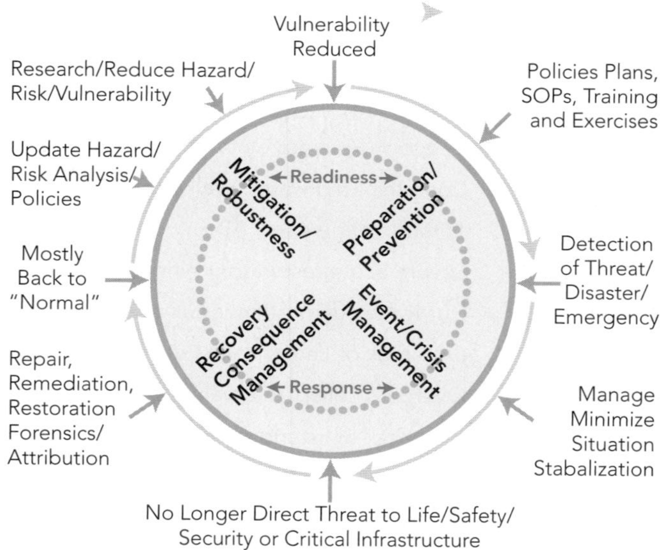

SOP refers to standard operating procedures.
Etkin, D., Haque, E., Bellisario, L., & Burton, I. (2004). An assessment of natural hazards and disasters in Canada: A report for decision makers and practitioners. Retrieved from http://www.crhnet.ca/docs/Hazards_Assessment_Summary_eng.pdf. Reprinted with permission.

The risks associated with natural hazards need to be understood so that activities can be implemented that could prevent or reduce a natural hazard. Examples of prevention and mitigation are that although we cannot prevent car crashes, we can mitigate the results by designing automobiles with seat belts and air bags and insisting that young children be transported in safety car seats. Other examples are building a retaining wall to divert flood water away from a community, public awareness programs on disaster mitigation, elevating homes in areas prone to floods, placing electric cables underground to avoid accumulation of ice, and supporting actions with efforts to ensure effective building codes and proper land use. One specific example of disaster prevention and mitigation was the building of the Red River Floodway to protect the city of Winnipeg, Manitoba, from the pending effect of the Red River Basin. The floodway was supported by federal and provincial funding. When it was built in 1960, it cost approximately $60 million. It has been used at least 20 times, and in 1997 it is estimated to have saved at least $6 billion (Public Safety Canada, 2009). This is an example of prevention and mitigation as a measure to eliminate the risk and impact of a hazard and therefore prevent disasters before they can occur.

Community health nurses (CHNs) prevent and mitigate by advocating for safe environments. Based on their knowledge that disasters are both natural and human-made, they assess for and report environmental health hazards. For example, the CHN needs to be aware of and report unsafe equipment, faulty structures, and the beginning of disease epidemics such as measles or influenza.

In the prevention and mitigation stage, there can also be activities such as conducting research on risks and associated hazards; introducing changes to legislation that may be required to reduce the risks associated with the hazards; and public education activities, including warnings of possible disasters (Etkin et al., 2004). Prevention and mitigation activities help the community to reduce their disaster vulnerability. **Disaster vulnerability** refers to the chance that a disaster is likely to occur and considers the ability of a community to avoid or cope with potential disasters. Different communities can cope with certain hazards because of past experiences and related preparedness. For example, British Columbia handles snow avalanches better than most provinces would likely handle them, should this occur. Avalanches occur more commonly on the western coast of Canada than on the eastern coast, and British Columbia has the material and human resources prepared to deal with these hazardous events. Although eastern Ontario is accustomed to handling snow and ice conditions, the 1998 ice storm challenged the ability of many communities to cope with the magnitude of this event, so it became a disaster.

CHNs who are familiar with their community look out for possible risks and take appropriate actions. For example, while driving in a new subdivision that is experiencing rapid growth, a CHN notes that schoolchildren are crossing a busy street without any traffic lights or crossing guard. This CHN recognizes that there is potential for a disaster because children are required to cross the street to reach their school. The children frequently cross the street in large groups and are often distracted and not watching the traffic closely. The CHN takes action by contacting the school principal, the city councillor for that ward, and the police department to discuss the risks involved and identifies the need for preventive action. Frequently, CHNs are members of the municipal community planning groups for disaster prevention and mitigation. These committees are instrumental in identifying disaster risks in the community and initiating strategies to prevent the occurrence of disasters.

Disaster Preparedness

Stage 2 of the disaster management cycle is **disaster preparedness,** which refers to a readiness to respond to and manage a disaster situation and its consequences. Planning is the essential component in preparedness for a disaster (Etkin et al., 2004). The plan must be both realistic and simple. During the preparedness stage, emergency plans are developed, implemented, evaluated, and revised. Since the events of September 11, 2001, communities have become more skilled in developing plans to prepare for a disaster. They use education, team planning, and mock disaster events, and there is a clear assignment of responsibility to health care professionals in the community to design plans to reduce community vulnerability, develop disaster response plans, and provide training before any hazardous event. Most communities have emergency or disaster plans in place to deal with local disasters. Sometimes provincial or territorial governments become involved in assisting with the disaster management, through human or financial resources. The federal government contributes to the management of natural and human-made hazards and disasters when requested by a provincial or territorial government.

The PHAC (2010a) provides access to many documents that address the planning and also discuss anticipated individual, family, and community responses to the stress that is the result of a disaster and provides some community resources that would be of value to CHNs (see the Weblinks on the Evolve Web site). CHNs are a valuable resource at planning meetings for disaster preparedness because of their knowledge about the kind of responses that individuals, families, and communities may have during and after a natural or human disaster. CHNs are knowledgeable about appropriate community resources that will be required. One activity that CHNs could initiate would be the development of an emergency preparedness pamphlet to educate the public.

Personal Preparedness

Individuals and families need to be prepared for emergency and disaster situations since they may need to wait for up to 72 hours before emergency workers can reach them (Health Canada, 2006). In Canada, there is potential for a variety of natural disasters such as pandemic flu, power outages, and winter storms that may involve freezing rain or heavy snowfalls. Therefore, families need to be prepared for any type of natural or human disaster. Health Canada and other emergency preparedness agencies such as the Canadian Red Cross provide information such as checklists and tool kits to assist families to prepare for an emergency. Family emergency preparedness kits are easy and inexpensive to put together (Government of Canada, 2010). These disaster supply kits should include items such as first aid supplies, emergency blankets, flashlight, radio, medications, ice packs, nonperishable food and water sufficient for at least 72 hours, copies of each person's medical information, local emergency telephone numbers, copies of emergency plans, and copies of important documents such as driver's licences, birth certificates, and passports. Detailed recommendations for what needs to be included in a disaster supply kit are available from the Health Canada Web site "Preparing Your Family for an Emergency" (see Evolve Weblinks) and the Canadian Red Cross Web site "Be Prepared not Scared: Emergency Preparedness Begins with You," found in the Tool Box on the Evolve Web site. CHNs are an important resource to families in assisting them to be prepared for an emergency or disaster.

Professional Preparedness

Advance personal and family preparation can help ease some of the conflicts that arise and allow CHNs to attend to client needs sooner. CHNs may be asked to respond to a disaster situation; however, if they have not prepared their own plan to take care of their personal responsibilities, they may not be as prepared to attend to their professional responsibilities. Conflicts between family- and work-related duties are inevitable. For example, a CHN who is also the mother of a young child will not be able to participate fully, if at all, in disaster relief efforts until family arrangements have been made. CHNs assisting in disaster relief efforts need to be as healthy as possible, both physically and mentally, to serve clients, families, and other disaster victims. Sometimes, CHNs themselves are disaster victims. For example, during the SARS outbreak in Ontario, many nurses became disaster victims as a result of taking care of SARS clients. Refer to the "Evidence-Informed Practice" box for research study findings regarding the influence of SARS on health care workers.

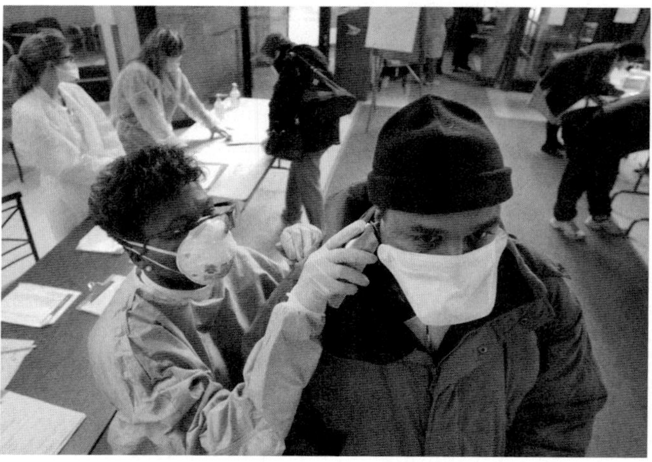

Nurses who are disaster victims themselves and need to provide care to others at the same time experience considerable stress. This was the experience of many nurses in major urban Canadian centres during the SARS epidemic in 2003.

CHNs need to be aware of and understand the disaster plans at their workplace and in their community. CHNs who are familiar with their workplace and community disaster plans are better able to participate in disaster drills and community mock disasters and when disasters occur. Adequately prepared CHNs will be leaders in a disaster and will assist others during the recovery phase.

All health care workers need to be certified in first aid and cardiopulmonary resuscitation. In addition, the **Centre for Emergency Preparedness and Response (CEPR)** (under the umbrella of the PHAC and responsible for coordinating services required to handle all health risk and security threats in Canada) provides a comprehensive program to train and certify health emergency response teams (HERTs) to enable them to respond to emergency situations in Canadian communities (PHAC, 2010a). The Office of Emergency Response Services (OERS) supports emergency health and social services nationally and internationally. It is responsible for the management of the National Emergency Stockpile System (NESS), which includes the various medical and pharmaceutical emergency supplies needed. The OERS manages quarantine officers at international airports in Canada and it also deploys the HERTs (PHAC, 2010b).

Evidence-Informed Practice

In early 2003, an outbreak of severe acute respiratory syndrome (SARS) started in China and Hong Kong (Parry, 2003). By the end of April 2003, 73 of the 144 SARS cases in Toronto involved health care workers (Booth et al., 2003; Dwosh, Hong, Austgardan, Herman, & Schabas, 2003). At the time of this study, there was a paucity of research examining the impact of SARS on staff working in hospitals that had few cases but were maintaining the strict precautions. A questionnaire was developed and distributed by the community hospital (an acute care facility in the Toronto area) to assess the impact of SARS on client care and on staff (managers, doctors, and nurses). Findings on how client care was affected were ranked differently by doctors and by nurses. Factors affecting client care were cancelled clinics and procedures, lack of visitors, fear of coming to the hospital, infection control, staff burnout, holding false ideas about safety precautions, poor communication about SARS, increased non-job duties related to SARS, and trouble concentrating on work. Although this study explored the impact on a variety of hospital staff, the discussion here presents study findings on the nurses as respondents only. The findings on the effect of SARS on the nurses in this study were that visitor restrictions were viewed as an important factor in affecting client care; nurses in outpatient settings had less direct client care than did nurses working in in-patient settings or in the emergency department; nurses reported increased burnout and perceived increased effects on job satisfaction; they reported that communication was not adequate (which contrasts with physicians' perceptions), especially in areas of being informed and in decision making; nurses relied on peer support to manage the stresses; and they perceived that infection control precautions were not strict enough.

The authors concluded that the impact of SARS was clearly different for nurses compared to other staff in a hospital setting. Therefore, they concluded that disaster planning must consider these differences in responses and coping mechanisms. The authors suggested that health care agencies, such as hospitals, need to establish mechanisms that will allow a response to nurses' concerns and also that will encourage participation by nurses in decision making.

Application for CHNs: CHNs need to be willing to participate on committees that are establishing disaster plans at the workplace so their knowledge and experience are shared at the prevention and mitigation stage of a disaster. When a disaster occurs, CHNs need to ensure they are represented on committees in their health care organization so they will be involved in decision making about client issues and issues affecting nursing.

Questions for Reflection & Discussion

1. What information should a disaster preparedness plan include as about how to address stresses that may be encountered by CHNs in a disaster?
2. What are some possible explanations for why hospital nurses may feel inadequately involved in decision making in emergency disaster preparedness?
3. How would you prepare a searchable question with reference to nursing in this study?

Reference: Tolomiczenko, G. S., Kahan, M., Ricci, M., Strathern, L., Jeney, J., Patterson, K., & Wilson, L. (2005). SARS: Coping with the impact at a community hospital. *Journal of Advanced Nursing, 50*(1), 101–110.

Community Preparedness

It is important for all disaster workers to work together cooperatively and with clear role definitions before a disaster and to use clear communication to set up and implement their community disaster plan. A solid disaster plan requires the talents, coordination, and cooperation of many different people and organizations, both in and outside the health profession, such as health care professionals, firefighters, police, coroners, municipal planners, teachers, educational institutions, business and community agencies, media, and volunteer groups. Knowing in advance exactly what is expected of each organization during an emergency or disaster gives the staff the opportunity to acquire necessary knowledge and to practise necessary skills beforehand (Gebbie & Qureshi, 2002). Most health care facilities have written disaster plans and require employees to perform annual mock disasters. An understanding of past disasters and of performance in mock disaster drills influences planning for future disasters. For example, reviews of real and simulated disasters may identify that the local community has not appropriately used the CHNs because of a lack of information about community health nursing roles. Mass casualty mock disasters are key parts of preparedness. Regardless of whether the mock disasters are carried out via a computer simulation or enacted in a realistic scenario, the objectives are as follows (Gebbie & Qureshi, 2002):

- To promote confidence
- To develop skills
- To coordinate activities
- To coordinate participants

A leader needs special skills in disaster management, including the ability to coordinate many organizations at one time. Terrorist events such as those of September 11, 2001, in the United States and others that followed; the contaminated water disaster in Walkerton, Ontario; and the outbreak of SARS in Toronto have all increased the awareness of the need to plan for a disaster and to require mock disasters. A great deal of information has been compiled on how to specifically plan for human-made disasters, which often occur with no forewarning. Part of planning for a bioterrorism attack is learning the symptoms of illnesses that are likely to be caused by infectious agents. For both natural and human-made disasters, there are often early warning signs. For example, signs of a tornado include hail, strong rain, and a green sky. Signs of a human-made disaster may not be as clear, but being aware of suspicious activities is important.

The community must have an adequate warning system and a backup evacuation plan to remove those individuals from areas of danger who hesitate to leave or who are unable to leave. Some people refuse to leave their homes because they are afraid that their possessions will be lost or destroyed by the disaster or from looting afterward. Law enforcement personnel or others in authority may have to speak directly to these reluctant residents to convince them to leave their homes and go to safer places. Also, some people mistakenly believe that experience with a particular type of disaster is enough preparation for the next one. People need to be convinced that predisaster warnings are official, serious, and personally important before they are motivated to take action. Some persons who are unable to leave are those with physical or mental illnesses or disabilities. A disaster plan needs to include how to safely evacuate these dependent persons and where to take them. Frequently, in disaster planning, large centres such as schools, hotels, universities, colleges, and arenas are considered as places for community residents to congregate.

In response to the newly emphasized need for disaster preparedness, the Government of Canada established Public Safety Canada (PSC) in 2003 to coordinate federal departments and agencies responsible for national security and safety of Canadians. The PSC works with several agencies to provide the following programs: Corrections, Crime Prevention, Emergency Management, Law Enforcement, National Security, and Policy Development Contribution Program (PDCP) (Public Safety Canada, 2010). Additional information can be found at the Public Safety Canada Weblink on the Evolve Web site. 

Most provinces and territories in Canada have an **Emergency Measures Organization (EMO)** that assumes the responsibility for developing, coordinating, and managing emergency response plans within the defined area. Initially, emergencies are managed by local municipalities—usually by hospitals, fire departments, and police. Should additional assistance be required, the provinces or territories assist. Assistance from the federal government is available if the emergency continues to escalate.

CHNs facilitate preparation in the community as part of the disaster preparedness team. CHNs need to review the disaster history of the community in which they work and live. They need to consider how past disasters have affected the health care delivery system, how particular organizations fit into the disaster plan, and what role they and others are expected to play in a disaster. CHNs also educate members of their community about how to prepare for a disaster, especially information that educates families on individual and family disaster preparedness.

CHNs help initiate or update an agency's disaster plan, provide educational programs and materials regarding disasters specific to an area, and organize disaster drills. CHNs also provide an updated record of vulnerable populations within the community. When calamity strikes, disaster workers need to know what kinds of populations they are attempting to assist. For example, if a tornado strikes a retirement village, the needs are quite different from those seen after a tornado hits a church filled with families or a centre for the physically challenged. In addition to sharing where special populations exist, CHNs educate disaster workers about the effects the disaster might have on them. CHNs need to review individual strategies, including available specific resources, in the event of an emergency.

The CHN who leads a preparedness effort can help recruit others within an organization who will help, if and when a response is required. Although there is no psychological profile of a disaster leader, those persons possessing self-awareness, flexibility, crisis and risk communication skills and have the ability to address mistakes without blaming would-be suitable leaders (Health Canada, 2007). The leader needs to know a great deal about the institution and be familiar with the individuals who work there. Persons with disaster management training, especially those who have served during real disasters, also make valuable members of any preparedness team.

CHNs fulfill many roles in the community. They need to understand what the available community resources will be after a disaster strikes and, most importantly, how the community will work together. A community-wide disaster plan serves as a roadmap for what "should" occur before, during, and after the response and the role of each participant in the plan. Disaster preparedness plans contribute to safer communities, reduce loss of life, and can reduce injuries.

Influenza Pandemic Preparedness

An **influenza pandemic** occurs when a change in the Influenza A virus takes place, causing the development of a new strain to which people have little or no immunity. As a result, a worldwide outbreak of influenza can occur, called an influenza pandemic (World Health Organization [WHO], 2009). A pandemic influenza ("flu") is one example of an impending natural disaster for which emergency disaster preparedness is essential. There has been global planning to monitor, report, and coordinate activities when a pandemic influenza is identified. It could start in any country in the world, and it is thought that it will spread very rapidly to other countries. The effects of a pandemic influenza will be more serious than the usual effects of the yearly influenza that is now experienced; a comparison of an ordinary influenza (flu) and an influenza pandemic can be found in Appendix 11. One of the challenges is that no one can predict with certainty the full effects of this influenza; but, based on past history, it is predicted to be a major human health threat. For further information on communications and the use of various tools to facilitate communication in a pandemic, refer to the Government of Ontario Web site "Health Sector Crisis Communications Toolkit" found in the Tool Box on the Evolve Web site.

In response to the likelihood of the pandemic influenza occurring in Canada, the Canadian Pandemic Influenza Plan has been developed. It is predicted that between 4.5

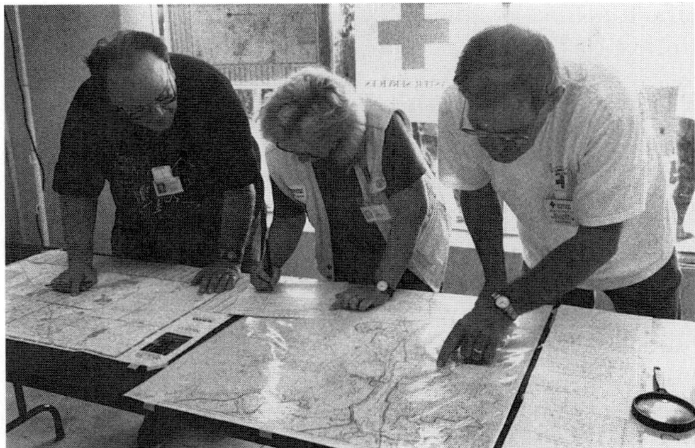
Understanding the community's disaster plan is a key role for community health nurses who seek greater involvement in disaster management.

and 10.6 million people in Canada will get this disease, with 2.5 million people requiring outpatient care and many requiring hospitalization, and that 11,000 to 58,000 people will die (PHAC, 2006b). Huston (2004) describes the pandemic influenza to likely be "1,000 times worse than SARS" (p. 184). Federal, provincial, territorial, and local disaster plans are coordinated with mechanisms established so that the communication of accurate information can occur rapidly in response to an outbreak (Huston, 2004; Johnson, Bone, & Predy, 2005; Tam, Sciberras, Mullington, & King, 2005). The PHAC (2006a) has outlined the following pandemic preparedness activities: maintain the Canadian Pandemic Influenza Plan; organize for pandemic vaccine production; develop and test a prototype vaccine from the influenza strain; establish a national antiviral stockpile; manage a national emergency stockpile system; provide international leadership on pandemic preparedness; assist countries affected by the avian influenza to develop their ability to respond; conduct research to promote the global response to pandemic influenza; monitor and release timely information to provinces and territories; perform ongoing surveillance for influenza; provide ongoing support and maintenance of quarantine services in major cities where international airports are located; and increase public awareness of influenza. For further information, refer to the PHAC's "Pandemic Preparedness Activities" Weblink on the Evolve Web site. This site provides information on the steps taken at the federal government level in collaboration with provincial and territorial governments to protect Canadians from a possible influenza pandemic. The "Ethical Considerations" box deals with a potential influenza pandemic.

Since the SARS outbreak, many reports have been written outlining recommendations to improve Canada's public health system, specifically in its ability to respond effectively and efficiently to outbreaks of communicable diseases that threaten the health of Canadians. One of the outcomes of the report was the establishment of the Public Health Agency of Canada (PHAC) in 2004. This agency and the creation of enhanced monitoring and surveillance systems (PHAC, 2008) have recently affected the role of public health nurses (PHNs) as Canada mobilized resources in response to the arrival of the influenza A H1N1 virus (also initially referred to as the "swine flu") and the pandemic alert period when a new influenza virus subtype was detected in Mexico.

In April 2009, PHAC sent out a media release to Canadian public health units/authorities stating that the WHO, the United States Centers for Disease Control (CDC), and the government of Mexico were reporting that an unusual influenza-like illness had been identified in Mexico and in travellers arriving from Mexico. Provincial and territorial laboratories were requested to send samples of the unidentified influenza virus from

ETHICAL CONSIDERATIONS

You are a CHN working in a rural community. You have been visiting an elementary school where the principal is concerned about an increased number of absent students. The principal also indicates that many students have flu-like symptoms and the parents are refusing to seek medical attention for these children.

Ethical principles that apply to the above scenario:

- *Respect for autonomy in relation to informed decision making.* CHNs recognize that capable persons may place a different weight on individualism and may choose to follow a family's values rather than community values in decision making.
- *Beneficence.* CHNs provide care directed first and foremost toward the health and well-being of the person, family, or community in their care.
- *Respect for autonomy.* CHNs build trustworthy relationships as the foundation of meaningful communication, recognizing that building these relationships involves a conscious effort. Such relationships are critical to understanding people's needs and concerns.
- *Providing safe, compassionate, competent, and ethical care* (CNA *Code of Ethics*). During a natural or human-made disaster, including a communicable disease outbreak, CHNs have a duty to provide care using appropriate safety precautions.

Question to Consider

1. Using the above ethical principles and values, what is the CHNs' responsibility in relation to this situation?

individuals with severe respiratory illness of unknown cause to the National Microbiology Laboratory (NML) in Winnipeg. Canada's chief public health officer also requested that Canadians returning from Mexico contact their health care provider if they were experiencing symptoms of respiratory illness (PHAC, 2009a). Before the end of April 2009, the Canadian NML had confirmed 13 cases in four provinces of the recently identified influenza A H1N1 virus as the same virus that had originated in the Mexican population and had also been identified in the United States. Public Health Canada issued Travel Health Alert Notices to airlines advising travellers to Mexico of the health risk, and Travel Health Warnings were released to the public through a variety of media strategies, requesting that they postpone nonessential travel to Mexico.

At the end of April 2009, the WHO announced that the pandemic alert level related to this influenza A H1N1 virus had moved from phase 4 to phase 5, meaning that human-to-human spread of the virus had gone from small clusters and localized outbreaks to one or more large clusters and outbreaks confirmed in at least two countries. The WHO uses phases in its approach to national preparedness and response plans to pandemics to assist countries in their emergency preparedness and planning for pandemics. In response to the shift in pandemic phase, public health authorities initiated a number of strategies to mitigate and contain the outbreak according to the direction provided by the PHAC of Canada and in accordance with the emergency and pandemic plan for their region. Dependent on the health unit or health authority, some of the PHN functions included enhancing surveillance, meeting specific case-reporting criteria, and sharing guidelines with health care providers related to screening patients who present with influenza-like illnesses and following specific protocols for lab testing and reporting results. As well, some PHNs were engaged in disseminating important information through a variety of mass media channels to the public that included the Travel Health Warning information, information focusing on proper handwashing, cough etiquette, and advising the public to stay home if they were experiencing specific signs and symptoms of flu. Some PHN roles also included working in call centres to respond to the surge in phone calls from the community requesting more information on the H1N1 virus. For further information on the pandemic periods, pandemic phases, and public health nursing activities, refer to Table 16-3. More specific timelines for the H1N1 virus for 2009 are outlined in Box 16-1.

PHN Roles During the H1N1 Outbreak

Important health notices for health care professionals are provided by the Chief Medical Officer of Health and the Emergency Management Branch to ensure consistent, accurate, and current information is received in a timely manner to assist in local emergency planning. PHNs use this information as well as access additional information found on the Canadian governmental Web sites in their role of developing and delivering accurate, relevant, and consistent messaging to the public and health care practitioners. These sites include the three PHAC Web sites: "Frequently Asked Questions—H1N1 Flu Virus," "Surveillance: Deaths Associated with H1N1 Flu Virus in Canada," and "Get the Facts on the H1N1 Flu Virus" found in the Weblinks on the Evolve Web site.

TABLE 16-3 Pandemic Influenza and Public Health Nursing Activities

Pandemic Periods	Pandemic Phases	Public Health Nurse (PHN) Activities
Interpandemic Period Could be outbreaks in animals or birds that are low risk to humans	Phase 1 No new influenza strains are identified in humans.	• PHNs working in all areas of public health actively participate in education and training opportunities related to possible roles they may be redeployed to from their day-to-day business on a regular basis (often annually) as part of emergency preparedness and response education as required by their provincial/territorial health unit or authority and Federal Emergency Preparedness and Response System. • PHNs who work in infectious disease control division review current publications and surveillance literature from PHAC as well as participate in routine human influenza surveillance and monitoring and seasonal influenza vaccine program.
	Phase 2 A circulating animal influenza virus subtype poses a substantial risk of human disease.	• Preparation and updating of educational materials for the general public focused on risks, risk avoidance, universal and respiratory hygiene etiquette, and information on how to reduce transmission if in need of seeking health care. • Preparation of materials for health care sector, reinforcing recommendations for management of clients with respiratory illnesses and need for access to masks for coughing clients. • Preparation of media articles and workshop materials, updating of infection control procedures and community contact lists, development of current fact sheets and updating of Web page information to keep public and health professionals informed of status of influenza in their community and related risk avoidance or self-care strategies. Development of packages for specific at-risk populations (new parents, seniors, etc.) or cultural groups, including the use of translation services or community leaders to ensure messages related to accessing health care services, risk reduction, and self-care are presented in a culturally sensitive and appropriate manner. • Promotion and provision of educational sessions to workplaces, schools, health sector, and community organizations on need for business continuity planning for potential pandemic.
Pandemic Alert Period Human outbreaks of a new influenza strain	Phase 3 A new influenza virus subtype is detected in humans. There may be isolated cases of human-to-human spread with close contact.	• PHNs are notified by the PHAC and the territorial/provincial/regional health authorities of current infection control precautions and guidelines that are to be relayed to confirmed cases, their contacts and caregivers, and health professionals that focus on the testing, isolation, and treatment of confirmed cases and their contacts either in self-isolation at home or in health care setting as containment strategy. • PHNs are trained and commit to follow reporting procedures using provincial and federal databases and monitoring systems as directed by the PHAC and their respective health authorities. • PHNs may provide information to health professionals related to appropriate provincial public health laboratory for client samples to be tested and distribute antivirals in clinical settings. • PHNs may coordinate laboratory testing by referring clients and health professional to appropriate public health or designated provincial laboratories, reporting results from physicians and labs electronically, and arranging transportation to the National Microbiology Laboratory for confirmation of positive test results.

(Continued)

TABLE 16-3 Pandemic Influenza and Public Health Nursing Activities—Cont'd

Pandemic Periods	Pandemic Phases	Public Health Nurse (PHN) Activities
	Phase 4 Small clusters of human-to-human spread are reported but the virus does not spread easily. Outbreaks are localized.	• PHNs receive and review information daily (guidelines, protocols, notifications, incubation, communicability, and transmission) from the PHAC and provincial/territorial health authorities through Web-based surveillance and monitoring systems and direct e-mail notification to health units. Educational materials are developed and resources distributed based on this information to health care sectors and public. • PHNs continue to follow federal (PHAC) and provincial/territorial health authority directives for reporting cases and contact follow-up information that may have changed or enhanced reporting criteria (may refer them to Fluwatch.ca or PHAC information for health professionals on Influenza Pandemic Plan). Also, in Ontario the "Important Health Notice" published by the Ministry of Health and Long-Term Care is a good resource for updates and directives for PHNs.
	Phase 5 Larger clusters are reported but human-to-human spread is still localized. Virus is spreading more easily but is not fully transmissible.	• PHNs continue to provide updated infection control information electronically or by phone or fax to health professionals in long-term care, clinical settings, physicians' offices, the hospital sector, and individuals being cared for at home or in a residential setting related to self-care and isolation at home or in hospital; includes instructions on what to do if the individual health status worsens. • PHNs receive guidelines and report criteria from the PHAC and provincial/territorial health authorities to assist them in monitoring and reporting on all identified individuals who receive antiviral drugs related to symptoms, compliance, and adverse reactions. • PHN role now also focuses on the active surveillance of close contacts where possible. The PHN through phone calls, letters, and possibly home visits identifies, monitors, and provides all contacts with written/verbal information on protective measures (hygiene and respiratory etiquette, signs, and symptoms), what to do if they experience symptoms, and how to safely seek medical attention with minimal exposure or contact with others. • PHNs work with additional public health staff that may include health educators, health promotion officers, health protection and infection control staff, and communication specialists to develop and distribute information via Web pages, media notices (radio, TV, newspaper), electronic notices, information forums, letters, and faxes to health care professionals and community clients related to protective measures, respiratory etiquette, handwashing, and access and use of antivirals to contain spread. As well, PHNs know the importance of keeping the public and health care providers aware that antivirals are effective only if used within 48 hours of onset of symptoms and, due to the potential for limited amounts available, would inform them of priority groups to receive the antiviral as identified by federal and provincial health authorities (PHAC).

SOURCE: Adapted from Public Health Agency of Canada. (2006). *The Canadian pandemic influenza plan for the health sector.* Retrieved from www.phac-aspc.gc.ca/cpip-pclcpi/hl-ps/index-eng.php.

BOX 16-1 Timelines for H1N1 Virus in 2009

- March 18: First cases in Mexico
- April 25: WHO declares a public health emergency of international concern
- April 26: The United States declares a public health emergency
- April 27: WHO increases the pandemic alert level to phase 4, indicating sustained human-to-human transmission
- April 28: PHAC issues a travel health warning, recommending that travellers from Canada postpone elective or nonessential travel to Mexico until further notice
- April 29: WHO increases the pandemic alert level to phase 5, indicating widespread human infection and imminent pandemic
- April 29: Canada provides laboratory testing support to Mexico
- April 30: WHO refers to new influenza virus as influenza A (H1N1)
- May 6: Genetic makeup of H1N1 flu virus decoded
- May 18: PHAC lifts travel health warning to Mexico
- June 11: WHO increases the pandemic alert level to phase 6, indicating that a global pandemic is under way
- June 29: First case of oseltamivir-resistant H1N1 flu virus reported (Denmark)
- July 1: WHO renames novel influenza virus as Pandemic (H1N1) 2009
- July 3: First reported case of acquired oseltamivir-resistant H1N1 flu virus (Hong Kong)
- July 13: WHO releases recommendations on pandemic (H1N1) 2009 vaccines
- July 21: First Canadian case of oseltamivir-resistant H1N1 flu virus reported (Quebec)
- September 16: Canada announces H1N1 vaccine rollout sequencing
- October 23: Canada officially enters second wave of Pandemic (H1N1) 2009

SOURCE: Community Hospital Infection Control Association (CHICA-Canada). (2009). *Links and resources: Pandemic (H1N1) 2009 virus.* Retrieved from www.chica.org/links_swineflu.html.

In May 2009, Canada launched a mass media campaign to inform the public about measures to take to reduce their risks of getting the flu and Public Health continued to increase surveillance and case management. Plans were put into place by PHAC to ensure the National Antiviral Stockpile could be mobilized and discussions were initiated with government-contracted drug manufacturers to begin the process of developing and producing a vaccine. Protocols and guidelines were developed and disseminated by health experts from provincial, territorial, and the health care sector to mitigate potential impacts on the health care sector if the virus became more virulent and the outbreak escalated in the community. In June 2009, the WHO raised the H1N1 pandemic alert to phase 6 and entered the pandemic period based on sustained community-level outbreaks in more than three countries across two WHO regions. Fortunately, most countries reported moderate illnesses globally with most clients recovering at home without treatment. In Canada over the summer of 2009, the PHAC stopped counting individual cases of persons with H1N1 but monitored for unusual clusters, the severity of outbreaks, hospitalizations, and patterns and trends in community spread and deaths from H1N1. Guidance documents were developed and distributed to various health care sectors as well as guidelines for schools, summer camps, daycares, and caregivers. In October, 2009 Canada approved the H1N1 vaccine and its distribution to all provinces and territories. For further information, refer to the "Health Canada Approves Pandemic H1N1 Flu Vaccine for Canadians" Weblink on the Evolve Web site.

Table 16-3 outlines the pandemic periods and phases for all pandemic influenzae as identified by WHO and also includes the main PHN activities associated with the phases. Further information on the pandemic influenza plan for the health care sector is available at the PHAC Weblink, "The Canadian Pandemic Influenza Plan for the Health Sector" on the Evolve Web site.

All provinces and territories have an influenza pandemic preparedness plan. These plans are available and included on the Government of Canada Pandemic Preparedness Web site (see the Weblinks on the Evolve Web site). The Canadian Pandemic Influenza Plan provides federal direction to the provinces or territories and municipal government levels for planning for when a pandemic influenza occurs. In Ontario, provincial planning addresses areas such as roles, responsibilities, and frameworks for decision making; goals, strategies, and planning assumptions; system-wide issues, activities, and tools; public health measures; infection prevention control and occupational health and safety; health human resource planning; ensuring availability of material resources; and communications (Ontario Ministry of Health and Long-Term Care, 2008). The following questions indicate some of the areas that the Ontario pandemic influenza plan addresses:

1. What are the roles and responsibilities of the different governmental levels?
2. What are the goals?
3. Which strategies are to be used?
4. What are the assumptions underlying the goals and strategies?
5. Which surveillance activities are currently in place to monitor for pandemic influenza?
6. Which surveillance activities are to be used when a pandemic outbreak occurs?
7. Which vaccines will be purchased? How? Where from? Where will they be stockpiled?
8. Which antiviral medications will be purchased by the province? How? Where from? Where will they be stockpiled?
9. What public health measures will be used to manage pandemic influenza and protect the public?
10. What occupational health and safety measures are planned to (a) protect health personnel and (b) ensure the adequacy of equipment and supplies?
11. What are the roles and steps to be taken by each sector in the health system to respond to pandemic influenza?

Although these questions were developed in reference to the Ontario pandemic influenza preparedness plan, similarities are found in other provincial and territorial pandemic influenza preparedness plans.

Although there are national, provincial or territorial, and municipal pandemic preparedness plans, when the pandemic influenza occurs, all health care operations will be managed at the local or regional level (Tam et al., 2005). The local public health infrastructure needs to be prepared to lead and respond to emergencies, as well as maintaining core functions (Johnson et al., 2005). Many workplaces and other institutions such as universities are developing their own pandemic influenza preparedness plans. These plans also need to be documented and shared with local pandemic influenza preparedness planning teams to ensure a coordinated disaster management plan. As well, the Canadian Nurses Association is working with Health Canada to explore strategies to strengthen the role of nursing in disaster management at national, provincial or territorial, and municipal levels (Canadian Nurses Association, 2006).

Locally, mechanisms need to be in place for ill persons and their families to receive needed medical care. Public health units or health authorities in municipalities are taking the lead role in preparing and managing the emergencies related to infectious diseases (Johnson et al., 2005). Public health units or health authorities locally and regionally will "maintain core functions and … lead and support health sector responses to emergencies" (Johnson et al., 2005, p. 412). Some of the core public health functions that are recommended include surveillance activities; preparation for full-scale vaccine programs that would include ensuring that vaccine supplies and staff for mass immunization clinics are available; and specific public health measures such as reviewing and updating all influenza educational materials and ensuring that resources will be available to handle the many tasks that will be required in a pandemic influenza situation (e.g., case finding, isolation of cases, immunization clinics, and tracking) (Huston, 2004).

CHNs need to continually monitor the latest information on the pandemic planning and activities. Available resources may vary in communities. One resource used in Ontario by health care professionals is a monthly newsletter published by the Ontario Ministry of Health and Long-Term Care called *The Pandemic Planner* (avail-

CRITICAL VIEW

1. **a)** What are the types of natural disasters for which your community is at risk?

   b) What is the role of the public health nurse in the disaster preparedness plan in your community?

2. What are your provincial or territorial and municipal pandemic influenza preparedness plans?

CRITICAL VIEW

1. How can you protect yourself and your family from a pandemic influenza?
2. **a)** What pandemic influenza plans do (i) your community and (ii) your educational institution have?

   b) What roles have been identified for health professionals, including nursing students, within the pandemic influenza plan as described in question 2a?

able in the Evolve Weblinks). This resource provides the latest information on the federal, provincial or territorial, and local initiatives. Resources are also available for workplaces to address pandemic planning. For information on this planning, refer to the Canadian Centre for Occupational Health and Safety Weblink "Pandemic Planning" on the Evolve Web site.

Disaster Response

Stage three of the disaster management cycle is **disaster response,** which refers to activities that are carried out by emergency response teams consisting of police, firefighters, medical personnel, and others during and following a disaster. This is the time when the emergency plans are implemented. The community residents need to listen to the radio and television to obtain the most current information on the steps to be taken. Depending on the type and severity of a disaster, residents may be advised to remain in their homes and use their emergency kits and supplies or may be directed to certain facilities for safe shelter.

The physical and emotional effects of disasters on people in a community depend on factors such as the type, cause, and location of the disaster; magnitude and extent of damage; duration; and amount of warning provided. For example, no one may die in an earthquake, but the structural damage to buildings and the continuous aftershocks may last for weeks and cause intense psychological stress. In addition, the longer it takes for structural repairs and other cleanup, the longer the psychological effects can last. In the United States and Canada, the terrorist attacks of September 11, 2001, created extreme anger and grief but also led to a huge increase in compassion. Twenty-five Canadians died in this disaster. In Canada, people responded by donating money and volunteering to assist the rescue and cleanup efforts. In the United States, thousands of people helped by rescuing victims from the buildings, donating blood, and donating money. Within 1 month of the attack, an estimated US$757 million in cash contributions and hundreds of truckloads of goods had been donated to help the families of victims and rescue workers (Yates, 2001).

It is important to be aware that individuals react to the same disaster in different ways, depending on their age, cultural background, health status, social support structure, and general ability to adapt to crises. Box 16-2 describes common reactions of adults and children to disasters. Initial reactions of victims can include fear, distress, anxiety, anger, numbness, difficulty concentrating, and difficulty making decisions (PHAC, 2005). Disturbances in bodily functions, such as gastrointestinal upsets, diarrhea, and nausea and vomiting, are also common (PHAC, 2005). Additionally, there may be fear

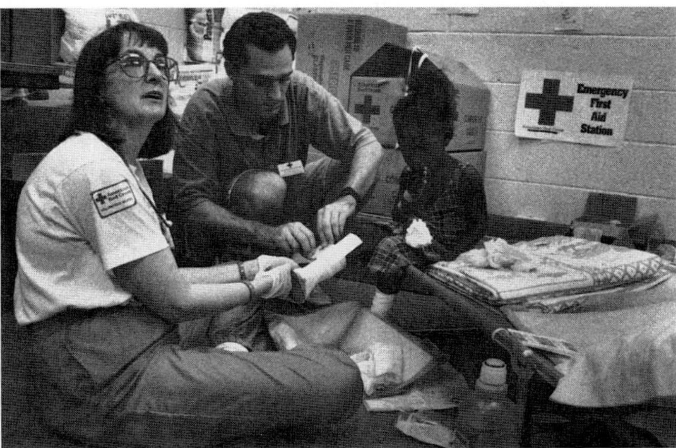

The effects of a disaster can be disruptive.

BOX 16-2 Common Reactions to Disasters

Adults

- Extreme sense of urgency
- Panic and fear
- Disbelief
- Disorientation and numbness
- Reluctance to abandon property
- Difficulty in making decisions
- The need to help others
- Anger
- Blaming and scapegoating
- Delayed reactions
- Insomnia
- Headaches
- Apathy and depression
- Sense of powerlessness
- Guilt
- Moodiness and irritability
- Jealousy and resentment
- Domestic violence

Children

- Regressive behaviours (bedwetting, thumbsucking, crying, clinging to parents)
- Fantasies that disaster never occurred
- Nightmares
- School-related problems, including an inability to concentrate and a refusal to go back to school

of leaving home or loved ones, and fear of travelling (PHAC, 2005).

During disasters, there may be an exacerbation of an existing chronic disease. For example, the emotional stress of being a disaster victim may make it difficult for people with diabetes to control their blood sugar levels. Grief results in harmful effects to the immune system. It reduces the function of cells that protect against viral infections and tumours. Hormones that are produced by the body's flight-or-fight mechanism also play a role in mediating the effects of grief. The effects on young children can be especially disruptive. They can resort to regressive behaviours such as sucking their thumb, wetting their bed, crying, and clinging to parents (PHAC, 2005) or have nightmares. Box 16-3 lists other populations at risk for severe disruption from a disaster. For further information, refer to the PHAC Weblink "Responding to Stressful Events," on the Evolve Web site. Additionally, refer to the Department of National Defence Weblink, which discusses the role of the Canadian military in disaster relief, including the Disaster Assistance Response Team (DART).

Role of the CHN in Disaster Response

Once rescue workers arrive at the scene, plans for triage should begin immediately. **Triage** is the process of separating casualties and allocating treatment on the basis of the victims' potential for survival. Varying priorities are assigned by the triage team. Accurate information, acquired through assessment, facilitates rapid rescue and recovery. These assessments help match available resources to a population's emergency needs. For example, assessments in sudden-impact disasters, such as tornadoes and earthquakes, are more concerned with ongoing hazards, injuries and deaths, shelter requirements, and clean water. Assessments in gradual-onset disasters, such as famines, are most concerned with mortality rates, nutritional status, immunization status, and environmental health.

Ongoing assessments or surveillance reports by CHNs are just as important as initial assessments. Surveillance reports indicate the continuing status of the affected population and the effectiveness of ongoing relief efforts. CHNs continue to inform relief managers of needed resources. Surveillance continues into the recovery phase of a disaster. CHNs need to recognize that rescue workers experience psychological stress during and after a disaster (Morren, Dirkzwager, Kessels, & Yzermans, 2007). The degree of workers' stress depends on the nature of the disaster, their role in the disaster, individual stamina, and other environmental factors. Environmental factors include noise, inadequate workspace, physical danger, and stimulus overload, especially exposure to death and trauma. For further information, refer to Health Canada's *Preparing and Responding to Workplace Trauma: A Manager's Handbook* (listed in the Weblinks on the Evolve Web site).

BOX 16-3 Populations at Greatest Risk for Disruption After a Disaster

- Persons with disabilities
- Persons living on a low income, including the homeless
- Persons who do not understand the local language
- Persons living alone
- One-parent families
- Persons new to the area
- Institutionalized persons or those with chronic mental illness
- Previous disaster victims or victims of traumatic events
- Persons who are not citizens or legally documented immigrants
- Substance abusers

Shelter Management

Shelters are generally the responsibility of the local Red Cross chapter, although in massive disasters the military may be used to set up "tent cities" for the masses who need temporary shelter. Because of their comfort in delivering aggregate health promotion, disease prevention, and emotional support, CHNs make ideal shelter managers and team members. Although physical health needs are the priority initially, especially among older adults and the chronically ill, many of the predominant problems in shelters revolve around stress. The shock of the disaster itself, loss of personal possessions, fear of the unknown, living in proximity to total strangers, and even boredom can cause stress.

Nurses working in shelters can use the following commonsense approaches to help victims deal with stress (American Red Cross, 2002):

- Listen to victims tell and retell their feelings about the disaster and their current situation.
- Encourage victims to share their feelings with one another if it seems appropriate to do so.
- Help victims make decisions.

LEVELS OF PREVENTION

Related to Disaster Management

PRIMARY PREVENTION

Community health nurses participate with community committee members in developing a disaster management plan for the community.

SECONDARY PREVENTION

Community health nurses participate in assessing disaster victims and are involved in triage for care.

TERTIARY PREVENTION

Community health nurses participate in home visits to uncover dangers that may cause additional injury to victims or cause other problems (e.g., house fires from unsafe use of candles).

- Delegate tasks (e.g., reading, crafts, playing games with children) to teenagers and others to help combat boredom.
- Provide the basic necessities (food, clothing, rest).
- Try to recover or get needed items (prescription glasses, medications).
- Provide basic compassion and dignity (e.g., privacy when appropriate and if possible).
- Refer a client to a mental health counsellor if the situation warrants.

Highly trained mental health counsellors, such as psychologists, psychiatrists, clinical social workers, and nurses, are always available in large-scale disasters. They are important members of any disaster team, no matter what the level of disaster, and their services need to be used as often as necessary.

During a disaster, the Canadian Red Cross may open shelters for those affected by the disaster and provide food and lodging to families and emergency workers (Canadian Red Cross, 2006). CHNs may be involved with a variety of activities such as providing first aid, food preparation, record keeping, and maintaining a safe environment.

Disaster Recovery

Stage four of the disaster management cycle is disaster recovery. **Disaster recovery** refers to activities that focus on rebuilding to predisaster or near-predisaster conditions and on community safety so that the risk of a recurrence of the disaster is reduced. This is when there is recovery from the physical, psychological, and financial damage. Cleanup, repair, and rebuilding occur in the community. Disaster victims may need community assistance to rebuild their lives and learn to deal with all losses encountered as a result of the disaster.

This stage is the best time to start thinking about the lessons learned from the disaster and to consider actions that will decrease vulnerability and mitigate future disasters (Etkin et al., 2004). This is also when the public and politicians have heightened awareness and openness to consider prevention strategies (Etkin et al., 2004). Therefore, there is often a willingness to implement mitigation activities to reduce or avoid future similar disasters. Also, disaster plans are reviewed and revisions are made.

Disaster recovery efforts are expensive, and the costs are growing because of the number of people involved and the amount of technology that must be restored. The economic impact of natural disasters is found in data and financial cost estimates on Canadian disasters from the beginning of the twentieth century (Etkin et al., 2004). Usually, the government takes the lead in rebuilding efforts, whereas the business community tries to provide economic support. Many other organizations help with rebuilding efforts, such as religious groups and community service organizations.

The role of CHNs in the disaster recovery phase is to partner with community disaster team members to evaluate the consequences of the disaster. CHNs provide information about what resources are available and accessible in order to facilitate individual and community recovery. Community cleanup efforts can cause many physical and psychological problems such as lifting heavy objects that may result in back injury and an increased occurrence in gastrointestinal infections due to poor water quality. CHNs need to continue to teach proper body mechanics, proper hygiene, make sure immunization records are current, monitor for the environmental health hazards (physical, chemical, biological, ergonomic, and psychological), and initiate required actions.

It is important to be alert for environmental health hazards during the recovery phase of a disaster. During home visits, CHNs may uncover situations such as a faulty housing structure or lack of water or electricity. Objects that have been blown into the yard by a tornado or that floated in from a flood may be dangerous and must be removed. Case finding and referral are critical during the recovery phase and may continue for a long time. CHNs and community organizations partner with the victims of a disaster and provide supportive environments.

Being prepared for a disaster is of major importance to how disasters are managed. Refer to the Canadian Red Cross Weblink "Integrating Emergency Management and High-Risk Populations" (on the Evolve Web site). This Web site presents a report of a project examining how the at-risk Canadian population was included in emergency management at all governmental levels. Disaster planning does not guarantee that the management of a disaster will always go as planned but it does contribute to minimizing the negative physical, psychological, social, and economic impacts related to the disaster. CHNs have many of the necessary skills required to deal with a disaster and need to ensure that they are prepared to respond to a disaster and work with their community to meet the challenges of disaster management. 

STUDENT EXPERIENCE

As a nursing student, you have been assigned to a secondary school for your community health nursing clinical experience.

1. Write down your thoughts and beliefs about violence in schools. Questions to consider: In general, how do you feel about school shootings and school violence? Why do you think such violence occurs? What warning signs might violent school-aged children demonstrate? How do you think violence in schools can be prevented?
2. Locate research articles identifying what is known about school violence in Canada.
3. Based on your research findings, outline a teaching package that could be implemented in the school.

REMEMBER THIS!

- The number of disasters, both human-made and natural, continues to increase, as does the number of people affected by them.
- In Canada and other countries, school violence, a human-made disaster, has increased in intensity and magnitude.
- The cost of recovery from a disaster has risen sharply because of the amount of technology that must be restored.
- Personal preparedness involves individuals and families preparing for a disaster.
- Professional preparedness involves an awareness and understanding of the disaster plan at work and in the community.
- Canadians need to prepare for a pandemic influenza outbreak, a natural disaster, which is a highly infectious disease with the potential for catastrophic outcomes.
- CHNs are increasingly getting involved in disaster prevention and mitigation, disaster planning, disaster response, and disaster recovery through their local health unit or health authority or government.
- Helping clients maintain a safe environment and advocating for environmental safety measures in the community are key roles for the CHN during all phases of disaster management.
- It is important for CHNs to know about available community resources, especially for vulnerable populations, during the preparedness stage of disaster management to ensure smoother response and recovery stages.
- People in a community react differently to a disaster depending on the type, cause, and location of the disaster; its magnitude and extent of damage; its duration; the amount of warning that was provided; and previous exposures to disasters.
- People react differently to disasters depending on factors such as their age, cultural background, health status, social support structure, and general adaptability to crisis.
- The stress experienced by CHNs is compounded if they are both the victims and caregivers in a disaster.
- A key attribute in aiding disaster victims is flexibility.
- A human disaster requires a different disaster management response than a natural disaster.
- The stage of disaster known as disaster recovery occurs as all involved agencies pull together to restore the economic and civic life of the community.

REFLECTIVE PRAXIS

Case Study

Paula, a public health nurse (PHN) in a medium-size public health department in Forest Ridge, was called to serve on her first municipal disaster assignment. Her disaster skills were tested when a tornado hit the next city and its surrounding areas. Paula left Forest Ridge to help manage an elementary-school cafeteria shelter in the tornado hit zone.

The devastation that Paula saw en route to the school had a negative effect on her. Assigned to help with client intake, she patiently listened to the disaster victims, referred many of the most distraught clients to the mental health counsellor, and set priorities for other needs as they arose. For example, she found that many of her clients had left their medications behind and needed therapy. Other needs included diapers and formulas for infants, prescription eyeglasses, and clothing. As the days went on, the stress level in Paula's shelter grew. The crowded living conditions and lack of privacy took its toll on the shelter residents. Around the tenth day of her assignment, Paula began to experience pounding headaches and had difficulty concentrating. She thought she would be fine, but the mental health counsellor said that she was experiencing a stress reaction.

1. Which of the following actions would probably be the most useful for Paula to take?
   a) Share her feelings with the on-site mental health counsellor on a regular basis
   b) Call home to share her feelings with family members
   c) Meet the needs of her clients to the best of her ability and accept the fact that stress is a part of the job
2. What community resources would likely be involved in this disaster?

Answers are on the Evolve Web site at http://evolve.elsevier.com/Canada/Stanhope/community/.

What Would You Do?

1. If you thought a pandemic influenza might affect your community, what steps would you take to adequately prepare for the possible disaster? What steps would you take to ensure safety and preparedness for your family and for the clients for whom you care? Whose help would you enlist? To whom would you go for advice?
2. Assume that your community has the potential to be hit by a tornado. List the groups that would be most vulnerable. What steps could you take in advance to reduce their vulnerability? What community resources are available?

TOOL BOX

evolve

The Tool Box contains useful instruments that can be applied in community health nursing practice. These related resources are found either in the appendices at the back of this book or on the Evolve Web site at http://evolve.elsevier.com/Canada/stanhope/community/.

Appendices

- Appendix 11: What You Should Know About an Influenza Pandemic

Tools

Canadian Red Cross. *Be Prepared, Not Scared: Emergency Preparedness Begins with You.*
This is a disaster preparedness guideline for families and individuals on how to prepare an emergency survival kit and what to do during and after a disaster. The site includes checklists to assist in preparation.

Government of Ontario. *Health Sector Crisis Communications Toolkit.*
This tool kit contains information on the communications that need to occur in a pandemic situation. Various grids, logs, and checklists are provided to facilitate communication during a pandemic.

WEBLINKS

evolve

Direct links to these resources can be found on the text's accompanying Evolve Web site at http://evolve.elsevier.com/Canada/Stanhope/community.

Campbell, A. *The SARS Commission—Spring of Fear: Final Report.* Toronto: Ontario Ministry of Health and Long-Term Care. This document provides the executive summary and the final report by Mr. Justice Archie Campbell of the Ontario Superior Court of Justice, who was appointed commissioner by the Government of Ontario to investigate the introduction and spread of SARS under the *Health Protection and Promotion Act.*

Canadian Centre for Emergency Preparedness. This Canadian voluntary organization provides information on disaster management, principles and practices, research results, and a listing of the educational institutions that provide disaster risk-management courses.

Canadian Centre for Occupational Health and Safety. Pandemic Planning. This site has information on and links to a multitude of sites from across Canada that provide information relevant to the workplace about planning for a pandemic.

Canadian Red Cross. *Integrating Emergency Management and High-Risk Populations: Survey Report and Action Recommendations.* This is the report of a project that examined how the at-risk Canadian population was included in emergency management at all governmental levels. A framework is described for emergency management of the at-risk population. Recommendations to further develop emergency management measures for high-risk populations are included.

Department of National Defence. This Canadian site discusses the role of the Canadian military in disaster relief, including the Disaster Assistance Response Team (DART).

Government of Canada. *SafeCanada.ca—Emergencies and Disasters.* This site provides detailed information about national disasters and emergency plans across Canada, such as fire prevention, earthquake preparedness, pandemic preparedness, and bioterrorism.

Government of Canada. ***SafeCanada.ca—Pandemic Preparedness.*** This site contains many Web connections containing information pertaining to pandemic preparedness. Some of the sites identify preparedness plans for different provinces, and some of the sites provide general information.

Government of Canada. ***SafeCanada.ca—School Violence.*** This site contains many links to various resources across Canada pertaining to violence in Canadian schools.

Health Canada. ***Health Canada Approves Pandemic H1N1 Flu Vaccine for Canadians.*** This is the announcement by Health Minister Leona Aglukkaq on the plans to administer the H1N1 vaccine to Canadians. The national recommendations are included.

Health Canada. ***Preparing and Responding to Workplace Trauma: A Manager's Handbook.*** This handbook assists managers to work with employees who have experienced a traumatic workplace event as well as to support community members during or after a major traumatic event.

Health Canada. ***Preparing Your Family for an Emergency.*** This site provides basic information on getting ready for an emergency and provides excellent Web links for more detailed information on emergency preparation and response.

Ontario Ministry of Health and Long-Term Care. ***The Pandemic Planner.*** This site provides current and past issues of the Ontario Ministry's monthly newsletter for health professionals provide information on influenza pandemic planning.

Public Health Agency of Canada. ***The Canadian Pandemic Influenza Plan for the Health Sector.*** This site provides information on the Canadian plan for a pandemic influenza for the health sector and includes information such as public education, public health management of persons with symptoms of influenza, and management of contacts of cases and outlines strategies to control the disease in the community.

Public Health Agency of Canada. ***Emergency Response Services.*** This site provides links to a vast array of documents that assist with emergency planning and mitigation such as emergency food services and emergency preparedness guide.

Public Health Agency of Canada. ***Frequently Asked Questions—H1N1 Flu Virus.*** This site provides general information on the H1N1 flu virus, use of vaccines and antivirals for treatment, as well as activities to protect from the H1N1 virus and its management with specific populations such as Aboriginal peoples.

Public Health Agency of Canada. ***Get the Facts on the H1N1 Flu Virus.*** This site provides general information, such as information on the symptoms and care of someone with the H1N1 virus. Information is provided on specific groups such as Aboriginals and pregnant women. A map is provided to allow access to specific H1N1 information about provincial and territorial management of the H1N1 flu virus.

Public Health Agency of Canada. ***Pandemic Preparedness Activities.*** This site provides information on the steps taken at the federal government level in collaboration with provincial and territorial governments to protect Canadians from a possible influenza pandemic.

Public Health Agency of Canada. ***Responding to Stressful Events.*** This eight-page online brochure identifies typical reactions of families, children, and teens and discusses stress-management strategies and community resources.

Public Health Agency of Canada. ***Surveillance: Deaths Associated with the H1N1 Flu Virus in Canada.*** This site provides updates on the latest deaths reported for each province and territory associated with the H1N1 flu virus.

Public Safety Canada. Programs. The site provides links to the programs offered by this agency, which was organized to protect Canadians and assist them in handling emergencies, promoting community safety, and dealing with crime.

Registered Nurses' Association of Ontario. ***SARS Unmasked: Final Report on the Nursing Experience with SARS in Ontario.*** This document is an extensive report on nurses' experiences and emotions due to the SARS outbreak, provides a chronological development of SARS, talks about lessons learned, and provides recommendations for changes in a failing health care system.

Royal Roads University. ***Disaster and Emergency Management.*** This resource provides Weblinks for national and international organizations and associations that are involved with disaster management, as well as links for disaster planning tools.

REFERENCES

ABC News. (2010). *Haiti earthquake: Why so much damage?* Retrieved from http://abcnews.go.com/Technology/HaitiEarthquake/haiti-shallow-earthquake-magnified-damage-californias-san-andreas/story?id=9562379.

American Red Cross. (2002). *Disaster mental health services: An overview*(ARC Pub No 3077-2A).Washington, DC: Author.

Booth, C. M., Matukas, L., Tomlinson, G., Rachlis, A., Rose, D., Dwosh, H., & Detsky, A. S. (2003). Clinical features and short-term outcomes of 144 patients with SARS in the greater Toronto area. *Journal of the American Medical Association, 289*, 2801–2809.

Campbell, A. (2006). *The SARS Commission—Spring of fear: Final report*. Retrieved from http://www.health.gov.on.ca/english/public/pub/ministry_reports/campbell06/campbell06.html.

Canadian Nurses Association. (2006). Highlights from the 2005 CNA annual report. *Canadian Nurse, 102*(5), 24–33.

Canadian Paediatric Society. (2006). *Submission to the standing committee on finance on the 2006 pre-budget consultations*. Retrieved from http://www.cps.ca/ENGLISH/Advocacy/Reports/2006FinanceCommittee_Pre-BudgetSubmission.pdf.

Canadian Red Cross. (2006). *What we do during disasters*. Retrieved from http://www.redcross.ca/article.asp?id=000302&tid=025.

Community Hospital Infection Control Association (CHICA-Canada). (2009). *Links and resources: Pandemic (H1N1) 2009 virus*. Retrieved from http://www.chica.org/links_swineflu.html.

Dwosh, H. A., Hong, H. H., Austgardan, D., Herman, S., & Schabas, R. (2003). Identification and containment of an outbreak of SARS in a community hospital. *Canadian Medical Association Journal, 168*(11), 1415–1420.

Etkin, D., Haque, E., Bellisario, L., & Burton, I. (2004). *An assessment of natural hazards and disasters in Canada: A report for decision makers and practitioners*. Ottawa: Environment Canada.

Foreign Affairs and International Trade Canada. (2010). *Summative evaluation of start's global peace and security fund—Haiti*. Retrieved from http://www.international.gc.ca/about-a_propos/oig-big/2009/evaluation/gpsf_fpsm_haiti09.aspx?lang=eng.

Gebbie, K. M., & Qureshi, K. (2002). Emergency and disaster preparedness: Core competencies for nurses—what every nurse should but may not know. *American Journal of Nursing, 102*(1), 46–51.

Government of Canada. (2010). *Preparing a family emergency kit in plain English*. Retrieved from http://www.getprepared.gc.ca/index-eng.aspx.

Health Canada. (2006). *It's your health: Preparing your family for an emergency*. Retrieved from http://www.hc-sc.gc.ca/iyh-vsv/life-vie/emerg-urg_e.html.

Health Canada. (2007). *Preparing for the stress of disasters and mass emergencies—Federal emergency responders: Organizational actions to reduce and manage stress and support employees*. Retrieved from http://www.hc-sc.gc.ca/ewh-semt/pubs/occup-travail/actions-mesures/stress-eng.php.

Historica Foundation of Canada. (2010). *The Canadian encyclopedia*. Retrieved http://www.thecanadianencyclopedia.com/index.cfm?PgNm=TCE&Params=A1ARTA0002313.

Huston, P. (2004). Commentary: Thinking locally about pandemic influenza. *Canadian Journal of Public Health, 95*(3), 184–185.

Johnson, M., Bone, E., & Predy, G. (2005). Taking care of the sick and scared: A local response in pandemic preparedness. *Canadian Journal of Public Health, 96*(6), 412–414.

Jones, R. L. (2009). *Canadian disasters: An historical survey*. Retrieved from http://web.ncf.ca/jonesb/DisasterPaper/disasterpaper.html.

Krawchuk, C. (2003). *Federal report: Learning from SARS renewal of public health in Canada*. Retrieved from http://www.cbc.ca/news/background/SARS/SARS_report.htm.

Library and Archives Canada. (2006). *SOS! Canadian disasters*. Retrieved from http://www.collectionscanada.ca/sos/002028-1300-e.html.

McCready, J. (2004). *Ice storm 1998: Lessons learned*. Retrieved from http://www.treecanada.ca/cufc6/proceedings/papers/McCready.pdf.

Mildon, B. (2004). In the wake of SARS: Structures and strategies. *Community Health Nurses Association of Canada Newsletter, 6*(3), 1–3, 10–16.

Morren, M., Dirkzwager, A. J. E., Kessels, F. J. M., & Yzermans, J. (2007). *The influence of a disaster on the health of rescue workers: A longitudinal study*. Retrieved from http://www.cmaj.ca/cgi/content/full/176/9/1279?maxtoshow=&HITS=10&hits=10&RESULTFORMAT=&fulltext=morren&andorexactfulltext=and&searchid=1&FIRSTINDEX=0&sortspec=relevance&resourcetype=HWCIT.

Natural Resources Canada. (2009). *Natural hazards*. Retrieved from http://atlas.nrcan.gc.ca/site/english/maps/environment/naturalhazards/1.

Ontario Ministry of Health and Long-Term Care. (2008). *Ontario health plan for an influenza pandemic*. Retrieved from http://www.health.gov.on.ca/english/providers/program/emu/pan_flu/ohpip2/preface.pdf.

Parry, J. (2003). China is still not open enough about SARS, says WHO. *British Medical Journal, 326*, 1055.

Public Health Agency of Canada. (2005). *Responding to stressful events: Taking care of ourselves, our families and our communities*. Retrieved from http://www.phac-aspc.gc.ca/publicat/oes-bsu-02/comm-eng.php.

Public Health Agency of Canada. (2006a). *The Canadian pandemic influenza plan for the health sector*. Retrieved from http://www.phac-aspc.gc.ca/cpip-pclcpi/pdf-e/cpip-eng.pdf.

Public Health Agency of Canada. (2006b). *Highlights from the Canadian pandemic influenza plan for the health sector: Preparing for an influenza pandemic, the Canadian perspective*. Retrieved from http://www.phac-aspc.gc.ca/cpip-pclcpi/hl-ps/index.html.

Public Health Agency of Canada. (2008). *Fact sheet: Progress achieved since SARS.* Retrieved from http://www.phac-aspc.gc.ca/sars-sras-gen/sars0308-eng.php.

Public Health Agency of Canada. (2009). *Flu watch.* Retrieved from http://www.phac-aspc.gc.ca/fluwatch/09-10/w41_09/index-eng.php.

Public Health Agency of Canada. (2010a). *Centre for Emergency Preparedness and Response.* Retrieved from http://www.phac-aspc.gc.ca/cepr-cmiu/index-eng.php.

Public Health Agency of Canada. (2010b). *Emergency response services.* Retrieved from http://www.phac-aspc.gc.ca/emergency-urgence/index-eng.php.

Public Safety Canada. (2008). *An emergency management framework for Canada.* Retrieved from http://www.publicsafety.gc.ca/prg/em/emfrmwrk-eng.aspx.

Public Safety Canada. (2009). *About disaster mitigation.* Retrieved from http://www.publicsafety.gc.ca/prg/em/ndms/aboutsnac-eng.aspx#typ.

Public Safety Canada. (2010). *Programs.* Retrieved from http://www.publicsafety.gc.ca/prg/index-eng.aspx.

Raholm, M., Arman, M., & Rehnsfeldt, H. (2008). The immediate lived experience of the 2004 tsunami disaster by Swedish tourists. *Journal of Advanced Nursing, 63*(6), 597–606.

Registered Nurses' Association of Ontario. (2004). *SARS unmasked: Final report on the nursing experience with SARS in Ontario.* Retrieved from http://www.rnao.org/Storage/24/1891_SARS_Report_June_04.pdf.

Tam, T., Sciberras, J., Mullington, B., & King, A. (2005). Fortune favours the prepared mind: A national perspective on pandemic preparedness. *Canadian Journal of Public Health, 96*(6), 406–408.

Tolomiczenko, G. S., Kahan, M., Ricci, M., Strathern, L., Jeney, J., Patterson, K., & Wilson, L. (2005). SARS: Coping with the impact at a community hospital. *Journal of Advanced Nursing, 50*(1), 101–110.

The University of British Columbia. (2003). *SARS, West Nile and monkey pox.* Retrieved from http://www.communityaffairs.ubc.ca/talkofthetown/2003/fall/sars.html.

Veenema, T. G. (2003). Essentials of disaster planning. In T. G. Veenema (Ed.), *Disaster nursing and emergency preparedness for chemical, biological, and radiological terrorism and other hazards.* New York: Springer.

World Health Organization. (2009). *Current WHO phase of pandemic alert.* Retrieved from http://www.who.int/csr/disease/avian_influenza/phase/en/.

Yates, J. (2001, October 6). Gifts, letters piling up at N.Y. relief centers. *Chicago Tribune,* A1.

CHAPTER 17

Communicable and Infectious Disease Prevention and Control

KEY TERMS

acquired immunity 532
acquired immunodeficiency syndrome (AIDS) 553
active immunization 532
anthrax 528
chlamydia 548
common vehicle 533
communicable disease 531
communicable period 533
directly observed therapy (DOT) 564
disease 533
elimination 531
emerging infectious diseases 528
environment 532
eradication 531
gonorrhea 548
hantavirus pulmonary syndrome (HPS) 528
hepatitis A virus (HAV) 555
hepatitis B virus (HBV) 556
hepatitis C virus (HCV) 556
herd immunity 532
HIV antibody test 564
horizontal transmission 533
incubation period 533
infection 533
infectiousness 532
natural immunity 532
partner notification 564
passive immunization 532
resistance 532
severe acute respiratory syndrome (SARS) 534
surveillance 534
vaccine 532
vector 533
vertical transmission 533

See Glossary on page 593 for definitions

OBJECTIVES

After reading this chapter, you should be able to:

1. Discuss the past and current effect and threats of infectious diseases on society.
2. Explain how the elements of the epidemiological triangle interact to cause infectious diseases.
3. Identify the determinants of health that affect communicable diseases, infectious diseases, and sexually transmitted infections (STIs).
4. Provide examples of infectious disease–control interventions at the three levels of prevention.
5. Define *surveillance* and discuss the functions and elements of a surveillance system.
6. Discuss the factors contributing to newly emerging or re-emerging infectious diseases.
7. Discuss issues related to obtaining and maintaining appropriate levels of immunization against vaccine-preventable diseases.
8. Describe the agents associated with food-borne illness and explain the appropriate prevention measures.
9. Describe the natural history of human immunodeficiency virus (HIV) infection and relevant client education at each stage.
10. Discuss the clinical signs of communicable diseases, infectious diseases, HIV, hepatitis, and STIs.
11. Identify groups that are at greatest risk and explain specific considerations for HIV, STIs, hepatitis, and tuberculosis.
12. Describe community health nursing actions to prevent and care for people who experience communicable, parasitic, and infectious diseases.
13. Apply appropriate community health nursing assessment and interventions for communicable, parasitic, and infectious diseases.

CHAPTER OUTLINE

Knowledge about the risk of communicable and infectious diseases has changed dramatically in recent years. Concern about communicable and infectious diseases requires that community health nurses (CHNs) stay current about communicable disease guidelines. This chapter presents an overview of the communicable and infectious diseases and sexually transmitted infections (STIs) with which CHNs deal most often and their nursing management, including primary, secondary, and tertiary prevention. These diseases are often acquired through behaviours that can be avoided or changed. For this reason, community health nursing interventions have focused on disease prevention. Prevention can take the form of vaccine administration (as for hepatitis A and B), early detection (for tuberculosis [TB]), or teaching clients about abstinence or safer sex (for STI prevention). Although not all infectious diseases are directly communicable from person to person, the terms *infectious diseases* and *communicable diseases* are used interchangeably throughout this chapter.

HISTORICAL PERSPECTIVES

In 1900, communicable diseases were the leading causes of death in Canada. Improved nutrition, vaccines, and antibiotics have put an end to the epidemics that once ravaged entire populations. In 1926, TB caused 7% of all deaths in Canada; by 1990, less than 1% of deaths occurred due to TB (Lung Association, 2006a). In the early 1900s, in Canada, the underlying belief that TB treatment had to occur on an in-patient basis led to the establishment of numerous sanatoriums and specialized TB units in hospitals. The minimum length of in-patient treatment was 1 year, but many clients were treated in-house for a longer period. Over the 15-year period between 1938 and 1953, the number of beds assigned for the treatment of TB rose from 9,000 to over 19,000 (Lung Association, 2006b). Antimicrobial drugs were discovered for the effective treatment of TB in 1948, and from that time until the late 1970s, the number of cases of TB took a downward trend and, therefore, sanatoriums were gradually phased out. By the 1980s, the downward trend levelled off. Refer to the Saskatchewan Lung Association Web site for historical information on TB and Canada's role in fighting TB, both found in the Weblinks on the Evolve Web site.

Currently, in Canada, because of the aggressive treatment of TB, the number of new cases and the number of people dying from this disease is smaller than in similar countries; however, we need to remain vigilant in the surveillance of this disease. In January 2006, a strategic plan to stop TB internationally, called The Global Plan to Stop TB 2006–2015, was announced. The World Health Organization (WHO) secretariat is coordinating this plan with more than 400 partner organizations, including the World Bank and Canadian and U.S. foreign aid agencies. Refer to Table 17-1 for facts about tuberculosis in Canada. For further information about TB in Canada, such as its case reporting and its treatment, refer to the Public Health Agency of Canada (PHAC) Web site titled *Tuberculosis in Canada* (in the Tool Box on the Evolve Web site). TB cases most often occur in large urban centres such as Toronto, Montreal, and Vancouver.

TABLE 17-1 Facts on TB in Canada in 2006 and 2007

Tuberculosis in Canada 2006	Tuberculosis in Canada 2007
New active and relapsed TB reported cases were 1,619 (5.0/100,000)	New active and relapsed TB reported cases were 1,548 (4.7/100,000)
Nunavut reported highest rate at 157.9/100,000 cases	Nunavut reported highest rate at 99.6/100,000 cases
Prince Edward Island had no reported cases	Prince Edward Island had no reported cases
British Columbia, Ontario, and Quebec, the provinces making up 76% of Canada's population, reported 73% of the total cases	British Columbia, Ontario, and Quebec, the provinces making up 75% of Canada's population, reported 75% of the total cases
17% of the total cases were in persons 35–44 years of age, accounting for the largest number of the total cases	18% of the total cases were in persons 35–44 years of age, accounting for the largest number of the total cases
64% of the cases were foreign-born persons	66% of the cases were foreign-born persons
12% of the cases were Canadian-born non-Aboriginals	11% of the cases were Canadian-born non-Aboriginals
20% of the cases were Canadian-born Aboriginals	20% of the cases were Canadian-born Aboriginals
62% of the cases were diagnosed with pulmonary TB	65% of the cases were diagnosed with pulmonary TB

SOURCE: Adapted from Public Health Agency of Canada. (2009). *Tuberculosis in Canada, 2006.* Retrieved from http://www.phac-aspc.gc.ca/publicat/2009/tbcan06/index-eng.php; and Public Health Agency of Canada. (2009). *Tuberculosis in Canada, 2007: Pre Release.* Retrieved from http://www.phac-aspc.gc.ca/publicat/2008/tbcanpre07/index-eng.php.

Appendix 12 (Non-Vaccine-Preventable Diseases) provides other information about TB, such as epidemiology, mode of transmission, incubation period, indicators, time of occurrence, and nursing considerations.

There has been a general decrease in the number of reported cases in the past 10 years, with most of this decrease being in the Canadian-born non-Aboriginal population. In 2007, when compared to 2006 TB cases, there was a decrease of 6.3% and the case rate decreased by 7.2%. Since statistics have been recorded in Canada pertaining to TB records, the case rate reached the lowest in 2007 (PHAC, 2009h). In comparison with other TB rates globally, the WHO estimates that approximately 9 million new TB cases occur yearly (WHO, 2009e). It is estimated that in the European region alone, the hourly TB incidence rate is 49 TB cases and 7 deaths (WHO, 2009e). To explore specific information about TB for European countries, refer to the WHO Web site *Tuberculosis in the European Region* (found in the Evolve Weblinks).

With advanced control of communicable diseases and as individuals live longer, chronic diseases—heart disease, cancer, and stroke—have replaced infectious diseases as the leading causes of death. In fact, each year in Canada, the majority of deaths occur from the following noncommunicable diseases: cardiovascular conditions, cancer, diabetes, and respiratory conditions (Shah, 2003; Vollman, Anderson, & McFarlane, 2008). However, infectious diseases have not vanished. Organisms once susceptible to antibiotics are becoming increasingly drug resistant and may result in vulnerability to diseases no longer thought to be a threat. And in the twenty-first century, infectious diseases have become a means of terrorism.

Emerging infectious diseases are those in which the incidence has actually increased in the past two decades or has the potential to increase in the near future. These emerging diseases may include new or known infectious diseases. Consider the following examples: (1) Ebola virus, a mysterious new killer with a frightening mortality rate that sometimes reaches 90%, has no known treatment and has no recognized reservoir in nature; (2) human immunodeficiency virus (HIV) and acquired immunodeficiency syndrome (AIDS), not a new disease, but the resultant immunocompromise is largely responsible for the rising numbers of previously rare opportunistic infections such as cryptosporidiosis, toxoplasmosis, and *Pneumocystis* pneumonia; (3) West Nile virus (WNV), which is new in this country and is transmitted mainly by WNV-infected mosquitoes; (4) **anthrax,** an acute disease caused by the spore-forming bacterium *Bacillus anthracis,* which is highly resistant to disinfection and environmental destruction and may remain in contaminated soil for many years; (5) avian influenza virus, a contagious viral infection that most often affects birds but can infect mammals; (6) the H1N1, which is a new strain of influenza virus that is transmissible to humans and for which humans have developed little or no immunity—therefore, there could be a rapid spread of the disease, resulting in a worldwide outbreak, referred to as an *influenza pandemic*; and (7) cryptococcal disease, a rare but treatable fungal infection that has emerged on Vancouver Island, British Columbia (British Columbia Centre for Disease Control, 2005).

New killers are emerging, and old familiar diseases are taking on different, more virulent characteristics. Consider the following recent developments. Legionnaires' disease and toxic shock syndrome, unknown in the mid-twentieth century, have become part of our common vocabulary. The identification of infectious agents causing Lyme disease and Ehrlichiosis has led to two new tick-borne diseases becoming an area of concern.

Hantavirus pulmonary syndrome (HPS), also referred to as hantavirus disease, is an infectious disease caused by the hantavirus that begins with flu-like symptoms that can become life-threatening when the virus affects the lungs and causes respiratory problems (Canadian Centre for Occupational Health & Safety, 2008). In Canada, deer mice *(Peromyscus maniculatus)* are the principal carriers of HPS. Infected mice shed the virus in fresh urine, droppings, and saliva. Humans become infected from the inhalation of the virus if exposed to heavily contaminated materials in which mice have nested. Also, but less frequently, ingestion of contaminated food or water by humans can lead to HPS. Seldom are people infected as a result of having been bitten by a mouse. In Canada, between 2000 and 2004, 12 cases of HPS were diagnosed, with these cases being reported in Alberta and Saskatchewan (PHAC, 2006b).

Necrotizing fasciitis, most commonly referred to as flesh-eating disease, is a severe condition that has a high fatality rate. A skin injury usually precedes the development of the disease. Most frequently, the bacteria causing the disease are group A streptococci (GAS). This condition is common in temperate zones and semitropics, although rare cases have occurred in Canada. Health Canada (2006a) estimates there are between 90 and 200 cases per year, with a fatality rate of 20 to 30%. Since January 2005, this disease has been included under surveillance by Health Canada.

Consumption of improperly cooked hamburgers and unpasteurized apple juice and unpasteurized milk contaminated with a highly toxic strain of *Escherichia coli* (O157:H7) can cause illness and death. One of the most common medical problems, persistent diarrhea, can be the result of travel to underdeveloped countries. The occurrence is often due to lower standards of water quality, sanitation, and food preparation. Although travellers may take particular hygiene, food, and water precautions, these actions have a limited effectiveness in preventing the development of persistent diarrhea due to parasitic and bacterial pathogens.

In 1996, the fear that "mad cow disease" (bovine spongiform encephalopathy [BSE]) could be transferred to humans through beef consumption led to the slaughter of thousands of British cattle and a ban on the international sale of British beef. The organism was identified in Canada in 1993 in a beef cow that had been brought into Canada from Britain in 1987. The disease also appeared in the United States in 2003, when a BSE-infected animal was imported from Canada. BSE has been reported in many countries, including several in Europe as well as Japan, the United States, and Israel. Since 1990, BSE has been a reportable disease in Canada (Canadian Food Inspection Agency, 2009a). Based on this surveillance, four cases were found in Canadian beef. The first case occurred in May 2003, with two cases in January 2005 and one case in 2009 (Canadian Food Inspection Agency, 2005; 2009a). Numerous measures have been taken to prevent further cases and the spread of BSE, such as surveillance programs, feeding product controls, and cattle identification programs. The cartoon illustrates that BSE had a high profile in the media during the most recent outbreak.

New-variant Creutzfeldt-Jakob disease (nvCJD), which attacks the brain with fatal results, is the disease hypothesized but not yet proven to result from eating beef infected with the transmissible agent that causes BSE. This disease is a reportable disease in Canada. Figure 17-1 identifies the current and predicted CJD cases in Canada by province and territory. In Canada, the number of suspected cases of CDJ from 1997 to May 2009 were 971, and the deaths from CJD from 1999 to May 2009 were 357 (PHAC, 2009a). This data is updated frequently. For the latest updates, refer to the PHAC Web site titled *Creutzfeldt-Jakob Disease* found in the Weblinks on the Evolve Web site.

In 1999, the first Western hemisphere activity of West Nile Virus (WNV), a mosquito-transmitted illness that can affect livestock, birds, and humans, occurred in New York City. The first confirmed human cases of WNV were in Ontario and Quebec in 2002. In 2007, in Canada, 2,015 confirmed WNV infections were reported with 12 deaths (Norris, 2009). The numbers of reported cases of WNV were Saskatchewan (1,285), Manitoba (578), Alberta (318), British Columbia (19), Ontario (12), Quebec (2) and Nova Scotia (1) (Norris, 2009). In 2008, in Canada there was marked decrease in the number of cases with 36 confirmed human infections and 2 deaths (Norris, 2009). As of October 2010, there were five reported cases in the year 2010 of WNV.

In early 2003, severe acute respiratory syndrome (SARS), a previously unknown disease of undetermined etiology and with no definitive treatment, was first reported in China and Hong Kong. In March 2003, the first Canadian cases were reported. The infected persons were identified as Canadians returning from Hong Kong. The WHO and Health Canada worked collaboratively to monitor and control the SARS outbreak in Canada (until the establishment of the PHAC in September 2004). Further information about SARS was provided in Chapter 16.

In Canada, the PHAC includes the Centre for Infectious Disease Prevention and Control, a Centre for Chronic Disease Prevention and Control, and the Pandemic Preparedness Secretariat (PPS), as well as a Travel Health site. The PPS was established in the spring of 2006 due to the global concern about avian and pandemic influenzas.

Worldwide, infectious diseases account for approximately one-third (approximately 17 million) of deaths globally (Global IDEA Scientific Advisory Committee, 2004). Approximately 6 million deaths worldwide result

Bovine spongiform encephalopathy (BSE), severe acute respiratory syndrome, and West Nile virus are infectious diseases that have had a high profile in Canada in recent years.

SOURCE: Steve Nease, 05/23/03. Reprinted with permission.

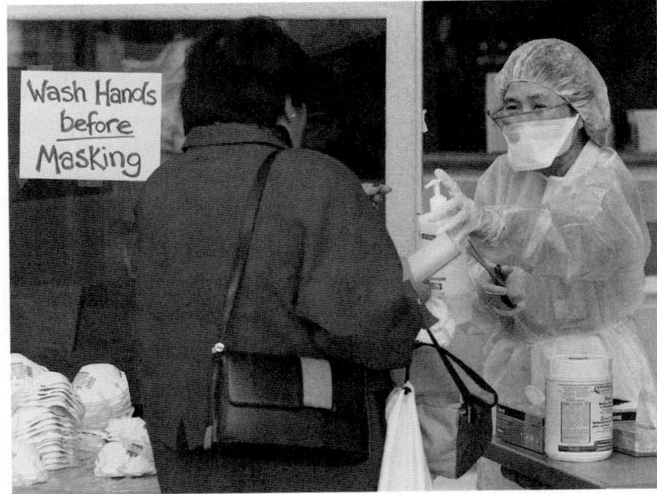

The occurrence of severe acute respiratory syndrome in 2003 heightened awareness of the enormous financial and human cost due to a lack of readiness for this type of outbreak.

FIGURE 17-1 Cases of Creutzfeldt-Jakob Disease in Canada by Province and Territory, 2009

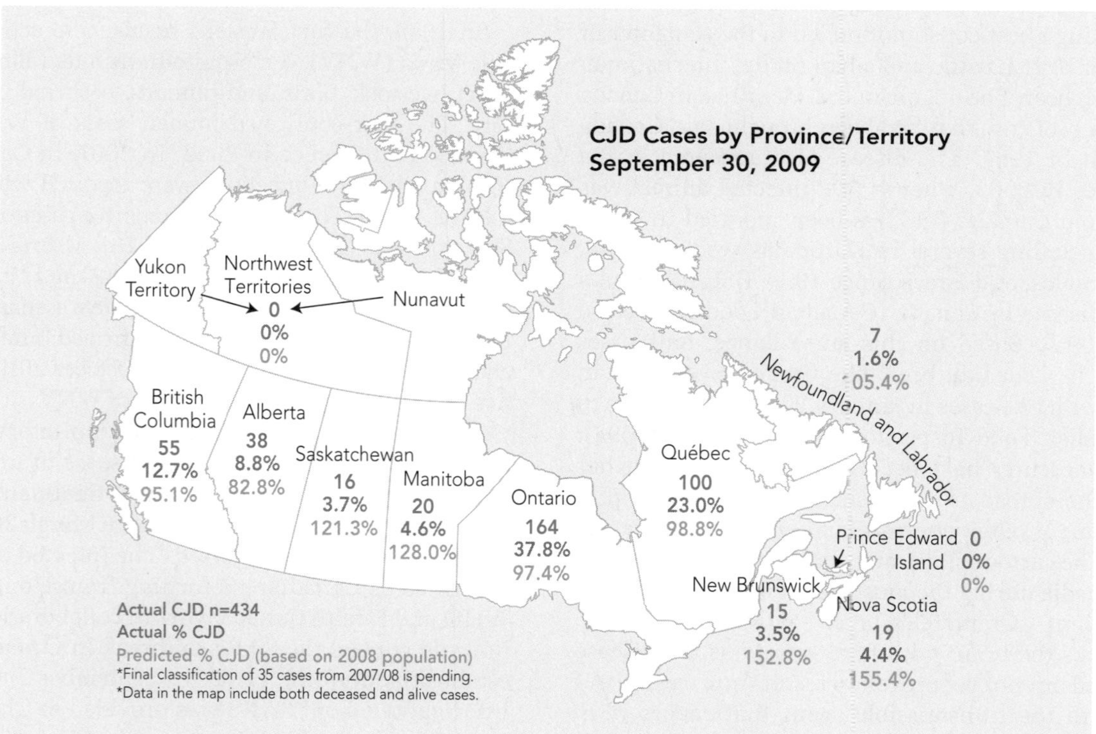

SOURCE: Public Health Agency of Canada. (2009). *Referrals of suspected CJD reported to CJD-SS, Creutzfeldt-Jakob Disease Surveillance System Statistics*. Retrieved from http://www.phac-aspc.gc.ca/hcai-iamss/cjd-mcj/cjdss-ssmcj/stats-eng.php#ref.

from HIV and AIDS, TB, and malaria, and there are approximately 11 million child deaths worldwide mainly from other infectious diseases (Global IDEA Scientific Advisory Committee, 2004). With increased opportunities for travel to underdeveloped countries, there has been an increase in the incidence of certain infectious diseases, such as malaria and hepatitis. Infectious diseases continue to present varied, multiple, and complex challenges to all health care providers. CHNs need to know about these diseases to effectively participate in diagnosis, treatment, prevention, and control.

CRITICAL VIEW

Refer to the following Web site to answer the questions below:

http://www.humansecurity-chs.org/finalreport/English/chapter6.pdf

1. a) What is the relationship between diseases and poverty globally? Provide examples to support your discussion.

   b) What are the barriers related to the control of infectious diseases globally?

2. What are some examples of health inequities globally?

DETERMINANTS OF HEALTH

Several determinants affect health, illness, health promotion, and disease prevention. There are associations between the determinants of health and communicable and infectious diseases and STIs. For example, poverty and low literacy may lead to social exclusion of individuals because they have limited access to health services and programs for communicable and infectious diseases. Gender is a factor in the incidence and prevalence of several STIs. The CHN role is to create a supportive environment—for example, through providing information sessions and accessible health services such as clinics. The "Determinants of Health" box on the next page identifies some of the determinants.

CRITICAL VIEW

1. The pandemic influenza is often compared with the Spanish influenza. What are the similarities and differences between these two strains?
2. How would you differentiate between the avian influenza and the pandemic influenza?

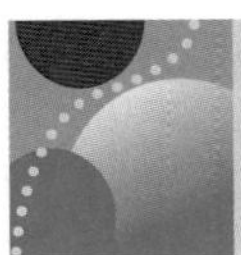

Determinants of Health
Communicable, Infectious, and Sexually Transmitted Infections

- In Canada, approximately 242,500 persons are infected with hepatitis C (HCV), with approximately 8,000 of these new infections occurring in 2007 (PHAC, 2009c). It has been found that one in five persons in Canada who experienced HCV is an immigrant who has difficulties with access to health care (Remis, cited in Sherman et al., 2007). As a chronic disease, HCV places a substantial economic burden on Canadians (Sherman et al., 2007).
- In Canada, over 4 million persons obtain their drinking water from private wells, and these wells can become contaminated from poor construction, improper location, or if surface water is contaminated (Health Canada, 2008).
- In Canada, approximately 11 million persons annually experience food-related illnesses (PHAC, 2010a). Canadians with weakened immune systems such as the very young, pregnant, or older adults are more likely to experience more severe symptoms and require the help of a health professional (PHAC, 2010a).
- Globally, approximately 55,000 people die of rabies annually and approximately 95% of these deaths are in Asia and Africa (WHO, 2009a).
- Seventy-two percent of all reported cases of syphilis occur in men ages 30 to 59 years (PHAC, 2008a).
- Twenty-eight percent of youth between the ages of 15 and 17 years reported being sexually active, compared to 80% of young adults 20–24 years of age having reported being sexually active, with both groups having reported having more than one sexual partner in the previous year (Statistics Canada, 2005). Sexuality issues are one aspect of adolescent development (Gender and Health Collaborative Curriculum Project, 2008), and sexual intercourse is one component of sexuality.
- Over 66% of all reported cases of chlamydia in Canada occurred in females, with the predominant age group being 15 to 24 years (PHAC, 2008a). This high prevalence rate of chlamydia infections in females is not acceptable (Sex Information and Education Council of Canada [SIECCAN], 2009).
- Approximately 60% of all reported cases of gonorrhea in Canada occurred in males (PHAC, 2008a). The research evidence consistently demonstrates that condom use significantly reduces the occurrence of chlamydia, gonorrhea, and other STIs (SIECCAN, 2009).

COMMUNICABLE DISEASES

Communicable disease can be prevented and controlled. The goal of prevention and control programs is to reduce the prevalence of a disease to a level at which it no longer poses a major public health problem. In some cases, diseases may even be eliminated or eradicated. The goal of **elimination** is to remove a disease from a large geographical area such as a country or region of the world.

CRITICAL VIEW

1. What other determinants of health could have relevance to communicable and infectious diseases and sexually transmitted infections?
2. What are the implications of the determinants of health and having communicable or infectious diseases or sexually transmitted infections on equity, social justice, health disparities, and empowerment?

Eradication is the permanent elimination of a disease worldwide. The WHO officially declared the global eradication of smallpox on May 8, 1980 (WHO, 1999). After the successful eradication of smallpox, the eradication of other communicable diseases became a realistic goal.

Agent, Host, and Environment

A **communicable disease** is a disease of human or animal origin caused by an infectious agent. Its transmission depends on the successful interaction of the infectious agent, the host, and the environment, the factors that make up the epidemiological triangle (see Chapter 3). Changes in the characteristics of any of the factors may result in disease transmission. Consider the following examples. Antibiotic therapy may not only eliminate a specific pathological agent, it may also alter the balance of normally occurring organisms in the body. As a result, one of these agents overruns another, and disease, such as a yeast infection, occurs. HIV performs its deadly work not by directly poisoning the host but by destroying the host's immune reaction to other disease-producing agents. Individuals living in the temperate climate of Canada do not contract malaria at home, but they may become infected if they change their environment by travelling to a climate where malaria-carrying mosquitoes thrive. As these examples illustrate, the balance among agent, host, and environment is often precarious and may be unintentionally disrupted. In the twenty-first century, the potential results of such disruption require attention as advances in science and technology, destruction of natural habitats, explosive population growth, political instability, and a worldwide transportation network combine to alter the balance among the environment, people, and the agents that produce disease.

Agent Factor

Four main categories of infectious agents can cause infection or disease: bacteria, fungi, parasites, and viruses. The individual agent may be described by its ability to cause disease and by the nature and the severity of the disease. *Infectivity, pathogenicity, virulence, toxicity, invasiveness,* and *antigenicity,* terms commonly used to characterize infectious agents, are defined in Box 17-1.

Host Factor

A human or animal host can harbour an infectious agent. The characteristics of the host that may influence the spread of disease are host resistance, immunity, herd immunity, and infectiousness. **Resistance** is the ability of the host to withstand infection, and it may involve natural or acquired immunity. **Natural immunity** refers to species-determined, innate resistance to an infectious agent. For example, coyotes in Saskatchewan rarely contract rabies. **Acquired immunity** is the resistance acquired by a host as a result of previous natural exposure to an infectious agent. Having measles once protects against future infection. Acquired immunity may be induced by active or passive immunization. **Active immunization** refers to the immunization of an individual by the administration of an antigen (infectious agent or **vaccine** [a preparation of killed microorganisms, living attenuated organisms, or living fully virulent organisms]) to stimulate active response by the host's immunological system and is usually characterized by the presence of antibodies produced by the individual host and therefore provides complete protection against the specific disease. Vaccinating children against childhood diseases is an example of inducing active immunity. **Passive immunization** refers to immunization through the transfer of a specific antibody from an immunized individual to a nonimmunized individual, such as the transfer of antibodies from mother to infant or the administration of an antibody-containing preparation (immune globulin or antiserum). Passive immunity from immune globulin is almost immediate but short-lived. It is often induced as a stopgap measure until active immunity has time to develop after vaccination. Examples of commonly used immune globulins include those for hepatitis A, rabies, and tetanus.

Herd immunity refers to the immunity of a group or community. It is the resistance of a group of people to the invasion and spread of an infectious agent. Herd immunity is based on the resistance of a high proportion of individual members of a group to infection. It is the basis for increasing immunization coverage for vaccine-preventable diseases. Higher immunization coverage will lead to greater herd immunity, which in turn will block the further spread of the disease. For example, the national immunization campaign for the administration of the H1N1 vaccine was an effort to achieve herd immunity.

Infectiousness is a measure of the potential ability of an infected host to transmit the infection to other hosts. It reflects the relative ease with which the infectious agent is transmitted to others. Individuals with measles are extremely infectious; the virus spreads readily via airborne droplets. A person with Lyme disease cannot spread the disease to other people (although the infected tick can).

BOX 17-1 Six Characteristics of an Infectious Agent

1. *Infectivity:* The ability to enter and multiply in the host
2. *Pathogenicity:* The ability to produce a specific clinical reaction after infection occurs
3. *Virulence:* The ability to produce a severe pathological reaction
4. *Toxicity:* The ability to produce a poisonous reaction
5. *Invasiveness:* The ability to penetrate and spread throughout a body tissue
6. *Antigenicity:* The ability to stimulate an immunological response

Environment Factor

In the context of communicable and infectious diseases, the **environment** refers to all that is external to the human host, including physical, biological, social, and cultural factors. These environmental factors facilitate the transmission of an infectious agent from an infected host to other susceptible hosts. Reduction in communicable disease risk can be achieved by altering these environmental factors. Using mosquito nets and repellants to avoid insect bites, installing sewage systems to prevent fecal contamination of water supplies, and washing utensils after contact with raw meat to reduce bacterial contamination are all examples of altering the environment to prevent disease.

Modes of Transmission

Infectious diseases can be transmitted horizontally or vertically. **Vertical transmission** is the passing of an infection from parent to offspring via sperm, placenta, milk, or contact in the vaginal canal at birth. Examples of vertical transmission are transplacental transmission of HIV and syphilis. **Horizontal transmission** is the person-to-person spread of infection through one or more of the following four routes: direct or indirect contact, common vehicle, airborne, or vector borne. Most STIs are spread by direct sexual contact. Enterobiasis, or pinworm infection, can be acquired through direct contact or indirect contact with contaminated objects such as toys, clothing, and bedding. **Common vehicle** refers to the transportation of the infectious agent from an infected host to a susceptible host via food, water, milk, blood, serum, saliva, or plasma. Hepatitis A can be transmitted through contaminated food and water; hepatitis B can be transmitted through contaminated blood. Legionellosis and TB are both spread via contaminated droplets in the air. A **vector** is a nonhuman organism, often an insect, that either mechanically or biologically plays a role in the transmission of an infectious agent from source to host. For example, a vector can be an arthropod, such as a tick or mosquito, or other invertebrate, such as a snail, that can transmit the infectious agent by biting or depositing the infective material near the host.

Disease Development

Exposure to an infectious agent does not always lead to an infection. Similarly, infection does not always lead to disease. Infection depends on the infective dose, the infectivity of the infectious agent, and the immunocompetence of the host. It is important to differentiate infection and disease, as clearly illustrated by the HIV/AIDS epidemic. **Infection** refers to the state produced by the invasion of a host by an infectious agent. Infection involves the entry, development, and multiplication of the infectious agent in the susceptible host. Such infection may or may not produce clinical signs. **Disease** refers to the presence of abnormal alterations in the structure or functioning of the human body that fits within the medical model. It is one of the possible outcomes of infection, and it may indicate a physiological dysfunction or pathological reaction. For example, individuals who test positive for HIV are infected, but if they do not exhibit clinical signs, they are not considered at that time to have the disease. If individuals test positive for HIV and also exhibit clinical signs of AIDS, they are infected and have the disease.

Incubation period and *communicable period* are not synonymous. **Incubation period** is the time interval between the invasion by an infectious agent and the first appearance of signs and symptoms of the disease. The incubation periods of infectious diseases vary from between 2 and 4 hours for staphylococcal food poisoning to between 10 and 15 years for AIDS. **Communicable period** is the interval during which an infectious agent may be transferred directly or indirectly from an infected person to another person. The period of communicability for influenza is 3 to 5 days after the clinical onset of symptoms. Hepatitis B–infected persons are infectious many weeks before the onset of the first symptoms and remain infective during the acute phase and chronic carrier state, which may persist for life.

Disease Spectrum

Persons with infectious diseases may exhibit a broad spectrum of disease that ranges from subclinical infection to severe and fatal disease. Those with subclinical or nonapparent infections are important from the public health point of view because they are a source of infection but may not be receiving the care that those with a clinical disease receive. They should be targeted for early diagnosis and treatment. Those with a clinical disease may exhibit localized or systemic symptoms and mild to severe illness. The final outcome of a disease may be recovery, death, or something in between, including a carrier state; complications requiring an extended hospital stay; or disability requiring rehabilitation.

At the community level, the disease may occur in endemic, epidemic, or pandemic proportion. *Endemic* refers to the constant presence of a disease within a geographical area or a population. For example, pertussis is endemic in the United States. *Epidemic* refers to the occurrence of a disease in a community or region in excess of normal expectancy. Although people tend to associate large numbers with epidemics, even one case can be termed *epidemic* if the disease was considered previously eliminated from that area. For example, one case of polio, a disease considered eliminated from Canada, would be considered epidemic. *Pandemic* refers to an epidemic occurring worldwide and affecting large populations. HIV/AIDS is both epidemic and pandemic as the number of cases is growing rapidly across various regions of the world. SARS emerged as an infectious disease and an example of a pandemic. In February 2003, the world learned of a mysterious respiratory disease primarily infecting travellers and health care workers in Southeast Asia (Katz & Hirsch, 2003). Thought at first to be a form of influenza, this illness was soon recognized as an atypical and sometimes deadly pneumonia, transmitted easily through close contact and seemingly unresponsive to treatment with antibiotics and antiviral medications. Initially confined to mainland China, this disease of unknown etiology and no respect for national borders spread to Hong Kong and then quickly to Hanoi, Singapore, and Toronto, prompting the WHO in 2003 to release a rare emergency travel advisory that heightened the surveillance of clients with atypical pneumonia around the globe (WHO, 2011). Intense international investigation revealed that **severe acute respiratory syndrome (SARS),** as this illness came to be called, was associated with a new strain of coronavirus. Between March 15 and April 15, 2003, 36 clients were diagnosed with SARS at the Queen Mary Hospital in Hong Kong (Tiwari et al., 2003). Common symptoms included cough, dyspnea, malaise, and fever. By the end of July 2003, more than 8,000 cases with more than 800 deaths had been reported to the WHO from approximately 30 countries (WHO, 2003). A very large number of individuals infected by SARS can be traced back to unrecognized cases in hospitals, suggesting that prompt identification and isolation of symptomatic people are the keys to interrupting transmission. There is no vaccine or cure for SARS.

A more recent pandemic was declared worldwide, known as H1N1 (swine flu), and was discussed in Chapter 16. See the "Ethical Considerations" box, below, about safety precautions during a communicable disease outbreak.

ETHICAL CONSIDERATIONS

"During a human-made or natural disaster, including a communicable disease outbreak, nurses have a duty to provide care using appropriate safety precautions" (CNA, 2008, p. 46). This raises ethical concerns for CHNs who might be worried about the adequacy of safety precautions.

Ethical principles that apply to the prevention and control of communicable and infectious diseases are these:

- *Distributive justice.* To do with fairness. There should be a fair distribution of the benefits and burdens in society based on the needs and contributions of its members.
- *Beneficence.* CHNs have general obligations to perform actions that maintain or enhance the dignity of clients whenever those actions do not place undue burden on the health care providers.

Question to Consider

1. What are the CHN's ethical responsibilities in preventing the spread of HINI to populations at risk, such as persons newly infected with HIV?

SURVEILLANCE OF COMMUNICABLE DISEASES

Surveillance is a systematic and ongoing observation and collection of data concerning disease occurrence to describe phenomena and detect changes in frequency or distribution. It gathers the *who, when, where,* and *what;* these elements are then used to answer *why.* A good surveillance system systematically collects, organizes, and analyzes current, accurate, and complete data for a defined disease condition. The resulting information is promptly released to those who need it for effective planning, implementation, and evaluation of disease prevention and control programs. Infectious disease surveillance incorporates and analyzes data from a variety of sources. Box 17-2 lists 10 commonly used data elements.

List of Reportable Diseases

All provinces and territories in Canada are required to report communicable diseases. In order to facilitate and monitor specific communicable diseases, a reporting mechanism is in place. The list of notifiable or reportable diseases in Canada is shown in Box 17-3. Table 17-2 shows PHAC's statistics for notifiable diseases by province for June 2007.

Primary, Secondary, and Tertiary Prevention

The three levels of prevention in community health are *primary, secondary,* and *tertiary.* In prevention and control of infectious disease, primary prevention seeks to reduce the incidence of disease by preventing it before it happens, and in this, government often provides assistance. Many interventions at the primary

BOX 17-2 Ten Basic Elements of Surveillance

1. Mortality registration
2. Morbidity reporting
3. Epidemic reporting
4. Epidemic field investigation
5. Laboratory reporting
6. Individual case investigation
7. Surveys
8. Use of biological agents and drugs
9. Distribution of animal reservoirs and vectors
10. Demographic and environmental data

BOX 17-3 Nationally Notifiable Infectious Diseases

- Acute flaccid paralysis
- Acquired immunodeficiency syndrome
- Amebiasis
- Anthrax
- Botulism
- Brucellosis
- Campylobacteriosis
- Chancroid
- Chicken pox
- Chlamydia, genital
- Cholera
- Creutzfeldt-Jakob disease
- Cryptosporidiosis
- Cyclosporiasis
- Diphtheria
- Giardiasis
- Gonococcal ophthalmia neonatorum
- Gonorrhea
- Group B streptococcal disease of the newborn
- Hantavirus pulmonary syndrome
- Hepatitis A
- Hepatitis B
- Hepatitis C
- Hepatitis non-A, non-B
- Human immunodeficiency virus
- Influenza, laboratory confirmed
- Invasive group A streptococcal disease
- Invasive *Haemophilus influenzae* type b disease
- Invasive meningococcal disease
- Invasive pneumococcal disease
- Legionellosis
- Leprosy
- Listeriosis (all types)
- Malaria
- Measles
- Meningitis, other bacterial
- Meningitis, pneumococcal
- Meningitis, viral
- Mumps
- Paratyphoid
- Pertussis
- Plague*
- Poliomyelitis
- Rabies
- Rubella
- Rubella, congenital
- Salmonellosis
- Shigellosis
- Smallpox
- Syphilis, all
- Syphilis, congenital
- Syphilis, early latent
- Syphilis, early symptomatic (primary and secondary)
- Syphilis, other
- Tetanus
- Trichinosis
- Tuberculosis
- Tularemia
- Typhoid
- Verotoxigenic *Escherichia coli*
- Viral hemorrhagic fevers (Crimean-Congo, Ebola, Lassa, Marburg)
- West Nile virus asymptomatic infection
- West Nile virus fever
- West Nile virus neurological syndromes
- West Nile virus unclassified or unspecified
- Yellow fever*

* The notifiable disease database has never received a report of plague or yellow fever.

SOURCE: Adapted from Public Health Agency of Canada. (2003). *Notifiable diseases on-line*. Retrieved from http://dsol-smed.phac-aspc.gc.ca/dsol-smed/ndis/list_e.html#tab1.Reprinted with permission of the Minister of Public Works and Government Services Canada, 2010.

level, such as federally supplied vaccines and "no shots, no school" immunization laws, are population based because of public health mandate. CHNs deliver many of these childhood immunizations in public and community health settings, check immunization records in daycare facilities, and monitor immunization records in schools. The goal of secondary prevention is to prevent the spread of disease once it occurs. Activities centre on rapid identification of potential contacts to a reported case. Contacts may be (1) identified as new cases and treated or (2) determined to be possibly exposed but not diseased and appropriately treated

TABLE 17-2 Notifiable Diseases by Province for June 2007 (Preliminary)

Disease	Nfld.	PEI	NS	NB	Que.	Ont.**	Man.	Sask.	Alta.	BC	YT	NWT	Nvt.**	June 2007	Jan. to June 2007	Jan. to June 2006
Diseases Preventable by Routine Vaccination																
Acute flaccid paralysis*																
Diphtheria																
Invasive *Haemophilus influenzae* type B disease										2		1		4	11	9
Hepatitis B	2		1		45					4				52	289	321
Measles					47									47	57	10
Mumps	1		25	30	8		2		2	3				71	447	26
Pertussis			2	1	8		1		5	59				76	242	1,186
Poliomyelitis																
Rubella					1		1							2	4	2
Congenital rubella syndrome																
Tetanus															2	1
Sexually Transmitted and Blood-Borne Pathogens																
Acquired immunodeficiency syndrome*																
Chlamydia, genital	42	11	130	101	1026		373	237	827	759	13	77		3,596	23,304	33,594
Creutzfeldt-Jakob disease																10
Gonorrhea	1		5	2	103		114	80	170	90	1	10		576	3,493	5,254
Hepatitis C	7	5		7	164		19	39	61	199	1	1		503	3,553	6,290
Human immunodeficiency virus infection*																
Syphilis, congenital															4	4
Syphilis, infectious†					17		1		13	18				49	390	842
Syphilis, other				1	9		3	1		11				25	182	931

Diseases Transmitted by Direct Contact and Respiratory Routes														
Chicken pox	19			5				8			1	33	171	424
Group B streptococcal disease of the newborn							1 1		1 1			2 2	7 7	31 31
Hantavirus pulmonary syndrome								1				1	1	3
Influenza, laboratory confirmed*														
Invasive group A streptococcal disease	2		4	3	27	2		21	21		2	82	496	632
Invasive pneumococcal disease	1			2	54	8	12	36	41		3	157	1357	1,493
Legionellosis					11							11	20	35
Leprosy					1								1	2
Invasive meningococcal disease	1				5				3			9	99	111
Tuberculosis*														
Enteric Food- and Water-borne Diseases														
Botulism													3	2
Campylobacteriosis	3	3	9	22	213	25	32	111	199		1	618	2575	4,038
Cholera									1			1	4	
Cryptosporidiosis				2	4	1	1	9	3			20	116	207
Cyclosporiasis			2		2				10			14	31	70
Giardiasis	2	2	5	12	65	6	7	35	59	2	1	196	1,104	1,818
Hepatitis A				1	8	1		1	2			13	95	2,16
Salmonellosis	1		7	12	77	15	6	64	66			248	1,463	2,584
Shigellosis					9	1		5	16			31	213	349
Typhoid								2	4			6	32	85
Verotoxigenic *Escherichia coli*	1			1	14	9	3	29	15		1	73	208	346

(Continued)

TABLE 17-2 Notifiable Diseases by Province for June 2007 (Preliminary)—Cont'd

Disease	Nfld.	PEI	NS	NB	Que.	Ont.	Man.	Sask.	Alta.	BC	YT	NWT	Nvt.*	June 2007	Jan. to June 2007	Jan. to June 2006
Vector-Borne and Other Zoonotic Diseases																
Brucellosis					1									1	3	2
Malaria				2	7				8	4				21	89	168
Plague																
Rabies															1	
Yellow fever																
Bioterrorism Agents																
Anthrax																
Smallpox																
Tularemia								1						1	7	3
Viral hemorrhagic fevers																

* The number of cases are shown at the end of the year only.
** No data received for June 2007.
† Includes syphilis primary, secondary, and early latent.

Source: Public Health Agency of Canada. (2007). *Notifiable diseases by province for June 2007 (preliminary)*. Notifiable Diseases Section, Surveillance and Risk Assessment Division/Centre for Infectious Disease Prevention and Control. Retrieved from http://www.phac-aspc.gc.ca/bid-bmi/dsd-dsm/ndmr-rmmdo/pdf/2007/jun07.pdf. Reprinted with permission of the Minister of Public Works and Government Services Canada, 2010.

with prophylaxis. Public health disease control laws also assist in secondary prevention because they require investigation and prevention measures for individuals affected by a communicable disease report or outbreak. These laws can extend to the entire community if the exposure potential is deemed great enough, as could happen with an outbreak of smallpox or epidemic influenza. Much of the communicable disease surveillance and control work in Canada is performed by CHNs. Tertiary prevention works to reduce complications and disabilities through treatment and rehabilitation.

Role of CHNs in Prevention

Prevention is at the centre of community health nursing practice. Examples of such involvement include delivery of immunizations for vaccine-preventable diseases, especially childhood immunization, and the monitoring of immunization status in clinic, daycare, school, and home settings. CHNs work in communicable disease surveillance and control, teach and monitor blood-borne pathogen control, and advise on prevention of vector-borne diseases. They teach methods for responsible sexual behaviour, screen for STIs, conduct contact tracing for STIs, and provide HIV counselling, testing, and follow-up. They screen for TB, identify TB contacts, and deliver directly observed TB therapy (DOT) in the community, discussed later in the chapter.

Vaccine-Preventable Diseases

Vaccines are one of the most effective methods of preventing and controlling communicable diseases. Diseases such as polio, diphtheria, pertussis, and measles, which previously occurred in epidemic proportions, are now controlled by routine childhood immunization. They have not, however, been eradicated, so children need to be immunized against these diseases. In Canada, immunization is strongly recommended but not compulsory in that choices can be made by parents to not have their children immunized; however, their children will not be permitted to attend school should there be a disease outbreak. Many infants and toddlers, the group most vulnerable to these potentially severe diseases, do not receive scheduled immunizations on time despite the availability of free vaccines. CHNs who work in regions where groups obtain exemption from immunization on religious or health belief grounds, where immunization is incomplete, or where international visitors are frequent need to be especially alert for communicable disease cases and the need for prompt outbreak control among particularly susceptible populations. Communicable diseases in all age groups can best be prevented through the use of vaccines. Refer to Table 17-3 for a detailed description of the vaccine-preventable communicable diseases. The routine immunization recommended for children in Canada is found in Appendix E-5 on the Evolve Web site. For some diseases, booster doses are required throughout the lifespan. The *Canadian Immunization Guide* (PHAC, 2006a) can be found at the PHAC Weblink on the Evolve Web site.

LEVELS OF PREVENTION

RELATED TO INFECTIOUS DISEASE INTERVENTIONS

Primary Prevention

To prevent the occurrence of disease, the role of the CHN is to

- Provide counselling for individuals on prevention of sexually transmitted infections (STIs)
- Provide immunization such as influenza vaccine, tetanus boosters, and Pneumovax
- Provide safe food-handling information
- Provide community education about prevention of communicable diseases in well populations
- Notify contacts about their exposure to a reportable communicable disease
- Advocate for public policy on the prevention of water contamination

Secondary Prevention

To prevent the spread of disease, the role of the CHN is to

- Screen for tuberculosis in health care workers
- Conduct partner notification for STIs
- Offer clinics for testing for human immunodeficiency virus
- Advocate for the availability for required screening services

Tertiary Prevention

To reduce complications and disabilities through treatment and rehabilitation, the role of the CHN is to

- Initiate and monitor therapy (e.g., initiate directly observed therapy for tuberculosis treatment)
- Identify community resources for supportive care (e.g., funds for purchasing medications)
- Refer to self-help support groups
- Promote behaviour change to minimize risk factors (e.g., adolescents with STIs)

CRITICAL VIEW

1. a) Should influenza vaccination be mandatory for community health nurses? Explain.
   b) What is the evidence for and against immunization?
2. a) How would you explain immunizing agents to parents?
   b) How would you address parental concerns about immunization?

Refer to the following Web site to compare your answers to the questions:

http://www.caringforkids.cps.ca/immunization/index.htm

Influenza

Influenza ("flu") is a viral respiratory infection often indistinguishable from the common cold or other respiratory diseases. The most important factors to note about influenza are its epidemic nature and the mortality that may result from pulmonary complications, especially in older adults. There are three types of influenza viruses: A, B, and C. Type A is usually responsible for large epidemics, whereas outbreaks from type B are more regionalized; type C epidemics are less common and usually result in only mild illness. Influenza viruses often change in the nature of their surface appearance or their antigenic makeup. Types B and C are fairly stable viruses, but type A changes constantly. Minor antigenic changes are referred to as *antigenic drift,* and they result in yearly epidemics and regional outbreaks. Major changes such as the emergence of new subtypes are called *antigenic shift;* these occur only with type A viruses. Antigenic shift and drift lead to epidemic outbreaks every few years and pandemic outbreaks every 10 to 40 years. The preparation of influenza vaccine each year is based on the best possible prediction of what type and variant of virus will be most prevalent that year. Because of the changing nature of the virus, yearly immunization is necessary and is given in the early fall before the influenza season begins. Influenza shots do not always prevent infection, but they do result in milder disease symptoms, especially in healthy population groups. Annually in Canada, between 2,000 and 8,000 persons die of seasonal influenza (flu) and related complications (PHAC, 2010b). For further information about seasonal influenza refer to Table 17-3.

In the spring of 2009, the H1N1 flu virus (human swine influenza) surfaced in North America (see Chapter 16). This flu virus differs from the seasonal flu virus in that it is a new strain and most persons do not have a natural immunity. Consequently, it has potential to cause serious illness. The H1N1 vaccine was developed and available to all Canadians in the fall of 2009. The Canadian Public Health Agency (CPHA) urged that all Canadians be immunized against H1N1 because "the scientific evidence is clear: the important benefits the vaccine offers far outweigh any potential risks" (CPHA, 2009a). In the initial phase of the H1N1 immunization program, priority vaccinations were targeted for administration to the following groups: children between the ages of 6 months and 5 years; persons in close contact with and caregiving for infants under 6 months of age or immunocompromised individuals; individuals residing in remote communities; health care workers involved with the delivery of essential health services; and persons under 65 years of age with a chronic illness (CPHA, 2009b). In June 2009, WHO declared the H1N1 flu as a pandemic influenza (WHO, 2009a). Further information on the H1N1 flu virus can be found in Table 17-3, at the PHAC Web site *Your H1N1 Preparedness Guide*, and at the Health Canada Web site *Health Concerns: Influenza (flu)* found in the Weblinks on the Evolve Web site. Both resources provide influenza information for health care professionals and consumers.

Smallpox, a severely acute highly contagious disease caused by the variola virus found worldwide, has been eradicated since 1979 (WHO, 2009d). In the 1950s, approximately 50 million cases of smallpox occurred globally each year; however, due to vaccination, this number fell to between 10 and 15 million in the late 1960s (WHO, 2009d). A global campaign to eradicate this deadly and disfiguring disease resulted in its complete eradication. In 1980, the WHO declared that smallpox had been globally eradicated, and immunization for smallpox was terminated (WHO, 2009d). The only documented existing virus sources are preserved and secured at the Centers for Disease Control and Prevention in Atlanta and a research institute in Novosibirsk, Russia. Supplies of smallpox vaccine are located in the United States and maintained by the WHO. Several countries, including Canada, are negotiating with pharmaceutical companies to produce additional vaccine to be used in a bioterrorism situation should it arise. Despite threats of bioterrorism, there are no plans to reintroduce universal smallpox immunization with the existing vaccine because of potential side effects. Many health care providers have never seen smallpox; however, they have seen the distinctive scar left on so many shoulders of those who have had the vaccination. The emergence of one case of smallpox would need to be recognized immediately because people are not immunized and one case of smallpox would be considered a global epidemic.

TABLE 17-3 Vaccine-Preventable Infectious Diseases*

Disease	Epidemiology	Mode of Transmission	Incubation Period	Indicators	Time of Occurrence	Nursing Considerations
Diphtheria	From 1986 to 2004 there have only been between 2 and 5 annual cases of diphtheria in Canada. Most of those cases occurred in young adults 20 years of age or older who did not have adequate protection (PHAC, 2007c).	Toxigenic strains of *Corynebacterium diphtheriae* cause the disease. The organism (both toxigenic and nontoxigenic strains) may be harboured in the nasopharynx, skin, and other sites of asymptomatic carriers. Transmission is most often spread by respiratory means.	2–5 days, with range of 1–10 days	Formation of a greyish membrane in the respiratory tract with surrounding inflammation, which may lead to respiratory obstruction		Investigate reported cases and initiate control measures for outbreaks, and use every opportunity to immunize.
Haemophilus influenzae type B	In 2004, the incidence of reported cases was 0.3 per 100,000 (81 cases). From 1986 to 1993, the number of cases reported varied from 100 to 650 cases per year. In 1993, the Hib vaccine became incorporated into the childhood vaccination routine. As a result, the number of cases has dropped per year (PHAC, 2007d).	Infection enters the body through the nose or mouth; bacteria are spread by respiratory droplets and by direct contact with discharges from the nose or mouth of an infected person (Alberta Health and Wellness, 2005).	2–4 days	Most commonly associated with bacterial meningitis but can also cause pneumonia and inflammation of the skin, joints, bone, throat, and heart. Acute-onset fever, vomiting, and lethargy in 50 to 55%. Can also cause epiglottitis, pneumonia, bacteremia, and other complications		Educate regarding the importance of immunization, especially in young children.
Hepatitis A	Between 1990 and 2004, the number of reported cases of HAV infection ranged from 3,562 in the year 1991 to 396 in 2003, representing rates of (10.8/100,000–1.2/100,000 population). Since the vaccine in 1996, there have been no major outbreaks of this disease and the number of new annual cases has steadily declined (PHAC, 2007e).	Refer to Appendix 13.	15–50 days, with an average of 20–30 days	Refer to Appendix 13.	Little seasonal variation	Educate regarding importance of immunization. Refer to Appendix 13.

(Continued)

TABLE 17-3 Vaccine-Preventable Infectious Diseases*—Cont'd

Disease	Epidemiology	Mode of Transmission	Incubation Period	Indicators	Time of Occurrence	Nursing Considerations
Hepatitis B	In Canada, the incidence of hepatitis B is approximately 2.3 per 100,000 people. Twice as many men are affected as women. Those most affected are in the 30- to 39-year-old age bracket (PHAC, 2007f).	Refer to Appendix 13.	45–160 days; average 120 days	Refer to Appendix 13.	Little seasonal variation	Educate regarding importance of immunization. Refer to Appendix 13.
Influenza	It is estimated that 10 to 25% of the Canadian population is affected by the influenza virus yearly (Health Canada, 2006a). Of these, more than 4000 die each year of related complications. Hardest hit is the older adult population (Health Canada, 2009).	Transmitted by airborne respiratory droplets entering into nose or mouth or through direct contact with eyes and touching contaminated surfaces	1–4 days, with an average of 2 days	Influenza typically starts with headache, chills, and cough, followed rapidly by fever, anorexia, muscle aches, fatigue, running nose, sneezing, watery eyes, and throat irritation. Nausea, vomiting, and diarrhea may occur, especially in children (PHAC, 2010b).	Usually runs from November to April	Counsel regarding measures to prevent spread of influenza. Monitor outbreaks and educate regarding the importance of yearly immunization.
Measles (red measles, rubeola)	The incidence of measles dropped dramatically between 2000 and 2002 when the number of cases decreased from 199 to 6. Seven cases occurred in 2004 because of Canadians not being immunized (PHAC, 2009f). In early 2010, 44 measles cases were confirmed in British Columbia in unvaccinated persons (British Columbia Centre for Disease Control, 2010).	Transmitted by droplet spread or direct contact with nasal or throat secretions of infected persons; less commonly by airborne spread or indirect contact with freshly infected articles. In closed areas, infections have been documented for up to 2 hours after source of infection has been removed; one of the most readily transmitted	7–18 days after contact with person with red measles; fever and cough usually occur 3–4 days prior to the rash. Rash fades in 4–7 days (Alberta Health Services, 2008).	An acute disease with prodromal fever, conjunctivitis, cough, and Koplik's spots on the buccal mucosa. Red blotchy rash appears in 3–7 days, beginning on the face and head and becoming generalized, lasting 3–7 days. Leukopenia occurs; other symptoms include anorexia, diarrhea, lymphadenopathy, and otitis media. More severe in infants and adults. Systemic infection; primary		Investigate reported cases and initiate control measures for outbreaks; use every opportunity to immunize. Certain groups such as infants and adults become more severely ill when infected with red measles.

		diseases. Extremely communicable from slightly before the prodromal period to 4 days after appearance of rash; minimal after the second day of rash		site of infection is the respiratory epithelium of the nasopharynx. Bacterial superinfection; case fatality rate may be as high as 25% but usually <0.5% in Canada (PHAC, 2009f)		
Meningococcal infection (meningitis)	Between 1985 and 2001, an average of 305 cases were reported annually. Children under 1 year of age and 15- to 19-year-olds are the most affected (PHAC, 2005a).	Transmitted by airborne droplets or by direct contact with respiratory secretions	3–4 days, with a range of 2–10 days	Sudden onset of fever, headache, and stiff neck, often accompanied by other symptoms, such as nausea, vomiting, photophobia, and altered mental status	Disease occurs year round, but there is seasonal variation, with the majority of cases occurring in the winter months.	Identify and monitor high-risk groups for outbreaks. Educate regarding importance of immunization.
Mumps	Since the vaccination program, the annual number of reported cases has greatly decreased; however, there continues to be localized outbreaks usually in under-vaccinated communities (PHAC, 2007g).	Respiratory transmission by inhaling airborne droplets of infected person or direct contact with objects contaminated with infected saliva	14–24 days	Chills, headache, anorexia, general malaise, fever, swelling, and tenderness of one or more salivary glands. Deafness may occur in less than one to five cases per 100,000 persons; it is usually transient but may be permanent.	Disease occurs year round, but is most frequent in late winter and early spring.	Counsel pregnant women that mumps infection during the first trimester of pregnancy may increase the rate of spontaneous abortion. Educate regarding the importance of immunization.
Pertussis (whooping cough)	Immunization has helped to decrease the incidence of pertussis; however, outbreaks still do occur (PHAC, 2007h).	Respiratory transmission by inhaling airborne droplets of infected person	5–21 days	First stage can last 1–2 weeks and includes a runny nose, sneezing, low-grade fever, and a mild cough. Second stage usually lasts 1–6 weeks, but can last up to 10 weeks.		Monitor for outbreaks and educate regarding immunization.

(Continued)

TABLE 17-3 Vaccine-Preventable Infectious Diseases*—Cont'd

Disease	Epidemiology	Mode of Transmission	Incubation Period	Indicators	Time of Occurrence	Nursing Considerations
				Characteristic symptom is a series of rapid coughs, at the end of which the client has a prolonged inhaling effort characterized by a high-pitched whoop. May turn blue and vomit Third stage may last for months. Cough usually disappears after 2–3 weeks, but paroxysms may recur with any subsequent respiratory infection.		
Pneumo-coccal infections	In the <5-year age group, there were an estimated 15 deaths, 65 cases resulted in meningitis, and 700 cases caused bacteremia; pneumonia occurred in 2,200 individuals who needed hospitalization and in 9,000 who did not (Health Canada, 2006b).	Bacteria are spread by direct oral contact, such as kissing; by inhaling airborne respiratory droplets from the nose or throat of infected persons; or indirectly through articles soiled with respiratory discharges involving secretions from the nose.	1–3 days	Pneumococcal pneumonia: abrupt onset of fever, shaking, chills, chest pain, coughs with sputum production, shortness of breath, rapid breathing and heart rate, and weakness Pneumococcal meningitis: sudden onset of high fever, lethargy or coma, nausea and vomiting, and a stiff neck. Fever, vomiting, and convulsions may be the first symptoms in young children (PHAC, 2003b). Acute otitis media: often caused by pneumococci bacteria, demonstrated by ear pain or red bulging tympanic membrane	Winter and early spring	Identify and educate high-risk groups regarding importance of immunization.

Poliomyelitis (polio)	Canada was declared to be polio free in 1994 after certification from the Pan American Health Organization (PHAC, 2009d).	Transmission occurs via the fecal–oral route (PHAC, 2009d).	6–20 days	Fever, mild headache, sore throat, constipation, fatigue, and stiff neck are usual symptoms and flaccid paralysis of the legs may occur (PHAC, 2009d).	Continue surveillance for possible cases. Educate regarding the importance of vaccination.
Rabies	Between 1985 and 1999, no human cases of rabies were reported in Canada. From 1925 to 1985, 22 people died from rabies, and in the year 2000, one person died in Canada (PHAC, 2007i)	Transmitted through close contact with saliva of infected animals, most often by a bite, scratch, or licks on broken skin or mucous membranes, such as the eyes, nose, or mouth. In very rare cases, person-to-person transmission has occurred when saliva droplets were dispersed in the air (PHAC, 2008c). Injury to the upper body or face poses the greatest risk of transmission.	Can be as short as 5 days or as long as several years, usually taking 20–60 days	First symptoms usually nonspecific, influenza-like symptoms—fever, tiredness, headache—may last for a few days. Acute stage, which quickly follows, demonstrates anxiety, confusion, insomnia, agitation, hallucinations, and hyperactivity (furious rabies) or paralysis (dumb rabies). Acute period usually ends after 2–10 days. Complete paralysis develops followed by coma. Without intensive care, death occurs during the first 7 days of illness (PHAC, 2008c).	Provide counselling to clients who are travelling to areas with an increased incidence of rabies. Educate regarding the steps to take to decrease personal risk of rabies. Educate regarding post-exposure treatments and monitoring.
Rubella (German measles)	In Canada, rubella is not very common, with usually fewer than 30 cases of rubella being reported annually (PHAC, 2005b). Those who have not been immunized can cause rubella outbreak clusters (PHAC, 2007j).	Respiratory transmission by inhaling nasal droplets	12–23 days	General malaise, runny nose, cough, painless, rose-coloured spots on the roof of the mouth, conjunctivitis, swollen tender lymph nodes on back of neck or under the ears, rash that begins on	Rubella is highly contagious (PHAC, 2005b). It is recommended that rubella vaccine not be given to children under 12 months of age or to pregnant women.

(Continued)

TABLE 17-3 Vaccine-Preventable Infectious Diseases*—Cont'd

Disease	Epidemiology	Mode of Transmission	Incubation Period	Indicators	Time of Occurrence	Nursing Considerations
				face and neck and then spreads to trunk, arms, and legs, which joins together to form patches. Older girls or women may develop pain and swelling in joints.		It is recommended that the vaccine be administered to all female adolescents and to women of child-bearing age (advise to avoid pregnancy for 1 month after vaccination) (PHAC, 2005b). Counsel pregnant women about congenital rubella syndrome (CRS). CRS can result in miscarriages, stillbirths, and fetal malformations. 85% of CRS cases occur with infection in the first trimester; this is very rare after the twentieth week of pregnancy (PHAC, 2007h).
Tetanus (lockjaw)	Due to immunization programs, cases of tetanus have decreased. During 1980–2004, annual reported cases of tetanus range from 1 to 10 with an average of 4 per year. The last death in Canada from tetanus occurred in 1997 (PHAC, 2007k).	Transmitted usually when a skin wound becomes contaminated by a bacterium called *Clostridium tetani*, found in soil and animal feces	3–21 days	Stiffness of jaw (lockjaw); restlessness; dysphagia; headache; fever; sore throat; chills; muscle spasms; stiffness in neck, arms, and legs; painful muscle contractions; and convulsions		Assess and educate regarding the importance of immunization.

Varicella (chicken pox)	50% of Varicella cases usually occur in children before the age of 5 years. Adults have the highest case fatality rates (30 deaths/100,000 cases); infants (7 deaths/100,000 cases); and children and youth 1–19 years of age (1–1.5 deaths/100,000 cases (PHAC, 2007l).	Spread by direct contact with virus shed from skin lesions, oral secretions, or airborne route. Period of infection is 1 to 2 days before onset of the rash and lasts until all lesions are crusted over.	10—21 days, usually 14—16	Fever, abdominal pain, sore throat, headache, general malaise 1–2 days before rash. Rash begins as small, red, flat spots and develops into itchy, thin-walled blisters, usually less than one-quarter inch wide, filled with clear fluid and a red base. They appear over 2–4 days. The blister breaks, leaving open sores, which finally crust over to become dry, brown scabs.	Investigate cases and initiate control measures for outbreaks and educate regarding immunization.

PHAC = Public Health Agency of Canada.
*Note: Data are Canadian unless otherwise specified.

Sources: Health Canada, 2006b; Health Canada, 2009; PHAC, 2005a; PHAC, 2005b; PHAC, 2006a; PHAC, 2007c; PHAC, 2007e; PHAC, 2007f, PHAC, 2007g; PHAC, 2007h; PHAC, 2007i; PHAC, 2007j; PHAC, 2007k; PHAC, 2007l; PHAC, 2009f.

CRITICAL VIEW

Immunization has dramatically decreased measles cases in Canada. Prior to the availability of measles vaccine, most children contracted the disease. Measles in Canada now occurs sporadically, mostly because of Canada's high standard of childhood immunization programs for vaccine-preventable communicable diseases.

1. What kinds of questions might families ask the community health nurse about vaccination?
2. How would you respond to these family questions?

Non–Vaccine-Preventable Diseases

Non–vaccine-preventable diseases are diseases that cannot be prevented by vaccination. TB, a non–vaccine-preventable disease, is of concern globally, and discussion follows. Many of the food- and water-borne illnesses (e.g., *Salmonella, E. coli*) and diseases transmitted by vectors (WNV, Lyme disease) are discussed later.

Tuberculosis

Tuberculosis (TB) is a mycobacterial disease caused by *Mycobacterium tuberculosis* and is transmitted by airborne droplets. There are different types of TB, such as pulmonary TB, ocular TB, genitourinary TB, miliary/disseminated TB, and bone and joint TB. TB can be active or latent. Reactivation of latent infections is more common in immunocompromised persons, cigarette smokers, underweight and undernourished persons, persons with diabetes mellitus, and those with silicosis (PHAC, 2007a). For most Canadians, the risk of developing TB is very low. However, in 2007 there were approximately 1,547 new cases of TB reported in Canada, so it is important to know the symptoms and how to minimize risk (Ontario Lung Association, 2009). The following groups in Canada are at increased risk of developing TB: those who travel to and from countries where TB is endemic; First Nations peoples living in communities with a high prevalence of TB; homeless persons; residents of some long-term care facilities or persons in correctional facilities; health care workers; and persons with weakened immune systems such as alcoholics, diabetics, those infected with HIV, and older adults (Health Canada, 2006d). Some of the roles of the PHAC in relation to TB are data collection and analysis of reported cases in order to improve TB prevention and control and monitoring through surveillance of drug resistance nationally to TB.

Screening, diagnosis, and management of TB are well outlined in the *Canadian Tuberculosis Standards,* 2007, which is available online and is listed in the Tool Box on the Evolve Web site. CHNs may administer and interpret TB skin tests, collect specimens, monitor medications, and provide education and support when necessary; therefore, familiarity with the current TB guidelines is paramount. An additional resource for health care providers, titled *Tuberculosis for Health Care Providers,* is included in the Tool Box on the Evolve Web site. It covers epidemiology, screening, diagnosis, treatment, and management of TB.

Sexually Transmitted Infections

Previously, the diseases included under *sexually transmitted infections (STIs)* were referred to as *sexually transmitted diseases,* and sometimes the terms are sometimes used interchangeably. The incidence or number of new cases of some STIs, such as syphilis, has been declining, while the incidence of others, such as herpes simplex and chlamydia, is increasing. Also, the actual rates of STIs may be twice the reported rate. In Canada, since 1997, there has been a steady increase in the numbers of reported cases of STIs, with chlamydia being the most common, gonorrhea the second most common, and syphilis the least common (Cropp, Latham-Caranico, Stebben, Wong, & Duarte-Franco, 2007). **Chlamydia** is an STI caused by the organism *Chlamydia trachomatis,* which causes infection of the urethra and cervix. Infections may be asymptomatic and, if untreated, result in severe morbidity. **Gonorrhea** is an STI caused by a bacterium, *Neisseria gonorrhoeae,* resulting in inflammation of the urethra and cervix and dysuria, or it may result in no symptoms. These diseases have long-term health effects, and CHNs need to be knowledgeable about STIs. The common STIs are listed in Table 17-4. The PHAC Web site *Sexually Transmitted Infections (STI): Sexual Health Facts and Information for the Public* provides valuable information on STIs in Canada and can be found at the Evolve Weblinks. The *Canadian Guidelines on Sexually Transmitted Infections* (listed in the Tool Box on the Evolve Web site) provide a reference for professionals with additional new information in the 2008 revision on at-risk populations—that is, vulnerable populations. The PHAC Web site *The FACTS on the Safety and Effectiveness of HPV Vaccine* (found in the Evolve Weblinks) provides answers to the many questions about the HPV vaccine.

Generally, community health nursing considerations for all STIs would include the need for diagnosis and confidential treatment for any person, regardless of age; public education about the indicators of STIs, mode of transmission, and the importance of early treatment and follow-up; reporting; and contact tracing follow-up.

TABLE 17-4 Common Sexually Transmitted Infections

Sexually Transmitted Infection	Epidemiology	Mode of Transmission	Incubation Period	Indicators	Nursing Considerations
Chlamydia	Rates have been rising since 1997, with over 65,000 cases reported in 2006. The 15- to 24-year-old age group is responsible for over 66% of reported cases. There is probably underreporting because the disease is asymptomatic in a number of individuals (PHAC, 2008a).	Oral, vaginal, or anal sex	2–6 weeks	Females: Genital discharge, burning feeling while urinating, lower abdominal pain, pain during sex, and abnormal vaginal bleeding Males: Burning when voiding, urethral itch, urethral discharge (milky or watery), and pain or swelling in testicles. Often individuals are asymptomatic.	Counsel clients regarding risk factors such as the following: • Having sexual contact with a chlamydia-infected partner. • Having a new sexual partner or more than two sexual partners in the past year. • Having had a previous STI. • Having had sexual exposure to vulnerable populations. Prevention of chlamydia: • Encourage clients to practise safer sex. • Screen vulnerable populations (e.g., injection drug users, incarcerated individuals, sex trade workers, street youth, etc.). • Assess, treat, and counsel partners of infected individuals. • Provide specific screening, treatment, and counselling for pregnant women in the high-risk population. Follow-up: • Infected individuals require specific follow-up and education (refer to STI guidelines).

(Continued)

TABLE 17-4 Common Sexually Transmitted Infections*—Cont'd

Sexually Transmitted Infection	Epidemiology	Mode of Transmission	Incubation Period	Indicators	Nursing Considerations
Genital herpes	Annual incidence in Canada is not known; however, it is increasing globally with country variations. It is more commonly acquired by females (PHAC, 2008a).	Most commonly spread by direct contact with open sores, usually during genital, oral, or anal sex. Although it is rare, pregnant women can pass this infection to their baby during or after childbirth. Herpes infection in infants can be life-threatening.	2–21 days; average of 6 days	Tingling or itching in the genital area, painful blisters, fever, and general malaise Females: Sores may occur on the vagina, on the cervix, inside or near the vagina, on the genitals, near the anus, or on the thighs and buttocks; tender lumps in the groin Males: Sores on the penis, around the testicles, near the anus, and on thighs and buttocks; tender lumps in the groin Both males and females can get sores in the mouth or in the genital area after oral sex with an infected person.	Counsel regarding the chronic aspects of the disease. Educate about the likelihood of recurring episodes, potential for infecting partner during asymptomatic periods, and care of infected area and type of clothing to wear, and that antiviral therapy may shorten the duration of lesions and prevent recurrent outbreaks. Counsel regarding safer-sex practices and informing past sexual partners.
Hepatitis B	See Table 17-3 and Appendix 13 (Viral Hepatitis Profiles)				
HIV/AIDS	It is estimated that 30% of individuals infected with HIV are not aware they have it. In 2000–2004, there was a rise in HIV cases in Canada by 20%. The largest category is males (homosexual and heterosexual), followed by women and intravenous drug users. Women made up 25% of cases in 2004, compared with 10% prior to 1995, and those aged 15–19 years had the largest increase in incidence rates. Aboriginal peoples also had an increasing rate of disease (PHAC, 2008a).	Exposure to blood or body fluids from an HIV-infected person by sexual contact, IV drug use, HIV-infected blood transfusions, perinatal mother-to-child transmission, or occupational exposure. Since 1985, improved blood product screening from donors has decreased HIV transmission by blood transfusions (PHAC, 2008a).	HIV: Can produce antibodies within 3 months. AIDS: Median time from acquiring HIV to the diagnosis of AIDS now exceeds 10 years (PHAC, 2008a).	Acute HIV: Fever, arthralgia or myalgia, rash, lymphadenopathy, sore throat, fatigue, headache, oral ulcers or genital ulcers, >5 kg weight loss, nausea, vomiting, and diarrhea Chronic HIV: Oral hairy leukoplakia, unexplained fever (>2 weeks), fatigue or lethargy, unexplained weight loss (>10% body weight), chronic diarrhea (>3 weeks), unexplained lymphadenopathy (usually generalized), cervical dysplasia, dyspnea and dry cough, loss of vision, recurrent or chronic candidiasis (oral, esophageal, vaginal), dysphagia (esophageal candidiasis), red–purple nodular skin or mucosal lesions (Kaposi sarcoma), encephalopathy, herpes zoster (especially if severe, multidermatomal, or disseminated), increased frequency or severity of mucocutaneous herpes simplex infection (PHAC, 2008a)	Screen and counsel high-risk populations; counsel pregnant mothers about the possibility of transmission to their child during pregnancy, at birth, or while breastfeeding; and offer HIV testing. Educate regarding safer sex, not sharing needles, using universal precautions, and informing past sexual partners.

Human papillomavirus (HPV)	Approximately 29% of young women are affected by HPV. Regular screening is effective in reducing rates of cervical cancer. It is one of the most common STIs (PHAC, 2008a).	Spread through sex, close skin-to-skin contact, or genital area contact with someone who is infected	2–3 months	Warts can appear in clusters like cauliflower. They can be raised or flat and size can vary. Women may present with warts on the vagina, anus, cervix, and vulva. Men can have them on the scrotum or penis. Warts can appear on the lips or mouth after oral sex. Warts may be itchy with discharge or bleeding.	Counsel clients regarding transmission through sexual contact and risk factors for disease. Educate about safer-sex practices and the need for regular Papanicolaou tests. Know the provincial/territorial schedule for administration of Gardasil and counsel clients accordingly.
Syphilis	Of the three nationally reported STIs, syphilis is the least common. However, rates continue to be on the rise, particularly in males. Rates from 1994 to 2000 were 0.4–0.6 per 100,000 people, whereas rates for 2002 were 1.5 per 100,000 (PHAC, 2008a).	Spread during oral, vaginal, or anal sex. Pregnant women with syphilis can transmit syphilis to their unborn child, sometimes causing birth defects and death.	1–13 weeks, but typically between 3 and 4 weeks	Primary stage: Painless sore appears on the penis, vulva, or vagina typically; nontender regional lymphadenopathy Secondary stage: Nonpruritic skin rash 6–12 weeks postinfection, commonly on palms or soles; fever, anorexia, general malaise, enlarged lymph nodes, mouth sores, inflammation of eyes; condylomata lata (raised areas) develop where mucous areas meet skin Latent stage: No symptoms but infection still present Tertiary stage: Cardiovascular syphilis—usually 10 to 25 years after infection—aneurysm, aortic valve leak Neurosyphilis: Benign tertiary syphilis—lumps appear on skin, organs, especially face, scalp, upper trunk and leg, or bones and leave scars	Counsel clients that all partners need to be notified according to the time frames outlined by the STI guidelines (PHAC, 2008a) and that there is a VDRL blood test available.
Trichomonas	Approximately one-quarter of women infected are asymptomatic. Annual prevalence in Canada is not known. Risk of HIV contraction increases with trichomonas (PHAC, 2008a).	Spread by sexual contact	4–28 days	Females: • Frothy, off-white or yellowish green vaginal discharge • Itching and irritation of the genital area • Vaginal odour • Pain during sex • Painful or frequent urination Males: Often asymptomatic Possible symptoms are as follows • Slight discharge from the penis • Burning sensation on urination • Irritation and redness of the head of the penis	Counsel regarding need for treatment of partner(s) (PHAC, 2008a). Educate about safe sex and the chance of increased early delivery or increased low birth weight.

(Continued)

TABLE 17-4 Common Sexually Transmitted Infections*—Cont'd

Pediculosis pubis (pubic lice) and scabies	Incidence of pubic lice and scabies has increased to pandemic numbers due to increased poverty, global travel, and increased sexual freedom (PHAC, 2008a).	Pubic lice: Spread by person-to-person contact, including sexual contact Scabies: Contact with mite-infected sheets, towels, or clothing	Pubic lice: Within a few days to 5 weeks Scabies: 2–6 weeks	Pubic lice: • Severe pruritus in the pubic area and later in all hairy areas. • Light brown insects the size of a pinhead may be seen. • Oval, whitish eggs may be seen on the hair. Scabies: • Severe pruritus in the pubic area • A rash with burrows between fingers; on wrists, abdomen, ankles, bend of elbows; or around genitals	Educate client to: • Avoid close body contact with others • Avoid scratching because it can lead to secondary infections • Obtain treatment to avoid transfer of infection • Wash clothes and bed linens in hot water or dry clean and press with a very hot iron • Freeze clothes, fabrics, or blankets or store them in an air-tight plastic bag for 2 weeks to destroy the insects and their eggs • Inform sex partner(s) and anyone who has shared bed sheets, clothing, or towels, even if they don't have an itch or rash, so that they can seek treatment. Topical medications are recommended. Clients may refer to pubic lice as "crabs."

AIDS = acquired immunodeficiency syndrome; HIV = human immunodeficiency virus; PHAC = Public Health Agency of Canada; STI = sexually transmitted infection; VDRL = Venereal Disease Research Laboratories.

SOURCE: Public Health Agency of Canada. (2008). *Canadian guidelines on sexually transmitted infections*. Retrieved from http://www.phac-aspc.gc.ca/std-mts/sti-its/pdf/sti-its-eng.pdf.

CRITICAL VIEW

The challenge of human papillomavirus (HPV) prevention is that condoms do not necessarily prevent infection. Warts may grow where barriers, such as condoms, do not cover, and skin-to-skin contact may occur. It is recommended that the Gardasil vaccine for HPV be administered to females before they become sexually active. In 2007, the National Advisory Committee on Immunization recommended administration of this vaccine to females between the ages of 9 and 26 years (PHAC, 2009b).

1. At what age do you think sexual health education should be initiated with a female child in order to administer the vaccine prior to the female becoming sexually active?
2. In your province or territory, what is the recommended immunization schedule for this vaccine?

Refer to the following Web site to compare your answers to the questions:

http://www.phac-aspc.gc.ca/std-mts/hpv-vph/fact-faits-vacc-eng.php

Human Immunodeficiency Virus (HIV) Infection

HIV infection and **acquired immunodeficiency syndrome (AIDS)** continue to have a significant political and social effect on society. AIDS is a syndrome that can affect the immune and central nervous systems and cause infections or cancers. It is caused by human immunodeficiency virus (HIV). The economic costs of HIV and AIDS result from premature disability and treatment, and many families become disrupted and lose creative and economic productivity.

It is estimated that approximately 58,000 Canadians were living with HIV/AIDS in 2006 (International Development Research Centre, 2009). Although globally AIDS has been an epidemic, HIV/AIDS infections have decreased due to prevention programs (WHO, 2009b). For information on HIV/AIDS globally and in Canada, refer to Boxes 17-4 and 17-5.

Many of the AIDS-related opportunistic infections are caused by microorganisms that are commonly present in healthy individuals but do not cause disease in persons with an intact immune system. These microorganisms proliferate in those with HIV and AIDS because of a weakened immune system. Opportunistic infections may be caused by bacteria, fungi, viruses, or protozoa. The

BOX 17-4 Some Global HIV/AIDS Information

- Many countries are making progress in addressing HIV/AIDS epidemics.
- The global epidemic, although stabilizing, is still at too high a level.
- Although the rate of new HIV infections is falling in many countries, globally there are increases in new infections in other countries.
- In 14 of 17 African countries with adequate survey data, the percentage of young pregnant women (ages 15–24) who are living with HIV has declined since 2000–2001.
- In 2007, approximately 370,000 children under 15 years of age were infected with HIV.
- Many young people between 15 and 24 years of age especially males, lack comprehensive information about avoiding exposure to the HIV virus.
- People who inject illegal drugs, homosexual men, and sex workers are disproportionately affected with HIV for all areas except Sub-Saharan Africa.
- Some recommended actions are to concentrate on societal factors contributing to HIV risk and vulnerability; deal with stigma and discrimination related to HIV; decrease gender disparities; and reverse the epidemic of HIV so that new infections can be prevented.
- In low- and middle-income countries, sex before age 15 is on the decline in all regions.
- By 2007, in low- and middle-income countries, the number of people who received antiretroviral medications had greatly increased.
- Children are less likely than adults to receive antiretroviral medicines.
- Women and children are most negatively affected by this HIV/AIDS epidemic.
- This epidemic is affecting the economic base of high-prevalence countries.
- In 2007, for the first time, the number of people globally living with HIV had decreased.

SOURCE: Adapted from UNAIDS. (2008). *2008 report on the global AIDS epidemic: Executive summary.* Retrieved from http://data.unaids.org/pub/GlobalReport/2008/JC1511_GR08_ExecutiveSummary_en.pdf.

BOX 17-5 Canadian HIV/AIDS Information

- The proportion of prevalent cases of HIV is increasingly occurring in women, a situation now referred to as the feminization of HIV.
- In the Public Health Agency of Canada's 2008 surveillance report, 17% of those diagnosed with HIV were women, which is a 21% increase from 2002.
- In 2007, for the first time, the number of newly diagnosed HIV cases decreased.
- Aboriginal peoples make up 7.5% of HIV cases in Canada.
- Exposure by women who inject illegal drugs is decreasing, while exposure of women to HIV has increased through heterosexual contact.
- HIV is on the rise in young women in Canada in the 10–29 age group, with more of these women being Aboriginal.
- Newly diagnosed clients who follow the treatment regime are likely to have a lifespan similar to the general population.
- HIV-positive women are at greater risk for human papilloma virus (HPV) infection, cervical cancer, and mental illness, especially depression and anxiety.

SOURCE: Nicholson, P. (2009). *Women and the changing face of HIV in Canada.* Women's Health Matters Network. Retrieved from http://www.womenshealthmatters.ca/resources/show_res.cfm?ID=43940.

most common opportunistic diseases are *Pneumocystis carinii* pneumonia and oral candidiasis. TB, an infection that is becoming more prevalent because of HIV infection, can spread rapidly among immunosuppressed individuals. Thus, HIV-infected individuals who live near one another, such as in long-term care facilities, prisons, drug treatment facilities, or other settings, must be carefully screened and deemed noninfectious before admission to such settings.

HIV is not transmitted through casual contact such as touching or hugging someone who has HIV infection. It is not transmitted by insects, coughing, sneezing, office equipment, or sitting next to or eating with someone who has HIV infection. Worldwide, the largest number of HIV infections result from heterosexual transmission. CHNs can educate about the modes of transmission and be role models for how to behave toward and provide supportive care for those with HIV infection. An understanding of how transmission does and does not occur helps family and community members feel more comfortable in relating to and caring for persons with HIV. Box 17-6 lists the modes of transmission for HIV.

BOX 17-6 Modes of Transmission of Human Immunodeficiency Virus (HIV)

HIV can be transmitted in the following ways:

- Sexual contact, involving the exchange of body fluids, with an infected person
- Sharing or reusing needles, syringes, or other equipment used to prepare injectable drugs
- Perinatal transmission from an infected mother to her fetus during pregnancy or delivery or to an infant when breastfeeding
- Transfusions or other exposure to HIV-contaminated blood or blood products, organs, or semen

The epidemiology, screening, diagnosis and management, treatment, and follow-up of HIV and additional information are well outlined by the PHAC (2008a) in the *Canadian Guidelines on Sexually Transmitted Infections,* 2008 edition, in the chapter titled "Human Immunodeficiency Virus (HIV) Infections," which is available online at the link provided in the Tool Box on the Evolve Web site. CHNs are mostly involved with screening and counselling, follow-up, and providing education and support when necessary; therefore, familiarity with the current HIV guidelines is crucial.

Because AIDS is a chronic disease, affected individuals continue to live and work in the community. They have bouts of illness interspersed with periods of wellness when they are able to return to school or work. When they are ill, much of their care is provided in the home. The CHN teaches families and significant others about personal care and hygiene, medication administration, routine practices and additional precautions to ensure infection control, and healthy lifestyle behaviours such as adequate rest, balanced nutrition, and exercise. (Refer to the PHAC's *Routine Practices and Additional Precautions for Preventing the Transmission of Infection in Health Care* Web site, listed in the Weblinks on the Evolve Web site.) HIV-infected children should attend school because the benefit of attendance far outweighs the risk of transmitting or acquiring infections.

A growing number of services are available for persons with HIV and AIDS. Voluntary and faith-based groups, such as community-based organizations or AIDS support organizations, have developed in some localities to address the many needs. Services include counselling, support groups, legal aid, personal care services, housing programs, and community education programs. CHNs collaborate with workers from community-based organizations in the client's home and may serve to advise these groups in their supportive work.

INFECTIOUS DISEASES

Infectious diseases can be spread by direct and indirect modes of transmission from host to host. The agent can be a virus, bacterium, parasite, or fungus. If untreated, these diseases are often fatal and the best approach is prevention. Examples to be discussed here are hepatitis, water-borne and food-borne diseases, vector-borne diseases, diseases of travellers, zoonoses, and parasitic diseases.

Hepatitis

Viral hepatitis refers to a group of infections that primarily affect the liver. These infections have similar clinical presentations but different causes and characteristics. Brief profiles of the types of hepatitis are presented in Appendix 13 (Viral Hepatitis Profiles). There are six types of viral hepatitis: hepatitis A, hepatitis B, hepatitis C, hepatitis D, hepatitis E, and hepatitis G (PHAC, 2004). The three most commonly occurring are hepatitis A virus, hepatitis B virus, and hepatitis C virus. (For specific information on the vaccines available in Canada for hepatitis infections, refer to the PHAC *Canadian Immunization Guide* [2006], listed in the Weblinks on the Evolve Web site.)

Hepatitis

Hepatitis A virus (HAV) is a virus most often transmitted through the fecal–oral route. Sources may be water, food, or sexual contact. The virus level in the feces appears to peak 1 to 2 weeks before symptoms appear, making individuals highly contagious before they realize they are ill. The clinical course of hepatitis A ranges from mild to severe and often requires prolonged

Evidence-Informed Practice

Liver cancer is a significant health problem in Asia, and it also occurs more frequently in the Chinese population living in North America. Little is known about disease prevention and control in the Chinese population in Canada. The purpose of this research was to determine the numbers of Chinese adult immigrants in Vancouver, B.C., who have had HBV testing and who have been vaccinated and to explore their knowledge about HBV. Data collection included a survey using a mailed questionnaire to Chinese households in Vancouver and a random selection of participants for interviews. A total of 504 participants were interviewed (217 men and 287 women). Of these participants, 366 were interviewed in Cantonese, 102 in Mandarin, and 36 in English. Fifty-seven percent of participants had previously had HBV testing; 38% had been vaccinated; and 6% were HBV carriers. There were fewer men than women who had been tested and vaccinated. The participants' educational levels were associated with HBV testing in women (the higher the education, the more likely the woman was tested). Shorter length of time in North America for both genders was also associated with HBV testing. Over 80% of participants knew that HBV could be spread by persons who are asymptomatic and that HBV can cause cirrhosis and liver cancer. However, there was some confusion over the route over HBV transmission—for example, fewer participants knew that hepatitis B is not transmitted via food (especially males in the sample) and is transmitted during sexual intercourse; approximately 50% did not know that HBV infection is lifelong.

Implications for CHNs: The findings of this study strongly suggest that targeted educational campaigns are needed for the Chinese immigrant population about the importance of testing and vaccination for hepatitis B. It is important for CHNs to involve members of the community in all educational campaigns. CHNs need to plan and implement educational campaigns that consider literacy levels, use of interpreters for language translation, and cultural interpretation.

Questions for Reflection & Discussion

1. What type of vaccination campaign would you introduce to encourage the Chinese immigrant population to receive the hepatitis B vaccination?
2. Why are vaccinations important for populations?
3. What recent evidence on vaccination in the Asian population of immigrants in Canada are you able to locate? Use the following key words: hepatitis B, Asian population, vaccination, health knowledge, practices, immigration.

REFERENCE: Hislop, T. G., Teh, C., Low, A., Li, L., Tu, S. P., Yasui, Y., & Taylor, V. M. (2007). Hepatitis B knowledge, testing and vaccination levels in Chinese immigrants to British Columbia, Canada. *Canadian Journal of Public Health, 98*(2), 125–129.

convalescence. Onset is usually acute with fever, nausea, lack of appetite, malaise, and abdominal discomfort, followed after several days by jaundice.

Although there has been a vaccine for this disease since 1995, hepatitis A infection remains one of the most frequently reported vaccine-preventable diseases. Persons most at risk for HAV infection are travellers to countries with high rates, children living in areas with high rates of HAV infection, injection drug users, men who have sex with men, and persons with clotting disorders or chronic liver disease.

Hepatitis A is found worldwide. In developing countries where sanitation is inadequate, epidemics are not common because most adults are immune from childhood infection. In countries with improved sanitation, outbreaks are common in daycare centres whose staff must change diapers, among household and sexual contacts of infected individuals, and among travellers to countries where hepatitis A is endemic. Box 17-7 lists recommendations for the administration of immune globulin for HAV.

Good sanitation and personal hygiene are the best means of preventing infection. People who travel often or for long periods in countries where the disease is endemic should receive the HAV vaccine. Hepatitis A is associated with the highest mortality and morbidity rates of any vaccine-preventable infection in travellers. Yet, many travellers do not get immunized, resulting in it being the most frequently occurring vaccine-preventable disease. Hepatitis B is also a disease associated with international travel. In Canada, Twinrix® is a vaccine that protects against hepatitis A and B.

BOX 17-7 Recommendations for Recipients of Administration of Immune Globulin for Hepatitis A Virus

- All household and sexual contacts of persons with hepatitis A virus (HAV)
- All staff of daycare centres if a case of HAV occurs among children or staff
- Household members whose diapered children attend a daycare centre where three or more families are infected
- Staff and residents of prisons or institutions for developmentally disabled persons, if they have close contact with persons with HAV
- Hospital employees if exposed to feces of infected clients
- Food-handlers who have a co-worker infected with HAV; restaurant patrons only in limited situations

Hepatitis B virus (HBV) is a virus transmitted through exposure to infected body fluids. Infection results in a clinical picture that ranges from a self-limited acute infection to fulminant hepatitis or hepatic carcinoma, possibly leading to death. The number of new cases of HBV in North America has been decreasing as a result of the use of HBV vaccine. The groups with the highest prevalence are users of injection drugs, persons with STIs or multiple sex partners, immigrants and refugees and their descendants who came from areas where there is a high endemic rate of HBV, health care workers, hemodialysis clients, inmates of long-term correctional institutions, and young adults (especially homeless adolescents) (PHAC, 2008b).

HBV infection can be prevented by immunization, prevention of nosocomial occupational exposure, and prevention of exposure via sex or injection drug use. Vaccination is recommended for persons with occupational risk, such as health care workers, and for children. Hepatitis B immune globulin is given after exposure to provide passive immunity and thus prevent infection.

Hepatitis C virus (HCV) is a virus transmitted through exposure to infected blood and body fluids. HCV infection was first identified in the late 1980s. This infection has been called "the silent stalker" since up to 70% of newly infected people experience no symptoms and it may take up to 30 years for symptoms to appear (Harkness, 2003; Health Canada, 2005). Primary prevention of HCV infection includes screening of blood products and donor organs and tissue; risk reduction counselling and services, including obtaining the sexual and injection drug-use history; and infection control practices. Secondary prevention strategies include testing of high-risk individuals, including those who seek HIV testing and counselling, and appropriate medical follow-up of infected clients. HCV testing should be offered to persons who received blood or an organ transplant before 1992, health care workers after exposure to blood or body fluids, children born to HCV-positive women, and persons who have ever injected drugs or been on dialysis. For further information on hepatitis C, refer to the Canadian AIDS Treatment Information Exchange (CATIE) Hepatitis C Toolkit listed in the Tool Box on the Evolve Web site. This tool kit is organized to search by topic or by format, and within the format search an additional tool kit titled *Chee Mamuk*, consisting of 22 fact sheets with information on hepatitis C prevention and treatment specific to Aboriginals.

Water- and Food-Borne Diseases

Water-borne pathogens usually enter water supplies through animal or human fecal contamination and frequently cause enteric disease. They include viruses, bacteria, and protozoans. HAV is probably the most publicized water-borne viral agent, although other viruses may also be transmitted by this route (enteroviruses, rotaviruses, and paramyxoviruses). The most important water-borne bacterial diseases are cholera, typhoid fever, and bacillary dysentery. However, other *Salmonella* types, *Shigella, Vibrio,* and various coliform bacteria, including *E. coli* O157:H7, may be transmitted in the same manner. In the past, the most important water-borne protozoans have been *Entamoeba histolytica* (amebic dysentery) and *Giardia lamblia,* but outbreaks of cryptosporidiosis in municipal water in the town of North Battleford, Saskatchewan, in April 2001, and *E. coli* in the town of Walkerton, Ontario, in May 2001, led government and nongovernmental groups to explore how best to safeguard municipal water supplies. Protozoans do not respond to traditional chlorine treatment as do enteric and coliform bacteria, and their small size requires special filtration.

Food-borne illness, or "food poisoning," is often categorized as food infection or food intoxication. Food infection results from bacterial, viral, or parasitic infection of food and includes salmonellosis, hepatitis A, and trichinosis. Food intoxication results from toxins produced by bacterial growth, chemical contaminants (heavy metals), and a variety of disease-producing substances found naturally in certain foods such as mushrooms and some seafood. Examples of food intoxications are botulism, mercury poisoning, and paralytic shellfish poisoning. Table 17-5 outlines some of the most common agents of food intoxication, their incubation period, associated food source, duration, and clinical presentation. Although it is not a hard-and-fast rule, food infections are associated with incubation periods of 12 hours to several days after ingestion of the infected food, whereas food intoxications become obvious within minutes to hours after ingestion. Botulism is a clear exception to this rule, with an incubation period of a week or more in adults. The term *ptomaine poisoning,* often used when discussing food-borne illness, does not refer to a specific causal organism.

Protecting the nation's food supply from contamination by all virulent microbes is a complex issue that would be incredibly costly and time consuming to address. However, much food-borne illness, regardless of causal organism, can be prevented easily through simple changes in food preparation, handling, and storage to destroy or denature contaminants and prevent their further spread. The WHO's *Ten Golden Rules for Safe Food Preparation* are presented in Box 17-8.

Salmonellosis is a bacterial disease. Although morbidity can be significant, death is uncommon except among pregnant women, infants, older adults, and persons who are immunocompromised (Canadian Food Inspection Agency, 2009d). The rate of infection is highest among infants and small children. The number of *Salmonella* infections reported annually is between 6,000 and 12,000 cases, and it is estimated that only a small number of cases are recognized clinically as they present as a stomach flu (Health Canada, 2006c).

Outbreaks occur commonly in restaurants, hospitals, nursing homes, and places where children are together. The transmission route is eating food derived from an infected animal or contaminated by the feces of an infected animal or person. Meat, poultry, and eggs are the foods most often associated with salmonellosis outbreaks. Animals are the common reservoir for the various *Salmonella* serotypes, although infected humans may also fill this role. Animals are more likely to be chronic carriers. Reptiles such as iguanas have been implicated as *Salmonella* carriers, along with pet turtles, poultry, cattle, swine, rodents, dogs, and cats. Person-to-person transmission is an important consideration in daycare and institutional settings.

E. coli O157:H7 belongs to the enterohemorrhagic category of *E. coli* serotypes that produce a strong cytotoxin that can cause a potentially fatal hemorrhagic colitis. This pathogen was first described in the 1990s in humans following the investigation of two outbreaks of illness that were associated with the consumption of hamburger from a fast-food restaurant chain. Undercooked hamburger has been implicated in several outbreaks, as have roast beef, alfalfa sprouts, unpasteurized milk and apple cider, municipal water, and person-to-person transmission in daycare centres. Infection with *E. coli* O157:H7 causes bloody diarrhea, abdominal cramps, and, infrequently, fever. Pregnant women, children, immunocompromised persons, and older adults are at the highest risk for clinical disease and complications (Canadian Food Inspection Agency, 2009b). Hemolytic uremic syndrome (HUS), a blood disorder, is seen in 15% of cases and may be fatal (Canadian Food Inspection Agency, 2009b). Hamburger often appears to be involved in outbreaks because the grinding process exposes pathogens on the surface of the whole meat to the interior of the ground meat, effectively mixing the exterior bacteria throughout the hamburger so that searing the surface no longer suffices to kill all bacteria. Tracking the contamination is complicated by the fact that hamburger is often made of meat ground from several sources. The best protection against this pathogen, as with most food-borne agents, is to thoroughly cook food before eating it.

Vector-Borne Diseases

Vector-borne diseases refer to illnesses for which the infectious agent is transmitted by a carrier, or vector, usually an arthropod (mosquito, tick, fly), either biologically or mechanically. With *biological transmission,* the vector is necessary for the developmental stage of the infectious agent. An example is the mosquitoes that

TABLE 17-5 Commonly Encountered Food Intoxications

Causal Agent	Incubation Period	Duration	Clinical Presentation	Associated Food/Source
Staphylococcus aureus	30 minutes–7 hours	1–2 days	Sudden onset of nausea, cramps, vomiting, and prostration, often accompanied by diarrhea; rarely fatal	All foods, especially those likely to come into contact with food-handlers' hands that may be contaminated from infections of the eyes and skin
Clostridium perfringens (strain A)	6–24 hours	1 day or less	Sudden onset of colic and diarrhea, sometimes nausea; vomiting and fever unusual; rarely fatal	Inadequate handling (preparation, storage, and reheating) of high-protein foods such as meats or high-starch foods such as cooked beans and gravies; food contaminated by soil, dust, sewage, and intestinal tracts of animals and humans; multiplication of organisms if exposed to low or no oxygen
Paralytic shellfish poisoning (PSP)	A few minutes–10 hours	2–3 days	Tingling sensation or numbness around lips that spreads to the face and neck; prickly sensation in the fingertips and toes, headache, dizziness. More severe cases have incoherent speech, prickly sensation in the arms and legs, loss of coordination of the limbs, weakness, rapid pulse, respiratory difficulties, temporary blindness, and nausea and vomiting. Extreme cases have respiratory muscle paralysis leading to respiratory arrest and death.	Seafood such as clams, oysters, and mussels, and the tomalley of lobster and crab
Listeria monocytogenes	24 hours–70 days	24–48 hours	Nausea, vomiting, cramps, diarrhea, severe headache, constipation, persistent fever, and in some cases meningitis, encephalitis, and septicemia may develop and can lead to death	Hot dogs; deli meats; soft and semi-soft cheeses if made from unpasteurized milk; paté and meat spreads; smoked seafood and fish; raw and undercooked meat, poultry, and fish
Clostridium botulinum	12–36 hours	Usually 2 hours–14 days and may be longer	Nausea, vomiting, fatigue; dryness in throat and nose to respiratory failure; central nervous system symptoms such as dizziness, double vision, headache, paralysis, and sometimes death	Improperly prepared home-canned low-acid fruits, vegetables, and juices plus salmon; infants under 1 year of age who have been given honey; Inuit population when consuming improperly prepared raw or parboiled meats from marine animals
Salmonella	12–72 hours	2–7 days	Nausea, vomiting, diarrhea, abdominal cramps, fever. It may be fatal in high-risk groups.	Eggs, poultry, unpasteurized milk, raw fruits and vegetables, sprouts, nuts, fish, shrimp, sauces and salad dressings, peanut butter, cocoa, chocolate
Escherichia coli (*E. coli*)	A few hours–10 days	7–10 days	Severe abdominal cramping, bloody diarrhea; if hemolytic uremic syndrome (HUS) may have seizures, strokes, may need blood transfusions and kidney dialysis	Ground beef, raw fruits and vegetables, including sprouts, unpasteurized dairy products or apple juice/cider; untreated water
Shigellosis	Immediately and up to 1 month later	12–50 hours after eating contaminated food	Flu-like symptoms such as nausea, vomiting, fever, diarrhea, stomach cramps	Consuming food or water contaminated by *Shigella*, such as salads, chopped turkey, raw oysters, deli meats, unpasteurized milk. Can be transferred by flies

SOURCES: Health Canada. (2003). *Assessment of the Canadian Food Inspection Agency's activities related to domestic ready-to-eat meat products.* Retrieved from http://www.hc-sc.gc.ca/fn-an/securit/eval/reports-rapports/report_cfia-rapport_acia-34-eng.php; Canadian Food Inspection Agency. (2009). *Salmonella food safety facts: Preventing food borne illness.* Retrieved from http://www.inspection.gc.ca/english/fssa/concen/cause/salmonellae.shtml; Canadian Food Inspection Agency. (2009). *E.coli 0157:H7 food safety facts: Preventing food borne illnesses.* Retrieved from http://www.inspection.gc.ca/english/fssa/concen/cause/ecolie.shtml; Canadian Food Inspection Agency. (2009). *Shigella food safety facts: Preventing food borne illnesses.* Retrieved from http://www.inspection.gc.ca/english/fssa/concen/cause/shige.shtml; Canadian Food Inspection Agency. (2009). *Food safety facts on paralytic shellfish poisoning (PSP).* Retrieved from http://www.inspection.gc.ca/english/fssa/concen/cause/pspe.shtml; Canadian Food Inspection Agency. (2008). *Food safety facts on Listeria.* Retrieved from http://www.inspection.gc.ca/english/fssa/concen/cause/listeriae.shtml.

BOX 17-8 Ten Golden Rules for Safe Food Preparation

1. Choose food processed for safety (avoid unpasteurized foods).
2. Cook food thoroughly (poultry, meat, and eggs are contaminated when raw and need to be cooked thoroughly).
3. Eat cooked food immediately (microbes start growing immediately as cooked foods cool).
4. Store cooked food carefully (to keep food over a period of time, either keep it hot—above 60°C—or cold—below 4°C).
5. Reheat cooked foods thoroughly to ensure a temperature of at least 70°C is evenly distributed in the food).
6. Avoid contact between raw foods and cooked foods (wash and/or use separate food-handling and storage equipment for raw and cooked foods).
7. Wash hands repeatedly (use soap and running water to wash hands prior to food preparation and after every interruption).
8. Keep all kitchen surfaces meticulously clean (use soap and water and clean wiping cloths for food preparation areas).
9. Protect foods from insects, rodents, and other animals (keep foods in storage containers at all times).
10. Use pure water (boil water if of questionable quality for adding to foods or making ice for drinks).

SOURCE: Adapted from World Health Organization. (n.d.). *The WHO golden rules for safe food preparation.* Retrieved from https://apps.who.int/fsf/goldenrules.htm

carry malaria. *Mechanical transmission* occurs when an insect simply contacts the infectious agent with its legs or mouth parts and carries it to the host. For example, flies and cockroaches may contaminate food or cooking utensils.

Vector-borne diseases encountered in some parts of Canada are those associated with ticks, such as Lyme disease *(Borrelia burgdorferi)* and Rocky Mountain spotted fever *(Rickettsia rickettsii)* (less common). CHNs who work with large immigrant populations or with international travellers may encounter malaria and dengue fever (traveller's disease), both carried by mosquitoes. For information on dengue fever, refer to the Public Health Agency of Canada Web site *Dengue Fever* (see the Evolve Weblinks). Most recently in the news, WNV is an example of endemic mosquito-borne viruses. There is a wealth of Web site resources through the PHAC on vector-borne diseases. CHNs need to be current in their knowledge of the incidence, prevalence, and patterns of these diseases and new ones occurring in Canada.

Measures for preventing exposure to ticks include reducing tick populations, avoiding tick-infested areas, wearing protective clothing when outdoors (long sleeves and long pants tucked into socks), using repellents, and immediately inspecting for and removing ticks when returning indoors. Researchers are looking at the effectiveness of using tick-killing acaricides in rodent bait boxes and at deer-feeding stations in areas where Lyme disease is highly concentrated. Ticks require a prolonged period of attachment (6 to 48 hours) before they start blood-feeding on the host; prompt tick discovery and removal can help prevent transmission of the disease. Ticks should be removed with steady, gentle traction on tweezers applied to the head parts of the tick. The tick's body should not be squeezed during the removal process to avoid infection that could be transmitted from resultant tick feces and tissue juices (PHAC, 2008d). When outdoors, permethrine sprayed on clothing and tick repellents containing diethyltoluamide (DEET) can offer effective protection; use of DEET should be avoided on children younger than 2 years because of reports of significant toxicity, including skin irritation, anaphylaxis, and seizures. For further information on Lyme disease, refer to the PHAC Web site *Lyme Disease,* listed in the Evolve Weblinks.

Diseases of Travellers

Individuals travelling outside Canada need to be aware of and take precautions against diseases to which they may be exposed. The diseases and the precautions depend on the individual's health status, the travel destination, the reason for travel, and the length of travel. Persons who plan to travel in remote regions for an extended period may need to consider rare diseases and take special precautions that would not apply to the average traveller. Consultation with public health officials can provide specific health information and recommendations for a given situation.

On return from travel abroad, travellers may bring back with them an unplanned souvenir in the form of disease. Therefore, a history of travel should always be closely considered. Even the apparently healthy returned traveller, especially one who was in a tropical country for some time, should undergo routine screening to rule out acquired infections. Likewise, refugees and immigrants may arrive with infectious disease problems ranging from helminthic infections to diseases of major public health significance such as TB, malaria, cholera, and hepatitis. CHNs need to be familiar with these diseases and other infectious diseases. The PHAC Web site *A–Z*

Infectious Diseases, found in the Evolve Weblinks, provides CHNs with information on infectious diseases.

Malaria

Worldwide, malaria is the most prevalent vector-borne disease, occurring in more than 100 countries. In Canada, the incidence of malaria is largely due to newcomers from countries where malaria is endemic and from a small percentage of Canadian travellers to these malaria-endemic areas. Immigrants and visitors from areas where malaria is endemic may become clinically ill after entering this country. CHNs need to be aware of this possibility.

Malaria prevention depends on protection against mosquitoes and appropriate chemoprophylaxis. Drug resistance is an increasing problem in combating malaria. Of the four causes of human malaria, *Plasmodium ovale* and *Plasmodium vivax* result in disease that can progress to relapsing malaria, and *P. vivax* is increasingly drug resistant. *Plasmodium falciparum* causes the most serious malarial infection and is highly drug resistant. Thus, decisions about antimalarial drugs must be tailored individually on the basis of the type of malaria in the specific area of the country to be visited, the purpose of the trip, and the length of the visit. The PHAC and WHO publish guides on the status of malaria and recommendations for prophylaxis on a country-by-country basis. At this time, no one drug or drug combination is known to be safe and efficacious in preventing all types of malaria. Antimalarials are generally started a week to several weeks before leaving Canada and are continued for 4 to 6 weeks after returning. Despite appropriate prophylaxis, malaria may still be contracted. Travellers should be advised of this fact and urged to seek immediate medical care if they exhibit symptoms of cyclical fever and chills up to 1 year after returning home.

Diarrheal Diseases

Travellers often suffer from diarrhea, so much so that colourful names, such as *Montezuma's revenge, turista,* and *Colorado quickstep,* exist in our vocabulary to describe these bouts of intestinal upset. Some of these diarrheas do not have infectious causes and may result from stress, fatigue, schedule changes, and eating unfamiliar foods. Acute infectious diarrheas are usually of viral or bacterial origin. *E. coli* probably causes more cases of traveller's diarrhea than all other infective agents combined. Protozoan-induced diarrheas such as those resulting from *Entamoeba* and *Giardia* are less likely to be acute, and they more commonly present once the traveller returns home. Travellers need to pay special attention to what they eat and drink.

As in this country, much food-borne disease abroad can be avoided if the traveller eats thoroughly cooked foods prepared with reasonable hygiene; eating foods from street vendors is not recommended. Trichinosis, tapeworms, and fluke infections, as well as bacterial infections, result from eating raw or undercooked meats. Raw vegetables may be a source of bacterial, viral, helminthic, or protozoal infection if they have been grown with or washed in contaminated water. Fruits that can be peeled immediately before eating such as bananas are less likely to be a source of infection. Dairy products should be pasteurized and appropriately refrigerated.

Water in many areas of the world is not potable (safe to drink), and drinking this water can lead to infection with a variety of protozoal, viral, and bacterial agents, including amoebae, *Giardia, Cryptosporidium,* and various coliform bacteria, and can also lead to hepatitis and cholera. Unless travelling in an area where the piped water is known to be safe, only boiled water (boiled for 1 minute), bottled water, or water purified with iodine or chlorine compounds should be consumed. Ice should be avoided because freezing does not inactivate these agents. If the water is questionable, choose coffee or tea made with boiled water, carbonated beverages without ice, beer, wine, or canned fruit juices.

Zoonoses

A *zoonosis* is an infection transmitted from a vertebrate animal to a human under natural conditions. The agents that cause zoonoses do not need humans to maintain their life cycles; infected humans have simply somehow managed to get in their way. Means of transmission include animal bites, inhalation, ingestion, direct contact, and arthropod intermediates. This last transmission route means that some vector-borne diseases may also be zoonoses. Other than vector-borne diseases, some of the more common zoonoses in Canada include toxoplasmosis *(Toxoplasma gondii),* cat-scratch disease *(Bartonella henselae),* brucellosis (*Brucella* species), listeriosis *(Listeria monocytogenes),* salmonellosis (*Salmonella* serotypes), and rabies (family Rhabdoviridae, genus *Lyssavirus*).

Rabies

One of the most feared of human diseases, rabies (formerly *hydrophobia*) has the highest case fatality rate of any known human infection—essentially 100%. Rabies is a significant public health problem worldwide (WHO, 2009c). Rabies in humans in Canada has greatly decreased since the availability of a vaccination for pets. Other carriers of rabies are raccoons, skunks, foxes, coyotes, and bats. Small rodents, rabbits and hares, and opossums rarely carry rabies. Epidemiological information should be consulted for information on the potential carriers for a given geographical region. When the virus spreads from wild to domestic animals, cats are often involved. Since 1924, 23 people have died of rabies in Canada (PHAC, 2007i). For the years 2000–2005, there were a total of 2,238 cases of confirmed animal rabies reported in Canada, with skunks accounting for 40% of the total cases (PHAC, 2007i). The best protection against rabies remains vaccinating domestic animals—dogs, cats, cattle, and horses. If an individual is bitten, the bite wound should be thoroughly cleaned with soap and water and a physician consulted immediately. Suspicion of rabies should exist if the bite is from a wild animal or an unprovoked attack from a domestic animal. Even when there is no suspicion of rabies, a physician should be contacted because tetanus and antibiotic prophylaxis may be indicated.

PARASITIC DISEASES

Parasitic diseases are more prevalent in developing countries than in developed countries such as Canada because of the tropical climate and inadequate prevention and control measures. A lack of cheap and effective drugs, poor sanitation, and a scarcity of funding lead to high reinfection rates even when control programs are attempted. Parasites are classified into four groups: nematodes (roundworms), cestodes (tapeworms), trematodes (flukes), and protozoa (single-celled animals). Nematodes, cestodes, and trematodes are all referred to as *helminths.*

CHNs and other health professionals need to be aware of the growing numbers of reported parasitic infections in Canada. Factors that may be contributing to this rise in detection are (1) international travel, (2) immigration of persons from developing countries, and (3) increased number of refugees (PHAC, 2002). Some common parasites that cause infections that a CHN might encounter are *Enterobius* (pinworm), *Giardia lamblia, Trichuris trichiura* (whipworm), *Ascaris lumbricoides* (roundworm), and *Taenia solium* (pork tapeworm).

Responsibilities for evaluating the risks of parasitic diseases in Canada and for conducting surveillance studies are undertaken by Health Canada's Blood-Borne Pathogens Division of the Bureau of Infectious Diseases, Centre for Infectious Disease Prevention and Control, PHAC. The maintenance of safe blood products is undertaken through evaluating risk and advising on policy direction and changes.

Correct diagnosis by CHNs and other health care workers allows the provision of appropriate treatment and client education for preventing and controlling parasitic infections. Diagnosis of parasitic diseases is based on a history of travel, characteristic clinical signs and symptoms, and the use of appropriate laboratory tests to confirm the clinical diagnosis. Knowing what specimens to collect, how and when to collect them, and what laboratory techniques to use are all important in establishing a correct diagnosis. Effective drug treatment is available for most parasitic diseases. The high cost of the drugs, drug resistance, and toxicity are some of the common therapeutic problems. Measures for prevention and control of parasitic diseases include early diagnosis and treatment, improved personal hygiene, safer-sex practices, community health education, vector control, and improvements in the sanitary control of food, water, and wastes.

THE CHN'S ROLE IN PROVISION OF PREVENTIVE CARE

From prevention to treatment, CHNs function as counsellors, educators, advocates, case managers, and primary care providers. Appropriate interventions for primary, secondary, and tertiary preventions are reviewed. The community health nursing process is used to care for clients with communicable diseases. CHNs are in an ideal position to affect the outcomes of communicable diseases, and their influence begins with primary prevention.

Primary Prevention

The goal of primary prevention is to keep people healthy and avoid the onset of disease. This begins with assessing for risk behaviour and providing relevant interventions on how to avoid infection. Health promotion includes education on healthy behaviours. To assess the risk of acquiring an infection, the CHN takes a history that focuses on potential exposure, which varies with the specific organism being studied and its mode of transmission. The specific questions that need to be asked of clients who are at risk for acquiring STIs can be especially challenging to them. The CHN needs to obtain a sexual history and history of injection drug use for clients and their partners. The sexual history provides information that could lead to the need for specific diagnostic tests, treatment modalities, and partner notification. It also facilitates the evaluation of risk factors and is necessary for the CHN to be able to provide relevant education for the client's lifestyle.

Assessing a client's risk of acquiring an STI should be done with all sexually active individuals. Such risk assessments should be included as baseline assessment data for those attending all clinics and those who receive school health, occupational health, public health, and home nursing services. To be most effective, the CHN obtaining a client's sexual history needs to do the following:

- Remain supportive and open to facilitate honesty
- Use terms the client will understand (be prepared to suggest multiple terms)
- Speak candidly so the client will feel comfortable talking

A thorough sexual history requires obtaining personal and sensitive information. It includes such information as the types of relationships, the number of sexual partners and encounters, and the types of sexual behaviours that are practised. The confidential nature of the information and how it will be used should be shared with the client to establish open communication and goal-directed interaction. Most clients feel uneasy disclosing such personal information. The CHN can ease this discomfort by remaining supportive and open during the interview to facilitate honesty about intimate activities. The CHN serves as a model for discussing sensitive information in a candid manner. When discussing precautions, direct and simple language needs to be used to describe specific behaviours. This encourages the client to openly discuss sexuality during this interaction and with future partners.

CHNs who are uncomfortable discussing topics such as sexual behaviour or sexual orientation are likely to avoid assessing risk behaviours with the client and may therefore compromise data collection. CHNs can gain confidence in conducting sexual risk assessments by understanding their own values and feelings about sexuality and realizing that the purpose of the interaction is to improve the client's health. The CHN's comfort in discussing sexual behaviour can be improved by using role-playing to practise assessments of sexual and injection drug-use behaviours and by contracting with clients to make behaviour changes.

Identifying the number of partners for sex and partners for injection drug use and the number of contacts with these partners provides information about the client's risk. The chance of exposure decreases as the number of partners decreases, so people in mutually monogamous relationships are at low risk for acquiring STIs. This information can be obtained by asking, "How many sex (or drug) partners have you had over the past 6 months?" It is important to avoid basing assumptions about the sexual partner(s) on the client's sex, age, ethnicity, or any other factor. Stereotypes and assumptions about who people are and what they do are common problems that keep interviewers from asking the questions that lead to obtaining useful information. For example, it should not be taken for granted that if a man is homosexual he has more than one partner. Be aware also that the long incubation of HIV and the subclinical phase of many STIs lead some monogamous individuals to assume erroneously that they are not at risk.

It is important to identify whether the person has sexual contact with men, women, or both. This information can be obtained by asking, "Do you have sex with men, women, or both?" This lets the client know that the CHN is open to hearing about these behaviours; in this way, the CHN is more likely to obtain information that is relevant to sexual practices and risk. Women who are exclusively lesbian are at low risk for acquiring STIs, but bisexual women may transmit STIs between male and female partners. In addition, it is possible for men to have sexual contact with other men and not label themselves as homosexual. Therefore, education to reduce risk that is aimed at homosexual men will not be heeded by men who do not see themselves as homosexual. In such situations, the CHN can ask, "When was the last time you had sex with another man?"

Certain sexual practices are more likely to result in exposure to and transmission of STIs. Dangerous sexual activities include unprotected anal or vaginal intercourse, oral–anal contact, and insertion of a finger or fist into the rectum. These practices introduce a high risk of transmission of enteric organisms or result in physical trauma during sexual encounters. The CHN can obtain information about sexual encounters by asking, "Can you tell me the kinds of sexual practices in which you engage? This will help determine what risks you may have and the type of tests we should do." Clients who engage in genital–anal, oral–anal, or oral–genital contact will need throat and rectal cultures for some STIs, as well as cervical and urethral cultures.

Drug use is linked to STI transmission in several ways. Drugs such as alcohol put people at risk because these drugs can lower inhibitions and impair judgement about engaging in risky behaviours. Addictions to drugs may cause individuals to perform sexual favours in order to acquire the drug or money to purchase the drug. This increases both the frequency of sexual contacts and the chances of contracting STIs. Thus, the CHN needs to obtain information on the type and frequency of drug use and the presence of risk behaviours. The administration of vaccines to prevent infection, such as for hepatitis A and C, is an example of primary prevention.

Interventions to prevent infection are aimed at preventing specific infections. These interventions can take several forms and include, for example, education on how to prevent infection or the availability of vaccines. For example, on the basis of the information obtained in the sexual history and risk assessment just described, the CHN needs to identify specific education and counselling needs of the client. The community health nursing interventions focus on contracting with clients to change behaviour and reduce their risk in regard to sexual practice.

Sexual abstinence is the best way to prevent STIs. However, for many people, sexual abstinence is not realistic, and teaching about how to make sexual behaviour safer is critical. Safer sexual behaviour includes masturbation, dry kissing, touching, fantasy, and vaginal and oral sex with a condom. If used correctly and consistently, condoms can prevent both pregnancy and STIs because they prevent the exchange of body fluids during sexual activity. Condoms are not always used correctly; thus, information about proper use of condoms and how to communicate with a partner is also necessary. The CHN has many opportunities to convey this information during counselling. Condom use may be viewed as inconvenient, messy, or decreasing sensation. Moreover, alcohol consumption may accompany sexual activity, which also may decrease condom use (PHAC, 2008a). The CHN can enable clients to become more skilled in discussing safer sex through role-modelling and practising communication skills through role play.

Female condoms can also be a barrier to body fluid contact and therefore protect against pregnancy and STIs. The main advantage of the female condom is that its use is controlled by the woman. Because it is made of polyurethane, it is also useful if a latex sensitivity develops to regular male condoms. Symptoms of latex allergy include penile, vaginal, or rectal itching or swelling after use of a male condom or diaphragm. The female condom consists of a sheath over two rings, with one closed end that fits over the cervix.

Clients should understand that it is important to know the risk behaviours of their sexual partners, including a history of injection drug use and STIs, bisexuality, and any current symptoms. This is because each sexual partner is potentially exposed to all the STIs of all the persons with whom the other partner has been sexually active.

Injection drug use is risky because the potential for injecting blood-borne pathogens, such as HIV and HBV, exists when needles and syringes are shared. During intravenous drug use, small quantities of drugs are repeatedly injected. Blood is withdrawn into the syringe and is then injected back into the user's vein. Individuals need to be advised against using injectable drugs and sharing needles, syringes, or other drug paraphernalia. If equipment is shared, it should be in contact with full-strength bleach for 30 seconds and then rinsed with water several times to prevent injecting bleach. People who inject drugs are difficult to reach for health care services. Effective outreach programs include using community peers, increasing accessibility of drug treatment programs combined with HIV testing and counselling, and long-term repeat contacts after completion of the program.

Because of the illegal nature of injectable drugs and the poverty associated with HIV, many people at risk have neither the inclination nor the resources to seek health care. CHNs need to work to establish programs within communities because the opportunities for counselling on the prevention of HIV and other STIs are increased by bringing services into the neighbourhoods of those at risk. Workers go into communities to disseminate information on safer sex, drug treatment programs, and discontinuation of drug-use or safer drug-use practices (e.g., using new needles and syringes with each injection). Some programs provide sterile needles and syringes, condoms, and literature about anonymous test sites.

Using primary prevention, CHNs educate healthy groups about the prevention of communicable diseases. Information about modes of transmission, testing, availability of vaccines, and early symptoms can be provided to groups in the community and can help prevent the spread of STIs and HIV. Effective and convenient places to hold these educational sessions include schools, businesses, and churches. When talking with groups about HIV infection, the CHN needs to discuss the following:

- The number of people who are diagnosed with AIDS
- The number infected with HIV
- Modes of transmission of the virus
- How to prevent infection
- Common symptoms of illness
- The need for a compassionate response to those afflicted
- Available community resources
- Content about other STIs since the mode of transmission (sexual contact) is the same
- Information on these diseases, including the distribution, incidence, and consequences of the infection for individuals and society

Evaluation is based on whether risky behaviour has changed to safe behaviour and, ultimately, whether illness is prevented. Condom use is evaluated for consistency if the client is sexually active. Other behaviours, such as abstinence or monogamy, can be evaluated for their implementation. At the community level, behavioural surveys can be done to measure reported condom use and condom sales, and measures of disease incidence and prevalence can be calculated to evaluate the effectiveness of intervention.

Secondary Prevention

Secondary prevention includes screening for diseases to ensure their early identification and treatment, and follow-up with contacts to prevent further spread. In general, client teaching and counselling need to include education about preventing self-reinfection, managing symptoms, and preventing the infection of others. People who have engaged in high-risk behaviours should be tested for HIV.

The 2008 *Canadian Guidelines on Sexually Transmitted Infections* clearly identify at-risk persons who should be offered HIV testing (these guidelines are available at the link listed in the Tool Box on the Evolve Web site).

HIV pretest and post-test counselling are an important part of care when the **HIV antibody test** is indicated. The ELISA test (enzyme-linked immunosorbent assay) is a laboratory procedure that detects HIV antibodies and is the test commonly used to screen blood for the presence of the HIV antibody. Clients must know that the antibody test is not diagnostic for AIDS but is indicative of HIV infection. Therefore, a positive ELISA test is confirmed using the Western blot test (a confirmatory test). The STI guidelines thoroughly outline the precounselling and postcounselling needed for persons with negative and positive antibody test results (PHAC, 2008a).

Partner notification, also known as *contact tracing,* is an example of a population-level intervention aimed at controlling communicable diseases. Partner notification programs usually occur in conjunction with reportable disease requirements and are carried out by most health units and health authorities. Partner notification is done by confidentially identifying and notifying individuals who have been exposed to persons who have reportable diseases. This could result in, for example, family members and close contacts of individuals with TB being tested by a Mantoux skin test.

Individuals diagnosed with a reportable STI are asked to provide the names and locations of their partners so that they can be informed of their exposure and obtain the necessary treatment. Clients may be encouraged to notify their partners and to encourage them to seek treatment. If the client agrees to do so, suggestions on how to tell partners and how to deal with possible reactions need to be explored. In some instances, clients may feel more comfortable if the CHN notifies those who are exposed. When clients are the ones who contact their partners about possible infection, the CHN contacts health care providers or clinics to verify that the exposed partners have been examined.

If the client prefers not to participate in notifying partners, the CHN contacts them—often by a home visit—and counsels them to seek evaluation and treatment. The client is offered literature describing treatment, risk reduction, and the clinic's location and hours of operation. The identity of the infected client who provides the names of partners for sex or injection drug use cannot be revealed. Maintaining confidentiality is critical with all persons with STIs but particularly with those who are HIV positive because discrimination may still occur.

Tertiary Prevention

Tertiary prevention can apply to many of the chronic viral STIs and TB. For viral STIs, much of this effort focuses on managing symptoms and psychosocial support regarding future interpersonal relations. Many clients report feeling contaminated, and support groups may be available to help clients cope with chronic STIs.

One tertiary intervention is **directly observed therapy (DOT)** programs for TB medication monitoring. The CHN observes and documents individual clients taking their TB drugs. When clients prematurely stop taking TB medications, there is a risk of the TB becoming resistant to the medications. This can affect an entire community of people who are susceptible to this airborne disease. Health professionals share in the responsibility of adhering to treatment, and DOT ensures that TB-infected clients have adequate medication. Thus, DOT programs are aimed at the population level to prevent antibiotic resistance in the community and to ensure effective treatment at the individual level. Many health units and health authorities have DOT home health programs to ensure adequate treatment. In the 2007 edition of the PHAC's *Canadian Tuberculosis Standards* (see Evolve Weblinks), refer to Chapter 6 and the section titled "Directly Observed Therapy" (2007a, pp. 120–122), which discusses the role of the health care worker who is frequently a CHN in the DOT process.

The management of AIDS in the home may include monitoring physical and emotional health status and referring the family to additional care services for maintaining the client in the home. Case management is important in all phases of HIV infection. It is especially important at this stage to ensure that clients have adequate services to meet their needs. This may include ensuring that medication can be obtained by identifying funding resources, maintaining infection control standards, reducing risk behaviours, identifying sources of respite care for caretakers, or referring clients for home or hospice care. Community health nursing interventions include teaching families about managing symptomatic illness by preventing deteriorating conditions such as diarrhea, skin breakdown, and inadequate nutrition.

The importance of teaching caregivers about infection control in home care is vital. Concerns about the transmission of HIV may be expressed by clients, families, friends, and other groups. Whereas fear may be expressed by some, others who care for loved ones with HIV may not take adequate precautions such as wearing gloves because of the concern about appearing as though they do not want to touch a loved one. Others may believe myths that suggest they cannot be infected by someone they love. Routine practices and additional precautions need to be taught to caregivers in the home setting. All blood and articles soiled with body fluids need to be handled as if they were infectious or contaminated by bloodborne pathogens. Gloves should be worn whenever hands will be expected to touch nonintact skin, mucous membranes, blood, or other fluids. A mask, goggles, and gown should also be worn if there is potential for splashing or spraying of infectious material during any care. All protective equipment should be worn only once and then disposed of. If the skin or mucous membranes of the caregiver come in contact with body fluids, the skin should be washed with soap and water and the mucous membranes should be flushed with water as soon as possible after the exposure. Thorough handwashing with soap and water—a major infection control measure—should be conducted whenever hands become contaminated and whenever gloves or other protective equipment (mask, gown) is removed. Soiled clothing or linen should be washed in a washing machine filled with hot water using bleach as an additive and should be dried on the hot-air cycle of a dryer.

Because many children receive their immunizations from their family physician, nurse practioners, or through their public health units or health authorities, CHNs play a major role in the effort to increase immunization coverage of infants and toddlers. Public health nurses track children known to be at risk for underimmunization and call or send reminders to their parents. They help avoid missed immunization opportunities by checking the immunization status of every young child encountered, whether the clinic or home visit is related to immunization or not. In addition, they organize immunization outreach activities in the community that deliver immunization services; provide answers to parents' questions and concerns about immunization; and educate parents about why immunizations are needed, about inappropriate contraindications to immunization, and about the importance of completing the immunization schedule on time.

CHNs are frequently involved at different levels of the surveillance system for all communicable and infectious diseases. They play important roles in collecting data, making diagnoses, investigating and reporting cases, and providing information to the general public. Examples of possible activities include investigating sources and contacts in outbreaks of pertussis in school settings or shigellosis in daycare; TB testing and contact tracing; collecting and reporting information pertaining to notifiable communicable diseases; and providing morbidity and mortality statistics to those who request them, including the media, the public, service planners, and grant writers.

STUDENT EXPERIENCE

All provinces and territories in Canada are required to report communicable diseases. In order to facilitate and monitor specific communicable diseases, a reporting mechanism is in place. The list of notifiable infectious diseases in Canada is shown in Box 17-3 on page 535.

1. Find the incidence of at least 10 of these notifiable diseases in your community.
2. How does this disease incidence compare with the provincial and national disease incidence?

REMEMBER THIS!

- The burden of infectious diseases is high in both human and economic terms. Preventing these diseases needs to be given high priority in our current health care system.
- The successful interaction of the infectious agent, host, and environment is necessary for disease transmission. Knowledge of the characteristics of each of these three factors is important in understanding the transmission, prevention, and control of these diseases.
- Effective intervention measures must be aimed at breaking the chain linking the agent, host, and environment. An integrated approach focused on all three factors simultaneously is an ideal goal to strive for but may not be feasible for all diseases.
- Health care professionals must constantly be aware of vulnerability to threats posed by emerging infectious diseases. Most of the factors causing the emergence of these diseases are influenced by human activities and behaviour.
- Communicable diseases are preventable. Preventing infection through primary prevention activities is the most cost-effective public health strategy.
- Health care professionals need to always apply infection control principles and procedures in the work environment. They need to strictly practise the universal blood and body fluid precautions strategy to prevent the transmission of HIV and other bloodborne pathogens.
- Effective control of communicable diseases requires the use of a multisystem approach focusing on improving host resistance, improving safety of the environment, improving public health systems, and facilitating social and political changes to ensure health for all people.
- Communicable disease prevention and control programs must move beyond providing drug treatment and vaccines. Health promotion and education aimed at changing client behaviour must be emphasized.
- CHNs play a key role in all aspects of prevention and control of communicable diseases. Close cooperation with other members of the interdisciplinary health care team needs to be maintained. Mobilizing community participation is essential to successful implementation of programs.
- Nearly all communicable diseases discussed in this chapter are preventable because they are transmitted through specific, known behaviours.
- In Canada, as of 1997, the rates of the three nationally reportable STIs (chlamydia, gonorrhea, and syphilis) have been steadily increasing.
- STIs affect certain groups in greater numbers. Factors associated with risk include being younger than 25 years, being a member of a minority group, residing in an urban setting, being impoverished, and substance abuse.
- It is important for CHNs to educate clients about ways to prevent communicable diseases.
- Many STIs do not produce symptoms in clients.
- Hepatitis A is often silent in children, and children are a significant source of infection to others.
- The emergence of multidrug-resistant TB has prompted the use of DOT in Canada and other countries to ensure adherence with drug-treatment regimens.
- Early detection of communicable diseases is important because it results in early treatment and prevention of additional transmission to others. Treatment includes effective medications, stress reduction, and proper nutrition.
- Partner notification, or contact tracing, is done by identifying, contacting, and ensuring the evaluation and treatment of persons exposed to infected sexual partners or infected partners from injectable drug use. Contact tracing is also conducted with TB and HAV.
- Most of the care (both home and outpatient) that is provided for HIV is done within the community setting, which reduces direct health care costs but increases the need for financial support of home and community health services.
- The goal of primary prevention is to keep people healthy and avoid onset of disease.
- Secondary prevention includes screening of diseases to ensure early identification and treatment, and follow-up of contacts to prevent further spread.
- Tertiary prevention involves rehabilitation and applies to many of the chronic diseases such as STIs and TB.

REFLECTIVE PRAXIS

Case Study 1

Li Ming had immigrated to Canada from Tibet with her father and brother after her mother's death. During a trip to the emergency room with a fever, hemoptysis, and cough, she was diagnosed with drug-resistant tuberculosis (TB) and placed in directly observed therapy (DOT), which meant a CHN from the local health unit or health authority had to witness her ingesting her medication daily. Ms. Ming found taking the medication a big problem; swallowing the pills caused her to gag. She was embarrassed to have to take them in front of a CHN, and that made the whole situation even harder. Fortunately, the rest of the family had negative Mantoux skin test results and needed to be tested only periodically.

Ms. Ming was thin but not emaciated. She spoke English well enough to communicate with the community health nurse, Rachel, who told her she could take her time swallowing the medication. They chatted each day about Ms. Ming's life in Tibet and her adjustment to Canada. Ms. Ming worked in a beauty salon washing hair. Although she was 25 years old, her father did not want her to date, and so she never had.

Rachel worked to decrease Ms. Ming's anxiety. She taught Ms. Ming some relaxation exercises that Ms. Ming was able to use. During the first week of visits, it took about an hour for the pills to be ingested. A month later, the pill-taking was down to 15 minutes and she no longer gagged.

1. a) Explain how you would prepare and administer a Mantoux test to Li Ming.

   b) Is the test diagnostic for TB? Explain.

   c) How would you interpret the TB test? Explain.

2. a) What is the two-step TB testing?

   b) When would the two-step TB test be performed?

3. If TB was suspected in one of the family members, what other tests would be performed?

4. Rachel is asked by a nursing colleague if the DOT therapy is known to be the best approach. Find an evidence-informed article that would assist Rachel in responding to her colleague. To assist with your literature, search *The International Journal of Tuberculosis and Lung Disease,* which contains recent articles on this topic. Other journals also cover this topic.

Answers are provided on the Evolve Web site at http://evolve.elsevier.com/Canada/Stanhope/community/.

This case study was created by Deborah C. Conway and modified by the Canadian authors.

Case Study 2

The rising numbers of foreign-born residents in communities that did not previously have large immigrant populations provide a challenge to those involved with communicable disease control, especially in outbreak situations. Language barriers, specific cultural practices, and undocumented status all contribute to opportunities for infection and present obstacles to prevention and control. It is common for diseases such as TB, brucellosis, measles, hepatitis B, and parasitic infections to originate in other countries and be diagnosed only after arrival in Canada. People coming from countries without, with newly established, or with poorly enforced vaccination programs may not be immunized. These people are particularly susceptible to infection in an outbreak situation. For example, many people coming from Latin America have not been immunized against rubella. Differences in cultural practices can lead to outbreaks of food-borne illness. Listeriosis outbreaks have been traced to the use of unpasteurized milk in cottage-industry cheese production.

In the face of a single infectious disease report or an outbreak situation, when working with communities whose members speak little English, it is vital to (1) have a means of communication, (2) be able to provide a culturally appropriate message, and (3) have an established level of trust. Ideally, these requirements are addressed before an outbreak occurs, allowing a prompt and efficient response when immediate action is needed.

1. Which one of the following would be a useful first step in building trust with a largely non–English-speaking immigrant community?

   a. Hold a health fair in the community

   b. Provide incentives to use health unit or health authority services

   c. Identify trusted community leaders such as spiritual leaders and ask for their help in developing a plan

   d. Distribute a brochure in the target community language

2. What might best encourage nonregistered newcomers to respond to a request to be immunized during an outbreak situation?

a. Use an already established public health program to provide interpreter services, making it clear that proof of immigration status is not required for services

b. Place a request in the newspaper in the language of the targeted individuals

c. Involve trusted community leaders in making the request

d. Emphasize to the individuals the severity of the consequences if immunization does not occur

3. What means of communication would work best when targeting largely non–English-speaking communities of recent immigrants?

a. Publish newspaper articles in target language

b. Request radio announcements in target language

c. Post fliers in target language in the community

d. Enlist trusted community leaders to make announcements

4. How would community health nurses best go about developing information to effectively reach a largely non–English-speaking community of recent immigrants?

a. Use the services of the local university or college communications department

b. Ask community leaders to work with translators and prevention specialists to develop messages using their own words

c. Hire a professional to translate an existing well-developed English-language brochure

d. Use brochures provided by the provincial or territory health unit or health authority

Answers are provided on the Evolve Web site at http://evolve.elsevier.com/Canada/Stanhope/community/.

Case Study 3

Yvonne is a 20-year-old woman who visits the Bridgewater and District Health Authority prenatal clinic. Examination reveals she is at 14 weeks' gestation. She is single but has been in a steady relationship for the past 6 months with Phil. She states that she has no other children. Yvonne agrees to have a test for human immunodeficiency virus (HIV) and the results come back positive.

Yvonne is shocked and emotionally distraught about the positive test results. Understanding that Yvonne will not be able to concentrate on all the questions and information that need to be covered, the CHN sets priorities regarding essential information to obtain and provide during this visit.

1. List the relevant factors to consider on the basis of this information.
2. What questions does the CHN need to ask with regard to controlling the spread of HIV to others?
3. What information is most important to give to Yvonne at this time?
4. What follow-up does the CHN need to arrange for Yvonne?

Answers are provided on the Evolve Web site at http://evolve.elsevier.com/Canada/Stanhope/community/.

What Would You Do?

1. To become familiar with the reportable diseases that are a problem in your community, look at how many cases have been reported during the past month, 6 months, and year. Contrast these numbers with federal and provincial or territorial statistics. How is your community different from or similar to these larger jurisdictions? If different, what environmental, political, or demographic features may contribute to this difference?
2. Review a variety of sources (such as the local paper and health unit or health authority reports available on the Internet) in your community to identify what infectious diseases are routinely encountered in the school-age population. Discuss risk factors for disease in school-age youths and the strategies employed to prevent infectious diseases in this age group. Outline school policies that would be needed for the prevention of infectious diseases in the student population.
3. Review the *Canadian Required Immunization Schedule* found in Appendix E-5 on the Evolve site. Identify the immunization program that is provided in your province or territory and identify the differences that exist, if any. Reflect on why the scheduling is different. e
4. Identify the number of reported cases of AIDS and the number of reported cases of HIV infection in your community and province or territory. How are the cases distributed by age, sex, and geographical location? How does this rate compare with the national average?
5. Identify counselling and support services that are available in your community for people with HIV, sexually transmitted infections, and infectious diseases. Identify any improvements or changes that you would recommend.

TOOL BOX

evolve

The Tool Box contains useful instruments that can be applied in community health nursing practice. These related resources are found either in the appendices at the back of this book or on the Evolve Web site at http://evolve.elsevier.com/Canada/Stanhope/community/.

Appendices

- Appendix 12: Non–Vaccine-Preventable Infectious Diseases
- Appendix 13: Viral Hepatitis Profiles
- Appendix E-5: Canadian Required Immunization Schedule

Tools

Canadian AIDS Information Treatment Information Exchange (CATIE). Hepatitis C Toolkit.
This tool kit contains comprehensive information and prevention resource materials on hepatitis C. The information is available in different formats such as videos, posters, tool kits, pamphlets, and wallet cards. The site contains a resource titled "Chee Mamuk" that outlines the impact hepatitis C has on Aboriginals; it provides 22 fact sheets with information on hepatitis C prevention and treatment.

Canadian Guidelines on Sexually Transmitted Infections.
This site provides a reference for professionals for the prevention and management of STIs with additional new information in the 2008 revision of the 2006 guidelines that now contains information on at-risk populations—that is, vulnerable populations.

Canadian Public Health Association. *Leading Together: Canada Takes Action on HIV/AIDS (2005–2010).*
This resource outlines a 5-year action plan that will facilitate implementation of strategies that can be used by many levels of government and other agencies across Canada to address HIV/AIDS in Canada.

Flu Prevention Checklist.
This one-page checklist from the PHAC provides tips on staying healthy and preventing the spread of seasonal influenza or pandemic influenza. An excellent Weblink is provided for additional information on influenza.

Public Health Agency of Canada (2007). *Canadian Tuberculosis Standards,* 6th edition.
This Web-based resource is primarily aimed at the general physician and public health nurse. Its intent is to inform the health care professional about the management and control of TB and contains clinical protocols and other reference information necessary in the management of TB. Several tables and charts make this edition user friendly.

***Tuberculosis for Health Care Providers,* 4th Edition.**
This 2009 Ontario Lung Association 32-page publication covers epidemiology, screening, diagnosis, treatment, and management of TB for health care providers.

WEBLINKS

evolve

Direct links to these resources can be found on the text's accompanying Evolve Web site at http://evolve.elsevier.com/Canada/Stanhope/community/.

Canada's Role in Fighting Tuberculosis. This site provides information about tuberculosis in Canada, its history, and its current status.

Canadian Pediatric Society. *Immunization.* This site provides current information on immunization specifically for families.

Health Canada. *Health Concerns: Influenza (Flu).* Information for health care professionals and consumers is found on this site. It has direct links for each province and territory and provides specific information such as eligibility, clinic locations, and vaccine availability.

Public Health Agency of Canada. *A-Z Infectious Diseases.* This site provides CHNs with information on infectious diseases, listed alphabetically. The infectious disease information covers areas such as disease description and symptoms, how the disease presents itself, disease occurrence, and disease transmission.

Public Health Agency of Canada. *Canadian Immunization Guide,* 7th Edition. The 2006 *Canadian Immunization Guide* provides all information required for the preparation and administration of immunization required for vaccine-preventable diseases. Part 2 discusses the specific consideration for the recommended immunization for infants, children, and adults.

Public Health Agency of Canada. *Dengue Fever.* This site provides information on the cause, the risk to travellers, disease severity, prevention, and treatment.

Public Health Agency of Canada. *The Facts on the Safety and Effectiveness of HPV Vaccine.* This site provides answers to some of the common questions about the HPV vaccine.

Public Health Agency of Canada. *Lyme Disease.* This site provides information on topics such as the emergence of Lyme disease in Canada, distribution and challenges of Lyme disease, and its treatment.

Public Health Agency of Canada. *Routine Practices and Additional Precautions for Preventing the Transmission of Infection in Health Care.* This site provides infection control measures such as handwashing and isolation techniques.

Public Health Agency of Canada. *Sexually Transmitted Infections (STI): Sexual Health Facts and Information for the Public.* The site provides statistics on the rates by age group, sex, and province for chlamydia, gonorrhea, and syphilis and information about sexual health and other STIs.

Public Health Agency of Canada. *Travel Health.* This site provides regularly updated information on the occurrences internationally on communicable and infectious diseases that may be encountered, with the recommended immunization schedules for travel as well as travel preparation advice.

Public Health Agency of Canada. *Your H1N1 Preparedness Guide.* This site explains the H1N1, indicators of the infection, prevention and treatment, and preparedness for a possible pandemic.

Saskatchewan Lung Association. *Canada's Role in Fighting Tuberculosis.* A historical perspective into TB in Canada is presented on this site, as well as how Canada is addressing this progressive disease.

World Health Organization. *Tuberculosis in the European Region.* The site gives specific information about TB for European countries and provides access to information on treatment, surveillance, monitoring, evaluation, and policy to control worldwide TB.

REFERENCES

Alberta Health Services. (2008). *Red measles (Rubeola)*. Retrieved from http://www.healthlinkalberta.ca/Topic.asp?GUID=%7BE3F9FDCC-D4EF-4A67-B9D9-0E16A7AE9FD5%7D.

Alberta Health and Wellness. (2005). *Public health notifiable disease management guidelines: Invasive Haemophilus influenzae type B*. Retrieved from http://www.health.alberta.ca/documents/ND-Haemophilus-Non-B.pdf.

British Columbia Centre for Disease Control. (2005). *Questions and answers for crytococcal disease*. Retrieved from http://www.shape.bc.ca/resources/pdf/crytococcal.pdf.

British Columbia Centre for Disease Control. (2010). *Measles outbreak in BC—latest case count*. Retrieved from http://www.bccdc.ca/resourcematerials/newsandalerts/healthalerts/MeaslesMarch30.htm.

Canadian Centre for Occupational Health & Safety. (2008). *Hantavirus*. Retrieved from http://www.ccohs.ca/oshanswers/diseases/hantavir.html.

Canadian Food Inspection Agency. (2005). *Bovine spongiform encephalopathy (BSE)*. Retrieved from http://www.inspection.gc.ca/english/anima/heasan/disemala/bseesb/bseesbfse.shtml.

Canadian Food Inspection Agency. (2008). *Food safety facts on Listeria*. Retrieved from http://www.inspection.gc.ca/english/fssa/concen/cause/listeriae.shtml.

Canadian Food Inspection Agency. (2009a). *Bovine spongiform encephalopathy (BSE) cases confirmed in Canada in 2009*. Retrieved from http://www.inspection.gc.ca/english/anima/disemala/rep/2009bseesbe.shtml.

Canadian Food Inspection Agency. (2009b). *E.coli 0157:H7 food safety facts: Preventing food borne illnesses*. Retrieved from http://www.inspection.gc.ca/english/fssa/concen/cause/ecolie.shtml.

Canadian Food Inspection Agency. (2009c). *Food safety facts on paralytic shellfish poisoning (PSP)*. Retrieved from http://www.inspection.gc.ca/english/fssa/concen/cause/pspe.shtml.

Canadian Food Inspection Agency. (2009d). *Salmonella food safety facts: Preventing food borne illness*. Retrieved from http://www.inspection.gc.ca/english/fssa/concen/cause/salmonellae.shtml.

Canadian Public Health Association. (2009a). *Canadian Public Health Association urges Canadians to get vaccinated against H1N1: Making complex decisions on immunization simpler with credible information*. Retrieved from www.cpha.ca/uploads/media/h1n1_clearinghouse_e.pdf.

Canadian Public Health Association. (2009b). *Pandemic H1N1: Fast facts for front-line clinicians*. Retrieved from http://www.cpha.ca/uploads/portals/idp/pandemic/h1n1_fast_fact_e.pdf.

Cropp, R. Y., Latham-Caranico, C., Stebben, M., Wong, T., & Duarte-Franco, E. (2007). What's new in management of sexually transmitted infections. *Canadian Family Physician, 53*(10), 1739–1741.

Gender & Health Collaborative Curriculum. (2008). *Gender and poverty*. Retrieved from http://www.genderandhealth.ca/en/modules/poverty/Poverty-adolescent-environment-01.jsp?r=.

Global IDEA Scientific Advisory Committee. (2004). Health and economic benefits of an accelerated program of research to combat global infectious diseases. *Canadian Medical Association Journal, 171*(10), 1203–1208.

Harkness, G. A. (2003). Hepatitis C: The "silent stalker". *American Journal of Nursing, 103*(9), 24–25.

Health Canada. (2003). *Assessment of the Canadian Food Inspection Agency's activities related to domestic ready-to-eat meat products.* Retrieved from http://www.hc-sc.gc.ca/fn-an/securit/eval/reports-rapports/report_cfia-rapport_acia-34-eng.php.

Health Canada. (2005). *Hepatitis C.* Retrieved from http://www.hc-sc.gc.ca/iyh-vsv/diseases-maladies/hepc_e.html.

Health Canada. (2006a). *Flesh-eating disease.* Retrieved from http://www.hc-sc.gc.ca/iyh-vsv/diseases-maladies/flesh-chair_e.html.

Health Canada. (2006b). *Pneumococcal vaccine.* Retrieved from http://www.hc-sc.gc.ca/hl-vs/iyh-vsv/med/pneum-eng.php.

Health Canada. (2006c). *Salmonella prevention: It's your health.* Retrieved from http://www.hc-sc.gc.ca/hl-vs/iyh-vsv/food-aliment/salmonella-eng.php.

Health Canada. (2006d). *Tuberculosis.* Retrieved from http://www.hc-sc.gc.ca/iyh-vsv/diseases-maladies/tubercu_e.html.

Health Canada. (2008). *Environmental and workplace health: Water treatment devices for disinfection of drinking water.* Retrieved from http://www.hc-sc.gc.ca/ewh-semt/pubs/water-eau/disinfect-desinfection-eng.php.

Health Canada. (2009). *It's your health: Influenza.* Retrieved from http://www.hc-sc.gc.ca/hl-vs/alt_formats/pacrb-dgapcr/pdf/iyh-vsv/diseases-maladies/flu-grippe-eng.pdf.

Hislop, T. G., Teh, C., Low, A., Li, L., Tu, S. P., Yasui, Y., & Taylor, V. M. (2007). Hepatitis B knowledge, testing and vaccination levels in Chinese immigrants to British Columbia, Canada. *Canadian Journal of Public Health, 98*(2), 125–129.

International Development Research Centre. (2009). *HIV/AIDS in Canada.* Retrieved from http://www.idrc.ca/en/ev-110951-201-1-DO_TOPIC.html.

Katz, J. R., & Hirsch, A. M. (2003). When global health is local health. *American Journal of Nursing, 103*(12), 75–79.

Lung Association (2006a). *Tuberculosis in Canada today: Resurgence.* Retrieved from http://www.lung.ca/tb/tbtoday/resurgence/.

Lung Association. (2006b). *Tuberculosis in Canada today: The sanatorium age.* Retrieved from http://www.lung.ca/tb/tbhistory/sanatoriums/.

Nicholson, P. (2009). *Women and the changing face of HIV in Canada.* Women's Health Matters Network. Retrieved from http://www.womenshealthmatters.ca/resources/show_res.cfm?ID=43940.

Norris, S. (2009). *West Nile Virus in Canada. In Brief. Parliamentary information and research service.* Retrieved from http://www2.parl.gc.ca/Content/LOP/ResearchPublications/prb0911-e.pdf.

Ontario Lung Association. (2009). *Tuberculosis for health care providers* (4th ed.). Retrieved from https://lung.healthdiary.ca/Guest/Product.aspx?IDS=yaQAZ%2f8w5Dph%2fsSJ8eILtw%3d%3d.

Public Health Agency of Canada. (2002). Blue ribbon committee on bloodborne parasitic diseases. *Canada Communicable Disease Report, 28*(S3). Retrieved from http://www.phac-aspc.gc.ca/publicat/ccdr-rmtc/02vol28/28s3/index.html.

Public Health Agency of Canada. (2003a). *Notifiable diseases on-line.* Retrieved from http://dsol-smed.phac-aspc.gc.ca/dsol-smed/ndis/list_e.html#tab1.

Public Health Agency of Canada. (2003b). *Notifiable diseases on-line: Meningitis pneumococcal.* Retrieved from http://dsol-smed.phac-aspc.gc.ca/dsol-smed/ndis/diseases/pneu_e.html.

Public Health Agency of Canada. (2004). *Bloodborne pathogens section: Viral hepatitis.* Retrieved from http://www.phac-aspc.gc.ca/hcai-iamss/bbp-pts/hep-eng.php.

Public Health Agency of Canada. (2005a). Guidelines for the prevention and control of meningococcal disease. *Canada Communicable Disease Report, 31S1*(6). Retrieved from http://www.phac-aspc.gc.ca/publicat/ccdr-rmtc/05pdf/31s1_e.pdf.

Public Health Agency of Canada. (2005b). *Travel health. Rubella.* Retrieved from http://www.phac-aspc.gc.ca/tmp-pmv/info/rubella-eng.php.

Public Health Agency of Canada. (2006a). *Canadian immunization guide* (7th ed.). Retrieved from http://www.phac-aspc.gc.ca/publicat/cig-gci/index-eng.php.

Public Health Agency of Canada. (2006b). *Hantavirus pulmonary syndrome.* Retrieved from http://dsol-smed.phac-aspc.gc.ca/dsol-smed/ndis/disease2/hantavirus-eng.php.

Public Health Agency of Canada. (2007a). *Canadian Tuberculosis standards* (6th ed.). Retrieved from http://www.phac-aspc.gc.ca/tbpc-latb/pubs/pdf/tbstand07_e.pdf.

Public Health Agency of Canada. (2007b). *Notifiable diseases by province for June 2007 (preliminary).* Retrieved from http://www.phac-aspc.gc.ca/bid-bmi/dsd-dsm/ndmr-rmmdo/pdf/2007/jun07.pdf.

Public Health Agency of Canada. (2007c). *Vaccine-preventable diseases: Diphtheria.* Retrieved from http://www.phac-aspc.gc.ca/im/vpd-mev/diphtheria-eng.php.

Public Health Agency of Canada. (2007d). *Vaccine-preventable diseases: Haemophilus influenzae type b.* Retrieved from http://www.phac-aspc.gc.ca/im/vpd-mev/hib-eng.php.

Public Health Agency of Canada. (2007e). *Vaccine-preventable diseases: Hepatitis A.* Retrieved from http://www.phac-aspc.gc.ca/im/vpd-mev/hepatitis-a_e.html.

Public Health Agency of Canada. (2007f). *Vaccine-preventable diseases: Hepatitis B.* Retrieved from http://www.phac-aspc.gc.ca/im/vpd-mev/hib-eng.php.

Public Health Agency of Canada. (2007g). *Vaccine-preventable diseases: Mumps.* Retrieved from http://www.phac-aspc.gc.ca/im/vpd-mev/mumps_e.html.

Public Health Agency of Canada. (2007h). *Vaccine-preventable diseases: Pertussis.* Retrieved from http://www.phac-aspc.gc.ca/im/vpd-mev/pertussis-eng.php.

Public Health Agency of Canada. (2007i). *Vaccine-preventable diseases: Rabies.* Retrieved from http://www.phac-aspc.gc.ca/im/vpd-mev/rabies-eng.php.

Public Health Agency of Canada. (2007j). *Vaccine-preventable diseases: Rubella.* Retrieved from http://www.phac-aspc.gc.ca/im/vpd-mev/rubella_e.html.

Public Health Agency of Canada. (2007k). *Vaccine-preventable diseases: Tetanus.* Retrieved from http://www.phac-aspc.gc.ca/im/vpd-mev/tetanus-eng.php.

Public Health Agency of Canada. (2007l). *Vaccine-preventable diseases: Varicella.* Retrieved from http://www.phac-aspc.gc.ca/im/vpd-mev/varicella-eng.php.

Public Health Agency of Canada. (2008a). *Canadian Guidelines on sexually transmitted infections.* Retrieved from http://www.phac-aspc.gc.ca/std-mts/sti-its/pdf/sti-its-eng.pdf.

Public Health Agency of Canada. (2008b). *Hepatitis B fact sheet*. Retrieved from http://www.phac-aspc.gc.ca/hcai-iamss/bbp-pts/hepatitis/hep_b-eng.php.

Public Health Agency of Canada. (2008c). *Rabies vaccine: Questions and answers on rabies*. Retrieved from http://www.phac-aspc.gc.ca/im/rabies-faq_e.html.

Public Health Agency of Canada. (2008d). *Ticks and Lyme disease*. Retrieved from http://www.phac-aspc.gc.ca/id-mi/tickinfo-eng.php.

Public Health Agency of Canada. (2009a). *Creutzfeldt-Jakob disease*. Retrieved from http://www.phac-aspc.gc.ca/hcai-iamss/cjd-mcj/cjdss-ssmcj/stats-eng.php#canada.

Public Health Agency of Canada. (2009b). *The FACTS on the safety and effectiveness of HPV vaccine*. Retrieved from http://www.phac-aspc.gc.ca/std-mts/hpv-vph/fact-faits-vacc-eng.php.

Public Health Agency of Canada. (2009c). *Management and treatment of chronic hepatitis C*. Retrieved from http://www.phac-aspc.gc.ca/hepc/faq-eng.php.

Public Health Agency of Canada. (2009d). *Poliomyelitis*. Retrieved from http://www.phac-aspc.gc.ca/tmp-pmv/info/polio-eng.php.

Public Health Agency of Canada. (2009e). *Referrals of suspected CJD reported to CJD-SS, Creutzfeldt-Jakob Disease Surveillance System Statistics*. Retrieved from http://www.phac-aspc.gc.ca/hcai-iamss/cjd-mcj/cjdss-ssmcj/stats-eng.php#ref.

Public Health Agency of Canada. (2009f). *Travel health. Measles*. Retrieved from http://www.phac-aspc.gc.ca/tmp-pmv/info/measles_e.html.

Public Health Agency of Canada. (2009g). *Tuberculosis in Canada 2006*. Retrieved from http://www.phac-aspc.gc.ca/publicat/2009/tbcan06/index-eng.php.

Public Health Agency of Canada. (2009h). *Tuberculosis in Canada 2007: Pre Release*. Retrieved from http://www.phac-aspc.gc.ca/tbpc-latb/pubs/tbcan07/index-eng.php.

Public Health Agency of Canada. (2010a). *The anatomy of a foodborne illness outbreak*. Retrieved from http://www.phac-aspc.gc.ca/fs-sa/anatomy-eng.php.

Public Health Agency of Canada. (2010b). *Influenza*. Retrieved from http://www.phac-aspc.gc.ca/influenza/index-eng.php.

Sex Information and Education Council of Canada (2009). Sexual health education in the schools. *Canadian Journal of Human Sexuality, 18*(1–2), 47–60.

Shah, C. P. (2003). *Public health and preventive medicine in Canada* (5th ed.). Toronto, ON: Elsevier Canada.

Sherman, M., Shafran, S., Burak, K., Doucette, K., Wong, W., Girgrah, N., & Deschênes, M. (2007). Management of chronic hepatitis C: Consensus guidelines. *Canadian Journal of Gastroenterology, 21*(Suppl. C), 25C–34C.

Statistics Canada (2005). Early sexual intercourse, condom use and sexually transmitted diseases. *The Daily*. Retrieved from http://www.statcan.gc.ca/daily-quotidien/050503/dq050503a-eng.htm.

UNAIDS. (2008). *2008 Report on the global AIDS epidemic: Executive summary*. Retrieved from http://data.unaids.org/pub/GlobalReport/2008/JC1511_GR08_ExecutiveSummary_en.pdf.

Vollman, A. R., Anderson, E. T., & McFarlane, J. (2008). *Canadian community as partner: Theory and multidisciplinary practice* (2nd ed.). Philadelphia, PA: Lippincott, Williams & Wilkins.

World Health Organization. (1999). *Smallpox eradication: Destruction of variola virus stocks. Fifty-second World Health Assembly*. Retrieved from http://ftp.who.int/gb/pdf_files/WHA52/ew5.pdf.

World Health Organization. (2009a). *Influenza A (H1N1): Pandemic alert phase 6 declared, of moderate severity*. Retrieved from http://www.euro.who.int/influenza/AH1N1/20090611_11.

World Health Organization. (2009b). *New HIV infections reduced by 17% over the past eight years*. Retrieved from http://www.who.int/mediacentre/news/releases/2009/hiv_aids_20091124/en/index.html.

World Health Organization. (2009c). *Rabies*. Retrieved from http://www.who.int/mediacentre/factsheets/fs099/en.

World Health Organization. (2009d). *Smallpox: Historical significance*. Retrieved from http://www.who.int/mediacentre/factsheets/smallpox/en/.

World Health Organization. (2009e). *Tuberculosis in the European region*. Retrieved from http://www.euro.who.int/tuberculosis.

World Health Organization. (n.d.). *The WHO golden rules for safe food preparation*. Retrieved from https://apps.who.int/fsf/goldenrules.htm.

CHAPTER 18

Applications in Working with Specific Aggregates

OBJECTIVES

After reading this chapter, you should be able to:

1. Describe the application of the community health nursing process to promote wellness in an Aboriginal community using a capacity-building approach.
2. Explain the phases of the capacity-building process and the means used to engage Aboriginal community members as community partners.
3. Select appropriate assessment methods and types of action based on cultural and ethical considerations.
4. Compare and contrast the application of risk reduction and capacity building approaches.
5. Identify the underlying concepts relevant to the application: the determinants of health, population-based practice, health promotion, risk reduction, chronic disease prevention and management, capacity building, teamwork, program planning, and evaluation and sustainability of health programming.
6. Analyze health concerns and community health nursing interventions.
7. Demonstrate reflective thinking about the application of community health nursing practice.

CHAPTER OUTLINE

Section A of this chapter was written by Alwyn Moyer and Elizabeth Diem. Section B was written by Bonnie Myslik.

This chapter provides an opportunity for application of and reflection on concepts that have been presented earlier in this textbook. It provides students with the opportunity to apply knowledge and skills acquired from working through the content presented in this textbook. Therefore, its format is different from that of the other chapters.

Section A of this chapter illustrates the use of the community health nursing process to develop a wellness program for an Aboriginal community in the fictitious town of "Northern." This section describes the application of a collaborative, community-based program planning process that incorporates strategies to build capacity to improve the health and wellness outcomes of First Nations women living in an urban community and on nearby reserves. Section A provides some background information on the community and the health issue, and describes the community assessment, planning, action, and evaluation of the wellness program. The information is provided from the perspective of two community health nurses, one of whom works at an Aboriginal wellness centre in the city; the other works at a health centre on the reserve.

Section B provides various mental health situations with which community health nurses may be actively involved. Community health nurses (CHNs) working with clients with mental health issues and mental illness are often referred to as *community mental health nurses* (CMHNs). Section B includes case studies, some of which present questions for reflection and response, and others that ask you to describe your reflective thinking. Reflective thinking is rational focused thinking about a situation that often results in decisions being made and evaluated based on knowledge and experience.

SECTION A: USING THE COMMUNITY HEALTH NURSING PROCESS WITH AN ABORIGINAL COMMUNITY

Background: Marina is a Master's prepared nurse and the Wellness Coordinator at the Aboriginal Wellness Centre in Northern, a city in Ontario. Her colleague, Anna, is the CHN in charge of the health centre on the largest reserve in the area. Marina and Anna are meeting Sarah, a fourth-year nursing student who is completing her community health clinical assignment. Marina is the preceptor, but Sarah will spend some time with Anna at the health centre and accompany her on monthly visits to the smaller and more remote reserves. Sarah is from the Mohawk Nation, whereas the First Nations in this region are Ojibwe and members of the Anishnabek Nation. Sarah grew up in an urban setting but has a mentor from the Aboriginal Nurses Association of Canada (ANAC) mentorship project (2009), who lives on a reserve. The purpose of this first meeting is to confirm the working arrangements and to introduce Sarah to the wellness project, which began last year. The meeting begins with Marina providing an overview of the initial community health assessment and planning process, which is ongoing. She explains that there are cycles within cycles of the community health nursing process.

COMMUNITY HEALTH ASSESSMENT

Northern is a well-established industrial city in northern Ontario, with a population of 100,000. The city is a major transportation hub for the region, which is rich in natural resources. In recent years, the forestry and mining industries have been depressed and are making a very slow recovery. The population is stagnant and many families have lost jobs. The city has a rich multicultural European heritage and is home to approximately 8,000 Aboriginal peoples, mainly First Nations. Several small reserves lie within a 200-km radius of the city. The many lakes and forests make this an ideal place for outdoor pursuits, but it is not as easy to maintain an active lifestyle through the long, cold winters.

Over the past year, the regional public health unit and the Aboriginal Wellness Centre have formed a network of community groups with a view to increasing access to health promotion and disease prevention opportunities for low-wage earners in the region. The community partners, all of whom have a common interest in physical activity programming, include community health and resource centres, recreational facilities, neighbourhood organizations, churches, schools, and local industry. To date, the network has identified several pre-existing initiatives relevant to physical activity:

- Advocacy for people on social assistance or receiving low wages
- A Healthy Babies Healthy Children program
- Walking programs in malls and seniors' centres with training of lay fitness instructors by the city's recreation department
- A lending program for pedometers at the public library
- Healthy Workplaces: Personalized health information on healthy eating, physical activity, smoking cessation, and stress management offered by several employers, including a large mining company

The network aims to promote physical activity to low-wage earners as a means of increasing wellness and preventing the onset of chronic diseases like diabetes. This strategy is informed by Canadian Community Health Survey data that confirm that people with higher incomes and education report better levels of health overall, are more likely to be physically active, are less likely to have diabetes and other chronic conditions, and live longer (Labonté, Muhajarine, Winquist, & Quail, 2009). Network members want to expand the reach of their programs to priority populations. In this area, the priority populations have been identified as Aboriginal communities, youth living independently, parents of young children, homeless and underhoused community members, and seniors living in isolated situations. Recently, the community partners received special project funding to develop strategies to increase physical activity in the Aboriginal population.

The public health unit compiled a community profile that compared urban and rural Aboriginal populations with the total urban population. They drew information from several sources: the 2006 Community profile and Aboriginal population profile for the Census Metropolitan Area (CMA) and public health unit (Statistics Canada, 2006a, 2006b) and the profiles of First Nations living on reserves in the region (Indian Northern Affairs Canada, 2010). To make comparison easier, the results were summarized in a table. Table 18-1 illustrates the type of information that might be gathered from the above-mentioned sources for the community of Northern. (For a tool kit providing "steps" and "tools" to facilitate the health assessment process in Canadian communities where mining is a major industry, see the Mining Watch Canada link in the Tool Box. For information on assessing the community health needs of First Nations and Inuit, see the Health Canada Weblink on the Evolve Web site.)

The profile of the urban community showed that 10,055, or 8.3% of the population, self-identified as Aboriginal in 2006 in the CMA. This is more than double the proportion of Aboriginal peoples (3.8%) in the Canadian population (Statistics Canada, 2006a). A breakdown of the figures showed that 7,420 (74%)

TABLE 18-1 Town of "Northern" Population Estimates, 2006

	Urban Community			Urban Aboriginal Profile			Rural Aboriginal Profile		
	Total	Male	Female	Total	Male	Female	Total	Male	Female
Total Population	122,910	59,885	63,025	10,055	4,655	5,400	2,014	1,062	953
<15	20,235	10,350	9,885	2,995	1,475	1,520	602	271	331
15-64	82,980	41,015	41,960	6,670	2,985	3,680	1,335	647	688
>64	19,680	8,515	11,165	385	200	190	77	44	33
Median age	42	41	41	26	23	28	24	21	26
% Aged 15 and over	84	83	84	70	68	72	72	69	73
Health Indicators									
Well-being									
Perceived health, very good or excellent	66,740 (54.3%)	(56.6%)	(53.9%)	5,571 (55.4%)	*	*	806 (40.0%)	*	*
Health Conditions									
Overweight or obese	72,640 (59.1%)	(70.9%)	(53.8%)	6,355 (63.2%)	*	*	1,470 (73.0%)	*	*
Health Behaviours									
Leisure-time physical activity, moderately active or active	73,992 (60.2%)	(62.6%)	(58.4%)	6,103 (60.7%)	*	*	429 (21.3%)	*	*
Personal Resources									
Sense of community belonging	90,585 (73.7%)	(80.5%)	(78.4%)	7,993 (79.5%)	*	*	1,621 (80.5%)	*	*

**Data not available*

identified as being First Nations; 2,375 (24%) as Métis, and the remainder (2%) identified as Inuit or mixed heritage.

The public health manager explained that it was difficult to find comparative health information on small communities. While several First Nations communities across the country have participated in Regional Health Surveys, access to the data is restricted to the participating community (Jeffery et al., 2006). This conforms to principles of ownership, control, access, and possession (OCAP) governing the collection and use of Aboriginal health information (First Nations Centre, 2009).

ABORIGINAL HEALTH STATUS

It is widely acknowledged that the health status of Aboriginal peoples in Canada falls below that of the general Canadian population, although it is difficult to find comparable statistics supporting this claim (Reading, 2009a, 2009b). The life expectancy for Registered Indian men is 70.4 years, compared with 64.4 years for Inuit men and 77 years for non-Aboriginal men; the life expectancy for Registered Indian women is 75.5 years, compared with 69.8 for Inuit women and 82 years for non-Aboriginal women (Reading, 2009b). (The data were collected in Canada during different time periods: non-Aboriginal Canadians between 2000 and 2002; Registered Indians in 2001; and Inuit from 1999 to 2003.) Furthermore, Aboriginal people have higher rates of many chronic and infectious diseases, such as tuberculosis and type 2 diabetes (Reading, 2009b). Indeed, the prevalence of diabetes mellitus in First Nations is considered to have reached epidemic proportions (Reading, 2009b). The 2001 Aboriginal Peoples Survey found a diabetes prevalence rate greater than 8% in First Nations people with legal Indian status living off reserve; the rate reached 11% on reserves that participated in this survey (Statistics Canada, 2004). This compared with a diabetes prevalence rate of 4.3% in the non-Aboriginal population. In 2005, the Canadian Community Health Survey (CCHS) found the rate had risen to 4.9% in Canadians aged 12 or older (Sanmartin & Gilmore, 2008). Corresponding data were not available for the Aboriginal population, but it is likely that the prevalence of diabetes has continued to rise in this population also.

Many explanations have been offered for the increased vulnerability of the Aboriginal population: biological susceptibility, rural and remote lifestyle, health practices (Minore & Katt, 2007), low socioeconomic status that limits access to the social determinants of health (Ling Yu & Raphael, 2004), and lack of culturally appropriate health promotion programs (Fletcher, McKennitt, & Baydala, 2007). Historically, the federal government has provided a limited range of health services to First Nations living on reserve. In more recent years, the policy has shifted to facilitating First Nations control of these health services with a view to building local capacity and more culturally appropriate health planning and delivery (Smith & Lavoie, 2008). However, most primary care and all secondary and tertiary care services are provided through provincially operated services (Minore & Katt, 2007), which tend to be less available in rural and remote parts of the country (Nagarajan, 2004). In addition to Aboriginal peoples being exposed to a high-risk physical and socioeconomic environment, Bartlett (2003) argues that the health discrepancies are a result of sustained contact with an external society that brought dramatically different cultural norms and practices, resulting in extreme stress for many generations of Aboriginal peoples. From this perspective, improving health will require concerted efforts to reverse the cultural, social, economic, and political impacts of colonization. (For further information on the health of the Aboriginal peoples, refer to the two Reading Weblinks on the Evolve Web site.)

STUDENT EXPERIENCE

As with many countries, Canada has found that Aboriginal population estimates vary according to how identity is determined—for example, through self-identification, registration, or other means, and by how the figures are derived. Between 1996 and 2006, the Aboriginal population in Canada grew by 45%, compared with a growth rate of 8% for the non-Aboriginal population.

1. What are some possible reasons for this rapid increase in the Aboriginal population and the implications for health care.

Work in groups of two to four. Visit the Statistics Canada Web site at http://www12.statcan.ca/english/census06/data/highlights/Aboriginal/index.cfm?Lang=E

Select one or two Census Metropolitan Areas in your province or territory (Table 1) with a population greater than 1,000. Go back to the 2006 Census: Data Products. Compare and contrast the information provided on your chosen communities in the 2006 Census, Aboriginal Population Profiles with that provided through the First Nation Profiles on the Indian and Northern Affairs Canada (INAC) Web site at http://pse5-esd5.ainc-inac.gc.ca/fnp/Main/Search/SearchFN.aspx?lang=eng.

2. What factors might strengthen health or contribute to the vulnerability of First Nations in your chosen communities.

PLANNING

The community network is guided by a vision of improving the health of the population by reducing inequities and increasing access and control over the factors that determine health—the social determinants such as economic resources, education, social support, and a clean physical environment. This approach is directed toward individuals who are essentially healthy as well as those at risk. By increasing resources for all, including subpopulations living under high-risk conditions, the group aims to increase the health and well-being of the whole population.

Network members subscribe to the view that health is a resource that enables people to "adapt to, respond to, or control life's challenges and changes" (Frankish, Green, Ratner, Chomik, & Larsen, 1996). They are committed to using strategies that build capacity, either as their main goal or as a means to an end (Labonté, Woodard, Chad, & Laverack, 2002; MacLellan-Wright et al., 2007). This entails working with strengths and maximizing the assets and resources of individuals, groups, and collectives to deal with life challenges and changes. Integral to strategies like community development and empowerment, community capacity building is about increasing the capabilities of people to articulate and address community health issues and to overcome barriers to achieve improved outcomes in the quality of their life. Community participation is an essential element of capacity-building approaches. In principle, community participation can range from the token involvement of a few individuals to collective action (Howard-Grabman, 2007); however, the research evidence suggests that the greater the involvement—for example, the whole community giving input into the planning and delivery of its health promotion programs—the greater the responsiveness to community needs (Bracht, Kingsbury, & Rissel, 1999).

The community network intends to build capacity on two levels. The partnership brings together organizations in the community to share skills and resources, identify opportunities for collaboration, and make plans to work together to strengthen the community. Complementing the community-level activities, the organizations will support capacity-building approaches at the individual level by involving the people using the services in the planning and evaluating of the services.

Primary Prevention: Health Promotion and Risk Reduction

Whenever possible, population-based practice focuses on primary prevention. This level of prevention includes promoting health and reducing risk. The network members have conducted a literature review to identify what factors to consider when developing the physical activity program to increase wellness and decrease the prevalence of type 2 diabetes. They understand that regular exercise can help a person feel stronger and fitter, have more energy, and feel more relaxed and sleep better. As well, sedentary lifestyles are a known risk factor for chronic health problems (Public Health Agency of Canada [PHAC], 2003). So, increasing physical activity has the potential to both promote health and reduce the risk of ill health. Risk reduction approaches hinge on knowing which factors increase the likelihood of specific chronic diseases. Some risk factors, such as age, sex, and genetic inheritance, are nonmodifiable. Others, such as body type (weight distribution) and activity levels, are potentially modifiable. A risk reduction approach entails identifying the at-risk population and tailoring interventions to inform susceptible people about the risks and preventive measures. For example, type 2 diabetes, the most common form of the disease, is increasing at higher than expected rates, attributable to an increased incidence of the condition and decreased mortality (Lipscombe & Hux, 2007). The Diabetes Prevention Program found that people at risk of developing this condition were able to cut their risk by 58% with moderate physical activity (30 minutes a day) and weight loss (5 to 7% of body weight, or about 15 lb). For people over age 60, the risk was cut by almost 71% (Diabetes Prevention Program Research Group, 2002). However, equal standards of access to preventive care must be achieved for risk reduction strategies to be effective with at-risk groups ("Targeting High-Risk," 2007). This speaks to the importance of using risk reduction strategies within capacity-building approaches that foster broad community participation.

Community Health Nurse Considerations Regarding Planning

The community health nurse shared the following observations at the network planning group:

- The network already has links with the Aboriginal community. One Aboriginal organization is represented on the planning group, and the professor representing the university department of kinesiology is Aboriginal.
- The Aboriginal Wellness Centre has many connections to the urban and rural Aboriginal community, and several staff members are Aboriginal. Over the last 3 years, the health centre on the reserve has built an effective working relationship with most of the chiefs and the band council. At least one member of staff attends the health committee meetings each quarter.
- The potential users of a walking program are not represented on the network; however, three women attending a well woman's clinic on the largest reserve have approached the health centre to set up an exercise class.

Reflective thinking: The CHN's reflective thinking is that the Aboriginal community is represented at the network level; however, it is necessary to ensure that all appropriate community stakeholders are able to contribute to planning.

- The wellness centre now offers group classes on healthy nutrition, which they would like to expand to include an exercise component, particularly if they could train volunteer leaders, as is the case in the mall walking programs.
- The urban mall walking program attracts only women. The community outreach workers at the Aboriginal Wellness Centre say their clients have not joined the program because it is on the outskirts of the city and because the people going there "are all dressed in fancy sports outfits."
- The special project funding will be sufficient to conduct a pilot project, the results of which can be used to seek additional resources.

Reflective Thinking: The CHN's reflective thinking is that the Aboriginal community would like to participate in an activity program but there are barriers to overcome. Offering a program on the reserve would show a response to the expressed need and would fit with the health centre's goal of expanding the primary prevention services to include more health promotion. The special project funding would allow the health centre to get much-needed help because the staff has limited time and resources.

After the CHN shared her observations and after much deliberation, the network decided to develop a 6-week wellness program for Aboriginal women on two sites: the largest reserve, which is closest to the city, and the Aboriginal Wellness Centre in the city, which provides services to First Nations living on and off reserve, Métis, and Inuit. They acknowledge the importance of more fully involving Aboriginal peoples, especially women, in the region in the planning process.

Preparing to Implement the Walking Program on the Reserve

The wellness coordinator (Marina) at the Aboriginal Wellness Centre leading the pilot project, assisted by the nurse in charge of the main health centre on the reserves (Anna). The student nurse, Sarah, who will be with them for 3 months, and two community health representatives (CHR) from the wellness centre, are assigned to the project. In addition, Anna has invited the three women who had first approached her about the exercise class to join the planning team. Anna, taking on the leadership role of facilitator and resource (Camiletti, 1996), welcomed everyone to the first meeting and made introductions. The group sat around a table so they could see each other and feel encouraged to talk and ask questions.

They began the meeting with a topic that would encourage participation: What would attract women to an exercise class? The three women from the reserve, Patsy, Darlene, and Shania, offered several reasons for their interest: to stay healthy; to get balance in their lives and set an example for their children; to lose weight; and to have something to do. They said that people like to be outdoors in the summer and walk a lot but there is not much to do in the winter on the reserve. Because of television, people are more sedentary than in the past. They felt that women would benefit from the regular social interaction and had a brainstorming session about what makes it easy and what makes it hard to keep fit.

Anna handed out copies of the *Handbook for Canada's Physical Activity Guide to Healthy Active Living*, which was developed by PHAC and the Canadian Society for Exercise Physiology to look at for ideas on what types of exercise to include. (This handbook can be accessed at the PHAC Weblink at the Evolve Web site.) Apologetically, she explained that efforts were underway to tailor the guide for First Nations, Inuit, and Métis (Young & Katzmarzyk, 2007). Sarah commented that she was pleased to see that her exercise group at the university had all the elements of a good fitness program—strength training, cardiovascular fitness, and balance. Everyone agreed that the handbook had some good ideas and that their planning group could determine which activities would be suitable for First Nations women in their community.

From there, the discussion turned to questions about how formal the program should be, where it would be held, and the best time of day and day of week. They identified two possible settings: the church hall, which was more central, and the health centre meeting room, which could provide child care on some days of the week. The question of whether to charge a small admission fee was also discussed. Anna explained that they had funding to run the exercise class and that she could help with the organization but did not have the skills or the time to run the group herself. One CHR, a trained fitness instructor, said she could lead the class if she had volunteers to help set up. Since there was a small fund to pay volunteers for their work, this might be an option. The CHR explained that they respected traditional practices with groups at the Aboriginal Wellness Centre, usually starting with a snack and an opening prayer and on some occasions there would be a smudging ceremony. They decided it would be best to ask the elders on the reserve for advice on these matters.

Anna summarized their discussion and proposed that they gather further information from the community. This would provide specific information about what women wanted in an exercise group and about what they did not want, which they could use to guide planning. At the same time, informing community members about their intentions would raise awareness in the exercise program and create interest. Everyone agreed to approach three Aboriginal women on the reserve and ask the following questions:

1. What types of physical activity (e.g., walking) have you participated in over the last 12 months? (Question on 2007–2008 Regional Health Survey [First Nations Centre, 2009; Jeffery et al., 2006])
2. What sort of exercises would you like to see included in the class?
3. Where would be the most convenient place to hold the exercise class—in the church hall or in the health centre?

To keep it simple, they decided they would record the answers in point form and give the notes to Sarah to summarize for the next meeting in 2 weeks' time.

At the second team meeting, Anna welcomed everyone and explained the task that day was planning the fitness class in more detail. They had three sources of information to look at:

1. The summary of the interviews with local Aboriginal women
2. An overview of best practices on increasing activity levels in adults (Canadian Cancer Society, Manitoba Division, 2008)
3. A review of patterns of physical activity, their determinants and consequences, and the results of various interventions designed to increase the physical activity of Aboriginal peoples in Canada and the United States (Young & Katzmarzyk, 2007)

Sarah presented a summary of the 12 completed interviews (note: The themes are based on a summary of incentives for attending a prenatal exercise program for urban Aboriginal women [Klomp, Dyck, & Sheppard, 2003]).

The key themes are listed below:

- The program should be for Aboriginal women only. It is better when you know other participants.
- People like it when there is food; it brings people together.
- Over half of the women said they would need child care.
- It is good to have time to talk to the exercise leader about the exercises, to find out if you are doing them properly; other suggestions were to include information on what to eat and possibly traditional healing practices.
- There should be time to socialize afterward.
- It is easier to exercise with music that has a good rhythm, music that gets you moving.
- It should not be too strenuous to start so everyone can keep up; they have to know how to do the exercises.

Anna explained that the review of best practices for increasing activity levels provided useful information on how to put together a program, but none of the studies on which the review was based had been conducted with an Aboriginal population. Nor was there sufficient information on program participants to assess applicability to this community (Canadian Cancer Society, Manitoba Division, 2008). One North American review found that relatively little is known about the patterns and levels of physical activity in Aboriginal populations or about the determinants and barriers to physical activity in different environmental and cultural contexts (Young & Katzmarzyk, 2007).

The planning group decided it would be best to use the identified needs as a guide. As well, they would consider using programs and strategies that had some claim to being effective, despite the incomplete information. They can see they have made progress and reason that if they build on strengths and work with the resources they have and in partnership with community members, they are more likely to develop a program that the community needs and wants. There is evidence that capacity-building approaches have been successful with Aboriginal communities (Fletcher et al., 2007). Across communities with unique histories, languages, cultural practices, and spiritual beliefs, Fletcher and colleagues found that interventions that used community-based participatory approaches appeared to be more successful in building capacity and creating and sustaining positive health outcomes than those that involved Aboriginals to a lesser degree, as consultants.

Anna then introduced the group to the Community Capacity Building Tool (CCBT) (PHAC, Alberta/NWT Region, 2008). The CCBT was designed to assist community-based health projects to integrate community capacity building into their work. The tool uses a definition of community capacity developed in Australia (Hawe, King, Noort, Jordens, & Lloyd, 2000; Hawe, Noort, King, & Jordens, 1997):

> *An approach to the development of sustainable skills, organizational structures, resources and commitment to health improvement in health and other sectors, to prolong and multiply health gains many times over. (New South Wales Health Department, 2001, p. i)*

Drawing on this definition, the CCBT identifies nine features of community capacity building:

1. Participation
2. Leadership

3. Community structures
4. Role of external support
5. Asking why
6. Obtaining resources
7. Skills, knowledge, and learning
8. Linking with others
9. Sense of community

Anna proposed that they use the tool to determine where their group is in the capacity-building process and what they need to do next. They focus on the first feature—Participation.

> *Participation is the active involvement of people in improving their own and their community's health and well-being. Participating in a project means the target population, community members, and other stakeholders are involved in project activities, such as making decisions and evaluation.* (PHAC, Alberta/NWT Region, 2008, p. 1)

Sarah recorded their answers to the accompanying questions and the phrase that best encapsulates their progress on the key questions. Likening it to a journey, they have to decide whether they have "Just started," are "On the road," "Nearly there," or "We're there."

- Have we actively involved community organizations? *On the road:* The project team is a subcommittee of a community-wide network of health, social services, and education groups with an interest in physical activity programming. Our first step in linking to the Aboriginal community organizations on the reserve will be to talk to the chief and council and get their support.
- Have we actively involved the priority community? *On the road:* Three members of our planning group live on the largest reserve in the area. One woman (Shania) is a member of the health committee and a member of the board of the urban Aboriginal Wellness Centre, so has a voice in decision making about health matters. We need to recruit Aboriginal women from the city and from the smaller reserves in the area. Also, we do not have representation from First Nations women in their middle years.
- Have we identified and overcome barriers to the priority group participating in project meetings? *On the road:* The project meetings are being held on the reserve to make it easy for First Nations women to attend. We cannot provide child care regularly, and transportation may be a barrier to participation for Aboriginal women from the city and from the smaller reserves.
- Are we using different methods to keep everyone informed about the project? *Just started:* The project team will communicate by e-mail and by word of mouth. They have not thought about how they will keep others informed.

After a brief look through the rest of the CCBT, they got into a discussion about the feature "Asking Why," which recommends using a community process to uncover the root causes of community issues. Shania commented: "Yes, it is more than not enough to do in our community. We want people to want to live here, young and old. We don't really get together much any more. When I was a girl, my family was active all year round, there was always something going on, we didn't exercise but we walked, went out on the land, danced, and had fun." Anna agreed, saying it is only through dialogue and sharing what we know with the community that we will find the right approach for this community. The group acknowledged the importance of community dialogue but felt they were not ready to go to the community yet. Anna suggested that they leave it for now and come back to it next time to avoid being overwhelmed. They decided to start the next meeting with a discussion on this topic. The CHR suggested using a Talking Circle, where everyone has an opportunity to contribute if they want to. The aim is to create an inclusive atmosphere so that everyone can have a voice; the purpose is not debate but to hear the different opinions (Muin'iskw & Crowfeather, 2009; Running Wolf & Rickard, 2003).

The remainder of the meeting was spent on beginning to shape the exercise class based on previously identified best practices for physical activity programming (Canadian Cancer Society, Manitoba Division, 2008). Their program would include two complementary components identified as effective (exercise sessions and small group education) and some strategies found to be effective (recommending regular brisk walking and putting emphasis on behavioural skill training). They agreed to the following:

- Offer exercise classes for 6 weeks, 2 sessions per week, modelled on the programs offered by the city.
- Include in each session a warm-up, cardio, and cool-down, with a mix of exercises to increase strength and flexibility.
- Invite the CHR from the Aboriginal Wellness Centre, a trained fitness instructor, to run the classes with help from Sarah and volunteers.
- Recruit volunteers to help set up equipment and organize social activities after class.
- Include 15 minutes of health information on topics selected by participants. Incorporate tools and techniques to take charge of health based on self-management concepts (Registered Nurses' Association of Ontario, 2010).
- Make it fun! Use music with a beat.

(For information on Aboriginal dance traditions across Canada, see the Carleton University *Native Dance* Weblink on the Evolve Web site.)

CRITICAL VIEW

1. The CCBT is designed to measure and describe the contribution of funded programs to community capacity building.
   a) How would you explain this tool to community members on your planning committee?
   b) One committee member tells you that the tool is too complicated and takes time away from delivering the program. How might you respond to this criticism?
2. Who else in the urban community might be interested in collaborating on a physical activity program for Aboriginal people?
   a) Think broadly. Add to Table 18-2 below, drawing on knowledge of your own community.
   b) The current partnership is mainly from the health sector. What other sectors might be interested in joining this alliance? What might they contribute? What might they gain? For example, the local high school is trying to increase levels of physical activity in all its students, boys and girls. It has many First Nations students. Also, it has a large gymnasium, which could be used.

TABLE 18-2 Inventory of Urban Community Programs and Activities That Support Healthy Lifestyles

Program Type	Urban Community Organization
Walking programs Mall & seniors' centres	City recreation department
Fitness classes/swimming	YM-YWCA & fitness centres
Sports program	Universities and schools
Pedometers for lease	Main library
Camping, canoeing	Youth organizations (e.g., Boy Scouts, Girl Guides)
Skating	Municipal rinks, local rinks
Sponsored walks	Charities

STUDENT EXPERIENCE

Work in a group to complete one of the following:

1. How might you prepare to take part in an Aboriginal cultural experience such as a smudge ceremony?
2. Develop a 10-minute health information session for use in a physical activity program that incorporates a discussion of selected traditional healing practices.
3. a) An elder suggested that a medicine wheel (see Figure 18-1) be used to design the fitness program and offered to help with this. Log on to the Four Directions Interactive Teaching Web site at http://www.fourdirectionsteachings.com/main.html. After listening to the introduction, click on "Ojibwe" to hear the teachings on the medicine wheel.
   b) How might traditional knowledge and views be incorporated into a physical activity program? (For an example of using the medicine wheel in program planning, see the Ontario Aboriginal Diabetes Strategy Weblink on the Evolve Web site.)

FIGURE 18-1 Medicine Wheel

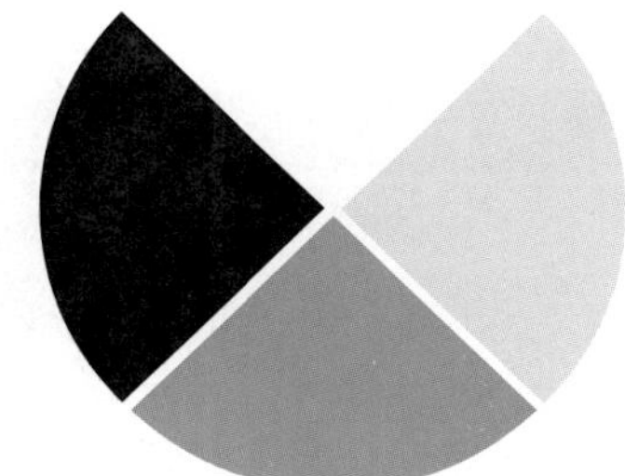

CRITICAL VIEW

Marina has noticed that Sarah is able to explain her work when they meet one on one but seems reluctant to present the same ideas at the group planning meetings. Marina wants Sarah to practise her leadership skills at these meetings. She wonders whether Sarah's hesitation to speak is a personal characteristic or whether there are cross-cultural influences at play. Having read the framework for First Nations, Inuit, and Métis nursing, Marina is intrigued by the emphasis on providing a culturally safe environment for learning (ANAC, 2009). Traditionally, nurses have been encouraged to be sensitive to cultural influences on health behaviour and respect different ways of knowing. However,

(Continued)

CRITICAL VIEW—Cont'd

some argue that culture is socially constructed, arising within a historical context and maintained by complex power relationships, which are not readily visible and can serve to marginalize people (Gray & Thomas, 2006; Smith, Edwards, Varcoe, Martens, & Davies, 2006; Smylie, Williams, & Cooper, 2006). They argue that it is not sufficient to merely accommodate differences because it can perpetuate inequities. They recommend that nurses question how cultural differences have arisen, what purpose they serve, and how they are perpetuated in order to take action and provide a health care environment where different cultures can feel safe and begin to shape a system responsive to their needs.

1. How might Marina convey her observations to Sarah and provide a culturally safe environment to explore this situation?
2. A grocery store in the city wants to donate day-old doughnuts to the physical activity program. Discuss the pros and cons of accepting this offer.

ACTION AND EVALUATION

Anna provided a progress report to the network meeting in town. Shania, Susan, and the CHR attended the meeting for information and to get to know the partners. Anna had put together their ideas in a logic model, described below. The logic model (see Table 18-3) identifies three components to the program: partnership building, skill development, and physical activity classes. It also links the main activities under each component with the intended results. This overview is intended to help everyone concerned to understand how the program is supposed to work. It will also guide actions and allow different people to be involved in the delivery of the program without losing direction (Health Canada, 1996).

Evaluation Report

The physical activity program—Walk the Talk—was delivered over 6 weeks in the early fall, almost as planned but with one or two adjustments to accommodate delays and unexpected findings from the initial focus group. An interim program evaluation was conducted after the final session. The findings from this evaluation provided

TABLE 18-3 Physical Activity Program Logic Model

Community Capacity Building to Increase Wellness in an Aboriginal Community			
Components	**Partnership Building**	**Skill Development**	**Physical Activity Classes**
Priority group	Urban and rural community groups and organizations	First Nations women living on and off reserve	First Nations women, aged 25–70, living on reserve
Activities	Build partnerships with urban and rural groups and organizations to encourage physical activity	Recruit women to project steering committee and build skills: • Organizational skills • Exercise leadership skills	Recruit 10–15 participants: • Advertisements in community store, • Community radio, and • Word of mouth
	Engage community groups: a) On reserve: • Presentation to chief and council • Community information session b) Urban	Engage women in project steering-group activities: • Arrange meetings at convenient time and place • Encourage participation by being friendly and informal • Seek feedback on what works and what does not	Eliminate or reduce barriers to participation: • Offer sessions in an easily accessible location, at minimal cost to participants • Provide opportunity for socialization • Conduct a focus group with participants to identify needs, interests, and the perceived barriers to participation • Customise the program to the needs of women on the reserve

TABLE 18-3 Physical Activity Program Logic Model—Cont'd

Community Capacity Building to Increase Wellness in an Aboriginal Community			
Components	**Partnership Building**	**Skill Development**	**Physical Activity Classes**
	Develop communication strategy to keep community partners informed	Train women as exercise leaders	Engage women in a 6-week, 2-hour/week fitness program that • Builds fitness and skills • Provides health information (e.g., nutrition, proper footwear, traditional practices), and • Is fun
Process indicators	Community participation • Number and type of community meetings • Number of organizations or sectors involved	Planning team established • Number of Aboriginal women on planning team • Meetings every 2–4 weeks, documented in minutes	Fitness program in progress • Number of women recruited • Number of women participating per session
Short-term outcomes		• Perceived benefit to being a member of the steering group and training as exercise leader and suggestions for improvement (focus group)	Participants have • Increased engagement in a regimen of physical activity • Increased awareness of risk factors for poor health and chronic disease such as diabetes (low level of physical activity and poor nutrition) Program tailored to needs: Number and description of: • Customizing strategies • Barriers identified and addressed
Intermediate outcomes		Community leaders: • Women with necessary skills to sustain physical-activity initiatives in their respective communities	Participants: • Increased participation in physical activity • Reduced social isolation
Long-term outcomes	• Increased fitness and well-being of community members • Decreased risk factors for chronic disease • Increased community capacity • Environment supportive of members being physically active		

feedback on the program and a baseline measurement on physical activity levels for the second session (see Table 18-4).

The evaluation plan was derived from the logic model but took into consideration that the program was being implemented in stages and that some components might take longer to implement than others. The planning group determined the questions that were important to answer at this point:

1. Was the First Nations community engaged in decision making about the program?
2. Was the physical activity program implemented as planned?

3. How were barriers to access identified and resolved?
4. To what extent did the program achieve its goals?

The planning group identified indicators of success for each question and located or developed tools to gather the required information.

In keeping with the capacity-building intent of the program, the Aboriginal women on the planning group were involved in designing the evaluation. In addition, they helped to gather and interpret the data, and played a key role in presenting the findings to the fitness group and at a community meeting. The results of the evaluation are summarized by question in Table 18-4.

The lessons learned and recommendations for future programs were shared with the health committee and at a community meeting. One unanticipated result from the physical activity program generated much discussion. Two or three participants had arranged to walk together on the weekends. They used the pedometers provided by the exercise group to keep track of their mileage, and the gadgets

TABLE 18-4 Walk the Talk Program Evaluation Plan

Question	Project Activity/Indicator of Success	Evaluation Tool	Who Has the Information?
Was the First Nations community engaged in decision making about the program?	• Three First Nations women were recruited to the planning group and participated in the development and evaluation of the program. • The women represented two First Nations community organizations (health committee and school board). • The women said they found the steering group meetings long at times but felt they had been able to contribute more with each meeting and were satisfied with the decision-making process. • Women from the reserve were consulted on the design of the activity program. • Community leaders were kept informed about the project.	• Steering group minutes • Steering group meeting evaluation	Steering group chair • The minutes record meeting attendance, key discussion points, outcomes, and action items. • At the end of each meeting, the chair sought feedback on the meeting, going around the table. Everyone preferred this to completing an evaluation form (Diem & Moyer, 2005).
Was the physical activity program implemented as planned?	• The classes were advertised in the store and on the radio but most people heard about them from their friends and family.	• Poster • Radio announcement • Registration feedback	Steering group chair • Recruitment successes and challenges were tracked and recorded in the meeting minutes.
	• The CHR led the classes with assistance from the nursing student and two First Nations women recruited and paid as volunteer helpers. • Twelve women registered for the classes; 9 of the women completed the session; 3 women had dropped out by week 3, one because her child was ill, the others because they found the exercises too strenuous. • The exercise portion of the class was followed as planned. Different types of exercises were added for variety, e.g., dance routines. • The social gatherings after class were well attended.	• Exercise class record	CHR/project coordinator • The CHR tracks the number of women attending each session and make notes of any changes to the program.

TABLE 18-4 Walk the Talk Program Evaluation Plan—Cont'd

Question	Project Activity/Indicator of Success	Evaluation Tool	Who Has the Information?
Were the barriers to access identified and addressed?	• The results of the focus group at the end of week 1 were used to tailor the program. • The main barrier to participation was identified as the lack of child care. Women were encouraged to bring their children to the class but it meant they might have to temporarily leave the group to attend to them. Once or twice a sitter was available.	• Focus group summary of barriers • Steering group minutes • Program adaptation	Project coordinator Steering group chair
Did the program achieve its goal?	• At the 6-week focus group (9 participants), women said they felt they had benefited from the group and were more active. • They found the health information sessions interesting, appreciated the attempts to bring in traditional practices, and suggested additional topics for discussion. • All women said the social activities were enjoyable and kept them coming back.	Focus group summary	Project coordinator

CHR = Community health representative.

had generated a lot of interest from families. Everybody wanted one! Before long, there was talk about a "community walk" around the lake. The old path around the lake had become overgrown, so the community planned to get together one weekend to clear it. The exercise group was a small beginning, but it was starting to bring the community together and build in sustainability.

CRITICAL VIEW

1. Compare the capacity-building approach to the *Canadian Community Health Nursing Standards of Practice* and the values and beliefs (Appendix 1). What is the same? What is different?
2. a) Select a health promotion model, theory, or framework from Chapter 4 of this textbook.
   b) What are the implications of using this model, theory, or framework for the physical activity program described above.
3. What are examples of one or two focus group questions that might be used to generate discussion about tailoring physical activity to cultural needs.

SECTION B: MENTAL HEALTH STORIES FOR REFLECTION AND DISCUSSION

The first part of this chapter dealt with applying community health nursing skills to improve the wellness of a specific aggregate—a Canadian Aboriginal community. In this next section, we will focus on applying community health nursing skills, particularly reflective thinking, to situations involving the aggregate of persons with mental health challenges. Some of the following case studies pertaining to mental illness have questions, and other case studies ask for reflection.

DEINSTITUTIONALIZATION

Deinstitutionalization of individuals with mental health conditions has been part of mental health reform. One of the community mental health nurse's (CMHN) clients who has schizophrenia lives in a residence specializing in the care of mentally ill clients. The residence is located in a small suburban area where there has been an influx of young families with children. There have not been any incidents involving the residents, who use local services along with other members of the community. Unfortunately, local residents have recently begun to actively lobby to have the mental health residence removed from its current location.

1. Discuss the issues that may be affecting this community's current action.
2. What are the broad implications of this community's action for the individuals who live in this residence?
3. What strategies could the CMHN and her employer use to advocate for the continued integration of mentally ill clients in the community?

MENTAL ILLNESS AND THE FAMILY

Nancy, 35 years of age, is married with two young children. She was diagnosed with bipolar illness 10 years ago and has been stable with medication therapy and ongoing psychiatric care.

She and her husband recently moved into the area and were seeking primary health care. An application to a local family health team resulted in her husband and children being accepted. However, the physician at the clinic declined her application, stating that her care was too complex and he would not be able to accept her into the practice. Nancy reports what has occurred to her CMHN.

1. Discuss the ongoing effects of the stigma of mental illness and its potential impact on Nancy's care.
2. What are some possible impacts of Nancy's illness on family roles and functions?
3. What opportunities exist for the mental health nurse to intervene in this situation?
4. Discuss "shared care" as a strategy to increase the comfort and skill of primary health care providers in providing mental health care.
5. What would be the advantages and disadvantages of an interdisciplinary/interprofessional team approach in this client situation? Support your answer(s).

MENTAL HEALTH ISSUES IN YOUNG ADULTHOOD

Ayana, 20 years old, is a first-year university student from Ethiopia, studying business. A roommate brings her to the Canadian Mental Health Association, concerned about her recent change in behaviour. She hasn't been to classes or showered in 2 weeks and has been staying in her bedroom with the curtains closed. Her roommate also described some peculiar behaviour, including mumbling and peeking out through the curtains.

1. What are some possible medical and psychiatric diagnoses that the CMHN might consider?
2. What questions in the history should be asked of Ayana and her roommate to validate the CMHN nursing hunches?
3. Since Ayana's family does not live in the country, the CMHN takes her to the local emergency department where she is "cleared" of any medical illness. A psychiatrist assesses her briefly but is unable to admit her to hospital due to lack of beds and places her on a waiting list for admission, which may take over a week. What plans should the CMHN make for the care of this young woman in the interim? Be specific.
4. What community resources should the CMHN refer Ayana to?
5. In this situation, how could the CMHN apply the Ottawa Charter strategies of strengthening community action and building healthy public policy?

HOMELESSNESS AND MENTAL HEALTH ISSUES

Hank is a 64-year-old Aboriginal man who has been living on the streets in a large urban centre for the last 5 years. He lost his job as a truck driver and remained unemployed. His wife divorced him and left him penniless. Hank comes to the street health clinic with an open ulcer on his right lower leg. His affect is flat; he has little to say and merely grunts yes or no to questions. His blood pressure is elevated at 208/102. Hank, without any regular primary health care, has two immediate health care concerns. The CHN conducts a holistic biopsycho-socioenvironmental assessment of Hank's health.

1. What other priorities does the CHN identify?
2. What are the social determinants of health having an impact on Hank's health?
3. In reference to the *Canadian Community Health Nursing Standards of Practice,* what are the relevant CHN interventions?
4. Considering the social determinants of health, what are the opportunities for advocating for Hank's health and his overall situation?

WORKING WITH A COMMUNITY GROUP EXPERIENCING MENTAL HEALTH ISSUES

Salim, a CMHN at a mental health agency, has been assigned to develop and facilitate a substance abuse recovery support group for an 8-week period, offered four times a year. The target population includes clients, ages 20 to 65, who experience depression or bipolar disorder and substance abuse. Enrollment will be limited to 15 participants per group. The CMHN, although experienced in dealing with mental illness, has limited experience leading group sessions.

1. What strategies can the CMHN use to engage members of this newly formed group?
2. What partners might the CMHN involve in working with this group? Explain why this would be important.
3. What can the CMHN do to promote group effectiveness?
4. According to the Consumer Survivor Initiative, what are the individual benefits of participation in this type of therapy?

STUDENT EXPERIENCE

Patrick, 33 years old, was referred to the mental health clinic by his CHN, who is one of the mental health professionals at the local branch of the Canadian Mental Health Association (CMHA).

Reflective Thinking: I wonder if the CHN involved Patrick in the decision making about this referral? I wonder about Patrick's level of functioning and his capacity to be involved?

When he was initially referred, he was homeless and without any financial resources. He had sustained a head injury 10 years ago, causing him to lose his previous job as a factory worker due to gait instability and cognitive impairment, placing him in a very vulnerable position.

Reflective Thinking: Unemployment and poverty contribute to homelessness.

He was living from couch to couch with people who would take him in.

Reflective Thinking: This type of homelessness is often referred to as hidden homelessness.

He had no sustainable income and was not aware of how to access assistance.

Reflective Thinking: Possible feelings of helplessness.

He had subsequently developed a major depression. The CHN recognized that mental health issues can be the result of poor living conditions, poverty, and inability to access appropriate health care. Acting as an advocate for Patrick, the CHN helped him find temporary housing at a local institution, food from the local food bank, and clothing from a local service agency

Reflective Thinking: These are social determinants of health that a CHN can assist with.

An application was completed for social assistance and, eventually, a disability pension.

Reflective Thinking: If he has money, then his food insecurity may no longer be an issue and he may be able to find affordable housing.

The CHN referred him for intensive case management with CMHA and ongoing counselling. He was referred to the primary health care clinic to rule out any physical illness and also to psychiatry to begin antidepressant therapy. Physiotherapy and occupational therapy were also engaged in dealing with his physical disabilities.

Reflective Thinking: How long will all these referrals take? Were the steps of the referral process followed? Who will fulfill the case manager role? I wonder if an interdisciplinary/interprofessional or multidisciplinary team approach will be used? Without the intervention of the CHN in dealing with Patrick's complex care needs, he would likely have succumbed to his vulnerable status, living homeless, in a large urban centre.

1. Carefully read the above client situation, focusing on the examples of *Reflective Thinking.*
2. Review the following three client situations (**Situations 1, 2, and 3**).
3. Identify your *Reflective Thinking* for each of these client situations.
4. Share your *Reflective Thinking* with your classmates.

Situation 1. Janine, 36 years old, with no primary health care provider, came to the clinic to be interviewed as a new client. Her primary diagnosis was clinical depression. Her husband and three children, who are very healthy, had been accepted by another physician in the community. However, this physician advised Janine that he could not accept her as a patient because her care was "too complicated." The Primary Health Care Nurse Practitioner accepted her to the family health team clinic and encouraged her family to move to this new practice as well. This decision was based on the knowledge that individuals who have mental health issues are vulnerable to destabilization without appropriate medical and psychiatric care. The stigma of mental illness also complicates the individual's ability to participate

(Continued)

STUDENT EXPERIENCE—Cont'd

in society. She was quite relieved, although she had been understandably upset that she had been refused care due to her mental illness. She felt that having her family stay with the previous primary health care provider would only make her worry about the quality of care they would receive, particularly if they needed complex care, considering that the physician had admitted that he did not want to provide care to complicated cases.

What is your reflective thinking?

Situation 2. Charlene, a 42-year-old female, was accepted to the primary health care clinic after referral from the CMHN of the local branch of CMHA. Charlene, who has been divorced twice, is the single mother of two teenage daughters. In spite of several hospitalizations over the years, with severe episodes of both mania and depression, she had managed to keep her family together and provide support to her daughters with some help from her mother, who lived at a distance. Although receiving financial disability support due to her illness, she did work 2 days per week at a residence for individuals incapacitated by severe and persistent mental illness. She found this work gratifying as she shared her compassion and experience with these individuals. Two years after Charlene's initial referral, she came to the office to report that her eldest daughter was demonstrating symptoms of mania. She was subsequently diagnosed with bipolar disorder. There were many exacerbations, hospitalizations, varying levels of adherence to a therapeutic regimen, and chaos in their home. Within a year after this, her daughter became pregnant and gave birth to a beautiful baby girl. While a happy event on one level, it created further distress in an already stressed family. Finally, a year later, the youngest daughter began exhibiting all the signs of bipolar disorder, with the diagnosis confirmed for her as well. Charlene, with the ongoing support of the CMHN from the CMHA along with regular visits to the physician, psychiatrist, nurse practitioner, and social worker of the primary health care team, maintained a sense of balance during the stressful periods of her life. Charlene credits the interdisciplinary/interprofessional team approach for her success in maintaining her family, engaging in meaningful work, and achieving balance in her mental health.

What is your reflective thinking?

Situation 3. A Mexican Mennonite family, consisting of the mother Agatha, father Jacob, and six children ranging in ages from 2 months to 18 years of age, moved to Canada for employment. Agatha had not been coping well since her parents were killed in a tragic car accident 2 years earlier, and was experiencing low motivation and mood, which seriously affected her ability to care for herself and her family. The local Mennonite community social meeting place provides space for the local community nursing agency case manager to come and assist families in accessing health care. Jacob came with Agatha to discuss her current health. The case manager conducted a health assessment and made a referral to the local health care centre for access to primary health care. A referral was also made by the case manager to the local CMHA branch for mental health assessment and access to intensive case management by a CMHN and counselling. Additional referrals were made to local community programs such as the public health program for Healthy Babies and parenting classes. The physician, in collaboration with a nurse practitioner at the primary health care clinic, after ensuring that there were no medical illnesses such as hypothyroidism or anemia, which might aggravate or imitate depression and anxiety, ordered antidepressant and anti-anxiety medications. The community nursing agency case manager maintained contact with the CMHN from the CMHA in planning care and coordinating referrals until Agatha's mental health became stable and the family's situation improved. Access to primary health care, specialized mental health services, and community programs was crucial in improving the health status and quality of life for Agatha and her family.

What is your reflective thinking?

TOOL BOX

evolve

The Tool Box contains useful instruments that can be applied in community health nursing practice. These related resources are found either in the appendices at the back of this book or on the Evolve Web site at http://evolve.elsevier.com/Canada/Stanhope/community/.

Appendices

- Appendix 1: Canadian Community Health Nursing Standards of Practice

Tools

Mining Watch Canada. *Mining and Health: A Community-Centred Health Assessment Toolkit.* This community-centred health assessment tool kit is the result a project to facilitate the assessment of the health of a community for communities that have mining as one of their major industries. The tool kit provides "steps" and "tools" that will facilitate the health assessment process.

WEBLINKS

evolve

Direct links to these resources can be found on the text's accompanying Evolve Web site at http://evolve.elsevier.com/Canada/Stanhope/community.

Carleton University. *Native Dance.* This site provides information on the Native dance Web project, which is a diverse dialogue on culture, history, and traditional knowledge with Aboriginal cultural partners, educational institutions, government, and private industry. "With over 100 videos of original footage, and over 900 new images, Native Dance contains a wealth of information on Dance Traditions from coast to coast in Canada." Menus are provided to choose videos for visually experiencing Native dance.

Health Canada. *Community Health Needs Assessment: A Guide for First Nations and Inuit Health Authorities.* This site provides general information for planners working with First Nations and Inuit communities to conduct a community health needs assessment. It describes how to plan, implement, evaluate, and share findings of a community health assessment. This guide is intended for use with First Nations and Inuit communities that are planning to take over responsibility for their own health programming and develop programs that are consistent with community values and beliefs.

Indian and Northern Affairs Canada (INAC). *First Nation Profiles Interactive Map.* This site is an interactive site that provides users the opportunity to click on a dot for a specific First Nations community to get connected to First Nation community information.

Ontario Aboriginal Diabetes Strategy. One of the strategies on this site is to provide a comprehensive and coordinated approach to diabetes prevention and management. This Web site provides some statistics on the prevalence of diabetes in Aboriginal peoples in Ontario.

Public Health Agency of Canada. *Handbook for Canada's Physical Activity Guide to Healthy Active Living.* This handbook was developed in partnership with the Canadian Society for Exercise Physiology. New guidelines are anticipated in early 2011. This handbook provides information about the importance of physical activity along with exercises and suggestions on how to lead a healthy active life.

Reading, J. *The Crisis of Chronic Disease Among Aboriginal Peoples: A Challenge for Public Health, Population Health and Social Policy.* A life course approach is described, focusing on the determinants of health to explore risk factors for diseases in Canadian Aboriginal peoples. The burden of various chronic diseases in Aboriginal peoples is also discussed.

Reading, J. *A Life Course Approach to the Social Determinants of Health for Aboriginal Peoples.* This site provides information on the disparities experienced by Aboriginal peoples and their cumulative influence on health. As well, it provides information on the prevalence and impact of chronic diseases such as tuberculosis, cardiovascular diseases, diabetes mellitus, and cancer in Aboriginal peoples.

REFERENCES

Aboriginal Nurses Association of Canada. (2009). *Cultural competence and cultural safety in nursing education. A framework for First Nations, Inuit and Métis nursing. Making it happen: Strengthening First Nations, Inuit and Métis health human resources*. Ottawa: Aboriginal Nurses Association of Canada.

Bartlett, J. G. (2003). Involuntary cultural change, stress phenomenon and Aboriginal health status. *Canadian Journal of Public Health, 94*(3), 165–166.

Bracht, N., Kingsbury, L., & Rissel, C. (1999). A five-stage community organization model for health promotion: Empowerment and partnership strategies. In N. Bracht (Ed.), *Health promotion at the community level: New advances* (2nd ed., pp. 83–104). Thousand Oaks, CA: Sage.

Camiletti, Y. A. (1996). A simplified guide to practising community-based/community development initiatives. *Canadian Journal of Public Health, 87*(4), 244–248.

Canadian Cancer Society, Manitoba Division. (2008). *Information package for evidence-informed interventions: Effective community and primary care physical activity interventions for adults*. Retrieved from http://www.cancer.ca/Manitoba/Prevention/MB-Knowledge%20Exchange%20Network/~/media/CCS/Manitoba/Files%20List/English%20files%20heading/pdf%20not%20in%20publications%20section/KEN%20-%20Adults%20Community-based%20Physical%20Activity_567321662.ashx.

Diabetes Prevention Program Research Group. (2002). Reduction in the incidence of type 2 diabetes with lifestyle intervention or metformin. *New England Journal of Medicine, 346*(6), 393–403.

Diem, E., & Moyer, A. (2005). *Community health nursing projects: Making a difference*. Philadelphia, PA: Lippincott Williams & Wilkins.

First Nations Centre. (2009). *Health information, research and planning: An information resource for First Nations health planners*. Ottawa: National Aboriginal Health Organization. Retrieved from http://www.naho.ca/firstnations/english/documents/HealthInformationResearchandPlanning_001.pdf.

Fletcher, F., McKennitt, D., & Baydala, L. (2007). Community capacity building: An Aboriginal exploratory case study. *Pimatisiwin: A Journal of Aboriginal and Indigenous Community Health, 5*(2), 9–32.

Frankish, C. J., Green, L. W., Ratner, P. A., Chomik, T., & Larsen, C. (1996). *Health impact assessment as a tool for population health promotion and public policy*. Vancouver: Institute of Health Promotion Research, University of British Columbia.

Gray, D. P., & Thomas, D. (2006). Critical reflections on culture in nursing. *Journal of Cultural Diversity*, 13(2), 76–82.

Hawe, P., King, L., Noort, M., Jordens, C., & Lloyd, B. (2000). *Indicators to help with capacity building in health promotion* (No. SHPN: 990099). North Sydney, NSW: Australian Centre for Health Promotion. Better Health Good Health Care.

Hawe, P., Noort, M., King, L., & Jordens, C. (1997). Multiplying health gains: The critical role of capacity-building within health promotion programs. *Health Policy, 39*, 29–42.

Health Canada. (1996, 2001-12-08 [Revised: April 17, 2000]). *Population health approach—Guide to project evaluation: A participatory approach*. Retrieved from http://www.phac-aspc.gc.ca/ph-sp/resources-ressources/guide/index-eng.php?option=print.

Howard-Grabman, L. (2007). *Demystifying community mobilization: An effective strategy to improve maternal and newborn health*. Washington, DC: US Agency for International Development's ACCESS Program.

Indian and Northern Affairs (INAC). (2010). *First nation profiles*. Retrieved from http://pse5-esd5.ainc-inac.gc.ca/fnp/Main/index.aspx?lang=eng.

Jeffery, B., Abonyi, S., Hamilton, C., Bird, S., Denechezhe, M., Lidguerre, T., & Whitecap, Z. (2006). *Community health indicators toolkit*. University of Regina and University of Saskatchewan. Retrieved from http://www.uregina.ca/fnh/Combined%20Domains%20-%20Jun-07.pdf.

Klomp, H., Dyck, R. F., & Sheppard, S. (2003). Description and evaluation of a prenatal exercise program for urban Aboriginal women. *Canadian Journal of Diabetes, 27*(3), 231–238.

Labonté, R., Muhajarine, N., Winquist, B., & Quail, J. (2009). *Healthy populations: A report of the Institute of Wellbeing*. Toronto: Institute of Wellbeing. Retrieved from http://www.ciw.ca/Libraries/Documents/HealthyPopulation_DomainReport.sflb.ashx.

Labonté, R., Woodard, G. B., Chad, K., & Laverack, G. (2002). Community capacity building: A parallel track for health promotion programs. *Canadian Journal of Public Health, 93*(3), 181–182.

Ling Yu, V., & Raphael, D. (2004). Identifying and addressing the social determinants of the incidence and successful management of type 2 diabetes mellitus in Canada. *Canadian Journal of Public Health, 95*(5), 366–368.

Lipscombe, L. L., & Hux, J. E. (2007). Trends in prevalence, incidence, and mortality in Ontario, Canada 1995–2005: A population-based study. *The Lancet, 369*(9563), 750–756.

MacLellan-Wright, M. F., Anderson, D., Barber, S., Smith, N., Cantin, B., Felix, R., & Raine, K. (2007). The development of measures of community capacity for community-based funding programs in Canada. *Health Promotion International, 22*(4), 299–306.

Minore, B., & Katt, M. (2007). Aboriginal health care in Northern Ontario. *Institute for Research on Public Policy Choices, 13*(6), 3–19.

Muin'iskw (Jean), Crowfeather, D. (2009). *Mik'maw spirituality—Talking circles*. Retrieved from http://www.muiniskw.org/pgCulture2c.htm.

Nagarajan, K. V. (2004). Rural and remote community health care in Canada: Beyond the Kirby Panel Report, the

Romanow Report and the federal budget of 2003. *Canadian Journal of Rural Medicine*, *9*(4), 245–251.

New South Wales Health Department. (2001). *A framework for building capacity to improve health* (No. SHPN: 990226). Sydney: New South Wales Health Department.

Public Health Agency of Canada. (2003). *The benefits of physical activity*. Retrieved from http://www.phac-aspc.gc.ca/pau-uap/fitness/benefits.html#2.

Public Health Agency of Canada. (2009). *Handbook for Canada's physical activity guide to healthy living*. Retrieved from http://www.phac-aspc.gc.ca/hp-ps/hl-mvs/pag-gap/pdf/handbook-eng.pdf.

Public Health Agency of Canada, Alberta/NWT Region. (2008). *Community capacity building tool*. Retrieved from http://www.phac-aspc.gc.ca/canada/regions/ab-nwt-tno/documents/CCBT_English_web_000.pdf.

Public Health Agency of Canada & Canadian Society for Exercise Physiology. (2002). *Handbook for Canada's physical activity guide to healthy active living*. Retrieved from http://www.phac-aspc.gc.ca/pau-uap/fitness/pdf/handbook_e.pdf.

Reading, J. (2009a). *A life course approach to the social determinants of health for Aboriginal peoples*. Retrieved from http://www.parl.gc.ca/40/2/parlbus/commbus/senate/com-e/popu-e/rep-e/appendixAjun09-e.pdf.

Reading, J. (2009b). *The crisis of chronic disease among Aboriginal peoples: A challenge for public health, population health and social policy*. Retrieved from http://www.cahr.uvic.ca/docs/ChronicDisease%20Final.pdf.

Registered Nurses' Association of Ontario (RNAO). (2010). *Strategies to support self-management in chronic conditions: Collaboration with clients*. Toronto, Canada: RNAO.

Running Wolf, P., & Rickard, J. A. (2003). Talking circles: A Native American approach to experiential learning. *Journal of Multicultural Counseling and Development*, *31*, 39–43.

Sanmartin, C., & Gilmore, J. (2008). Diabetes: Prevalence and care practices [Electronic Version]. Catalogue no. 82-003-XPE. *Health Reports*, *19*, 5. Retrieved from http://www.statcan.gc.ca/pub/82-003-x/2008003/article/10663-eng.pdf.

Smith, D., Edwards, N., Varcoe, C., Martens, P. J., & Davies, B. (2006). Bringing safety and responsiveness into the forefront of care for pregnant and parenting Aboriginal people. *Advances in Nursing Science Philosophy and Ethics*, *29*(2), E27–E44.

Smith, R., & Lavoie, J. (2008). First Nations health networks: A collaborative system approach to health transfer. *Health Care Policy*, *4*(2), 101–112.

Smylie, J., Williams, L., & Cooper, N. (2006). Culture-based literacy and Aboriginal health. *Canadian Journal of Public Health*, *97*(Suppl. 2), S21–S25.

Statistics Canada. (2004). *A profile of Canada's North American Indian population with legal Indian Status*. Ottawa: Statistics Canada. Retrieved from http://www.aboriginalroundtable.ca/sect/stscan/NAI_Status_e.pdf.

Statistics Canada. (2006a). *Table 1. Aboriginal identity population by age groups, median age and sex and Table 3. Aboriginal identity population, 2006 counts, percentage distribution, percentage change and sex. Aboriginal Peoples Highlight Tables, 2006 Census*. from http://www12.statcan.ca/english/census06/data/highlights/Aboriginal/index.cfm?Lang=E.

Statistics Canada. (2006b). *2006 community profiles*. Retrieved from http://www12.statcan.gc.ca/census-recensement/2006/dp-pd/prof/92-591/index.cfm?Lang=E.

Targeting high-risk populations in the fight against diabetes. (2007). *The Lancet*, *369*(9563), 716.

Young, T. K., & Katzmarzyk, P. T. (2007). Physical activity of Aboriginal people in Canada. *Canadian Journal of Public Health*, *98*, 148–160.

Glossary

Absolute homelessness Refers to those people who are perpetually homeless, sometimes referred to as the chronic homeless.

Absolute poverty Individuals and families who are unable to financially meet their basic needs for the necessities of life such as food, clothing, and shelter.

Accountability Answering to someone (client, profession, and society) for one's own professional actions with another; acting in a manner consistent with professional responsibilities and standards of practice.

Acid rain A pollutant found in the environment, consisting of unusually acidic precipitation caused by emissions of sulphur dioxide and nitrogen oxides.

Acquired immunity The resistance acquired by a host as a result of previous natural exposure to an infectious agent; may be induced by passive or active immunization.

Acquired immunodeficiency syndrome (AIDS) A syndrome that can affect the immune and central nervous systems and cause infections or cancers. It is caused by human immunodeficiency virus (HIV).

Action research A systematic study of practice interventions.

Active immunization The immunization of an individual by the administration of an antigen to stimulate active response by the host's immunologic system, resulting in complete protection against a specific disease.

Advocacy Actions one undertakes on behalf of another and are taken to influence decision makers, in communities and governments, to support a policy or cause that is health promoting.

Ageism The term used for discrimination toward older people because of their age.

Agent Causative factor invading a susceptible host through an environment favourable to produce disease, such as a biological or chemical agent; part of the epidemiological triangle.

Aggregate Groups within a population.

Aging The total of all changes that occur in a person with the passing of time.

Allophones People whose first language is neither French or English.

Analytical epidemiology A form of epidemiology that investigates causes and associations between factors or events and health.

Anthrax An acute disease caused by the spore-forming bacterium *Bacillus anthracis.*

Assessment A systematic appraisal of type, depth, and scope of health concerns as perceived by clients, health providers, or both.

Asset mapping Capturing community-based initiatives such as community development, strategic planning, and organizational development.

Behavioural risk The pattern of personal health habits that defines individual and family health status.

Beneficence A principle that is complementary to nonmaleficence and requires that we "do good." We are limited by time, place, and talents in the amount of good we can do. We have general obligations to perform those actions that maintain or enhance the dignity of other persons whenever those actions do not place an undue burden on health care providers. Health care professionals have special obligations of beneficence to clients.

Best practices The application of best available evidence to improve practice.

Bioethics A branch of ethics that applies the knowledge and processes of ethics to the examination of ethical problems in health care.

Biological risk A potential health danger for a person who may be prone to certain illnesses because of inherited genetics or family lifestyle patterns.

Built environment Anything physical in the environment that is built or produced by humans.

Canadian Nurses Association (CNA) A national association for registered nurses in Canada whose role is to advocate for nursing and health issues.

Canadian Public Health Association (CPHA) A national organization founded in 1912 to facilitate interdisciplinary efforts to promote health for Canadians.

Canadian Red Cross A national organization founded to reduce human suffering through various health, safety, and disaster-relief programs in affiliation with the International Red Cross.

Capacity building A process that relies strongly on collaboration and partnerships. Building capacity ensures that partners develop the skills and resources required to hold programs together, thereby increasing their chances for long-term success.

Care coordination An essential indirect function that involves linking clients with services.

Care planning The CHN and clients working together to provide adequate health care service at home.

Case fatality rate The proportion of persons diagnosed with a specific disorder who die within a specified period of time.

Case management Linking clients with services and providing direct nursing services including teaching, counselling, screening, and immunizing.

Case manager A CHN who works to enhance continuity and provide appropriate care for clients whose health concerns are actually or potentially chronic and complex.

Centre for Emergency Preparedness and Response (CEPR) A federal government agency under the jurisdiction of the Public Health Agency of Canada. This centre is responsible for coordinating services required to handle all health risk and security threats in Canada.

Certification A mechanism, usually by means of written examination, that provides an indication of professional competence in a specialized area of practice.

Change agent A nursing role that facilitates change in client or agency behaviour to more readily achieve goals. This role stresses gathering and analyzing facts and implementing programs.

Change partner A nursing role that facilitates change in client or agency behaviour to more readily achieve goals. This role includes the activities of serving as an enabler-catalyst, teaching problem-solving skills, and being an advocate.

Chlamydia A sexually transmitted infection caused by the organism *Chlamydia trachomatis,* which causes infection of the urethra and cervix. Infections may be asymptomatic and if untreated result in severe morbidity.

Circular communication Communication between people where each person influences the behaviour of the other.

Client Refers to individuals, families, groups or aggregates, communities, populations, or society.

Climate change A change in weather patterns over time in a geographic area that is related to changes in the amount of greenhouse gases; can be the result of natural or human-made causes or created by humans.

Coalition Groups who share a mutual issue or concern and join forces to attain a common goal in reference to addressing the issue.

Code of ethics A framework of moral standards that delineate a profession's values, goals, and obligations.

Collaboration The commitment of two or more partners such as agency, client, or professional who are in a power-sharing partnership.

Collaborative client-centred practice The active involvement of health care professionals from various disciplines working together collaboratively to improve client health outcomes.

Commendations Praises from the health professional to the family for patterns in behaviour that are family strengths within the family unit.

Common vehicle Transportation of the infectious agent from an infected host to a susceptible host via water, food, milk, blood, serum, saliva, or plasma.

Communicable disease A disease of human or animal origin caused by an infectious agent and resulting from the transmission of that agent from an infected person, animal, or inanimate source to a susceptible host. Infectious disease may be communicable or noncommunicable (e.g., tetanus is infectious but not communicable).

Communicable period The interval during which an infectious agent may be transferred from an infected source directly or indirectly to a new host.

Communitarianism Refers to abstract, universal principles that are not an adequate basis for moral decision making. History, tradition, and concrete moral communities should be the basis of moral thinking and action.

Community In the context of community health nursing, people and the relationships that emerge among them as they develop and commonly share agencies, institutions, and a physical environment; members may be defined in terms of geography or special interests.

Community capacity An approach used by CHNs that identifies and works with community strengths to promote a positive view of the community.

Community competence Linked to community problem-solving ability and empowerment. A competent community is able to use its problem-solving abilities to identify and deal with community health issues.

Community development A process whereby community members identify health concerns/issues affecting their community that require development of capacity-building skills to bring about realization of the needed change; improving the health of the community by engaging the community in working toward community-identified needs.

Community forums A meeting, such as a townhall meeting, in which involved parties can gain an understanding of a particular issue of concern to them; they do not include decision making.

Community health Meeting collective needs by identifying health concerns and strengths and managing behaviours within the community and between the community and the larger society.

Community health assessment The process of thinking critically about the community and getting to know and understand the community client as partner. Assessments help identify community health concerns and identify strengths and resources.

Community health concerns Are actual, potential, or possible health challenges within a target population with identifiable contributing factors in the environment.

Community health nursing An umbrella term that includes community health nurses working in a variety of practice areas, such as public health, home health, occupational health, and others.

Community health strengths Resources available to meet a community health concern.

Community mobilization The use of community capacity to bring about change through an action plan, usually developed and implemented with community partners.

Community partnership A collaborative decision-making process participated in by community members and professionals. It is crucial because community members and professionals who are active participants in such a process have a vested interest in the success of efforts to improve the health of their community.

Comprehensive services Health services that focus on more than one health problem or concern.

Confidentiality A situation in which the professional is obligated to not disclose specific client information.

Consequentialism An approach in which the right action is the one that produces the greatest amount of good or the least amount of evil in a given situation.

Contracting Making an agreement between two or more parties; involves a shift in responsibility and control toward a shared effort by client and professional as opposed to an effort by the professional alone. It is a vital component of all nurse–client relationships.

Corrections nurse Registered nurse who works in correctional facilities providing community health nursing interventions that include direct care, health promotion, disease prevention, inmate advocacy, and crisis intervention.

Cultural awareness Self-examination and in-depth exploration of one's own beliefs and values as they influence behaviour.

Cultural blindness A denial of diversity and the inability to recognize the uniqueness of individual clients.

Cultural competence A combination of culturally congruent behaviours, practice attitudes, and policies that allows nurses to work effectively in cross-cultural situations.

Cultural interpretation Provided by an interpreter, interpretation of the spoken word along with additional information about the culture

Cultural knowledge The information necessary to provide nurses with an understanding of the organizational elements of cultures and to provide effective nursing care.

Cultural nursing assessment A systematic way to identify the beliefs, values, meanings, and behaviours of people while considering their history, life experiences, and the social and physical environments in which they live.

Cultural safety Gaining an understanding of others' health beliefs and practices so that one's actions demonstrate working toward equity and the avoidance of discrimination. There is a recognition of and respect for cultural identity so that power balance exists between the health care provider and client recipient.

Cultural skill The effective integration of cultural knowledge and awareness to meet client needs.

Culture A set of beliefs, values, and assumptions about life that are widely held among a group of people and that are transmitted across generations.

Culture shock The feeling of helplessness, discomfort, and disorientation experienced by an individual attempting to understand or effectively adapt to another cultural group that differs in practices, values, and beliefs. It results from the anxiety caused by losing familiar sights, sounds, and behaviours.

Data collection The process of acquiring existing, readily available information or developing new information about the community and its health.

Data gathering The process of obtaining existing, readily available data.

Data generation The process of developing data that do not already exist, through interaction with community members, individuals, families, or groups. The data are frequently qualitative rather than numerical.

Database The combination of the gathered and generated data.

Demonstration project A project funded externally to promote the testing of ideas and hunches.

Denial A primary symptom of addiction to substances. Methods of denial include the following: lying about use, minimizing use patterns, blaming or rationalizing, intellectualizing, changing the subject, using anger or humour, and "going with the flow."

Deontology An ethical theory that bases moral obligation on duty and claims that actions are obligatory irrespective of the good or bad consequences that they produce. Because humans are rational, they have absolute value. Therefore, persons should always be treated as ends in themselves and never as mere means.

Descriptive epidemiology A form of epidemiology that describes a disease in terms of what, who, where, when, and why.

Determinants of health Factors that influence the risk for or distribution of health outcomes. They are income and social status, social support networks, education, employment and working conditions, social environments, physical environments, personal health practices and coping skills, healthy child development, biology and genetic endowment, health and social services, gender, and culture.

Directly observed therapy (DOT) A system of providing medications for persons with tuberculosis infection in which the client is monitored for taking the medication to maximize adherence to the treatment.

Disaster Any human-made or natural event that causes destruction and devastation that cannot be relieved without assistance.

Disaster preparedness A readiness to respond to and manage a disaster situation and its consequences.

Disaster prevention and mitigation Ongoing activities aimed at minimizing or eradicating risks of natural or human-made disasters before the disasters occur.

Disaster recovery Activities that focus on rebuilding to predisaster or near-predisaster conditions and on community safety so that the risk of a recurrence of the disaster is reduced.

Disaster response Activities that are carried out by emergency response teams consisting of police, firefighters, medical personnel, and others during and following a disaster.

Disaster vulnerability The chance that a disaster is likely to occur; considers the ability of a community to avoid or cope with potential disasters.

Discharge planning A nursing strategy or action to prevent health concerns from arising following discharge.

Disease The presence of abnormal alterations in the structure or functioning of the human body that fits within the medical model.

Disease course The identifiable progression of disease.

Disease prevention Refers to the activities taken by the health sector to prevent the occurrence of disease, to detect and stop disease development in those at risk, and to reduce the negative effects once a disease is established.

Distribution The pattern of a health outcome in a population; the frequencies of the outcome according to various personal characteristics, geographical regions, and time.

Distributive justice Requires that there be a fair distribution of the benefits and burdens in society based on the needs and contributions of its members. This principle requires that, consistent with the dignity and worth of its members and within the limits imposed by its resources, a society must determine a minimal level of goods and services to be available to its members. For community and public health professionals, this principle takes on considerable importance.

District nursing A system in early public health nursing in which a nurse was assigned to each district in a town to provide a wide variety of health services to needy people.

Diversity In the cultural context includes consideration of similarities and differences.

Downstream thinking Looking at individual health concerns and treatments without considering the sociopolitical, economic, and environmental variables. It is curative focused.

Dyke, Eunice A pioneer in public health nursing in Ontario who worked for the Toronto Department of Public Health starting in the early 1900s.

Ecological study A study that bridges descriptive and analytical epidemiology.

Ecomap Represents the family's interactions with other groups and organizations, accomplished by using a series of circles and lines.

Economic risk Determined by the relationship between family financial resources and the demands on those resources.

Educator A community health nurse who teaches clients or staff for the purpose of facilitating learning.

Elimination Focuses on removing a disease from a large geographical area such as a country or region of the world.

Emergency Measures Organization (EMO) A provincial or territorial organization that develops, coordinates, and manages all emergencies and disasters. There are provincial and territorial variations in the naming of these organizations.

Emerging infectious diseases Diseases in which the incidence has increased in the past two decades or has the potential to increase in the near future.

Empowerment A process that is used to actively engage the client to gain greater control and involves political efficacy, improved quality of community life, and social justice.

Enabling In the context of health promotion, taking action with clients to empower them by using resources so clients gain control over their health and environment in order to improve their health.

Endemic The rate of disease, injury, or other condition that is usually present in a population.

Engagement The beginning of the interview process with a family, where the focus is on the establishment of the nurse–client relationship.

Environment Part of the epidemiological triangle; all those factors internal and external to the client that constitute the context in which the client lives and that influence and are influenced by the host and agent interactions; the sum of all external conditions affecting the life, development, and survival of an organism.

Environmental epidemiology The study of the effect on human health of physical, chemical, and biological factors in the external environment.

Environmental health The achievement of health and wellness and the prevention of illness and injury from the exposure to physical and/or psychosocial environmental hazards.

Environmental justice From a population health perspective, efforts to reduce the impact of health inequalities and socioeconomic marginalization of persons resulting from environmental conditions affecting adequate nutrition, shelter, sanitation, and safe working conditions.

Environmental scan Assesses both the internal and external environments and is frequently used by researchers to assess population health issues; by organizations to develop, evaluate, and revise programs; and by policy makers to address social, economic, technological, and political issues.

Environmental standards Governmental guidelines or rules that impose limits on the amount of pollutants or emissions produced.

Epidemic A rate of disease clearly in excess of the usual or expected frequency in that population.

Epidemiological triangle A simple model that depicts the often-complex relationships among the agent, host, and environment.

Epidemiology Study of the distribution and factors that determine health-related states or events in a population and the use of this information to control health problems.

Equality Equal rights under the law, such as security, voting rights, freedom of speech and assembly, and the extent of property rights; also includes access to education, health care, and other social goods such as economic good and fundamental political rights, and equal opportunities and obligations; involves the whole society.

Equity In the context of health care, all persons will have the opportunity through equal access to reach full health potential.

Eradication The irreversible termination of all transmission of infection by extermination of the infectious agents worldwide.

Ethical decision making The component of ethics that focuses on the process of how ethical decisions are made. It involves making decisions in an orderly process that considers ethical principles, client values and abilities, and professional obligations.

Ethical dilemmas Puzzling moral problems in which a person, group, or community can envision morally justified reasons for both taking and not taking a certain course of action.

Ethical issues Moral challenges facing the nursing profession.

Ethics A branch of philosophy that includes both a body of knowledge about the moral life and a process of reflection for determining what persons ought to do or be, regarding this life.

Ethnicity Shared feeling of peoplehood among a group of individuals. It represents the identifying characteristics of culture (e.g., race, religion, national origin).

Ethnocentrism A type of cultural prejudice in which one believes that one's own cultural group is the best, is preferred, and is superior to others.

Ethnography Used to understand a culture from the emic perspective.

Evaluation The appraisal of the effects of some organized activity or program. Provision of information through formal means, such as criteria, measurement, and statistics, for making rational judgements necessary about outcomes of care.

Evidence-informed practice Combining the best evidence from research with clinical practice, knowledge and expertise, and client preferences or choices when making clinical decisions.

Experimental or intervention studies Include interventions to test preventive or treatment measures, techniques, materials, policies, or drugs. Community or clinical trials are examples of such studies conducted in community health.

Faith communities Distinct groups of people who acknowledge specific faith traditions and gather in churches, cathedrals, synagogues, or mosques.

Family Two or more individuals who depend on one another for emotional, physical, or financial support. Members of a family are self-defined.

Family caregiving Assisting clients to meet their basic needs and providing direct care such as personal hygiene, meal preparation, medication administration, and treatments.

Family crisis A situation whereby the demands of the situation exceed the resources and coping capacity of the family.

Family demographics The study of the structure of families and households and the family-related events, such as marriage and divorce, that alter the structure through their number, timing, and sequencing.

Family functions Behaviours or activities performed to maintain the integrity of the family unit and to meet the family's needs, individual members' needs, and society's expectations.

Family health A dynamic, changing, relative state of well-being that includes the biological, psychological, sociological, cultural, and spiritual factors of the family system.

Family nursing Nurses and families working together to ensure the success of the family and its members in adapting to responses to health and illness.

Family nursing assessment A comprehensive family data-collection process used to identify the health concerns facing the family. It is the cornerstone for family nursing interventions. Family strengths are emphasized as the building blocks for interventions.

Family nursing theory A theory whose function is to characterize, explain, or predict phenomena (events) evident within family nursing.

Family resiliency The ability of family members to cope with expected and unexpected stressors.

Family strengths Positive family behaviours or qualities that contribute to the health of families.

Family structure The characteristics and demographics (gender, age, number) of individual members who make up family units.

Family systems nursing model The Calgary Family Assessment Model focuses on the family unit as client and consists of a structural, developmental, and functional assessment of the family.

Feminine ethic A belief in the morality of responsibility in relationships that emphasize connection and caring.

Feminist ethics Knowledge and critique of classical ethical theories developed by men and women; it entails knowledge about the social, cultural, political, economic, environmental, and professional contexts that insidiously and overtly oppress women as individuals or within a family, group, community, or society.

Feminists Women and men who hold a world view advocating economic, social, and political statuses for women that are equivalent to those of men.

Focus group A group of individuals residing in the community who share their beliefs, opinions, and experiences about a selected discussion topic.

Forensic nurses Registered nurses who have additional education in forensic science in order to provide specialized care to persons who have experienced trauma or death from violence, criminal activity, or traumatic accidents.

Functional families Family units that provide autonomy and are responsive to the particular interests and needs of individual family members.

Genogram A pictorial illustration of three generations of family members with gender and age, their relationships, health status, and mortality.

Gerontological nursing The specialty of nursing concerned with assessment of the health and functional statuses of older adults, planning and implementing health care and services to meet the identified needs, and evaluating the effectiveness of such care.

Gerontology The specialized study of the processes of aging.

Global health A field of study, research, and practice that places a priority on improving health and achieving equity in health for all people worldwide.

Goals Generally broad statements of desired outcomes. The end or terminal point toward which intervention efforts are directed.

Gonorrhea A sexually transmitted infection caused by a bacterium, *Neisseria gonorrhoeae,* resulting in inflammation of the urethra and cervix and dysuria, or it may result in no symptoms.

Grounded theory A qualitative research method used for theory development.

Group A collection of two or more individuals in face-to-face interactions with a common purpose(s) and who are in an interdependent relationship.

Group process How a group as a unit is working and how group members interact with one another.

Hantavirus pulmonary syndrome (HPS) A respiratory disease, often fatal, that has struck young people.

Harm reduction Strategies such as implementing policies or programs to decrease the adverse health consequences of substance use often not requiring abstinence.

Harm reduction model A health care approach to address substance abuse problems by reducing the harm associated with drugs without requiring that all drug use cease.

Hazardous waste Any waste material that poses actual or potential harm to the environment and to humans.

Health A resource for everyday living that is holistic and includes physical, social, and personal capabilities, with health being viewed positively.

Health disparities The wide variations in health services and health status among certain population groups defined by specific characteristics.

Health enhancement A health promotion strategy that is used to increase health and resiliency to promote optimal health and well-being (the client can be at any point on the risk continuum).

Health inequities The principal causes of the disparities that are usually not within the typical domain of health, such as the social determinants; these social, economic, cultural, and political inequities result (directly or indirectly) in health disparities.

Health literacy Having the knowledge and skills to access, understand, evaluate, and communicate information and to make informed health decisions so as to promote, maintain, and improve health.

Health ministries Activities and programs in faith communities directed at improving the health and well-being of individuals, families, and communities across the lifespan.

Health program Consists of a variety of planned activities to address the assessed health concerns of clients over time and builds on client strengths in order to meet specific goals and objectives.

Health program evaluation process The systematic process of appraising all aspects of a program to determine its impact.

Health program implementation process The systematic process of appraising all aspects of a program to determine its impact.

Health program management Addresses health issues of populations and consists of four steps: assessing, planning, implementing, and evaluating a health program, in partnership with the client.

Health program planning process An organized approach to identifying and choosing interventions to meet specified goals and objectives that address client health concerns.

Health promotion The process of enabling people to increase control over the determinants of health and thereby improve their health.

Health protection Focuses on health maintenance by dealing with the immediate health risks.

Health risk appraisal The process of identifying and analyzing an individual's prognostic characteristics of health and comparing them with those of a standard age group, thereby providing a prediction of a person's likelihood of prematurely developing the health problems that have high morbidity and mortality in this country.

Health risk reduction The application of selected interventions to control or reduce risk factors and minimize the incidence of associated disease and premature mortality.

Health risks Factors that determine or influence whether disease or other unhealthy results occur.

Health surveillance "The tracking and forecasting of any health event or health determinant through the collection of data, and its integration, analysis and interpretation into surveillance products, and the dissemination of those surveillance products to those who need to know" (Network for Health Surveillance in Canada cited in Shah, 2003, p. 89).

Healthy community A community in which "people, organizations, and local institutions work together to improve the social, economic, and environmental conditions that make people healthy—the determinants of health" (Rural Communities Impacting Policy, 2006, p.1).

Healthy public policy A policy that is developed with the intent to have a positive effect on or to promote health in populations.

Hepatitis A virus (HAV) A virus that is transmitted by the fecal–oral route. The clinical course of hepatitis A ranges from mild to severe and often requires prolonged convalescence. Onset is usually acute, with fever, nausea, lack of appetite, malaise, and abdominal discomfort, followed after several days by jaundice.

Hepatitis B virus (HBV) A virus that is transmitted through exposure to infected body fluids. Infection results in a clinical picture that ranges from a self-limited acute infection to fulminant hepatitis or hepatic carcinoma, possibly leading to death.

Hepatitis C virus (HCV) A virus that is transmitted through exposure to infected blood and body fluids. Hepatitis C virus infection may present with such mild symptoms that it goes unrecognized.

Herd immunity Immunity of a group or community. The resistance of a group of people to the invasion and spread of an infectious agent.

Hidden homelessness Refers to those persons who may be sleeping in their vehicles and/or use the couch or other temporary sleeping cot at a friend's home.

HIV antibody test A laboratory test ELISA (enzyme-linked immunosorbent assay) that detects HIV antibodies.

Holistic care Care concerned with the body, mind, and spirit relationships of persons in an environment that is always changing.

Home visit Provision of community health nursing care where the client resides.

Horizontal transmission The person-to-person spread of infection through one or more of the following routes: direct or indirect contact, common vehicle, airborne, or vector borne.

Hospice Palliative system of health care for terminally ill persons. It can take place in the home with family involvement under the direction and supervision of health professionals, especially the home care nurse. Hospice care takes place in the hospital when severe complications of terminal illness occur or when the family becomes too exhausted to fulfill commitments.

Hospice care The delivery of palliative care of the very ill and dying, offering both respite and comfort.

Host A living species (human or animal) capable of being infected or affected by an agent.

Human-made disasters Destruction or devastation caused by humans.

Hypothesizing The development of a hunch based on information collected about the family that the community health nurse decides to explore further.

Illness An individual's personal experience of, perception of, and reaction to a disease whereby they are unable to function at their desired "usual" level.

Immigrant A person who has chosen to live in Canada and has been accepted by the Government of Canada and may apply for permanent residency.

Implementation Carrying out a plan that is based on careful assessment of health concerns. The fourth phase of the community health nursing process, which involves the work and activities aimed at achieving the goals and objectives. Implementation efforts may be made by the person or group who established the goals and objectives, or they may be shared with or even delegated to others.

Incidence rate The frequency or rate of new cases of an outcome in a population; provides an estimate of the risk of disease in that population over the period of observation.

Incubation period The time interval beginning with invasion by an infectious agent and continuing until the organism multiplies to sufficient numbers to produce a host reaction and clinical symptoms.

Indoor air quality A measure of the breathable air inside a habitable structure or conveyance. A measure of the chemical, physical, or biological contaminants in indoor air.

Infection The state produced by the invasion of a host by an infectious agent. Such infection may or may not produce clinical signs.

Infectiousness A measure of the potential ability of an infected host to transmit the infection to other hosts.

Influenza pandemic Occurs when a change in the Influenza A virus takes place, causing the development of a new strain against which people have little or no immunity.

Informant interviews Directed conversation with selected members of a community about community members or groups and events; a direct method of assessment.

Injury prevention Using strategies to help populations and individuals to prevent and reduce the risk of injury.

Interdependent The involvement among different groups or organizations within the community that are mutually reliant upon each other.

Interdisciplinary collaboration A working agreement in which health team members carefully analyze their role and work together to determine the best plan for a client's care.

Interdisciplinary team Team, often referred to as interprofessional, containing members with expertise from a variety of disciplines such as nurses, social workers, dietitians, physiotherapists, and physicians and that includes the client in the assessment, planning, implementation, and evaluation of client care.

Interpretation The process by which a spoken or signed message in one language is relayed, with the same meaning, in another language.

Intervention activities Means or strategies by which objectives are achieved and change is effected.

Intradisciplinary team In community health nursing, nurses working with other nurses.

Knowledge exchange Researchers and decision makers collaboratively problem solving so that research is planned, developed, disseminated, and applied.

Leadership Complex concept that consists of behaviours that guide or direct members and determine and influence group action; in a group context, the ability to influence and direct others; includes acts that assist the group to meets its goal(s) and influence group actions to maintain the group.

Linguistic interpretation Interpretation of the spoken word only.

Menopause A developmental stage in which the levels of the hormones estrogen and progesterone change in a woman's body.

Meta-analysis A technique that results in a summary statistic of the results when studies are comparable.

Metropolitan Life Insurance Company A life insurance company that also provided home nursing services for its beneficiaries and their families starting in 1909.

Monitoring The periodic or continuous surveillance or testing to determine the level of compliance with statutory requirements and/or pollutant levels in various media or in humans, plants, and animals.

Morals Shared and generational societal norms about what constitutes right or wrong conduct.

Morbidity The number of reported cases or occurrence of disease in a population.

Mortality The number of deaths in a population due to a disease.

Multiculturalism A belief that promotes recognition of diversity of citizens with respect to their ancestry and supports acceptance and belonging.

Multidisciplinary team Team made up of members who have expertise from a variety of disciplines such as nurses, social workers, dietitians, physiotherapists, and physicians working independently who come together to make client-based decisions.

Natural disasters Destruction or devastation caused by natural events.

Natural history of disease The course or progression of a disease process from onset to resolution.

Natural immunity Species-determined innate resistance to an infectious agent.

Negative predictive value Proportion of persons with a negative test who are disease free.

Neglect A lack of services that are necessary for the physical and mental health of an individual by the individual or a caregiver.

Newcomer A person who arrives in a new country to settle there for a variety of reasons and with a variety of background experiences.

Nightingale, Florence An English nurse who is credited with establishing nursing as a discipline.

Nonmaleficence A principle, according to Hippocrates, that requires that we do no harm. It is impossible to avoid harm entirely, but this principle requires that health care professionals act according to the standards of due care, always seeking to produce the least amount of harm possible.

Nonpoint source A diffuse pollution source (i.e., without a single point of origin or not introduced into a receiving stream from a specific outlet). The pollutants may be carried off the land by storm water. Examples of nonpoint sources are traffic, fertilizer or pesticide runoff, and animal wastes.

Nurse entrepreneur A CHN, a registered nurse who is self-employed in the provision of nursing services to clients in the home or in a variety of settings, such as workplaces, government agencies, not-for-profit agencies, and private businesses; may be generalists (e.g., a primary health care nurse practitioner working in an independent practice) or specialists (e.g., a nurse offering foot-care clinics).

Nurse practitioner A CHN, a registered nurse with a minimum of baccalaureate-level academic preparation and advanced practice nursing education, usually at a master's degree level.

Objectives A precise behavioural statement of the achievement that will accomplish partial or total realization of a goal; includes the date by which the achievement is expected to be completed.

Occupational and environmental health history Contains questions that provide the data necessary to rule out or confirm job-induced conditions and health concerns.

Occupational health nursing A specialty area within community health nursing with a focus on disease prevention, including rehabilitation and health promotion activities in the workplace.

Operational health planning A process that is used on a smaller scale and starts with a specific objective in relation to health program planning.

Outcome evaluation Makes a judgement about the results of a program. Also, it can be referred to as summative evaluation.

Outcomes The results or impact of program interventions.

Outpost nurse A CHN, a registered nurse who works in remote outpost communities.

Outrage The emotional public response to the perception of risk related to an environmental issue and where trust in authorities is weak.

Palliative care Alleviating the symptoms of, meeting the special needs of, and providing comfort for dying clients and their families by the CHN.

Pandemic A worldwide outbreak of an epidemic disease based on the rate of disease, injury, or other condition that exceeds the usual level in the population and is widespread geographically.

Parish nurses CHNs who respond to health and wellness needs within the faith context of populations of faith communities and are partners with the church in fulfilling the mission of health ministry.

Parish nursing A community-based and population-focused professional nursing practice with faith communities to promote whole-person health to its parishioners, usually focused on primary prevention.

Participant observation Conscious and systematic sharing in the life activities and occasionally in the interests and activities of a group of persons; observational methods of assessment; a direct method of data collection.

Participatory action research An action-oriented research technique used to develop client-centred interventions and services and to influence policy.

Partner notification A population-level intervention aimed at controlling communicable diseases that involves identifying and locating contacts of persons who have been diagnosed with a transmissible disease to notify them of exposure and encourage them to seek medical treatment.

Partnership A relationship between individuals, groups, or organizations, in which the partners are actively working together in all stages of planning, implementation, and evaluation.

Passive immunization Immunization by a transfer of a specific antibody from an immunized person to one who is not immunized.

Pastoral care staff Faith community leaders, including clergy, nurses, and educational and youth ministry staff.

PEEST An analysis of *p*olicies, *e*conomic climate, *e*nvironmental factors, *s*ocial (population and lifestyle trends) factors, and *t*echnological factors affecting a situation.

Person in need of protection A person who cannot return to his or her country because of personal safety reasons and has been given protection by the Government of Canada.

Phenomenology A qualitative research method used to understand the meaning of the lived experience.

Point epidemic A concentration in space and time of a disease event, such that a graph of frequency of cases over time shows a sharp point, usually suggestive of a common exposure.

Point source A stationary location or fixed facility from which pollutants are discharged; any single identifiable source of pollution (e.g., a pipe, ditch, ship, ore pit, factory smokestack).

Poisons Toxic substances that cause injury, illness, or death to humans and other organisms.

Population A large group or collection of people who share one or more personal or environmental characteristics.

Population health Determining the health of a population using the determinants of health and the health status indicators as measurements of health.

Population-focused practice Directs community health nursing practice with an emphasis on improving health inequalities to a defined population or aggregates compared with individual-level care.

Positive predictive value The proportion of persons with a positive screening or diagnostic test who do have the disease (the proportion of "true positives" among all who test positive).

Poverty Having insufficient financial resources to meet basic living expenses.

Precautionary principle Principle that suggests that when credible doubt exists, action should be on the side of caution.

Prejudice Negative attitudes about a person or group without factual data.

Prevalence rate Identifies the number of persons in a population who have a disease or experienced an event at a specific period.

Primary care Provides the first contact between individuals and the health care system and usually refers to the curative treatment of disease, rehabilitation, and preventive measures.

Primary caregiver The health care professional who is primarily responsible for providing for health care needs of clients.

Primary health care A model defined as essential health care based on practical, scientifically sound, and acceptable methods and technology made universally accessible to individuals and families in the community through their full participation and at a cost that the community and country can afford to maintain at every stage of their development, in the spirit of self-reliance and self-determination. Primary health care is comprehensive and addresses social justice and equity issues.

Primary prevention A type of intervention or activity that seeks to prevent disease from the beginning—before people have a disease; relates to the natural history of a disease.

Primordial prevention Activities to prevent risk factors for health issues from ever occurring through changes in the socioeconomic status of society.

Principlism An approach to problem solving in bioethics that uses the principles of respect for autonomy, beneficence, nonmaleficence, and distributive justice as the basis for organization and analysis.

Process evaluation An evaluation of a program or activity while it is in development. Also, it can be referred to as formative evaluation.

Proportion A type of ratio that shows the relationship between the total number and the frequency of occurrence in the case of a particular health event.

Proportionate mortality ratio The proportion of all deaths due to a specific cause.

Protective factors Variables, such as individual characteristics, family support systems, and environmental supports, that assist in managing the stressors associated with being at risk.

Psychoactive drugs Drugs that can alter emotions and are used for enjoyment in social and recreational settings and for personal use to self-medicate physical or emotional discomfort.

Public health What society collectively does to ensure that conditions exist in which people can be healthy; a scientific discipline that includes the study of epidemiology, statistics, and assessment as well as program planning and policy development.

Public health nursing Community health nursing with a distinct focus on and scope of practice; requires a specific knowledge base. Public health nursing is built on the blending of nursing and the discipline of public health. It is a practice that involves primary, secondary, and tertiary prevention, with a main focus on primary prevention, health surveillance, and at-risk populations. Public health nurses are employed by government agencies to deliver core public health services.

Qualitative research A research methodology that explores human experiences. It uses words, text, or themes rather than numbers to describe the experiences.

Quantitative research A research methodology that tests hypotheses and uses numbers to describe relationships, differences, and cause–effect interactions among variables.

Race Primarily a social classification that relies on physical markers such as skin colour to identify group membership. Individuals may be of the same race but of different cultures.

Racially visible People of colour. Synonym for the term *visible minority.*

Racism A prejudice in which one cultural group perceives itself to be superior to another cultural group.

Randomized controlled trials Research method to test the efficacy and safety of interventions. They must have a random sample, manipulation, and a control group.

Rate A measure of the frequency of a health event in a defined population during a specified period.

Rathbone, William A British philanthropist who founded the first district nursing association in Liverpool, England. With Florence Nightingale, he advocated for district nursing throughout England.

Referral process A systematic problem-solving approach involving a series of actions that help clients use resources for the purpose of resolving needs.

Refugee A person who has come to Canada, without choice, as a result of having to leave his or her country because of fear of persecution or war; also may include those living in a refugee camp.

Relative poverty Individuals and families whose income is considerably less than that of their peers.

Reliability The precision of a measuring instrument that depends on its consistency from one time of use to another and its accuracy.

Resiliency The ability of people to successfully cope when faced with a threat or hardship.

Resistance The ability of a host to withstand infection. It may involve natural or acquired immunity.

Respect for autonomy Based on human dignity and respect for individuals, autonomy requires that individuals be permitted to choose those actions and goals that fulfill their life plans unless those choices result in harm to another.

Risk The probability that a specific health problem will develop in a client because of exposure to certain factors within a specified period of time.

Risk assessment Qualitative and quantitative evaluation of the risk posed to human health and/or the environment by the actual or potential presence and/or use of specific pollutants.

Risk avoidance A disease prevention strategy that is used to avoid health problems and to remain at low risk level (the client is at no or low risk on the continuum).

Risk communication The exchange of information about health or environmental risks among, for example, risk assessors and managers, the general public, news media, and interest groups.

Risk factors Variables that create stress and therefore challenge the client's health status.

Risk management The reduction of risks by selecting and implementing strategies informed by the risk assessment process.

Risk reduction A disease prevention strategy that is used to reduce or alter health problems so the disease is detected and treated early to prevent moving to high risk level (the client is at low to moderate risk).

Rural Defined either in terms of the geographical location and population density or the distance from or time needed to commute to an urban centre.

Screening The application of a test to persons who are at risk for a certain condition but do not manifest any symptoms.

Secondary analysis An analysis using previously gathered data.

Secondary prevention Intervention that seeks to detect disease early in its progression (early pathogenesis) before clinical signs and symptoms become apparent in order to make an early diagnosis and begin treatment; relates to the natural history of a disease.

Sensitivity The extent to which a test identifies those individuals who have the condition being examined.

Setting for practice The community for the community health nurse.

Severe acute respiratory syndrome (SARS) A previously unknown disease of undetermined etiology and no definitive treatment that was reported in early 2003; it was associated with a new strain of coronavirus.

Sexual assault A term used instead of *rape;* refers to the following three levels—sexual assault, sexual assault with a weapon, and aggravated sexual assault.

Sexual assault nurse examiner (SANE) A CHN, a registered nurse who has completed specialized education in forensic science. They assume a wide range of roles and responsibilities in response to the physical, emotional, and psychological needs of persons who have experienced sexual assault, regardless of age or gender; they provide crisis intervention, assess injuries, provide pregnancy prevention by offering the morning-after pill, test for and treat STIs, and collaborate with community partners.

Sheltered homelessness Refers to those persons who need to use emergency shelters, either occasionally or regularly, for sleeping purposes.

Sink Any process, activity, or mechanism that removes a greenhouse gas, an aerosol, or a precursor of a greenhouse gas from the atmosphere.

Social determinants of health "The economic and social conditions that shape the health of individuals, communities, and jurisdictions as a whole. . . . Social determinants of health are about the quantity and quality of a variety of resources that a society makes available to its members" (Raphael, 2009, p. 3).

Social justice The fair distribution of society's benefits and responsibilities and their consequences. It focuses on the relative position of one social group in relation to others in society as well as on the root causes of disparities and what can be done to eliminate them.

Social risks Risky social situations that can contribute to the stressors experienced by families. If adequate resources and coping processes are not available, breakdowns in health can occur.

Society Systems that incorporate the social, political, economic, and cultural infrastructure to address issues of concern.

Specificity The extent to which a test identifies those individuals who do not have the disease or condition being examined.

Stereotyping The basis for ascribing certain beliefs and behaviours about a group to an individual without giving adequate attention to individual differences.

Strategic health planning Involves matching client needs, client and provider strengths and competencies, and resources.

Subjective poverty Individuals and families who perceive that they have insufficient income to meet their expenses.

Subpopulations Aggregates within the larger population.

Surveillance A systematic and ongoing observation and collection of data concerning disease occurrence to describe phenomena and detect changes in frequency or distribution.

Survey Method of assessment in which data from a sample of persons are reported to the data collector.

Sustainability The maintenance and continuation of established community programs.

SWOT A method of analysis which identifies strengths (S), weaknesses (W), opportunities (O), and threats (T) involved in a project or venture.

Systematic review A summary of the research evidence that relates to a specific question and to the effects of an intervention.

Team A specialized group working toward a common goal or activity.

Telehealth Health information sent from one site to another by electronic communication; the delivery of health care services over distance.

Telenurse A CHN who is a registered nurse with specific nursing knowledge and skill that includes enhanced assessment skills and strong clinical knowledge necessary to provide nursing service to clients using only information technology such as the telephone.

Termination phase When the purpose of the visit has been accomplished, the CHN reviews with the family what has occurred and what has been accomplished. This phase provides a basis for evaluating whether further home visits are needed or referrals to community resources are required.

Tertiary prevention Treatment and rehabilitation interventions that begin once the disease is obvious; the aim is to interrupt the course of the disease, reduce the amount of disability that might occur, and begin rehabilitation; relates to the natural history of a disease.

Testicular self-examination Self-examination of the testicles to assess for any unusual lumps or bumps.

Three *Ds* *D*ementia (progressive intellectual impairment), *d*epression (mood disorder), *d*elirium (acute confusion).

Transition The movement from one developmental or health stage or condition to another that may be a time of potential risk for families.

Translation The written conversion of one language into another.

Triage The process of separating casualties and allocating treatment based on the victims' potential for survival.

Upstream thinking A "big picture" approach. Community health nurses using upstream thinking would consider the determinants of health and other relevant economic, political, and environmental factors that may influence the health of the client.

Urban Geographical areas described as nonrural and having a higher population density.

Utilitarianism An ethical theory based on the weighing of morally significant outcomes or consequences regarding the overall maximizing of good and minimizing of harm for the greatest number of people.

Vaccine A preparation of killed microorganisms, living attenuated organisms, or living fully virulent organisms that is administered to produce or artificially increase immunity to a particular disease.

Validity The accuracy of a test or measurement; how closely it measures what it claims to measure. In a screening test, validity is measured by sensitivity and specificity.

Values Beliefs about the shared worth or importance of what is desired or esteemed within a society.

Vector A nonhuman organism, often an insect, that either mechanically or biologically plays a role in the transmission of an infectious agent from source to host.

Veracity Telling the truth; it is the nurse's duty to tell the truth. Veracity promotes trust in the nurse–client therapeutic relationship.

Vertical transmission The passing of an infection from parent to offspring via sperm, placenta, milk, or contact in the vaginal canal at birth.

Violence Those nonaccidental acts, interpersonal or intrapersonal, that result in physical or psychological injury to one or more persons. It can be physical, psychological, sexual, financial, or spiritual abuse.

Virtue ethics Asks, "What kind of person should I be?"; its goal is to enable persons to flourish as human beings.

Virtues Acquired, excellent traits of character that dispose humans to act in accord with their natural good.

Visible minority A term used by Statistics Canada to describe people of colour, that is, people who are neither Caucasian nor Aboriginal.

Visiting nurse associations Agencies staffed by nurses who provide care where the client needs it and most often in the home.

Visiting nurses CHNs who provide care wherever the client may be—home, work, or school.

Vulnerable populations Those groups who bear a greater "burden" of illness and distress than other groups.

Wald, Lillian The first public health nurse in the United States and an influential social reformer. One notable contribution was founding the Henry Street Settlement in New York.

Web of causation (also known as the web of causality) Complex interrelations of factors interacting with each other to influence the risk for or distribution of health outcomes.

Windshield survey Can be conducted by walking or driving through a community; it is an observational method used as a part of a community health assessment.

Women's health Health promotion, health protection or disease prevention, and health maintenance in adult women.

Work–health interactions The influence of work on health shown by statistics on illnesses, injuries, and deaths associated with employment.

Work-site walk-through An assessment of the workplace conducted by the CHN, specifically an occupational health nurse.

List of Appendices

APPENDIX 1

Canadian Community Health Nursing Standards of Practice

The Canadian Community Health Nursing Standards of Practice:

- define the scope and depth of community nursing practice
- establish criteria or expectations for acceptable nursing practice and safe, ethical care
- support ongoing development of community health nursing
- promote community health nursing as a specialty
- provide the foundation for certification of community health nursing as a specialty by the Canadian Nurses Association
- inspire excellence in and commitment to community nursing practice

All community health nurses are expected to know and use these standards when working in any of the areas of practice, education, administration, or research. Nurses in clinical practice will use the standards to guide and evaluate their own practice. Nursing educators will include the standards in course curricula to prepare new graduates for practice in community settings. Nurse administrators will use them to direct policy and guide performance expectations. Nurse researchers will use these standards to guide the development of knowledge specific to community health nursing.

Nurses may enter community health nursing as new practitioners and require experience and opportunities for additional learning and skill development to help them develop their practice. The *Community Health Nursing Standards of Practice* become basic practice expectations after 2 years of experience. The practice of expert community health nurses will extend beyond these standards.

STANDARD 1: PROMOTING HEALTH

Community health nurses view health as a dynamic process of physical, mental, spiritual, and social well-being. Health includes self-determination and a sense of connection to the community. Community health nurses believe that individuals and communities realize hopes and satisfy needs within their cultural, social, economic, and physical environments. They consider health as a resource for everyday life that is influenced by circumstances, beliefs, and the determinants of health. Social, economic, and environmental health determinants include (Health Canada, 2000):

- income and social status
- social support networks
- education
- employment and working conditions
- social environments
- physical environments
- biology and genetic endowment
- personal health practices and coping skills
- healthy child development
- health services
- gender
- culture

Community health nurses promote health using the following strategies: (a) health promotion, (b) prevention and health protection, and (c) health maintenance, restoration, and palliation. They recognize they may need to use these strategies together when providing care and services. This standard incorporates these strategies from the frameworks of primary health care (World Health Organization, 1978), the Ottawa Charter for Health Promotion (World Health Organization, 1986) and the Population Health Promotion Model (Health Canada, 2000).

A) Health Promotion

Community health nurses focus on health promotion and the health of populations. Health promotion is a mediating strategy between people and their environments. It is a positive, dynamic, empowering, and unifying concept based in the socioenvironmental approach to health.

It recognizes that basic resources and conditions for health are critical for achieving health. The population's health is closely linked with the health of its members and is often reflected first in individual and family experiences from birth to death. Community health nurses also consider sociopolitical issues that may be underlying individual and community problems.

Healthy communities and systems support increased options for well-being in society.

The community health nurse

1. Collaborates with individual, community, and other stakeholders to do a holistic assessment of assets and needs of the individual or community.
2. Uses a variety of information sources to access data and research findings related to health at the national, provincial, territorial, regional, and local levels.
3. Identifies and seeks to address root causes of illness and disease.
4. Facilitates planned change with the individual, community, or population by applying the Population Health Promotion Model.
    - Identifies the level of intervention necessary to promote health.
    - Identifies which determinants of health require action or change to promote health.
    - Uses a comprehensive range of strategies to address health-related issues.
5. Demonstrates knowledge of and effectively implements health promotion strategies based on the Ottawa Charter for Health Promotion.
    - Incorporates multiple strategies: promoting healthy public policy, strengthening community action, creating supportive environments, developing personal skills, and reorienting the health system.
    - Identifies strategies for change that will make it easier for people to make healthier choices.
6. Collaborates with the individual and community to help them take responsibility for maintaining or improving their health by increasing their knowledge, influence, and control over the determinants of health.
7. Understands and uses social marketing, media, and advocacy strategies to raise awareness of health issues, place issues on the public agenda, shift social norms, and change behaviours if other enabling factors are present.
8. Helps the individual and community to identify their strengths and available resources and take action to address their needs.
9. Recognizes the broad impact of specific issues on health promotion such as political climate and will, values and culture, individual and community readiness, and social and systemic structures.
10. Evaluates and modifies population health promotion programs in partnership with the individual, community, and other stakeholders.

B) Prevention and Health Protection

The community health nurse applies a range of activities to minimize the occurrence of diseases or injuries and their consequences for individuals and communities. Governments often make health protection strategies mandated programs and laws for their overall jurisdictions.

The community health nurse

1. Recognizes the differences between the levels of prevention (primary, secondary, tertiary).
2. Selects the appropriate level of preventive intervention.
3. Helps individuals and communities make informed choices about protective and preventive health measures such as immunization, birth control, breastfeeding, and palliative care.
4. Helps individuals, groups, families, and communities to identify potential risks to health.
5. Uses harm reduction principles to identify, reduce, or remove risk factors in a variety of contexts, including the home, neighbourhood, workplace, school, and street.
6. Applies epidemiological principles when using strategies such as screening, surveillance, immunization, communicable disease response and outbreak management, and education.
7. Engages collaborative, interdisciplinary, and intersectoral partnerships to address risks to individual, family, community, or population health and to address prevention and protection issues such as communicable disease, injury, and chronic disease.
8. Collaborates on developing and using follow-up systems in the practice setting to ensure that the individual or community receives appropriate and effective service.
9. Practices in accordance with legislation relevant to community health practice (e.g., public health legislation and child protection legislation).
10. Evaluates collaborative practice (personal, team, and intersectoral) for achieving individual and community outcomes such as reduced communicable disease, injury, chronic disease, or impacts of a disease process.

C) Health Maintenance, Restoration and Palliation

Community health nurses provide clinical nursing care, health education, and counselling to individuals, families, groups, and populations whether they are seeking to maintain their health or dealing with acute, chronic, or terminal illness. Community health nurses practice in health centres, homes, schools, and other community-based settings. They link people to community resources and coordinate or facilitate other care needs and supports. The activities of the community health nurse may range from health screening and care planning at an individual level to intersectoral collaboration and resource development at the community and population level.

The community health nurse

1. Assesses the health status and functional competence of the individual, family, or population within the context of their environmental and social supports.
2. Develops a mutually agreed upon plan and priorities for care with the individual and family.
3. Identifies a range of interventions including health promotion, disease prevention, and direct clinical care strategies (including palliation), along with short- and long-term goals and outcomes.
4. Maximizes the ability of an individual, family, or community to take responsibility for and manage their health needs according to resources and personal skills available.
5. Supports informed choice and respects the individual, family, or community's specific requests while acknowledging diversity, unique characteristics, and abilities.
6. Adapts community health nursing techniques, approaches, and procedures as appropriate to the challenges in a particular community situation or setting.
7. Uses knowledge of the community to link with, refer to, or develop appropriate community resources.
8. Recognizes patterns and trends in epidemiological data and service delivery and initiates strategies for improvement.
9. Facilitates maintenance of health and the healing process for individuals, families, and communities in response to significant health emergencies or other community situations that negatively impact health.
10. Evaluates individual, family, and community outcomes systematically and continuously in collaboration with individuals, families, significant others, community partners, and other health practitioners.

STANDARD 2: BUILDING INDIVIDUAL AND COMMUNITY CAPACITY

Building capacity is the process of actively involving individuals, groups, organizations, and communities in all phases of planned change to increase their skills, knowledge, and willingness to take action on their own in the future. The community health nurse works collaboratively with the individual or community affected by health-compromising situations and with the people and organizations that control resources. Starting where the individual or community is, community health nurses identify relevant issues, assess resources and strengths, and determine readiness for change and priorities for action. They take collaborative action by building on identified strengths and involving key stakeholders such as individuals, organizations, and community leaders. They work with people to improve the determinants of health and make it easier to make the healthier choice.

Community health nurses use supportive and empowering strategies to move individuals and communities toward maximum autonomy.

The community health nurse

1. Works collaboratively with the individual, community, other professionals, agencies, and sectors to identify needs, strengths, and available resources.
2. Facilitates action in support of the five priorities of the Jakarta Declaration to
    - promote social responsibility for health
    - increase investments for health development
    - expand partnerships for health promotion
    - increase individual and community capacity
    - secure an infrastructure for health promotion
3. Uses community development principles.
    - Engages the individual and community in a consultative process.
    - Recognizes and builds on the readiness of the group or community to participate.
    - Uses empowering strategies such as mutual goal setting, visioning, and facilitation.
    - Understands group dynamics and effectively uses facilitation skills to support group development.
    - Helps the individual and community to participate in the resolution of their issues.
    - Helps the group and community to gather available resources to support taking action on their health issues.

4. Uses a comprehensive mix of community and population-based strategies such as coalition building, intersectoral partnerships, and networking to address concerns of groups or populations.
5. Supports the individual, family, community, or population to develop skills for self-advocacy.
6. Applies principles of social justice and engages in advocacy to support those who are not yet able to take action for themselves.
7. Uses a comprehensive mix of interventions and strategies to customize actions to address unique needs and build individual and community capacity.
8. Supports community action to influence policy change in support of health.
9. Actively works with health professionals and community partners to build capacity for health promotion.
10. Evaluates the impact of change on individual or community control and health outcomes.

STANDARD 3: BUILDING RELATIONSHIPS

Community health nurses build relationships based on the principles of connecting and caring. Connecting involves establishing and nurturing relationships and a supportive environment that promotes the maximum participation and self-determination of the individual, family, and community. Caring involves developing empowering relationships that preserve, protect, and enhance human dignity. Community health nurses build caring relationships based on mutual respect and understanding of the power inherent in their position and its potential impact on relationships and practice.

One of the unique challenges of community health nursing is building a network of relationships and partnerships with a wide variety of relevant groups, communities, and organizations. These relationships happen within a complex, changing, and often ambiguous environment with sometimes conflicting and unpredictable circumstances.

The community health nurse

1. Recognizes her or his personal beliefs, attitudes, assumptions, feelings, and values about health and their potential effect on interventions with individuals and communities.
2. Identifies the individual and community beliefs, attitudes, feelings, and values about health and their potential effect on the relationship and intervention.
3. Is aware of and uses culturally relevant communication when building relationships. Communication may be verbal or nonverbal, written or graphic. It may involve face-to-face, telephone, group facilitation, print, or electronic methods.
4. Respects and trusts the ability of the individual or community to know the issue they are addressing and solve their own problems.
5. Involves the individual, family, and community as an active partner to identify relevant needs, perspectives, and expectations.
6. Establishes connections and collaborative relationships with health professionals, community organizations, businesses, faith communities, volunteer service organizations, and other sectors to address health-related issues.
7. Maintains awareness of community resources, values, and characteristics.
8. Promotes and supports linkages with appropriate community resources when the individual or community is ready to receive them (e.g., hospice or palliative care, parenting groups).
9. Maintains professional boundaries in often long-term relationships in the home or other community settings where professional and social relationships may become blurred.
10. Negotiates an end to the relationship when appropriate (e.g., when the client assumes self-care or when the goals for the relationship have been achieved).

STANDARD 4: FACILITATING ACCESS AND EQUITY

Community health nurses embrace the philosophy of primary health care. They collaboratively identify and facilitate universal and equitable access to available services. They collaborate with colleagues and with other members of the health care team to promote effective working relationships that contribute to comprehensive client care and optimal client care outcomes.

They are keenly aware of the impact of the determinants of health on individuals, families, groups, communities, and populations. The practice of community health nursing considers the financial resources, geography, and culture of the individual and community.

Community health nurses engage in advocacy by analyzing the determinants of health and influencing other sectors to ensure their policies and programs have a positive impact on health. Community health nurses use advocacy as a key strategy to meet identified needs and enhance individual and community capacity for self-advocacy.

The community health nurse

1. Assesses and understands individual and community capacities including norms, values, beliefs, knowledge, resources, and power structures.
2. Provides culturally sensitive care in diverse communities and settings.
3. Supports individuals and communities in their choice to access alternate health care options.
4. Advocates for appropriate resource allocation for individuals, groups, and populations to support access to conditions for health and health services.
5. Refers, coordinates, or facilitates access to services in the health sector and other sectors.
6. Adapts practice in response to the changing health needs of the individual and community.
7. Collaborates with individuals and communities to identify and provide programs and delivery methods that are acceptable to them and responsive to their needs across the life span and in different circumstances.
8. Uses strategies such as home visits, outreach, and case finding to ensure access to services and health-supporting conditions for potentially vulnerable populations (e.g., persons who are ill, elderly, young, poor, immigrants, or isolated or have communication barriers).
9. Assesses the impact of the determinants of health on the opportunity for health for individuals, families, communities, and populations.
10. Advocates for healthy public policy by participating in legislative and policy-making activities that influence health determinants and access to services.
11. Takes action with and for individuals and communities at the organizational, municipal, provincial, territorial, and federal levels to address service gaps and accessibility issues.
12. Monitors and evaluates changes and progress in access to the determinants of health and appropriate community services.

STANDARD 5: DEMONSTRATING PROFESSIONAL RESPONSIBILITY AND ACCOUNTABILITY

Community health nurses work with a high degree of autonomy when providing programs and services. Their professional accountability includes striving for excellence, ensuring that their knowledge is evidence based and current, and maintaining competence and the overall quality of their practice. Community health nurses are responsible for initiating strategies that will help address the determinants of health and generate a positive impact on people and systems.

Community health nurses are accountable to a variety of authorities and stakeholders as well as to the individual and community they serve. This range of accountabilities places them in a variety of situations with unique ethical dilemmas. One dilemma might be whether responsibility for an issue lies with the individual, family, community, or population or with the nurse or the nurse's employer. Other dilemmas include the priority of one individual's rights over the rights of another, individual, or societal good; allocation of scarce resources; and quality versus quantity of life.

The community health nurse

1. Takes preventive or corrective action individually or in partnership to protect individuals and communities from unsafe or unethical circumstances.
2. Advocates for societal change in support of health for all.
3. Uses nursing informatics (including information and communication technology) to generate, manage, and process relevant data to support nursing practice.
4. Identifies and takes action on factors which affect autonomy of practice and quality of care.
5. Participates in the advancement of community health nursing by mentoring students and new practitioners.
6. Participates in research and professional activities.
7. Makes decisions using ethical standards and principles, taking into consideration the tension between individual versus societal good and the responsibility to uphold the greater good of all people or the population as a whole.
8. Seeks help with problem solving as needed to determine the best course of action in response to ethical dilemmas, risks to human rights and freedoms, new situations, and new knowledge.
9. Identifies and works proactively—through personal advocacy and participation in relevant professional associations—to address nursing issues that will affect the population.
10. Contributes proactively to the quality of the work environment by identifying needs, issues, and solutions; mobilizing colleagues; and actively participating in team and organizational structures and mechanisms.
11. Provides constructive feedback to peers as appropriate to enhance community health nursing practice.

12. Documents community health nursing activities in a timely and thorough manner, including telephone advice and work with communities and groups.
13. Advocates for effective and efficient use of community health nursing resources.
14. Uses reflective practice to continually assess and improve personal community health nursing practice.
15. Seeks professional development experiences that are consistent with current community health nursing practice, new and emerging issues, the changing needs of the population, the evolving impact of the determinants of health, and emerging research.
16. Acts upon legal obligations to report to appropriate authorities any situations of unsafe or unethical care provided by family, friends, or other individuals to children or vulnerable adults.
17. Uses available resources to systematically evaluate the availability, acceptability, quality, efficiency, and effectiveness of community health nursing practice.

REFERENCES

Health Canada. (2000). *Population health approach*. Retrieved from http://www.hc-sc.gc.ca/hppb/phdd/approach/index.html.

World Health Organization. (1978). *Alma-Ata 1978: Report of the international conference on primary health care*. Geneva: Author.

World Health Organization, Canadian Public Health Association, Health and Welfare Canada. (1986). *The Ottawa charter for health promotion*. Ottawa: Canadian Public Health Association.

APPENDIX 2

CNA Position Statement: "Interprofessional Collaboration"

CNA POSITION

The Canadian Nurses Association (CNA) believes that the people of Canada are entitled to a health system with the capacity to help them meet both their physical and their mental health needs—whether those needs are illness prevention, early detection, treatment, rehabilitation or recovery. Further, the association believes that the responsiveness of the health system can be strengthened through effective collaboration among health professionals.

CNA believes that respecting the following six principles, as outlined in *The Principles and Framework for Interdisciplinary Collaboration in Primary Health Care,*[1] will facilitate collaboration among professions and professionals:

1. Focus on the Patient/Client

The needs of individual patients and clients must be the focus of health services. Health professionals work together to optimize the health and wellness of each individual and involve the individual in decision-making about his/her health. Individuals and their families are actively engaged in the prevention, promotion and management of health problems. Health professionals respect that personal health information must be kept confidential.

2. Population Health Approach

Using assessments of the demographics and health status of a community will ensure the relevance of health services, including the identification of appropriate health professions. Trends in the health of the population are tracked to assess the impact of the services offered.

3. Quality Care and Services

Health professionals work together to identify and assess research evidence as a basis for identifying treatment and management of health problems. Health outcomes are continuously evaluated to track the effectiveness and appropriateness of services.

[1](Enhancing Interdisciplinary Collaboration in Primary Health Care [EICP], 2005)

4. Access

The right service is provided at the right time, in the right place and by the right care provider. Geographic barriers are minimized. Service delivery is respectful of age, gender, culture, language, religion and lifestyle of patients/clients.

5. Trust and Respect

Each profession brings its own set of knowledge and skills—the result of education, training and experience—to collaborative health services. Each professional contributes to an individual's health. Shared decision-making, creativity and innovation allow providers to learn from each other and enhance the effectiveness of their collaborative efforts.

6. Communication

Active listening and effective communication skills facilitate both information sharing and decision-making.

To support and sustain interprofessional collaboration, CNA believes that eight structural elements[2] must also be present:

1. The planning, recruitment, education and workplace to support human resources
2. Long-term funding allocations that support the necessary infrastructure and information technology requirements of interprofessional collaboration
3. Liability insurance framework for interprofessional teams
4. Regulatory framework that recognizes the decision-making processes and roles within interprofessional collaboration
5. Information technology and infrastructure
6. Standards that guarantee both inter-operability and access by appropriate professionals to electronic health records

[2](EICP, 2005)

7. Governance and management structures
8. Planning and evaluation frameworks and assessment tools to measure the performance of interdisciplinary collaborative practices that are supported by ongoing research and surveillance.

BACKGROUND

As a partner in the Enhancing Interdisciplinary Collaboration Project, CNA contributed to the development of *The Principles and Framework for Interdisciplinary Collaboration in Primary Health Care,* which describes the effectiveness of service integration to the health of Canadians:

> *The range and complexity of factors that influence health and well-being, as well as disease and illness, require health professionals from diverse health professions to work together in a comprehensive manner. For example, individuals need health information, diagnosis of health problems, support for behavioural change, immunization, screening for disease prevention and monitoring of management plans for chronic health problems. Working together, the combined knowledge and skills of health professionals become a powerful mechanism to enhance the health of the population served.*
>
> *Working together can take various forms. At the simplest level, health professionals consult their patients/clients and, when appropriate, each other about the services needed by their patients/clients. In more complex situations, health professionals work more closely, identifying (together with patients/clients) what services are needed, who will provide them and what adjustments need to be made to the health management plan. The number and type of service health professionals depend on the nature of the health issue and the availability of resources. This is a dynamic process that responds to changing needs.*[3]

Canada has a history of effective interprofessional collaboration in community health centres, and chronic disease management teams have been in operation for many years in regions across Canada. Research on the experiences of these sites as well as consultation with providers has identified the barriers and enablers to interprofessional collaboration.

Approved by the CNA Board of Directors, November 2005

[3](EICP, 2005)

REFERENCES

Enhancing Interdisciplinary Collaboration in Primary Health Care. (2005). *The principles and framework for interdisciplinary collaboration in primary health care.* Ottawa: Author. Retrieved from http://www.eicp-acis.ca/en/principles/sept/EICP-Principles%20and%20Framework%20Sept.pdf.

Additional References Consulted:

Canadian Association of Occupational Therapists, Canadian Dietetic Association, Canadian Nurses Association, & Canadian Physiotherapy Association. (1996). *Integrated health human resources development: An inventory of activity in Canada.* Ottawa: Integrated Health Human Resources Development Project.

Canadian Association of Social Workers. (2003, March). *Canadian Association of Social Workers: Social policy principles.* Retrieved from http://www.casw-acts.ca/advocacy/socialpolicy_e.pdf.

Canadian Centre for Analysis of Regionalization and Health (2003, November). *CCARH Newsletter.* Saskatoon, SK: Author.

Canadian Health Services Research Foundation. (2003). *Choices for change: The path for restructuring primary healthcare services in Canada.* Retrieved from http://www.chsrf.ca/final_research/commissioned_research/policy_synthesis/pdf/choices_for_change_e.pdf.

Canadian Medical Association & Canadian Nurses Association. (1996). *Working together: A joint CNA/CMA collaborative practice project: HIV/AIDS example.* Ottawa: Authors.

Canadian Pharmacists Association. (2004). *Pharmacists and primary health care.* Retrieved from http://www.pharmacists.ca/content/about_cpha/whats_happening/cpha_in_action/pdf/primaryhealth2a.pdf.

Canadian Psychological Association. (2000). *Strengthening primary care: The contribution of the science and practice of psychology.* Retrieved from http://www.cpa.ca/primary.pdf.

College of Family Physicians of Canada. (2000). *A prescription for renewal.* Retrieved from http://www.cfpc.ca/English/cfpc/communications/health%20policy/primary%20care%20and%20family%20medicine/default.asp?s = 1.

Dieleman, S. L., Farris, K. B., Feeny, D., Johnson, J. A., Tsuyuki, R. T., & Brilliant, S. (2004). Primary health care teams: Team members' perceptions of the collaborative process. *Journal of Interprofessional Care, 18*(1), 75–78.

Dietitians of Canada. (2001). *The role of the registered dietitian in primary health care.* Retrieved from http://www.dietitians.ca/news/downloads/role_of_RD_in_PHC.pdf.

Gagné, M. A. (2005). *Advancing the agenda for collaborative mental health care in Canada.* [Report prepared for the Canadian Collaborative Mental Health Initiative]. Retrieved from http://www.ccmhi.ca/en/products/documents/EN_AdvancingAgenda_paper.pdf.

Hasselback, P., Saunders, D., Dastmalchian, A., Alibhai, A., Boudreau, R., Chreim, S., et al. (2002). *The Taber Integrated Primary Care Project: Turning vision into reality*. Retrieved from http://www.chsrf.ca/final_research/ogc/pdf/hasselback_final.pdf.

Kachala, E. (2004). *Building a primary health care infrastructure in Halton-Peel: Planning for the future*. [Final report of the Primary Health Care Task Force]. Retrieved from http://www.dhcarchives.com/protected/uploaded/publication/PRIMARY%20HEALTH%20CARE%20FINAL%20REPORTWEB.pdf.

King, N., & Ross, A. (2004). Professional identities and interprofessional relations: Evaluation of collaborative community schemes. *Social Work in Health Care, 38*(2), 51–72.

Klaiman, D. (2004). Increasing access to occupational therapy in primary health care. *Occupation Therapy Now, 6*(1), 14–18. Retrieved from http://www.caot.ca/default.asp?pageid=1031.

Leatt, P., Pink, G. H., & Guerriere, M. (2000). Towards a Canadian model of integrated healthcare. *Healthcare Papers, 1*(2), 13–35.

Marriott, J., & Mable, A. L. (2000). *Opportunities and potential: A review of international literature on primary health care reform and models*. Ottawa: Health Canada.

Nolte, J. (2005). *Enhancing interdisciplinary collaboration in primary health care in Canada*. [Report]. Retrieved from http://www.eicp.ca/en/resources/pdfs/Enhancing-Interdisciplinary-Collaboration-in-Primary-Health-Care-in-Canada.pdf.

Sicotte, C., D'Amour, D., & Moreault, M. P. (2002). Interdisciplinary collaboration within Quebec community health care centres. *Social Science and Medicine, 55*(6), 991–1003.

Working Group on Interdisciplinary Primary Care Models, Advisory Committee of Interprofessional Practitioners (1997). *Interdisciplinary primary care models*. Ottawa: AGIP [Final report].

Source: Canadian Nurses Association. Retrieved from http://www.cna-aiic.ca/CNA/documents/pdf/publications/PS84_Interprofessional_Collaboration_e.pdf.

CNA Backgrounder: "Social Determinants of Health and Nursing: A Summary of the Issues"

APPENDIX 3

WHAT'S THE ISSUE?

In all countries, it is well-established that poorer people have substantially shorter life expectancies and more illnesses than the rich. This phenomenon has been observed since at least the nineteenth century when Chadwick (1965) investigated the health of the working classes in Victorian England.

Two contemporary British studies have been very influential in their documentation of the relationship between socioeconomic factors and health status. The Whitehall civil service study compared the health status of individuals over time with their position in a well-defined job hierarchy. Those lower in the hierarchy experienced three times the risk of death from heart disease, stroke, cancer, gastrointestinal disease, accident, and suicide compared with those at the top of the hierarchy. These differences could not be explained by differences in medical care.

The Secretary of State for Health in Britain was concerned about why—30 years after the establishment of the National Health Service (which made health services available to all, regardless of income)—significant differences in mortality between social classes persisted. The Black Report, released in 1980 (Townsend, Davidson, & Whitehead, 1992) concluded that these differences in health status were not the result of individual differences, but rather of structural differences in the way members of these different classes led their lives. This included a wide range of factors such as income, employment and working conditions, housing, education, nutrition, stress and violence—what we now consider the social determinants of health.

Social determinants of health have a significant impact on the predisposition of individuals and groups to illness, as well as the way in which they experience and recover from illness. It is critical that nurses understand the impact of these factors on the individuals and groups that they work with, and include these factors in their assessments. This information may affect the choice of intervention and the need for other community resources. At a broader level, nurses can use their experience to advocate for progressive policies that address the social determinants of health.

WHY IS THIS ISSUE IMPORTANT?

How This Issue Relates to the Health of Canadians

Genetics and traditional risk factors, such as activity, diet and tobacco use, are not the best predictors of whether we stay healthy or become ill. Some of the best predictors of adult-onset diabetes, heart attack, stroke and many other diseases are social determinants.

> *Social determinants of health are the economic and social conditions that influence the health of individuals, communities and jurisdictions as a whole. Social determinants of health determine whether individuals stay healthy or become ill (a narrow definition of health). Social determinants of health also determine the extent to which a person possesses the physical, social and personal resources to identify and achieve personal aspirations, satisfy needs and cope with the environment (a broader definition of health). Social determinants of health are about the quantity and quality of a variety of resources that a society makes available to its members* (Raphael, 2004, p. 1).

A wealth of evidence supports this idea that the socioeconomic circumstances of individuals and groups have at least as much—and often more—influence on health status as medical care and personal health behaviours. The World Health Organization identifies the following as some of the most important social determinants of health (Wilkinson & Marmot, 2003):

Poverty

- Absolute poverty (not being able to access basic resources such as food and shelter) has a profound effect on health status. People living on the streets suffer the highest risk of premature death. In addition to the direct effects of being poor, an individual's health can be compromised by living in neighbourhoods with high concentrations of unemployment, poor housing, a poor environment and limited access to services (Wilkinson & Marmot, 2003).

- Canada has made little progress in addressing the issue of poverty. In 2000, 14.7% of Canadians were poor, which is a higher percentage than in pre-recession 1989 (13.9%). Seniors are the only group for which the poverty rate decreased during this period (moving from 22.5% to 16.4%) (Curry-Stevens, 2004).
- Child poverty in Canada increased during the 1990s, from 14.7% in 1989 to 15% in 2004, representing one in six children (Curry-Stevens, 2004).
- There is a graded relationship between household income and emotional and behavioural problems in childhood—the lower the household income, the higher the incidence of these problems (Canadian Institute of Child Health, 2004).
- Income is thought to affect health in these ways:
    - material deprivation removes the prerequisites for healthy development such as shelter, food, warmth, and the ability to participate in society,
    - living on low income causes psychosocial stress, which damages people's health, and
    - low income limits people's choices and works against desirable changes in behaviour (Raphael, 2004).

Economic Inequality

- Economic inequality (the gap between the richest and poorest in a society) may be an even more significant social determinant of health than absolute poverty. As the gap between rich and poor widens, health status declines (Auger, Raynault, Lessard, & Choinière, 2004; Raphael, 2002).
- Family incomes have become more polarized in Canada. The proportion of middle-income families (earning between $30,000 and $59,999/year) decreased by 17% relative to other income groups in the period from 1980 to 2000. "Well-off" families (between $60,000 and $99,999/year) also decreased by 6.1% relative to other income levels. At the same time, the ranks of the working poor ($5,000 to $19,999) and the very rich (above $150,000) rose substantially—by 23% and 95.5% respectively—relative to other income groups (Curry-Stevens, 2004).

Social Status

- People with less social standing usually run at least twice the risk of serious illness and premature death as those with more. This is an effect that is not limited to the poor, but extends across all strata of society (Wilkinson & Marmot, 2003).

Stress

- Social and psychological circumstances can cause long-term stress. Continual anxiety, insecurity, low self-esteem, social isolation, and lack of control over work and home life have powerful effects on health, especially on the cardiovascular and immune systems. Individuals experiencing long-term stress are more vulnerable to conditions such as infections, diabetes, high blood pressure, heart attack, stroke, depression, and aggression (Wilkinson & Marmot, 2003).

Education and Care in Early Life

- The foundations of adult health are laid before birth, in infancy, and in early childhood. Poor fetal development is a risk for health in later life. For example, low birth weight has been linked to higher risk of diabetes (Wilkinson & Marmot, 2003). Low birth weight is more than twice as common for women with low incomes (9%) compared to women with higher incomes (4%) (Canadian Institute of Child Health, 2004).
- Infancy and early childhood are critical stages of physical, mental and emotional development. Insecure emotional attachment and low levels of stimulation can lead to reduced readiness for school and problem behaviour. High-quality child care can mitigate against such inadequacies. It can provide intellectual and social stimulation that promotes cognitive development and social competence. The positive effects of high-quality childcare persist into later life, especially in lower-income children (Friendly, 2004).
- Good health-related habits, such as eating sensibly and exercising, are strongly influenced during early childhood.
- The public school system in Canada has played an important role in preparing young people for the future. This system has been under stress in recent years due to budget cutbacks, labour conflicts and pressure to address increased needs such as special education. If this universal system is not able to respond to such challenges successfully, an important pillar in the Canadian social structure will be threatened, which will impact on the health of Canadian children (Ungerleider & Burns, 2004).

Social Exclusion

- Social exclusion denies individuals the opportunity to participate in the activities normally expected of members of their society. There is evidence of growing social exclusion in Canadian society, particularly for Aboriginal people, non-European immigrants and people of colour.

- Aboriginal people and people of colour are more than twice as likely to live in poverty and three times as likely as the average Canadian to be unemployed, despite their level of qualifications (Galabuzi, 2004).

Employment and Job Security

- Although having a job is generally better for health than being unemployed, stress at work has an important impact on health. Having little control over one's work is associated with increased risk of low back pain, cardiovascular disease and depression (Wilkinson & Marmot, 2003).
- Longer and more unpredictable hours, combined with already high and rising job demands are particularly likely to cause stress and anxiety in families where both partners work, and for single-parent families. More than one-third of 25- to 44-year-old women who work full-time and have children at home report that they are severely time-stressed, and the same is true of one in four men. Twenty-six percent of married fathers, 38% of married mothers, and 38% of single mothers report severe time stress, with levels of severe stress rising by about 20% between 1992 and 1998 (Statistics Canada, 1999).
- Unemployed people and their families often experience great psychological and financial problems. They are substantially at increased risk of premature death (Wilkinson & Marmot, 2003).
- Job insecurity has been shown to increase depression, anxiety and heart disease. Only one-half of all working Canadians has a single, full-time job that has lasted 6 months or more. Less than half of non-unionized workers have access to employer-sponsored benefits and pensions. The percentage of Canadians in full-time permanent jobs has dropped from 67% in 1989 to 63% in 2000. For many Canadians, work has become precarious (Polanyi, Tompa, & Foley, 2004).

Social Support

- Social support helps give people the emotional and practical resources they need to get through life. Social isolation and exclusion are associated with increased rates of premature death, depression, higher levels of pregnancy complications and higher levels of disability from chronic illness (Wilkinson & Marmot, 2003).

Food Security

- A well-balanced diet and an adequate supply of nutritious food are essential elements for good health. Shortage of food and lack of variety cause malnutrition and a range of deficiency diseases. Overeating contributes to cardiovascular disease, diabetes, cancer, obesity and cavities (Wilkinson & Marmot, 2003).
- *Food insecurity* is defined as the inability to acquire or consume an adequate diet quality or sufficient quantity of food in socially acceptable ways. One in ten Canadian households (representing three million people and 678,000 children) experience food insecurity (McIntyre, 2004).

How This Issue Relates to the Functioning of the Health Care System

In 1996, Statistics Canada estimated that 23% of years of life lost from all causes prior to age 75 could be attributed to income differences (Raphael, 2004). The two diseases where the links to social determinants have been investigated most thoroughly are heart disease and diabetes.

Cardiovascular Disease

- Heart disease and stroke are the leading killers of Canadians, responsible for 40,000 deaths every year—over one-third of all Canadian deaths. These diseases account for 18% of hospital patient days. The total combined cost to the Canadian economy of heart disease and stroke is estimated to be $18.5 billion per year (Heart & Stroke Foundation, 2003).
- Income differences account for 6,366 additional premature deaths from cardiovascular disease (Raphael, 2001).

Diabetes

- It is estimated that two million Canadians have diabetes and the rate of incidence is rising. Diabetes is one of the eight leading causes of hospitalization, accounting for close to 300,000 admissions per year. Diabetes costs the Canadian economy an estimated $13.2 billion every year (Canadian Diabetes Association, 2004).
- There has been a huge increase in mortality due to diabetes in low-income communities in Canada. Low-income Canadians face higher risks of diabetes than average Canadians, particularly females (four times higher risk) and Aboriginals (three to five times higher risk) (Ling Yu & Raphael, 2004).

WHY IS THIS ISSUE IMPORTANT TO NURSES?

Working on the front lines of the health care system, nurses see the impact of the social determinants of health every day. They see individuals and groups of people who are more susceptible to illness, who experience more complications, or whose recovery process is much longer. If they ask the right questions during their assessment process, nurses will often find links between these people and issues such as low income, high levels of stress, job insecurity, food insecurity, poor housing, and social isolation. Even if they do know about these issues, nurses often feel powerless to address them.

Despite mounting evidence for the role of social determinants on health status, much of the focus for prevention and management of diseases such as diabetes and heart disease remains highly medicalized. Our system is really about sick care, not health care. The emphasis is on identifying high-risk individuals who are urged to seek medical attention where a healthy provider will screen for biomedical risk factors, prescribe medication (if necessary), advise adopting a healthy lifestyle, and then monitor the disease. Research has placed a similar focus on the identification of individual risk factors, as opposed to structural or societal issues. As well, government policies and programs have emphasized individual responsibility for health almost exclusively (Ling Yu & Raphael, 2004).

Addressing social determinants of health requires a shift in some of the prevailing thinking about health. It requires people to realize that the health system has an important—but limited—role in addressing health. It also requires people to challenge some of the ideas they may have about poverty, equity and social justice. These are not individual issues, but structural ones.

What do we do, as a society, to address the social determinants of health? The forces of globalization and changing economic policies force many people into precarious employment where they cannot earn enough to support themselves and their families. Recessions and systematic budget cutting over the past 20 years have decimated health, social and educational infrastructures across the country. In addition, we like to think we live in an egalitarian society but, in fact, some groups, such as visible minorities, new Canadians, Aboriginal people and single-parent families, face substantial economic and social barriers that have significant impacts on health. Confronting these issues is a big challenge that means addressing some of our most fundamental values.

Sweden and Finland have taken progressive national approaches to address social determinants of health. Building on these examples, Raphael (2004) advocates that Canada take action in three key areas:

- Develop policies to reduce the incidence of low income (including increasing minimum wages and improving pay equity)
- Develop policies to reduce social exclusion (including progressive taxation to reduce inequalities in income, measures to protect the rights of minority groups, and employment policies that preserve and create jobs)
- Develop policies to restore and enhance Canada's social infrastructure (including strategies to ensure access to pharmaceuticals and dental care, a national child care strategy, and strengthened health and social services)

The social determinants of health are not external to their work in the health system; indeed, they are the very foundation of a healthy society. The *Ottawa Charter for Health Promotion* (World Health Organization [WHO], 1986) outlines the prerequisites of health as peace, shelter, education, food, income, a stable eco-system, sustainable resources, social justice and equity. Canadians will not be able to achieve the health goals we set as a society—and nurses and other health professionals will not be able to achieve the success they seek in their individual work with patients—until we make it a priority to address social determinants.

WHAT HAS THE CNA DONE TO ADDRESS THIS ISSUE?

CNA participates on a variety of national coalitions and committees that address the social determinants of health:

- CNA is a partner of **Child and Family Canada,** which provides quality, credible resources on children and families.
- CNA is a member of the **National Children's Alliance.**
- CNA staff served on the **Expert Advisory Board** of the **Children's Health Team,** which reported to the **Commission for Environmental Cooperation.**
- CNA is a member of the **Environmental Health Coalition.**
- CNA is a member of the **Canadian Coalition for Green Health Care.**
- CNA is a member of the **Canadian Coalition for Public Health in the 21st Century.**

CNA has developed policy papers and position statements that address the social determinants of health including:

- Position statement, *The Environment as a Determinant of Health*
- Joint policy statement with the Canadian Medical Association, *Environmentally Responsible Activity in the Health Sector*

WHAT CAN NURSES DO ABOUT THIS ISSUE?

Nurses can play an important role to address social determinants of health by working on their individual practices, helping to reorient the health care system, and advocating for healthy public policies:

Individual Nursing Practice

- Understand the impact of social determinants on the health of your patients.
- Include questions on social determinants—for example, income, housing, food security, social support—in your assessments of patients.
- Consider social determinants in your treatment and follow-up plans. For example, determine whether patients are financially able to access recommended programs such as physiotherapy. If not, try to help the patient to access financial assistance to make these programs accessible.
- If you work with disadvantaged communities, help people with common health issues to understand the link to social determinants, and to organize to take action.
- Know that community and health resources are available to your clients.

Reorienting the Health Care System

- Ensure that health promotion programs go beyond lifestyle and behaviour to take social determinants into account. For example, physical activity programs should be designed so that fees and transportation are not barriers to participation. When access to nutritious food is an issue, refer people to programs such as community gardens and collective kitchens.
- Encourage health departments to take a social determinants approach, including considering the impact of economic inequalities and poverty.
- Advocate for universal access to basic health programs such as dental care and pharmacare.

Healthy Public Policies

- Speak from experience. Use stories from your patients to help advocate for policies that address social determinants of health.
- Make decision-makers aware of the research on links between socioeconomic factors and health.
- Look at how structural issues of class, race and gender affect the way in which populations experience health problems, and develop initiatives that address these issues. For example, Aboriginal people are at very high risk of diabetes, yet this is being treated largely as an individual lifestyle issue. Research shows that issues like poverty, housing, employment and food security in this population need to be addressed before real progress in dealing with this and other health and social issues can be made.

WHERE CAN YOU GO FOR FURTHER INFORMATION?

- Dr. Dennis Raphael's Web site at York University has many reports and publications on social determinants of health and a link to the SDOH listserv (quartz.atkinson.yorku.ca/QuickPlace/draphael/Main.nsf/h_Toc/add17a118af948d985256cd900682d5b/?OpenDocument).
- Genuine Progress Index for Atlantic Canada (www.gpiatlantic.org)
- Public Health Agency of Canada (www.phacaspc.gc.ca/ph-sp/phdd/whatsnew.html)
- World Health Organization Commission on Social Determinants of Health (www.who.int/social_determinants/en)

FURTHER READING

Canadian Institute for Child Health. *The health of Canada's children—A CICH profile: Low birth weight.* Retrieved from www.cich.ca/PDFFiles/ProfileFactSheets/English/LBWEng.pdf.

Edwards, P. (2004). *The social determinants of health: An overview of the implications for policy and the role of the health sector.* Retrieved from http://www.phac-aspc.gc.ca/phsp/phdd/overview_implications/01_overview.html.

Health Canada. (2003). *Diabetes in Canada* (2nd ed.). Retrieved from http://www.phac-aspc.gc.ca/publicat/dic-dac2/english/01cover_e.html.

Khalema, N. E. (2005, March). *Who's healthy? Who's not? A social justice perspective on health inequities. Cross links.* Retrieved from www.chps.ualberta.ca/publications/cross_links/Khalema-CrossLinks-Mar2005.pdf.

Minnesota Health Improvement Partnership Social Conditions and Health Action Team. (2001). *A call to action: Advancing health for all through social and economic change.* Retrieved from http://www.health.state.mn.us/divs/chs/mhip/action.pdf.

Raphael, D. (2003). Bridging the gap between knowledge and action on the societal determinants of cardiovascular disease: How one community hit—and hurdled—the lifestyle wall. *Health Education, 103*(3), 177–189.

Spencer, N. (2003). Social, economic and political determinants of child health. *Pediatrics, 112*(3), 704–706.

REFERENCES

Auger, N., Raynault, M. F., Lessard, R., & Choinière, R. (2004). Income and health in Canada. In D. Raphael (Ed.), *Social determinants of health: Canadian perspectives.* Toronto: Canadian Scholar's Press, Inc.

Canadian Diabetes Association. (2004). *The prevalence and costs of diabetes.* Retrieved from www.diabetes.ca/Section_about/prevalence.asp.

Canadian Institute of Child Health. (2004). *The health of Canada's children—A CICH profile: Income inequity.* Retrieved from http://www.cich.ca/PDFFiles/ProfileFactSheets/English/Incomeinequity.pdf.

Chadwick, E. (1965). *Report on the sanitary condition of the labouring population of Great Britain, 1842.* Edinburgh: Edinburgh University Press.

Curry-Stevens, A. (2004). Income and income distribution. In D. Raphael (Ed.), *Social determinants of health: Canadian perspectives.* Toronto: Canadian Scholars' Press, Inc.

Friendly, M. (2004). Early childhood education and care. In D. Raphael (Ed.), *Social determinants of health: Canadian perspectives.* Toronto: Canadian Scholars' Press, Inc.

Galabuzi, G.-E. (2004). Social exclusion. In D. Raphael (Ed.), *Social determinants of health: Canadian perspectives.* Toronto: Canadian Scholars' Press, Inc.

Heart and Stroke Foundation. (2003). *The growing burden of heart disease and stroke in Canada, 2003.* Retrieved from http://ww2.heartandstroke.ca/images/English/Heart_Disease_EN.pdf.

Ling Yu, V., & Raphael, D. (2004, September/October). Identifying and addressing the social determinants of the incidence and successful management of type 2 diabetes mellitus in Canada. *Canadian Journal of Public Health, 95*(5).

McIntyre, L. (2004). Food Insecurity. In D. Raphael (Ed.), *Social determinants of health: Canadian perspectives.* Toronto: Canadian Scholars' Press, Inc.

Polanyi, M., Tompa, E., & Foley, J. (2004). Labour market flexibility and worker insecurity. In D. Raphael (Ed.), *Social determinants of health: Canadian perspectives.* Toronto: Canadian Scholars' Press, Inc.

Raphael, D. (2001). *Inequality is bad for our hearts: Why low income and social exclusion are major causes of heart disease in Canada.* Toronto: North York Heart Network.

Raphael, D. (2002). *Social determinants of health: Why is there such a gap between our knowledge and its implementation?.* Retrieved from http://www.medanthro.net/academic/topical/ryerson.ppt#1.

Raphael, D. (2004). Introduction to the social determinants of health. In D. Raphael (Ed.), *Social determinants of health: Canadian perspectives.* Toronto: Canadian Scholars' Press, Inc.

Statistics Canada. (1999, November 9). General social survey: Time use. *The Daily.* Retrieved from http://www.statcan. ca/Daily/English/991109/td991109.htm.

Townsend, P., Davidson, N., & Whitehead, M. (Eds.), (1992). *Inequalities in health: The Black report and the health divide.* London: Penguin Books.

Ungerleider, C., & Burns, T. (2004). The state and quality of Canadian public education. In D. Raphael (Ed.), *Social determinants of health: Canadian perspectives.* Toronto: Canadian Scholars' Press, Inc.

Wilkinson, R., & Marmot, M. (Eds.). (2003). *Social determinants of health: The solid facts.* Copenhagen: World Health Organization. Retrieved from www.who.dk/document/E81384.pdf.

World Health Organization. (1986). *Ottawa Charter for Health Promotion.* Geneva: Author, October 2005 BG 008.

Source: Canadian Nurses Association. (2005). Retrieved from http://www.cna-nurses.ca/CNA/documents/pdf/publications/BG8_Social_Determinants_e.pdf.

Ethics in Practice for Registered Nurses: Social Justice in Practice

APPENDIX 4

Consider the following scenarios:

- Tara, a public health nurse in a rural community, has just learned that the town's hospital is slated for closure. Losing the hospital would be a real blow to the community, which is already experiencing various health-related issues and social problems.
- Shakira, who works in a nursing home, begins to notice the frail condition of some of the elderly spouses who regularly visit their loved ones. It occurs to her that many of them are low-income persons who lack social supports.
- Gordon works in an emergency department where he observes student nurses being treated poorly, and he sometimes experiences oppressive behaviour himself. He feels that such events are abusive and that his work environment is rapidly becoming "toxic."

INTRODUCTION

The above scenarios highlight some of the experiences relating to the issue of social justice that nurses may encounter in their everyday practice. What can these nurses do to address the situations in which they find themselves? How can the *Code of Ethics for Registered Nurses* support and guide them?

The 2008 revision of the Canadian Nurses Association (CNA) *Code of Ethics for Registered Nurses* reflects nursing's interest and involvement in social justice. The code is now presented in two parts, with dimensions of social justice reflected in each. Part I sets out the seven primary values and corresponding ethical responsibilities that registered nurses in Canada are expected to uphold. Part II contains 13 statements describing ethical endeavours that nurses may undertake to address social inequities affecting health and well-being (see Box A4-1). As the code states, "Although these endeavours are not part of nurses' core ethical responsibilities, they are part of ethical practice and serve as a helpful motivational and educational tool for all nurses" (CNA, 2008, p. 2). Nurses who have little familiarity with the concept of social justice may not have a clear vision of the relevance of part II of the code to their own practice. The purpose of this paper is therefore to enhance nurses' understanding of social justice and to help raise their awareness of how the code can guide them in social justice endeavours.

In the following paragraphs the concept of social justice is explained and its importance to nursing outlined. A brief discussion of reasons for the growing interest in social justice and the determinants of health follows. Finally, three scenarios are offered as examples of how these ideas might translate into concrete nursing actions. It is recognized that not all nurses will take leadership roles in addressing social justice issues; however, many can be involved in other ways, as demonstrated in the scenarios. These scenarios have been developed to demonstrate how nurses might act locally, given that many nurses are not involved in international efforts related to social justice. The scenarios are meant to reflect everyday practice and to show how small changes can have large effects.

WHAT IS SOCIAL JUSTICE?

Social justice means the fair distribution of resources and responsibilities among the members of a population, with a focus on "the relative position of one social group in relationship to others in society as well as on the root causes of disparities and what can be done to eliminate them" (CNA, 2006, p. 7). When the concept of social justice is applied to health and health care, the term *resources* is taken to mean not just direct services but also other facets of life that can have a positive effect on health, such as food security, adequate housing, gainful employment and acceptable working conditions, adequate income, adequate education, social inclusion and the presence of a social safety net (Ervin & Bell, 2004; McGibbon, Etowa & McPherson, 2008; Raphael, 2004; World Health Organization, 2008). Collectively, these are known as the *social determinants of health*, defined in the CNA code of ethics as "factors in the social environment, external to the health care system, that exert a major and potentially modifiable influence on the health of populations" (CNA, 2008, p. 28). Taking action for social justice means attempting to reduce system-wide differences that disadvantage

BOX A4-1 Ethical Endeavours from the Code of Ethics

Part II of the *Code of Ethics for Registered Nurses* is reproduced here. To download a free copy of the complete code, visit www.cna-aiic.ca.

Part II: Ethical Endeavours

There are broad aspects of social justice that are associated with health and well-being and that ethical nursing practice addresses. These aspects relate to the need for change in systems and societal structures in order to create greater equity for all. Nurses should endeavour as much as possible, individually and collectively, to advocate for and work toward eliminating social inequities by:

i. Utilizing the principles of primary health care for the benefit of the public and persons receiving care.

ii. Recognizing and working to address organizational, social, economic and political factors that influence health and well-being within the context of nurses' role in the delivery of care.

iii. In collaboration with other health care team members and professional organizations, advocating for changes to unethical health and social policies, legislation and regulations.

iv. Advocating for a full continuum of accessible health care services to be provided at the right time and in the right place. This continuum includes health promotion, disease prevention and diagnostic, restorative, rehabilitative and palliative care services in hospitals, nursing homes, home care and the community.

v. Recognizing the significance of social determinants of health and advocating for policies and programs that address these determinants.

vi. Supporting environmental preservation and restoration and advocating for initiatives that reduce environmentally harmful practices in order to promote health and well-being.

vii. Working with individuals, families, groups, populations, and communities to expand the range of health care choices available, recognizing that some people have limited choices because of social, economic, geographic or other factors that lead to inequities.

viii. Understanding that some groups in society are systemically disadvantaged, which leads to diminished health and well-being. Nurses work to improve the quality of lives of people who are part of disadvantaged and/or vulnerable groups and communities, and they take action to overcome barriers to health care.

ix. Advocating for health care systems that ensure accessibility, universality and comprehensiveness of necessary health care services.

x. Maintaining awareness of major health concerns such as poverty, inadequate shelter, food insecurity and violence. Nurses work individually and with others for social justice and to advocate for laws, policies and procedures designed to bring about equity.

xi. Maintaining awareness of broader global health concerns such as violations of human rights, war, world hunger, gender inequities and environmental pollution. Nurses work individually and with others to bring about social change.

xii. Advocating for the discussion of ethical issues among health care team members, persons in their care, families and students. Nurses encourage ethical reflection, and they work to develop their own and others' heightened awareness of ethics in practice.

xiii. Working collaboratively to develop a moral community. As part of the moral community, all nurses acknowledge their responsibility to contribute to positive, healthy work environments.

certain groups and prevent equal access to determinants of health and to health care services.

Understandings of social justice are largely influenced by feminist and critical social theories, which focus on the negative effects of oppression of any kind. By extension, then, social justice in health care also means working to prevent oppressive practices such as discrimination against individuals on the basis of gender, sexual orientation, age or any other social factor that might affect health and well-being (Boutain, 2005; McGibbon et al., 2008). From that we can see that social justice (or injustice) can arise in one-to-one interactions between a nurse and a patient or client and among health care providers themselves. These ideas will be explored in the following paragraphs.

WHY IS SOCIAL JUSTICE A NURSING CONCERN?

In its publication on social justice, CNA (2006, p. 7) noted that "all societies suffer from broad, systematic inequities and oppression" that can have a negative impact on the health of individuals and communities. According to Boutain (2005, p. 404), "If societal relationships based on racial, ethnic, gender and economic status are more equal, population health indicators between diverse groups become more stable, nationally and globally," potentially resulting in more positive outcomes.

Canada is not immune to unequal social relationships. The Canadian Council on Social Development (n.d.) reports that as of 2004 about 3.5 million Canadians were living in poverty, including 865,000 children under the age of 18, with rates highest among female lone-parent families. Poverty rates were highest overall in British Columbia (14.2%), and lowest in Prince Edward Island (6%). In 2005 about 5% of the Canadian population relied on welfare. There were important regional differences in welfare income across provinces: in 2005 a single employable person in New Brunswick received \$3,201, while in Newfoundland and Labrador payments were \$7,189. That same year, only British Columbia increased welfare income for those with disabilities. And according to Campaign 2000 (2007), one in four First Nations children living in First Nations communities lives in poverty, while one in two children in recent immigrant families lives in poverty.

These Canadian statistics are shocking, but global data reveal an even more disturbing picture. Tables on the Global Issues Web site show that at least "80% of humanity lives on less than \$10 a day" and "over three billion people live on less than \$2.50 per day" (Shah, 2008). In a recent report on social justice and determinants of health, the World Health Organization (2008) concluded that because of social inequities, it will take international efforts and massive political will to improve the health conditions of much of the world's population.

What, then, is nursing's role with regard to social justice? It is becoming apparent that social justice should play a significant role in nursing practice (Bekemeier & Butterfield, 2005; Fahrenwald, Taylor, Kneipp & Canales, 2007). As Falk-Rafael (2005, p. 222) has pointed out, "Nurses practice at the intersection of public policy and personal lives; they are, therefore, ideally situated and morally obligated to include socio-political advocacy in their practice." This may certainly be reflected in international efforts, but it is important to note that social justice does not always present as a broad socio-political activity. It is also part of daily practice. Striving to overcome oppression and discrimination wherever they are encountered in the health care system is important in nursing (Varcoe, 2004). The nursing values of "providing safe, compassionate competent and ethical care," "promoting health and well-being" and "preserving dignity" outlined in part I of the *Code of Ethics for Registered Nurses* support this belief. Since fostering the health and well-being of patients or clients requires creation of a healing environment (Marck, 2004), it follows that nurses should endeavour to ensure that no individual receiving care feels discriminated against or oppressed in any way. In particular, "promoting health and well-being" (CNA, 2008) requires nurses to ensure that those who need nursing care are treated with respect and that disparities arising as a result of background and social status are acknowledged and minimized to the extent possible. Promoting social justice thus becomes foundational to every nursing encounter.

WHY NOW IN NURSING?

Social justice has been considered central to public health nursing since its beginning (Ervin & Bell, 2004; Krieger & Birn, 1998) and has long been a core tenet of mental health nursing as well. In the early 1900s nurse activists such as Lillian Wald and Lavinia Dock were vocal in their insistence that societal inequities had to be addressed if the mental and physical health of the population were to improve. They promoted a vision of health as a societal concern (Bekemeier & Butterfield, 2005). However, as individualism and autonomy became more important in North America, health came to be understood as a matter of individual responsibility (Boutain, 2005). At the same time the bulk of health care dollars was being directed toward institutionalized illness care rather than health promotion. Most nurses in Canada were educated in hospital schools, where the focus was on caring for the sick, and issues of population health and social justice were seldom, if ever, discussed, except in university courses on public health.

Now, however, the focus in Canadian health care is shifting. The report of the Commission on the Future of Health Care in Canada (2002) (widely known as the Romanow Report) and that of the Premier's Advisory Council on Health in Alberta (2002) (also known as the Mazankowski Report) recognized that the current system places a great deal of emphasis on technology and illness care, which does not necessarily increase the overall health of the population. Both reports suggested that more attention must be paid to the social determinants of health. Although the reports were criticized for continuing to place too much responsibility on the individual rather than society, they did acknowledge that inequities in access to health care exist and that population (and individual) health is strongly influenced by societal structures and the social determinants of health. As a result, health care reform is now paying more attention to social justice issues (Butler-Jones, 2004).

Another change has been in nursing education, which in Canada now takes place primarily in universities and colleges. A vital feminist influence has been evident in much nursing research and scholarship, and there is consequently a growing recognition, both nationally and internationally, of the influence of oppression, marginalization and social exclusion on health and well-being (Fitzpatrick, 2003). Globalization, defined as "a process of closer interaction of human activity" (Davidson, Meleis, Daly & Douglas, 2003, p. 163), is increasing rapidly and has resulted in a greater awareness of the ways in which socio-political disparities can affect each of us. Nurse scholars have suggested that nurses can and should be involved in seeking solutions to social justice problems because their knowledge and numbers (Davidson et al., 2003; Falk-Rafael, 2005) make them ideally suited to take both individual and collective action. World problems such as climate change and natural disasters point to important links between health and environment and the need for directed action. Issues of violence and hunger are present in Canada and across the globe. As a result of these various forces there has been a strong call to increase attention to social justice in undergraduate nursing curricula (Fahrenwald et al., 2007; Reimer Kirkham, Van Hofwegen & Hoe Harwood, 2005; Schim, Benkert, Bell, Walker & Danford, 2006; Vickers, 2008).

It is becoming increasingly clear that social justice matters. The Canadian health care system is poised for change, with more emphasis to be placed on determinants of health and primary health care (Health Canada, 2004). CNA's publication on social justice states that "social justice is a means to an end as well as an end in itself" (2006, p. 2). It is a means to an end because social justice is necessary for individual and population health, including the health of nurses themselves, and to the health care system as a whole. It is an end unto itself because a just society is a better society. Consequently, Canadian nurses are being called more urgently to the pursuit of social justice.

SOCIAL JUSTICE AND ETHICAL PRACTICE

Both parts I and II of the code of ethics (CNA, 2008) contain statements about social justice. In part I, values such as "preserving dignity" and "promoting justice" speak to the importance of safeguarding human rights and having a non-judgemental, non-discriminative stance toward those receiving care. Part II, the ethical endeavours, suggests aspects of nursing that "relate to the need for change in systems and societal structures in order to create greater equity for all" (p. 20) both nationally and internationally. It draws nurses' attention to broader, global issues such as war, violence and hunger, and encourages nurses to consider taking action individually and collectively, to the extent of their ability, to address social injustice wherever it arises.

In the following paragraphs three scenarios are presented as examples of how a nurse in everyday practice can work for social justice. The first example describes a situation in which a nurse has a concern about health care services in a rural community. The second scenario involves a nurse's actions with respect to access to services for a vulnerable group. The third example involves social justice with an acute care organization. Each scenario is followed by reflections on how the nurse might respond, using the *Code of Ethics for Registered Nurses* for guidance. It is important to recognize that a nurse may not feel able, for a variety of reasons, to take the lead in these types of situations. However, all nurses should recognize the importance of joining in to whatever extent they can.

SCENARIO 1: RURAL HEALTH AND ACCESS TO SERVICES

As a public health nurse, Tara was starting to feel overwhelmed by some of the health-related problems in her rural community. The town itself was experiencing growing problems of domestic violence and substance abuse, apparently precipitated by the closure of the town's sawmill and widespread unemployment. As well, health statistics from the neighbouring aboriginal reserve were truly shocking. Access to clean water on the reserve was limited, as contamination had been discovered in a number of water wells. Infant mortality was much higher than the national average, there had been a startling number of youth suicides over the past year, and the incidence of type 2 diabetes was reaching epidemic proportions. The local aboriginal council had made several attempts to draw government attention to their plight, but despite some promises, nothing had been done. To top it all off, the town's hospital was slated for closure. The hospital in the next town, 70 kilometres away, was to become the care centre for the community.

Losing the local hospital would be a real blow to the community, especially to low-income elderly persons without transportation, who made up a large part of the community's population.

Tara felt angry just thinking about how unfair it was that those living in rural areas did not have the same access to health care or the same attention to their health needs as those living in cities. Here, the ratio of health care providers to population was dismal. A variety of identified health concerns were not being addressed, and now things would get even worse. As a nurse, Tara felt she should take some kind of action. The whole situation was simply not acceptable!

The *Code of Ethics for Registered Nurses* offers support for Tara in taking action on her concerns. The code says that part of ethical practice is "working with individuals, families, groups, populations and communities to expand the range of health care choices available, recognizing that some people have limited choices because of social, economic, geographic or other factors that lead to inequities" (p. 21, item vii). As a public health nurse, Tara would have the skills to help build the community's capacity to take action on what are effectively social justice issues.

She should start by establishing what nurses, other health care providers and members of the community think about the problem. She could point out some of the inequities that she has observed: the lack of services for health promotion, the environmental problems such as water quality, the social issues arising because of lack of employment opportunities, the health statistics for the reserve and the existing and impending restriction of access to health care. She could also point out that those most likely to be harmed by the government's decision to close the hospital are more vulnerable members of society who, for reasons that often also arise from social injustice, are reluctant or incapable of expressing their views and therefore may benefit from nurse advocates. In this way, Tara would be helping others in "recognizing the significance of social determinants of health" (p. 20, item v). Tara could also point out to her nursing colleagues that the *Code of Ethics for Registered Nurses* suggests that "in collaboration with other health care team members and professional organizations, [nurses advocate] for changes to unethical health and social policies, legislation and regulations" (p. 20, item iii).

Nurses and members of the community who are also concerned about the issues could then work with Tara to create an action plan for engaging more community support, which would coincide with the code's statement about "maintaining awareness of major health concerns... [and working] individually and with others for social justice" (p. 21, item x). They might start with a community forum to identify general concerns and possible courses of action. Other community health service providers might be encouraged to become involved, as they would have the credibility to "advocat[e] for a full continuum of accessible health care services to be provided at the right time and in the right place" (p. 20, item v). Nurses could offer to work with the community members in whatever strategies they might devise. For example, they might want to meet with government officials to request reversal of the decision to close the hospital. The code urges "advocating for policies and programs that address [social] determinants [of health]" (p. 201, item v), so the nurses might collaborate with aboriginal leaders to create more political awareness of health issues on the reserve. Together, they could host community presentations on health-related topics to raise public awareness, and they could organize a letter-writing campaign. They might decide to alert local and regional media, such as newspapers and radio, to the disparities in health and health care on the reserve and in the rural community in general. Framing the problems as social justice issues might help to gain the attention of decision-makers.

Nurses living and working in a community have the skills and knowledge to improve the health of that community and to help build its capacity to take action. Taking political action is one way in which to make a difference. The code suggests that "nurses work individually and with others for social justice and to advocate for laws, policies and procedures designed to bring about equity" (p. 21, item x). Reforms in health care are expected to lead to greater emphasis on primary care (Health Canada, 2004), which may radically change the role of nursing. In preparation for such change it is essential that nurses embrace the idea that "advocating for health care systems that ensure accessibility, universality and comprehensiveness of necessary health care services" (CNA, 2008, p. 21, item ix) is a nursing concern. "As the largest group of health professionals in Canada, nurses have the power to promote and lobby for equity in the health care system" (McGibbon et al., 2008, p. 27).

The next scenario describes a situation that might be more familiar to nurses working in long-term care. Here, a nurse is challenged to address issues arising from inadequate services to support healthy aging.

SCENARIO 2: SUPPORTING HEALTHY AGING

Shakira was administering medications to Mr. Yanitsky, a long-term care resident in the Berryville Nursing Home, when his wife of 66 years came into the room. Shakira noticed that Mrs. Yanitsky was looking increasingly frail and seemed to be losing weight. When she inquired about Mrs. Yanitsky's health, she was told, "I'm fine, dear, but I had a little fall yesterday and I'm feeling a bit bruised and sore today."

Shakira took a closer look and noticed a large bruise on Mrs. Yanitsky's hand and a bump on her forehead. She asked, "Do you mind showing me your bruises? I'm a little worried about you." Mrs. Yanitsky responded by pulling up her sweater and showing Shakira her back, which was, indeed, bruised and sore-looking, and she seemed to have pain each time she breathed. Shakira suspected broken ribs. Even more startling was how thin the woman was. Her ribs and spine stood out plainly under her skin.

Shakira asked Mrs. Yanitsky if she had visited the doctor after the fall and was told, "Oh no, dear. I haven't had time, have I? And it's such a bother to try to get to the doctor. I'm not as spry as I used to be. It's hard to make the appointment because I don't hear very well on the telephone, and I don't drive anymore, so I have to take the bus. It's hard enough to get here to visit my husband. I'm fine, though. Really. Don't worry about me. I'm a tough old bird!"

Later in the afternoon Shakira spoke to the doctor and asked if it would be possible to organize an x-ray for Mrs. Yanitsky. The doctor replied that there really wasn't any mechanism to do that through the long-term care centre; instead, the patient would have to go to the emergency department. That got Shakira thinking. She knew that Mrs. Yanitsky would never go to emergency on her own. She also thought about some of the other elderly persons who were regular visitors and recalled that she had often seen signs of increasing frailty in those who visited their loved ones regularly. It occurred to her that many of them were lacking support. She broached the subject with Marlene and Anita, the other nurses who regularly worked the day shift. They, too, had made the same kinds of observations and had worried about their visitors. Most were elderly, and many had reduced financial circumstances, so were less able to arrange for access to services they might need. As they talked, the nurses began to speculate on what, if anything, they should do about the situation.

Part II of the *Code of Ethics for Registered Nurses* encourages the nurses in this scenario to take action, "understanding that some groups in society are systematically disadvantaged, which leads to diminished health and well-being. Nurses work to improve the quality of lives of people who are part of disadvantaged and/or vulnerable groups and communities, and they take action to overcome barriers to health care" (p. 21, item viii). In this scenario, the vulnerable are those low-income elderly persons who have difficulty accessing health care services. With the growing emphasis on primary care and health promotion, working to help this group is part of nurses' ethical practice.

There are many actions that Shakira and her colleagues might take. To start with, they could get together with their manager to identify any community supports with whom they could partner. If none exist, they might suggest a monthly health clinic to be run out of the long-term care centre. If the community is interested in establishing such a clinic, the nurses could assist in organizing a "citizen's action group" to act as a steering committee for the initiative, with the objective of developing and submitting a funding proposal to government. Involving patients and family members, such as Mr. and Mrs. Yanitsky, would be an important step in identifying needs and generating ideas. From the patients and visitors themselves, the nurses might well obtain useful ideas for establishing the clinic; they might also identify people with skills in raising public awareness and funds. An important part of the proposal would be to emphasize the cost-effectiveness of the initiative: in helping to prevent illness, such a clinic could save money over the long term. Some features of the clinic might be assessment by a gerontological nurse practitioner; home follow-up by a registered nurse for such things as falls prevention, living conditions and social supports; assessment of nutritional status by a dietitian; mobile x-ray services; provision of blood test services by a laboratory technician; and assessment of social circumstances (such as finances) by a social worker. The nurses might even suggest starting a program like Meals on Wheels or a dining club through the long-term care centre. Such a proactive stance would go a long way to reducing the health inequities of this vulnerable population.

In considering their options, the nurses would be drawing on their experience in long-term care, their nursing knowledge about the determinants of health, their awareness of the importance of illness prevention and their skills in facilitating community action. Like Tara, the nurse in scenario 1, they can make a difference. Undertaking the ethical endeavour of "advocating for a full continuum of accessible health care services to be provided at the right time and in the right place" (p. 20, item iv) could extend their practice in an interesting and challenging way and might enhance their work life. Addressing social justice concerns can be personally satisfying, as well as ethical.

In the next scenario, one nurse decides to take action toward creating a healthier work environment by recognizing that social justice affects students and staff, as well as patients.

SCENARIO 3: CREATING A MORAL COMMUNITY

Gordon had been working in the emergency department for about a year. He had just had a disagreement with the medical head of the department, who had ordered what Gordon thought might be an incorrect dose of a medication. He understood that unusual doses are sometimes required, but as a professional he felt he had to check. When he asked the physician about the dose, she glared at him and asked sarcastically, "And when did you complete medical school?" She then walked away without answering his question. Gordon felt that his query should not have elicited rudeness on the physician's part. However, he had observed that she frequently acted disrespectfully toward nurses.

Later, Gordon was working with Charlie, a young man who had been involved in a motorcycle accident and who required removal of the gravel embedded in his skin. It was an uncomfortable procedure, and Gordon offered Charlie some analgesic, which was refused. Gordon had just gotten started when Charlie cursed and took a swing at him, connecting with the side of his head and almost knocking him off his feet. Gordon advised Charlie that his actions were unacceptable and left the cubicle to seek assistance. This was not the first time that Gordon had been hit by a patient while working in this emergency department. The incident reinforced for Gordon the fact that this issue of physical violence against nurses in his department needed to be addressed.

At the end of this shift, walking through the unit, Gordon heard another nurse yelling at a student, "I don't know what it is with you people. Don't you know anything? Get out of my sight. You're just useless." The student's eyes filled with tears, and she turned away. It was the second time on this shift alone that Gordon had seen this particular nurse treating a student with contempt. Gordon decided that something had to be done. His workplace was rapidly becoming a "toxic" environment.

In this scenario, the primary issue is one of social justice because the practices that Gordon has observed are oppressive and/or violent, with the result that the work environment is becoming negative and unhealthy. The code of ethics has much to say about the issues identified. Part I states that "Nurses have a responsibility to conduct themselves according to the ethical responsibilities outlined in this document... in what they do and how they interact with persons receiving care... and other members of the health care team" (p. 8). Part I also requires nurses to "prevent and minimize all forms of violence" (p. 9). An ethical endeavour described in part II is "working collaboratively to develop a moral community. As part of the moral community, all nurses acknowledge their responsibility to contribute to positive, healthy work environments" (p. 21, item xiii). Gordon is justified in taking action about his concerns as part of practising ethically.

If Gordon were to go to the literature, he would discover that what he has observed has been termed "lateral violence," a form of bullying aimed at dominating or silencing nurses (Center for American Nurses, 2008; Griffin, 2004). It has been suggested that nurses who have experienced oppression may go on to oppress others because they lack self-esteem (Vickers, 2008). In one Canadian study, nurses admitted that how they felt about themselves influenced the degree to which they practised ethically; they also reported that they sometimes treated patients, students and colleagues "in ways that were not supportive and at times were even demeaning" (Rodney, Hartrick Doane, Storch, & Varcoe, 2006, p. 26). Another form of oppression experienced by nurses is physical violence against them, which has become an international concern (Luck, Jackson, & Usher, 2008) and is increasing in incidence (Whelan, 2008). Nurses have been reported to be at greater risk of physical violence in the workplace than even prison guards or police (St-Pierre & Holmes, 2008). Devising strategies to counter this violence is of concern to nurses and managers alike and is one way in which social justice can be enacted.

In the scenario just described, the behaviour of both the physician who was rude to Gordon and the nurse who was hard on the student could be considered examples of lateral violence, although some authors have suggested that lateral violence occurs only among nurses themselves, with bullying or domination by physicians being a common cause (Sheridan-Leos, 2008). Charlie's (successful) attempt to hit Gordon is also a form of bullying. The escalating level of both kinds of violence toward nurses and students is a symptom of an unhealthy workplace.

Gordon has several options and selecting among them will require an analysis of the situation using the values and ethical endeavours set out in the code of ethics. First, he might consider what it is that makes a physician feel justified in treating a nurse badly. He might turn to the literature for insights into how to manage power relationships in nursing. He could also explore ways in which conflict situations might be managed. He might then approach the physician to discuss how they can improve their professional working relationship, with the shared goal of safe patient care. This requires considerable moral courage, because challenging another, particularly within a hierarchical structure, can be difficult. Moral courage means having the courage or strength of will to act on one's beliefs. Gordon can support his actions by referring to the code of ethics, which encourages him to work toward a more healthy work environment.

Similarly, Gordon may want to talk to his nursing colleague about her behaviour toward students. The code is very precise about the need for nurses to treat students in a respectful manner and to provide them with mentorship and guidance (p. 14, item D10, and p. 19, item G9). The code also specifies that "nurses refrain from judging, labelling, demeaning, stigmatizing and humiliating behaviours toward persons receiving care, other health care professionals and each other" (p. 17, item F2); this principle should be extended to students, who also deserve to be treated with respect. In this way, Gordon would be encouraging his colleague to reflect on her actions and would be "advocating for the discussion of ethical issues among health care team members," as the code of ethics suggest (p. 21, item xii).

It might also be necessary to consider whether the problem is more systemic. From the scenario, it appears that the culture of the emergency department may permit, and even implicitly support, oppression of nurses and students, as no one has openly criticized the physician and nurse for their behaviour. If this is the case, Gordon may wish to approach his unit manager about his concerns. It may be advisable for the unit manager to address the problem in a more public forum such as a staff meeting, indicating that there will be no tolerance for such aggression. The actions of the staff could also be addressed through quality assurance processes. In addition, the unit manager could work through the hospital's administrative structure for development and approval of policies against lateral violence. The clinical ethics committee could also act as a resource in clarifying values and beliefs at individual and institutional levels. If no action is taken on the issue, and if the situation does not improve, Gordon could be justified in taking his concerns to senior hospital management. If the seriousness of the situation escalates and no measures are taken, Gordon could make inquiries to the appropriate provincial or territorial regulatory bodies, which might choose to investigate the inappropriate behaviour as unethical practice.

Gordon could similarly approach his unit manager about the incident with Charlie, the patient, suggesting that the issue of physical violence against nurses needs to be addressed. Such aggression is unacceptable, and institutions should have in place zero-tolerance policies that protect the safety of nurses. If the institution does not have such a policy, then Gordon might ask the unit manager to take the concerns forward. If there is a policy and it is not being enforced, then again, this becomes an issue for those at higher levels of authority. In the past, many nurses have accepted that some level of violence is to be expected in their jobs (Whelan, 2008), but acts of violence such as that demonstrated by Charlie are simply unacceptable. A strong awareness of social justice as a right not just of patients but also of nurses will help the nurses in Gordon's department to be strong in demanding support for a secure, safe work environment. The *Code of Ethics for Registered Nurses* indicates that one ethical endeavour that nurses might undertake is "recognizing and working to address organizational, social, economic and political factors that influence health and well-being within the context of nurses' role in the delivery of care" (p. 21, item ii).

Gordon should not expect to address his concerns alone but could exhibit ethics leadership by encouraging his nursing colleagues to oppose violence and bullying in any form; he could also enlist the aid of the clinical educator. She or he could be asked to develop educational sessions to help nurses become more alert to these issues—that is, to recognize them as instances of unacceptable behaviour or unethical practice and to devise strategies to work against them (Griffin, 2004). Gordon and his colleagues could also work on ways to change what Daiski (2004, p. 43) has called "disempowering relationships." A concerted effort on the part of nurses, who greatly outnumber other health care providers, could have a great effect on the moral community in the unit and throughout the institution.

Social justice should not be the responsibility of a single individual; it must also be reflected in the ethos or ethics environment of health care structures and institutions. All staff members should be included in discussions as a way of promoting a positive culture of collaboration in the workplace.

CONCLUSION

Social justice plays a significant role in nursing and nursing education. The *Code of Ethics for Registered Nurses* emphasizes the importance of social justice in everyday nursing practice, as well as in socio-political action at national and international levels. In this paper, three scenarios have been used to demonstrate how nurses might work within their communities, their institutions and their departments to enhance attention to social justice for patients and staff. Whether they are involved in direct care, administration, education, research or policy development, it is useful for nurses to reflect on how social justice issues relate to their daily practice. The questions in Box A4-2 may prove helpful to nurses in this respect.

The scenarios in this paper offer just a few examples of how nurses might take action at the local level, but the code also suggests that nurses consider taking whatever opportunity they can, individually and collectively, to address issues occurring within a global context, such as violence, hunger and poverty (CNA, 2008, p. 21, item xi).

Many opportunities exist for nurses to learn about social justice issues. The Web sites of provincial, territorial, national and international nursing organizations offer helpful resources. Attending nursing conferences, such as those organized by CNA and the International Council of Nurses, is another way to strengthen awareness of social justice issues. The International Centre for Nursing Ethics also sponsors an annual conference where nurses can learn about some of the issues arising in other parts of the world and ways in which nurses have taken action to reduce social inequities. Canadian Nurses Interested in Ethics, an affiliate of CNA, is another forum where nurses can share information and discuss issues (http://cniethics.ca).

BOX A4-2 Reflecting on Social Justice, the Social Determinants of Health, and Inequities in Access

Practice

- Does my practice area offer sessions on social justice, the SDH (social determinants of health) and inequities in access (e.g., the relationship between postnatal outcomes and unemployment or between seniors' health and the cost of home heating)?
- Do I routinely associate client "non-compliance" with the possibility that the client has no money for transportation or prescribed treatments?
- Is lack of action on my part a form of discrimination?

Education

- Do I incorporate social justice, the SDH, and inequities in access in my teaching of the specialty areas (e.g., the relationships between cardiac outcomes, race, gender)?
- Does my institution offer faculty training on social justice and health?
- Is lack of action on my part a form of discrimination?

Research

- Am I encouraged to ask research questions that address the issues of marginalized peoples?
- What steps do I take to ensure diverse participants and perspectives are included in my sample?
- Do I use appropriate research methods (e.g., participatory engagement) to study inequities in health care?

Management and Policy

- Does my workplace implement policies that explicitly address social justice, the SDH and inequities in access? Are these policies reviewed regularly?
- What happens when I apply the CNA social justice gauge (2006) to the policy documents of my workplace? Of my political party?
- How does my political party perform on social justice issues such as child poverty and homelessness?

SOURCE: McGibbon, Etowa, & McPherson, 2008, p. 26.

Considerable information related to social justice is also available from the Internet. The following are just a few examples of these sources:

- Information about the World Health Organization's Commission on Social Determinants of Health can be found at www.who.int/social_determinants/en/.
- The Public Health Agency of Canada has a social determinants of health department, and a search of the agency's Web site (www.phac-aspc.gc.ca/index-eng.php) yields over 1,600 articles, position statements and other documents, with links.
- The Canadian Council for International Co-operation (www.ccic.ca/e/home/index.shtml) has considerable information on social justice initiatives.

Clearly, the nursing profession is becoming more aware of the importance of social justice issues at all levels, from global health to population health, individual care and nurses' rights. This awareness of social justice as an important part of ethical nursing practice is essential as we move toward a more enlightened, more just and more sustainable health care system and a more humane and equitable world. Canadian nurses can be part of this movement for change and, with knowledge and determination, can make a difference. Health for all is a goal that nurses can understand and a goal toward which they should be prepared to work as part of everyday ethical practice.

REFERENCES

Bekemeier, B., & Butterfield, P. (2005). Unreconciled inconsistencies: A critical review of the concept of social justice in 3 national nursing documents. *Advances in Nursing Science, 28*(2), 152–162.

Boutain, D. M. (2005). Social justice as a framework for professional nursing. *Journal of Nursing Education, 44*, 404–407.

Butler-Jones, D. (2004). *Key principles. Primary health reform and public health.* [Web pages revised 2005] Ottawa: Public Health Agency of Canada. Retrieved from www.phac-aspc.gc.ca/publicat/prm_spr/2_e.html.

Campaign 2000. (2007). *It takes a nation to raise a generation: Time for a national poverty reduction strategy. 2007 report card on child and family poverty in Canada.* Toronto: Author. Retrieved from www.campaign2000.ca/rc/rc07/2007_C2000_NationalReportCard.pdf.

Canadian Council on Social Development (n.d.). Economic security: Poverty. Ottawa: Author. Retrieved from www.ccsd.ca/factsheets/economic_security/poverty/ccsd_es_poverty.pdf.

Canadian Nurses Association. (2006). *Social justice... a means to an end, an end in itself.* Ottawa: Author.

Canadian Nurses Association. (2008). *Code of ethics for registered nurses.* Ottawa: Author.

Center for American Nurses. (2008, June, July, August). The Center for American Nurses calls for an end to lateral violence and bullying in nursing work environments: New position statement offers information and recommended strategies. *Oklahoma Nurse, 16.*

Commission on the Future of Health Care in Canada. (2002). *Building on values: The future of health care in Canada—Final Report.* Ottawa: Author.

Daiski, I. (2004). Changing nurses' dis-empowering relationship patterns. *Journal of Advanced Nursing, 48,* 43–50.

Davidson, P. M., Meleis, A., Daly, J., & Douglas, M. (2003). Globalisation as we enter the 21st century. *Contemporary Nurse, 15,* 162–174.

Ervin, N. E., & Bell, S. E. (2004). Social justice issues related to the uneven distribution of resources. *Journal of the New York State Nurses Association, 35*(1), 8–13.

Fahrenwald, N. L., Taylor, J. Y., Kneipp, S. M., & Canales, M. K. (2007). Academic freedom and academic duty to teach social justice: A perspective and pedagogy for public health nursing faculty. *Public Health Nursing, 24*(2), 190–197.

Falk-Rafael, A. (2005). Speaking truth to power: Nursing's legacy and moral imperative. *Advances in Nursing Science, 28*(2), 212–223.

Fitzpatrick, J. J. (2003). Social justice, human rights, and nursing education [Editorial]. *Nursing Education Perspectives, 24,* 65.

Griffin, M. (2004). Teaching cognitive rehearsal as a shield for lateral violence: An intervention for newly licensed nurses. *Journal of Continuing Education in Nursing, 35,* 257–263.

Health Canada. (2004). *Primary health care and health system renewal.* Retrieved from http://www.hc-sc.gc.ca/hcs-sss/prim/renew-renouv-eng.php.

Krieger, N., & Birn, A. (1998). A vision of social justice as the foundation of public health: Commemorating 150 years of the spirit of 1848. *American Journal of Public Health, 88,* 1603–1606.

Luck, L., Jackson, D., & Usher, K. (2008). Innocent or culpable? Meanings that emergency department nurses ascribe to individual acts of violence. *Journal of Clinical Nursing, 17,* 1071–1078.

Marck, P. (2004). Ethics for practitioners: An ecological framework. In J. L. Storch, P. Rodney, & R. Starzomski (Eds.), *Toward a moral horizon: Nursing ethics for leadership and practice* (pp. 232–247). Toronto: Pearson Education Canada.

McGibbon, E., Etowa, J., & McPherson, C. (2008). Health-care access as a social determinant of health. *Canadian Nurse, 104*(7), 23–27.

Premier's Advisory Council on Health. (2002). *A framework for reform.* Edmonton: Government of Alberta.

Raphael, D. (Ed.), (2004). *Social determinants of health: Canadian perspectives.* Toronto: Canadian Scholars' Press.

Reimer Kirkham, S., Van Hofwegen, L., & Hoe Harwood, C. (2005). Narratives of social justice: Learnings in innovative clinical settings. *International Journal of Nursing Education Scholarship, 2*(1). Article 28. Retrieved from www.bepress.com/ijnes/vol2/iss1/art28.

Rodney, P., Hartrick-Doane, G., Storch, J., & Varcoe, C. (2006). Toward a safer moral climate. *Canadian Nurse, 10*(8), 24–27.

Schim, S. M., Benkert, R., Bell, S. E., Walker, D. S., & Danford, C. (2006). Social justice: Added metaparadigm concept for urban health nursing. *Public Health Nursing, 24*(1), 73–80.

Shah, A. (2008). *Poverty facts and stats.* Retrieved from www.globalissues.org/article/26/poverty-facts-and-stats.

Sheridan-Leos, N. (2008). Understanding lateral violence in nursing. *Journal of Oncology Nursing, 12,* 399–403.

St-Pierre, I., & Holmes, D. (2008). Managing nurses through disciplinary power: A Foucaldian analysis of workplace violence. *Journal of Nursing Management, 16,* 352–359.

Varcoe, C. (2004). Widening the scope of ethical theory, practice, and policy: Violence against women as an illustration. In J. L. Storch, P. Rodney, & R. Starzomski (Eds.), *Toward a moral horizon: Nursing ethics for leadership and practice* (pp. 414–432). Toronto: Pearson Education Canada.

Vickers, D. A. (2008). Social justice: A concept for undergraduate nursing curricula? *Southern Online Journal of Nursing Research, 8*(1). Retrieved from www.snrs.org/publications/SOJNR_articles2/Vol08Num01Art06.html.

Whelan, T. (2008). The escalating trend of violence toward nurses. *Journal of Emergency Nursing, 34,* 130–133.

World Health Organization. (2008). *Health equity through action on the social determinants of health.* Geneva: Author.

SOURCE: Canadian Nurses Association. (2009). *Ethics in practice for registered nurses: Social justice in practice.* Ottawa: Author. Retrieved from http://www.cna-aiic.ca/CNA/documents/pdf/publications/Ethics_in_Practice:April_2009_e.pdf.

APPENDIX 5

Declaration of Alma-Ata

The International Conference on Primary Health Care, meeting in Alma-Ata this twelfth day of September in the year nineteen hundred and seventy-eight, expressing the need for urgent action of all governments, all health and development workers, and the world community to protect and promote the health of all the people of the world, hereby makes the following Declaration:

I

The Conference strongly reaffirms that health, which is a state of complete physical, mental, and social wellbeing, and not merely the absence of disease or infirmity, is a fundamental human right and that the attainment of the highest possible level of health is a most important worldwide social goal, whose realization requires the action of many other social and economic sectors in addition to the health sector.

II

The existing gross inequality in the health status of the people, particularly between developed and developing countries and within countries, is politically, socially, and economically unacceptable and is therefore of common concern to all countries.

III

Economic and social development, based on a new international economic order, is of basic importance to the fullest attainment of health for all and to the reduction of the gap between the health status of developing and developed countries. The promotion and protection of the health of the people are essential to sustained economic and social development and contribute to a better quality of life and to world peace.

IV

The people have the right and duty to participate individually and collectively in the planning and implementation of their health care.

V

Governments have a responsibility for the health of their people, which can be fulfilled only by the provision of adequate health and social measures. In the coming decades a main social target of governments, international organizations, and the whole world community should be the attainment by all peoples of the world by the year 2000 of a level of health that will permit them to lead a socially and economically productive life. Primary health care is the key to attaining this target as part of development in the spirit of social justice.

VI

Primary health care is essential health care based on practical, scientifically sound, and socially acceptable methods and technology made universally accessible to individuals and families in the community through their full participation and at a cost that the community and country can afford to maintain at every stage of their development in the spirit of self-reliance and self-determination. It forms an integral part both of the country's health system, of which primary health care is the central function and main focus, and of the overall social and economic development of the community. It is the first level of contact for individuals, the family, and the community with the national health system bringing health care as close as possible to where people live and work, and it constitutes the first element of a continuing health care process.

VII

Primary health care

1. Reflects and evolves from the economic conditions and sociocultural and political characteristics of the country and its communities and is based on the application of the relevant results of social, biomedical, and health services research and public health experience;
2. Addresses the main health problems in the community, providing promotive, preventive, curative, and rehabilitative services accordingly;
3. Includes at least education concerning prevailing health problems and the methods of preventing and controlling them; promotion of food supply and proper nutrition; an adequate supply of safe water and basic sanitation; maternal and child health care, including family planning; immunization against the major infectious diseases; prevention and control of locally endemic diseases; appropriate treatment of common diseases and injuries; and provision of essential drugs;
4. Involves, in addition to health sector, all related sectors and aspects of national and community development, in particular agriculture, animal husbandry, food industry, education, housing, public works, communication, and other sectors; and demands the coordinated efforts of all those sections;

5. Requires and promotes maximum community and individual self-reliance and participation in the planning, organization, operation, and control of primary health care making fullest use of local, national and other available resources; and to this end, develops through appropriate education the ability of communities to participate;
6. Should be sustained by integrated, functional, and mutually supportive referral levels, leading to the progressive improvement of comprehensive health care for all, and giving priority to those most in need;
7. Relies, at local and referral levels, on health workers, including physicians, nurses, midwives, auxiliaries, and community workers, as applicable, as well as on traditional practitioners as needed, suitably trained socially and technically to work as a health team and to respond to the expressed health needs of the community.

VIII

All governments should formulate national policies, strategies, and plans of action to launch and sustain primary health care as part of a comprehensive national health system and in coordination with other sectors. To this end, it will be necessary to exercise political will, to mobilize the country's resources, and to use available external resources rationally.

IX

All countries should cooperate in a spirit of partnership and service to ensure primary health care for all people because the attainment of health by people in any one country directly concerns and benefits every other country. In this context the joint WHO-UNICEF report on primary health care constitutes a solid basis for the further development and operation of Primary Health Care throughout the world.

X

An acceptable level of health for all the people of the world by the year 2000 can be attained through a fuller and better use of the world's resources, a considerable part of which is now spent on armaments and military conflicts. A genuine policy of independence, peace, détente, and disarmament could and should release additional resources that could well be devoted to peaceful aims and in particular to the acceleration of social and economic development of which primary health care, as an essential part, should be allotted its proper share.

SOURCE: World Health Organization. (1978). *Primary health care: Report of the International Conference on Primary Health Care,* Alma-Ata, USSR, Sept 6–12, 1978, Geneva: WHO.

APPENDIX 6

Ottawa Charter for Health Promotion

The first international Conference on Health Promotion, meeting in Ottawa this 21st day of November, 1986, hereby presents this charter for action to achieve Health for All by the year 2000 and beyond.

This conference was primarily a response to growing expectations for a new public health movement around the world. Discussions focused on the needs in industrialized countries, but took into account similar concerns in all other regions. It built on the progress made through the Declaration on Primary Health Care at Alma Ata, the World Health Organization's Targets for Health for All document, and the recent debate at the World Health Assembly on intersectoral action for health.

HEALTH PROMOTION

Health promotion is the process of enabling people to increase control over, and to improve, their health. To reach a state of complete physical, mental, and social well-being, an individual or group must be able to identify and to realize aspirations, to satisfy needs, and to change or cope with the environment. Health is, therefore, seen as a resource for everyday life, not the objective of living. Health is a positive concept emphasizing social and personal resources, as well as physical capacities. Therefore, health promotion is not just the responsibility of the health sector, but goes beyond healthy life-styles to well-being.

Prerequisites for Health

The fundamental conditions and resources for health are peace, shelter, education, food, income, a stable eco-system, sustainable resources, social justice and equity. Improvement in health requires a secure foundation in these basic prerequisites.

Advocate

Good health is a major resource for social, economic and personal development and important dimension of quality of life. Political, economic, social cultural, environmental, behavioural, and biological factors can all favour health or be harmful to it. Health promotion action aims at making these conditions favourable through *advocacy* for health.

Enable

Health promotion focuses on achieving equity in health. Health promotion action aims at reducing differences in current health status and ensuring equal opportunities and resources to *enable* all people to achieve their fullest health potential. This includes a secure foundation in a supportive environment, access to information, life skills and opportunities for making healthy choices. People cannot achieve their fullest health potential unless they are able to take control of those things which determine their health. This must apply equally to women and men.

Mediate

The prerequisites and prospects for health cannot be ensured by the health sector alone. More importantly, health promotion demands coordinated action by all concerned: by governments, by health and other social and economic sectors, by non-governmental and voluntary organizations, by local authorities, by industry and by the media. People in all walks of life are involved as individuals, families and communities. Professional and social groups and health personnel have a major responsibility to *mediate* between differing interests in society for the pursuit of health. Health promotion strategies and programmes should be adapted to the local needs and possibilities of individual countries and regions to take into account differing social, cultural, and economic systems.

HEALTH PROMOTION ACTION MEANS:

Build Healthy Public Policy

Health promotion goes beyond health care. It puts health on the agenda of policymakers in all sectors and at all levels, directing them to be aware of the health consequences of their decisions and to accept their responsibilities for health.

Health promotion policy combines diverse but complementary approaches including legislation, fiscal measures, taxation and organizational change.

It is coordinated action that leads to health, income and social policies that foster greater equity. Joint action contributes to ensuring safer and healthier goods and services, healthier public services, and cleaner, more enjoyable environments.

Health promotion policy requires the identification of obstacles to the adoption of healthy public policies on non–health sectors, and ways of removing them. The aim must be to make the healthier choice the easier choice for policymakers as well.

Create Supportive Environments

Our societies are complex and interrelated. Health cannot be separated from other goals. The inextricable links between people and their environment constitutes the basis for a socio-ecological approach to health. The overall guiding principle for the world, nations, regions and communities alike, is the need to encourage reciprocal maintenance—to take care of each other, our communities and our natural environment. The conservation of natural resources throughout the world should be emphasized as a global responsibility.

Changing patterns of life, work and leisure have a significant impact on health. Work and leisure should be a source of health for people. The way society organizes work should help create a healthy society. Health promotion generates living and working conditions that are safe, stimulating, satisfying and enjoyable.

Systematic assessment of the health impact of a rapidly changing environment—particularly in areas of technology, work, energy production and urbanization—is essential and must be followed by action to ensure positive benefit to the health of the public. The protection of the natural and built environments and the conservation of natural resources must be addressed in any health promotion strategy.

Strengthen Community Action

Health promotion works through concrete and effective community action in setting priorities, making decisions, planning strategies and implementing them to achieve better health. At the heart of this process is the empowerment of communities, their ownership and control of their own endeavours and destinies.

Community development draws on existing human and material resources in the community to enhance self-help and social support, and to develop flexible systems for strengthening public participation and direction of health matters. This requires full and continuous access to information, learning opportunities for health, as well as funding support.

Develop Personal Skills

Health promotion supports personal and social development through providing information, education for health and enhancing life skills. By so doing, it increases the options available to people to exercise more control over their own health and over their environments, and to make choices conducive to health.

Enabling people to learn throughout life, to prepare themselves for all of its stages and to cope with chronic illness and injuries, is essential. This has to be facilitated in school, home, work and community settings. Action is required through educational, professional, commercial and voluntary bodies, and within the institutions themselves.

Reorient Health Services

The responsibility for health promotion in health services is shared among individuals, community groups, health professionals, health service institutions and governments. They must work together towards a health care system which contributes to the pursuit of health.

The role of the health sector must move increasingly in a health promotion direction, beyond its responsibility for providing clinical and curative services. Health services need to embrace an expanded mandate which is sensitive and respects cultural needs. This mandate should support the needs of individuals and communities for a healthier life, and open channels between the health sector and broader social, political, economic, and physical environment components.

Reorienting health services also requires stronger attention to health research as well as changes in professional education and training. This must lead to a change of attitude and organization of health services, which refocuses on the total needs of the individual as a whole person.

MOVING INTO THE FUTURE

Health is created and lived by people within the settings of their everyday life; where they learn, work, play, and love. Health is created by caring for oneself and others, by being able to take decisions and have control over one's life circumstances, and by ensuring that the society one lives in creates conditions that allow the attainment of health by all its members.

Caring, holism and ecology are essential issues in developing strategies for health promotion. Therefore, those involved should take as a guiding principle that, in each phase of planning, implementation and evaluation of health promotion activities, women and men should become equal partners.

Commitment to Health Promotion

The participants of this conference pledge:

- to move into the arena of healthy public policy, and to advocate a clear political commitment to health and equity in all sectors;
- to counteract the pressures towards harmful products, resource depletion, unhealthy living conditions, and environments, and bad nutrition; and to focus attention on public health issues such as pollution, occupational hazards, housing and settlements;
- to respond to the health gap within and between societies, and to tackle the inequities in health produced by the rules and practices of these societies;
- to acknowledge people as the main health resource; to support and enable them to keep themselves, their families and friends healthy through financial and other means, and to accept the community as the essential voice in matters of its health, living conditions and well-being;
- to reorient health services and their resources towards the promotion of health; and to share power with other sectors, other disciplines and most importantly, with people themselves;
- to recognize health and its maintenance as a major social investment and challenge; and
- to address the overall ecological issue of our ways of living.

The conference urges all concerned to join them in their commitment to a strong public health alliance.

Call for International Action

The Conference calls on the World Health Organization and other international organizations to advocate the promotion of health in all appropriate forums and to support countries in setting up strategies and programmes for health promotion.

The Conference is firmly convinced that if people in all walks of life, nongovernmental and voluntary organizations, governments, the World Health Organization and all other bodies concerned join forces in introducing strategies for health promotion, in line with the moral and social values that form the basis of this charter, Health for All by the year 2000 will become a reality.

This charter for action was developed and adopted by an international conference, jointly organized by the World Health Organization, Health and Welfare Canada and the Canadian Public Health Association. Two hundred and twelve participants from 38 countries met from November 17 to 21, 1986, in Ottawa, Canada to exchange experiences and share knowledge of health promotion.

The Conference stimulated an open dialogue among lay, health and other professional workers, among representatives of governmental, voluntary and community organizations, and among politicians, administrators, academics and practitioners. Participants coordinated their efforts and came to a clearer definition of the major challenges ahead. They strengthened their individual and collective commitment to the common goal of Health for All by the Year 2000.

This charter for action reflects the spirit of earlier public charters through which the needs of people were recognized and acted upon. The charter presents fundamental strategies and approaches for health promotion which the participants considered vital for major progress. The conference report develops the issues raised, gives concrete examples and practical suggestions regarding how real advances can be achieved, and outlines the action required of countries and relevant groups.

The move towards a new public health is now evident worldwide. It was reaffirmed not only by the experiences but by the pledges of Conference participants who were involved as individuals on the basis of their expertise. The following countries were represented: Antigua, Australia, Austria, Belgium, Bulgaria, Canada, Czechoslovakia, Denmark, Eire, England, Finland, France, German Democratic Republic, Federal Republic of Germany, Ghana, Hungary, Iceland, Israel, Italy, Japan, Malta, Netherlands, New Zealand, Northern Ireland, Norway, Poland, Portugal, Romania, St. Kitts-Nevis, Scotland, Spain, Sudan, Sweden, Switzerland, Union of Soviet Socialist Republic, United States of America, Wales, and Yugoslavia.

Source: World Health Organization. (1986). *Ottawa Charter for Health Promotion* (p. 5). Retrieved from http://www.who.int/healthpromotion/conferences/previous/ottawa/en/.

Giger and Davidhizar's Transcultural Assessment Model

APPENDIX 7

CULTURALLY UNIQUE INDIVIDUAL

1. Place of birth
2. Cultural definition
   What is...
3. Race
   What is...
4. Length of time in country (if appropriate)

COMMUNICATION

1. Voice quality
   A. Strong, resonant
   B. Soft
   C. Average
   D. Shrill
2. Pronunciation and enunciation
   A. Clear
   B. Slurred
   C. Dialect (geographical)
3. Use of silence
   A. Infrequent
   B. Often
   C. Length
      (1) Brief
      (2) Moderate
      (3) Long
      (4) Not observed
4. Use of non-verbal
   A. Hand movement
   B. Eye movement
   C. Entire body movement
   D. Kinesics (gestures, expression, or stances)
5. Touch
   A. Startles or withdraws when touched
   B. Accepts touch without difficulty
   C. Touches others without difficulty
6. Ask these and similar questions:
   A. How do you get your point across to others?
   B. Do you like communicating with friends, family, and acquaintances?
   C. When asked a question, do you usually respond (in words or body movement, or both)?
   D. If you have something important to discuss with your family, how would you approach them?

SPACE

1. Degree of comfort
   A. Moves when space invaded
   B. Does not move when space invaded
2. Distance in conversations
   A. 0 to 18 inches
   B. 18 inches to 3 feet
   C. 3 feet or more
3. Definition of space
   A. Describe degree of comfort with closeness when talking with or standing near others
   B. How do objects (e.g., furniture) in the environment affect your sense of space?
4. Ask these and similar questions:
   A. When you talk with family members, how close do you stand?
   B. When you communicate with co-workers and other acquaintances, how close do you stand?
   C. If a stranger touches you, how do you react or feel?
   D. If a loved one touches you, how do you react or feel?
   E. Are you comfortable with the distance between us now?

SOCIAL ORGANIZATION

1. Normal state of health
   A. Poor
   B. Fair
   C. Good
   D. Excellent
2. Marital status
3. Number of children
4. Parents living or deceased?
5. Ask these and similar questions:
   A. How do you define social activities?
   B. What are some activities that you enjoy?
   C. What are your hobbies, or what do you do when you have free time?
   D. Do you believe in a Supreme Being?
   E. How do you worship that Supreme Being?
   F. What is your function (what do you do) in your family unit/system?
   G. What is your role in your family unit/system (father, mother, child, advisor)?

H. When you were a child, what or who influenced you most?
I. What is/was your relationship with your siblings and parents?
J. What does work mean to you?
K. Describe your past, present, and future jobs.
L. What are your political views?
M. How have your political views influenced your attitude toward health and illness?

TIME

1. Orientation to time
   A. Past-oriented
   B. Present-oriented
   C. Future-oriented
2. View of time
   A. Social time
   B. Clock-oriented
3. Physiochemical reaction to time
   A. Sleeps at least 8 hours a night
   B. Goes to sleep and wakes on a consistent schedule
   C. Understands the importance of taking medication and other treatments on schedule
4. Ask these and similar questions:
   A. What kind of timepiece do you wear daily?
   B. If you have an appointment at 2 PM, what time is acceptable to arrive?
   C. If a nurse tells you that you will receive a medication in "about a half hour," realistically, how much time will you allow before calling the nurse's station?

ENVIRONMENTAL CONTROL

1. Locus-of-control
   A. Internal locus-of-control (believes that the power to affect change lies within)
   B. External locus-of-control (believes that fate, luck, and chance have a great deal to do with how things turn out)
2. Value orientation
   A. Believes in supernatural forces
   B. Relies on magic, witchcraft, and prayer to affect change
   C. Does not believe in supernatural forces
   D. Does not rely on magic, witchcraft, or prayer to affect change
3. Ask these and similar questions:
   A. How often do you have visitors at your home?
   B. Is it acceptable to you for visitors to drop in unexpectedly?
   C. Name some ways your parents or other persons treated your illnesses when you were a child.
   D. Have you or someone else in your immediate surroundings ever used a home remedy that made you sick?
   E. What home remedies have you used that worked? Will you use them in the future?
   F. What is your definition of "good health"?
   G. What is your definition of illness or "poor health"?

BIOLOGICAL VARIATIONS

1. Conduct a complete physical assessment noting:
   A. Body structure (small, medium, or large frame)
   B. Skin colour
   C. Unusual skin discolorations
   D. Hair colour and distribution
   E. Other visible physical characteristics (e.g., keloids, chloasma)
   F. Weight
   G. Height
   H. Check lab work for variances in hemoglobin, hematocrit, and sickle cell phenomena if Black or Mediterranean
2. Ask these and similar questions:
   A. What diseases or illnesses are common in your family?
   B. Describe your family's typical behaviour when a family member is ill.
   C. How do you respond when you are angry?
   D. Who (or what) usually helps you to cope during a difficult time?
   E. What foods do you and your family like to eat?
   F. Have you ever had any unusual cravings for
      (1) White or red clay dirt?
      (2) Laundry starch?
   G. When you were a child, what types of foods did you eat?
   H. What foods are family favourites or are considered traditional?

NURSING ASSESSMENT

1. Note whether the client has become culturally assimilated or observes own cultural practices.
2. Incorporate data into plan of nursing care:
   A. Encourage the client to discuss cultural differences; people from diverse cultures who hold different views can enlighten nurses.
   B. Make efforts to accept and understand methods of communication.
   C. Respect the individual's personal need for space.
   D. Respect the rights of clients to honour and worship the Supreme Being of their choice.
   E. Identify a clerical or spiritual person to contact.
   F. Determine whether spiritual practices have implications for health, life, and well-being (e.g., Jehovah's Witnesses may refuse blood and blood derivatives;

an Orthodox Jew may eat only kosher food high in sodium and may not drink milk when meat is served).

G. Identify hobbies, especially when devising interventions for a short or extended convalescence or for rehabilitation.

H. Honour time and value orientations and differences in these areas. Allay anxiety and apprehension if adherence to time is necessary.

I. Provide privacy according to personal need and health status of the client. (NOTE: The perception of and reaction to pain may be culturally related.)

J. Note cultural health practices.
   (1) Identify and encourage efficacious practices.
   (2) Identify and discourage dysfunctional practices.
   (3) Identify and determine whether neutral practices will have a long-term ill effect.

K. Note food preferences.
   (1) Make as many adjustments in diet as health status and long-term benefits will allow and that dietary department can provide.
   (2) Note dietary practices that may have serious implications for client.

SOURCE: Davidhizar, R. E., & Giger, J. N. (1998). *Canadian transcultural nursing: Assessment and intervention.* St. Louis, MO: Mosby.

APPENDIX 8

Community-as-Partner Model

The community-as-partner model was developed to illustrate public health nursing as a synthesis of public health and nursing. The model, originally titled *community-as-client,* has evolved to incorporate the philosophy that nurses work with communities as partners. This is congruent with what was learned about how communities (and people, for that matter) change and grow best, that is, by full involvement and self-empowerment, not by imposed programs and structures.

The model's "heart" is the assessment wheel (Figure A8-1), which depicts that the people actually are the community—the core elements. Without people there is no community, and it is the people (their demographics, values, beliefs, history) that are of interest to the public health nurse. Surrounding the people, and integral with them, are the identified eight subsystems of a community. These subsystems (physical environment, education, safety and transportation, politics and government, health and social services, communication, economics, and recreation) both affect and are affected by the people. To understand this interaction, one must understand each subsystem; therefore, incorporate its assessment into assessment of the people.

The "wheel" (actually the entire community, including the people and subsystems) is shown with broken lines between each subsystem to show that these are not discrete, but that all subsystems affect each other. Within the community are lines of resistance, those "strengths" that defend against stressors (e.g., a school-based program to prevent teen violence); identifying strengths in the community is as important as identifying "problems." Surrounding the community are lines of defense, depicted in the model as "flexible" and "normal" to indicate that there are two types of defense: one is the usual (normal) "health" of a community and the other is more dynamic (flexible) and changes more rapidly. Two illustrations may assist in clarifying these lines. The flexible line of defense may be a temporary response to a stressor. For instance, an environmental stressor such as flash flooding or a major fire may call into play resources from within the community and from surrounding areas; these resources are considered the flexible lines of defense. The normal line of defense is the usual level of health a community has reached over time. Examples of normal lines of defense include the immunization rate, adequate housing, or access to Meals-on-Wheels for shut-ins; all of these contribute to the health of the community.

Stressors affect the community and may be of the community or from outside the community. Either way, the community's response to stressors is mitigated by its overall health state, that is, by the strength of its lines of resistance and defense. Knowing these strengths is one purpose of the community assessment. In the analysis phase of the nursing process, the nurse will weigh the stressor and the degree of reaction it causes in order to describe a community nursing diagnosis that, in turn, will give direction to goals and interventions. One method for stating the community nursing diagnosis is to state the "problem" as the degree of reaction (from which the goal is derived) and the "as related to" as stressors ("causes" that help define needed interventions). Using this method, an example of a community nursing diagnosis might be as follows: High rate of tuberculosis (the problem, the degree of reaction) related to poor hygiene and sanitation, crowded living conditions, poverty, and consumption of raw milk (stressors) as manifested by open garbage, and poor ventilation; an average of 5.6 persons per household; and sale of raw milk for income (the "data" collected in your assessment).

Think for a moment how each subsystem contributes to the health of the community. The nurse can see how an inadequate infrastructure, such as lack of modern sewage treatment or unemployment, can affect the health of all of the citizens.

Many models exist to provide a framework for assessing a community. This systems model gives one other way to describe a community. Working with the community is a vital and challenging task for nurses. Using a model wherein the community is viewed as a partner will help formulate community-focused interventions and promote the health of the entire community.

Elizabeth T. Anderson, RN, FAAN, DrPH
Professor and Chair, Department of Community Health and Technology
University of Texas School of Nursing at Galveston
University of Texas Medical Branch
Galveston, Texas

FIGURE A8-1 The Community Assessment Wheel, the Assessment Segment of the Community-as-Partner Model

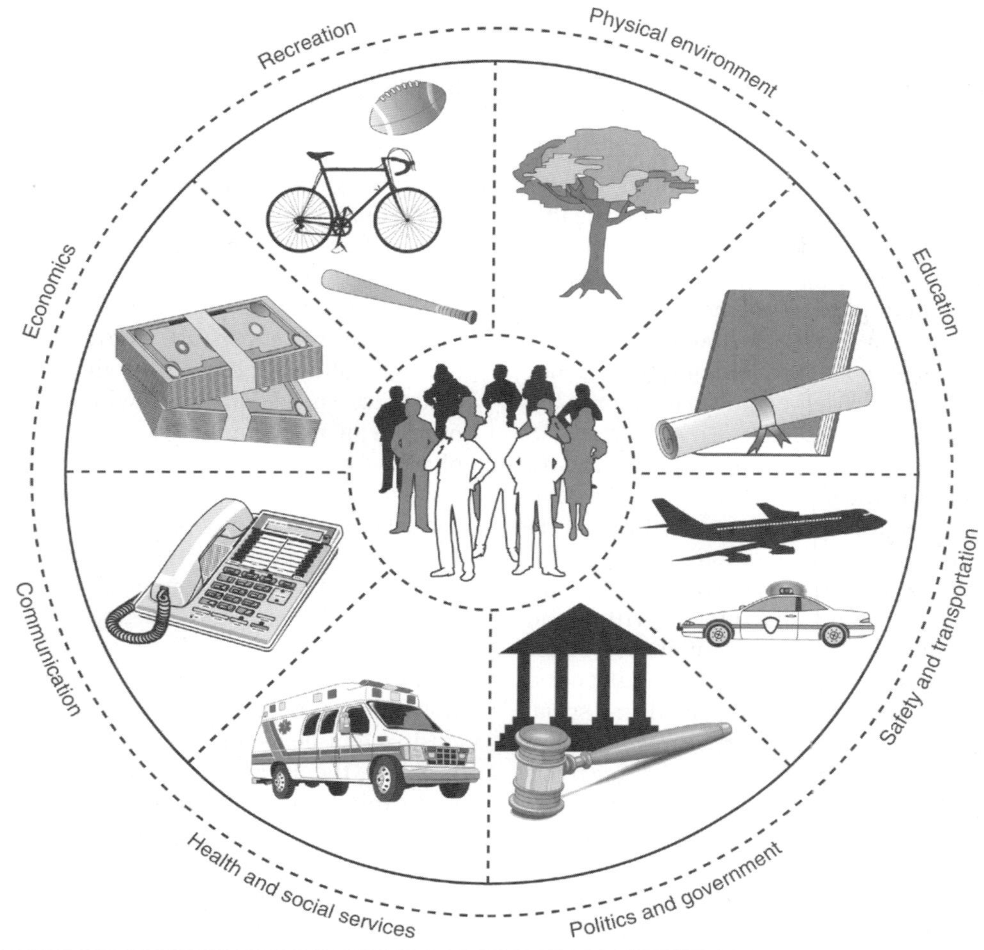

Source: Anderson E. T., & McFarlane, J. (2000). Community-as-partner theory and practice in nursing (3rd ed.). Philadelphia, PA: Lippincott, Williams & Wilkins.

The Calgary Family Assessment Model and the Calgary Family Intervention Model

APPENDIX 9

ASSESSING THE NEEDS OF THE FAMILY: THE CALGARY FAMILY ASSESSMENT MODEL

Family assessment is essential to providing adequate family care and support. To help families adjust to acute and chronic illness, nurses need to understand the family unit, what the illness means to the family members, what the illness means to family functioning, how the family has been affected by the illness, and the support the family requires (Neabel, Fothergill-Bourbonnais, & Dunning, 2000). Box A9-1 lists families who should be especially considered for a family assessment. During an assessment, the nurse, client, and family collaboratively engage in conversation to systematically collect information and reflect on issues important to the client's well-being at this particular time.

The Calgary Family Assessment Model (CFAM) is a framework nurses may use in order to do a thorough family assessment (Wright & Leahey, 2000). It has received wide recognition, and faculties and schools of nursing around the world have adopted it. The International Council of Nurses recognizes it as one of the four leading family assessment models in the world (Schober & Affara, 2001). The CFAM focuses on three major categories of family life: (1) the structural dimension, (2) the developmental dimension, and (3) the functional dimension. Each category has several subcategories; however, not all subcategories are relevant to all families (see Figure A9-1). The nurse must decide, on a family-by-family basis, which subcategories are relevant at each point in time. Using too many subcategories may overwhelm a nurse with data; using too few may distort a family's strengths or problems. The model provides a framework to draw from during discussions about family issues.

Structural Assessment

The structural dimension of the family includes the following:

- *Internal structure*—The people who are included in the family and how they are connected to each other
- *External structure*—The relationships the family has with people and institutions outside of the family
- *Context*—The whole situation or background relevant to the family

Internal Structure

The internal structure of the family—its composition and connections among family members—can be further divided into six subcategories: composition, gender, sexual orientation, rank, order, subsystems, and boundaries.

Composition

Composition refers to the individual members who form the family. The family composition is not limited to the traditional nuclear family and may include various family forms. It is important to note whether there have been any recent additions or losses to the family composition.

> Questions to Ask the Family: *Who is in your family? Does anyone else live with you, for example, grandparents, boarders? Has anyone recently moved out, married, or died? Is there anyone else you think of as a family member who is not biologically related?*

Gender

Gender is the set of beliefs about or expectations of male and female behaviour and experiences. These beliefs are fundamental to male and female relationships and are influenced by culture, religion, and family. It is useful to understand how males and females in a particular family may view the world differently.

> Questions to Ask the Family: *How have your parents' ideas about masculinity and femininity affected your own? Do you have expectations of your children based on their gender? Is the division of labour in your family based on gender roles?*

Sexual Orientation

Included here are heterosexual, homosexual, bisexual, and transgendered orientations. Heterosexism, a belief that privileges male–female bonding over other types of bonding, is a form of bias that can affect families and

BOX A9-1 Families Who Should Be Considered for a Family Assessment

Families who may benefit most from a family assessment include those who:

- Are experiencing emotional, physical, or spiritual suffering or disruption caused by a family crisis (e.g., acute or end-of-life illness, injury, death)
- Are experiencing emotional, physical, or spiritual suffering or disruption caused by a developmental milestone (e.g., birth, marriage, child leaving home)
- Define an illness or problem as a family issue (e.g., the impact of chronic illness on the family)
- Have a child or adolescent whom they identify as having difficulties (e.g., school phobia, fear of cancer treatment)
- Are experiencing issues that are serious enough to jeopardize family relationships (e.g., terminal illness, substance abuse)
- Have a family member who is about to be admitted to the hospital for psychiatric or mental health treatment
- Have a child who is about to be admitted to the hospital

SOURCE: Wright, L. M., & Leahey, M. (2009). *Nurses and families: A guide to family assessment and intervention* (4th ed., p. 5). Philadelphia, PA: F. A. Davis.

health care providers. Discrimination of sexual orientation continues to be an issue in North American society. Unless it is particularly relevant to the client or family's presenting concern, the nurse does not usually ask questions about sexual orientation but is careful when asking general questions to avoid stereotyping or making assumptions.

Rank Order

The order of children by age and gender is called *rank order*. The birth order, gender, and distance in age between siblings are important factors to consider because they may influence roles and behaviours. Also important is the child's characteristics and the family's idealized "program" for the child (going to school, college, university, work, getting married, etc.).

> Questions to Ask the Family: *How many children are there in your family? What are the ages of the children? Do you have expectations of the eldest that are different from those for the younger children?*

Subsystems

Subsystems are smaller groups of relationships within a family. Subsystems can be created based on generation, interests, skills, or gender. For example, a family could have a sibling subsystem, a husband–wife subsystem, and a parent–child subsystem. Each family member usually belongs to several subsystems, and in each subsystem, they play a different role, use different skills, and have a different level of power. For example, a teenager behaves differently with her younger sister from how she does with her father. Adapting to the demands of different subsystems is a necessary skill for each family member.

> Questions to Ask the Family: *What are your family's subgroups? Are there frequent disagreements among and between subgroups? If your family had more or fewer subgroups, what effect do you think that might have?*

Boundaries

Boundaries define family subsystems and distinguish one subsystem from another. They define how members participate in each subsystem. For example, a child in a parent–child subsystem may be given certain responsibilities and power but not be expected to be involved with family decision making. Boundaries can be weak, rigid, or flexible, and they change over time as family members age or are gained or lost.

> Questions to Ask the Family: *Whom do you talk with if you feel happy? Whom do you talk with if you feel sad? Are there any "unwritten" rules in the family about topics that are never to be discussed with someone outside of the family?*

External Structure

External structure refers to the connections that family members have to those outside of the family. There are two subcategories to external structure: extended family and larger systems.

Extended Family

Extended family includes the family of origin and present generation and step-relatives. How each member sees self as an individual, yet also as part of the family, is a critical structural area for assessment. The nurse should note whether family members make many references to the extended family during the interview.

> Questions to Ask the Family: *Where do your parents live? How often do you have contact with them and/or your brothers and sisters? Which family members do you see or speak with regularly? To which relatives are you closest?*

FIGURE A9-1 Branching Diagram of the CFAM

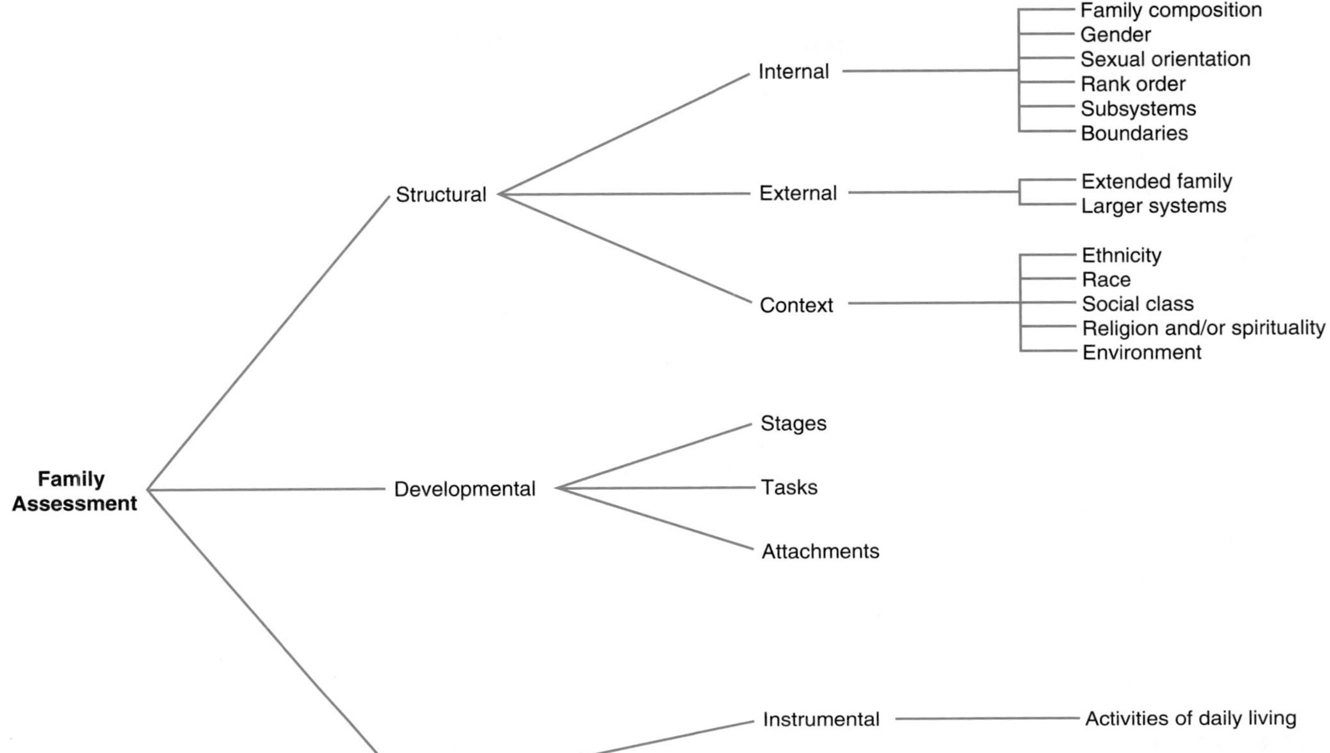

SOURCE: Wright, L. M., & Leahy, M. (2009). *Nurses and families: A guide to family assessment and intervention* (5th ed., p. 48). Philadelphia, PA: F. A. Davis.

Larger Systems

Larger systems are groups with whom the family has meaningful contact. Groups include health care providers, work, church, school, friends, and social agencies, such as public welfare, child welfare, foster care, and courts. Usually, contact with such larger systems is helpful. However, some families have difficult relationships with individuals from these groups, which can create stress for the family.

Questions to Ask the Family: *What agency professionals are involved with your family? How many agencies regularly interact with you? How is this involvement helpful or unhelpful?*

Context

Context refers to the situation or background relevant to the family. A family can be viewed in the context of ethnicity, race, social class, spirituality and religion, and environment.

Ethnicity

Ethnicity, which is the concept of a family's cultural and ethnic heritage, is an important influence on family interaction. Ethnicity often influences a family's function, structure, perspectives, values, health beliefs, and philosophies. Cultural and ethnic heritage can affect, for example, religious practices, child-rearing practices, recreational activities, and nutrition. Members of one ethnic group may subscribe to differing beliefs, traditions, and restrictions, even within the same generation.

Questions to Ask the Family: *Do you think of your family as having a strong ethnic identity? Has your ethnic background influenced your health care? Could you tell me about ethnic traditions you practise? How are your practices similar or different from those suggested by our health clinic?*

Race

Race (biological characteristics such as skin and hair colour) influences individual and group identification and is closely connected to ethnicity. Family members' interactions among themselves and with health care professionals are influenced by racial attitudes, stereotypes, and discrimination. If ignored, these influences can harm the nurse and family's relationship.

Questions to Ask the Family: *If you and I were of the same race, would our conversation be different? If so, how?*

Social Class

Social class is shaped by education, income, and occupation. Each class has its own values, lifestyles, and behaviours that influence family interaction and health care practices.

Questions to Ask the Family: *What is your job, and how many hours a week do you work? Does anyone in the family work shifts? How does that influence your family functioning? What level of education have you completed? Does your family have economic problems at this time?*

Religion and Spirituality

Religion or religious beliefs, rituals, and practices can influence a family's ability to cope with or manage an illness or health concern (Wright, 2004). Spirituality is often an underused resource in family work.

Questions to Ask the Family: *Are you involved in a church, temple, mosque, or synagogue? Would you discuss a family problem with anyone from your place of worship? Do you consider your spiritual beliefs a resource?*

Environment

The *family environment* refers to the larger community, neighbourhood, and home. Environmental factors that may affect family functioning include availability or lack of adequate space and of access to schools, daycare, recreation, and public transportation.

Questions to Ask the Family: *What are the advantages and disadvantages of living in your neighbourhood? What community services does your family use? What community services would you like to learn about?*

Structural Assessment Tools

The CFAM encourages nurses to create genograms and ecomaps to help document and understand the structure of a family and its contact with outside individuals and organizations. A *genogram* is a sketch of the family structure and relevant information about family members (see Figure 12-4 in Chapter 12). Some agencies have genogram forms, but genograms can also be sketched on other forms, such as admission forms or Kardex cards. The genogram becomes part of the documentation about the client and family. In some facilities, the information is collected on admission and then hung at the client's bedside, serving as a visual reminder to all health care professionals involved with the client to think about the family. An *ecomap* is a sketch of the family's contact with persons outside of the family (see Figure 12-5 in Chapter 12). The family members who share the household are depicted in the centre of the ecomap, and various important extended family members or larger systems are sketched in to show their relationship to the family. Nurses draw genograms and ecomaps for families with whom they will be involved for more than 1 day. Information for brief genograms and ecomaps can be gleaned from family members during the structural assessment. The most essential information for genograms includes data about age, occupation or school grade, religion, ethnicity, and current health status of each family member. For a brief genogram, the nurse focuses only on information that is relevant to the family and the health problem.

Developmental Assessment

Families, like individuals, change and grow over time. Although families are all unique, they tend to go through certain stages that require the family to adjust, adapt, and change roles. Each developmental stage presents challenges and includes tasks that need to be completed before the family can successfully move on to the next stage. Family development is more than the concurrent development of children and adults. It is the interaction between an individual's development and the phase of the family developmental life cycle that can be significant for family functioning. Therefore, in addition to understanding family structure, nurses should understand the developmental life cycle of each family.

In their model of family life stages, McGoldrick and Carter (1982, Carter and McGoldrick, 1999) described the emotional aspects of lifestyle transition and the changes and tasks necessary for the family to proceed developmentally (see Table A9-1). The nurse can use this model to promote behaviours to achieve essential tasks and help families prepare for transitions. It should be noted that the model presented in Table A9-1 does not address diverse family forms, such as blended families, one-parent families, families without children, or common-law partners.

TABLE A9-1 Stages of the Family Life Cycle

Family Life Cycle Stage	Emotional Process of Transition: Key Principles	Second-Order Changes in Family Status Required to Proceed Developmentally
1. Leaving home; single young adults	Accepting emotional and financial responsibility for self	1. Differentiation of self from family of origin 2. Development of intimate peer relationships 3. Establishment of self regarding work and financial independence
2. The joining of families through marriage; the new couple	Commitment to new system	1. Formation of marital system 2. Realignment of relationships with extended families and friends to include spouse
3. Families with young children	Accepting new members into the system	1. Adjusting marital system to make space for child(ren) 2. Joining in childrearing, financial, and household tasks 3. Realignment of relationships with extended family to include parenting and grandparenting roles
4. Families with adolescents	Increasing flexibility of family boundaries to include children's independence and grandparents' frailties	1. Shifting of parent–child relationships to permit adolescents to move in and out of system 2. Refocus on midlife marital and career issues 3. Beginning shift toward caring for older generation
5. Launching children and moving on	Accepting a multitude of exits from and entries into the family system	1. Renegotiation of marital system as a dyad 2. Development of adult–adult relationships between grown children and their parents 3. Realignment of relationships to include in-laws and grandchildren 4. Dealing with disabilities and death of parents (grandparents)
6. Families in later life	Accepting the shifting of generational roles	1. Maintaining own and couple functioning and interests in face of physiological decline; exploration of new familial and social role options 2. Support for a more central role of middle generation 3. Making room in the system for the wisdom and experience of the elderly, supporting the older generation without overfunctioning for them 4. Dealing with loss of spouse, siblings, and other peers and preparing for own death; life review and integration

SOURCE: Developed by Carter, B., & McGoldrick, M. (Eds.). (1999). The expanded family life cycle: Individual, family and social perspective. In L. Wright & M. Leahy. (2009). *Nurses and families: A guide to family assessment and intervention* (5th ed.). (p. 292). Philadelphia, PA: F. A. Davis.

Functional Assessment

A functional assessment focuses mainly on how family members interact and behave toward each other. The nurse assesses how family members function by closely observing their interactions. There are two subcategories of family functioning: instrumental and expressive functioning.

Instrumental Functioning

Instrumental functions are the normal activities of daily living, such as preparing meals, sleeping, and attending to health needs. For families with health problems, these activities often become a challenge. Roles often change as family members cope with illness and disability in the family.

> Questions to Ask the Family: *Who is usually responsible for housekeeping and child care? Do other family members help with these tasks? Does anyone in the family require help with activities of daily living? Who usually provides this help?*

Expressive Functioning

Expressive functioning refers to the ways in which people communicate. Illness and disability often alter expressive functioning within the family. A diagnosis may cause intense feelings of anxiety or grief, both within the person being diagnosed and within other family members. Nurses should encourage families to explore their understanding of illness and how it impacts their lives. There are 10 subcategories of expressive functioning: emotional, verbal, nonverbal, and circular communication; problem solving; roles; influence; beliefs; and alliances and coalitions.

Emotional Communication

Emotional communication refers to the range and types of feelings that are expressed by the family. Most families express a wide range of feelings. However, families with problems often have rigid patterns with a narrow range of emotional expression. For example, a family coping with a father's diagnosis of cancer may be consumed by anxiety and not express optimism or hope for the future. Family roles and gender may affect expression of emotions.

> Questions to Ask the Family: *How can you tell when each member of your family is happy, sad, or under stress? How do you express happiness, sadness, or stress?*

Verbal Communication

The nurse should observe a family's verbal communication, focusing on the meaning of the words in terms of the relationship. Is communication among family members clear and direct, or is it vague and indirect? The nurse should also ask family members their opinions about how well the family communicates.

> Questions to Ask the Family: *Which family member communicates most clearly? How might your family members communicate with each other more effectively?*

Nonverbal Communication

Nonverbal communication consists of messages conveyed without words, including body language, eye contact, gesturing, crying, and tone of voice.

> Questions to Ask the Family: *How do you think your daughter feels when your son rolls his eyes while she is talking? Who shows the most distress when talking about dad's drinking?*

Circular Communication

Circular communication refers to communication between family members that is reciprocal; that is, each person influences the behaviour of the other. Circular communication can be adaptive or maladaptive. For example, an adaptive communication pattern is when a parent comforts the child because the child cries. Because the parent responds to the child, the child feels safe and secure. An example of a maladaptive communication pattern is when a parent criticizes a teenager for not phoning home. The teenager is angry for being criticized and avoids the parent. Because the teenager avoids the parent, the parent becomes angrier and criticizes more.

> Questions to Ask the Family: *You mentioned that your teenage daughter does not phone home. What do you do then? How do you think that affects her?*

Problem Solving

Problem solving refers to how a family thinks about actions to take to resolve difficult situations.

> Questions to Ask the Family: *Who first notices problems? How does your family tend to deal with problems? Is one member more proactive than others about solving problems?*

Roles

Roles are established patterns of behaviour for family members, often developed through interactions with others. Formal roles include those of mother, husband, friend, and so forth. Informal roles can include, for example, those of "the softy," "the angel," or "the scapegoat."

> Questions to Ask the Family: *Who is the "good listener" in your family? Who is "the angel"?*

Influence

Influence refers to methods of affecting or controlling another person's behaviour. Influence may be instrumental (the use of privileges as reward for behaviour, e.g., the promise of candy, computer time), psychological (the use of communication to influence behaviour, e.g., praise, admonishment), or corporal (the use of body contact, e.g., hugging, hitting).

Questions to Ask the Family: *What method does your mom use to get Noreen to go to bed at the right time? How does your grandma get Luis to attend school when he refuses to?*

Beliefs

Beliefs are individual- and family-held fundamental ideas, values, opinions, and assumptions (Wright, Watson, & Bell, 1996). Beliefs influence behaviour and how the family adapts to illness. For example, if a family believes that vaccinations may cause long-term disabilities, the parents may decline vaccinating an infant.

Questions to Ask the Family: *What do you believe is the cause of your husband's depression? What do you believe would be the effect on your chronic pain if you choose to participate in that treatment?*

Alliances and Coalitions

Alliances and coalitions involve the directionality, balance, and intensity of relationships among family members or between families and nurses.

Questions to Ask the Family: *If the children are playing well together, who would most likely start them fighting? Who would stop them from fighting?*

FAMILY INTERVENTION: THE CALGARY FAMILY INTERVENTION MODEL

After the assessment, the nurse needs to intervene to help families meet their needs. A range of nursing interventions can be offered to families. Some, such as parent education and caregiver support, are general; others are specific and require therapeutic communication and family interviewing skills. The ultimate goal is to help family members discover solutions that reduce or alleviate emotional, physical, and spiritual suffering. Whether caring for a client with the family as context or directing care to the family as client, nursing interventions aim to increase family members' abilities in certain areas, to remove barriers to health care, and to do things that the family cannot do for itself. The nurse guides the family in problem solving, provides practical services, and conveys a sense of acceptance and caring by listening carefully to family members' concerns and suggestions.

Nurses must tailor their interventions to each family and the chosen domain of family functioning. The nurse must remember that each family is unique. As well, nurses can only offer interventions to the family. They should not instruct or insist on a particular kind of change or way of family functioning.

The Calgary Family Intervention Model (CFIM) is a companion model to the CFAM and can be used as a guide for family intervention (Wright & Leahey, 2009). The CFIM focuses on promoting and improving family functioning in three domains: cognitive (thinking), affective (feeling), and behavioural (doing). Interventions may affect functioning in any or all of the three domains. For example, the clinic nurse informs a wife that her husband who has amyotrophic lateral sclerosis is still capable of large gross motor movement and suggests that he could help with chores in the house, such as bringing the laundry upstairs. This intervention challenges the wife's thinking that her husband is incapable of work, influences the wife to feel less depressed over her husband's declining physical capacity, and leads to the wife changing her behaviour by including her husband when doing other household chores.

The CFIM recommends many nursing practices that promote family functioning, including asking interventive questions, offering commendations, providing information, validating emotional responses, encouraging illness narratives, supporting family caregivers, and encouraging respite.

Asking Interventive Questions

One of the simplest but most effective ways that nurses can help families is by engaging in a conversation with families and asking them questions. Questions lead the family to reflect on their situation, clarify their opinions and ideas, and understand how they are affected by their family member's illness or condition. By hearing their own responses to questions, family members can better understand themselves and each other, and perhaps discover new solutions. Interventive questions also provide important information to the nurse.

There are two types of interventive questions: linear and circular questions (Tomm, 1987, 1988). Linear questions provide the nurse with information about a client or family. They explore a family member's descriptions or perceptions of a problem. For example, when exploring a couple's perceptions of their daughter's anorexia nervosa, the nurse could begin with linear questions:

"When did you notice that your daughter had changed her eating habits?" "Why do you think she stopped eating normally?" These questions inform the nurse of the young woman's eating patterns and illuminate family perceptions or beliefs about eating patterns.

Circular questions help determine changes that could be made in a client's or family's life. They help explain a problem. For example, with the same family, the nurse could ask, "Who is most worried about Cheyenne's anorexia?" "How does Mother show that she's worrying the most?" Circular questions help the nurse understand relationships between individuals, beliefs, and events and provide valuable information to help create change. In this way, circular questions often make new cognitive connections, paving the way for different family behaviours. Whereas linear questions may imply that the nurse knows what is best for the family, circular questions facilitate change by inviting the family to discover their own answers. Linear questions tend to target specific yes-or-no answers, thereby limiting the options for the family. For example, "Have you tried time-out to discipline your 3-year-old?" An alternative circular question might be, "Which type of discipline seems to work best for your 3-year-old?"

Several types of circular questions exist, and each can affect the cognitive, affective, and behavioural domains. These types include difference questions, behavioural effect questions, hypothetical or future-oriented questions, and triadic questions (Wright & Leahey, 2009; see Table 12-5 in Chapter 12).

Offering Commendations

Families do not always view their own system as one that has inherently positive components. The nurse can help the family become aware of its own unique strengths, thereby increasing its potential and capabilities. A *commendation* is a statement that emphasizes strengths or abilities of the family. While spending time with the family, the nurse may observe many instances in which the family displays positive attributes. It is important to acknowledge these to the family so that the family members can appreciate their own resiliency. By commending a family's strengths and competencies, nurses can offer family members a new view of themselves. The nurse should look for patterns of behaviour to commend, rather than a single occurrence. For example, the nurse may say, "Your family is showing much courage in living with your wife's cancer for 5 years," or "I'm very impressed with how the family worked together during the crisis." Families coping with chronic, life-threatening, or psychosocial problems frequently feel hopeless in their efforts to overcome or live with the illness. Therefore, nurses can never offer too many truthful commendations. In a study of families experiencing chronic illnesses, families reported that the nursing team's commendations were "an extremely important facet of the process" (Robinson, 1998).

Family strengths include clear communication, adaptability, healthy child-rearing practices, support and nurturing among family members, and the use of crisis for growth. The nurse can help the family focus on these strengths instead of its problems and weaknesses.

Providing Information

Families need information from health care professionals about developmental issues, health promotion, and illness management, especially if the illness is complex (Levac, Wright, & Leahey, 2002; Robinson, 1998). Accurate and timely information is essential for the family to make decisions and cope with difficult situations. One of the roles the nurse will need to adopt is that of an educator. Health education is a process by which information is shared by nurse and client in a two-way fashion. Family and client needs for information may be recognized through direct questioning, but they are generally far more subtle. The nurse may recognize that the father is fearful of cleaning the newborn's umbilical cord area or that an older adult woman is not using her cane safely. Respectful communication is required. Often, the subtle needs for information can be approached by saying, "I notice you are trying to not touch the umbilical cord area; I see that a lot." Or, "You use the cane the way I did before I was shown a way to keep from falling or tripping over it; do you mind if I show you?" When the nurse assumes a humble position instead of coming across as an authority on the subject, this attitude often decreases the client's defences and invites the client to listen without feeling embarrassed.

Validating or Normalizing Emotional Responses

Validation of intense emotions can alleviate feelings of isolation and loneliness and help family members make the connection between a family member's illness and the family's emotional response. For example, after a diagnosis of a life-shortening illness, families frequently feel out of control or frightened. It is important for nurses to validate these strong emotions and to reassure families that they will adjust and learn new ways to cope.

Encouraging Illness Narratives

Too often, clients and family members are encouraged to talk only about the medical aspects of their illness rather than the emotional aspects. An illness narrative is the person's story of how the illness affects his or her whole being, including the emotional, intellectual, social, and spiritual dimensions. Hearing the illness narrative helps the nurse understand the person's strengths and challenges. This information enables the nurse to offer commendations acknowledging the client's abilities. Many people also find that the telling of their story helps them better understand themselves, their experience, and their family's experience.

The need to communicate what it is like to live with individual, separate experiences, particularly the experience of illness, is powerful in human relationships (Nichols, 1995; Wright, 2004). Frequently, nurses believe that listening entails an obligation to "fix" whatever concerns or problems are raised. However, showing compassion and offering commendations is usually more therapeutic or helpful than offering solutions to problems (Bohn, Wright, & Moules, 2003; Hougher Limacher, 2003; Hougher Limacher & Wright, 2003; Moules, 2002).

Encouraging Family Support

Nurses can enhance family functioning by encouraging and assisting family members to listen to each other's concerns and feelings. This assistance can be particularly useful if a family member is embracing some constraining beliefs when a loved one is dying or has died (Wright & Nagy, 1993). For example, a family may believe that talking with the ill person about death and dying would hasten the person's death.

Supporting Family Caregivers

Family members are often afraid of becoming involved in the care of an ill member without a nurse's support. One way the nurse can best provide family care is through supporting family caregivers. Without adequate preparation or support, caregiving can be stressful, causing a decline in the health of the caregiver and the care receiver or even the development of abusive relationships.

Despite its demands, caregiving can be a positive and rewarding experience (Picot, Youngblut, & Zeller, 1997). Whether it is one spouse caring for the other or a child caring for a parent, caregiving is an interactional process. The interpersonal dynamics between family members influence the ultimate quality of caregiving. Thus, the nurse can play a key role in helping family members develop better communication and problem-solving skills to build the relationships needed for successful caregiving.

Researchers have identified variables, such as caregiver and care recipient expectations of one another, that influence caregiving quality. Carruth (1996) has studied the concept of reciprocity, in which care recipients acknowledge the importance of the caregiver's help to share, which contributes to a caregiver's perception of self-worth. When the caregiver knows that the care recipient appreciates his or her efforts and values the assistance provided, the caregiving relationship is healthier and more satisfying. When caregiver and client solve problems together, overprotection or oversolicitous behaviour can be avoided. Clients feel in control of their care and responsible for care decisions. The caregiver also feels very positive and enjoys the caregiving experience (Isaksen, Thuen, & Hanestad, 2003).

Encouraging Respite

Nurses should encourage respite for caregivers, who may feel guilty about needing or wanting to withdraw from the caregiving role. Caregivers may not recognize their needs for respite. Sometimes, an ill person may be encouraged to accept another person's temporary assistance so that the caregiving family members can take a break. Whatever the situation, the nurse should remember that each family's need for respite varies.

Providing care and support for family caregivers often involves using available family and community resources for respite. A caregiving schedule is useful when all family members participate, extended family members share any financial burdens posed by caregiving, and distant relatives send cards and letters communicating their support. However, it is imperative for the nurse to understand the relationship between potential caregivers and care recipients. If the relationship is not a supportive one, community services may be a resource for both the client and family.

Use of community resources might include locating a service required by the family or providing respite care so that the family caregiver has time away from the care recipient. Services that may be beneficial to families include caregiver support groups, housing and transportation services, food and nutrition services, housecleaning, legal and financial services, home care, hospice, and mental health resources. Before referring a family to community resources, it is critical that the nurse understands the family's dynamics and knows whether support is desired or welcomed. Often, a family caregiver resists help, feeling obligated to be the sole source of support to the care recipient. The nurse must be sensitive to family relationships and help caregivers understand the normality of caregiving demands.

Source: Potter, P. A., Perry, A. G., Ross-Kerr, J. C., & Wood, M. J. (Eds.). (2009). *Canadian fundamentals of nursing* (4th ed., pp. 280–288). Toronto, ON: Mosby.

REFERENCES

Bohn, U., Wright, L. M., & Moules, N. J. (2003). A family systems nursing interview following a myocardial infarction: The power of commendations. *Journal of Family Nursing, 9*(2), 151–165.

Carruth, A. K. (1996). Development and testing of the caregiver reciprocity scale. *Nursing Research, 45*, 92–97.

Carter, B., & McGoldrick, M. (Eds.). (1999). *The expanded family life cycle: Individual, family and social perspectives* (3rd ed.). Boston: Allyn & Bacon.

Hougher Limacher, L. (2003). *Commendations: The healing potential of one family systems nursing intervention.* Unpublished doctoral thesis. Calgary, Alberta: University of Calgary.

Hougher Limacher, L., & Wright, L. M. (2003). Commendations: Listening to the silent side of a family intervention. *Journal of Family Nursing, 9*(2), 130–135.

Isaksen, A. S., Thuen, F., & Hanestad, B. (2003). Patients with cancer and their close relatives: Experiences with treatment, care, and support. *Cancer Nursing, 26*(1), 68–74.

Levac, A. M. C., Wright, L. M., & Leahey, M. (2002). Children and families: Models for assessment and intervention. In J. Fox (Ed.), *Primary health care of infants, children, and adolescents* (2nd ed., pp. 10–19). St. Louis, MO: Mosby.

McGoldrick, M., & Carter, E. (1982). The stages of the family life cycle. In F. Walsh (Ed.), *Normal family processes.* New York: Guilford Press.

Moules, N. J. (2002). Nursing on paper: Therapeutic letters in nursing practice. *Nursing Inquiry, 9*(2), 104–113.

Neabel, B., Fothergill-Bourbonnais, F., & Dunning, J. (2000). Family assessment tools: A review of the literature from 1978–1997. *Heart & Lung, 29*, 196–209.

Nichols, M. P. (1995). *The lost art of listening.* New York: Guilford Press.

Picot, S. J. F., Youngblut, J., & Zeller, R. (1997). Development and testing of a measure of perceived caregiver rewards in adults. *Journal of Nursing Measurement, 5*, 33–52.

Robinson, C. A. (1998). Women, families, chronic illness, and nursing interventions: From burden to balance. *Journal of Family Nursing, 4*(3), 271–290.

Schober, M., & Affara, F. (2001). *The family nurse: Frameworks for practice.* Geneva, Switzerland: International Council of Nurses.

Tomm, K. (1987). Interventive interviewing: Part II. Reflexive questioning as a means to enable self-healing. *Family Process, 26*, 167–183.

Tomm, K. (1988). Interventive interviewing: Part III. Intending to ask lineal, circular, strategic or reflexive questions. *Family Process, 27*, 1–15.

Wright, L. M. (2004). *Spirituality, suffering, and illness: Ideas for healing.* Philadelphia: F. A. Davis.

Wright, L. M., & Leahey, M. (2000). *Nurses and families: A guide to family assessment and intervention* (3rd ed.). Philadelphia: F. A. Davis.

Wright, L., & Leahey, M. (2009). *Nurses and families: A guide to family assessment and intervention* (5th ed.). Philadelphia, PA: F. A. Davis.

Wright, L. M., & Nagy, J. (1993). Death: The most troublesome family secret of all. In E. Imber Black (Ed.), *Secrets in families and family therapy* (pp. 121–137). New York: W. W. Norton.

Wright, L. M., Watson, W. L., & Bell, J. M. (1996). *Beliefs: The heart of healing in families and illness.* New York: Basic Books.

CNA Position Statement: "Nurses and Environmental Health"

APPENDIX 10

CNA POSITION

The environment is an important determinant of health and has a profound impact on why some people are healthy and others are not.[1]

The Canadian Nurses Association (CNA) *Code of Ethics for Registered Nurses* supports registered nurses' engagement in environmental health issues as part of their work for social justice. The code suggests that as part of ethical practice, registered nurses may undertake the ethical endeavours of "supporting environmental preservation and restoration and advocating for initiatives that reduce environmentally harmful practices in order to promote health and well-being" and "maintaining awareness of broader global health concerns such as... environmental pollution."[2]

Canadians trust nurses[3] and value their expertise.[4] CNA believes that the public expects nurses to be aware of and know how to promote Canadians' health in the context of environmental health issues. This is accomplished through nurses' roles in clinical practice, education, research, administration and policy. Given that some populations "are more vulnerable to environmental risks as a result of physical differences, behaviours, location and/or control over their environment," nurses must be particularly strong advocates for these populations.[5]

The role of nurses in environmental health includes:

- assessing and communicating risks of environmental hazards to individuals, families and communities;
- advocating for policies that protect health by preventing exposure to those hazards and promoting sustainability; and
- producing nursing science, including interdisciplinary research, related to environmental health issues.

[1]This position statement does not address health care work environments. For positions on this topic, please see Joint CNA/CFNU Position Statement on Practice Environments: *Maximizing Client, Nurse and System Outcomes,* 2006.

[2](Canadian Nurses Association [CNA], 2008a, pp. 20–21).

[3]Unless otherwise stated, *nurse* or *nursing* refers to any member of a regulated nursing category, i.e., a registered nurse, licensed/practical nurse, registered psychiatric nurse or nurse practitioner. This definition reflects the current situation in Canada whereby nurses are deployed in a variety of collaborative arrangements to provide care.

[4](EKOS, 2007).

[5](Health Canada, 2008).

Understanding and applying environmental health principles should be a part of every nurse's practice. Still, many nurses do not feel adequately prepared to engage in policy issues related to environmental health.[6] CNA values the work that nurse leaders, educators and students are doing to integrate and bolster nursing knowledge and skills related to environmental health, and advocates for continued inclusion of environmental health concepts in basic and continuing nursing education, strengthened where necessary and taught in both academic and workplace settings. Rather than taught as a specialized area of practice, environmental health can be integrated into all areas of nursing practice.

Nurses are valuable contributors as principal investigators and as co-investigators in interdisciplinary environmental health research. Their increased participation in nursing science related to environmental health issues supports all areas of nursing practice and ensures that nursing perspectives are incorporated.

Human health depends on the health of the environment, and CNA values actions that prevent or reduce harm to the environment. CNA expects that as nurses become more aware of environmental health issues, they will increasingly focus on reducing the environmental impact of the health setting in which they work and their personal activities, and thus promote environmental sustainability.

CNA endorses the use of the *precautionary principle* as a fundamental tenet of practices that affect the environment. The precautionary principle proposes that "where there are threats of serious or irreversible damage, lack of full scientific certainty shall not be used as a reason for postponing cost-effective measures to prevent environmental degradation."[7]

Protecting human health and preventing disease and death must be the first priority for environmental legislation and regulations. All levels of government in Canada have a responsibility to manage environmental hazards through various governance instruments. Nurses and nursing organizations must work with governments to improve environmental policy and to advocate for healthy public policies.

Finally, CNA believes that intersectoral and interdisciplinary collaboration, within and outside of the health system, is crucial to nurses' work in environmental health.

[6](CNA, 2008b).

[7](United Nations, 1992).

BACKGROUND

In 2004, the World Health Organization (WHO) defined environmental health as addressing "those aspects of human health, including quality of life, that are determined by physical, chemical, biological, social, and psychosocial factors in the environment. It also refers to the theory and practice of assessing, correcting, controlling, and preventing those factors in the environment that can potentially affect adversely the health of present and future generations."[8]

WHO has recently revised this definition; however, the earlier definition is useful in guiding nursing practice in environmental health because it includes determinants of health that nurses already routinely address (biological, social and psychosocial factors, including income inequity) and adds others they may not (physical and chemical factors). Its use supports the view that addressing environmental health enhances work in which nurse are already engaged, rather than introducing a new specialty area. It also provides specific guidance for areas of nursing intervention (assessing, correcting, controlling and preventing) that are part of theories and conceptual frameworks used by nurses.

The connections between health and the environment, including air, water and food quality, are well known. Canadians' health is affected by poor outdoor air quality (resulting in increases in mortality and morbidity from both cardiovascular and respiratory diseases), chemicals (implicated as a cause of cancer, endocrine disruption, reproductive toxicity and neurotoxicity, among other health effects)[9] and toxic waste. More recently, our understanding has broadened to include other environmental influences on health such as housing quality, waste disposal, road safety and noise.[10] Canada has also felt the effects of global threats to health, such as ozone depletion, air pollution and soil erosion. Climate change has affected the health of Canadians through increases in exposure to vector-borne disease (such as West Nile virus infection), higher incidence of water- and food-borne illnesses, more frequent extreme weather events and severe heat waves.[11] Workplaces can also be a source of significant environmental exposure, through biological, chemical, radiological or physical hazards that affect indoor air and the health of workers.[12]

Nurses are uniquely qualified to bring information to the public on protection from environmental exposures. They have the assessment skills and scientific background to identify potential hazards, and the communication skills to explain the exposure, and how to reduce its risk, in an understandable way.

Nurses have a history of advocating for patients and for other issues of public policy such as women's suffrage, sanitation, birth control and women's rights;[13] they have recently advocated for environmental health issues such as regulations restricting pesticide and tobacco use.[14] Other issues nurses are currently involved with are climate change, through advocating for clean air regulations, and environmental social justice, through addressing disparities in wealth among nations. Nurses are also taking action at work and in their personal lives by reducing greenhouse gas emissions and wastes; using, and encouraging others to use, less toxic products; increasing the use of reusable and recyclable products; and moving away from consumerism toward an understanding of the impact that our resource use and waste production has on global well-being.

Nursing education, including basic and continuing education, enables nurses to consider environmental factors that may be contributing to poor health; understand environmental hazards and their impact on health; understand the role of individuals and communities in providing good stewardship of the environment; make recommendations about how to reduce or prevent exposures to environmental hazards; and conduct research on environmental health issues.

Nursing research in environmental health focuses on identifying environmental exposures that pose a risk to human health, and evaluating the effectiveness of nursing interventions designed to reduce their impact; this involves assessing which populations are most vulnerable to what exposures, and which strategies are most effective in reducing their risk.

WHO has calculated that the impact of environmental hazards on health is heaviest among poor and vulnerable populations in developing countries. Within developed countries, vulnerable populations, including families living in poverty, migrant workers and visible minority groups, are more likely to be exposed to environmental hazards at home, in their community and at work.[15] In addition, children, wherever they live, are especially vulnerable "because they have no control over their prenatal and postnatal environments, including the quality of the air they breathe, the water they drink, the food they eat, and their place of residence."[16] In Canada, residents of First Nations communities are particularly at risk of health problems related to unsafe drinking water,

[8](World Health Organization, 2004).
[9](Wigle, 2003).
[10](Myres & Betke, 2002).
[11](Health Canada, 2005).
[12](Guenther & Hall, 2007).

[13](Lewenson, 2006).
[14](Registered Nurses' Association of Ontario, 2006; 2007).
[15](Prüss-Üstün & Corvalán, 2006).
[16](Wigle, 2003).

lack of adequate sanitation and substandard housing.[17] Northern Inuit are also affected significantly.

The *Canadian Environmental Protection Act* employs the precautionary principle and other environmental protection principles.[18] Although the precautionary principle was developed to protect the environment, it can also be used to guide health protection activities. For nurses, applying the precautionary principle means that risk reduction activities with individuals, families and communities should focus on minimizing exposures to environmental hazards through advocacy, risk communication and recognized occupational and public safety controls, even where there is not scientific certainty of the harmful health effects of exposure.

Associations in Canada and the United States have developed environmental health principles for nurses. The American Public Health Association released a set of principles for public health nurses; the Canadian Occupational Health Nurses Association has standards for the occupational health nurse on their website that address environmental health; and the American Nurses Association has environmental health principles for nurses.[19]

[17](Health Canada, 2000).

[18](Government of Canada, 1999).

[19](American Nurses Association, 2007; American Public Health Association, 2005; Canadian Occupational Health Nurses Association, 2003).

REFERENCES

American Nurses Association. (2007). *ANA's principles of environmental health for nursing practice with implementation strategies*. Washington, DC: Author.

American Public Health Association. (2005). *Environmental health principles for public health nursing*. Washington, DC: Author.

Canadian Nurses Association. (2008a). *Code of ethics for registered nurses*. Ottawa: Author.

Canadian Nurses Association. (2008b). *Nurses and environmental health: Survey results*. Ottawa: Author.

Canadian Occupational Health Nurses Association. (2003). *Occupational health nursing practice standards*. Toronto: Author. Retrieved from www.cohna-aciist.ca/pages/content. asp?catid=10&catsubid=5.

EKOS. (2007). *Public view of environmental health issues and nursing: A qualitative study*. Unpublished paper prepared for CNA.

Government of Canada. (1999). *Canadian Environmental Protection Act*. Ottawa: Minister of Justice. Retrieved from http://laws.justice.gc.ca/en/C-15.31/.

Guenther, R., & Hall, A. G. (2007, May 31). Healthy buildings: Impact on nurses and nursing practice. *OJIN: The Online Journal of Issues in Nursing, 12*(2). Retrieved from www.nursingworld.org/ojin.

Health Canada. (2000). *A statistical profile on the health of First Nations in Canada*. Ottawa: Author. Retrieved from http://www.hc-sc.gc.ca/fnih-spni/pubs/gen/stats_profil_e.html.

Health Canada. (2005). *Your health and a changing climate: Information for health professionals*. Ottawa: Health Canada.

Health Canada. (2008). *Vulnerable populations*. Retrieved from www.hc-sc.gc.ca/ewh-semt/contaminants/vulnerable/index-eng.php.

Lewenson, S. B. (2006). A historical perspective on policy, politics and nursing. In D. J. Mason, J. K. Leavitt, & M. W. Chaffee (Eds.), *Policy and politics in nursing and health care* (pp. 21–33). St. Louis, MO: W. B. Saunders.

Myres, A., & Betke, K. (2002). Healthy environments = Healthy people. *Health Policy Research Bulletin 4*, 5–8. Ottawa: Health Canada.

Prüss-Üstün, A., & Corvalán, C. (2006). *Preventing disease through healthy environments: Towards an estimate of the environmental burden of disease*. Geneva: World Health Organization.

Registered Nurses' Association of Ontario [RNAO]. (2006). *Action on tobacco control: Action kit for RNs*. Retrieved from www.rnao.org/Storage.asp? StorageID=637.

RNAO. (2007). *Creating a healthier society: RNAO's challenge to Ontario's political parties; Building Medicare's next stage, focusing on prevention*. Retrieved from www.rnao.org/Storage/29/2398_RNAO_Election_Platform_2007.pdf.

United Nations. (1992). *Rio declaration on environment and development (principle 15)*. Rio de Janeiro: United Nations Conference on Environment and Development, June 3–14. Retrieved from www.unep.org/Documents.Multilingual/Default.asp?DocumentID=78&ArticleID=1163.

Wigle, D. (2003). *Child health and the environment*. New York: Oxford University Press.

World Health Organization. (2004). *Protection of the human environment*. Retrieved from www.who.int/phe/en as quoted in Frumkin, H. (2005). *Environmental health: From global to local*. New York: John Wiley and Sons.

SOURCE: Canadian Nurses Association. (2009). *Position Statement: Nurses and environmental health*. Ottawa: Author. Retrieved from http://www.cna-aiic.ca/CNA/documents/pdf/publications/PS105_Nurses_Env_Health_e.pdf.

What You Should Know About an Influenza Pandemic

APPENDIX 11

Ordinary Influenza (Flu)	Influenza Pandemic
Seasonal influenza happens every year.	An influenza pandemic happens only two or three times a century.
Seasonal influenza is usually around from November to April and then stops.	An influenza pandemic usually comes in two or even three waves several months apart. Each wave lasts about 2 months.
About 10% of Ontarians get ordinary seasonal influenza each year.	About 35% of Ontarians may get the influenza over the course of the full outbreak.
Most people who get seasonal influenza will get sick, but they usually recover within a couple of weeks.	About half of the people who get influenza during a pandemic will become ill. Most will recover, but it may take a long time. And some people will die.
Seasonal influenza is hardest on people who do not have a strong immune system: the very young, the very old, and people with certain chronic illnesses.	People of any age may become seriously ill with influenza during a pandemic. This depends on the virus.
In a normal influenza season, up to 2,000 Ontarians die of complications from influenza, such as pneumonia.	During an influenza pandemic, Ontario would see many more people infected and possibly many more deaths.
There are annual influenza shots that will protect people from seasonal influenza.	There is no existing vaccine for an influenza pandemic. It will take 4 to 6 months after the pandemic starts to develop a vaccine.
There are drugs that people can take to treat seasonal influenza.	These same drugs may also help people, but we will not know their full effectiveness until the virus is identified.

Source: Modified from the Web site of the Emergency Management Unit (EMU) of the Government of Ontario. Retrieved from http://www.health.gov.on.ca/english/public/program/emu/pan_flu/pan_flu_mn.html.

Non–Vaccine-Preventable Infectious Diseases

APPENDIX 12

Disease	Epidemiology	Mode of Transmission	Incubation Period	Indicators	Time of Occurrence	Nursing Considerations
Avian influenza (AI)	There have been no confirmed cases of human infection in Canada. The World Health Organization reports that there have been a total of 442 laboratory confirmed cases of AI with 262 deaths (WHO, 2009).	Human infection with the H5N1 virus is rare. It is thought that humans acquire the infection when they come into direct contact with an infected bird or its feces (WHO, 2007). This is especially possible during slaughter, butchering, or preparing the bird for consumption.	Incubation period can range from 2–8 days and possibly as long as 17 days (WHO, 2006)	Symptoms can resemble those of human influenza: fever, cough, aching muscles, sore throat, eye infections, and serious respiratory infections, including pneumonia. It is an aggressive virus that results in rapid deterioration and has a high fatality rate.		Counsel individuals who will be travelling to areas where there are outbreaks of the disease. Provide education to high-risk groups and general population regarding prevention measures. Identify possible cases and report to the appropriate authority.
Creutzfeldt-Jakob disease (CJD)	CJD has been found in all developed nations. The incidence ranges from 1 to 2 per million people per year. In Canada this statistic is comparable (PHAC, 2009b).	Not known to spread by contact from person to person or by the airborne or respiratory route; however, transmission can occur during invasive medical interventions.	Incubation period can extend up to 30 years	Progressive dementia including confusion and memory loss; progressive unsteadiness and clumsiness; visual disturbances such as dizziness, double vision, and blurriness; and muscle twitching, fatigue, and a variety of other neurological symptoms. Affected person is usually mute and immobile in the last stages; in most cases, death occurs within a few months of onset of symptoms. This disease always results in death as there is no treatment.		Educate public regarding indicators of the disease.
Hantavirus	Western Canada has the highest incidence with the first human case reported in 1994. Fifty cases have been reported in Western Canada. This is a serious illness with over 50% of those who get the disease dying (Canadian Centre for Occupational Health and Safety, 2008).	Direct contact with rodents or their droppings or inhalation in areas with large number of rodent droppings. No person-to-person transfer has been found. Hantavirus is found in urine, feces, and saliva of rodents. Workers in agricultural or rural settings (e.g., farmers, grain handlers) are at the highest risk.	3–60 days; average is 14–30 days	Fever, chills, headache; may develop gastrointestinal symptoms. Five days after onset of symptoms, cough and shortness of breath develop—this may be severe within hours due to pulmonary edema and deterioration of cardiopulmonary function.	Often occurs in spring	Provide information and education to the public regarding potential infection with virus when in contact with rodents or their droppings. Educate target groups about preventive measures.

HIV and AIDS	See Table 17-4.					
Lyme disease	Not a reportable disease in Canada. The PHAC monitors cases in all provinces and territories, but the number of human cases reported annually has a wide variation, so identifying trends is difficult. Most commonly found in Southern and Eastern Ontario, Southeastern Manitoba, Nova Scotia, and Southern BC (PHAC, 2006).	The bacterium that causes Lyme disease is normally carried in mice, squirrels, birds, and other small animals. The bacterium is transmitted to ticks when they feed on these infected animals and then to humans through the bites of the infected ticks.	3–32 days after tick exposure	Three stages: **First stage:** Red spot or rash at site of tick bite (erythema migrans), fatigue, chills, fever, headaches, joint pain, and swollen lymph nodes **Second stage:** Occurs if disease is left untreated and can last for months. Development of erythema migrans on other areas of the body; central and peripheral nervous system disorders, e.g., Bell's palsy, heart arrthythmias, arthritis and arthritic symptoms, and feelings of extreme fatigue **Third stage:** Chronic arthritis, neurological symptoms, i.e., problems with memory, speech, and sleep	Summer and early fall	Educate public regarding preventive measures that can be taken when entering into a possible tick-infested area. Educate public about what action to take in the event of being bitten by a tick. Assist in the surveillance of the disease.
Malaria	Canada has approximately 400 cases annually of malaria, with a high of 1,036 cases reported in 1997. It is thought to be underreported by approximately 50 to 70%; thus, the true number of cases is probably much higher (PHAC, 2004).	Transmitted to humans through a bite of an infected female mosquito. Very rarely, it can also be transmitted by transfusion with infected blood, or by shared needle use, or from a mother to her unborn child.	Varies, from 7–30 days	Fever and influenza-like symptoms such as headache, nausea, vomiting, muscle pain, malaise, shaking and chills, and spleen enlargement. *Plasmodium falciparum* can cause cerebral malaria leading to delirium, confusion, seizure, coma, kidney or respiratory failure, and even death.		Provide information for travellers who are visiting malaria-affected regions. Educate regarding measures that can be undertaken for prevention. Educate regarding symptoms of disease so that individuals can recognize if they may have become infected.

(*Continued*)

Disease	Epidemiology	Mode of Transmission	Incubation Period	Indicators	Time of Occurrence	Nursing Considerations
Noroviruses	In 1998–2001, fewer than 100 outbreaks were reported. Since 2002, there have been 300–400 outbreaks annually. Increased number of cases and improved reporting have likely contributed to this higher number (PHAC, 2005).	Found in the stool or vomit of infected individuals while they are ill and up to at least 3 days after recovery. May be contagious for as long 2 weeks after recovery. Infection can occur by direct contact with a person who is ill or has recently been ill or through indirect contact by touching surfaces contaminated with the virus, such as door handles, or by eating contaminated food or drinking contaminated water.	24–48 hours (median in outbreaks 33–36 hours), but cases can occur within 12 hours of exposure	Nausea, vomiting, diarrhea, and stomach cramps, Sometimes, people may have a low-grade fever, chills, headache, muscle aches, and fatigue. The illness often begins suddenly, about 24 to 48 hours after exposure.		Educate public regarding the importance of preventive measures such as handwashing. Monitor the number of cases occurring in the area.
Severe acute respiratory syndrome (SARS)	In Canada, a total of 438 cases were reported as of September 3, 2003. There was a mix of 251 probable cases and 187 suspect cases; WHO reported 41 deaths (PHAC, 2003).	Direct contact with an infected person's secretions or body fluid	10 days	Fever, body aches, headache, and respiratory symptoms—cough, shortness of breath, difficulty breathing, or pneumonia		Educate public regarding indicators of SARS. Provide information and education about prevention and spread of the virus. Use vigilance in the assessment of possible cases and report any suspicions immediately.

Tuberculosis (TB)	In 2007, in Canada the rate of TB was 4.7 per 100,000 population. The rate for New Brunswick and Nova Scotia was uner 1 per 100,000 population. Prince Edward Island had no reported cases of TB. The largest number of recorded cases was in the 35–44-year age range, and those 65 years of age and older also had high rates. Nunavut reported the highest incidence (99.2 per 100,000 population) (PHAC, 2009a).	Airborne transmission from infected person	Varies from weeks to years	Cough lasting 2 weeks or longer, especially with hemoptysis, fever, weight loss, night sweats, and anorexia		Identify high-risk groups and provide information and education. Provide information for travellers who may visit high-risk areas.
West Nile virus	As of September 2006, there were 110 cases of West Nile virus in humans in Canada. There were 24 cases in Alberta, 10 in Saskatchewan, 49 in Manitoba, and 27 in Ontario. There have been no deaths associated with the virus (PHAC, 2009c).	Transmission by bite of a mosquito that has ingested the blood of infected birds	2–15 days	Infected individuals may be asymptomatic or have only mild symptoms. Symptoms vary but include fever, headaches, body aches, mild rash, and swollen lymph nodes. Individuals with weakened immunity can develop more serious conditions such as meningitis, encephalitis, or acute flaccid paralysis.		Educate public regarding measures to undertake to avoid being bitten by mosquitoes. Identify high-risk areas and reinforce need for preventive measures.
Anthrax	No reported cases for humans. Usually, livestock are infected through eating food contaminated with the anthrax spores (Canadian Food Inspection Agency, 2009).	Transmission by inhalation (pulmonary), ingestion (gastrointestinal) or skin contact (cutaneous) (Canadian Food Inspection Agency, 2009)	1–7 days; usually 2–5 days	Skin infection: small painless bump that blisters and then develops an ulcer with a black centre. This is the most common type of infection. Stomach infection: fever, loss of appetite, vomiting, and diarrhea Lung infection: fever, sore throat, and general malaise, followed by dyspnea after several days. This is the most serious type of infection.		

(Continued)

Disease	Epidemiology	Mode of Transmission	Incubation Period	Indicators	Time of Occurrence	Nursing Considerations
Clostridium difficile	165 clients died in Quebec hospitals between August and December 2004 after contracting *C. difficile*. Other complications resulted in 399 clients being admitted to ICU and 126 undergoing a colectomy (Eggerston, 2005).	Direct contact with feces or objects contaminated with feces	1–10 days	Watery diarrhea, fever, anorexia, nausea, and abdominal pain		Educate and reinforce proper handwashing techniques as prevention in general public and in occupational settings, especially health care.

AIDS = acquired immunodeficiency syndrome; CFIA = Canadian Food Inspection Agency; HIV = human immunodeficiency virus; ICU = intensive care unit; PHAC = Public Health Agency of Canada; WHO = World Health Organization.

REFERENCES

Canadian Centre for Occupational Health and Safety (2008). *Hantavirus*. Retrieved from http://www.ccohs.ca/oshanswers/diseases/hantavir.html.

Canadian Food Inspection Agency (2009). *Anthrax*. Retrieved from http://www.inspection.gc.ca/english/anima/disemala/anthchar/anthcharfse.shtml.

Eggerston, L. (2005). Infectious disease; Quebec reports *C. difficile* mortality statistics. *Canadian Medical Association Journal*, 173(2). Retrieved from http://www.ncbi.nlm.nih.gov/pmc/articles/PMC1174844/pdf/20050719s00019p139.pdf.

Public Health Agency of Canada (2003). *Canadian SARS numbers*. Retrieved from http://www.phac-aspc.gc.ca/sars-sras/cn-cc/20030903_e.html.

Public Health Agency of Canada (2004). *Malaria*. Retrieved from http://www.phac-aspc.gc.ca/media/advisories_avis/mal_faq-eng.php.

Public Health Agency of Canada (2005). *Noroviruses fact sheet*. Retrieved from http://www.phac-aspc.gc.ca/id-mi/norovirus-eng.php.

Public Health Agency of Canada (2006). *Lyme disease fact sheet*. Retrieved from http://www.phac-aspc.gc.ca/id-mi/lyme-fs_e.html.

Public Health Agency of Canada (2009a). *Tuberculosis in Canada 2007: Pre Release*. Retrieved from http://www.phac-aspc.gc.ca/tbpc-latb/pubs/tbcan07/index-eng.php.

Public Health Agency of Canada (2009b). *Creutzfeldt-Jakob Disease*. Retrieved from http://www.phac-aspc.gc.ca/hcai-iamss/cjd-mcj/cjdss-ssmcj/stats-eng.php#canada.

Public Health Agency of Canada (2009c). *West Nile Virus MONITOR. West Nile Virus National Surveillance Reports: 2009*. Retrieved from http://www.phac-aspc.gc.ca/wnv-vwn/nsr-rns2009-eng.php.

World Health Organization (2006). *Avian influenza ("bird flu")*. Retrieved from http://www.who.int/mediacentre/factsheets/avian_influenza/en/.

World Health Organization (2007). *Avian influenza frequently asked questions*. Retrieved from http://www.who.int/csr/disease/avian_influenza/avian_faqs/en/index.html#whyso.

World Health Organization (2009). *Cumulative number of confirmed cases of Avian Influenza A/(H5N1) reported to WHO*. Retrieved from http://www.who.int/csr/disease/avian_influenza/country/cases_table_2009_09_24/en/index.html.

APPENDIX 13

Viral Hepatitis Profiles*

	Hepatitis A (HAV)	Hepatitis B (HBV)	Hepatitis C (HCV)	Hepatitis D (HDV)	Hepatitis E (HEV)	Hepatitis G
Incubation period in days	Range: 15–50 Average: 30	Range: 40–180 Average: 74	Range: 17–175 Average: 45	Range: 14–43 Average: 28	Range: 15–60 Average: 40	Unknown
Mode of transmission	• Fecal–oral • Water borne • Sexual contact with infected blood (rare)	• Blood borne • Sexual contact with infected blood • Exposure to infected sharps • Mother-to-newborn child at birth (vertical)	• Blood borne • Sexual (rare, but happens if presence of infected blood) • Mother-to-newborn child at birth (vertical) • Sharing personal items	• Most often by exposure to contaminated needles • Household • Rarely by sexual contact	• Fecal–oral	• Blood borne • Sharing personal items • Mother-to-newborn child at birth (vertical) • Sexual contact with infected blood
Incidence in Canada	2.9 cases per 100,000 persons	4.2 cases per 100,000 persons	10–20 cases per 100,000 persons	Extremely low	Rarely seen in Canada	1–4% of the Canadian blood donor population
Persons at risk	• Food handlers • Injection drug users • Travellers and workers in developing countries • Prisoners • Household contacts of persons who have HAV • Hemophiliacs	• Injection drug users sharing needles • Persons who "snort" drugs • Those who have unprotected sex with multiple partners • Homosexual and bisexual males • Immigrants from countries where virus is prevalent • Prisoners • Hemophiliacs	• Recipients of blood products or organs prior to 1990 • Injection drug users sharing needles • Persons who "snort" drugs • Hemodialysis clients • Those who receive tattoos or body piercing done with unsterile equipment	• Injection drug users sharing needles • Persons who "snort" drugs • Those who have unprotected sex with multiple partners • Homosexual and bisexual men • Immigrants from countries where virus is prevalent • Prisoners	• Those living in subtropical areas • Those with low SES, living in areas where virus is prevalent • People on maintenance dialysis • Injection drug users • People who have other viral blood-borne infections • Travellers to areas where the virus is prevalent	• Recipients of blood and blood products • Hemodialysis clients • Injection drug users sharing drug use equipment • Those who receive tattoos, acupuncture, or body piercing with unsterile equipment • Clients with impaired immune response

(Continued)

	Hepatitis A (HAV)	Hepatitis B (HBV)	Hepatitis C (HCV)	Hepatitis D (HDV)	Hepatitis E (HEV)	Hepatitis G
		• Hemodialysis clients • Health care and emergency care workers	• Those who have sex with an HCV carrier • Babies born to mothers who have HCV • Health care workers	• Hemophiliacs • Hemodialysis clients • Health care and emergency care workers		• Prostitutes • Homosexual and bisexual males
Chronic carrier state	No	Yes	Yes	Yes	No	Yes
Indicators	• Acute onset • Fever • Nausea • Lack of appetite • Malaise • Abdominal discomfort • Jaundice	• Mild influenza-like symptoms • Fever • Nausea • Extreme lethargy • Joint pain • Jaundice	• Fatigue • Anorexia • Malaise • Weight loss • Right-sided pain • Occasional jaundice	• Mild influenza-like symptoms • Fever • Nausea • Extreme lethargy • Joint pain • Jaundice	• Jaundice • Uneasiness • Loss of appetite • Abdominal pain • Inflammation of the liver	
Method of diagnosis	Serological test (anti-HAV), viral isolation	Serological test (HBsAg), viral isolation	Serological test (anti-HCV)	Serological test (anti-HDV), liver biopsy	Serological tests (anti-HEV)	None currently
Sequelae	No chronic infection	Chronic liver disease; liver cancer	Chronic liver disease; liver cancer	Chronic liver disease; liver cancer	No chronic infection	Rare or may not occur
Vaccine availability	Yes, vaccination recommended for preschool children, travellers to endemic regions, men who have sex with men	Yes, vaccination recommended for infants, individuals with exposure risks, men who have sex with men	No	No	No	No
Control and prevention	Personal hygiene, proper sanitation	Pre-exposure vaccination, reduction of risk behaviours for exposure	Screening of blood and organ donors; reduction of risk behaviours for exposure	Pre-exposure or post-exposure prophylaxis for HBV	Protection of water systems from fecal contamination	Unknown

	Hepatitis A (HAV)	Hepatitis B (HBV)	Hepatitis C (HCV)	Hepatitis D (HDV)	Hepatitis E (HEV)	Hepatitis G
Nursing considerations	• Educate client about mode of transmission and preventive measures • Recommend prophylactic immune globulin when there is exposure through close contact with an infected individual or contaminated food or water	• Recognize chronic HBV symptoms: • Anorexia • Fatigue • Abdominal pain • Hepatomegaly • Jaundice • Educate client about mode of transmission and preventive measures	• Assess high-risk clients for presence of HCV • Offer blood testing as indicated • Educate client about mode of transmission and preventive measures	• Educate client about mode of transmission and preventive measures	• Educate client about mode of transmission and preventive measures	• Educate client about mode of transmission and preventive measures

HBsAg = Hepatitis B surface antigen; *SES* = socioeconomic status.

**Note:* Data are Canadian unless otherwise specified.

SOURCE: Modified from Stanhope, M., & Lancaster, J. (2010). *Foundations of nursing in the community: Community-oriented practice*. St. Louis, MO: Mosby Elsevier; with additional information from Public Health Agency of Canada. (2004). *Blood borne pathogens section: Viral hepatitis.* Retrieved from http://www.phac-aspc.gc.ca/hcai-iamss/bbp-pts/hep-eng.php.

Photo Credits

CHAPTER 1

p. 3, From Wilson, S. F., & Giddens, J. F. (2001). *Health assessment for nursing practice* (2nd ed.). St. Louis: Mosby; **p. 22**, CP/Toronto Star/Rick Madonik.

CHAPTER 2

p. 47, Saskatchewan Archives Board (R-A13590-3); **p. 48**, Toronto Star Archives; **p. 49**, Courtesy Glenbow Archives, NA-3956-1; **p. 51**, Glenbow Archives, NA-3445-17; **p. 51**, Glenbow Archives, NA-3283-2; **p. 51**, Saskatchewan Archives Board (R-A11751); **p. 52**, Courtesy Glenbow Archives, NA-3956-2.

CHAPTER 3

p. 63, Courtesy Gloria Viverais-Dresler & Heather Jessup-Falcioni; **p. 84**, Courtesy Nancy Horan, SANE.

CHAPTER 4

p. 113, © photoGartner/iStockphoto.com; **p. 113**, CP/Richard Lam; **p. 123**, Jupiter Images; **p. 138**, © Her Majesty the Queen in Right of Canada, represented by the Minister of Health (2005).

CHAPTER 5

p. 157, Courtesy Heather Jessup-Falcioni and Gloria Viverais-Dresler.

CHAPTER 6

p. 170, Eric Gevaert/Shutterstock; **p. 175**, Courtesy Gloria Viverais-Dresler and Heather Jessup-Falcioni; **p. 177**, CP/Frank Gunn.

CHAPTER 7

p. 189, Glenbow Archives, NA-1960-1; **p. 205**, Richard Thornton/Shutterstock; **p. 211**, © Tony Freeman/PhotoEdit.

CHAPTER 8

p. 221, Jenny Solomon/Shutterstock; **p. 222**, Jupiter Images; **p. 242**, Emin Kuliyev/Shutterstock; **p. 246**, Courtesy Gloria Viverais-Dresler & Heather Jessup-Falcioni.

CHAPTER 9

p. 269, Jean Schweitzer/Shutterstock.

CHAPTER 10

p. 300, Courtesy Gloria Viverais-Dresler & Heather Jessup-Falcioni.

CHAPTER 11

p. 318, Debra Brash/Victoria Times Colonist; **p. 338**, From Stanhope, M., & Lancaster, J. (2006). *Foundations of nursing in the community* (2nd ed., p. 449). St. Louis: Mosby.

CHAPTER 12

p. 371, © Mark Richards/PhotoEdit; **p. 383**, © Michael Newman/PhotoEdit.

CHAPTER 13

p. 416, Stanhope, M., & Lancaster, J. (2006). *Foundations of nursing in the community* (2nd ed.). St. Louis: Mosby; **p. 420**, Carolina K. Smith, M.D./Shutterstock; **p. 422**, From Stanhope, M., & Lancaster, J. (2006). *Foundations of nursing in the community* (2nd ed.). St. Louis: Mosby; **p. 431**, Wouter van Caspel/iStockPhoto.

CHAPTER 14

p. 449, Courtesy Gloria Viverais-Dresler & Heather Jessup-Falcioni.

CHAPTER 15

p. 470, Natalia Bratslavsky/iStockPhoto; **p. 470**, Natalia Bratslavsky/iStockPhoto; **p. 487**, Reprinted from Stanhope, M., & Lancaster, J. (2004). *Community & public health nursing* (6th ed., p. 635). St. Louis: Elsevier/Mosby, with permission.

CHAPTER 16

p. 506, A. S. Zain/Shutterstock; **p. 508**, CP/J.P. Moczulski; **p. 511**, Courtesy American Red Cross. All rights reserved in all countries; **p. 517**, Courtesy American Red Cross. All rights reserved in all countries.

CHAPTER 17

p. 529, Steve Nease, 05/23/03. Reprinted with permission; **p. 529**, CP/Keven Frayer.

Index

Page numbers followed by *f* indicate figures; *t*, tables; *b*, boxes.

D

E